QUICK REFERENCE TO INTERNAL MEDICINE: OUTLINE FORMAT

QUICK REFERENCE TO INTERNAL MEDICINE: OUTLINE FORMAT

Roger C. Bone, M.D.
President and Chief Executive Officer
Professor of Medicine
The Medical College of Ohio
Toledo, Ohio
and former
Chairman, Department of Internal Medicine and
Dean, Rush Medical School
Rush-Presbyterian-St. Luke's Medical Center
West Congress Parkway
Chicago, Illinois

Robert L. Rosen, M.D.
Associate Chair, Department of Medicine
Rush-Presbyterian-St. Luke's Medical Center
West Congress Parkway
Chicago, Illinois

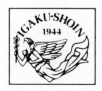

IGAKU-SHOIN   NEW YORK • TOKYO

Published and distributed by

IGAKU-SHOIN Medical Publishers, Inc.
One Madison Avenue, New York, New York 10010

IGAKU-SHOIN Ltd.,
5-24-3 Hongo, Bunkyo-ku, Tokyo 113-91.

Library of Congress Cataloging-in-Publication Data

Quick reference to internal medicine : outline format / Roger C. Bone,
    editor ; Robert L. Rosen, associate editor.
        p.   cm.
    Includes bibliographical references and index.
    ISBN 0-89640-229-0
    1. Internal medicine—Outlines, syllabi, etc.   I. Bone, Roger C.
II. Rosen, Robert L.
    [DNLM: 1. Internal Medicine—outlines.   WB 18 Q6 1994]
RC59.Q53   1994
616'.002'02—dc20
DNLM/DLC
for Library of Congress   93-25286
                                                                   CIP

ISBN: 0-89640-229-0   (New York)
ISBN: 4-260-14229-1   (Tokyo)

Printed and bound in the U.S.A.

10 9 8 7 6 5 4 3 2 1

Preface

QUICK REFERENCE TO INTERNAL MEDICINE:
Outline Format
Medical knowledge is accumulating these days at an exponential rate. One need only examine current textbooks on internal medicine to confirm this. Many are massive multivolume tomes that daunt the health-care professional who frequently seeks a succinct, up-to-date answer to a medical question.

It was this need among clinicians for a practical, comprehensive, authoritative source of swift information in internal medicine that gave rise to the concept embodied in *QUICK REFERENCE TO INTERNAL MEDICINE: Outline Format.*

The novel use of the outline format permits faster access and more rapid assimilation of medical information. The addition of a thumb-index permits swifter location of key medical data in 14 general sections devoted to General Internal Medicine, Allergy and Immunology, Cardiology, Pulmonary Medicine, Critical Care and Emergency Medicine, Infec-

tious Diseases, Digestive Diseases, Hematology, Oncology, Nephrology, Rheumatology, Endocrinology, Neurology, and Geriatric Medicine.

QUICK REFERENCE TO INTERNAL MEDICINE: Outline Format is the only internal medicine reference book available written in an all-inclusive outline format. The time-pressed reader will appreciate the quick access and retrieval of applicable clinical information.

The aim of this book is to provide information within fingertip reach of physicians in all specialties, interns, residents, medical students, nurses, and all other health-care professionals who require prompt answers to clinical problems. *QUICK REFERENCE TO INTERNAL MEDICINE: Outline Format* will also serve as a useful aid in preparing for board certification examinations.

Roger C. Bone, M.D.
Robert L. Rosen, M.D.

Acknowledgment

On behalf of my Associate Editor, Robert L. Rosen, M.D., I would like to thank Carol Sanes-Miller and Alfred B. Lord for their efforts in the production of this book. I would also like to thank Gene Kearn, Senior Medical Editor at Igaku-Shoin Medical Publishers, who helped us immensely with the conception and production of this book. Without him and the dedicated and persistent staff, this book could not have been published. I believe that we have produced an excellent text which should be a useful and lasting resource.

Roger C. Bone, M.D.

Contributors

Richard Abrams, M.D.
Assistant Professor of Medicine
Department of Internal Medicine
Section of General Internal Medicine
Rush-Presbyterian-St. Luke's Medical Center
Chicago, Illinois

Solomon S. Adler, M.D., F.A.C.P.
Professor of Medicine
Department of Internal Medicine
Director, Special Morphology Laboratory
Section of Hematology
Rush-Presbyterian-St. Luke's Medical Center
Chicago, Illinois

Kenning M. Anderson, M.D., Ph.D.
Assistant Professor of Medicine
Department of Internal Medicine
Section of Medical Oncology
Rush-Presbyterian-St. Luke's Medical Center
Chicago, Illinois

Susan Arendt, M.S., R.D.
Food and Nutrition Services
Rush-Presbyterian-St. Luke's Medical Center
Chicago, Illinois

John D. Bagdade, M.D.
Professor of Medicine
Department of Medicine
Section of Endocrinology/Metabolism
Rush-Presbyterian-St. Luke's Medical Center
Chicago, Illinois

David Baldwin, Jr., M.D.
Assistant Professor of Medicine
Department of Medicine
Section of Endocrinology/Metabolism
Rush-Presbyterian-St. Luke's Medical Center
Chicago, Illinois

Robert A. Balk, M.D.
Associate Professor of Medicine
Department of Medicine
Section of Pulmonary and Critical Care Medicine
Rush-Presbyterian-St. Luke's Medical Center
Chicago, Illinois

John T. Barron, M.D., Ph.D.
Assistant Professor of Medicine
Assistant Attending Physician
Director, Cardiac Metabolism Unit
Medical Director, Heart Failure and

Cardiac Transplantation Program
Rush-Presbyterian-St. Luke's Medical Center
Chicago, Illinois

Evan M. Barton, M.D.
Professor of Medicine
Department of Internal Medicine
Section of Rheumatology
Rush-Presbyterian-St. Luke's Medical Center
Chicago, Illinois

David A. Bennett, M.D.
Assistant Professor of Neurology
Department of Neurology
Rush-Presbyterian-St. Luke's Medical Center
Chicago, Illinois

Constance A. Benson, M.D.
Associate Professor of Medicine
Department of Medicine
Section of Infectious Disease
Rush-Presbyterian-St. Luke's Medical Center
Chicago, Illinois

Joseph Bick, M.D.
Clinical Instructor in Medicine
Department of Medicine
Section of Infectious Disease
Rush-Presbyterian-St. Luke's Medical Center
Chicago, Illinois

Joel A. Block, M.D.
Assistant Professor of Medicine
Department of Internal Medicine
Section of Rheumatology
Rush-Presbyterian-St. Luke's Medical Center
Chicago, Illinois

Philip D. Bonomi, M.D.
Professor of Medicine
Department of Internal Medicine
Section of Medical Oncology
Rush-Presbyterian-St. Luke's Medical Center
Chicago, Illinois

Roger C. Bone, M.D.
President and Chief Executive Officer
Professor of Medicine
The Medical College of Ohio
Toledo, Ohio
and former
Chairman, Department of Internal Medicine and
Dean, Rush Medical School
Rush-Presbyterian-St. Luke's Medical Center
Chicago, Illinois

Melanie Brandabur, M.D.
Instructor
Department of Neurology

Rush-Presbyterian-St. Luke's Medical Center
Chicago, Illinois

Steven Brint, M.D.
Assistant Professor of Neurology
Department of Neurology
University of Illinois School of Medicine
Chicago, Illinois

Michael D. Brown, M.D.
Assistant Professor
Department of Internal Medicine
Section of Digestive Diseases
Rush-Presbyterian-St. Luke's Medical Center
Chicago, Illinois

Calvin R. Brown, M.D.
Assistant Professor of Medicine
Department of Internal Medicine
Section of Rheumatology
Rush-Presbyterian-St. Luke's Medical Center
Chicago, Illinois

Thomas A. Buckingham, M.D.
Associate Professor of Medicine
Department of Internal Medicine
Section of Cardiology
Rush-Presbyterian-St. Luke's Medical Center
Chicago, Illinois

Jack Bulmash, M.D.
Assistant Professor of Medicine
Department of Internal Medicine
Section of Geriatrics
Rush-Presbyterian-St. Luke's Medical Center
Chicago, Illinois

James E. Calvin, M.D.
Associate Professor of Medicine
Department of Internal Medicine
Section of Cardiology
Rush-Presbyterian-St. Luke's Medical Center
Chicago, Illinois

Robert Wells Carton, M.D., M.A.
Professor Emeritus
Department of Religion and Health and
Department of Medicine
Rush-Presbyterian-St. Luke's Medical Center
Chicago, Illinois

Larry Casey, M.D., Ph.D.
Associate Professor of Medicine
Department of Internal Medicine
Section of Pulmonary and Critical Care Medicine
Rush-Presbyterian-St. Luke's Medical Center
Chicago, Illinois

John R. Charter, M.D.
Professor of Medicine
Department of Radiology

Rush-Presbyterian-St. Luke's Medical Center
Chicago, Illinois

Michael G. Chez, M.D.
Department of Pediatrics
Section of Child Neurology
Lutheran General Medical Center
Park Ridge, Illinois

Vidyasagar Chodimella, M.D.
Research Associate
Department of Internal Medicine
Section of Pulmonary Medicine
Rush-Presbyterian-St. Luke's Medical Center
Chicago, Illinois

Jan Clarke, M.D.
Assistant Professor of Medicine
Department of Internal Medicine
Section of Geriatrics
Rush-Presbyterian-St. Luke's Medical Center
Chicago, Illinois

Melody A. Cobleigh, M.D.
Associate Professor of Medicine
Department of Internal Medicine
Section of Medical Oncology
Rush-Presbyterian-St. Luke's Medical Center
Chicago, Illinois

Edmond Ray Cole, Ph.D.
Professor of Biochemistry
Associate Professor of Medicine
Unit Director, Clinical Coagulation Laboratory
Rush-Presbyterian-St. Luke's Medical Center
Chicago, Illinois

Cynthia Comella, M.D.
Assistant Professor of Internal Medicine
Departments of Internal Medicine and Neurology
Rush-Presbyterian-St. Luke's Medical Center
Chicago, Illinois

Andrew C. Dixon, M.D.
Director, Intensive Care Unit
Penobscot Respiratory
Bangor, Maine

Arcot Dwarakanathan, M.D.
Assistant Professor of Medicine
Department of Medicine
Section of Endocrinology/Metabolism
Rush-Presbyterian-St. Luke's Medical Center
Chicago, Illinois

Matthew G. Fleming, M.D.
Assistant Professor of Dermatology
Departments of Dermatology and Pathology
Rush-Presbyterian-St. Luke's Medical Center
Chicago, Illinois

Judith E. Frank, M.D.
Instructor
Department of Internal Medicine
Section of Rheumatology
Rush-Presbyterian-St. Luke's Medical Center
Chicago, Illinois

Walter Fried, M.D.
Professor of Medicine
Department of Internal Medicine
Section of Hematology
Rush-Presbyterian-St. Luke's Medical Center
Chicago, Illinois

Henri Frischer, M.D., Ph.D.
Professor of Medicine and Professor of
    Pharmacology
Department of Internal Medicine Section of
    Hematology, and Department of Pharmacology
Director, Section of Blood Genetics and
    Pharmacogenetics
Rush-Presbyterian-St. Luke's Medical Center
Chicago, Illinois

Daniel R. Ganger, M.D.
Assistant Professor of Medicine
Department of Internal Medicine
Rush-Presbyterian-St. Luke's Medical Center
Chicago, Illinois

Howard M. Gebel, Ph.D.
Associate Professor
Departments of Immunology/Microbiology and
    General Surgery
Rush-Presbyterian-St. Luke's Medical Center
Chicago, Illinois

Anita Gewurz, M.D.
Assistant Professor
Departments of Immunology/Microbiology
Department of Pediatrics
Rush-Presbyterian-St. Luke's Medical Center
Chicago, Illinois

Paul Glickman, M.D.
Associate Professor of Medicine
Department of Internal Medicine
Section of Rheumatology
Rush-Presbyterian-St. Luke's Medical Center
Chicago, Illinois

Eric Gluck, M.D.
Assistant Professor of Medicine
Department of Internal Medicine
Associate Director, Respiratory Care
Section of Pulmonology
Rush-Presbyterian-St. Luke's Medical Center
Chicago, Illinois

William E. Golden, M.D.
Director, Division of General Internal Medicine
University of Arkansas for Medical Sciences
Little Rock, Arkansas

Mitchell Goldman, M.D.
Clinical Instructor of Medicine
Department of Medicine
Section of Infectious Disease
Rush-Presbyterian-St. Luke's Medical Center
Chicago, Illinois

Larry J. Goodman, M.D.
Associate Professor of Medicine
Department of Medicine
Section of Infectious Disease
Rush-Presbyterian-St. Luke's Medical Center
Chicago, Illinois

Stephanie A. Gregory, M.D.
Professor of Medicine
Department of Internal Medicine
Associate Director, Section of Hematology
Rush Cancer Institute
Rush-Presbyterian-St. Luke's Medical Center
Chicago, Illinois

Paul K. Hanashiro, M.D.
Associate Professor of Medicine
Department of Internal Medicine
Director, Emergency Services
Rush-Presbyterian-St. Luke's Medical Center
Chicago, Illinois

Alan A. Harris, M.D.
Professor of Medicine
Department of Medicine
Section of Infectious Disease
Rush-Presbyterian-St. Luke's Medical Center
Chicago, Illinois

Charlotte A. Harris, M.D.
Assistant Professor of Medicine
Department of Internal Medicine
Section of Rheumatology
Rush-Presbyterian-St. Luke's Medical Center
Chicago, Illinois

Jules E. Harris, M.D.
The Samuel G. Taylor, III, Professor of Medicine
Department of Internal Medicine
Section of Oncology
Rush-Presbyterian-St. Luke's Medical Center
Chicago, Illinois

Mary K. Hayden, M.D.
Assistant Professor of Medicine
Department of Medicine
Section of Infectious Disease

Rush-Presbyterian-St. Luke's Medical Center
Chicago, Illinois

Michael W. Heniff, M.D.
Instructor of Medicine
Department of Medicine
Section of Pulmonary and Critical Care Medicine
Rush-Presbyterian-St. Luke's Medical Center
Chicago, Illinois

Judith Heyworth, M.D.
Assistant Professor of Medicine
Department of Internal Medicine
Section of Geriatrics
Rush-Presbyterian-St. Luke's Medical Center
Chicago, Illinois

Rebecca Hoffman, M.D.
Instructor
Department of Internal Medicine
Section of Allergy and Immunology
Rush-Presbyterian-St. Luke's Medical Center
Chicago, Illinois

Susan Hou, M.D.
Assistant Professor
Department of Internal Medicine
Section of Nephrology
Rush-Presbyterian-St. Luke's Medical Center
Chicago, Illinois

John P. Huff, M.D., Ph.D.
Assistant Professor of Medicine
Department of Internal Medicine
Section of Geriatrics
Rush-Presbyterian-St. Luke's Medical Center
Chicago, Illinois

Joseph J. Jares, III, M.D.
Instructor of Medicine
Department of Neurological Sciences
Rush-Presbyterian-St. Luke's Medical Center
Chicago, Illinois

Donald M. Jensen, M.D.
Associate Professor
Department of Internal Medicine
Chief, Subsection of Hepathology
Rush-Presbyterian-St. Luke's Medical Center
Chicago, Illinois

Judd Jensen, M.D.
Midwest Associates in Neurology
Oak Park, Illinois

C.R. Kannan, M.D.
Associate Professor of Medicine
Rush-Presbyterian-St. Luke's Medical Center
Chairman, Division of Endocrinology

Cook County Hospital
Chicago, Illinois

Edward H. Kaplan, M.D.
Assistant Professor of Medicine
Department of Internal Medicine
Section of Oncology
Rush-Presbyterian-St. Luke's Medical Center
Chicago, Illinois

Richard Karrel, M.D.
Assistant Professor
Department of Internal Medicine
Section of Psychiatry
Rush-Presbyterian-St. Luke's Medical Center
Chicago, Illinois

Robert Katz, M.D.
Associate Professor of Medicine
Department of Internal Medicine
Section of Rheumatology
Rush-Presbyterian-St. Luke's Medical Center
Chicago, Illinois

Harold Kennedy, M.D.
Professor of Medicine
Department of Internal Medicine
Section of Cardiology
Rush-Presbyterian-St. Luke's Medical Center
Chicago, Illinois

Harold A. Kessler, M.D.
Professor of Medicine
Department of Medicine
Section of Infectious Disease
Rush-Presbyterian-St. Luke's Medical Center
Chicago, Illinois

Lloyd W. Klein, M.D.
Associate Professor of Medicine
Co-Director, Cardiac Catheterization Laboratory
Director, Interventional Cardiology
Rush-Presbyterian-St. Luke's Medical Center
Chicago, Illinois

William H. Knospe, M.D.
Elodia Kelm Professor of Hematology and
    Professor of Medicine
Department of Internal Medicine
Section of Hematology
Rush-Presbyterian-St. Luke's Medical Center
Chicago, Illinois

Stephen Korbet, M.D.
Associate Professor of Medicine
Department of Medicine
Section of Nephrology
Rush-Presbyterian-St. Luke's Medical Center
Chicago, Illinois

Kenneth Kortas, Pharm.D.
Clinical Pharmacist
Department of Medicine
Section of Infectious Disease
Rush-Presbyterian-St. Luke's Medical Center
Chicago, Illinois

Ludwig Kornel, M.D., Ph.D.
Professor of Medicine and Biochemistry
Department of Medicine
Section of Endocrinology/Metabolism
Rush-Presbyterian-St. Luke's Medical Center
Chicago, Illinois

Lawrence Layfer, M.D.
Associate Professor of Medicine
Department of Internal Medicine
Section of Rheumatology
Rush-Presbyterian-St. Luke's Medical Center
Chicago, Illinois

Paul Evans Later, M.D.
Instructor
Department of Nephrology
Rush-Presbyterian-St. Luke's Medical Center
Chicago, Illinois

Jerrold B. Leikin, M.D.
Associate Professor of Medicine
Department of Internal Medicine
Director, Rush Poison Control Center
Associate Director, Emergency Services
Rush-Presbyterian-St. Luke's Medical Center
Chicago, Illinois

James Levin, M.D.
Clinical Instructor in Medicine
Department of Medicine
Section of Infectious Disease
Rush-Presbyterian-St. Luke's Medical Center
Chicago, Illinois

Stuart Levin, M.D.
Professor of Medicine
Department of Medicine
Rush-Presbyterian-St. Luke's Medical Center
Chicago, Illinois

William Leslie, M.D.
Assistant Professor of Medicine
Department of Internal Medicine
Section of Medical Oncology
Rush-Presbyterian-St. Luke's Medical Center
Chicago, Illinois

Edmund J. Lewis, M.D.
Professor of Medicine
Department of Internal Medicine
Section of Nephrology

Rush-Presbyterian-St. Luke's Medical Center
Chicago, Illinois

Philip R. Liebson, M.D.
Professor of Medicine
Senior Attending Physician
Director, Echocardiography Laboratory
Consultant, Preventive Cardiology
Rush-Presbyterian-St. Luke's Medical Center
Chicago, Illinois

Sarah T. Lincoln, M.D.
Assistant Professor of Medicine
Department of Internal Medicine
Section of Medical Oncology
Rush-Presbyterian-St. Luke's Medical Center
Chicago, Illinois

Thomas F. Lint, Ph.D.
Professor
Department of Immunology/Microbiology
Rush-Presbyterian-St. Luke's Medical Center
Chicago, Illinois

Jeffrey M. Lisowski, M.D.
Assistant Professor of Medicine
Department of Medicine
Section of Infectious Disease
Rush-Presbyterian-St. Luke's Medical Center
Chicago, Illinois

James E. Macioch, D.O.
Assistant Professor of Medicine
Assistant Attending Physician
Associate Director, Echocardiography Laboratory
Rush-Presbyterian-St. Luke's Medical Center
Chicago, Illinois

Catherine M. MacLeod, M.D., F.R.C.P.(C), F.A.C.P., F.C.P.
Assistant Professor of Pharmacology and Internal
    Medicine
Departments of Pharmacology and Internal
    Medicine
Section of Infectious Disease
Rush-Presbyterian-St. Luke's Medical Center
Chicago, Illinois

Theodore Mazzone, M.D.
Associate Professor of Medicine
Department of Internal Medicine
Section of Endocrinology
Rush-Presbyterian-St. Luke's Medical Center
Chicago, Illinois

Rajalaxmi McKenna, M.D.
Associate Professor of Medicine
Department of Internal Medicine
Section of Hematology
Unit Director

Platelet Function, Radiohematology, and Venous
    Thrombosis Diagnostic Laboratories
Rush-Presbyterian-St. Luke's Medical Center
Chicago, Illinois

Margaret A. McLaughlin, M.D.
Assistant Professor
Department of Internal Medicine
Section of General Internal Medicine
Rush-Presbyterian-St. Luke's Medical Center
Chicago, Illinois

Bruce C. McLeod, M.D.
Professor of Medicine
Department of Internal Medicine and Pathology
Section of Hematology
Director, Apheresis Unit
Rush-Presbyterian-St. Luke's Medical Center
Chicago, Illinois

Lynn Meisles, M.D.
Department of Internal Medicine
Section of Rheumatology
Rush-Presbyterian-St. Luke's Medical Center
Chicago, Illinois

Steven L. Meyers, M.D.
Instructor
Department of Neurological Sciences
Rush-Presbyterian-St. Luke's Medical Center
Chicago, Illinois

Margaret Michalska, M.D.
Clinical Instructor of Medicine
College of Medicine
Department of Internal Medicine
Section of Rheumatology
University of Illinois
Chicago, Illinois

Donald A. Misch, M.D.
Assistant Professor of Psychiatry
Department of Psychiatry and Health Behavior
Medical College of Georgia
Augusta, Georgia

James Moy, M.D.
Assistant Professor of Pediatrics
Department of Immunology/Microbiology
Section of Pediatrics
Rush-Presbyterian-St. Luke's Medical Center
Chicago, Illinois

Christopher G. Murlas, M.D.
Associate Professor of Medicine
Department of Medicine
Section of Pulmonary Medicine
Rush-Presbyterian-St. Luke's Medical Center
Chicago, Illinois

Joan C. Murray, M.D.
Instructor of Medicine
Department of Neurology
Rush-Presbyterian-St. Luke's Medical Center
Chicago, Illinois

Linda Ray Murray, M.D., M.P.H.
Attending Physician
Division of Occupational Medicine
Department of Medicine
Cook County Hospital
Chicago, Illinois

Hassan Najafi, M.D.
John Ben Professor of Surgery and Chairman
Senior Attending Physician
Department of Cardiovascular-Thoracic Surgery
Rush-Presbyterian-St. Luke's Medical Center
Chicago, Illinois

Yousef N. Nawas, M.D.
Assistant Professor of Medicine
Department of Internal Medicine
Section of Pulmonology
Rush-Presbyterian-St. Luke's Medical Center
Chicago, Illinois

Jeffrey A. Nelson, M.D.
Assistant Professor of Medicine
Department of Medicine
Section of Infectious Disease
Rush-Presbyterian-St. Luke's Medical Center
Chicago, Illinois

Gretajo Northrop, M.D., Ph.D.
Associate Professor of Medicine
Department of Medicine
Section of Endocrinology/Metabolism
Rush-Presbyterian-St. Luke's Medical Center
Chicago, Illinois

Jack Ohringer, M.D.
Assistant Professor of Medicine
Department of Medicine
Section of Digestive Diseases
Rush-Presbyterian-St. Luke's Medical Center
Chicago, Illinois

Lee Ann Onder
Quality Assurance
Cleveland Clinic
Cleveland, Ohio

Mark Overton, M.D.
Assistant Professor of Medicine
Department of Internal Medicine
Section of Geriatrics
Rush-Presbyterian-St. Luke's Medical Center
Chicago, Illinois

Janis Orlowski, M.D.
Assistant Professor of Medicine
Department of Internal Medicine
Section of Nephrology
Rush-Presbyterian-St. Luke's Medical Center
Chicago, Illinois

Ritwick Panicker, M.D.
Senior Fellow
Fred Hutchinson Cancer Research Center
University of Washington School of Medicine
Seattle, Washington

Joseph E. Parrillo, M.D.
James B. Herrick Professor of Medicine
Chief, Section of Cardiology
Chief, Section of Critical Care Medicine
Rush-Presbyterian-St. Luke's Medical Center
Chicago, Illinois

Edward L. Passen, M.D.
Assistant Professor of Medicine
Department of Medicine
Section of Cardiology
Rush-Presbyterian-St. Luke's Medical Center
Chicago, Illinois

William Piccione, Jr., M.D.
Assistant Professor of Surgery
Assistant Attending Physician
Surgical Director, Heart Transplantation Program
Department of Cardiovascular-Thoracic Surgery
Rush-Presbyterian-St. Luke's Medical Center
Chicago, Illinois

Serge J.C. Pierre-Louis, M.D.
Assistant Professor
Department of Neurological Sciences
Rush-Presbyterian-St. Luke's Medical Center
Chicago, Illinois

Bennett Plotnick, M.D.
Assistant Professor
Department of Internal Medicine
Section of Digestive Diseases
Rush-Presbyterian-St. Luke's Medical Center
Chicago, Illinois

Jovan M. Popovich, M.D.
Fellow, Section of Rheumatology
Department of Medicine
Rush-Presbyterian-St. Luke's Medical Center
Chicago, Illinois

John C. Pottage, Jr., M.D.
Associate Professor of Medicine
Department of Medicine
Section of Infectious Disease
Rush-Presbyterian-St. Luke's Medical Center
Chicago, Illinois

G. Wendell Richmond, M.D.
Director of Clinical Services, Allergy and Clinical
    Immunology Program
Associate Professor
Departments of Immunology/Microbiology,
    Internal Medicine, and Pediatrics
Rush-Presbyterian-St. Luke's Medical Center
Chicago, Illinois

Andrew Ripeckyj, M.D.
Assistant Professor
Department of Psychiatry
Rush-Presbyterian-St. Luke's Medical Center
Chicago, Illinois

Barry J. Riskin, M.D.
Instructor
Department of Neurology
Rush-Presbyterian-St. Luke's Medical Center
Chicago, Illinois

Roger Rodby, M.D.
Assistant Professor of Medicine
Department of Internal Medicine
Section of Nephrology
Rush-Presbyterian-St. Luke's Medical Center
Chicago, Illinois

Robert L. Rosen, M.D.
Associate Chair
Department of Medicine
Section of Pulmonary Medicine
Rush-Presbyterian-St. Luke's Medical Center
Chicago, Illinois

Howard Rosenblate, M.D.
Associate Professor
Department of Internal Medicine
Section of Digestive Diseases
Rush-Presbyterian-St. Luke's Medical Center
Chicago, Illinois

Robert S. Rosenson, M.D.
Assistant Professor of Medicine
Director, Preventive Cardiology
Section of Cardiology
Rush-Presbyterian-St. Luke's Medical Center
Chicago, Illinois

Steven Rothschild, M.D.
Assistant Professor
Department of Family Practice
Section of Geriatrics
Rush-Presbyterian-St. Luke's Medical Center
Chicago, Illinois

David B. Rubin, M.D.
Associate Professor
Department of Medicine
Section of Pulmonary Medicine

Department of Therapeutic Radiology
Director, Section of Radiation Biology
Rush-Presbyterian-St. Luke's Medical Center
Chicago, Illinois

Will G. Ryan, M.D.
Professor of Medicine
Department of Medicine
Section of Endocrinology/Metabolism
Rush-Presbyterian-St. Luke's Medical Center
Chicago, Illinois

Seymour M. Sabesin, M.D.
Josephine Dyrenforth Professor of Medicine
Department of Medicine
Director, Section of Digestive Diseases
Rush-Presbyterian-St. Luke's Medical Center
Chicago, Illinois

Samuel Saltzberg, M.D.
Assistant Professor of Medicine
Department of Medicine
Section of Pathology
Rush-Presbyterian-St. Luke's Medical Center
Chicago, Illinois

Delphin Santos, M.D.
Instructor
Department of Internal Medicine
Section of Rheumatology
Rush-Presbyterian-St. Luke's Medical Center
Chicago, Illinois

Richard J. Sassetti, M.D.
Professor
Departments of Internal Medicine and Pathology
Section of Hematology
Director, Blood Center
Rush-Presbyterian-St. Luke's Medical Center
Chicago, Illinois

Gary L. Schaer, M.D.
Associate Professor of Medicine
Associate Attending Physician
Director, Cardiac Catheterization Laboratories
Section of Cardiology
Rush-Presbyterian-St. Luke's Medical Center
Chicago, Illinois

John Schaffner, M.D.
Associate Professor
Department of Internal Medicine
Chief, Subsection of Gastroenterology
Rush-Presbyterian-St. Luke's Medical Center
Chicago, Illinois

Thomas J. Schnitzer, M.D.
Professor of Medicine
Department of Internal Medicine
Chief, Section of Rheumatology

Rush-Presbyterian-St. Luke's Medical Center
Chicago, Illinois

John Segreti, M.D.
Associate Professor of Medicine
Department of Medicine
Section of Infectious Disease
Rush-Presbyterian-St. Luke's Medical Center
Chicago, Illinois

Jeffrey Semel, M.D.
Assistant Professor of Medicine
Department of Medicine
Section of Infectious Disease
Rush-Presbyterian-St. Luke's Medical Center
Chicago, Illinois

John L. Showel, M.D.
Associate Professor of Medicine
Department of Internal Medicine
Sections of Medical Oncology and Hematology
Rush-Presbyterian-St. Luke's Medical Center
Chicago, Illinois

Michael R. Silver, M.D.
Assistant Professor of Medicine
Director, Respiratory Care Unit
Section of Pulmonary and Critical Care Medicine
Rush-Presbyterian-St. Luke's Medical Center
Chicago, Illinois

David Simon, M.D.
Assistant Professor of Medicine
Department of Medicine
Section of Infectious Disease
Rush-Presbyterian-St. Luke's Medical Center
Chicago, Illinois

Sheldon Sloan, M.D.
Assistant Professor of Medicine
Department of Internal Medicine
Section of Gastroenterology
Rush-Presbyterian-St. Luke's Medical Center
Chicago, Illinois

Michael C. Smith, M.D.
Assistant Professor
Department of Neurology
Rush-Presbyterian-St. Luke's Medical Center
Chicago, Illinois

Jeffrey R. Snell, M.D.
Assistant Professor of Medicine
Department of Internal Medicine
Associate Director, Coronary Care Unit
Section of Cardiology
Rush-Presbyterian-St. Luke's Medical Center
Chicago, Illinois

Debra Syeluga, Ph.D., R.D.
Assistant Professor of Medicine
Department of Internal Medicine
Section of Medical Oncology
Rush-Presbyterian-St. Luke's Medical Center
Chicago, Illinois

J. Peter Szidon, M.D.
Professor of Medicine
Department of Medicine
Section of Pulmonary Medicine
Rush-Presbyterian-St. Luke's Medical Center
Chicago, Illinois

Samuel G. Taylor IV, M.D.
Professor of Medicine
Department of Internal Medicine
Section of Medical Oncology
Rush-Presbyterian-St. Luke's Medical Center
Chicago, Illinois

Charles R. Thomas, Jr., M.D.
Assistant Professor of Medicine
Department of Medicine
Division of Oncology
Research Fellow
Division of Experimental Biology
Department of Radiation Oncology
University of Washington School of Medicine
Seattle, Washington

Larry Thomas, Ph.D.
Assistant Professor
Department of Immunology/Microbiology
Rush-Presbyterian-St. Luke's Medical Center
Chicago, Illinois

Gordon M. Trenholme, M.D.
Professor of Medicine
Department of Medicine
Rush-Presbyterian-St. Luke's Medical Center
Chicago, Illinois

Michael Uzer, M.D.
Assistant Professor of Medicine
Department of Internal Medicine
Section of Digestive Diseases
Rush-Presbyterian-St. Luke's Medical Center
Chicago, Illinois

Denise Verges, M.D.
Instructor
Department of Internal Medicine
Section of Rheumatology
Rush-Presbyterian-St. Luke's Medical Center
Chicago, Illinois

Annabelle S. Volgman, M.D.
Assistant Professor of Medicine

Department of Medicine
Director of the Electrophysiology Service
Section of Cardiology
Rush-Presbyterian-St. Luke's Medical Center
Chicago, Illinois

Denise C. Weaver, M.D.
Clinical Instructor in Medicine
Section of Infectious Disease
Rush-Presbyterian-St. Luke's Medical Center
Chicago, Illinois

Steven B. Wilkinson, M.D.
Instructor
Department of Neurology
Rush-Presbyterian-St. Luke's Medical Center
Chicago, Illinois

Wayne C. Williamson, M.D.
Assistant Professor of Medicine
Department of Internal Medicine
Section of General Internal Medicine
Rush-Presbyterian-St. Luke's Medical Center
Chicago, Illinois

Janet M. Wolter, M.D.
Professor of Medicine
Department of Internal Medicine
Section of Medical Oncology
Rush-Presbyterian-St. Luke's Medical Center
Chicago, Illinois

Robert B. Wright, M.D.
Assistant Professor
Department of Neurological Sciences
Rush-Presbyterian-St. Luke's Medical Center
Chicago, Illinois

Syed Zaidi, M.D.
Assistant Professor
Department of Internal Medicine
Section of Digestive Diseases
Rush-Presbyterian-St. Luke's Medical Center
Chicago, Illinois

Howard Zeitz, M.D.
Associate Professor of Medicine
Department of Internal Medicine
Rush-Presbyterian-St. Luke's Medical Center
Chicago, Illinois

Contents

Contents

SECTION 1

General Internal Medicine

CHAPTER 1

Preventive Health Care and the Periodic Health Examination

Margaret A. McLaughlin, M.D.

I. General Historical Background

A. The idea of using preventive interventions to benefit asymptomatic patients has been popular for most of the twentieth century.

1. Doctors affiliated with life insurance companies began to advocate periodic health examinations in the early 1900s.

2. Advocacy of periodic examinations was based on the following premises:

a. Asymptomatic individuals may have organic disease.

b. Periodic health examinations can detect early disease.

c. Morbidity and mortality can be reduced by the early detection of disease.

3. Although the effects of periodic examinations on morbidity and mortality were largely unknown and unproven, the notion of every individual having a periodic health examination became widely accepted.

B. Over the last 20 years, increasing emphasis has been placed on the importance of demonstrating the effectiveness of proposed preventive interventions before endorsing their use.

C. Currently, it is generally agreed that periodic health examinations incorporating preventive interventions are useful in asymptomatic individuals under the following circumstances:

1. The *frequency* and *content* of the examination are tailored to the patient's age, sex, and individual health risks.

2. Recommended interventions are supported by adequate evidence of clinical effectiveness.

D. Careful analysis of available preventive interventions has shifted the emphasis of the periodic health examination.

1. Screening of asymptomatic individuals is no longer advocated for many diseases.

2. Counseling and patient education have become recognized as valuable interventions, particularly in addressing personal health practices.

II. Classification of Preventive Care

Defined by where in the course of the disease the preventive intervention occurs.

A. Primary prevention

1. An intervention in an asymptomatic individual to prevent a pathological process from occurring.

2. Example—routine immunizations.
B. Secondary prevention
    1. An intervention in an asymptomatic individual with an established but presymptomatic pathological process.
    2. For the preventive intervention to be of value, treatment of the disease in the asymptomatic period must be more beneficial than treatment delayed until the appearance of symptoms.
    3. Example—screening for breast cancer via mammography.
C. Tertiary prevention
    1. An intervention in a symptomatic individual with established disease to prevent complications from the disease and disability.
    2. Example—prophylaxis against pneumocystis pneumonia in patients with acquired immunodeficiency syndrome (AIDS).
    3. Will not be covered further in this chapter.

III. **Types of Preventive Intervention**
A. Screening tests
    1. A test or examination procedure used to identify asymptomatic individuals needing further attention.
    2. When performed in the context of the clinical encounter, this activity is referred to as *case finding* (as opposed to mass screening at schools, health fairs, places of employment, etc.).
    3. Examples—blood pressure check, cholesterol determination, mammogram.
B. Counseling
    1. A patient receives information and advice about behaviors to reduce the risk of subsequent illness or injury.
    2. Examples—advice to stop smoking and encouragement to use a seat belt.
C. Immunization
    1. Vaccines and immunoglobulins taken to prevent infectious diseases.
    2. Example—tetanus booster shot.
D. Chemoprophylaxis
    1. Drugs or biologically active substances taken by patients to reduce the risk of developing a disease.
    2. Examples—postmenopausal estrogen replacement, low-dose aspirin in individuals with risk factors for myocardial infarction.

IV. **Determining the Effectiveness of Preventive Interventions**
Whether a particular preventive intervention is effective depends on the characteristics of the target disease, the properties of the intervention itself, and the population selected for the intervention.
A. Effectiveness of screening tests
    1. Characteristics of target diseases for which screening is beneficial
        a. Impact on the length or quality of life is significant.
        b. Prevalence is sufficient to warrant screening in asymptomatic individuals.
        c. Efficacious treatment is available.
        d. Treatment during the asymptomatic phase is more beneficial than treatment delayed until symptoms appear.
    2. Special methodological problems in evaluating screening tests
        a. Lead-time bias—early detection may increase the time from diagnosis to death (giving the appearance of longer survival) without actually prolonging life.
        b. Length bias—screening may identify a disproportionate number of slowly progressive cases of a disease.
    3. Characteristics of screening tests which determine efficacy
        a. Accuracy—measured by four indices: sensitivity, specificity, positive predictive values, and negative predictive values (see Chapter 7).
        b. Reliability—the ability of a test to obtain the same result when repeated.
    4. Population selection for effective screening—total benefit to society depends on the epidemiological characteristics of the target disease.
    5. Potential adverse effects of screening tests must be taken into consideration.
        a. Physical complications from the test procedure.
        b. Economic costs.
        c. Consequences of diagnostic errors (false-negative and false-positive results).
B. Effectiveness of counseling
    1. Counseling must be effective in bringing about desired behavioral changes.
    2. Changing personal behavior must improve the patient's outcome.
C. Effectiveness of immunizations and chemoprophylaxis
    1. Intervention must provide protection against the desired disease.

2. The financial cost must not be prohibitive.

3. The potential benefit must outweigh the potential risk of adverse consequences.

V. Quality of the Evidence Establishing the Effectiveness of Preventive Interventions

A rating system was developed by the Canadian Task Force on the Periodic Health Examination and has been used more recently by the U.S. Preventive Services Task Force. General ratings range between I and III, with more weight given to study designs that are less subject to bias and misinterpretation. Designs are ranked in decreasing order of importance:

A. I.   Randomized controlled trials

B. II-1. Nonrandomized controlled trials

C. II-2.

   1. Cohort studies

   2. Case-control studies

D. II-3.

   1. Comparisons between multiple time series

   2. Uncontrolled experiments

E. III. Descriptive studies and expert opinion

VI. Selected Groups Which Have Established Preventive Care Guidelines

A. Frame and Carlson

   1. Initial recommendations were published in 1975.

   2. Reviewed interventions to prevent common diseases.

   3. Made sex- and age-specific recommendations for preventive practices.

   4. Recommendations were updated in 1986.

B. Breslow and Somers

   1. Recommendations were published in 1977.

   2. Suggested a "lifetime health-monitoring program" for preventive practices.

C. Canadian Task Force (CTF) on the Periodic Health Examination

   1. Initial recommendations were published in 1979.

   2. Established by the Canadian government to determine how periodic health examinatiosn could improve the health of Canadians.

   3. Developed a highly structured and scientific process to identify diseases which might be preventable and to review continually the strength of the evidence supporting various preventive interventions.

   4. Identified the need to individualize recommendations based on risk factors.

5. Periodically updates recommendations.

D. American Cancer Society (ACS)

   1. Initial recommendations were published in 1980.

   2. Developed recommendations for the early detection of cancer in asymptomatic individuals.

   3. Recommendations were updated in 1988.

E. Medical Practice Committee of the American College of Physicians (ACP)

   1. Initial recommendations were published in 1981.

   2. Stated that annual physical examinations in low-risk, asymptomatic individuals could not be justified.

   3. Suggested that periodic examinations be individualized.

F. U.S. Preventive Services Task Force (USPSTF)

   1. Recommendations were published in 1989.

   2. Recommendations covered preventive services for 60 target conditions.

   3. Review process was similar to that used by the CTF and focused on the need for scientific, unbiased evidence to support recommendations.

G. Numerous medical specialty organizations, professional organizations, government health agencies, and others periodically make recommendations.

VII. Selected Preventive Care Guidelines: The History and Physical Examination

A. Height and weight

   1. USPSTF recommends routine measurement and evaluation as general screening.

   2. Optimal frequency is left to clinical discretion.

B. Blood pressure measurement

   1. Uniformly endorsed in all major preventive care guidelines for general screening.

   2. Recommended frequency varies somewhat (every 1–5 years), but most agree that blood pressure should be checked at every visit to a physician, irrespective of the reason for the visit.

C. Visual activity

   1. USPSTF recommends yearly evaluation in persons 65 years of age and older.

D. Hearing assessment

   1. USPSTF recommends yearly evalua-

tion based on history in persons 65 years of age and older. CTF recommends earlier evaluation if indicated by the history.

2. CTF and USPSTF both recommend screening in persons exposed to excessive noise levels.

E. Oral cavity examination
1. CTF recommends yearly screening in persons 65 years of age and older, while the USPSTF recommends against general screening. ACS recommends periodic screening (every 1–3 years, depending on age) in all adults.
2. Both CTF and USPSTF recommend an examination in adults with a history of tobacco use, and USPSTF recommends an examination in adults with excessive alcohol exposure.

F. Thyroid palpation
1. ACS recommends periodic examination in all adults.
2. USPSTF recommends periodic examination in adults who have a history of upper body irradiation.

G. Complete skin examination
1. ACS recommends periodic screening in all adults, while CTF and USPSTF recommend against screening.
2. CTF, USPSTF, and others recommend periodic exmination in those with risk factors for skin cancer.

H. Breast examination by clinician
1. CTF, USPSTF, ACP, and ACS recommend yearly examination in women 40 years of age and older; ACS recommends examination every 3 years in women aged 20–40.
2. Examination is recommended at an earlier age for those with risk factors for breast cancer (starting at 18 to 35 years of age, depending on the source of the recommendation).

I. Bimanual pelvic examination
1. ACS recommends examination every 1–3 years for women under age 40 and yearly for women over age 40.
2. USPSTF recommends against screening examinations.

J. Testicular examination
1. ACS recommends examination every 3 years for men under age 40 and yearly for men over age 40.
2. CTF and USPSTF recommend examination in men at increased risk for testicular cancer.

K. Digital rectal examination for prostatic cancer
1. ACS recommends yearly examinations in men aged 40 and over for general screening.
2. CTF and USPSTF make no recommendation on rectal examinations.

VIII. **Selected Preventive Care Guidelines: Laboratory Tests**
A. Nonfasting cholesterol
1. USPSTF and ACP recommend general screening every 5 years in adults aged 18 and older (ACP: until age 70).
2. More frequent screening is recommended in persons with known lipid abnormalities or additional risk factors for cardiovascular disease.

B. Fasting glucose
1. CTF, USPSTF, and ACP recommend against general screening.
2. All three recommend screening in some individuals with additional risk factors.

C. Hemoglobin measurement (for iron deficiency anemia)
1. CTF and USPSTF recommend against measurement for general screening purposes.

D. Thyroid function testing
1. CTF, USPSTF, and ACP recommend against general screening.

E. Urine Analysis
1. USPSTF recommends screening for bacteriuria (which ACP and CTF recommend against) in persons aged 60 and over. In addition, it recommends screening for hematuria and proteinuria in this age group.
2. Additional screening is recommended by CTF and USPSTF in some high-risk groups.

F. Resting electrocardiogram and exercise stress test
1. CTF, USPSTF, and ACP all recommend against general screening.
2. USPSTF recommends testing in some individuals who either have additional risk factors for cardiovascular disease or who engage in special activities.

G. Chest radiograph
1. CTF, USPSTF, ACP, and ACS all recommend against screening in low- and high-risk (smokers) individuals.

H. Mammography
I. CTF and ACP recommend yearly examinations in women aged 50 and over for general screening.

J. USPSTF recommends examinations every 1–2 years between the ages of 50 and 75 for general screening.

K. ACS recommends examinations every 1–2 years for women aged 40–50 and yearly examinations after the age of 50 for general screening.

L. CTF, USPSTF, and ACP all recommend starting yearly examinations in younger women (aged 35–40, depending on the group making the recommendation) with risk factors for breast cancer.

M. Papanicolaou smear
   1. CTF, USPSTF, ACP, and ACS all recommend obtaining smears at least every 3 years (initiating the test with the onset of sexual activity) in younger women after obtaining two or three normal annual smears.
   2. CTF increases the interval between smears to 5 years after the age of 36 and recommends continuing the test until age 74.
   3. ACP and USPSTF recommend continuing smears until the age of 65, or until later if there is no documentation of consistently normal cytology in the previous 10 years.
   4. Smears are recommended more frequently than every 3 years for women at higher risk for cervical cancer.
   5. Recommendations are for women who are or have been sexually active.

N. Stool examination for occult blood
   1. ACP and ACS recommend yearly screening in individuals aged 50 and over.
   2. CTF and USPSTF do not recommend screening in this age group but do suggest screening of certain high-risk individuals, starting at 45 to 50 years of age.

O. Sigmoidoscopy
   1. ACP and ACS recommend general screening every 3–5 years in individuals aged 50 and older.
   2. CTF and USPSTF make no recommendation for general screening in this age group.
   3. CTF and USPSTF recommend screening in high-risk individuals. The ACS recommends more frequent screening in high-risk individuals than in the general population.

IX. **Selective Preventive Care Guidelines—Counseling**
   A. The USPSTF has concluded that patient counseling by practitioners offers great opportunities to prevent illness.
   B. Recommendations were made for counseling in a number of areas.
      1. Diet (calories, fat, fiber, calcium, etc.)
      2. Physical activity and exercise
      3. Sexual practices
         a. Contraception
         b. Reducing the risk of sexually transmitted diseases
      4. Smoking
      5. Alcohol
      6. Drugs
      7. Injury prevention
         a. Motor vehicle accidents
         b. Fires
         c. Injuries from violence
         d. Falls in the elderly
         e. Back injuries
      8. Dental hygiene

Bibliography

American Cancer Society: *Summary of Current Guidelines for the Cancer-Related Checkup: Recommendations*. Atlanta, American Cancer Society, 1988.

Canadian Task Force on the Periodic Health Examination: The periodic health examination. *Can Med Assoc J* 121:1193–1254, 1979; 130:1278–1285, 1984; 134:724–727, 1986; 138:618–626, 1988; 141:209–216, 1989.

Eddy DM (ed): *Common Screening Tests*. Philadelphia, American College of Physicians, 1991.

Hayward RS, Steinberg EP, Ford DE, et al: Preventive care guidelines: 1991. *Ann Intern Med* 114:758–783, 1991.

U.S. Preventive Services Task Force: *Guide to Clinical Preventive Services: An Assessment of The Effectiveness of 169 Interventions*. Baltimore, Williams & Wilkins, 1989.

CHAPTER 2

Perioperative Medical Evaluation

William E. Golden, M.D.
Wayne C. Williamson, M.D.

I. **Overview**
   A. Internists perform many consultations to assess preoperative surgical risks and to manage medical complications of perioperative patients.
   B. The aging of the U.S. population and the development of new procedures have expanded geriatric surgery and have changed the demographics of the operating room.
   C. Consultants must assess the risks and benefits of a planned procedure for a particular patient.
   D. Anticipation of and preparation for complications of the intraoperative period such as the physiologic effects of anesthesia, fluid shifts, or blood loss, in addition to the expected morbidities of a particular surgical procedure, are paramount when dealing with patients who have a variety of preexisting medical conditions.
   E. Invasive cardiac monitoring and new pharmacologic anesthetic agents help patients at increased cardiopulmonary risk to tolerate operative interventions.
   F. A holistic general internal medicine evaluation is effective. Organ-specific consultations may be inefficient.

II. **Consultations**
   A. Goals
      1. Reduce perioperative morbidity and mortality.
      2. Maximize the management of responsive medical conditions.
      3. Identify unalterable conditions to enable the anesthesiology team to plan care.
      4. Perform postoperative surveillance to help the surgeon manage complications and avoid catastrophic complications leading to prolonged hospitalization.
   B. Techniques
      1. Respond to requests for consultation in a timely fashion.
      2. Understand the goals of the consulting surgeon.
      3. Write clear, brief notes and recommendations.
      4. Perform a risk assessment.
      5. Never "clear" a patient.
         a. This term has no meaning.
         b. Can imply a guarantee of a good outcome.
      6. Communicate directly with the surgeon when unexpected problems are identified.

7. Clarify if you may or are expected to write orders on specific aspects of patient management.
8. Urge consulting surgeons to admit frailer patients at midday or arrange for them to be seen in advance as outpatients to avoid hurried and incomplete evaluations.

III. Anesthesia

Anesthetic techniques and agents can cause significant changes in preload, myocardial contractility, autonomic responsiveness, and pulmonary functional residual capacity.

A. General

Inhalational—halothane, isoflurance, enflurane, nitrous oxide *Narcotic*—morphine, fentanyl, sufentanil

1. All inhaled anesthetics have a direct depressant effect on the myocardium. Cardiac output is maintained via reflex sympathetic stimulation and peripheral vasodilatation.
2. General anesthesia lowers functional residual capacity (FRC).
3. Narcotic techniques with the morphine congeners have minimal adverse cardiac effects, enabling complex procedures in patients with poor cardiovascular reserve.

B. Regional (spinal, epidural)

Overall mortality and morbidity are comparable to those of general anesthesia. In certain procedures regional techniques may reduce blood loss and the risk of thromboembolism. With regional blocks, one must consider the pain of tourniquets used in lower extremity surgery.

1. Spinal
   a. Has pulmonary effects similar to those of general anesthesia.
   b. Loss of FRC and promotion of atelectasis.
   c. Vasodilation leading to drop in preload.
2. Epidural
   a. Allows persistence of analgesia in the postoperative period; with an epidural catheter in place, repeated doses of epidural opiates can be administered postoperatively.
   b. Nerve blocks of the extremities and sacrum
      (1) Minimal cardiopulmonary effects
      (2) Useful in frail patients (e.g., elderly diabetics with foot ulcers.)

IV. Perioperative Risk

A. Goldman and Detsky indexes provide a good overview of the components of surgical risk. No absolute point totals are involved in deciding whether to perform surgery. The points indicate the relative risk of the procedure.
B. The most important component of these indexes is uncontrolled heart failure.
C. Risks can be identified and sometimes altered. If they are unalterable, the surgeon, anesthesiologist, and patient must decide if the benefits of surgery outweigh the risks.
D. Consultations can help manage postoperative morbidity in patients with unalterable, increased risk.
E. *Cardiac risk factors in noncardiac surgery (Goldman)*

Factor	Points
S_3 gallop or jugular venous distention	11
Myocardial infarction (MI) within the last 6 months	10
Rhythm other than sinus or premature atrial contractions (PACs) on preoperative ECG	7
5 PVCs per minute	7
Age over 70	5
Emergency operation	4
Intraperitoneal, intrathoracic, or aortic operation	3
Important aortic stenosis by clinical examination	3
Poor general medical condition	3

F. *Modified index of cardiac risk factors (Detsky)*

Factor	Points
Coronary artery disease	
MI within the last 6 months	10
MI more than 6 months preoperatively	5
Canadian Cardiovascular Society angina grading	
Class III	10
Class IV	20
Unstable angina within the last 6 months	10
Alveolar pulmonary edema	
Within 1 week	10

Factor	Points
Alveolar pulmonary edema	
Any history	5
Suspected critical aortic stenosis	20
Arrhythmias	
Rhythm other than sinus or PACs	5
Over 5 PVCs per minute any time preoperatively	5
Poor general medical condition	5
Age over 70	5
Emergency operation	10

G. New indices of morbidity are being developed.
   1. Current methods screen out few elective cases.
   2. New methods needed to predict postoperative morbidity.

V. **Preoperative Evaluation and Laboratory Tests**
   A. History, physical examination, and type of surgery should guide evaluation.
   B. Basic recommendations
      1. Minimal laboratory tests (e.g., hematocrit) needed for young, healthy patients.
      2. Recommended for most older surgical patients
         a. Complete blood count.
         b. Electrolytes, creatinine, glucose, serum transaminase.
         c. Electrocardiogram.
         d. Chest x-ray.
      3. Recommended for some patients
         a. Urinalysis and urine culture for arthroplasty patients.
         b. Prothrombin time and partial thromboplastin time in patients with a history of bleeding or a medical condition which increases the risk of coagulopathy.
         c. Baseline arterial blood gases for patients with chronic obstructive pulmonary disease (COPD).
         d. Pulmonary function tests useful in patients with severe COPD and in those scheduled for thoracotomy.
         e. Dipyrimidole thallium stress tests useful in patients who need major vascular surgery.
         f. Serum albumin determination to assess nutritional status in debilitated patients. It can predict a prolonged

postoperative course and difficulties with fluid management.

VI. **Preoperative Cardiovascular Risk**
   A. Coronary artery disease
      1. Fifty percent of patients 80 years old have occult coronary artery disease.
      2. Stable angina mildly increases risk.
      3. Unstable angina should be evaluated and treated.
      4. Stress tests and cardiac catheterization should be reserved for patients with angina of uncertain severity. Dipyrimidole thallium stress tests useful in patients who are unable to exercise.
      5. MI increases the cardiac risk, which declines with time and is stable 6 months after the MI.
      6. Invasive intraoperative monitoring (arterial line, Swan-Gantz catheterization) and morphine congeners (fentanyl, sufentanil) lower the risk and mortality of surgery in the first 6 months after infarction.
      7. Avoid surgery unless a true emergency occurs in the first 30 days after an infarction.
   B. Congestive heart failure
      1. Uncontrolled heart failure is the most significant and possibly remediable risk factor.
      2. Control of heart failure usually requires several days of therapy.
      3. Major surgery is feasible with invasive monitoring and morphine congeners in patients with serious cariomyopathy.
   C. Valvular heart disease
      1. General considerations
         a. Bacterial endocarditis prophylaxis is warranted for:
            (1) Prosthetic heart valves
            (2) Congenital malformations
            (3) Rheumatic heart disease
            (4) Mitral valve prolapse with insufficiency
            (5) Idiopathic hypertrophic sub-aortic stenosis
            (6) Patients with a previous history of endocarditis
         b. Not needed solely for patients with previous coronary artery bypass surgery
      2. Aortic stenosis
         a. Severe aortic stenosis is an independent risk factor for perioperative cardiac death. Preload loss on induction may provoke fatal cardiac arrest. Re-

cent literature demonstrates reduced risk with careful technique.
- b. If severe aortic stenosis is suspected, Doppler echocardiography should be performed to assess the valvular gradient.
- c. Patients with severe aortic stenosis should have valve replacement before elective surgery.

D. Carotid artery disease and cerebrovascular disease
1. Bruits
   - a. Bruits are not necessarily indicative of the presence or severity of carotid artery disease.
   - b. *Asymptomatic* bruits do not need evaluation preoperatively. They are a marker for diffuse atherosclerosis. They do not increase the risk of stroke. Noninvasive tests may indicate severe disease that might benefit from endarterectomy at some future time.
2. Transient ischemic attacks
   - a. Patient should have a full medical workup prior to elective surgery.
   - b. Carotid endarterectomy for significant lesions takes precedence over other noncardiac surgical procedures.
3. Strokes
   - a. Delay all surgery for at least 2 weeks following an acute cerebrovascular accident (preferably for 6 weeks unless an emergency exists).

E. Hypertension
1. Patients with poorly controlled preoperative hypertension may have hypertensive surges during:
   - a. Anesthesia induction
   - b. Visceral traction
   - c. Postoperative pain
2. Hypertension is not a major risk factor unless diastolic pressure above 110 mmHg.
3. Several days of control is recommended prior to a nonemergency procedure in patients with preoperative diastolic blood pressure above 120 mmHg.
4. Consider diuretics, α-blockers, or calcium channel blockers for rapid control (over hours to several days) in Afro-American patients.
5. In some patients in whom hypertension is poorly controlled, relative volume depletion may be present because of compen-

satory vasoconstriction. These patients can have great lability of hypertension with anesthetics because of alterations of autonomic tone.
6. Medications should be given on the day of surgery with minimal water (especially β-blockers and calcium channel blockers).
7. The only contraindications to elective surgery are untreated pheochromocytoma, coarctation of the aorta, and use of guanethidine.

VII. **Preoperative Pulmonary Risk**
A. COPD
1. No pulmonary function test value is prohibitive unless the planned procedure involves lung resection.
2. Risk-benefit analysis is especially important for patients with severe COPD.
3. Bronchodilators are helpful and should be in the therapeutic range preoperatively.
4. Control of preoperative pulmonary infections is important in reducing postoperative morbidity.
5. Complete pulmonary function tests are not mandatory but may help document risks in severe cases or in patients facing thoracotomy or lung resection.
6. Arterial blood gas determinations provide useful baselines for postoperative management of severe COPD.
7. Although various opinions have been published, most clinicians believe that cigarette smoking should be stopped several weeks prior to surgery.

B. Asthma
1. Assess disease stability and severity.
2. Perioperative airway manipulation and secretion production can exacerbate stable disease.
3. Maintain or maximize medications if the patient is unstable preoperatively.
4. Start steroids the night prior to surgery in patients with severe or unstable disease.

VIII. **Perioperative Diabetes Care**
A. Long-standing diabetes can increase the perioperative risk.
1. Autonomic neuropathy can promote cardiovascular instability and delayed gastric emptying.
2. Peripheral neuropathy can promote soft tissue injury in the bedridden or sedated patient.

3. Microvascular disease can increase the cardiac risk.

B. Poor diabetes control is associated with:
1. Delayed wound healing.
2. Increased risk of wound infection.

C. Basic management strategies
1. Check glucose control on admission. If glucose is uncontrolled, check stat levels the day of surgery. Use regular insulin to adjust glucose levels.
2. Stable type 1 and type 2 diabetics can be given one-half of their morning insulin and a D5 drip the day of surgery.
3. Oral agents should be held the day of surgery.
4. Early morning surgery avoids the problem of awkward glucose management.
5. Check glucose levels intraoperatively if surgery lasts more than 2 hr.
6. Brittle diabetics may benefit from frequent intraoperative glucose checks and an insulin drip.
7. All diabetics should have their glucose checked on arrival at the recovery room.
8. Sliding-scale insulin orders and glucose checks every 6–8 hr are preferred in all NPO postoperative diabetics. Restore the usual medication schedule depending on the dietary intake.
9. Postoperative tube feedings in diabetic patients are best managed with NPH insulin in equal doses every 12 hr.

IX. Postoperative Cardiac Management
A. Cardiac disease
1. MI
   a. Rarely occurs intraoperatively.
   b. Can occur up to 5 days postoperatively.
   c. Often silent. Presents as arrhythmia, congestive heart failure, or weakness.
2. Congestive heart failure
   a. Consider acute MI.
   b. Review the perioperative fluid history.
   c. Mild failure expected in postoperative very elderly patients (>85 years).
B. Hypertension
1. Assess for secondary causes:
   a. Pain
   b. Inappropriate cuff size
   c. Fluid overload
   d. Emergence from anesthesia
   e. Airway obstruction
2. Sample regimens for NPO hypertensive patients

a. Intravenous Aldomet—onset of effect delayed for several hours. Used for maintenance.
b. Transdermal clonidine—single patch lasts 1 week. Requires 36- to 48-hr skin saturation to achieve therapeutic loading if there are no previous drug levels.
c. Intravenous labetalol—good chronotropic and vasodilatory response for rapid, gentle blood pressure control in acute situations.

C. Arrhythmias
1. Always consider new MI.
2. New-onset atrial fibrillation is often transient and requires only rate control. Consider possible pulmonary embolism if the clinical setting is suggestive.
3. Premature ventricular beats are a common side effect of inhaled anesthetic agents and are often transient in the immediate postoperative period. Review the electrolyte status.
4. Sinus and junctional bradycardia are common side effects of anesthetic agents.
5. Sinus and junctional tachycardia can be seen with anesthetic agents. Assess volume and blood status. Consider sepsis, embolism, pain, and anxiety.

X. Postoperative Pulmonary Problems
A. Atelectasis (common cause of fever)
1. Incentive spirometry is the effective prophylaxis and treatment.
B. Pneumonia
1. Fairly rare complication.
2. Bronchitis is more frequent.
3. Treat increased sputum production with oral antibiotics unless an infiltrate is present in the chest x-ray. This usually requires intravenous antibiotics for hospital-acquired infection.
C. Asthma and COPD exacerbation
1. Use inhaled bronchodilators pre- and postoperatively.
2. Employ intravenous steroids with deterioration or brittle disease.

XI. Perioperative Thyroid Disease
A. Hyperthyroidism
1. Cancel elective surgery until the patient is euthyroid.
2. Start oral antithyroid drugs and β-blockers; treat for 10–14 days. Monitor free T_4.
3. Potassium iodide (Lugol's solution) with above medications will help avoid thyroid

storm if emergency surgery is required. Stress doses of steroids indicated in the treatment of thyroid storm.

B. Hypothyroidism
   1. Mild cases may not require treatment preoperatively.
   2. Severe cases may be associated with
      a. Intraoperative hypotension or hypothermia.
      b. Congestive heart failure.
      c. Gastrointestinal complications (ileus, constipation).
      d. Hypoventilation with problem in weaning from mechanical ventilation
      e. Obtundation.

XII. Perioperative Thromboembolism

A. Subcutaneous heparin is sufficient for most patients except those undergoing orthopedic and urologic procedures.
B. External pneumonic compression and low-dose warfarin may be helpful in orthopedic and urologic procedures.
C. Hip surgery without prophylaxis results in a 2% rate of fatal pulmonary embolus.
D. Postoperative ventilation-perfusion scans may be inconclusive due to the presence of atelectasis.
E. Duplex venous Doppler ultrasounds or venograms are useful for the diagnosis of postoperative deep venous thrombosis (DVT).
F. DVT must be treated with heparin followed by coumadin for 30–90 days.

XIII. Diagnostic Aspects of Postoperative Fever
Consider
   A. Atelectasis
   B. Pneumonitis
   C. Phlebitis
   D. Venous thrombosis
   E. Abscess
   F. Wound infection
   G. Bacteremia

   H. Resolving hematoma or seroma
   I. Drug reaction
   J. Hepatitis
   K. Blood transfusion
   L. Urinary tract infection
   M. Ileus

Bibliography

Boucher BA with Witt WO, Foster TS. The postoperative adverse effects of inhalational anesthetics. *Heart Lung* 5:63–69, 1986.

Cygan R, Waitskin H. Stopping and restarting medications in the perioperative period. *J Gen Intern Med* 2:270–283, 1987.

Detsky AI, Abrams HB, McLaughlin JR, et al. Predicting cardiac complications in patients undergoing noncardiac surgery. *J Gen Intern Med* 1:211–219, 1986.

Eagle KA, Boucher CA. Cardiac risk of noncardiac surgery. *N Engl J Med* 321:1330–1332, 1992.

Elliot MJ, Gill GV, Home PD, et al. A comparison of two regimens for the management of diabetes during open heart surgery. *Anesthesiology* 60:364–368, 1984.

Freeman WK, Gibbons RJ, Shub C. Preoperative assessment of cardiac patients undergoing noncardiac surgical procedures. *Mayo Clin Proc* 64:1105–1117, 1989.

Golden W, Lavender RC. Perioperative medical considerations, in Myers EM, Suen JY (eds): *Cancer of the Head and Neck*, ed 2. New York, Churchill Livingstone, 1989 pgs 101–120.

Goldman L, et al. Multifactorial index of cardiac risk in noncardiac surgical procedures. *N Engl J Med* 297:845–850, 1977.

Kaplan EB, Sheiner LB, Boeckmann AJ, et al. The usefulness of preoperative laboratory screening. *JAMA* 253:3576–3581, 1985.

Mohr DN, JeH, JK. Preoperative evaluation of pulmonary risk factors. *J Gen Intern Med* 3:277–287, 1988.

Prys-Roberts C, Meloche R, Foex P. Studies of anesthesia in relation to hypertension I. Cardiovascular responses of treated and untreated patients. *Br J Anesth* 43:122–137, 1971.

Role of carotid endarterectomy in asymptomatic carotid stenosis stroke. A Veterans Administration cooperative study: *Stroke* 17:534–539, 1986.

CHAPTER 3

Medical Ethics

Robert Wells Carton, M.D., M.A.

I. Definition

Medical ethics is concerned with the moral principles and rules which should obtain in the care of the sick and in the resolution of biomedical dilemmas.

II. Scope

While medical ethics applies to human actions anywhere in a medical or biological context, experience has shown that the insights of this discipline are more likely to be needed in certain situations:

A. Reproduction, including contraception, abortion, population control, surrogate motherhood, in vitro fertilization, management of the impaired newborn.

B. Genetics, including gene therapy and genome mapping.

C. Transplantation of tissues and organs.

D. Mental health situations, including behavior control.

E. Experimentation, including experimentation on human adults and children, recombinant DNA research, and experimentation on animals.

F. Life support, euthanasia, assisted suicide, and other tissues associated with death and allowing the patient to die.

G. Health care policy, including the distribution of health care.

H. Relationships of health care professionals with patients and their families, with colleagues, and with the public.

III. Principles of Medical Ethics

The principles of medical ethics have been derived from a variety of sources in philosophy and religion. The main philosophical sources are consequentialist ethics (How can I maximize the good?) and deontological ethics (What ought I do?). In the United States, medical ethics has been influenced by the Judeo-Christian ethical tradition. From this background, the following principles have evolved:

A. *Autonomy* The principle of respect for autonomy states that every competent person should be able to decide personally what medical treatment or other manipulations to undergo. The concepts of patient competence and informed consent are associated with the idea of autonomy.

1. Competence implies the following:

   a. Legal competence. The patient should be of a proper age for decision making. If this is the case, then a patient is considered *legally* competent until a court has declared him or her incompetent.

    b. Clinical competence. To be clinically competent, the patient should be able to understand the risks and benefits of a procedure to which he or she is giving assent. Clinical competence is judged by a physician.

  2. Informed consent should be obtained before patients are subjected to procedures of any magnitude. Informed consent is approval which a competent patient gives voluntarily after disclosure of the nature of a proposed action.

    In the United States today, the principle of patient autonomy is widely respected to the extent that its use does not impinge on the legitimate interest of the state. Autonomy is consonant with the American tradition of individualism. It allows for the expression of diverse personal values in a pluralistic society.

B. *Beneficence* The principle of beneficence appears in the Hippocratic Oath, in which the physician states: "I will follow that method of treatment which I consider for the benefit of my patients." This principle of maximizing the patient's good is sometimes separated from the principle of *nonmaleficence*, which is also present in the Hippocratic Oath: "[I will] abstain from whatever is deleterious and mischievous." But maximizing good and minimizing evil can be thought of as positive and negative qualities on the same scale. Here they are both included under the one principle of beneficence.

C. *Justice* The principle of justice implies that people should be treated fairly and as they deserve. This principle is relevant to almost every professional relationship with people into which a physician enters. On a micro scale, it implies that the physician should be fair in dealing with colleagues or with patients and their families. This is the justice of medical practice. On a macro scale, justice in the biomedical sphere is concerned with distribution of medical care throughout society.

  1. *Distributive justice* is the quality of fair or equitable allocation of resources. A major controversy in the practice of medicine at the present time focuses on the proper distribution of medical services. The question is: How should medical goods and services be distributed throughout the U.S. population in such a way that people are properly cared for without undue strain on the economy or on the resources of families?

IV. Application of Principles to Specific Situations

A. The moral problems listed in Section II can be approached using the principles of respect for autonomy, beneficence, and justice. As an example, consider the question of withdrawing ventilator support from a patient with progressive incurable illness who is also in respiratory failure (see Section II, F). The principle of *autonomy* directs that the patient's wishes should govern if the patient is competent. If the patient is not competent, a surrogate speaking for the patient will be able to approve or disapprove of the proposed action. According to the principle of *beneficence*, physicians should not injure the patient by withdrawing life support unless by doing so they act to relieve the patient of a situation which has become unduly burdensome and from which no recovery is deemed possible. The principle of *justice* may be invoked in two ways, depending on the scale:

  1. On a micro scale, the patient's physician, as his or her advocate, will work to see that the humanity of the patient is respected and that the patient receives all benefits to which he or she is entitled as a sick person.

  2. On a macro scale, societal agencies (courts, legislatures, etc.) may allocate resources, including those devoted to life support, in such a way as to maximize the good of society as a whole.

B. Application of ethical principles requires that the rights of others and of society be respected. These interpersonal and societal rights are represented by *laws*. Currently in the United States, the law applied to medical ethical dilemmas is almost entirely state law. Physicians encountering medical ethical problems should have a working knowledge of the applicable laws in the state in which they practice. Actions in this area must be taken within the framework prescribed by the relevant law.

C. Use of the principles of respect for autonomy, beneficence, and justice is generally necessary when approaching a medical ethical dilemma. But it may not be sufficient. These principles may not provide a determinate answer to the moral question being asked. The patient or surrogate may have been approached based on these three principles and still ask, "Doctor, what should I do?" In this case the physician must be prepared to give advice, based on his or knowledge of the patient's value structure. A consensual decision in many of the areas of medical ethics will reflect the deepest convictions of the patient and his or her family, as well as the ability of the physician and other members of the health care team to analyze the realities of the situation.

Bibliography

Aaron H, Schwartz WB: Rationing health care: The choice before us. *Science* 247:418–422, 1990.

Beauchamp TL, Childress JF: *Principles of Biomedical Ethics*, ed 3. New York, Oxford University Press, 1989.

Bone RC, Rackow EC, Weg JG: Ethical and moral guidelines for the initiation, continuation, and withdrawal of intensive care. *Chest* 97:949–958, 1990.

Walters L, Kahn TJ (eds): *Bibliography of Bioethics*, Vols 1–16. Washington, DC, Kennedy Institute of Ethics, Georgetown University, 1975–1990.

Chapter 4

Alcohol and Substance Abuse/Chemical Dependency

Richard Karrel, M.D.

I. **Definition of Chemical Dependency**
Chemical dependency (CD), the addiction to alcohol or other mood-altering chemicals, is a chronic, progressive, relapsing, and potentially fatal disease that affects all races, all socioeconomic strata, and both genders. CD is one of the leading causes of death and disability in the world; it is characterized by:
  A. Compulsive use of mood-altering chemicals despite adverse consequences (familial, medical, behavioral, social, professional, spiritual, emotional).
  B. Loss of control: periodic and/or continuous inability to control the use of mood-altering chemicals.
  C. Preoccupation with obtaining mood-altering chemicals.
  D. Chemical tolerance
    1. Increased dosage is needed to achieve the same effect, or a lessened effect is achieved with the same dosage.
    2. Some drugs do not induce tolerance (e.g., hallucinogens, marijuana).
  E. Chemical withdrawal
    1. Typical withdrawal syndrome—predictable display of symptoms/signs when the dose is abruptly reduced or discontinued. It is eliminated by administering the same chemical or by replacing it with a chemical of the same or a similar drug classification.
    2. There is an atypical withdrawl syndrome for some drugs (e.g., marijuana).
  F. Denial—defense mechanism characteristic of addiction. Marked by rationalization and by minimization of chemical usage and adverse consequences.
  G. Relapse—period(s) of usage following prolonged chemical abstinence.
II. **Etiology of Chemical Dependency**
  A. Biogenetic predisposition toward alcoholism
    1. Allelic association of the human dopamine D1 receptor gene.
    2. Family, twin, and adoption studies reveal a possible genetic predisposition.
  B. Endorphin-locus ceruleus hypothesis in opiate addiction
    1. Idiopathic/preexisting endorphin dysregulation may predispose individuals to addiction.
    2. Acquired endorphin dysregulation with

prolonged abuse may create an addictive process.

C. Self-medication hypothesis—explains chemical use but not compulsivity and loss of control.

D. Family, environment, and lifestyle influences—may explain chemical use but not compulsivity and loss of control.

III. **Drug Classification, Cross-Addiction, and Drug Substitution**

A. Classification of agents producing chemical dependency

1. Sedative-hypnotics—alcohol, benzodiazepines, barbiturates
2. Opiates—heroin, morphine, codeine, propoxyphene, methadone
3. Stimulants—cocaine, amphetamines, ephedrine, phenylephrine
4. Plants and cannabinols—marijuana, hashish, hash oil
5. Hallucinogens—lysergic acid diethylamide (LSD), phencyclidine (PCP), mescaline, psilocybin, amphetamines
6. Solvents—aerosol sprays, glue, gasoline, toluene

B. Cross-addiction—those addicted to one drug are, by definition, addicted to all drugs belonging to that class, and are predisposed to addiction to all classes of mood-altering drugs.

C. Drug substitution—substitution of drugs in the same or a different class to continue addiction.

IV. **Denial**

All individuals suffering from CD engage in denial, the primary sign of CD, and:

A. Minimize—quantity used, frequency, adverse consequences.

B. Rationalize—use, adverse consequences.

C. Believe—that they are in control of their usage.

V. **Alcohol and Drug History**

Patients who are intoxicated or suffering acute withdrawal may be unable or unwilling to give detailed alcohol and drug histories. CD patients are distrustful and have problems with judgment, rejection, and authority. Strict confidentiality must be ensured. To obtain a history, ascertain the age of first use, periods of use, and drug of choice, when problems first appeared due to drug use; patterns of use, frequency, amount, and last use; any prior detoxification; and any prior treatment. Also determine:

A. Failures at abstinence—has the patient ever tried to quit or cut down?

B. Blackouts—has the patient suffered amnesia during or after use?

C. Adverse consequences

1. Divorce, separation, job loss due to use, driving citations.
2. Medical problems related to alcohol or drug use.

D. Loss of control

1. Has the patient used chemicals to become intoxicated in order to escape from life situations/circumstances?
2. Has the patient ever been told that he or she drinks/uses chemicals too much or too often?
3. Has the patient ever accidentally overdosed, become sick, hallucinated, or suffered seizures?
4. Has the patient attempted to limit use but failed?

E. Compulsive use—does the patient gulp, sneak, hide, or stash?

F. Withdrawal—has the patient suffered hangovers, tremors, shakes, seizures, hallucinations, etc.?

G. Emotional consequences—has the patient ever experienced remorse, shame, or guilt from drinking/using chemicals?

VI. **Alcohol**

Alcohol is a central system (CNS) depressant, general anesthetic, sedative-hypnotic, and toxic solvent that is totally miscible in water. It is more frequenty abused than any other drug.

A. Epidemiology—alcoholism affects an estimated 15 to 20 million Americans.

1. Health-related costs in United States exceed $100 billion per year.
2. Alcohol is involved in most deaths due to suicide, homicide, motor vehicle accidents, overdoses, drowning, and trauma.
3. Alcoholism is a major cause of liver disease; peptic ulcer disease; pancreatitis; cardiovascular, hematopoietic, endocrine, nutritional, and nervous system diseases.
4. From 12 to 30% of all urban hospital medical/surgical inpatients screen positively for alcoholism on admission.
5. Fetal alcohol syndrome is the number one cause of mental retardation in the United States.

B. Intoxication—an initial small dose stimulates the CNS; with repeated doses, CNS depression occurs.

C. Effects—depend on the blood alcohol level;

Table 4-1. Blood Alcohol Levels of Intoxication

1. Mild to moderate [<100 mg/dl (0.10%)]
2. Legal intoxication [100–150 mg/dl (0.10–0.15%)]
   a. Altered cognition
   b. Personality and behavioral alterations
3. Moderate [150–199 mg/dl (0.15–0.19%)]
   a. Incoordination, nausea, vomiting
   b. Confusion
   c. Gait disturbance
4. Moderate to severe [200–299 mg/dl (0.20–0.29%)]
   a. Dysarthria
   b. Sensory dysfunction
   c. Visual disturbances
5. Severe [300–399 mg/dl (0.30–0.39%)]
   a. Hypothermia, hypoglycemia
   b. Poor muscle control, poor recall
   c. Convulsions
6. Potentially lethal [>400 mg/dl (0.40%)]
   a. Loss of consciousness, decreased reflexes
   b. Respiratory failure and death

they include euphoria, altered thought processes, incoordination, hypothermia, respiratory failure, and death (see Table 4-1).

D. Alcohol withdrawl syndrome—comprised of any or all of the following, which may occur sequentially or coincidentally:
   1. Minor withdrawal symptoms (6–10 hr after the last drink)—anxiety, mild agitation, tachycardia, tremor, gastrointestinal discomfort, hypertension.
   2. Severe withdrawal symptoms (8–24 hr after the last drink)—grand mal seizures, usually self-limited. Focal seizures signify CNS complications (meningitis, head injury, etc.). Patients with comorbid conditions and those with a history of severe withdrawal are more likely to suffer severe withdrawal.
   3. Hallucinations (8–24 hr after the last drink), usually visual (rats, bugs, spiders), sometimes auditory, rarely olfactory (which can be an ominous sign).
   4. Delirium tremens (12–72 hr after the last drink)—severe agitation, hallucinations, diaphoresis, hyperthermia, tremor, profound confusion, electrolyte imbalance, convulsions, potential cardiovascular collapse; 12% mortality rate if untreated.
   5. Post–acute withdrawal syndrome—may last for periods ranging from weeks to

months; consists mainly of agitation, insomnia, irritability, cravings, anxiety, and headaches.
E. Pharmacological treatment of alcohol withdrawal syndrome
   1. Most patients require no treatment or only symptomatic care (mild sedation).
   2. Multivitamin therapy—100 mg thiamine, immediately (before glucose is administered) and daily for 3 days to prevent and/or treat Wernicke-Korsakoff syndrome.
   3. Fluid, glucose, and electrolyte replacement and maintenance.
   4. Long-acting benzodiazepine—diazepam (10–30 mg) orally, intramuscularly, or intravenously every 2 hr as needed for agitation. Taper the dosage over 5–7 days until the patient is drug free.
      a. Sedative-hypnotics—recommended for their combination of sedative and anticonvulsant effects.
      b. Barbiturates—avoided due to their hepatic metabolic degradation rates and narrow toxic-therapeutic ratios.
   5. Convulsions controlled with sedative-hypnotics.
   6. Hallucinations controlled with haloperidol (intramuscularly, 2 mg every 4 hr as needed) and Cogentin (2 mg/day) to prevent the extrapyramidal effects of haloperidol.
   7. Delirium tremens managed with sedation; cardiac monitoring; temperature control; electrolyte, glucose, and fluid replacement; maintenance therapy.
   8. Clonidine, valproic acid, β-blockers, and carbamazepine have been given, with varying degrees of success.

VII. Sedative-Hypnotics
Sedative-hypnotic drugs act on the CNS and are used as muscle relaxants, anti-anxiety agents, and anticonvulsants. Physical dependency and significant withdrawal symptoms are common and can follow abuse or chronic therapeutic use.
A. Agents in this group include barbiturates, benzodiazepines, meprobamate, glutethimide, methyprylon, and methaqualone.
B. Physical dependency can result from low-dose therapeutic use (> 6 months), high therapeutic doses (> 30 days), and/or high-dose abuse (> 30 days).
C. Benzodiazepine intoxication—low toxicity unless ingested with other CNS depressants

(e.g., alcohol). Symptoms include slurred speech, incoordination, hyporeflexia, confusion, ataxia, horizontal nystagmus, and respiratory depression.

D. Sedative-hypnotic withdrawal syndrome—severity is related to the dose and length of usage.
 1. Types of withdrawal
  a. Acute major withdrawal (in high-dose sedative-hypnotic abusers)
   (1) Usually begins 1–2 days after the last dose of short-acting benzodiazepines or 2–4 days after the last dose of long-acting benzodiazepines (either may begin as long as 9 days after the last dose). Initial symptoms progress and worsen.
   (2) Symptoms/signs—anxiety, tremor, hypertension, agitation, panic, irritability, insomnia, nightmares, muscle spasms, hyperreflexia, seizures, delirium, hyperpyrexia, death.
   (3) Duration of maximal withdrawal symptoms
    (a) Long-acting—symptoms usually peak at 8 days and last for 2 weeks.
    (b) Short-acting—symptoms usually peak at 2–5 days and last for 8–9 days.
  b. Acute minor withdrawal (low-dose use for > 6 months)
   (1) Symptoms/signs
    (a) Begin 1 day after the last dose and consist mainly of anxiety, insomnia, muscle spasms, psychosis, panic, tachycardia, and hypertension.
    (b) May wax and wane in cycles separated by 2–10 days.
  c. Chronic withdrawal (low or high doses for > 6 months)
   (1) Chronic symptoms may begin 9–20 days after the last dose and may last for 15–45 days.
   (2) Symptoms/signs—depression, agitation, insomnia, nightmares, anorexia, emotional lability.
 2. Treatment of sedative-hypnotic withdrawal
  a. Outpatient who is physically dependent on low-dose benzodiazepines but still in control of usage—slow, step-wise reduction of dose. Propranolol may be instituted on the fifth day of withdrawal and continued for 2 weeks to control tachycardia, hypertension, and anxiety.
  b. Hospital detoxification for those at risk for major sedative-hypnotic withdrawal syndrome—use phenobarbital substitution:
   (1) Convert sedative-hypnotic to phenobarbital dosage (Table 4-2).
   (2) Divide into four doses, administered orally (no more than 500 mg/day).
   (3) Reduce the dosage by 30 mg/day.
   (4) Check for sustained horizontal nystagmus, slurred speech, and ataxia before giving each dose. Withhold the dose if one sign is present; withhold the next two doses if all signs are present.

VIII. Opiates
Opiates are narcotic analgesics that produce a classic withdrawal pattern. Heroin is viewed as the prototype, although methadone, codeine, hydrocodone, and oxycodone are also commonly abused.
 A. Opiate intoxication
  1. Mild to moderate—miosis, lethargy, dysarthria, apathy, euphoria.
  2. Severe—miosis, hypotension, depressed respiration, decreased consciousness, pulmonary edema, hypothermia, respiratory arrest.
 B. Medical complications
  1. Intravenous—acquired immunodeficiency syndrome (AIDS), hepatitis, systemic infections, pulmonary complications, cellulitis, tetanus, thrombophlebi-

Table 4-2. Dose Equivalents of Phenobarbital (30 mg)

Generic Drug	Dose (mg)
Diazepam	10
Alprazolam	1
Lorazepam	2
Oxazepam	10
Chlordiazepoxide	25
Pentobarbital	100
Secobarbital	100
Meprobamate	400
Methaqualone	300
Glutethimide	250

tis, bacteremia, endocarditis, organ abscesses, meningitis.

2. Oral—in combination with acetaminophen use, may cause liver damage.

C. Acute withdrawal—influenze-like syndrome, not life-threatening but protracted and uncomfortable.

1. Anticipatory stage (3–4 hr after the last dose)—fear of withdrawal, anxiety, drug craving, drug-seeking behavior.

2. Early stage (8–10 hr after the last dose)—anxiety, nausea, diaphoresis, rhinorrhea, lacrimation, dilated pupils, abdominal cramps, drug-seeking behavior, insomnia, photophobia, myalgias.

3. Peak stage (1–2 days after the last dose, lasts for 7–10 days)—severe anxiety, tremor, restlessness, agitation, panic, piloerection, diarrhea, muscle spasms, increased blood pressure, tachycardia, chills, intense drug-seeking behavior, arthralgias, myalgias, headaches, yawning.

4. Protracted withdrawal (1–6 months)—hypotension, bradycardia, apathy, lethargy, anorexia, opiate craving.

D. Treatment of withdrawal

1. Most patients can be detoxified in a safe, supportive, structured, nurturing environment.

2. Those with a history of moderate to severe opiate withdrawal also require pharmacological withdrawal treatment.

   a. Clonidine regimen (preferred)—0.2 mg orally every 4–6 hr for 24 hr, then 0.8–1.2 mg/day for 7–10 days, then tapered over 3–5 days.

      (1) Common side effect—postural hypotension.

      (2) Clonidine suppression of withdrawal usually requires long-acting benzodiazepines for 5–7 days to reduce agitation, anxiety, and insomnia.

   b. Clonidine reigmen (alternate)—transdermal no. 2 patch. Two patches for the patient < 70 kg; three pathes for the patient > 70 kg. With clonidine, (give 0.2 orally every 6 hr for 48 hr.)

      (1) Leave patches in place for 7 days.

      (2) If the patient is withdrawing from methadone, leave the patch in place for 10 days.

   c. Methadone regimen

      (1) Outpatient methadone detoxifica-

tion not recommended; high failure rate and lack of structure/control.

      (2) Inpatient detoxification—administer methadone in 5-mg increments over 24 hr to suppress acute physical withdrawal signs. Rarely, > 20 mg/day is needed. Then reduce by 5 mg/day increments.

3. Experimental pharmacological treatments

   a. Levomethadyl acetate—methadone congener; has a longer duration of action, fewer sedative effects, and low abuse potential.

   b. Lofexidine (α_2-agonist), guanfacine (α_2-agonist), guanabenz (long-acting α_2-agonist), delta sleep-inducing peptide (DSIP), interferon, calcium channel inhibitors for efficacy in opiate withdrawal.

E. Long-term pharmacological treatment—naltrexone (long-acting opiate antagonist), 150 mg orally every 3 days. Block euphoric effects. Given after 5–7 days of abstinence to avoid acute withdrawal.

F. Experimental long-term pharmacological treatment—buprenorphine hydrochloride, a partial agonist-antagonist.

IX. Cocaine and CNS Stimulants

Cocaine dependency represents the most severe form of addiction. It produces an imbalance of neurochemicals, particularly dopamine. Cocaine dependency causes more drug deaths than any other chemical except alcohol. Amphetamines, potent sympathomimetic and CNS stimulate drugs produce almost the same effects as cocaine (i.e., intoxication, addiction, withdrawal).

A. Cocaine ("lady", "snow", "crack") is a powerful CNS stimulant, local anesthetic, vasoconstrictor, and sympathomimetic.

1. Routes of administration

   a. Intranasal—CNS effect achieved in 5 min, with a 15- to 20-min peak stimulus, followed by a progressive crash over 1–2 hr.

   b. Intravenous—CNS effect achieved in 7 sec, with a 2- to 5-min peak stimulus, followed by a progressive crash over 20 min.

   c. Inhalation (smoking)—CNS effect achieved in < 7 sec, with a 2- to 5-min peak stimulus, followed by a progressive crash over 20 min.

d. Mucosal—effectively absorbed through any mucosal surface, including oral, rectal, and vaginal surfaces.

2. Medical complications
    a. Cardiovascular—life-threatening arrhythmias, acute myocardial infarction, angina, cardiac arrest, cardiovascular accident, malignant hypertension, aortic dissection, AIDS.
    b. Pulmonary—"crack lung," asthma, pneumomediastinum, pneumothorax, pulmonary edema, congestive heart failure, respiratory failure.
    c. Miscellaneous—convulsions, status epilepticus, malignant hyperthermia, nasal perforation, retinal artery occlusion.

3. Acute cocaine intoxication—euphoria, elation, mydriasis, talkativeness, hyperactivity, flight of ideas, convulsions, CNS medullary depression, death.

4. Chronic cocaine intoxication—irritability, paranoia, suspicion, fatigue, dysphoria, anhedonia, illusions, delusions, paranoid ideations, hallucinations, paranoid psychosis, anorexia, exhaustion, collapse.

5. Cocaine withdrawal syndrome—hyperphagia, drug craving, apathy, depression, anhedonia, intense fatigue, hypersomnia or insomnia, chills, confusion, dreaming, postcocaine psychosis.

6. Pharmacological treatment of cocaine withdrawal—required for patients who do not respond to a supportive, structured, nurturing environment alone.
    a. Combination of bromocriptine (a dopamine agonist) and desipramine (an antidepressant)—relative success achieved in reducing drug craving, depression, and anhedonia.
        (1) Bromocriptine—2.5 mg qid, tapered daily; discontinue on day 18.
        (2) Desipramine—50 mg at bedtime, increased daily to 250 mg by day 12; continue for 8 months.
    b. Bromocriptine alone—varying degrees of success.
    c. Desipramine alone—action is too slow.
    d. Experimental drugs for reducing cravings/withdrawal depression—amantadine (a dopamine releaser), levodopa, carbidopa, phenelzine, trazodone, calcium channel blockers.

7. Some patients may require psychiatric intervention for severe depression or postcocaine psychosis.

B. Amphetamines and chemically related sympathomimetics
    1. Methamphetamine ("speed", "crystal"), dextroamphetamine, methylphenidate, phenmetrazine, phentermine, chlorphentermine.
    2. Routes of administration, acute and chronic intoxication, and medical and psychiatric complications similar to those of cocaine.
    3. Treatment of acute withdrawal
        a. Most patients respond well to a supportive, structured, nurturing environment.
        b. Some patients may require psychiatric intervention for severe depression or continued postamphetamine psychosis.

X. **Hallucinogens and Psychedelic Drugs**
The drugs in this class produce hallucinations and gross perceptual distortions. They profoundly alter mood, thought, and behavior.

A. Drugs
    1. Lysergic acid diethylamide (LSD)
        a. The prototype hallucinogen, referred to as "acid."
        b. Used more by adolescents than by adults.
        c. Routes of administration—oral, intranasal, parenteral.
        d. Intoxication—onset within 5–10 min; peak effects achieved at 30–90 min; effects usually last for 12 hr, possibly with chronic effects lasting for days.
        e. CNS effects—euphoria, anxiety, panic, visual hallucinations, agitation, distortions of existing stimuli, "bad trips," violence.
        f. Physical effects—dilated pupils; anisocoria; facial flushing; piloerection; elevated blood pressure, pulse rate, temperature.
        g. Associated effects—flashbacks, recurrence of imagery post-drug use; may appear years after use or may represent the normal memory process.
    2. Phencyclidine (PCP)—a common street drug ("hog", "dust"), usually combined with other drugs (cocaine, marijuana, amphetamines).
        a. Routes of administration—oral, intra-

nasal, parenteral, inhalation (smoking).

   b. Effects occur immediately after injection or smoking.

   c. Intoxication

     (1) Cardinal signs—horizontal, vertical, rotary nystagmus; hypertension.

     (2) Other signs—sedation, agitation, catatonia, dystonia, convulsions, paranoid psychosis, violent behavior, coma, respiratory depression.

  3. Hallucinogenic amphetamines—methamphetamines and their derivatives (e.g., "ecstacy," "adam," "XTC").

   a. Highly addictive, commonly abused "designer" drugs.

   b. Effects—hallucinations, perceptual changes, illusions, object distortions, hypertension, diaphoresis, hypertonicity, ventricular fibrillation, death.

  4. Other commonly abused drugs in the class—psilocybin, mescaline, cannabinols, cocaine.

B. Hallucinogen and psychedelic drug withdrawal treatment

  1. No characteristic withdrawal syndrome.

  2. Withdrawal treated most effectively with supportive care—reality testing, nurturing, structured environment, mild sedation.

  3. Prolonged psychotic episodes require major tranquilizers, psychiatric consultation.

XI. Chemical Dependency Treatment

All patients suffering from CD need formal addiction treatment in an inpatient and/or outpatient setting. The ultimate goal of therapy is for patients to remain totally abstinent from all mood-altering chemicals.

A. Inpatient treatment

  1. Required for certain types of patients

   a. Those needing medical support to withdraw from physiological addiction.

   b. Emotionally or medically unstable individuals.

   c. Those capable of harming themselves or others.

  2. Structured treatment program designed to:

   a. Safely detoxify and stabilize.

   b. Confront the patient's denial system.

   c. Identify relapse triggers and teach relapse prevention techniques to support lifelong abstinence and recovery.

B. Outpatient treatment—recommended for emotionally and medically stable patients who are not suffering acute withdrawal syndrome.

C. Continuing care

  1. Relapse prevention program of individual and family support, self-help meeting attendance, 12-step recovery program.

  2. Ongoing individual and/or family psychotherapy and/or addiction counseling may be required.

D. Treatment for dual-diagnosis patients

  1. An estimated 15% of all patients suffering from CD also suffer from a major psychiatric illness.

  2. An estimated 50% or more of all CD patients also suffer from a characterological illness.

  3. Patients should be treated for both diagnoses, with priority given to total abstinence from all mood-altering chemicals.

Bibliography

Louria DB, Hensle T, Rose J: The major medical complications of heroin addiction. *Ann Intern Med* 67(1):1–21, 1967.

Moore R, Bone LR, Geller G, et al: Prevalence, detection and treatment of alcoholism in hospitalized patients. *JAMA* 261(3):403–407, 1989.

Sellers EM, Kalant H: Alcohol intoxication and withdrawal. *N Engl J Med* 294(14):757–762, 1976.

Smith DE, Wesson DR: Benzodiazepine dependency syndromes. *J Psychoactive Drugs* 15(1–2):85–95, 1983.

CHAPTER 5

Principles of Occupational Health

Linda Rae Murray, M.D., M.P.H.

I. Scope of the Field
  A. Occupational health involves the physical and emotional, health and safety of workers.
    1. In the United States there are approximately 100 million workers, all of whom have potential hazards onthe job.
  B. About 10,000 physicians practice occupational medicine full- or part-time. Fewer than 1,000 are formally trained or board certified in the field.
  C. The distribution of occupational illness in the United States as of 1988 is given in Table 5-1.

II. Recognizing Hazards
  A. Reasons why occupational and environmental diseases are difficult to recognize
    1. Work processes and potential exposure are generally not familiar to health care workers.
    2. Diseases produced by occupational and environmental exposure resemble diseases with other etiologies.
    3. Diseases produced by occupational exposure often have multifactorial etiologies.
    4. There is rarely a pathognomonic marker for occupational disease.
    5. There is frequently a long latency period between exposure and the manifestation of disease.
  B. Types of hazards (Table 5-2)
    1. Biological hazards
      a. Hazards in the work environment
        (1) Poison ivy, poison oak
        (2) Snakes, spiders
        (3) Fungi and bacteria (e.g., contamination of cutting fluids in metal-working processes, leptospirosis among agricultural and sewage workers)
      b. Hazards in work processes
        (1) Animal or plant product processes (e.g., anthrax, brucellosis)
      c. Hazards in the health care industry (e.g., tuberculosis, hepatitis, cytomegalovirus)
    2. Chemical hazards—tens of thousands of chemicals are introduced in the workplace each year; we have toxicological data on only a tiny fraction of them.
    3. Dust and mineral hazards (e.g., silica, coal, asbestos)
    4. Physical hazards
      a. Hypothermia
      b. Heat stress

Table 5-1. Percent of Occupational Illness by Category in the Private Sector, 1988

Type	Percent
Repetitive trauma	48
Skin	24
Lung disease (other than dusts)	7
Physical agents	7
Poisoning	2
Lung disease (dusts)	1
All other	11

Source: Bureau of Labor Statistics.

      c. Noise

      d. Vibration

      e. Electrical, lightning, and thermal burns

      f. Ionizing and nonionizing radiation

   5. Ergonomic hazards

      a. Worker/task fit

      b. Worker/tool fit

   6. Psychosocial hazards

      a. Absence of adequate protection of workers' rights

      b. Lack of control of work tasks

      c. Shift work, especially night work

  C. Process-related hazards

   1. Specific processes expose workers to typical hazards, which often combine and produce synergistic effects.

   2. Knowledge of the processes and exposures to be expected, as well as diseases seen in those workers, is essential to the practice of occupational medicine.

   3. Examples

      a. *Abrasive blasting* (surface treatment with high-velocity sand, steel shot, pecan shells, glass, or aluminum oxide): hazards include silica, noise, and lead poisoning.

      b. *Degreasing* (removes dirt and grease, using chemicals): hazards include explosions, solvent vapors, phosgene, and methyl chloride.

Table 5-2. Types of Hazards

Biological hazards
Chemical hazards
Dust and mineral hazards
Physical hazards
Ergonomic hazards
Psychosocial hazards

      c. *Electroplating* (coating of materials with thin layers of metal such as nickel, gold, silver, or cadmium): hazards include acid mists and hydrogen cyanide.

      d. *Machining* (metals, plastic, and wood worked and shaped with lathes, drills, and milling machines): hazards include dusts, cutting oils, mists, solvents, and metals.

      e. *Welding and metal cutting* (joining or cutting metals by heating them to molten or semimolten state): hazards include noise, heat, infrared and ultraviolet radiation, metal fumes, and other gases.

  D. Target organs

   Another way of looking at occupational diseases is to consider the occupational etiologies for renal disease, hemopoietic disorders, reproductive disorders, and so on.

III. Leading Work-Related Diseases and Injuries (Table 5-3)

  A. Occupational lung diseases—the major route of entry of occupational hazards

   1. Asphyxiant

      a. Simple respiratory asphyxiants replace oxygen in ambient air (e.g., nitrogen, methane, carbon dioxide: heavier than air; may build up in confined spaces)

      b. Chemical respiratory asphyxiants interfere with normal respiratory process

         (1) Carbon monoxide

            (a) Ubiquitous product of combustion

            (b) Preferentially binds to hemoglobin, decreasing the oxygen-carrying capacity of blood

         (2) Cyanide salts

            (a) Used in tanning, electroplating, photographic processes

Table 5-3. The 10 Leading Work-Related Diseases and Injuries

1. Occupational lung disease
2. Musculoskeletal injuries
3. Occupational cancers (other than lung cancer)
4. Occupation injuries (amputations, fractures, eye loss, lacerations, and traumatic deaths)
5. Cardiovascular disorders
6. Disorders of reproduction
7. Neurotoxic disorders
8. Noise-induced hearing loss
9. Dermatologic conditions
10. Psychological disorders

Source: National Institute for Occupational Safety and Health.

(b) Disable the cytochrome oxidase system, leading to metabolic asphyxiation

   (3) Hydrogen sulfide

     (a) Found in tanneries, sewage plants, rubber industry, petroleum refineries

     (b) Causes respiratory paralysis

2. Direct irritant damage

  a. Highly soluble gases and fumes

    (1) Usually damage the upper airways by causing direct chemical damage (e.g., ammonia)

  b. Moderately soluble gases and fumes

    (1) More likely to affect the entire respiratory tract

    (2) Causes parenchymal damage and pulmonary edema (e.g., chlorine)

  c. Slightly soluble gases and fumes

    (1) Often cause pulmonary edema with prolonged exposure (e.g., welding fumes, ozone, metal fumes including cadmium, mercury, nickel)

3. Production of fibrosis (see Section 4)

4. Constriction of airways through an allergic response (see Section 4)

5. Oncogenesis (primary lung cancer) (see Section 4)

B. Musculoskeletal injuries

1. Most frequently reported occupational disorder

2. Musculoskeletal disorders (from all causes) are the second most frequent cause of all disabilities after circulatory system disorders.

  a. For the working population (ages 18–64), musculoskeletal disorders are the number one cause of disability.

3. Cumulative trauma disorders

  a. Characteristics

    (1) Insidious onset

    (2) Few radiological or laboratory features

    (3) Persistent or recurrent pain, fatigue

    (4) Decline in work performance
     Examples: Meat processors may make 12,000 cuts of one motion per day; data entry clerks typically type 20,000 keystrokes an hour; assembly line workers may have to lift the shoulder and work above head level up to 7,500 times a day.

  b. Stages

    (1) Stage one

     (a) Fatigue and pain during work that improve with rest

     (b) Usually resolves within weeks to months

     (c) Usually reversible

    (2) Stage two

     (a) Fatigue and pain increase

     (b) Persist for longer periods (months)

     (c) Reduced capacity for repetitive work

     (d) Sleep disturbances often an early signal

    (3) Stage three

     (a) Fatigue and pain at rest

     (b) Chronic pain often present

     (c) Difficulty in performing nonoccupational tasks as well

     (d) Sleep disturbances

     (e) Disruption of social life

     (f) Often severe psychological stress

4. Law back syndrome

  a. Accounts for 25% of lost time from work due to material handling problems

  b. Can be correlated with acute injury in only 15% of workers

C. Occupational cancers (other than lung)

D. Occupational Injuries

1. No good sources of data are available for occupational injuries, according to the National Academy of Sciences.

2. Occupational fatalities: in the private sector, must be reported to the Occupational Safety and Health Administration (OSHA) within 24 hr.

  a. Audits have shown that one-third of occupational fatalities are missed.

  b. Estimates range from 6,000 to 12,000 deaths annually.*

3. Estimates of other types of injuries

  a. Fractures: 400,000

  b. Amputations: 21,000

  c. Eye injuries: 1 million

  d. Occupationally related back pain: 1 million

E. Cardiovascular disorders—leading cause of death in the United States

1. Arrhythmias—solvents, both halogenated

---

*Assuming a low estimate: 25 workers die on the job each work day.

and nonhalogenated, have been implicated.

   a. Agents that sensitize the myocardium to the effects of catecholamines

     (1) Halogenated solvents (1,1,1-trichloroethane and trichlorethylene) often used in degreasing operations

     (2) Chlorofluorocarbons (e.g., freon) used as refrigerants, propellants

   b. Agents that compromise the oxygen supply to the cardiac muscle

     (1) Carbon monoxide: ubiquitous in industrial settings

     (2) Methylene chloride: metabolized to carbon monoxide in the body (used in strippers, degreasers)

2. Ischemic heart disease

   a. Coronary heart disease

     (1) Carbon disulfide: workers have 2.5–5-fold increased risk of death from coronary heart disease.

     (2) Chronic carbon monoxide exposure

   b. Nonatheromatous heart disease

     (1) Nitrates (especially ethylene glycol and nitroglycerin) cause sudden death in ammunition workers

3. Myocardial injury

   a. Arsenic, cobalt, lead

4. Peripheral arterial occlusive disease

   a. Vibration syndrome, particularly leading to Raynaud's disease from hand tools

F. Disorders of reproduction—poorly understood

1. Basic epidemiology

   a. 7% of live-born babies are low birth weight

   b. 3% of live-born babies have major congenital malformations

   c. 20% of all pregnancies end in spontaneous abortion

2. Male reproductive dysfunction

   a. Lead—suppresses testicular secretion and central axis suppresion

   b. Estrogen—causes central axis suppression

   c. 1,2-Dibromo-3-chloropropane (DBCP)—causes testicular atrophy in rats; may decrease sperm counts in human males

3. Female reproductive dysfunction

   a. Reduced fertility (proposed mechanisms)

     (1) Suppression of ovulation (e.g., narcotics, stress)

     (2) Premature menopause (e.g., radiation, alkylating agents, inorganic mercury, organophosphate pesticides)

     (3) Spontaneous abortion (e.g., organoalides, cadmium, copper, lead, estrogens)

4. Fetotoxicity (animal evidence)

     (1) Selected examples: arsenic, benzene, DDT, ethylene oxide (used in hospital sterilization equipment), lead, polychorinated biphenyls (PCBs), thallium

5. Teratogenicity (animal evidence)

     (1) Selected examples: acrylonitrile, arsenic, benzene, chromium, endrin, tellurium, vinyl chloride

6. Transplacental carcinogens (animal evidence)

   a. Selected examples: arsenic, benzopyrene, diethyl-Stilbestrol, vinyl chloride

G. Neurotoxic disorders (selected)

1. Acute psychosis or marked emotional instability linked to carbon disulfide, manganese, mercury, toluene

2. Ataxic gait—acrlyamide, chlordane, kepone, DDT, manganese, methyl mercury, methyl-*n*-butly ketone (MBK), methyl chloride, toluene

3. Bladder neuropathy—linked with dimethylaminopropionitrile (DMAPN)

4. Impaired psychomotor function—carbon disulfide, lead, mercury, organophosphate insecticides, perchloroethylene and other solvents, styrene

5. Mixed sensorimotor neuropathy—acrylamide, arsenic, carbon disulfide, carbon monoxide, DDT, *n*-hexane, MBK, mercury

6. Seizures—lead, organic mercurials, organochlorine insecticides, organotin compounds

H. Noise-induced hearing loss

1. Widespread—21–29% of workers are estimated to suffer significant hearing loss at 90 dB over a 40-year working life; approximately 5–15% will have significant hearing loss at 85 dB.

2. Acoustical trauma—head trauma, explosions, and noises > 150 dB can rupture the tympanic membrane, and fracture or dislocate the ossciles of the middle ear.

3. Noise-induced hearing loss
   a. Acute—a temporary threshold shift caused by metabolic fatigue
   b. Chronic—gradual loss of hearing, typically in the frequency range of 3,000–6,000 Hz
4. Nonauditory effects of noise—not well studied, but endocrine changes and increased blood pressure are some of the suspected effects.

I. Dermatologic conditions
   1. Contact dermatitis
      a. Irritant contact dermatitis (about 80% of all contact dermatitis)
         (1) Commonly caused by soaps, detergents, and other cleaners that dissolve skin lipids and keratin.
      b. Allergic contact dermatitis (about 20% of all contact dermatitis)
         (1) Cell-mediated immune response which on reexposure causes an inflammatory reaction.
         (2) Selected sensitizers: rubber accelerators, antioxidants, metal salts (nickel, gold, chromium, cobalt), plastics process (epoxy resins), animal dander, urine, saliva.
   2. Occupational acne
      a. Obstruction of hair follicles
         (1) Chronic exposure to fats and oils, especially cutting oils.
         (2) Mechanical pressure (e.g., acne lesions on buttocks and other pressure areas in truck drivers)
      b. Chloracne—occurs after systemic exposure to chlorinated hydrocarbons (particularly dioxins and PCBs)
   3. Pigmentation disorders
      a. Stains—many chemicals and dyes bind to the keratin layer in the skin (e.g., dyes, heavy metals, tanning process)
      b. Hyperpigmentation:
         (1) Furnace workers and others chronically exposed to heat have dark, mottled skin
         (2) Arsenic, tetracycline, polyaromatic hydrocarbons
      c. Vitiligo—photographic chemicals (e.g., hydroquinone), phenols (used in resins and germicides)
   4. Skin cancer
      a. Ultraviolet radiation—affects outdoor workers and agricultural workers exposed to sunlight
      b. Ionizing radiation—affects health workers, uranium miners
   5. Other skin disorders
      a. Alopecia can be caused by thallium, sodium borate, chloropene dimers, ionizing radiation, and trauma.
      b. Cuts, lacerations, and burns can occur in a wide variety of jobs.

J. Psychological disorders
   1. Unemployment and underemployment
      a. Most prevalent occupational diseases in the United States
      b. Linked to increased gastrointestinal complaints, stress, sleep disorders, increased blood pressure
   2. Shift work and night work
      a. Sleep disturbances
         (1) Some studies show that workers on evening and night shifts have more accidents than other workers.
      b. Health complaints
         (1) Gastrointestinal complaints (some studies show increased rates of peptic ulcer disease and gastric acid)
      c. Psychosocial effects
         (1) Increased stress
         (2) Loss of social interactions

IV. **Taking an Occupational History**
   A. Brief occupational history
      1. Where do you work now?
      2. What type of work have you done most often in your life?
      3. Have you been exposed to anything that you think might affect your health?
   B. Complete occupational history
      1. Ask about parent's jobs and childhood exposures
      2. Chronological history of all jobs (including part-time, seasonal, and second jobs)
         a. Size of plant, shift worked, whether the plant is unionized
         b. Description of the job: determine exactly what the patient does
            (1) Body mechanics
            (2) Pace of work
            (3) Machines and equipment used
            (4) Overview of entire production process
         c. Potential exposures to hazards
            (1) Biological
            (2) Chemical (solvents, pesticides, etc.)
            (3) Dust and minerals (heavy metals, silica)
            (4) Physical hazards

(a) Heat/cold
(b) Noise/vibration
(c) Ionizing and nonionizing radiation
(5) Ergonomic conditions
   (a) Worker-tool fit
   (b) Lighting
   (c) Pace of work
   (d) Design of tasks
(6) Psychosocial hazards
   (a) Worker's rights in workplace (is there union protection?)
   (b) Level of worker's control over job tasks
   (c) Shift work/night work
d. Protective methods
   (1) Engineering controls
   (2) Ventilation
   (3) Personal protection equipment (e.g., gloves, aprons, goggles, respirators)
   (4) Medical surveillance (if any)
3. Discussion of symptoms—any relation to time, day of week, days off, change with vacation, relation to specific areas or processes, similar symptoms in coworkers
4. Environmental hazards
   a. Industrial or other sources of hazards at home
   b. Jobs of other household members
   c. Hazardous waste incidents
   d. Work around the home/yard
   e. Hobbies
   f. Seat belt use
   g. Presence of firearms

Bibliography

Adams, RM: *Occupation Skin Disease*. New York, Grune & Stratton, 1983.

Haddad LM, Winchester J: *Clinical Management of Poisoning and Drug Overdose*, ed 2. Philadelphia, WB. Saunders, 1990.

LaDou J: *Occupational Medicine*. Norwalk, CT, Appleton & Lange, 1990.

Levy BS, Wegman DH (eds): *Occupational Health: Recognizing and Preventing Work-Related Disease*, ed 2. Boston, Little, Brown, 1988.

Monk TH: Shiftwork performance. *Occup Med State of the Art Rev* 5:183–198, 1990.

Hathaway GJ, Proctor NH, Hughes JP, Fischman ML: *Proctor and Hughes Chemical Hazards of the Workplace* ed 3. New York: Van Nostrand Reinhold 1991.

Rom WN: *Environmental and Occupational Medicine*, ed 2. Boston, Little, Brown, 1992.

Rosenstock L, Cullen M: *Clinical Occupational Medicine*. Philadelphia, WB. Saunders, 1986.

US Department of Labor, Bureau of Labor Statistics: *Occupational Injuries and Illnesses in the United States, 1988*. Washington, D.C. Bulletin No. 2366. August 1990.

CHAPTER 6

Dermatology

Matthew G. Fleming, M.D.

I. **Introduction: The Approach to the Dermatologic Patient**

The history and physical examination of a dermatologic patient differ somewhat from their counterparts in general medicine. Points deserving emphasis in a dermatologic setting follow.

A. History
1. Course of illness: time of onset, site of onset, duration of disease, pattern of spread.
2. Symptoms: Usually itching, rarely pain or burning. Many dermatoses are asymptomatic.
3. Prior treatment. Topical corticosteroids may blunt the characteristic morphology of the disease, while other topicals may result in a contact dermatitis superimposed on the original dermatosis.
4. Drug exposure.
5. Past dermatologic history. Many dermatoses are chronic.
6. Environmental exposures. Exposures from work, hobbies, cosmetics, jewelry, plants, and clothing must be evaluated in a patient with contact dermatitis. Some dermatoses, such as lupus erythematosus, are exacerbated by exposure to sunlight. Inter-

personal contacts and foreign travel are important factors in infectious diseases.
7. Family history. Psoriasis, atopic dermatitis, melanoma, and several other diseases may run in families.

B. Physical examination
Dermatologic lesions may be described using the following terms.
1. Types of lesion
a. Primary lesions
Primary lesions are those present when the dermatosis first appears.
(1) Macule: a nonpalpable alteration in skin color less than 1 cm in diameter
(2) Patch: a nonpalpable alteration in skin color more than 1 cm in diameter
(3) Papule: a palpable elevation less than 1 cm in diameter
(4) Nodule: a palpable elevation more than 1 cm in diameter.
(5) Tumor: a large nodule
(6) Plaque: an elevated, broad lesion
(7) Vesicle: an accumulation of fluid within the skin less than 0.5 cm in diameter

(8) Bulla: an accumulation of fluid more than 0.5 cm in diameter

b. Secondary lesions

Secondary lesions result from alteration of the primary lesions by patient manipulation or by wound healing and other homeostatic processes. Secondary lesions include erosions, ulcers, crusting, lichenification, and scarring. An erosion results from loss of all or part of the viable epidermis, while an ulcer extends into the dermis.

Lichenification is thickening of the skin with accentuation of skin markings, resulting from prolonged scratching or rubbing.

c. Characteristics of the lesions such as scaling, erythema (redness), hypopigmentation, and hyperpigmentation should be noted.

II. A Brief Review of Topical Medications Used in Dermatology

A. Topical corticosteroids

Topical corticosteroids are the mainstay in the treatment of inflammatory dermatoses. Many are available, spanning a broad potency range (Table 6-1). Local complications such as striae and atrophy are more likely with the more potent steroids, especially when used for prolonged periods. The face, genitals, and intertriginous areas are most likely to suffer these complications, so only group V or weaker steroids should be used in these areas. Suppression of the hypothalamic-pituitary-adrenal axis may occur with some of the group I (superpotent) topical steroids. To avoid this problem, it is essential to follow the manufacturer's recommendations concerning the maximum allowable duration and area of treatment.

Topical steroids are available in cream, ointment, gel, and lotion forms. Lotions and gels are suitable for the scalp, while creams and ointments are used elsewhere. Ointments are stronger than creams but creams are more cosmetically acceptable, especially on the hands and face.

B. Antibacterials

1. Benzoyl peroxide, and erythromycin and clindamycin lotions and gels, are used primarily for acne and occasionally for other disorders such as folliculitis.

2. Bacitracin is effective against gram-positive organisms.

Table 6-1. Potency Ranking of Commonly Used Topical Corticosteroids

I: Highest potency
  Temovate (clobetasol propionate) cream and ointment
  Diprolene cream and ointment (betamethasone dipropionate)
  Ultravate (halobetasol propionate)
  Psorcon (diflorasone diacetate)

II: High potency
  Lidex (fluocinonide) cream, ointment, solution, and gel
  Topicort (desoximetasone) cream, ointment, and gel
  Diprosone (betamethasone diproprionate) ointment
  Halog (halcinonide) cream, ointment, and solution

III: Aristocort (triamcinolone acetonide) ointment, 0.1%
  Diprosone (betamethasone diproprionate) cream
  Valisone (betamethasone valerate) ointment

IV: Intermediate potency
  Westcort (hydrocortisone valerate) ointment
  Cordran (fluandrenolide) ointment, 0.05%
  Kenalog (triamcinolone acetonide) cream, 0.1%
  Synalar (fluocinolone acetonide) ointment, .025%

V: Westcort (hydrocortisone valerate) cream
  Valisone (betamethasone valerate) cream
  Cordran (fluandrenolide) cream, 0.05%
  Locoid (hydrocortisone butyrate) cream
  Diprosone (betamethasone diproprionate) lotion

VI: Low potency
  Tridesilon (desonide) cream
  DesOwen (desonide) cream
  Aclovate (alclometasone dipropionate) cream and ointment
  Synalar (fluocinolone acetonide) solution

VII: Lowest potency
  Hydrocortisone cream, ointment, and lotion

Source: Modified from Stoughton RB, Cornell RC: Review of superpotent topical corticosteroids. *Semin Dermatol* 6:73, 1987. Used with permission.

3. Bacitracin-polymyxin B ointment is effective against some gram-negative organisms, including *Pseudomonas*, as well as

against gram-positive organisms. Triple antibiotic ointments contain neomycin, which extends the gram-negative coverage but is a contact sensitizer.

4. A new topical antibiotic, mupirocin, is a highly effective therapy for impetigo.

C. Antifungals

1. Polyene antifungal: nystatin. Useful only for candidiasis.

2. Imidazole antifungals: miconazole, clotrimazole, econazole, ketoconazole, oxiconazole. Useful for dermatophytes and candida.

3. Allylamine antifungal: naftidine. A new class of antifungals useful for dermatophytes and candida.

D. Emollients

Emollients are useful for ordinary dry skin (xerosis), for ichthyosis, and as adjunctive therapy for eczema, especially atopic dermatitis. Many emollient lotions and creams are available over the counter. Lachydrin lotion, which contains lactic acid at 5% or 12% concentrations, is especially effective.

III. **Selected Common Dermatoses of Special Interest to the Generalist**

A. Psoriasis

1. Psoriasis is a chronic disorder characterized by erythematous, indurated plaques covered by a thick white scale with a distinctive distribution.

2. The etiology is largely genetic; psoriasis has an heritability of approximately 90%.

3. Pathophysiology

a. Increased epidermal proliferation.

b. Abnormal arachidonic acid metabolism, leading to overproduction of cyclooxygenase metabolites such as leukotriene B_4, a potent neutrophil chemotaxin.

c. Overproduction by keratinocytes of inflammatory cytokines, incluidng interleukins-1, -6, and -8.

d. Morphologic and functional abnormalities of dermal capillaries.

4. Diagnosis

a. History

Psoriasis may begin at any age, but there are two broad peaks in the age distribution curve: at approximately 20 and 55 years of age.

b. Clinical signs and physical findings

Lesions are red papules and plaques with micaceous scale, characteristically distributed on the elbows, knees, scalp, and lumbosacral area. The palms and soles, intergluteal cleft, and glans penis may also be involved. The nails are involved in about 30% of cases, with pitting, yellow discoloration, and subungual hyperkeratosis. Variants of psoriasis include guttate, pustular, and erythrodermic forms.

c. Diagnostic tests

Skin biopsy—Specific findings are not always encountered.

5. Differential diagnosis

Psoriasis may be confused with seborrheic dermatitis, chronic eczema, secondary syphilis, pityriasis rubra pilaris, and some drug eruptions.

6. Treatment

Treatment must be highly individualized. Limited disease may be treated with emollients and topical medications containing corticosteroids, coal tar, or anthralin. More extensive disease may require ultraviolet phototherapy and/or systemic treatment with methotrexate or retinoids.

7. Prognosis

Psoriasis is a chronic, relapsing disease.

B. Seborrheic dermatitis

1. Definition

Seborrheic dermatitis is an eczematous dermatitis which affects areas rich in sebaceous glands: the face, scalp, and sternal region.

2. Etiology

Unknown. A commensal yeast, *Pityrosporum ovale*, may play a role. Seborrheic dermatitis is common and unusually severe in patients with acquired immunodeficiency syndrome (AIDS).

3. Pathophysiology

Unknown

4. Diagnosis

a. History

Seborrheic dermatitis is most common in infancy, adolescence, and early and mid-adulthood.

b. Clinical signs and physical findings

There are dull red patches covered by greasy, yellowish scale, most commonly on the nasolabial folds, eyebrows, scalp, and periauricular area.

c. Diagnostic tests

Clinical features are distinctive, although the histology usually is not, so biopsy is rarely performed.

5. Differential diagnosis
Seborrheic dermatitis is rarely confused with psoriasis, chronic eczema, pityriasis rosea, or tinea versicolor.

6. Treatment
Topical corticosteroids and, for the scalp, shampoos containing tar, selenium sulfide, or zinc pyrithione.

7. Prognosis
Seborrheic dermatitis is chronic.

C. Stasis dermatitis
1. Definition
Stasis dermatitis is an eczematous dermatitis which results from incompetence of leg veins.

2. Etiology
Venous hypertension, sometimes as a sequela of deep venous thrombosis.

3. Pathophysiology
The increased pressure is transmitted from the veins to the capillary beds, where it causes transudation of fibrinogen. A pericapillary fibrin cuff forms. The cuff interferes with diffusion between the capillary and interstitium, compromising tissue nutrition and oxygenation.

4. Diagnosis
a. History
Stasis dermatitis is most common in elderly individuals, especially women. Patients with sickle cell anemia often develop the disease prematurely.

b. Clinical signs and physical findings
Characteristically, the medial lower leg just above the malleolus is affected. There is erythema, scaling, and a brownish discoloration reflecting hemosiderin deposition. Ulceration occurs in severe cases. Varices are often associated.

c. Diagnostic tests
None

5. Differential diagnosis
Stasis dermatitis must be distinguished from fungal infections and from other eczematous dermatitides affecting the lower legs, especially contact dermatitis.

6. Treatment
Low- to midpotency topical corticosteroids are helpful in treating the eczematous components. Support stockings and leg elevation facilitate venous return. Therapy of ulcers is difficult, and a discussion is beyond the scope of this text.

7. Prognosis
The eczematous dermatitis is chronic but can be controlled. Ulcerations, at best, clear slowly with treatment and, at worst, are intractable and progressive.

D. Dermatophytosis
1. Definition
Dermatophytosis is a superficial fungal infection caused by fungi belonging to the genera *Microsporum*, *Trichophyton*, and *Epidermophyton*. Dermatophytosis is subdivided, according to the site of the infection, into tinea pedis (foot), tinea manuum (hand), tinea cruris (groin), tinea corporis (other nonhairy sites), tinea capitis (scalp), and tinea unguium (nails).

2. Etiology
Trichophyton rubrum, *T. tonsurans*, *Epidermophyton floccosum*, and *Microsporum canis* are the species most often responsible for human disease. The first three are anthropophilic organisms (transmitted from person to person); the last is zoophilic (transmitted by animals, especially cats). Hydration and occlusion of the skin (e.g., by shoes) facilitate infection. AIDS patients often develop florid dermatophytosis.

3. Pathophysiology
The dermatophytic fungi grow within the keratinized layer of the skin, the stratum corneum, and within the hair.

4. Diagnosis
a. History
Patients with tinea capitis are often found to have an affected family member.

b. Clinical signs and physical findings
(1) Tinea capitis is most often noninflammatory, presenting with patches of scaling and alopecia. Inflammatory tinea capitis is associated with erythema, abscess formation, scarring alopecia, and lymphadenopathy.
(2) Tinea pedis most commonly presents with scaling, maceration, and fissuring in the toe webs. It may also present with diffuse scaling of the soles in a "moccasin" distribution. The vesicular type of tinea pedis is least common.
(3) Tinea manuum usually presents with diffuse scaling of one or, less commonly, both palms. Frequently

there is fine scaling in the skin creases.

(4) Tinea corporis and tinea cruris produce erythematous, scaly plaques. The border of the lesion is often prominent because of increased scaling or erythema, papules, or vesicles. There may be central clearing (ringworm).

(5) Tinea unguium affects the toenails more commonly than the fingernails. The most common type is distal subungual onychomycosis, which begins at the free edge of the nail and spreads proximally, producing subungual hyperkeratosis and a whitish or yellowish discoloration of the nail.

c. Diagnostic tests

When scales are scraped from the lesion and digested with 10% potassium hydroxide (KOH) with gentle heating, the keratinocytes are dissolved and fungal hyphae may be visible. If the KOH examination is negative, the scales should be cultured on a medium such as Sabouraud's agar.

5. Differential diagnosis

Noninflammatory tinea capitis may be confused with seborrheic dermatitis or dandruff, while inflammatory tinea capitis is often confused with pyoderma. Tinea cruris may be confused with intertrigo. Tinea unguium may be confused with psoriasis.

6. Treatment

Treatment usually consists of a topical imidazole antifungal such as econazole. Oral griseofulvin is usually necessary for tinea capitis and tinea unguium. Oral ketoconazole may be used to treat organisms resistant to griseofulvin.

7. Prognosis

The prognosis is favorable except for tinea unguium, where there is a high relapse rate.

Cutaneous Manifestations of Systemic Disease

I. Connective Tissue Diseases

A. Lupus erythematosus

1. In *discoid* lupus erythematosus, lesions are most common on the head and consist of well-defined, erythematous plaques with adherent scale and plugged follicles. Older lesions display atrophy, scarring, and hypo- and hyperpigmentation. Approximately 10% of patients who present initially with discoid cutaneous disease will ultimately develop systemic lupus erythematosus.

2. In *systemic* lupus erythematosus, lesions consist of ill-defined, erythematous, edematous patches, without scaling, atrophy, or altered pigmentation. A malar location is classic, but lesions may be widespread; they are more common on sun-exposed areas.

3. In *subacute* lupus erythematosus, two types of lesions may occur: psoriasiform and annular plaques.

B. Dermatomyositis

Lesions are erythematous to violaceous, somewhat edematous patches, which typically involve the upper eyelids and extensor extremities. *Gottron papules* may be seen over the knuckles. Most but not all studies have found an association in adults between dermatomyositis and malignancy. On average, about 15% of patients had a malignancy.

C. Scleroderma

1. Morphea

There are localized areas of induration, which may be surrounded by violaceous erythema. Variants include guttate, linear, frontoparietal, and generalized types.

2. Systemic sclerosis

Raynaud's phenomenon is usually the initial manifestation. Then swelling, induration, and ultimately atrophy and sclerosis begin on the hands and spread proximally. The face is also usually involved. Systemic sclerosis, but not morphea, is associated with systemic disease.

II. Acquired Immunodeficiency Syndrome

A. An acute, mononucleosis-like illness sometimes follows the initial infection with human immunodeficiency virus (HIV) after 2 to 5 weeks. In about 50% of cases this illness is associated with a rash. The rash resembles other viral exanthems. Lesions are morbilliform and favor the trunk. The extremities, face, and oral mucosa may also be involved; vesicles and pustules occur occasionally.

B. Patients with more advanced HIV infection are at increased risk for many common dermatoses, including seborrheic dermatitis, candidiasis, superficial fungal infection, warts, scabies, and molluscum contagiosum. These dermatoses may have unusually florid presentations in this setting.

C. Some dermatoses are common in AIDS patients but rare or nonexistent in immunocompetent invididuals and may therefore have significance for diagnosis.
 1. Kaposi's sarcoma
 2. Disseminated and chronic herpes
  Chronic perianal ulcers in AIDS patients are usually due to herpes simplex but may be caused by cytomegalovirus. Herpes zoster is common and may disseminate.
 3. Oral hairy leukoplakia
  This is caused by Epstein-Barr virus and presents as a white, corrugated plaque on the side of the tongue.
 4. Disseminated fungal infections, especially cryptococcosis and histoplasmosis
 5. "Papular eruption of AIDS"
  A variably pruritic, papular eruption on the head, neck, and upper trunk occurs in about 20% of patients.
 6. Generalized pruritus

III. Endocrine Disease
 A. Diabetes
  1. Diabetic dermopathy
   Erythematous papules, most commonly on the shins, evolve into atrophic, hyperpigmented patches.
  2. Bullosis diabeticorum
   Rather large, noninflammatory blisters arise suddenly on the distal extremities, then slowly heal.
  3. Necrobiosis lipoidica diabeticorum
   Atrophic, indurated, yellowish, telangiectatic plaques develop on the shins and occasionally elsewhere. Two-thirds of these patients are diabetic.
 B. Graves' disease
  The skin is warm and dry. The hair may be thinned. Pretibial myxedema may be associated. This presents with indurated plaques on the shins, sometimes extending to the calves or dorsal feet.
 C. Hypothyroidism
  The skin is rough and dry; the face is edematous.

IV. Leukocytoclastic Vasculitis
 A. Leukocytoclastic vasculitis (LCV) is the most common form of cutaneous vasculitis. It is a neutrophilic, necrotizing vasculitis affecting the small vessels of the skin and internal organs. LCV is frequently divided into Henoch-Schonlein purpura (HSP), seen in children and young adults, and hypersensitivity angiitis, which may occur at any age but is most common between 30 and 60 years of age.

 B. Triggers for LCV
  1. Infection
   a. Bacterial: streptococcal pharyngitis, dental abcess, etc. Streptococcal pharyngitis is an important cause of HSP.
   b. Viral, especially hepatitis B
  2. Drugs
  3. Collagen vascular disease
  4. Malignancy
  5. Idiopathic
 C. The pathomechanism involves immune complex deposition in the postcapillary venules.
 D. Clinical signs
  1. The earliest cutaneous lesions are erythematous macules and papules which quickly become purpuric. Urticarial plaques and ulcers also may occur. Lesions favor the arms and especially the legs.
  2. Systemic manifestations include nephritis, arthralgia, arthritis, abdominal pain, and gastrointestinal bleeding. Neurologic, pulmonary, and cardiac involvement are uncommon in HSP but may occur in hypersensitivity angiitis.
  3. Diagnostic tests should include throat culture, antistreptolysin-O titer, urinalysis, stool guaiac test, complete blood count, antinuclear antibody, rheumatoid factor, hepatitis B surface antigen (HBsAg), cryoglobulin, serum protein electrophoresis, and total hemolytic complement. HSP is characterized by immunoglobulin A (IgA)-containing immune complexes in the skin and blood.
 E. Course and therapy
  1. HSP is self-limited. It lasts for 3 to 6 weeks, but there are recurrences in 40% of cases. Therapy is supportive in most cases. The use of corticosteroids is controversial; they are beneficial for joint and gastrointestinal disease but probably not for nephritis, which is the most serious complication.
  2. Hypersensitivity angiitis has a much more variable course and may be fatal. Therapy usually consists of systemic corticosteroids, but colchicine, dapsone, antihistamines, and antimetabolites are sometimes used. Colchicine, dapsone, and antihistamines do not benefit the systemic manifestations.

V. Internal Malignancy
 A. Cutaneous metastasis
  Cutaneous metastasis is relatively uncommon. At autopsy, about 3% of patients with visceral malignancy are found to have cutaneous involvement. In women, breast carcinoma is by

far the most common primary site of origin, while lung carcinoma is most common in men. Carcinomas of the colon, oral cavity, kidney, and stomach, as well as malignant melanoma, also may metastasize to the skin.

The metastasis frequently develops in skin adjacent to the primary. Because of its rich vasculature, the scalp is a common location for metastases from primaries which spread through the blood. Cutaneous metastases usually present as nodules, but metastatic breast cancer can produce lesions of the chest wall which resemble cellulitis (*inflammatory carcinoma*) or scleroderma (*cancer en cuirasse*).

B. Paraneoplastic syndromes associated with internal malignancy
1. Acanthosis nigricans
Velvety hyperpigmentation is seen in the flexures of the neck, axillae, groin, and antecubital fossae. Associations include malignancy, obesity, and endocrinopathies. Acanthosis nigricans may also be familial.
2. Uncommon paraneoplastic syndromes include necrolytic migratory erythema, superficial migratory thrombophlebitis, hypertrophic osteoarthropathy, and gyrate erythema.

C. Cutaneous manifestations of leukemia and lymphoma
1. Nonspecific
a. Generalized pruritus (in the absence of a visible dermatosis)
b. Exfoliative erythroderma
c. Eczematous or papular eruption
d. Urticaria
e. Herpes zoster
2. Specific
Specific manifestations result from infiltration of the skin by malignant lymphocytes. Specific cutaneous lesions occur in 17% of patients with non-Hodgkin's lymphoma. Lesions are papules, nodules, and plaques.

Cutaneous Drug Reactions

Cutaneous drug reactions are common, occurring in about 2% of hospital patients. Cellular immune mechanisms have been implicated in morbilliform drug eruption and erythema multiforme, while urticaria is mediated by type I or type III immune reactions. Therapy in all cases centers on the elimination of the causative drug. Obviously, this can be difficult to identify. Drugs started a week or two preceding the eruption, especially if known to be frequent causes of drug eruption, should be the prime suspects. (This interval can be much shorter, days or even minutes, if there have been earlier courses of therapy with the same drug.) There are several clinicopathologic types of drug eruption.

VI. **Morbilliform Drug Eruption**
A. Frequent causes
Ampicillin, phenylbutazone, gold, sulfonamides, and gentamicin are especially likely to cause a morbilliform drug eruption. Many other drugs have also been implicated.
B. Clinical morphology
Lesions are erythematous macules and papules which may become confluent. The trunk and proximal extremities, especially where subject to pressure, are preferred sites. The face is generally spared.
C. Differential diagnosis
Viral exanthems may closely resemble a morbilliform drug eruption, both clinically and histologically. Acute graft-versus-host disease can usually be distinguished by early, relatively severe involvement of the palms and soles and by associated findings.
D. Therapy
Elimination of the causative drug and topical corticosteroids.
E. Prognosis
After elimination of the causative drug, the eruption often worsens for a few days and then slowly fades over 2 to 3 weeks. Even if the causative drug is continued, the eruption will usually resolve gradually, but progression to exfoliative dermatitis also may occur.

VII. **Erythema Multiforme (EM) and Toxic Epidermal Necrolysis (TEN)**
A. Frequent causes
Chlorpropamide, penicillins, phenothiazines, sulfonamides, and thiazides are frequent causes of EM. EM has other causes besides drugs, especially infections. Anticonvulsants, sulfonamides, penicillin derivatives, and nonsteroidal anti-inflammatory drugs are the most common cause of TEN, a variant of EM.
B. Clinical morphology
1. EM
Lesions are polymorphous and may include macules, papules, vesicles, and urticarial plaques. The target lesion is most characteristic and consists of a central papule (often dusky or surmounted by a vesicle) surrounded by a pale red ring and an outer dark red ring. The distribution is widespread but favors the distal volar ex-

tremities. There are erosions on the mucosae.

2. TEN

Diffuse skin tenderness and large, flaccid bullae are the initial mainfestations, followed by desquamation of large areas of skin.

C. Differential diagnosis

EM has a relatively distinctive clinical appearance. TEN may be confused with staphylococcal scalded skin syndrome and grade IV acute graft-versus-host disease.

D. Therapy

Therapy is supportive. TEN is best managed in a burn unit. The use of systemic corticosteroids for EM and TEN is controversial.

E. Prognosis

EM resolves within 6 weeks without sequelae. TEN is fatal in approximately 30% of cases. Sequelae include scarring, loss or dystrophy of hair and nails, and loss of visual acuity or even blindness.

VIII. Urticaria

A. Frequent causes

Antibiotics, salicylates, indomethacin, opiates, polypeptide hormones, and enzymes. Aside from drugs, there are many other possible causes of urticaria, including food or inhalant allergy, collagen vascular disease, infection, neoplasia, and physical factors (e.g., pressure, sunlight).

B. Clinical morphology

Urticaria produces broad, edematous, pruritic, pink plaques without scaling.

C. Differential diagnosis

Urticaria is relatively distinctive. Urticarial plaques which are violaceous or last for more than 24 hr should raise the possibility of urticarial vasculitis.

D. Therapy

Antihistamines antagonizing the H_1 receptor are the mainstay of therapy. Astemizole is a nonsedating antihistamine which is often effective. Occasionally it is necessary to add an H_2 blocker such as cimetidine.

E. Prognosis

Resolution usually occurs within a few weeks after use of the causative drug is stopped.

IX. Exfoliative Dermatitis

A. Frequent causes

Allopurinol, sulfonamides, hydantoins, sulfonylureas, gold compounds, and penicillins.

B. Clinical morphology

There is generalized erythema and scaling.

C. Differential diagnosis

Drugs cause only 10% of cases of exfoliative dermatitis. Other important causes include psoriasis, atopic dermatitis, contact dermatitis, mycosis fungoides, extracutaneous lymphoma, and internal cancer.

D. Therapy

Topical corticosteroids and supportive care.

E. Prognosis

If the causative drug is discontinued, the dermatitis will slowly resolve, but if it is continued, the dermatitis may persist indefinitely.

Bibliography

General References

Fitzpatrick TB, Eisen AZ, Wolff K, et al: *Dermatology in General Medicine*, ed 4. New York, McGraw-Hill, 1993.

Moschella SL, Hurley HJ: *Dermatology*, ed 3. Philadelphia, WB Saunders, 1992.

Rook A, Wilkinson DS, Ebling FJG, et al: *Textbook of Dermatology*, ed 4. Oxford, Blackwell Scientific Publications, 1986.

Introductory Texts

Fitzpatrick TB, Polano MK, Suurmond D: *Color Atlas and Synopsis of Clinical Dermatology*. New York, McGraw-Hill, 1983.

Orkin M, Maibach HI, Dahl MV: *Dermatology*. Norwalk, CT, Appleton & Lange, 1991.

Individual Topics

Arndt KA: *Manual of Dermatologic Therapeutics*, ed 4. Boston, Little, Brown, 1989.

Braverman IM: *Skin Signs of Systemic Disease*, ed 2. Philadelphia, WB Saunders, 1981.

Penneys NS: *Skin Manifestations of AIDS*. Philadelphia, JP Lippincott, 1989.

CHAPTER 7

Decision-Making in Clinical Practice

Richard Abrams, M.D.

I. **Interpretation of Diagnostic Tests**
   A. Normality
   Most tests yield results with values that fall along a continuous scale.
   1. When a test is performed on a population of normal individuals, the distribution of results is approximated by a normal curve.
      a. By definition, such a distribution has a mean and a standard deviation. The latter measures the degree of spread around the mean.
   2. Test results for 95% of the population lie within two standard deviations of the mean.
   3. Most laboratories define any value which is more than two standard deviations from the mean as abnormal, even though 5% of normal individuals have values that fall beyond that range.
      a. As the number of separate tests, n, increases, the likelihood that a healthy person will have n normal test results diminishes to $(0.95)^n$.
   4. Because of the phenemenon of regression toward the mean, abnormal test results from a normal person are less likely to be abnormal upon repeat testing.

   B. Test performance
   In order to interpret a test result, a method is needed to evaluate test performance (Figure 7-1).
   1. The true disease state of the patient is defined by the "gold standard" test.
      a. The gold standard test itself is frequently an imperfect test, and this causes most errors in evaluating test discrimination.
   2. The 2×2 table is obtained by applying both the index test and the gold standard procedure to each patient.
   3. The performance of a test can be characterized by its ability to detect true-positive and true-negative results.
      a. The sensitivity of a test (true-positive rate) is the likelihood that a diseased patient has a positive test.
      b. The specificity of a test (true-negative rate) is the likelihood that a nondiseased person has a negative test.
   C. Effect of prevalence on posttest probability of disease
   The interpretation of a test result depends on more than the test's performance; it is also

		True Disease State		
		Disease Present	**Disease Absent**	
Index Text	*Positive*	a	b	$a + b$
	Negative	c	d	$c + d$
		$a + c$	$b + d$	$a + b + c + d$

Sensitivity = $a/(a + c)$
Specificity = $d/(b + d)$
Predictive value of a positive test = $a/(a + b)$
Predictive value of a negative test = $d/(c + d)$

FIGURE 7-1. Performance of index and gold standard tests

determined by the prevalence of disease (also known as *pretest probability*) in the population being tested.
  1. The predictive value of a positive test is the fraction of patients with a positive test who also have disease.
  2. The predictive value of a negative test is the fraction of patients with a negative test who do not have disease.
  3. While the sensitivity and specificity are independent of the disease prevalence, the predictive value is critically dependent on it.
  4. Even if a test is very accurate, it may provide no new or useful information.
      a. It is necessary to evaluate whether the test results will change the estimation of the probability of disease or alter therapy.
  D. Trade-offs between sensitivity and specificity
  1. A receiver operator characteristic (ROC) curve expresses the relationship between sensitivity and specificity. It is used to describe the accuracy of a test over a range of cutoff values.
  2. The ROC curve may also be used to compare two tests for the same disease.
      a. A better test will have both a higher sensitivity and a higher specificity than a poorer test.

II. Decision Analysis
  A. This is a process for evaluating the optimal course of action when various clinical alternatives exist.
  1. It is not a method of diagnosis.
  B. The techique requires three steps:
  1. Creation of a decision tree
      a. A tree is a method of representing the important outcomes of a decision.
      b. Its creation is critically dependent on an unambiguous definition of the problem and on identification of decision alternatives.
  2. Determination of the probability of each outcome
      a. This is often based on the literature or on expert opinion.
      b. The probabilities apply to a specific patient rather than to the general patient.
  3. Assignment of a utility to each decision alternative
      a. A utility is a measure of the patient's relative preference for the outcome.
      b. Estimating utilities often requires subjective judgments.
  C. The preferred course of action is the one with the highest expected value.
  1. The expected value for each branch of the decision tree is calculated by multiplying its probability by its utility.
  2. The decision maker begins at the distal outcome nodes of the tree and uses their values to calculate each of the previous nodes until the root of the tree is reached.
  D. Sensitivity analysis is a method for testing the validity of a decision analysis.
  1. Estimates of probabilities and outcomes are varied, and then calculations are repeated to determine whether decision strategies would change.

III. Clinical Economics
  A. Economic concerns have become a growing concern in the health care field.
  1. Application of economic principles to medical practice does not mean that less money should be spent, but rather that the use of resources should become more efficient.
  2. Choices between alternative uses of re-

sources must consider both costs and outcomes.

B. Costs of medical care

1. Direct costs are the true costs of producing a service.

   a. A substantial portion of costs are for nonmedical services, such as transportation or lodging.

   b. Charges are set by the marketplace and may not reflect true costs.

2. Indirect costs are all costs of illness other than direct costs.

   a. These include the costs of loss of life or livelihood, as well as intangibles such as pain or grief.

3. Discounting is a method for calculating the present value of money which will be spent in the future.

   a. It is important to consider when the costs will be incurred, as a cost today is not equivalent to a cost in the future.

C. Economic analyses of medical care

A number of methods are used to describe decision alternatives by taking into account their costs. They are often used to make rules for allocating resources.

1. Cost-identification analysis looks strictly at the costs incurred because of a disease.

   a. This type of analysis is used to identify the diagnostic or treatment strategy with the lowest cost.

   (1) It assumes that the outcomes of the strategies are equivalent.

2. Cost-effectiveness analysis incorporates both cost and outcome.

   a. It considers the possibility of an improved outcome in exchange for increased use of resources.

   (1) It allows for comparison of alternative ways of treating a disease or using a resource.

3. Cost-benefit analysis puts costs and outcomes in the same terms.

   a. It allows for explicit decisions about the net benefit of a program.

   b. Its difficulty lies in placing a monetary value on health outcomes.

Bibliography

Eisenberg JM: Clinical economics: A guide to the economic analysis of clinical practice. *JAMA* 262:2879–2886, 1989.

Kassirer JP, Moskowitz AJ, Lau J, et al: Decision analysis: A progress report. *Ann Intern Med* 106:275–291, 1987.

Metz CE: Basic principles of ROC analysis. *Semin Nucl Med* 8:283–298, 1978.

Sox HC, Blatt MA, Higgins HC, et al: *Medical Decision Making*. Boston, Butterworths, 1988, pp 106–113.

CHAPTER 8

Quality Assurance

Robert L. Rosen, M.D.
Lee Ann Onder

I. Definition
A formal, systematic process of evaluating and monitoring the quality and appropriateness of patient care.
A. Assures appropriate, high-quality patient care
B. Provides a routine, systematic approach to measure the quality of care objectively
C. Identifies opportunities for improvement
D. Assists in the effective utilization of resources
E. Improves communication and awareness of patient care issues
F. Assists in staff credentialing and privileging

II. The 10 Steps of Quality Assurance
A monitoring and evaluation process that is endorsed by the Joint Commission on Accreditation of Healthcare Organizations (JCAHO) to provide a comprehensive and systematic approach to quality assurance.
A. Assign responsibility to an individual or group
   1. Activity must be taken seriously
   2. Authority to pursue the task must be present
B. Delineate scope of care or service(s) performed
C. Identify important aspects of care—high volume, high risk, or problem prone
D. Identify indicators (measurable variables) of structure, process, and/or outcome for each aspect of care
   1. Structure relates to the capacity for quality care, including physical resources and staff qualifications and quantity
   2. Process refers to how care is delivered, including treatment plans, indications for diagnostic or therapeutic approach, technical quality of procedures or care
   3. Outcomes is the result of a therapeutic intervention, including complications or adverse events, short-term responses to therapy, long-term health status of patients
E. Establish thresholds that will trigger further evaluation
   1. Threshold will vary for each indicator, depending on seriousness of issue
   2. Threshold should reflect both internal and external standards
F. Collect and organize data, comparing them with preestablished thresholds
G. Evaluate data for patterns or trends
H. Take actions to resolve problems by defining responsible person(s) and appropriate time frame

I. Assess response to interventions and document improvement

J. Communicate activities and actions to entire health care organization

III. **Examples of Medical Staff Quality Assurance Activities, as Suggested by JCAHO**

A. Departmental review follows a 10-step process

B. Surgical case review

1. Monitors and evaluates invasive procedures (tissue and nontissue)

2. Reviews procedures for appropriateness of care

3. Evaluates diagnostic discrepancies

C. Drug usage evaluation

1. Monitors and evaluates the prophylactic, therapeutic, and empiric use of drugs

2. Ensures that drugs are prescribed appropriately, safely, and effectively

D. Medical record review

1. Objectively evaluates physicians' performance

2. Guarantees complete, accurate, and timely documentation

E. Blood usage review

1. Evaluates appropriate usage of whole blood, blood components, and derivatives

2. Reviews all adverse transfusion reactions

3. Guarantees appropriate patient identification

F. Pharmacy and therapeutics committee

1. Develops and approves policies and procedures regarding selection, distribution, handling, use, and administration of drugs and diagnostic testing materials

2. Developes and maintains a drug formulary

3. Evaluates and approves protocols regarding investigational drugs

4. Defines and reviews all significant adverse drug reactions

Bibliography

The Joint Commission Accreditation Manual for Hospitals, Chicago. Joint Commission on Accreditation of Healthcare Organizations, 1991.

Jencks SF: Quality assurance. *JAMA* 263:2679–2681, 1990.

Lohr KN, Schroeder SA: A strategy for quality assurance in Medicare. *N Engl J Med* 322:707–712, 1990.

SECTION 2

Allergy and Immunology

Anaphylaxis

Rebecca Hoffman, M.D.

I. Definition

The term *anaphylaxis* is used specifically to denote an acute immunoglobulin E (IgE)-mediated, antigen-induced allergic reaction or more generally to describe a severe and abrupt reaction of unknown immunologic significance. Therefore it can be considered a clinical syndrome with multiple etiologic agents, a variety of signs and symptoms, and several mechanisms of pathogenesis.

II. Incidence

Data are generally unavailable for the overall incidence of specific antigen reactions.

A. Fatal anaphylaxis—0.4 case per million individuals per year.

B. Nonfatal—estimates range from 0.7 to 10%, depending on the etiology.

C. No increased risk with atopy.

D. Risk increases with the length and frequency of exposure to specific agents.

  1. Parenteral treatment is more likely than oral treatment to provoke anaphylaxis.

  2. Interrupted courses of therapy may induce anaphylaxis.

III. Etiology

Multiple agents include but are not limited to the following:

A. IgE-mediated

  1. Antibiotics—especially penicillins and their derivatives.

  2. Foods/food additives—most commonly legumes, nuts, shellfish, eggs, milk, metabisulfites.

  3. Therapeutic agents—allergen extracts, some muscle relaxants, steroids, some local anesthetics, vaccines, streptokinase, psyllium.

  4. Foreign proteins—insulin, L-asparaginase, chymopapain, protamine, adrenocorticotropic hormone (ACTH), heterologous serum, insect venoms, latex.

B. Non-IgE-mediated—may be due to immune complexes, complement, arachidonic acid metabolites, or direct histamine release.

  1. Radiocontrast media, (e.g., intravenous pyelogram dye)—may occur after use of oral or parenteral dyes.

  2. Infused blood/blood products.

3. Acetylated salicylates, benzoates, nonste-roidal anti-inflammatory agents, tartra-zine (FD&C yellow no. 5).
4. Opiates.
5. Curare, *d*-tubocurarine.
6. Pentamidine.
7. Methotrexate and other chemotherapeu-tic drugs.

C. Exercise-induced anaphylaxis—may or may not be associated with prior food ingestion.
D. Self-induced and hysterical reactions must be considered.
E. Idiopathic anaphylaxis is a diagnosis of ex-clusion.

IV. Pathophysiology

Clinical symptoms vary among patients but gen-erally involve multiple organ systems simulta-neously and occur within minutes after the introduction of a causative agent. Symptoms are due to chemical mediators such as histamine, leukotrienes, and prostaglandins released from basophils and mast cells.

A. Respiratory tract complications account for up to 70% of mortality. Signs and symptoms include hoarseness, a "lump in the throat" sensation, chest tightness, wheezing, rhini-tis, and laryngeal edema, which may lead to asphyxia.
B. Cardiovascular signs and symptoms include hypotension and vascular collapse with re-sultant arrhythmias and myocardial infarc-tion. Cardiovascular complications account for up to 25% of deaths from anaphylaxis.
C. Skin manifestations include urticaria, an-gioedema, pruritus, and generalized erythema.
D. Gastrointestinal signs and symptoms in-clude nausea, abdominal cramps, inconti-nence, and excessive vomiting and diarrhea.
E. Other common findings are a sense of im-pending doom, agitation, and disorienta-tion.
F. Death may occur within minutes if appro-priate therapy is not initiated immediately.

V. Diagnosis

Diagnosis of anaphylaxis is usually apparent and is based strictly on clinical signs and symp-toms in an appropriate clinical situation. Occa-sionally laboratory indications of systemic medi-ator release are indicated, such as serum tryptase levels.

VI. Differential Diagnosis

Because of the life-threatening nature of ana-phylaxis, in general one should treat for ana-phylaxis if there is any doubt about the diagno-sis. Other possibilities include:

A. Vasovagal reactions—these patients most likely have bradycardia, pallor, and dia-phoresis accompanying hypotension.
B. Myocardial infarction—chest pain usually predominates, with a paucity of skin and upper airway abnormalities.
C. Insulin reactions—usually only moderate hypotension and no skin or respiratory tract symptoms.
D. Other considerations are aspiration, seizure disorders, and hysterical reactions.

VII. Treatment

A. Acute therapy focuses on essential cardio-pulmonary resuscitation techniques and summoning emergency help immediately. The longer initial therapy is delayed, the greater the incidence of mortality. Further measures include:
1. Administration of 0.01 mg/kg aqueous epinephrine 1:1,000 (maximal dose, 0.3 to 0.5 mg) subcutaneously in two or three doses every 15–20 minutes.
   a. Patients on β-blocker therapy may ex-perience unopposed α-adrenergic stimulation with extreme hyperten-sion, so epinephrine should be given cautiously in low doses. Isoproterenol may be useful.
   b. For severe hypotension—dopamine, dobutamine, or IV epinephrine, 1:10,000, 1 ml slowly.
2. Place a tourniquet above the site of injec-tion of the causative agent or stop infusion of the causative agent as indicated. Loosen the tourniquet for 1 min every 3 min.
3. Give an H_1 blocker such as diphenhy-dramine, 1 mg/kg parenterally (IV or IM) up to 50 mg.
4. Fluids given intravenously, intubation or tracheotomy, pressor agents such as dopamine, and aminophylline may be indicated in individual cases.
5. Glucocorticoids are indicated in large doses (e.g., methylprednisolone, 60–120 mg IV every 6 hr) but will not affect the acute symptoms.

B. Prevention of anaphylactic episodes is the key to patient management.
1. If the offending agent is known, strict avoidance is indicated.
2. Patients should carry autoinjectable epi-nephrine at all times and understand the

need to seek medical attention immediately if a reaction occurs.

3. Evaluation of episodes with unknown triggers includes a complete medical history and physical exam, with attention to ingestants, temporal relationships of possible agents to symptoms, and other medical problems.

   a. Skin tests and challenges may provoke anaphylaxis but are indicated in some situations (e.g., insect venom sensitivity).

4. If a known anaphylactic agent is required for therapy, then desensitization must be done before therapy begins (e.g. penicillin) or pretreatment to prevent or lessen symptoms should be undertaken (e.g., radiocontrast media).

5. In the case of insect venom hypersensitivity, specific immunotherapy is indicated.

6. Health care personnel should be aware of agents that are common inducers of anaphylaxis and avoid prescribing unnecessary medications.

7. Patients should carry information on their persons regarding known anaphylactic sensitivities.

VIII. Prognosis

In general, the later the onset of initial symptoms, the less severe the episode. Recovery may take hours or may be prolonged, requiring hospitalization for several days. Complications such as myocardial infarction alter predictions for complete recovery.

Bibliography

Anaphylaxis

Middleton E: Anaphylaxis. In Wasserman SI, Marquardt DL (eds): 1365–1376

Sheffer AL: Anaphylaxis. *JACI* 75:227–233, 1985.

Sheffer AL: Anaphylaxis. *Insights Allergy* 5(3):1–7, 1990.

Rhinitis

James Moy, M.D.

I. Definition

Rhinitis is defined as inflammation of the mucous membranes of the nose. It may be divided into two broad categories: allergic and nonallergic.

A. Allergic rhinitis is characterized by symptoms of nasal pruritus, repetitive sneezing, watery rhinorrhea, and nasal congestion upon exposure to an inhaled allergen to which the patient can be demonstrated to be sensitive.
   1. Seasonal allergic rhinitis occurs most commonly in the spring and/or late summer/early fall.
   2. Perennial allergic rhinitis is primarily due to sensitivity to animal dander and/or insect (dust mite, cockroach) allergens.

B. There are numerous causes of nonallergic rhinitis.
   1. Eosinophilic, nonallergic rhinitis
   2. Vasomotor rhinitis
   3. Nasal polyposis
   4. Rhinitis medicamentosa
   5. Irritant rhinitis
   6. Neutrophilic rhinosinusitis
   7. Structural rhinitis
   8. Hormonal/endocrine

II. Etiology

A. Allergic rhinitis
   Immunoglobulin E (IgE)-mediated symptoms upon exposure to aeroallergens such as pollens, mold spores, animal proteins, and dust mites.

B. Nonallergic rhinitis
   1. The etiology of eosinophilic nonallergic rhinitis is unknown. This condition is sometimes associated with acetylsalicylic acid (ASA) sensitivity and rarely with Churg-Strauss syndrome.
   2. The etiology of vasomotor rhinitis is also unknown.
   3. The exact etiology of nasal polyposis is not known, although viral and bacterial infections and pollenosis have been proposed as possible causes.
   4. Rhinitis medicamentosa is the result of the chronic use of vasoconstricting nose sprays (intranasal α-adrenergic agonists) or the use of systemic drugs such as reserpine or pseudoephedrine.
   5. Irritant rhinitis symptoms are induced by stimulants (dusts or fumes) which are noxious to the nasal tissue. Examples in-

clude perfume, turpentine, and cigarette smoke.
6. Neutrophilic rhinosinusitis can be acute or chronic and is usually bacterial or viral, although spirochetal and fungal organisms have been reported in rare instances.
7. Structural rhinitis is most commonly due to septal deviation or rarely to choanal atresia/stenosis, trauma, cleft palate, and adenoid hypertrophy.
8. Hormonal/endocrine etiologies
   a. Pregnancy
   b. Thyroid disease
   c. Medications (oral contraceptives)

III. Pathophysiology
A. The IgE-mediated pathophysiology of allergic rhinitis consists of two phases: the early phase and the late phase.
1. The early phase (beginning within minutes after exposure to an allergen and lasting for 30 to 60) consists of IgE-mediated release of mast cell products such as histamine and leukotrienes, which results in mucosal edema from direct and reflex vasodilation, producing hypersecretion, pruritus, and sneezing.
2. The late phase (beginning approximately 3 to 4 hr following allergen exposure, reaching maximal intensity by 4 to 8 hr, and resolving in 12 to 24 hr) resembles more closely a chronic inflammation with an influx of eosinophils, neutrophils, and monocytes, which results in severe nasal congestion and mucous secretion.
B. The pathophysiology of all of the nonallergic rhinitides includes chronic nasal symptoms in the absence of any demonstratable IgE-mediated involvement. There is cellular infiltration (eosinophils, neutrophils, or basophils) of the nasal mucosa.

IV. Diagnosis
A. The diagnosis of allergic rhinitis is made by a history of nasal symptoms upon exposure to one or more aeroallergens. The allergen(s) may be determined by skin tests or by an in vitro procedure (radioallergosorbent test, or RAST) for assessing the presence of specific IgE antibodies to various allergens. On physical examination, the nasal mucosa is pale, wet, and edematous. The nasal turbinates are swollen and may completely occlude the nasal passageway. The only characteristic laboratory finding in allergic rhinitis is the presence of large numbers of eosinophils in a smear of the nasal secretions obtained duirng a symptomatic period.
B. A diagnosis of nonallergic rhinitis is made in the presence of nasal symptoms without any demonstratable relationship to an IgE-mediated process (see the list above).

V. Differential Diagnosis
A. Malignancies (tumors)
B. Wegener's granulomatosis
C. Foreign bodies
D. Cerebrospinal fluid rhinorrhea

VI. Treatment
A. The treatment of choice for allergic rhinitis is avoidance of the offending allergen. However, avoidance is not always possible. Pharmacologic agents for the treatment of allergic rhinitis include:
1. H_1 antihistamines (see chapter 14).
2. α-Adrenergic agents, topical or oral (e.g., pseudoephedrine, phenylpropanolamine).
3. Intranasal cromolyn spray.
4. Intranasal corticosteroid sprays.
5. In severe cases, oral steroids may be needed (e.g., prednisone, 20 mg every morning for 4 days).
6. If medications and environmental control of allergen exposure do not give adequate relief, immunotherapy (allergy shots) should be considered (see chapter 14).
B. The treatment of nonallergic rhinitis is more difficult.
1. A combination of antihistamines, oral decongestants, and/or corticosteroid sprays is effective in some cases of vasomotor and irritant rhinitis.
2. Topical (nasal sprays) and/or oral corticosteroids are used for nasal polyps. Antibiotics should be given for sinusitis, which is a frequent complication of nasal polyps.
3. Intranasal anticholinergic agents (atropine drops or ipratropium bromide) may be helpful in some cases of vasomotor rhinitis.

Bibliography

Middleton E: *Allergy: Principles and Practice* Edited by Elliot Middleton, et al. Ed 4. St. Louis, MO. C.V. Mosby Company 1993.

Patterson R: *Allergic Diseases: Diagnosis and Management.* Edited by Roy Patterson et al. Ed 4. Philadelphia, 1993.

Venom Reactions

Rebecca Hoffman, M.D.

Stinging insect allergy reactions may range from local induration and erythema at the sting site to anaphylaxis and death. The most common insects that cause these reactions are the apidae (honeybees and bumblebees), the vespidae (wasps, hornets and yellow jackets), and the fornicidae (fire ants and harvester ants).

I. Incidence

Surveys of several large population groups note the incidence of a systemic reaction from an insect sting to be 0.4–4% Death occurs in approximately 40 persons per year in the United States from insect sting allergy, through this number may be low due to additional unrecognized deaths from this cause.

II. Etiology

As noted, several groups of insects are responsible for the majority of insect venom allergic reactions.

A. Apidae (honeybees and bumblebees) generally sting only if provoked. The honeybee is the only stinging insect that leaves its stinger in the victim.

B. Vespidae (wasps, hornets, and yellow jackets) are more aggressive than bees and therefore will sting even if not provoked.

1. Wasps nest under roof eaves, behind shutters, and in shrubs and wood piles. They can be identified by their narrow, pinched waist and cigar-shaped abdomen.

2. Hornets build large, paper-like, football-shaped nests in trees or bushes in relatively exposed locations. They are identified by their yellow and black markings, narrow pinched waist, and short abdomen.

3. Yellow jackets come in frequent contact with man due to their nesting habits in the ground and in logs or wall crevices.

C. Formicidae (fire ants and harvester ants) are nonflying insects found predominantly in warmer climates (southeastern United States, Central and South America), except that harvester ants can be found as far north as Canada. They sting rather than bite. Their bite is used to hold on while they sting repeatedly, usually in a circular configuration, forming sterile pustules at the sting sites.

1. Fire ants are extremely aggressive and are the dominant stinging insect in the southeastern United States. Nests can be very large and are mobile, even floating down flooded rivers to new locations.

2. Harvester ants live in small colonies and nests that are conspicuous due to the large, bare patches of soil surrounding them. They do not rapidly swarm, but several species possess extremely potent venom.

III. Types of Reactions

Sting reactions range from mild local erythema to severe, life-threatening episodes. Unusual reactions such as serum sickness and encephalitis have been reported.

A. Anaphylaxis is the most serious consequence of stinging insect allergy. Most symptoms begin within 15 min of the sting and may include flushing, urticaria, pruritus, throat and chest tightness, wheezing, stridor, nausea, vomiting, diarrhea, and hypotension. The first exposure may result in anaphylaxis, though 5–40% of individuals have a history of a preceding large local reaction. Immunoglobulin E (IgE) antibody is responsible for triggering anaphylactic reactions.

B. Local reactions occur in nonallergic individuals and consist of mild swelling and erythema at the sting site that lasts for several hours. Fire ants sting in a characteristic circular pattern of pustules. Occasionally, more severe local reactions occur, with extension of swelling beyond the sting site that may involve one or more joints. These reactions usually last for 24–72 hr, and both IgE and IgG antibodies play a role in their occurrence.

C. Unusual or delayed reactions are less common. Neurologic and vascular symptoms such as vasculitis, serum sickness, neuritis, encephalopathy, and nephrosis may develop days to weeks after the sting and may be progressive. The pathogenesis is unknown. Toxic reactions due to the pharmacologic properties of the venoms may also be noted; these may be similar to anaphylactic symptoms.

IV. Venom Characteristics

Multiple components of venom have been identified; allergenic contents include phospholipase A1 & A2, hyaluronidase, phospholipase B, acid phosphatase, and melittin in apids and vespids. There is some degree of cross-reactivity between venoms of the same family, especially the vespids.

V. Diagnosis

The diagnosis is usually obvious if the patient knows that he has been stung and an immediate reaction develops. The difficulty comes in identifying which insect was responsible. As noted, fire ant stings have characteristic circular patterns and only honeybees leave the stinger in the victim; otherwise, identification is diffucult. If an adult has experienced a systemic reaction (anaphylaxis, shortness of breath, or generalized urticaria) skin testing or radioallergosorbent (RAST) testing is indicated. Children with systemic reactions limited to the skin have an extremely low incidence of severe reaction on resting and therefore are not candidates for testing or therapy.

A. Skin testing should be done to identify sensitivity in patients if possible. From 2 to 4 weeks must elapse between the time of the sting and testing.

B. RAST testing is less sensitive, and in approximately 15–20% of patients RAST will be negative, while skin tests are positive. However, in some patients, RAST testing is necessary (patients on chronic antihistamines or with severe skin disorders preventing skin testing).

VI. Treatment

A. Acute reactions should be treated according to their severity.

1. Anaphylaxis should be handled as for any other inciting event. The ABCs of cardiopulmonary resuscitation should be initiated immediately. Further measures include:

   a. Epinephrine, 0.01 mg/kg (1:1000 dilution) given SC up to 0.3 mg in children, 0.5 mg in adults. Repeat as necessary every 10–15 min.

   b. Diphenhydramine, 1 mg/kg po, IM, or IV, up to 50 mg in children or 100 mg in adults.

   c. Place a tourniquet above the site of the sting if it has occurred on an extremity; loosen the tourniquet every 5–10 min.

   d. Give IV fluids, vasopressors, aminophylline, and other measures as indicated.

   e. Corticosteroids (e.g., methylprednisolone, 40–60 mg IV) may be indicated for prolonged reactions.

2. Local reactions should be treated with application of cold packs to the sting site, oral antihistamines, and analgesics. Extremely large local reactions may benefit by the addition of oral steroids (e.g., prednisone, 20–40 mg daily for several days).

3. Unusual and toxic reactions may benefit

from steroid therapy, but since their etiology is unknown, therapy is empiric.

B. Prevention

Simple precautions will reduce the risk of subsequent stings.

1. All patients with a history of systemic or severe local reactions should carry autoinjectable epinephrine at all times and should wear proper identification describing their insect allergy.

2. Patients should avoid outdoor activities that may potentially disturb or attract stinging insects.

3. Patients should avoid "looking like a flower or smelling like a flower." This includes avoiding bright, colorful clothing, as well as perfumes and scented lotions, hair sprays, and sunscreens. White or tan clothing is preferable.

4. Removal of nests or hives should be done by a nonallergic person. Insect repellants may be helpful in deterring insects from rebuilding in the same area.

C. Immunotherapy

Over 95% of patients with a history of insect sting anaphylaxis are protected upon re-sting after venom immunotherapy. Therapy with purified venom extracts but not whole body extracts has been shown to protect against apid and vespid stings. Fire ant immunotherapy with either venom or whole body preparations is beneficial.

1. Indications

a. Adults with a history of a systemic reaction and positive skin or RAST tests should be treated with all appropriate venoms.

b. Children with a history of a systemic reaction not limited to the skin (only generalized urticaria or angioedema) and positive skin or RAST tests should be treated with all appropriate venoms.

c. Unusual or toxic reactions are not indications for venom immunotherapy.

2. Duration of therapy

Controversy exists regarding the length of venom immunotherapy needed to provide protection from subsequent stings. Current recommendations are for indefi-nite therapy, but recent studies suggest that 3 to 5 years of maintenance therapy is all that is necessary.

3. Mechanisms of protection from immunotherapy are thought to be due to a rise in venom-specific IgG and a decline in venom-specific IgE. However, specific levels of antibody to be attained through therapy are not yet known.

VII. Prognosis

A. Risk of testing and treatment

Less than 1% of insect-sensitive subjects experience systemic reactions from skin testing and approximately 10% of subjects undergoind immunotherapy experience systemic reactions, most of which are not severe. Given the severity of the problem being treated, this is an acceptable risk-benefit ratio. Venom immunotherapy is safe for use during pregnancy.

B. Benefits of therapy

Untreated adults who have experienced one anaphylactic reaction to a stinging insect have a 50–60% chance of recurrent anaphylaxis on re-sting. However, patients who have received appropriate immunization with venom have a repeat reaction rate of less than 2%. Children with severe systemic reactions not limited to the skin achieve similar protection. However, in many patients the stinging insect allergy may be self-limited. Until the true natural history of the disorder is determined, the full benefits of therapy will be unknown.

Bibliography

Insect Hypersensitivity

Barsky HE: Stinging insect allergy: avoidance, identification and treatment. *Postgrad Med* 82(3):157–162, 1987

Lockey RF: Immunotherapy for allergy to stinging insects (editorial). *N Engl J Med* 323:1627–1628, 1990.

Stafford CT, Rhoades RB, Bunker-Soler AL, et al: Survey of whole-body extract immunotherapy for imported fire ant- and other *Hymenoptera*-sting allergy. *JACI* 83:1107–1111, 1989.

Allergy: Principles and Practice Ed: E. Middleton, Jr., C. E. Reed, E. F. Ellis, N. F. Adkinson, Jr., J.W. Yunginger, St. Louis, MO 1988

Urticaria/Angioedema

James Moy, M.D.

I. Definition

Over 20% of the general population has suffered an eruption of urticaria at some point in their lives. Urticaria is characterized by the appearance of pruritic, erythematous, cutaneous elevations that blanch with pressure. Urticarial lesions are circumscribed, slightly elevated swellings that are usually multiple and vary in size. Individual lesions seldom last longer than 24 hr, although new lesions may appear every day. Angioedema is caused by pathologic alterations similar to those of urticaria, except that the swelling occurs in the deep dermis and subcutaneous tissue. In contrast to urticaria, angioedema has little or no associated pruritus.

II. Etiology

Urticaria/angioedema may be allergic, immunologic, or nonimmunologic. Considerations for the etiology of urticaria/angioedema include:

A. Foods and food additives
B. Drug reactions
C. Inhalant, ingestant, or contactant allergens
D. Physical urticarias
   1. Cold urticaria
   2. Cholinergic urticaria
   3. Dermographism
   4. Pressure urticaria
   5. Vibratory angioedema
   6. Solar urticaria
   7. Aquagenic urticaria
E. Transfusion reactions
F. Infections—bacterial, fungal, viral, helminthic
G. Chronic idiopathic urticaria/angioedema (> 6 weeks)

III. Pathophysiology

Vasoactive factors from various systems are thought to be potential mediators of urticaria and angioedema.

A. Mast cell release: histamine, prostaglandin D_2, leukotrienes C and D, platelet-activating factor, and kallikrein-like enzymes.
B. Activation of the complement system leads to release of the anaphylatoxins C3a, C4a, and C5a.
C. Activation of the Hageman factor–dependent pathway causes the release of bradykinin.
D. Mononuclear cells can produce and release histamine-releasing factors.

The pathophysiologic findings of urticaria are (1) erythema from dilatation of capillaries and venules; (2) wheal from increased permeability of blood vessels and leakage of serum into the extracapillary space; and (3) flare from dilatation of surrounding arterioles via an axonal reflex.

IV. Workup
A. Thorough history of all medications, including those sold over the counter (e.g., nonsteroidal anti-inflammatory drugs).
B. Elimination of suspected offending foods and/or additives. A complete elimination diet in which the patient is restricted to chicken, rice, and tap water for at least 72 hr is the best approach to identifying an ingestant as the etiology. If the urticaria resolves on the elimination diet, one or two foods may be added back to the diet daily, with careful observation for recurrence of symptoms.
C. Aeroallergen skin tests may be of some value in the rare case of urticaria secondary to an inhaled allergen.
D. There are specific tests for the physical urticarias (e.g., the ice cube test for cold urticaria).
E. Appropriate tests should be obtained if infection or systemic illness is suspected.
   1. Complete blood count
   2. Thyroid profile
   3. Erythrocyte sedimentation rate
   4. Antinuclear antibodies, complement profile
   5. Hepatitis profile
   6. Dental exam for caries
   7. Sinus films
   8. Stool for ova and parasites
   9. Skin biopsy
   10. Chest x-ray

V. Differential Diagnosis
A. Hereditary angioedema (see below).
B. Malignancies/angioedema with acquired C1 inhibitor deficiency.
C. Collagen vascular diseases
D. Urticaria pigmentosa/systemic mastocytosis
E. Thyroid disease

VI. Treatment
Elimination of the offending agent or treatment of the underlying illness is the optimal treatment. However, in 40% of acute urticaria and 80% of

chronic articaria, the etiology is not defined. Pharmacologic treatment includes antihistamines and, in severe cases, systemic corticosteroids.

VII. Hereditary Angioedema (C1 Inhibitor Deficiency)
A. Autosomal dominant
B. Incidence—1:1,000,000
C. There are two types:
   Type I: Markedly decreased synthesis of the protein (80% of cases)
   Type II: normal synthesis, but the protein is functionless (20% of cases)
D. Pathophysiology: Decreased C1 inhibitor (C1 INH) leading to uncontrolled production of C2b, the substrate for C2 kinin. C2 kinin acts like other kinins, causing angioedema. C1 INH also inhibits activated Hageman factor, kallikrein, and plasmin. Thus, it is also an important modulator of bradykinin generation. Due to uncontrolled primary pathway activation, C4 levels are low during attacks; thus, the C4 level is a valuable screening test.
E. Clinical course: Angioedema is episodic but may be life-threatening (laryngioedema). Symptoms of gastrointestinal edema are commonly seen. Episodes are usually secondary to physical trauma, although 45% of patients claim that anxiety triggered the episode. Lesions are never pruritic.
F. Therapy
   1. For acute episodes, give supportive care (i.e., airway management); ε-aminocaproic acid (Amikar) may be effective.
   2. Chronic treatment involves attenuated androgens (danazol or stanozolol), which increases synthesis of the C1 INH protein.

Bibliography

Middleton E: *Allergy: Principles and Practice.* Edited by Elliot Middleton, Jr. et al. ed 4. St. Louis, MO C.V. Mosby Company 1993.

Patterson R: *Allergic Diseases: Diagnosis and Management.* Edited by Roy Patterson et al. ed 4. Philadelphia 1993.

Roitt I: *Immunology.* Ivan M. Roitt, Jonathan Brostoff and David Male St. Louis, MO C.V. Mosby Company 1993.

CHAPTER **9-E**

Food Allergy

G. Wendell Richmond, M.D.

I. Problem

Ingestion of a food may result in an adverse reaction to a component of the food, whether it be a natural component or an additive.

A. Poorly defined terminology has led 20–30% of Americans to claim that they have self-diagnosed food "allergies". Standard nomenclature for adverse reactions to foods has been adopted by the American Academy of Allergy and Immunology (Table 9E-1).

B. Adverse reactions to foods may be categorized as either *food hypersensitivity* or *food intolerance* reactions.

1. Hypersensitivity reactions include all immunologically mediated reactions to foods; immunoglobulin E (IgE)-mediated reactions are best characterized.

a. Mast cells, bearing antigen-specific IgE, are prominently dispersed (10,000–20,000/cu mm) throughout the gastrointestinal mucosa; upon binding food antigen, histamine and other mediators (prostaglandins, leukotrienes, tryptase) are released, causing clinical symptoms.

b. A limited number of foods cause approximately 80% of IgE-mediated (allergic) reactions.

(1) Peanuts
(2) Nuts
(3) Egg
(4) Milk
(5) Shellfish
(6) Fish
(7) Soy
(8) Wheat

c. Food antigens inducing IgE-mediated disease are water-soluble, acid-stable, and proteolytically stable glycoproteins; lipids do not induce IgE-mediated reactions (e.g., patients with peanut allergy are not sensitive to 100% pure, non-peanut protein-contaminating peanut oil).

d. The prevalence of food allergy is approximately 6% in infants, 2% in children, and < 1% in adults.

e. Foods most likely to cease producing IgE-mediated reactions over time are milk, eggs, and soy.

Table 9E-1. Definitions of Terms for Adverse Food Reactions

1. Adverse reaction to a food	Clinically abnormal response caused by an ingested food or additive.
2. Food intolerance	General term describing an abnormal physiologic response to an ingested food or food additive that is nonimmunologic.
a. Food idiosyncrasy	Quantitatively abnormal response of a food product that differs from its physiologic or pharmacologic effect.
b. Food toxicity (poisoning)	Adverse effect caused by toxins expressed by the food itself or from microorganisms contaminating the food.
c. Pharmacologic food reaction	Adverse reaction as a result of a naturally derived or added chemical that produces a drug-like or pharmacologic effect.
d. Metabolic food reaction	Adverse reaction as a result of the effect of a food substance on metabolism of ingestion.
3. Food allergy (hypersensitivity)	Immunologic reaction resulting from ingestion of a food.
4. Food anaphylaxis	Classic allergic reaction to a food in which IgE and release of chemical mediators are involved.
5. Anaphylactoid reaction	Nonimmunologic mediated release of chemical mediators, resulting in a symptom complex resembling anaphylaxis.

Source: Adapted from the American Academy of Allergy and Immunology Committee on Adverse Reactions to Foods and National Institute of Allergy and Infectious Disease: *Adverse Reactions to Foods.* Publication No. 84-2442. Washington, DC: U.S. Department of Health and Human Services, Public Health Service, National Institutes of Health, July 1984. With permission.

2. Immune complex-mediated (Gell and Coombs type III) disease due to food antigens is uncommon.
   a. Milk-induced syndrome with pulmonary disease (Heiner's syndrome): recurrent pulmonary disease, gastrointestinal blood loss, iron deficiency anemia, serum precipitins to cow's milk protein.
   b. Food—anti-food antibody complexes are food sensitive and found in normal individuals.
3. Although they are immunologically mediated, there is no evidence that IgE-related events play a role in the pathophysiology of two gluten-sensitive diseases: gluten-sensitive enteropathy (celiac disease) and dermatitis herpetiformis.
C. Food intolerances account for the vast majority of adverse reactions to foods and are non-IgE mediated, nonimmunologic reactions.
   1. Pharmacologic food reactions (e.g., niacin-induced flushing, tyramine-induced headache).
   2. Metabolic food reaction (e.g., phenylalanine ingestion by phenylketonurics).
   3. Food idiosyncracy (e.g., lactose ingestion by lactase-deficient individuals).
   4. Food toxicity: the production or innate presence of a toxin within a food.

II. Differential Diagnosis

A. Reactions to additives and contaminants (food intolerance)
   1. Flavorings and preservatives
      a. Nitrates and nitrites (processed meats).
      b. Monosodium glutamate (flavor enhancer)
      c. Sulfiting agents (wine, dried apricots and raisins).
      d. Sodium benzoate, butylated hydroxyanisole (BHA), butylated hydroxytoluene (BHT) (preservatives in foods)
      e. Aspartame
   2. Dyes; tartrazine (FD&C yellow no. 5)
   3. Toxins
      a. Bacterial (botulism, *Staphylococcus aureus*).
      b. Fungal (aflatoxins, ergot)
      c. Seafood associated
         (1) Scrombroid poisoning (tuna, mackeral)—endogenous histamine levels are increased during improper storage.
         (2) Ciguantera poisoning (grouper, snapper, barracuda)
   4. Infectious agents
      a. Bacteria (*Salmonella, Shigella, Escherichia coli, Yersinia, Campylobacter*)
      b. Parasites (*Trichinella*)
      c. Virus (hepatitis)
   5. Accidental contaminents

   a. Heavy metals (cobalt, copper, mercury)
   b. Pesticides
B. Reaction to endogenous pharmacologic agents (food intolerance)
   1. Histamine (fish, cheese, beer, wine)
   2. Tyramine (cheese, avocado, banana, tomato)
   3. Serotonin (banana, tomato, pineapple juice)
   4. Caffeine (coffee, tea, soft drinks, cocoa)
   5. Theobromine (chocolate, tea)
   6. Phenylethylamine (chocolate)
   7. Alcohol
C. Gastrointestinal diseases
   1. Enzyme deficiencies
      a. Disaccharidase deficiency (lactase)
      b. Phenylketonuria
      c. Galactosemia
   2. Malignancy—carcinoid
   3. Structural abnormalities
      a. Hiatal hernia
      b. Pyloric stenosis
      c. Hirschsprung's disease
      d. Tracheoesophageal fistula
   4. Other
      a. Pancreatic insufficiency (cystic fibrosis)
      b. Cholecystitis
      c. Peptic ulcer disease

III. Focus of History and Physical Examination
A. Onset usually occurs within 5 to 30 min in IgE-mediated food reactions.
B. Initial symptoms due to IgE-mediated food reactions may include palatal or throat itching, nasal congestion, and throat tightness.
C. IgE-mediated food allergy reactions
   1. Generalized reactions
      a. Anaphylaxis
   2. Cutaneous reactions
      a. Urticaria/angioedema
      b. Atopic dermatitis
   3. Respiratory reactions
      a. Rhinoconjunctivitis
      b. Laryngeal edema
      c. Asthma
   4. Gastrointestinal reactions
      a. Nausea and abdominal pain
      b. Vomiting and diarrhea
      c. Colic

IV. Diagnostic Approach
A. History: Careful review of all ingestants (excluding tap water only) during 8 hr prior to the reaction
B. Elimination diet: Rice/chicken/lamb or Vivonex diet

   1. Elimination diet for 7–10 days; observe for clinical improvement.
   2. Add back one or two foods daily, with careful observation. If a food or constituent produces symptoms, avoidance for 3 weeks is followed by rechallenge; if the result is positive, further avoidance is warranted.
C. Puncture skin tests: indicated when a food antigen is suspected to cause IgE-mediated reaction. (Additives, preservatives, and coloring agents are not applicable.)
   1. If tests are negative: IgE-mediated food reaction is unlikely; challenge is rarely indicated.
   2. If tests are positive: strict avoidance diet is mandated for 3 weeks
      a. If unequivocal improvement occurs, continue the restricted diet.
      b. If improvement is equivocal and/or more than three foods are involved, perform a single-blind food challenge test in the office.
         (1) If the test is positive to one food, institute an appropriate elimination diet.
         (2) If the test is positive to more than one food:
            (a) Perform a double-blind, placebo-controlled (DBPC) food challenge.
            (b) DBPC food challenge is the gold standard study for food allergy.
            (c) If the DBPC challenge is positive, avoid the food.
         (3) Although there are few false-negative skin tests in food-allergic patients, false-positive skin tests are not uncommon.
D. In vitro antigen-specific IgE testing (radioallergosorbent test, RAST) is no more sensitive than skin testing and is more time-consuming and costly. Indicated in exquisitely food-sensitive patients, those with extensive skin disease, or those who cannot discontinue antihistamines.
E. Incremental dose challenge: non-immunologic food reaction (intolerance) sodium benzoate, tartrazine, sulfite, BHA, or BHT.
   1. No serologic studies or skin tests are available.
   2. Avoid foods containing a positive challenge constituent.
F. Sublingual food challenges and leukocyte cy-

totoxic testing, two controversial methods of food testing, have been shown to be neither reliable nor reproducible in controlled studies.

Adverse Reactions to Drugs

I. Definition

Adverse reactions to drugs occur in approximately 5% of hospitalized patients. Although the term *allergy* is generically used for those reactions, it implies an IgE-mediated mechanism which, in fact, infrequently explains the mechanism for the reaction.

A. Drug intolerance: the drug produces a known side effect at a dose lower than that tolerated by the general population.

B. Drug idiosyncrasy: a pharmacologically unexpected reaction to a drug.

C. Pseudoallergic drug reaction: a reaction that has the signs and symptoms of an allergic reaction but is not immunologically mediated; the reaction may occur during the initial dose of the drug.

1. Direct histamine release by a medication.
   a. Vancomycin
   b. Protamine
   c. Polymyxin B
   d. Codeine, morphine, meperidine
   e. Radiocontrast media
   f. D-Tubocurarine
   g. Pentamidine
   h. Deferoxamine
   i. Phytonadione (vitamin K)

2. Complement activation with the generation of anaphylatoxins C3a and C5a.
   a. Immune serum globulin; intramuscular preparations may contain 20% aggregated IgG that would activate complement if inadvertently given intravenously.
   b. Radiocontrast media.

3. Enzyme inhibitors
   a. Angiotensin-converting enzyme inhibitors have been associated with episodes of angioedema and cough.
   b. Nonsteroidal anti-inflammatory drugs (NSAIDS) may cause urticaria, angioedema, rhinosinusitis, or asthma.
      (1) All NSAIDS that block the cyclooxygenase pathway clinically cross-react with the prototypical drug acetylsalicylic acid (ASA); clinical cross-reactivity may approach 100% with agents like indomethacin and may occur to lesser degrees with other NSAIDS.
      (2) Weak inhibitors of the cyclooxygenase pathway rarely cause reactions; however, ASA reactors may have an adverse reaction to large doses of acetaminophen (extra-strength) or salsalate.
      (3) Shunting of arachidonate from the cyclooxygenase pathway to the lipoxygenase pathway, with the subsequent generation of leukotrienes C, D, and E, may be the basis for the intolerance.

D. Immunologically mediated drug reactions

1. Most drugs are low molecular weight chemicals and are poorly immunogenic. Covalent binding of the drug to a carrier protein (haptenation) results in a structure that is antigenic.
   a. Heptenation by highly reactive compounds (e.g., penicillins).
   b. Haptenation by metabolites of a drug; the parent drug is non-reactive (e.g., sulfonamides).
   c. Proteins from xenogeneic sources (e.g., horse, pig, cow) are complete antigens and produce an antibody response in all recipients.

2. Immunologically mediated drug reactions are categorized according to Gell and Coomb's classification.
   a. Type I (IgE-mediated): technically correct allergic drug reaction (e.g., penicillin, chymopapain, insulin, cisplatin).
      (1) Previous sensitization to the drug is required.
      (2) An immediate reaction occurs after subsequent exposure to a low concentration of the drug.
      (3) Clinical symptoms range from urticaria and angioedema to anaphylaxis.
   b. Type II (cytotoxic): antibody directed to an antigen on a specific cell (e.g., drug-induced anemia, neutropenia, thrombocytopenia).
      (1) The drug binds to the cell membrane; IgG or IgM anti-drug binds to the absorbed drug; complement activation results in cell lysis.
      (2) Associated with large doses of drug.
   c. Type III (immune complex): for example, sickness due to administration of foreign antisera.

d. Type IV (cell-mediated reaction): for example, neomycin-induced contact dermatitis.

II. Diagnosis

A. History

1. Listing of all medications administered immediately prior to and at the time of the reaction. Nonprescription medicinal agents must be included.

2. Determine the temporal relationship of the reaction to a suspected drug.

3. Define the symptom complex during the reaction (e.g., isolated cutaneous eruption, angioedema, erythema multiforme, Stevens-Johnson eruption, anaphylaxis).

4. Elicit a history of previous reactions to related drugs.

5. History of concurrent illness.

   a. Ampicillin rash in a patient with mononucleosis.

   b. Sulfamethoxazole rash in a patient with acquired immunodeficiency syndrome (AIDS)

B. Skin testing: detects IgE anti-allergen antibodies.

1. Skin testing is limited to a few drugs.

   a. Relevant antigenic determinants are poorly defined for the vast majority of drugs.

   b. Drugs are low molecular weight compounds (e.g., antibiotics), and are therefore poorly antigenic until covalently coupled with protein.

   c. Large molecular weight medications (e.g., insulin, chymopapain) may be suitable for skin testing.

2. Prototypic drug: penicillin

   a. The β-lactam ring is highly reactive with proteins; excellent hapten.

   b. Ninety-five percent of penicillin molecules are metabolized to the penicilloyl determinant (major determinant). Major determinant skin testing material is commercially available (benzyl penicilloyl polylysine, PPL).

   c. Five percent of penicillin is metabolized to penicilloate or penilloate derivatives (minor determinants). Currently, no minor determinant skin testing material is commercially available.

   d. A positive skin test to a major determinant identifies 80% of penicillin-allergic patients but misses 20% of patients sensitive to minor determinants.

   e. Anaphylaxis episodes are associated with positive skin tests for minor determinants.

   f. Predictive values of positive skin tests: 50–60% of patients have an immediate reaction upon reexposure to penicillin.

   g. Predictive value of negative skin tests.

      (1) Negative test when both PPL and a minor determinant are applied: < 1% of patients have an immediate reaction upon reexposure to penicillin.

      (2) Negative test when both PPL and freshly reconstituted Penicillin G are applied: < 5% of patients have an immediate reaction upon reexposure to penicillin.

   h. Penicillin skin testing only predicts an immediate reaction; it cannot predict non-IgE-mediated reactions (e.g., rash, Stevens-Johnson reaction, nephritis).

C. Incremental dose testing: applicable to some oral and parenteral medications. Patients are closely monitored as incremental concentrations of a suspected medication are administered. Dosing begins at subtherapeutic concentrations and proceeds to a full therapeutic dose (e.g., aspirin, local anesthetic).

D. In vitro assays of IgE anti-drug antibody (RAST): limited clinical usefulness at present due to inadequately defined relevant immunogenic determinants.

III. Management

A. Avoidance of the drug or class of drugs associated with the prior reaction; appropriate alternate therapy should always be initially considered.

1. Cross-reactivity between structurally similar compounds is most clearly typified by penicillin and cephalosporin.

   a. In vitro cross-reactivity is substantial between penicillin and first- and second-generation cephalosporins.

   b. Clinical evidence of cross-reactivity is approximately 8% in patients with a history of penicillin allergy given a cephalosporin. There is 1–2% cross-reactivity in patients with a positive penicillin history but a negative skin test.

   c. Immunologic responses to cephalosporin side chains appear more important than the response to the β-lactam epitope.

2. Cross-reactivity between penicillin and

monobactams has not been reported; in contrast, approximately 50% of penicillin-allergic patients have positive skin tests to imipenem, a carbapenem.

B. Desensitization: incremental increases in dose to the full therapeutic dose. The mechanism is debated; a graded histamine release with each subseuqent dose is the most convincing explanation.

1. Limited numbers of drugs have been studied. Penicillin serves as the prototype. Insulin and sulfonamide are other examples.
2. Parenteral and oral desensitization protocols have been defined. Due to the paucity of reported severe immediate reactions to oral administration of medications, oral desensitization, if applicable, is preferred. The penicillin oral protocol has been most closely studied and is the prototype of other protocols.
3. Desensitization precludes concern about an immediate reaction while the patient continues on medication.
   a. Desensitization to non-IgE-mediated immunologic reactions, however, does not occur (rash, nephritis, Stevens-Johnson reaction).
   b. Drug desensitization continues only when the drug is administered daily; once it is discontinued, the patient is again at risk of an immediate reaction.
4. Oral aspirin desensitization effectively induces a state of hyporesponsiveness in ASA-induced asthma, but it is ineffective in blocking ASA-induced urticaria.

C. Premedication
1. Premedication of patients with IgE-mediated reactions with corticosteroids and antihistamines unpredictably alters the course of an immediate reaction and cannot be relied on as a preventive measure.
2. Radiocontrast media reaction (pseudo-allergic reaction): occurs in 5–8% of all patients and in up to 35% of previous reactors. A life-threatening reaction occurs in 0.1% of all patients.

3. Premedication with corticosteroids and diphenhydramine decreases the reaction rate by at least 45% in previous reactors.
   a. Protocols vary but generally call for doses of steroid 1 to 2 hr prior to the procedure and either 7 and 13 hr or 12 hr prior to the procedure, with diphenhydramine given with the last does.
   b. Single doses of steroids given just prior to the procedure have been convincingly documented to provide no protection.

Bibliography for Adverse Reaction to Foods

Anderson JA, Sogin DD (eds): *Adverse Reactions to Foods.* American Academy of Allergy and Immunology and the National Institute of Allergy and Infectious Diseases. U.S. Department of Health and Human Services. NIH Publication No. 84-2442. July 1984.

Metcalfe DD (ed): Symposium proceedings on adverse reactions to foods and food additives. *J Allergy Clin Immunol* 78 pp 125–252, 1986.

Sampson HA: Adverse reactions to foods. In Middleton E, Reed CE, Ellis EF, et al (eds): *Allergy Principles and Practice.* St. Louis, CV Mosby, 1993, pp 1661–1686.

Simon RA, Stevenson DD: Adverse reactions to food and drug additives. In Middleton E, Reed CE, Ellis EF, et al (eds): *Allergy Principles and Practice.* St. Louis, CV Mosby, 1993, pp 1687–1704.

Bibliography for Adverse Reaction to Drugs

de Weck AL: Pharmacologic and immunochemical mechanisms of drug hypersensitivity. *Immunol Allergy Clin North Am* 11:461–474, 1991.

Gruchalla RS, Sullivan TJ: In vivo and in vitro diagnosis of drug allergy. *Immunol Allergy Clin North Am* 11:595–610, 1991.

Parker CW: Hapten immunology and allergic reactions in humans. *Arthritis Rheum* 24:1024–1036, 1981.

Sullivan TJ: Drug allergy. In Middleton E, Reed CE, Ellis EF, et al (eds): *Allergy Principles and Practice.* St Louis, CV Mosby, 1993, pp 1726–1746.

VanArsdel PP: Pseudoallergic drug reactions: Introduction and general review. *Immunol Allergy Clin North Am* 11:635–644, 1991.

CHAPTER 10

Immunodeficiency

G. Wendell Richmond, M.D.

I. **Definition**
Immunodeficiency diseases are a diverse group of disorders that, due to immune dysfunction, result in an increased susceptibility to recurrent infections.
   A. Altered immunologic responses are most commonly due to concomitant infections, malignancy, or therapeutic interventions and are termed *secondary immunodeficiencies*. (Table 10-1).
   B. Primary immunodeficiencies are generally considered to be congenital, although some complement and antibody deficiencies may begin during adulthood.
   C. Primary immunodeficiencies involving B lymphocytes, T lymphocytes, and complement systems have characteristic clinical presentations that should aid clinicians in evaluating the infection-prone patient.

II. **Classification**
   A. The World Health Organization has classified primary immunodeficiencies based on defects involving predominantly T cells, B cells, or both (Table 10-2).
   B. Deficiencies of each of the classical complement pathway components C1–C9 and the C1 control protein, C1 inhibitor, have been described, as well as deficiencies of the alternate complement components properidin and factor D.
   C. Factors H and I function to control C3 activation via the alternate pathway amplification loop. Deficiencies of these control components, like deficiencies of alternate pathway components, are rare.

III. **Etiology**
Many of the primary deficiencies are congenital, although some may be detected in the first to third decade.
   A. Most deficiencies have evidence of a genetic predisposition.
      1. T-cell immunodeficiencies are inherited in an X-linked (a subset of SCIDs, Wiskott-Aldrich syndrome, X-linked lymphroproliferative disease) or autosomal recessive mode (SCID, ataxia-telangiectasia, ADA deficiency, PNP deficiency, reticular dysgenesis).
      2. Patterns of inheritance of B-cell defects are often less clearly defined.
         a. X-linked: X-linked agamma-globulinemia; most patients have Ig deficiency with hyper-IgM.

Table 10-1. Secondary Immunodeficiencies

Age related
1. Prematurity
2. Aged

Infectious diseases
1. Human immunodeficiency virus (HIV) infection—acquired immunodeficiency syndrome (AIDS)
2. Cytomegalovirus
3. Congenital rubella
4. Epstein-Barr infection
5. Bacterial infections
6. Mycobacterial, fungal, parasitic infections

Malignancy/hematologic diseases
1. Leukemia
2. Lymphoma
3. Myeloma
4. Aplastic anemia

Surgery/trauma
1. Burns
2. Splenectomy

Immunosuppressive therapy
1. Radiation
2. Corticosteroids
3. Immunosuppressive drugs

Hereditary/metabolic diseases
1. Myotonic dystrophy
2. Down's syndrome
3. Sickle cell disease
4. Cystic fibrosis
5. Diabetes mellitus
6. Malnourishment
7. Uremia
8. Protein-losing enteropathy

Immune dysregulation
1. Systemic lupus erythematosus
2. Chronic active hepatitis
3. Graft-versus-host disease

Table 10-2. World Health Organization Classification of Primary Immunodeficiencies

Combined immunodeficiencies
1. Severe combined immunodeficiency (SCID)
   a. X-linked
   b. Autosomal recessive
2. Reticular dysgenesis
3. Adenosine deaminase (ADA) deficiency
4. Purine nucleoside phosphorylase (PNP) deficiency
5. Major histocompatibility complex (MHC) class II deficiency
6. MHC class I deficiency

Predominantly antibody deficiencies
1. X-linked agammaglobulinemia
2. X-linked agammaglobulinemia with growth hormone deficiency
3. Immunoglobulin (Ig) deficiency with increased M ("hyper-IgM" syndrome)
4. IgA deficiency
5. κ Chain deficiency
6. Selective deficiency of other immunoglobulin isotypes
7. Common variable immunodeficiency
8. Transient hypogammaglobulinemia of infancy

Other well-defined immunodeficiency syndromes
1. Wiskott-Aldrich syndrome
2. Ataxia-telangiectasia
3. DiGeorge syndrome (thymic hypoplasia)
4. Chronic mucocutaneous candidiasis
5. Hyper-IgE syndrome
6. X-linked lymphoproliferative disease

b. Autosomal recessive: some patients with IgA deficiency, immunoglobulin deficiency with hyper-IgM, common variable immunodeficiency (CVID).
c. Sporadic: CVID, immunodeficiency with thymoma, IgM deficiency, transient hypogammaglobulinemia of infancy, Ig deficiency with hyper-IgM.
3. Complement deficiencies are inherited in an autosomal recessive manner except for C1 inhibitor deficiency (autosomal dominant) and properidin deficiency (X-linked).

B. Differentiation defects
1. Defects of embryogenesis: Embryogenic arrest of third and fourth pharyngeal pouch development results in variable degrees of thymic and parathyroid hypoplasia and, rarely, aplasia (DiGeorge syndrome).
2. Defects in cell differentiation
   a. Patients with SCID have adequate stem cell precursors that fail to differentiate into thymocytes.
   b. B cells in patients with X-linked agammaglobulinemia (Bruton's disease) fail to differentiate from pre-B cells to B cells. The defect is related to the failure to synthesize a protein kinase, B cell progeniter kinase (BPK), encoded at a site on the proximal long arm of the X chromosome (Xq21.3–22).

c. The majority of patients with CVID have an intrinsic B-cell defect of Ig synthesis that cannot be overcome by combinations of B-cell activators.

C. Enzyme deficiencies
   1. ADA is an enzyme in the purine salvage pathway. Deficiency of ADA results in the accumulation of multiple purine products including deoxyadenosine. The latter is cytotoxic for both B and T lymphocytes, resulting in one form of autosomal recessive SCID.
   2. PNP converts inosine to hypoxanthine in the purine salvage pathway. Deficiency of this enzyme results in a profound T-cell defect with normal Ig levels.

D. Cellular immunoregulatory defects
   1. T-cell suppression of normal B-cell immunoglobulin synthesis (a common in vitro finding in CVID).
   2. Defects in providing adequate T-cell help necessary for Ig synthesis (rarely in CVID; transient hypogamma-globulinemia of infancy).
   3. Failure of T cells to provide an immunoglobulin class switch signal: Patients with Ig deficiency with increased IgM have defective expression of CD40 ligand (CD40L), a molecule expressed on activated T cells. The CD40 molecule is the CD40L receptor on B lymphocytes. When B–T lymphocytes communicate via a CD40–CD40L interaction, B cells proliferate and differentiate. Adding IL-4 results in an immunoglobulin class switch from IgM to IgE and from IgM to IgG and IgA in the presence of IL-10.

E. Homozygous deletion of genes
   1. Deletion of Ig heavy chain constant region genes in patients with IgA and IgG2 and IgG4 deficiencies with recurrent infections.
   2. Ig heavy chain constant region deletions have been detected, however, in individuals without recurrent infections.

IV. **Diagnosis**
   A. Clinical characteristics
      1. Predominantly T-cell or combined immunodeficiencies.
         a. DiGeorge syndrome
            (1) Hypocalcemic neonatal tetany, hypertelorism; low-set, prominent ears; micrognathia; anti-mongoloid slant of the eyes; cardiovascular abnormalities.
            (2) The variable extent of thymic and parathyroid hypoplasia results in varying degrees of disease severity. Patients with aplasia have severe neonatal disease. Some patients with less severe dysgenesis have more subtle T-cell defects, with onset occurring later in infancy.
            (3) Fulminant disease may develop after vaccination with live viral vaccines.
         b. Wiskott-Aldrich syndrome
            (1) X-linked disease.
            (2) The infant often presents with petechiae or bleeding episodes associated with thrombocytopenia and eczema.
            (3) Infections are initially bacterial but later are due to protozoan or viral pathogens.
            (4) Progressive T-cell deficiency with increasing age.
         c. Ataxia-telangiectasia
            (1) Cerebellar ataxia is often noted as the child begins to crawl or walk; ataxia usually is detectable by 5 years of age, and progressive deterioration is inevitable.
            (2) Telangiectasias, initially of the bulbar conjunctiva, later may involve multiple cutaneous sites.
            (3) Infections are predominantly bacterial or viral.
            (4) Patients have a markedly increased risk for the development of lymphorecticular malignancies.
         d. Chronic mucocutaneous candidiasis (CMCC)
            (1) Chronic candida infections involving the skin, nails, and mucous membranes.
            (2) Systemic candidal infections are rare.
            (3) CMCC is associated with various endocrinopathies (Table 10-3).
         e. X-linked lymphoproliferative disease
            (1) Fulminent lymphoproliferation occurs after an infection with Epstein-Barr virus (EBV).
            (2) Four patterns of involvement have been identified:
               (a) Progressively fatal EBV infection
               (b) B-cell lymphoma

(c) Hypogammaglobulinemia

(d) aplastic anemia

2. Predominantly immunoglobulin deficiencies

Antibody deficiency states, although representing multiple different defects of immunoglobulin synthesis, have common clinical characteristics (Table 10-3).

a. X-linked hypogammaglobulinemia (Bruton's disease)

(1) Recurrent infections begin after placentally transferred maternal IgG has been catabolized (by 6 months); most patients experience infections by the end of the first year of life.

(2) The clinical presentation, in addition to recurrent respiratory tract infections and otitis, may include pyoderma, arthritis, and meningitis.

(3) Lymphoid tissue is absent despite recurrent infections.

(4) Prolonged delays in diagnosis, estimated to be 3.5 years, lead to the development of bronchiectasis, due to recurrent lower respiratory tract infections.

(5) Viral infections are generally not problematic. Exceptions include:

(a) Enteroviral meningitis: life-threatening even with aggressive intrathecal and intravenous Ig therapy.

(b) Poliomyelitis: infection with the attenuated live virus used in oral polio vaccination programs.

(c) Hepatitis B antigenemia.

b. Common variable immunodeficiency (CVID)

(1) Onset at any age, beginning at 6 months. Most commonly diagnosed during the second and third decades of life.

(2) Recurrent sinopulmonary infections predominate clinically.

(3) Recurrent episodes of diarrhea are extremely common.

(a) *Giardia lamblia* is a common pathogen. It is difficult to detect by routine stool analysis, and endoscopy with jejunal biopsy is often required for diagnosis.

(b) A celiac-like enteropathy is often noted in CVID patients with diarrhea. A gluten-free diet may be beneficial in decreasing the severity of diarrheal disease.

(c) Lactose intolerance also contributes to gastro-intestinal symptoms.

(d) Diffuse lymphoid hyperplasia throughout the intestinal mucosa is termed *nodular lymphoid hyperplasia*.

(4) Autoimmune disease including pernicious anemia, autoimmune thyroid disease, autoimmune hemolytic anemia and thrombocytopenia, and alopecia are commonly identified in patients with CVID.

(5) Sarcoid-like granulomatous disease of the lung, liver, and spleen has been described.

(6) In contrast to patients with X-linked hypo-gammaglobulinemia, those with CVID may have marked lymphadenopathy.

(7) Patients with inadequately treated disease are at increased risk of developing lymphomas; those with pernicious anemia and achlorhydria are at increased risk of gastric carcinoma.

c. Isolated IgA deficiency

(1) Most IgA-deficient individuals are asymptomatic.

(2) Patients with recurrent sinopulmonary tract infections and IgA deficiency may have IgG2/IgG4 or IgG3 subclass deficiencies.

(3) IgA deficiency is associated with an increased risk of ulcerative colitis, Crohn's disease, gluten-sensitive enteropathy, and nodular lymphoid hyperplasia.

(4) Autoimmune diseases associated with IgA deficiency include rheumatoid arthritis, systemic lupus erythematosus, and juvenile rheumatoid arthritis.

(5) Atopic diseases occur five times more frequently in IgA-deficient individuals.

d. IgG subclass and lacunar deficiency

(1) IgG subclass quantitation must be interpreted in the context of age-matched levels.

(a) IgG2 levels may not reach adult levels until 12 years of age.

(b) IgG subclass levels are associated, in part, with the inheritance of IgG allotypes;

   (i) IgG2 has a single allotype: G2m(23).

   (ii) Seventy-five percent of a North American population is G2m(23) positive.

   (iii) The mean IgG2 levels in the G2m(23)-negative population are 63% of those of the G2m(23)-positive population.

(2) IgG1 deficiency usually results in hypogammaglobulinemia when Ig's are quantitated since it comprises 60–70% of the total IgG concentration.

(a) Predominant antibody response to protein and viral antigens.

(b) Usually associated with other subclass deficiencies.

(c) Clinical presentation is that of common variable immunodeficiency.

(3) IgG2, IgG3, and IgG4 deficiencies may present with normal IgG levels since they comprise 20–30, 8–10, and 1–5% of the total IgG concentration, respectively.

(a) Antibody responses to carbohydrate antigens are predominantly IgG2; therefore, sinopulmonary infections are typically encapsulated bacterial pathogens.

(b) IgG3 deficiency is reported to be the most common subclass deficiency in adults. It is often associated with other subclass deficiencies in symptomatic patients.

(c) IgG4 deficiency may be detected in up to 25% of the general population. Although it is reported to be associated with respiratory tract infections, the significance of a deficiency of this subclass is not clear.

(4) Patients with lacunar deficiencies have normal quantitative Ig and IgG subclass levels but have a defect in antibody responses to specific antigens, usually polysaccharides, resulting in sinopulmonary infections with encapsulated pyogenic bacteria.

e. Immunodeficiency with increased IgM (dysgammaglobulinemia with hyper-IgM).

(1) Marked male predominance; X-linked inheritance has been demonstrated in some families.

(2) Elevated IgM levels with deficient production of IgG and IgA.

(3) Recurrent sinopulmonary bacterial infections are associated with adenopathy and splenomegaly.

(4) Patients may occasionally develop neutropenia, hemolytic anemia, or thrombocytopenia.

(5) There is an increased risk of lympho-reticular malignancies.

f. Immunodeficiency with thymoma

(1) Recurrent sinopulmonary infections, characteristically with onset between 40 and 70 years of age.

(2) Panhypogammaglobulinemia is associated with thymoma (90% spindle cell, 10% malignant).

(3) Quantitation of peripheral blood B cells reveals markedly decreased numbers.

(4) Pure red cell aplasia occurs eight times more frequently than in patients with thymoma without humoral deficiency; myasthenia gravis is also more frequently noted.

(5) Surgical removal of the thymoma may result in improvement in red cell aplasia or myasthenia gravis; however, hypogammaglobulinemia fails to respond.

3. Complement deficiencies

a. Homozygous deficiencies of the early classical complement pathway components (C1, C2, C4) are associated with autoimmune diseases (systemic lupus erythematosus, discoid lupus erythematosus, glomerulonephritis).

b. Deficiency of C3, a component common to both the classical and alternate pathways, is associated with recurrent bacterial infections (predominantly pneumococcal), systemic lupus erythematosus, glomerulonephritis, and cutaneous vasculitis.

    c. Deficiencies of alternate pathway components (H, I, properidin) are less frequently described than classical component deficiencies and are generally associated with recurrent infections.

    d. Deficiency of the C1 inhibitor, a control protein that binds to activated C1, thereby inhibiting further complement activation, is associated with hereditary angioedema.

    e. Deficiencies of the terminal complement components (C5, C6, C7, C8) are associated with recurrent neisserial infections.

    f. Despite disease associations, many individuals with homozygous complement deficiencies have been described who are clinically well.

B. Laboratory diagnosis
  1. Screening assays
    a. Complete blood count with differential and platelet count.
    b. Quantitation of IgG, IgA, IgM, and IgE.
  2. Additional immunological evaluation
    a. Suspected antibody deficiency.
      (1) IgG subclass quantification.
      (2) Quantitation of antibody to specific antigens.
        (a) Isohemagglutinin titters (IgM anti-A, anti-B, or both): should be greater than 1:8 in all individuals except those with the AB blood group.
        (b) Tetanus, diphtheria (protein antigens).
        (c) Pneumococcal and *Haemophilus influenzae* B poly-saccharides (carbohydrate antigens).
        (d) Abnormal antibody titers to protein or carbohydrate antigens require immunization and repeat titers obtained 2–4 weeks later.
      (3) Quantitation of lymphocyte cell subsets (B, T, T-cell subsets).
    b. Suspected T-cell deficiency
      (1) Quantitation of lymphocyte cell subsets [B, T, T-cell subsets, natural killer (NK) cells].
      (2) Delayed hypersensitivity skin tests (candida, tetanus, purified protein derivative, trichophyton).

      (3) In vitro proliferation studies
        (a) Mitogens: phytohemagglutinen, concanavalin A
        (b) Antigens: tetanus
        (c) Allogeneic cells: mixed lymphocyte reaction
      (4) In neonates with cellular immunodeficiency, adenosine deaminase and purine nucleoside phosphorylase levels are determined from red blood cell samples.
    c. Suspected complement deficiency.
      (1) C3, C4 levels.
      (2) CH50: very low or undetectable value suggests complement deficiency.
    d. In cases of immunodeficiency where a secondary immunodeficiency due to the human immunodeficiency virus (HIV) is considered, routine HIV screening will require both antibody and antigen assays.

V. Treatment

A. T-cell deficiencies
  1. Bone marrow transplantation must be considered in severe T-cell deficiencies.
  2. Patients should *only* receive irradiated whole blood or blood products (3,000 R).
  3. Blood products should be from cytomegalovirus-negative donors.
  4. No immunizations with live virus vaccines should be given.
  5. Patients with DiGeorge syndrome respond to thymus transplantation.

B. B-cell deficiencies
  1. Ig replacement therapy.
    a. Intramuscular immunoglobulin: dose is 100 mg/kg every 2–4 weeks.
    b. Intravenous immunoglobulin
      (1) Dose is 400 mg/kg every 2–4 weeks.
      (2) Dosing and infusion intervals should be adjusted to maintain trough IgG levels at 550 ± 50 mg/dl.
      (3) Initial infusion rates should be reduced in patients with primary immunodeficiency diseases due to an increased likelihood of mild to moderate adverse reactions (e.g., 40–70 ml/hr).
      (4) Some patients with total absence of IgA may have anti-IgA antibodies. Infusion of blood products containing IgA may result in either anaphylactic or anaphylactoid reactions.

Therefore, if anti-IgA antibodies are detected, an intravenous Ig with low titers of IgA should be considered for infusion.

2. Antibiotic therapy
   a. Patients with an acute bacterial infection should initially receive an appropriate antibiotic for 24–48 hr prior to the infusion of intravenous Ig. This will reduce the likelihood of a phlogistic reaction upon Ig infusion.
   b. Patients with existing chronic purulent sinusitis or bronchiectasis when Ig replacement therapy is initiated may require appropriate antibiotic therapy to preclude further progression of disease.

3. Adjuvent therapy
   a. Chronic sinusitis, either poorly responsive to or rapidly recurrent after antibiotic therapy, requires a surgical evaluation.
   b. Diarrhea due to *G. lamblia* infestation is effectively treated with metronidazole, 250 mg three times daily for 5–7 days.

C. Complement deficiencies
1. Complement deficiencies associated with recurrent infections require therapy with appropriate antibiotics.
2. The advantage of replacing the missing complement component by administering fresh frozen plasma is unproven.
   a. Each complement component has a short half-life.
   b. The production of antibodies to the administered congenitally deficient protein limits its long-range effectiveness.
3. Immunization with polyvalent pneumococcal vaccine or tetravalent meningococcal vaccine is suggested in patients with C3–C8 deficiencies.

VI. Prognosis
A. T-cell deficiencies
1. Early detection and bone marrow replacement have enabled patients with a previously lethal disease to survive. Patients should do well if complications of graft-versus-host reactions are not too severe.
2. Patients with thymic aplasia (DiGeorge syndrome) have cellular reconstitution with thymus tissue transplants.
3. Patients with ataxia-telangiectasia (a progressive disease with prominent neurologic deterioration, increasing immunodeficiency) have a high incidence of non-Hodgkin's lymphoma.
4. SCID with ADA is the first genetic deficiency disease treated with gene therapy.

B. B-cell deficiencies
1. Early detection and adequate replacement of Ig deficiencies should allow a normal lifestyle and longevity.
2. Patients with CVID and X-linked lymphoproliferative disease are at increased risk of developing non-Hodgkin's lymphoma. Inadequate antibody replacement and frequent, recurrent infections may be predisposing factors for lymphomas in CVID.
3. Gastric carcinoma occurs rarely in patients with CVID and achlorhydria.
4. Patients with antibody deficiencies are susceptible to life-threatening enteroviral meningitis or encephalitis.

C. Complement deficiencies
1. Although 60–85% of patients with early primary pathway component deficiencies develop autoimmune disease, their prognosis is no different from that of their noncomplement-deficient counterparts.
2. Terminal pathway deficiencies predispose to meningococcal infections. Paradoxically, mortality rates from meningococcal infections in this population are lower than those in normocomplementemic patients.

Bibliography

Ammann AJ, Hong R: *Immunological Disorders in Infants and Children*, ed 3. Philadelphia, WB Saunders, 1989, pp 257–314.

Atkinson JP: Complement deficiency: Predisposing factor to autoimmune syndrome. *Am J Med* 85(Suppl 6A):45–47, 1988.

Figueroa JE, Densen P: Infectious diseases associated with complement deficiencies. *Clin Microbiol Rev* 4:359–395, 1991.

Frank MM: Complement: A brief review. *J Allergy Clin Immunol* 84:411–420, 1989.

Huston DP, Kavanaugh AF, Rohane PW, et al: Immunoglobulin deficiency syndromes and therapy. *J Allergy Clin Immunol* 87:1–17; 1991.

Ochs HD, Wedgwood RJP: *Immunological Disorders in Infants and Children*, ed 3. Philadelphia, WB Saunders, 1989, pp 226–256.

Rosen FS, Cooper MD, Wedgwood RJP: The primary immunodeficiencies. *N Engl J Med* 311:235–242, 300–310, 1984.

CHAPTER **11**

Immunopharmacology

Larry Thomas, Ph.D.

I. Introduction
  A. Immunopharmacology can be defined as the therapeutic control of signal transduction events, or their consequences, in immune and inflammatory cells.
  B. *Signal transduction* refers to the biochemical events that couple cellular activation and effect.
    1. Activation requires metabolically active cells and is initiated via specific cell receptors.
    2. Receptors are integral membrane proteins to which specific molecules, referred to as *ligands*, bind with high affinity. Examples of receptors are surface immunoglobulin on B lymphocytes, the T-cell antigen receptor (TCR/CD3 complex) on T lymphocytes, interleukin-2 (IL-2) receptors on T lymphocytes, C5a and leukotriene B4 receptors on granulocytes, and immunoglobulin E (IgE) receptors on basophils and mast cells.
    3. Mediator secretion, lymphocyte differentiation and proliferation, antibody production, and target cell killing are among the immune and inflammatory events governed by signal transduction.

II. Second Messengers
The second messengers of major importance in signal transduction are Ca^{2+}, inositol trisphosphate (IP3), diacylglycerol, and cyclic adenosine monophosphate (cAMP).
  A. Ca^{2+} is a necessary cofactor for the activation of many enzymes. The concentration of free Ca^{2+} in the cytosol increases as a result of the influx of external Ca^{2+} and the release of Ca^{2+} from intracellular stores.
    1. Ca^{2+} influx occurs through transmembrane proteins that act as on/off switches for ion permeability.
    2. Voltage-dependent Ca^{2+} channels in nerve and muscle tissue are activated by membrane depolarization.
    3. Receptor-operated Ca^{2+} channels in nonexcitable tissues are activated by ligand binding to specific receptors.
  B. Release of Ca^{2+} from intracellular stores is mediated by the formation of IP3.
    1. IP3 is produced by the action of phospholipase C on phosphatidylinositol bisphosphate in the cell membrane.
    2. Phospholipase C is a membrane-associated enzyme that becomes activated following ligand binding to surface receptors.

3. Receptor occupancy and phospholipase C activation are coupled by a guanine nucleotide-binding protein (G protein).

4. Occupancy of some receptors such as the TCR/CD3 complex is linked to activation of phospholipase C through tyrosine kinase-mediated phosphosylation.

C. Diacylglycerol is the second product generated by the phospholipase C-mediated cleavage of phosphatidylinositol bisphosphate.

1. Diacylglycerol, in combination with Ca^{2+}, activates protein kinase C.

2. Protein kinase C catalyzes the phosphorylation of numerous proteins at serine and threonine residues.

D. cAMP, through activation of protein kinase A, influences a multitude of biochemical pathways.

1. cAMP formation from ATP is catalyzed by adenyl cyclase, which is localized to the plasma membrane.

2. Activity of adenyl cyclase is regulated by ligand binding to surface receptors.

3. Occupancy of some receptors (e.g., β-receptors) causes increased adenyl cyclase activity, whereas occupancy of other receptors (e.g., muscarinic receptors) inhibits the activity.

4. Occupancy of either stimulatory or inhibitory receptors and changes in adenyl cyclase activity are coupled by distinct G proteins.

5. cAMP is rapidly inactivated to 5'-AMP by the enzyme cAMP phosphodiesterase, which in turn inactivates protein kinase A.

III. **Drugs that Influence Signal Transduction Events**

A. Ca^{2+} channel blockers

1. Compounds such as nifedipine or verapamil block voltage-dependent channels but have no effect on the receptor-operated channels that predominate on immune and inflammatory cells.

2. Cromolyn sodium inhibits IgE-mediated activation of mast cells by blockade of the receptor-operated channels. Cromolyn does not inhibit basophil activation.

B. Experimental drugs that interefere with IP3 and diacylglycerol formation, as well as protein kinase C activity, have been developed. However, none are currently available for therapeutic use.

C. Drugs that influence cAMP

1. Increases in adenyl cyclase activity, and

thus in cAMP, inhibit immune and inflammatory cell functions.

2. Receptors for the following ligands are linked to activation of adenyl cyclase.

   a. β-Agonists
   b. Histamine (H-2)
   c. Adenosine (A-2)
   d. Prostaglandin E2

3. With the exception of the β-agonists, the cAMP-mediated agents act primarily in a hormonal fashion.

4. Although β-agonists may inhibit cell activation, the primary therapeutic effect may derive from acting on β-2 receptors on bronchial smooth muscle.

5. Theophylline and aminophylline in high concentrations inhibit cAMP phosphodiesterase. However, they act therapeutically by blocking A-2 receptor-mediated bronchoconstrictor activity of adenosine.

IV. **Steroids and Nonsteroidal Drugs: Anti-inflammatory Activities**

The anti-inflammatory activities of steroids and nonsteroidals derive at least partially from their ability to block the generation of prostaglandins, thromboxane, and leukotrienes.

A. Arachidonic acid is liberated from membrane phospholipid by the enzyme phospholipase A2 following cell activation.

1. Arachidonic acid is metabolized via the cyclooxygenase pathway to prostaglandins, prostacyclin, and thromoboxane.

2. Alternatively, arachidonic acid is converted to leukotrienes B4, C4, D4, and E4 via the 5-lipoxygenase pathway.

B. Nonsteroidals inhibit the cyclooxygenase pathway and thus block formation only of the cyclooxygenase products.

C. Steroids indirectly inhibit phospholipase A2 activity and, consequently, block both the liberation and the metabolism of arachidonic acid.

1. Steroids do not directly inhibit phospholipase A2 activity.

2. Steroids bind to receptors in the cytoplasm and act on the nucleus to induce the synthesis of lipocortin, which blocks phospholipase A2 activity.

3. The degree to which lipocortin is responsible for the anti-inflammatory action of corticosteroids remains uncertain.

D. Specific inhibitors of 5-lipoxygenase, as well as specific antagonists of leukotrienes C4 and D4, are currently undergoing clinical trials.

V. Cyclosporins

A. Cyclosporin A is a potent immunosuppressant widely used in post-transplant therapy. Cyclosporin A inhibits Ca^{2+}-dependent T-lymphocyte activation.

B. Cyclosporin A does not act via a specific membrane receptor. Instead, cyclosporin A complexes with an intracellular isomerase, and the complex inhibits a specific phosphatase, calcineurin, required for expression of the interleukin-2 and other genes.

Suggested Reading

Berridge MJ: Inositol trisphosphate and calcium signaling. *Nature* 361:315–325, 1993.

Goldstein RA, Bowen DL, Fauci AS: Adrenal Corticosteroids. In Gallin JI, Goldstein IM, Snyderman R: *Inflammation: Basic Principles and Clinical Correlates, Second Edition.* New York, Raven Press, 1992, pp 1061–1081.

Schreiber SL, Crabtree GR: The mechanism of action of cyclosporin A and FK506. *Immunol. Today* 13:136–142, 1992.

CHAPTER 12

Transplantation

Howard M. Gebel, Ph.D.

I. Definition

A. *Solid organs:* The surgical replacement of a poorly functioning organ(s) in one subject (*recipient*) with a functional organ(s) from another individual (*donor*).

B. *Bone marrow:* The intravenous infusion of bone marrow (*stem cells*) obtained from a donor into a recipient whose own stem cells are no longer functional due either to disease or to the chemotherapy used to treat the disease.

II. Indications (Selected Examples)

A. Solid organs
1. Renal (end-stage renal disease)
   a. Diabetes
   b. Glomerulonephritis
2. Hepatic
   a. Primary biliary cirrhosis
   b. Biliary atresia
3. Cardiac
   a. Idiopathic cardiomyopathy
   b. Coronary artery disease
4. Other
   a. Lung (terminal respiratory failure); heart-lung (primary or secondary pulmonary hypertension); pancreas/islets of Langerhans (insulin-dependent diabetes); small bowel (trauma); inflammatory bowel disease

B. Bone marrow
1. Severe combined immunodeficiency
2. Aplastic anemia; thalassemia
   a. Chronic myelogenous leukemia
   b. Acute lymphoblastic leukemia

III. Types of Transplants

A. Autologous
The tissue (organ) donor and recipient are the same individual. Autologous transplants include:
1. Skin (burn victims)
2. Bone marrow (leukemia, lymphoma, breast cancer)

B. Allogeneic
The tissue (organ) donor and recipient are members of the same species.
1. Living related donor
   a. Parent (human leukocyte antigen, or HLA, haploidentical)
   b. Child (HLA haploidentical)
   c. Sibling
      (1) HLA identical
      (2) HLA haploidentical

(3) HLA nonidentical
2. Living unrelated donor: types of donors
    a. Spouse
    b. Friend
3. Cadaveric donor: types
    (*Note:* victim must be declared brain dead!)
    a. Gunshot wound victim
    b. Traffic accident victim
C. Xenogeneic
The tissue (organ) donor and recipient are members of different species.
1. Nonhuman primates
    The first heart transplants performed in humans were xenogeneic (nonhuman primates into humans). The survival of these transplants was quite short (hours to days), and a moratorium on such transplants was issued. More recently, a baboon heart was transplanted into a neonatal human female with extended (weeks) survival but ultimately was rejected.
2. Pigs
    The size, anatomy, and gestation time of pigs make them attractive candidates as xenogeneic organ donors. There are several problems; for example, humans have circulating anti-pig antibodies, which would likely cause immediate rejection of a pig organ graft by activating the complement cascade. New techniques in molecular biology, such as inserting a gene for decay accelerating factor into endothelial cells, are being used to determine whether these problems can be overcome. Xenogeneic transplants should continue to be considered experimental.
D. Artificial organs
Transplanted organs are mechanical, not human. They create many problems, including size, cost, and maintenance.

IV. **Factors Affecting the Success of Transplants**
A. Solid organs
1. Recipient factors
    a. Age of recipient (those < 50 years old have the best prognosis)
    b. Transplant status (i.e., primary graft or regraft: prognosis much better in primary graft recipient)
    c. Compliance with therapy
    d. Pretransplant transfusion
    e. Pretransplant immune status
        Preformed antibodies directed against the donor are a contraindication to renal allograft transplantation. Although liver transplants can be performed even in the presence of donor reactive antibodies, the long-term graft survival of such organs is poorer than that of patients transplanted with livers to which they have no pretransplant donor-directed antibodies.
2. Donor factors
    a. Warm/cold ischemia time
    b. Age (< 50 years old is best; however, this may be changing)
    c. Medical history
    d. Transfusion history
3. Other factors:
    a. HLA compatibility
        (1) Living related HLA-identical donor-recipient combinations have the best long-term allograft survival (kidneys).
        (2) Cadaveric donor kidneys that are completely HLA identical to the recipient (*six-antigen match*) have significantly enhanced long-term graft survival than donor-recipient combinations matched for fewer than four HLA antigens.
        (3) Center effects
            There are > 200 transplant centers around the world that submit their clinical results to a transplant registry. Centers are classified as excellent, good, or fair based on first-year graft survival. Center effects can be due to patient selection, physician experience, clinical follow-up, and other factors. The center effect raises important questions about how and where cadaveric kidneys should be distributed.
B. Bone marrow
1. Recipient factors
    a. Contributing disease and stage
    b. Age of patient (for many diseases, e.g., chronic myelogenous leukemia, the prognosis of a patient > 30 is much worse than for a patient < 30).
    c. HLA type (if the patient needs a living unrelated donor)
2. Donor factors
    a. HLA type
    b. Age
3. Other factors

a. Posttransplant infections
b. Graft-versus-host disease; see below

V. Complications

A. Immunologic rejection: solid organs
1. Hyperacute rejection
   a. Occurs within minutes to hours post-transplant.
   b. Antibody mediated; can usually be prevented by performing a pretransplant *crossmatch* with donor lymphocytes and recipient serum. If the donor lymphocytes react (i.e., are killed) by the recipient serum, the transplant is contraindicated.
   c. Graft immediately becomes soft, mottled, and blue.
2. Accelerated rejection
   a. Occurs within the first several days post-transplant.
   b. Antibody mediated; probably due to low-level donor reactive antibodies that were not detected in the lymphocyte crossmatch test. These antibodies can be detected by more sensitive crossmatch procedures such as *antiglobulin* and the *flow cytometric crossmatch*.
3. Acute rejection
   a. Occurs weeks to months posttransplant
   b. Cell mediated (T lymphocytes)
   c. Manifested as sudden decline in graft function
   d. Reversible with steroids, anti T-lymphocyte antibodies (*OKT3*)
4. Chronic rejection
   a. Progressive deterioration of graft function
   b. Irreversible
   c. Most likely due to long-standing immunologic assault (cellular and humoral) of the transplanted organ
B. Immunologic rejection: bone marrow
1. Graft-versus-host disease (GvHD)
   The transfused bone marrow often contains immunocompetent tissue which can recognize and react with recipient tissue. Target organs are the skin, liver, and intestine, and symptoms include severe rashes and diarrhea. GvHD can be fatal.
2. Failure to engraft
   Residual radioresistant cells in the recipient can be responsible for failed engraftment of donor marrow. This occurs more frequently in patients who are the recipients of T-cell-depleted marrow, suggesting that residual T cells in the donor marrow may aid engraftment. Unfortunately, residual T cells in the donor marrow also promote GvHD.
C. Infections
   Most common cause of death in transplant recipients. Infections can be bacterial (most common: *Staphylococcus aureus*), viral (cytomegalovirus), fungal (*Candida albicans*) or parasitic (*Pneumocystis carinii*). Transplant patients have an increased risk of infections due to their treatment with immunosuppressive drugs to prevent or reverse graft rejection.
D. Recurrence of original disease
   Common problem for both solid organ transplant recipients (e.g., complications of diabetes resulting in renal dysfunction) and bone marrow transplant recipients (relapse with the original disease such as chronic myelogenous leukemia).

VI. Treatment

A. Solid organs
1. Immunosuppressive drugs (currently in use)
   a. *Cyclosporine* (inhibits cytokine production by T lymphocytes, such as interleukin-2, or IL-2)
   b. *Prednisone* (anti-inflammatory; inhibits interleukin-1 production)
   c. *Antilymphocyte globulin* (an antiserum made in horses directed against human lymphocytes)
   d. *Azathioprine* (antiproliferative agent; purine analog)
   e. *OKT3* (monoclonal antibody directed against T lymphocytes)
2. Immunosuppressive drugs (experimental)
   a. FK506
   b. Deoxyspergualin
   c. Rapamycin
   d. Toxin-conjugated reagents (e.g., diphtheria A chain conjugated to IL-2. *Hypothesis:* The IL-2 component will bind to the IL-2 receptor expressing T cells (which are expressed only upon activation such as stimulation by a foreign tissue). The diphtheria toxin will then kill the cell.
3. Other approaches
   a. Total lymphoid irradiation

b. Dendritic cell depletion (*islets of Langerhans*)

c. Experimental techniques to promote graft acceptance without immunosuppressive drugs (induction of tolerance, e.g., donor-specific transfusions)

VII. Contraindications of Drugs

A. Increased susceptibility to life-threatening infections

B. Increased susceptibility to leukemia/lymphoma

C. Renal and hepatic toxicity (*cyclosporine*)

D. Lack of specificity of currently used drugs

VIII. Ethical Considerations

A. Living related

1. Risk of surgical procedure to donor

2. How consent is determined (particularly if the donor is a child)

3. Considering the conception of a child as a potential bone marrow donor for a child with a life-threatening illness curable only with a bone marrow transplant

B. Cadaveric

1. Distribution of HLA-typed kidneys

a. Should the center effect be considered?

b. Should a 6-year-old patient waiting for a second transplant receive an organ before a 15-year-old patient awaiting his first transplant?

c. Should recipients > 60 be considered as viable transplant candidates?

2. Sharing of kidneys as a national resource

Bibliography

Barry JM: Immunosuppressive drugs in renal transplantation. A review of the regimens. *Drugs* 44:554–556, 1993.

Chandler C, and Passaro E Jr: Transplant rejection. Mechanisms and treatment. *Arch Surg* 128:279–283, 1993.

Gjertson DW, Terasaki PI, Takemoto S, et al: National allocation of cadaveric kidneys by HLA matching. *N Engl J Med* 324:1032–1036, 1991.

Janeway CA (ed): *Current Opinion in Immunology* 4:545–581, 1992.

Terasaki PI (ed): Clinical Transplants 1991. Los Angeles, UCLA Tissue Typing Laboratory, 1991.

CHAPTER **13**

Recent Advances in the Laboratory Diagnosis of Immunologic Disorders: In Vitro Assays for Antigen Specific IgE and Tryptase

Anita Gewurz, M.D.

I. **New Methods**

Several new methods are available for the clinical evaluation of patients with known or suspected IgE-mediated diseases, including in vitro assays for allergen-specific IgE and measurement of serum tryptase in patients with possible anaphylaxis or mastocytosis.

A. Serologic testing for allergen-specific IgE (Allergosorbent test)

1. Principle: This test measures the binding of IgE in patient serum (or heparinized whole blood) to immobilized allergen using labeled anti-IgE antibody and various detection systems. Allergens available include various inhalants, foods, insect venoms, latex and certain drugs.

   a. Radioallergosorbent tests (RAST) use ^{125}I-labeled anti-IgE (Pharmacia Diagnostics, MAST Immuno-Systems or commercial laboratories).

   b. Enzyme-labeled anti-IgE kits are available from Kallestad, Ventrex, DRT Inc., 3M Diagnostics, Quidel, and Abbott Diagnostics or tests may be obtained from commercial laboratories.

2. Advantages

   a. Recommended for small children and persons with dermatographism, extensive skin disease, drug interference, or those in whom skin tests cannot be performed.

   b. Comparable in cost to skin tests, with less patient risk.

3. Disadvantages

   a. Allergosorbent tests that provide high specificity (few false negatives) may be 10–25% less sensitive than bioassays for specific IgE (skin testing or leukocyte histamine release). For this reason, they are *not* recommended for definitive diagnosis of anaphylactic sensitivity to venoms, food, or drugs.

   b. Modified scoring systems that increase sensitivity may generate more false positives.

   c. In vitro IgE techniques are more complex and time-consuming than skin tests.

   d. Inaccuracy may result if relevant allergenic determinants are not immobilized or are blocked by IgG or nonspecific IgE.

   e. Results from different commercial sources are difficult to compare.

4. Interpretation: Results are graded according

to the manufacturer's instructions, depending on the method used.

   a. Proper interpretation, particularly in the selection of allergens for testing and immunotherapy, depends on a careful patient history and physical examination, with accessory tests as indicated.

   b. Multiallergen panels, such as the Phadiatop Aeroallergen Screening RAST (Pharmacia Diagnostics) may be better than total IgE as a screening test for atopy.

B. Measurement of serum tryptase

   1. Principle: Anaphylaxis results from mast cell activation and release of mediators, including histamine and tryptase. Transient elevation of serum tryptase is a more sensitive and specific indicator of anaphylaxis than histamine, since tryptase is not as rapidly degraded or subject to exogenous elevation.

   2. Method: The test is performed by radioimmunoassay using frozen serum (see Bibliography).

   3. Indicators: Tryptase levels may provide useful diagnostic information in patients with unexplained or suspected anaphylaxis, particularly when the presentation is atypical, or when systemic mastocytosis is suspected.

   4. Interpretation

      a. Detection of increased serum tryptase in a serum obtained within 30 min to 4 hr of the acute event correlates closely with anaphylaxis, both IgE- and non-IgE-mediated. Levels are not increased in shock due to other causes.

      b. Baseline tryptase levels > 5 ng/ml are consistent with systemic mastocytosis.

Bibliography

Schwartz LB: Tryptase levels as an indicator of mast cell activation in systemic anaphylaxis and mastocytosis. *N Engl J Med* 316:1622–1626, 1987.

Shearer W: Specific diagnostic modalities: IgE, skin tests, and RAST. *J Allergy Clin Immunol* 84:1112–1118, 1989.

CHAPTER 14

Treatment of Allergic Diseases

Howard Zeitz, M.D.

I. Methods

There are three general ways to treat allergic diseases: environmental control, medication, and immunotherapy.

A. Environmental Control

1. The most effective therapy is to separate the patient from the allergen or the allergen from the patient.

2. For patients with food allergies, optimal treatment requires removal of the offending food from the diet.

3. For patients with contactant allergies (e.g., jewelry, cosmetics), optimal treatment requires elimination of the offending allergen.

4. For patients with occupational allergies, optimal treatment may require protective clothing and/or a respirator, air filtration, a new work assignment, or, if absolutely essential, a switch to a new job.

5. Optimal treatment for patients with disease caused by outdoor (seasonal) inhalant allergens (e.g., pollens, mold spores) includes air conditioning, especially for the sleeping room, to minimize exposure to these allergens.

6. Environmental control for patients who have symptoms caused by indoor (perennial) inhalant allergens (e.g., animals, feathers, mold spores, dust mites) may require several measures:

   a. Removal of pets from the household or, at the very least, from the sleeping room.

   b. Removal of pillows and comforters containing feathers.

   c. Control of dust mites via air filtration, protective bedding covers, frequent vacuuming, carpet removal, air filtration, and/or application of agents that inhibit mite growth in carpets and furniture.

   d. Application of antifungal agents, correction of construction defects that lead to mold growth, and/or a dehumidifier to reduce the moisture level needed by molds for growth.

B. Medication

1. Medications can be used by patients either to treat symptoms already present or to prevent the development of future symptoms.

2. *Antihistamines* are the most versatile of the medications. Treatment with an antihista-

mine can be helpful for most patients with itching, as well for many patients with ocular and nasal symptoms. Some patients with bronchial asthma also may benefit from treatment with an antihistamine.

a. *Traditional H1 blockers* all share the side effect of sedation in some treated patients; common agents include *brompheniramine, chlorpheniramine, cyproheptadine,* and *diphenhdramine.*

b. *Nonsedating H1 blockers*: newer antihistamines that induce sedation no more often than placebo; currently available agents include *astemizole, loratadine,* and *terfenadine.*

c. *Others:* used on rare occasions; examples include antidepressants with both H1 blocking activity and antidepressant activity, and H2 blockers (usually in combination with an H1 blocker) for treatment of chronic urticaria.

3. *Decongestants* can be used topically to relieve ocular erythema and congestion, or they can be used orally to relieve nasal congestion.

a. *Topical ocular agents:* common examples include *naphazoline* and *tetrahydrozoline.*

b. *Oral agents:* common examples include *pseudoephedrine* and *phenylpropanolamine.* These are available in rapid-onset and timed-release dosage forms.

4. *Bronchodilators* are used in the treatment of patients with bronchial asthma. They can be used preventively or to treat symptoms which are already present.

a. Agents which bind to the β-adrenergic receptor (commonly called β-*agonists*) are available in a variety of dosage forms, including liquids, tablets, solutions for injections, solutions for nebulization, and metered-dose inhalers. Frequently used compounds include *albuterol, metaproterenol, pirbuterol,* and *terbutaline.*

b. *Theophylline* also is available in a variety of dosage forms, including liquids, tablets, capsules, and solutions for intravenous administration. Because theophylline has a narrow therapeutic index (potential benefit versus potential toxicity), it is important to monitor continuous theophylline treatment with intermittent serum theophylline levels.

c. *Ipratropium bromide* is another bronchodilating agent. This synthetic agent with anticholinergic activity is available in only one dosage formulation: a metered-dose inhaler.

5. *Cromolyn sodium* is an anti-inflammatory medication that prevents allergic reactions by blocking the release of mediators from mast cells. This compound thereby blocks both the initial (immediate) phase and the subsequent late phase reaction, which together are responsible for the pathophysiology of the most common allergic diseases.

a. The oral dosage form works only within the gastrointestinal tract for patients with intestinal mastocytosis. Because there is no significant absorption, this dosage form is not useful for the treatment of any condition other than mastocytosis.

b. Patients with allergic rhinitis can be treated with a nasal aerosol at intervals throughout the day.

c. There are several dosage forms for the treatment of bronchial asthma: a metered-dose inhaler, an inhalational powder formulation, and a liquid preparation for nebulizer administration.

6. Nedocromil sodium is an anti-inflammatory medication currently available in a metered-dose formulation for the treatment of mild to moderate bronchial asthma. This compound can prevent reactions in a manner similar to if not identical with that of cromolyn sodium. In addition, this agent also has direct anti-inflammatory activity similar to that of corticosteroids.

7. *Topical corticosteroids* are used in the treatment of allergic disease when nonsteroidal medications do not provide sufficient relief.

a. A variety of topical steroid preparations (solutions, creams, and ointments) of varying potencies are available to treat allergic dermatoses.

b. Similarly, there are numerous ocular steroid solutions that can be used to treat allergic conjunctivitis.

c. Allergic rhinitis can be treated with several different nasal steroid aerosols, including *beclomethasone, flunisolide, triamcinolone,* and *dexamethasone,* administered via a metered-dose inhaler.

d. Bronchial allergies also can be treated with several different steroid aerosols, including *beclomethasone, flunisolide,* and *triamcinolone*, administered via a metered-dose inhaler.

8. *Systemic corticosteroids* are used primarily when topical steroids and nonsteroidal medications do not provide adequate relief of allergy symptoms.

   a. A variety of systemic steroid preparations (liquid, tablet, intramuscular, and intravenous) are available.

   b. When it is necessary to use these products, they can be used for only a few days (a *steroid burst*) if the symptoms are controlled easily.

   c. If continuing treatment is needed, side effects can be best avoided or minimized by administration in the morning, either on alternate days or (if necessary) daily.

   d. The preparation used most commonly is *prednisone*, which is metabolized in the liver to prednisolone (the active metabolite). *Prednisolone* is also available as a separate preparation, thereby bypassing the need for metabolic conversion of prednisone in the liver.

   e. A patient whose symptoms do not respond adequately to prednisone or prednisolone can be treated with a more potent steroid. These include (in order of increasing potency) *methylprednisolone* and a variety of fluorinated steroids such as *triamcinolone, dexamethasone,* and *betamethasone*.

C. Immunotherapy

   1. Immunotherapy should be used in conjunction with environmental control and medications taken at home.

   2. Formerly called *hyposensitization* or *desensitization*, immunotherapy should be given only in a medical care setting (e.g., outpatient office, health service, or clinic) with sufficient nurse and physician personnel and supplies to treat any adverse reactions.

   3. The goal of immunotherapy is to reduce the patient's sensitivity to one or more allergens by administering subcutaneous injections containing progressively stronger doses of allergen at regular intervals (usually once each week or every other week).

   4. Immunotherapy protocols have been developed for the treatment of allergic reactions caused by various inhalant allergens, including numerous pollens, mold spores, and dust mites. Treatment with extracts of other allergens (e.g., foods, animal proteins) has not yet been fully developed.

II. Summary

A. While some patients will respond to treatment with a single modality (environmental control *or* medication *or* immunotherapy), most patients will respond best to treatment which combines two or three modalities (environmental control *and/or* medication *and/or* immunotherapy).

B. The best approach to the treatment of allergic disease is to identify the *treatment program* which is best for the *individual* patient.

Bibliography

Callaghan B, Teo NC, Clancy L: Effects of the addition of nedocromil sodium to maintenance bronchodilator therapy in the management of chronic asthma. *Chest* 101:787–792, 1992.

Iliopoulos O, Proud D, Adkinson NF Jr, et al: Effects of immunotherapy on the early, late, and rechallenge nasal reaction to provocation with allergen: Changes in inflammatory mediators and cells. *J Allergy Clin Immunol* 87:855–866, 1991.

Platts-Mills TAE, Chapman MD: Dust mites: Immunology, allergic disease, and environmental control. *J Allergy Clin Immunol* 80:755–775, 1987. (Erratum, *J Allergy Clin Immunol* 82:841, 1988.)

Simons FER: H1-receptor antagonists: Clinical pharmacology and therapeutics. *J Allergy Clin Immunol* 84:845–861, 1989.

Weiner N: Norepinephrine, epinephrine and the sympathomimetic amines. In Gilman AG, Goodman LS, Rall TW, et al (eds): *Goodman and Gilman's The Pharmacological Basis of Therapeutics*. ed 7. New York, Macmillan, 1985, pp 145–180.

Welsh PW, Stricker WE, Chu CP, et al: Efficacy of beclomethasone nasal solution, flunisolide, and cromolyn in relieving symptoms of ragweed allergy. *Mayo Clin Proc* 62:125–134, 1987.

SECTION 3

Cardiology

CHAPTER 15

Approach to the Patient with Cardiovascular Disease

Harold Kennedy, M.D.

I. **Introduction**

Approaching the patient with cardiovascular disease is both simple and complex. While it is simple in that knowledge of the natural history of a disorder, its pathophysiology, and a basic diagnostic approach (history, physical examination, and diagnostic studies) are all that is required, it is complex in that there is a dazzling array of noninvasive and invasive diagnostic technologies (Table 15-1) which may be employed. This latter aspect demands a sound fund of knowledge of cardiovascular disease to be able to determine the sensitivity and specificity of a particular procedure in a specific population of patients to achieve a cost-effective approach. This is particularly true today, when cardiovascular diagnostic and therapeutic costs dominate the health care costs of most nations.

Figure 15-1 illustrates the time-tested approach to cardiovascular disease, but it has been modified to show that echocardiography/Doppler has replaced the chest x-ray as the visual examination of choice of the heart, and exercise/myocardial function studies (thallium, sestamibi, positron emission tomography) attest to the adequacy of cardiac metabolism, viability, and pathophysiologic function.

Table 15-2 presents the cardinal symptoms of cardiovascular disease in their relative order of frequency of presentation, while Table 15-3 presents the cardinal physical signs of cardiovascular disease. While a review of all the problems presenting to the cardiologist is beyond the scope of this chapter, an illustrative example relative to the complaint of chest pain is presented.

II. **Problem—Chest Pain**

Chest pain is a common complaint and must be characterized as to location, severity, quality, course of onset and offset, duration, precipitating and alleviating factors, and whether it is typical or atypical, to the examiner's knowledge. Although chest pains will overlap, the major considerations are angina pectoris, pleuritic pain, pericardial pain, chest wall pain, transmitted back pain, and gastrointestinal complaints.

III. **Differential Diagnosis of the Problem**

Only through careful firsthand history-taking experience will the physician be able to recognize typical and atypical historical patterns of chest pain. Nevertheless, the following salient characteristics are offered as a guide.

A. Angina pectoris—Indicative of myocardial ischemia usually secondary to atherosclerotic coronary artery disease. Characterized by a

Table 15-1.   Noninvasive and Invasive Diagnostic Tests

Noninvasive Diagnostic Tests

Electrocardiographic
  Standard electrocardiogram
  Vectorcardiogram
  Signal-averaged electrocardiogram
  Ambulatory (Holter) electrocardiogram
  Transtelephonic (intermittent) monitoring
Echocardiographic
  M-mode
  Two-dimensional (transthoracic)
  Transesophageal
  Doppler
Exercise Studies
  Standard exercise (treadmill, bicycle)
  Radionuclide studies
    Thallium
    Technetium gated blood pool
    Sestamibi
  Positron emission tomography
    Rubidium
    18-Deoxyglucose
Vascular Studies
  Doppler duplex scans
  Impedance plethysmography
  Tilt table testing

Invasive Diagnostic Tests

Catheterization
  Right heart hemodynamics
  Left heart hemodynamics
  Ultrasound intravascular scan
  Angioscopy
  Biopsy
Angiography (via catheterization)
  Ventricular angiograms
  Coronary angiograms
  Peripheral vascular angiograms
  Aortic arch angiograms
Electrophysiologic studies
  Programmed ventricular stimulation
  His bundle recording
  Atrial and ventricular pacing studies
  Tachycardia mapping studies

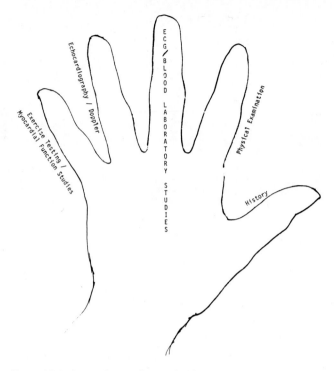

Figure 15-1 Approach to cardiovascular disease

activities; relieved by rest, withdrawal of precipitating factors, or nitroglycerin, usually within a matter of minutes (< 3 to 5 min).

B. Pericarditis—Pericardial pain is more likely to be left-sided or substernal, sharp in character, relieved by sitting and related to breathing.

C. Pleuritis—Pleuritic pain also tends to be localized and sharp, related to respiration and position, and aggravated by cough.

D. Costal-chondritis—Chest wall pain related to costal chondral inflammation of the left precordial area is long-lasting, and is associated with tenderness to pressure applied at a trigger area.

Table 15-2.   Cardinal Symptoms of Cardiovascular Disease

Chest pain
Dyspnea, orthopnea, paroxysmal nocturnal
  dyspnea, wheezing
Palpitations, dizziness, syncope
Edema, right upper abdominal fullness or
  tenderness (hepatomegaly)
Cough, hemoptysis
Fatigue, weakness
Muscular pain in extremities with exertion
  (intermittent claudication)
Cyanosis

dull, heavy, or burning discomfort of any severity; located substernally or precordially, with radiation to neck, shoulders, medial upper extremities, and infrequently to the back. Variable duration and severity; precipitated by exertion, mental stress, cold, and sexual activity; more common in morning hours with common in morning hours with normal

Table 15-3. Cardinal Physical Signs of Cardiovascular Disease

	Frequent	Infrequent
General habitus	Overweight Respiratory distress (coronary artery pulmonary disease) Asthenic, with skeletal abnormalities	Marfan's syndrome Turner's syndrome Cyanosis and clubbing
Head, eyes, ears, nose, throat	Fundiscopic (atrioventricular nicking) Sublingual vein Distension (long-standing right heart failure)	Roth spots Microaneurysms
Neck	Decreased carotid pulse (volume/upstroke) Carotid bruit Distended cervical veins (A and V waves at 45° elevation)	Deviated trachea Thyroid enlargement or nodule
Thorax	Abnormal Diameter AP ($\downarrow$ or $\uparrow$) Dullness, egophony Rales or rhonchi Pectus excavatum Pectus carinum	Thoracic asymmetry
Heart	Abnormal Point of Maximal Impulse (size, displaced) Parasternal lift (visible, palpable) Cardiomegaly (percussion) Precordial gallop (S_4, S_3) Murmurs (systolic, diastolic, continuous) Rubs or clicks	Epigastric area gallop Changes with posture or respiration
Abdomen	Right upper quadrant tenderness (peritoneal stretch of hepatic edema) Hepatomegaly Systolic bruit of aorta, iliacs, and femoral artery Ascites (shifting dullness)	Systolic bruit (renal artery) Palpable aortic aneurysmal dilatation
Genital		Inguinal hernia (secondary to chronic cough), scrotal edema
Extremities	Decreased systolic pulses (femoral, popliteal, posterior tibial, dorsal pedis) Systolic bruits Edema Skin coolness of distal extremities	Clubbing of fingers and toes
Skin	Dystrophic nail and skin changes of inferior extremities (diabetes) Dermatophytosis	Xanthelasma, xanthoma, or cyanosis
Neurologic	Evidence of Cardiovascular accident: Distal extremity loss of vibration, pain, and sensory function	

E. Gastrointestinal Disorders—Esophageal or upper gastrointestinal disorders can often result in referred substernal or epigastric discomfort or pain. Usually associated with symptoms of dyspepsia, often long-lasting, may be relieved by eructation or antacids, and usually unrelated to exercise.

IV. **Focus of the History and Physical Examination**
   A. Historical data: cardiac risk factors, chest pain characteristics, and other cardiovascular symptoms.
      1. History should identify the individual at risk of cardiac disease.
         a. Family history of cardiac disease.
         b. History of rheumatic fever or serious infectious disease.
         c. History of diabetes mellitus, hyperlipidemia, cigarette smoking, or alcohol abuse.
         d. Evidence of obesity or sedentary lifestyle.
      2. Describe chest pain characteristics.
         a. Precipitating factors—exertion, exercise, emotion, cold, coitus, or unpredictable pattern.
         b. Relieving factors—rest, cessation of activities, positional, use of nitroglycerin, and time of relief.
         c. Type of pain—dull, aching, burning, or heavy.
         d. Severity—mild, moderate, or severe. Describe if only a sensation of discomfort and not pain per se.
         e. Location—substernal, left precordial area, medial aspect of upper extremity (usually the left). Describe radiation to shoulder, side of neck, mandible, or elbows.
         f. Time pattern—angina is related directly to precipitating factors and occurs in close temporal relation. It is relieved, usually in minutes, by stopping the inciting factors and may be more commonly experienced in the morning hours because of circadian factors.
      3. Other cardiovascular symptoms may indicate the presence of cardiac disease or may be related to the chest pain.
         a. Palpitations—may indicate the presence of an arrhythmia which (depending on the rate and duration) may affect the chest pain.
         b. Dyspnea, orthopnea, paroxysmal nocturnal dyspnea—indicate elevated pulmonary capillary pressure often secondary to left ventricular failure or mitral valvular disease.
         c. Edema, fatigue, and weakness—reflect right ventricular failure, heart failure compensatory mechanisms, and decreased oxygen delivery to peripheral musculature.
         d. Decreased exercise tolerance—indicates an overall change in the individual's functioning cardiovascular system.
         e. Dizziness, syncope—may indicate rapid tachyarrhythmia or cardiac conduction system disease.
         f. Intermittent claudication—indicates the presence of severe peripheral atherosclerotic disease.
   B. Physical findings: general habitus; cardiac examination; peripheral vessels; thorax, abdominal exam, and peripheral extremities.
      1. General habitus can provide clues to underlying cardiac disease.
         a. Obesity indicates an inactive lifestyle and an increased saturated fat diet associated with atherosclerotic disease.
         b. Skeletal abnormalities of the thorax and spine suggest chronic obstructive pulmonary disease associated with cigarette smoking or connective tissue disorders and mitral valve prolapse.
      2. Cardiac examination focuses on inspection, palpation, percussion, and auscultation.
         a. Inspection usually reveals a normal precordium without abnormal lifts or a prominent maximal apical impulse.
         b. Palpation may disclose a sustained apical impulse over an enlarged area (more than one finger breadth) indicating left ventricular hypertrophy from an associated condition (e.g., hypertension).
         c. Percussion usually defines a normal left cardiac border unless it is end-stage coronary artery disease with cardiomegaly.
         d. Auscultation most commonly discloses an S_4 gallop or the apical systolic ejection murmur of functional mitral regurgitation or papillary muscle dysfunction. Moderate left ventricular impairment ($< 40\%$) or more end-stage disease is accompanied by an S_3 gallop.

3. Peripheral vessels may indicate evidence of the underlying atherosclerotic process.

   a. Carotid bruits may be asymptomatic or associated with complaints of dizziness or transient ischemic attack.

   b. Abdominal, iliac, and femoral bruits reflect atherogenesis of aorta, iliac, and femoral vessels.

   c. Decreased pulses of inferior or upper extremities reflect the obstructive nature of atherosclerotic occlusive disease.

4. Thorax and abdominal examinations can reflect secondary effects of myocardial failure from atherosclerotic coronary artery disease.

   a. Thorax examination may reveal rhonchi, rales, or wheezing secondary to pulmonary capillary wedge pressure elevation.

   b. Abdominal examination may disclose right upper quadrant tenderness, hepatomegaly, or ascites associated with congestive heart failure arising from coronary artery disease.

5. Peripheral extremities may demonstrate abnormalities associated with sequelae of coronary artery disease.

   a. Peripheral edema will result from combined left and right heart failure and compensatory heart failure neural (humoral mechanisms).

   b. Acrocyanosis or cyanosis may be associated with markedly impaired oxygen delivery to peripheral tissues.

   c. Dystrophic nail and skin changes may reflect atherosclerosis-induced loss of hair, impaired subcutaneous dermal changes, and susceptibility to dermatophytic infections.

V. Diagnostic Approach

The diagnostic approach should proceed from noninvasive to invasive studies when such confirmation or delineation is required.

A. Noninvasive diagnostic studies should be evaluated in a progressive manner, as indicated in Figure 15-1, being mindful of their relative cost effectiveness in an individual patient (age, sex, history, etc.).

1. A standard electrocardiogram (ECG) may show evidence of myocardial ischemia or its sequelae.

   a. Transient symmetrical T-wave inversions or ST-segment displacement during periods of chest pain are diagnostic of angina pectoris.

   b. Evidence of abnormal Q or QS waves indicates old myocardial infarction.

   c. Evidence of persistent ST or T-wave (with an ischemic pattern) abnormalities reflects subendocardial or non-Q-wave infarction or abnormal wall motion/aneurysm.

   d. High-peaked, symmetrical T waves may reflect early acute ischemia in specific myocardial diagnostic (anterior versus inferior) areas.

2. Chest x-ray findings depend on the chronicity and severity of underlying atherosclerotic cardiac disease.

   a. Early finding: if chest pain is the initial myocardial ischemic event, without previous myocardial damage, the chest x-ray may be normal without abnormality.

   b. Intermediate findings: if the patient has sustained previous myocardial damage (symptomatic or asymptomatic), the chest x-ray may show cardiomegaly and pulmonary venous congestion.

   c. Late findings: end-stage coronary artery disease is often associated with cardiomegaly, pulmonary venous congestion, and pleural or pericardial effusions.

3. Echocardiography is helpful in identifying the sequelae of previous coronary artery disease.

   a. Cardiac chamber enlargement can result from myocardial damage or papillary muscle dysfunction.

   b. Abnormal wall motion is usually asymmetric and nonglobal. It can result if transient ischemia is induced with exercise, dipyridamole, or adenosine.

   c. Rarely, imaging may disclose left main coronary artery disease.

4. Exercise testing is usually the most effective diagnostic test to define coronary artery disease–related chest pain.

   a. Standardized treadmill exercise protocols will induce chest pain, hemodynamic changes, and ECG ST-T changes of myocardial ischemia.

   b. Exercise testing can define functional exercise capacity to determine if the patient has cardiovascular impairment.

   c. Radionuclide exercise studies (thallium, technicium, sestamibi) can be used to examine the extent of myocardial ischemia and to define ischemia in patients suspected of having false-positive exercise ECG changes or ECG bundle branch block.

B. Invasive diagnostic studies may be necessary to render a definitive diagnosis for chest pain despite the pathophysiologic diagnostic capability of noninvasive studies. Nevertheless, rarely (e.g., syndrome X, variant angina pectoris), provocative testing in the catheterization laboratory may be necessary.

  1. Cardiac catheterization may reveal abnormal hemodynamic pressures, reflecting an underlying myocardial abnormality.

  2. Coronary and left ventricular angiography will provide visual evidence of the presence of atherosclerotic coronary artery disease or myocardial dysfunction. It may be used with ergonovine testing, pacing, or coronary flow reserve measurements.

Bibliography

Hurst JW: The physician's approach to the patient goals and cardiac appraisal. In Hurst JW, Schland RC (eds): *The Heart*, ed 7. New York, McGraw-Hill, 1990, 115.

Smith TW: Approach to the patient with cardiovascular disease. In Wynaarden JB, Smith LH (eds): *Cecil Textbook of Medicine*, ed 18. Philadelphia, WB Saunders, 1988, 175.

CHAPTER 16

Diagnostic Methods

Philip R. Liebson, M.D.
James E. Macioch, D.O.

I. Introduction

A. General diagnostic considerations

Beyond the history and physical examination, which can contribute much to the classification of cardiac disease and activity status, general diagnostic testing is frequently confirmatory rather than exploratory (Table 16-1).

1. Electrophysiologic activity

The electrocardiogram (ECG) is a routine test in hospital admission and in ambulatory patients above age 30. It may provide:

a. Prognostic information revealed by evidence of left ventricular hypertrophy or even nonspecific ST-T abnormalities, either of which increases the risk of cardiovascular mortality.

b. Evidence of conduction defects possibly not elucidated by physical examination (increased P-R interval, bundle branch blocks, hemiblocks).

c. Evidence of a prolonged Q-T interval, which may also be a risk factor in sudden cardiac death.

d. Abnormal Q waves (> 0.04 sec in leads I, II, III, AVL, AVF), presence of Q in V_1–V_4 which may suggest prior myocardial infarction or septal hypertrophy (hypertrophic cardiomyopathy).

2. General mechanical function/structure

There is no routine general diagnostic test for mechanical function, that is, a study which would be performed on entry into the hospital or in ambulatory patients similar to an ECG.

a. *The chest x-ray* is rarely a screening procedure for cardiac disease but is frequently ordered for general evaluation purposes. Nevertheless, cardiac information on the chest x-ray (posteroanterior, lateral) may include:

(1) Cardiac silhouette. Increased silhouette suggests chamber enlargement, usually left ventricular (LV) and/or right ventricular (RV), associated with heart failure, chronic valvular regurgitation, or pericardial infusion.

(2) Distribution of calcium occasionally seen in aortic knob in elderly patients with aortic sclerosis; of value if seen in area of aortic valve or mitral valve, possibly suggesting stenosis.

(3) Evidence of superior redistribution of pulmonary venous markings, suggesting increased left-sided filling pressure.

(4) Evidence of thoracic aortic aneurysm is occasionally discovered on x-ray in the elderly.

b. *Cardiac fluoroscopy* is now rarely utilized as a separate technique, but it still has some value in evaluation for the presence of pericardial calcification, associated with constrictive pericarditis and coronary artery calcification, which may indicate significant coronary artery disease.

c. Phonocardiography and external pulse recording may amplify and confirm physical findings and are valuable in differentiating the locations of murmurs and heart sounds.

3. Ischemic heart disease

Generally diagnosed initially by the history, but an *ECG* may be helpful. Aside from abnormalities referred to previously, marked S-T depressions in a few leads or diffuse S-T depressons in many leads may suggest not only ischemic heart disease but also a poor prognosis. No other general diagnostic tests are routinely indicated in patients without a history of coronary heart disease.

4. Risk of cardiovascular disease

Lipid profile (total cholesterol, LDL cholesterol, HDL-cholesterol, triglycerides) may be helpful in assessing the risk of coronary heart disease. Minimal testing in adults with no other risk factors should consist of a total cholesterol count every 5 years, beginning at age 20.

B. Patient with evidence of heart disease based on the history or physical examination.

1. Basic clinical testing

If there is evidence of possible heart disease, based on the history or physical examination, further testing beyond the studies discussed above (ECG, lipid profile, possible chest x-ray) should be pursued as follows:

a. Echocardiogram

Provides a comprehensive evaluation of the structure of the heart chambers, wall thickness, valves, and proximate vessels. Useful for diagnosis of left ventricular hypertrophy, a strong risk factor for cardiovascular mortality and

morbidity. A Doppler study provides information on valvular incompetence, shunts, and stenotic valvular gradients. Congenital malformations can be rapidly assessed, pericardial effusion diagnosed, and systolic performance determined. This test is mandatory if the chest x-ray shows an abnormal cardiac silhouette.

b. Ambulatory 24-hr ECG (Holter) monitoring

Useful for investigation of patients with "palpitations" or syncope. With appropriate calibration, it may also be used to determine S-T abnormalities consistent with myocardial ischemia.

c. Ambulatory 24-hr blood pressure monitoring

This relatively new technique is useful for evaluating circadian variation in blood pressure and for guiding antihypertensive therapy, especially in patients with orthostasis. Blood pressures are recorded every 15 min. This is primarily an outpatient technique, but it may be useful in selected hospitalized patients as well.

d. Exercise testing

This includes:

(1) Treadmill or bicycle for exercise stress.

(2) Injection of dobutamine, dipyridamole, or adenosine for pharmacologic stress testing

(3) Diagnosis evaluation by ECG, nuclear ^{201}Th or sestamibi (99M) for filling defects, ^{99m}Tc gated blood pool scans, or echocardiography for left ventricular function, the latter including segmental wall motion abnormalities.

(4) Studies are performed for investigation of coronary heart disease (ischemia), for exercise tolerance (for exercise prescription), and for prognostic significance (degree and distribution of ischemic abnormalities).

(5) Should be performed on all men over 35 and on all women over 40 who intend to embark on a moderate or stressful exercise program.

2. Second-level clinical testing

Beyond the echocardiogram, ambulatory

ECG, and blood pressure monitoring and exercise testing, more specialized testing may be necessary to elicit diagnostic and prognostic information. Key questions in determining the appropriateness of a test include:

- Does it have high predictive value for an accurate diagnosis?
- Is it cost effective?
- Can it provide prognostic information?

a. Cardiac catheterization and angiography

This technique provides information on:

(1) Direct pressures in the aorta, pulmonary artery, and cardiac chambers.

(2) Assessment of intercardiac or intervascular shunts.

(3) Left and right sided cardiac output.

(4) Silhouette visualization of cardiac chambers or arteries, using radiographic contrast to determine chamber size and to provide, evidence of valvular regurgitation or coronary artery constriction.

(5) Endomyocardial biopsy to evaluate histopathology.

Currently, cardiac catheterization remains a definitive approach for diagnosis of coronary artery disease, degree of shunting, and systolic performance of the LV.

b. Invasive electrophysiologic studies

Controlled electrical stimulation of the heart and electrophysiologic mapping in the catheterization laboratory, special care unit, or operating room has been a definitive comprehensive approach to assessment of the prognostic significance and efficacy of therapy for sick sinus syndrome, atrioventricular block, or serious ventricular arrhythmias. In some centers it is a mandatory procedure for evaluating any contemplated antiarrhythmic therapy in patients after cardiac arrest or sustained ventricular tachycardia not related to an acute myocardial infarction.

c. Computer Tomography (CT)

This x-ray technique provides outstanding tomographic imaging of the heart and blood vessels. Static CT imaging may allow accurate measurement and location of a cardiac mass, thrombus, pericardial effusion or pericardial thickening, aortic dissection, and tissue differences which may demonstrate amyloidosis, for example. Ultrafast CT with radiographic contrast injection allows evaluation of complex cardiac congenital abnormalities. The minimally invasive nature of this approach may make it suitable for use in infants and children. Coronary artery graft patency can be reasonably assessed without the need for cardiac catheterization.

d. Gated blood pool scans (MUGA)

Use of gamma emitting radio isotope (^{99m}Tc) allows precise determination of the left ventricular ejection fraction and is especially useful in evaluating the effect of exercise on the ejection fraction. This may be of prognostic significance for decisions on when to replace valves in chronic aortic or mitral regurgitation or for the need for intervention in coronary artery disease.

e. Magnetic resonance imaging (MRI)

This technique provides information on cardiovascular structure which may make it valuable for the diagnosis of aortic dissection, cardiac masses or ventricular aneurysms, and cardiac tissue characterization. It requires an extensive period in a metal-free environment, which prohibits imaging of patients who require support systems or whose bodies contain metal objects.

f. Positron emission tomography (PET)

Available in very few centers, this technique uses radioisotopes to evaluate regional myocardial metabolism, reflecting perfusion abnormalities. The technique may become an adjunct for assessing the presence of coronary artery disease in high-risk, asymptomatic patients, and for assessing the functional significance of stenosis in symptomatic patients and of myocardial viability after myocardial infarction. It may be a powerful tool to evaluate regional subendocardial ischemia when significant epicardial coronary artery disease has *not* been demonstrated by coronary angiography.

II. Phonocardiography and Noninvasive External Pulse Recordings

A. Phonocardiography
  1. Recording of the heart sounds and murmurs from the surface of the chest, used for:
     a. Timing of heart sounds.
     b. Demonstration of the effects of pharmacologic and physiologic maneuvers on the intensity and duration of murmurs and clicks.
  2. Simultaneous recordings of the ECG with a carotid pulse tracing, jugular venous pulse, or apex cardiogram.
  3. Indications include:
     a. Differentiation of ejection clicks from S_1, and S_4 gallops and demonstration of changes in the timing of clicks.
     b. Differentiation of aortic stenosis, mitral regurgitation murmurs, and evaluation of Austin Flint mitral stenosis murmurs.
     c. Differentiation of pulmonic from aortic flow murmurs.
     d. Timing of S_3 gallops, opening snaps.
     e. Timing of S_1, A_2, and P_2 for evaluation of external pulse recordings.
     f. Evaluation for continuous murmurs, that is, murmurs that go through the second sound.
  4. Significant findings
     a. Valsalva maneuver
        Valvular aortic stenosis versus hypertrophic subaortic stenosis. Murmur increases in subaortic stenosis and decreases in aortic stenosis during this maneuver.
     b. Aortic stenosis versus mitral regurgitation. Peripheral arterial dilatation increases the murmur of aortic stenosis and decreases the murmur of mitral regurgitation.
     c. Amyl nitrite increases pulmonic flow murmurs and decreases aortic flow murmurs. Peripheral arterial constriction increases left ventricular end-diastolic volume and early systolic murmur or click in mitral valve prolapse to a later point in systole.
B. Carotid pulse tracing
  1. Funnel attached to pulse transducer pressed over right internal carotid artery.
  2. For left ventricular ejection time indices.
  3. Demonstrates timing of second component of bifid pulse:
     a. Second pulse *before* incisura suggests subaortic stenosis.

     b. Second pulse *after* incisura suggests combined aortic regurgitation and valvular stenosis (bisferiens pulse).
  4. Upstroke prolonged in valvular aortic stenosis.
C. Jugular venous tracing
  1. Funnel attached to pulse transducer pressed into fossa above right clavicle.
  2. Exaggeration of A-wave signifies:
     a. Tricuspid stenosis.
     b. Right ventricular diastolic compliance abnormality.
     c. Periodic high-amplitude "cannon" A-wave in atrioventricular (AV) dissociation.
  3. Prominent V-wave in tricuspid regurgitation.
  4. Exaggerated y-descent in constrictive pericarditis (*square root sign*).
D. Apexcardiogram
  1. Patient in left lateral decubitus position; funnel attached to pulse transducer, placed over position of apex beat.
  2. a. O point = times with opening snap in mitral stenosis.
     b. F point of diastolic filling = times with left-sided S_3 gallop.
     c. Large A-wave is associated with left ventricular diastolic dysfunction.
     d. Bifid E-wave during ejection is associated with hypertrophic cardiomyopathy.
E. Systolic time intervals
  1. Used to evaluate LV performance.
     a. Preejection phase (PEP)/left ventricular ejection time (LVET) > 0.35 usually suggests LV dysfunction if there is no intraventricular conduction abnormality from beginning of QRS complex.
  2. PEP/LVET is accomplished by simultaneously recording ECG, carotid pulse (for LVET), and phonocardiogram (for A2).
  3. LVET = beginning of upstroke of carotid pulse to incisura—usually 240–360 msec.
     a. If > 360 msec, seen in aortic stenosis and very slow heart rates.
     b. If < 200, seen in severe LV dysfunction and very rapid heart rates.
  4. PEP = Q–A_2 interval (from simultaneous ECG and phonocardiogram)—LVET. This is increased in LV dysfunction.

III. **Echocardiography**
A. Technical description
  1. Echocardiography involves the transmission of ultrasound into the heart and large

proximal vessels and reception of reflected ultrasound signals by a transducer.

2. The transducer may be located over the chest or upper abdomen at certain sites (transthoracic):
   a. Left parasternal region.
   b. Over the apex (left axilla).
   c. Subxiphoid.
   d. Suprasternal.
   e. Right parasternal

3. The transducer may be inserted by an endoscope through the mouth into the esophagus (transesophageal). The modes of echocardiographic evaluation include M-mode/two dimensional and Doppler.
   a. M-mode/two-dimensional evaluates structural and motion characteristics of the cardiac walls, valves, and vessel walls.
   b. Doppler study evaluates velocity, direction, and distribution of blood flow in the cardiac chambers and proximal blood vessels.
      (1) Color Doppler provides sector visualization of blood flow distribution and direction. It is used to direct more specific pulsed or continuous wave Doppler evaluation.
      (2) Pulsed wave (PW) Doppler provides information on flow characteristics in relatively small areas of the heart and blood vessels. It is location specific but cannot quantify high velocities.
      (3) Continuous wave (CW) Doppler provides information on flow characteristics over a line from the transducer through the heart. It is spatially ambiguous but provides high-velocity information which can indirectly assess transvalvular and transseptal gradients.

4. The transducer is connected to an echocardiographic unit which sends out the electronic signal, converted by the transducer into ultrasound energy transmitted into the body. Return signals are received by the transducer and converted back to electronic signals, which in turn are converted in the echocardiographic unit into an image providing structure or velocity (Doppler information). The ECG is simultaneously recorded.

5. Data are stored on VCR tapes, strip charts, page prints, floppy disks, or hard disks.

6. Off-line analysis systems can be used for data analysis such as edge enhancement and quantitative evaluation.

7. Echocardiography is a painless, noninvasive technique, allowing frequent serial studies (transthoracic).

B. Indications
   1. Emergencies
      a. Pericardial effusions/tamponade.
      b. Acute congestive heart failure, cause unknown.
      c. Systemic or pulmonary embolic; rule out clot, vegetation, or tumor.
      d. Cardiogenic shock, low output: rule out valve obstruction.
      e. Rule our aortic dissection, thoracic aortic aneurysm.
   2. General
      a. Valve structure and function.
      b. Wall motion abnormalities.
      c. Global chamber function (systolic).
      d. Diastolic inflow characteristics (LV and RV).
      e. Congenital and acquired malformation and shunts.
      f. Pericardial disease.
      g. Characterization of cardiopathies.
      h. LV hypertrophy.
   3. Special indications for transesophageal study
      a. Aortic and mitral prosthetic valve regurgitation.
      b. Clots in left or right atrial appendage.
      c. Diagnosis of interatrial or interventricular septal defects.
      d. Evaluation of pulmonary veins near left atrium.
      e. Evaluation of thoracic aortic aneurysms, dissection, or atherosclerosis.
      f. Intraoperative evaluation of valvular or complex congenital heart disease repairs.
      g. Intraoperative evaluation of LV volume and function in patients with heart disease undergoing noncardiac surgery.
      h. Lack of transthoracic visualization.
   4. Stress echocardiography
      a. Evaluation of exercise-induced segmental left ventricular wall motion abnormalities as they relate to underlying coronary artery disease.
      b. Improves diagnostic accuracy in patients with equivocal standard exercise tests.

    c. Useful in management of postmyocardial infarction patients.

    d. Useful in management of postcoronary intervention patients (e.g., after percutaneous transluminal coronary angioplasty and after thrombolysis)

C. Potential findings

  1. Cardiac chambers (M-mode, two-dimensional)

    a. Clots, tumors

    b. Diastolic and/or systolic volume dimensions or areas, ejection fractions.

    c. Sludging of blood, suggesting incipient clotting.

  2. Cardiac walls (M-mode, two-dimensional)

    a. Thicknesses.

    b. Tissue characterization, calcification, fibrosis, scintillation appearance (amyloid).

    c. Differentiation among hypertrophic, dilated or restrictive cardiomyopathies.

  3. Cardiac structures (general) (two-dimensional)

    a. Relative positions.

    b. Shunts (Doppler or use of IV contrast injections of agitated saline or indocyanine green).

  4. Valves

    a. Structure and motion (M-mode, two-dimensional).

    b. Presence and degree of regurgitation (Doppler, including estimated gradients).

    c. Presence and degree of stenosis (Doppler, including estimated gradients).

    d. Stroke volume can be assessed by multiplying the transvalvular spatial velocity profile by the cross-sectional area of the corresponding chamber or vessel.

  5. Stress echocardiography

    a. Exercise-induced new LV wall motion abnormalities.

    b. Either a fall or no increase in global LV ejection fraction with exercise.

    c. Increase in LV volume with exercise.

  6. Structure of large vessels and malpositions

    a. Thoracic aorta.

    b. Pulmonary artery.

    c. Proximal pulmonary veins (transesophageal).

    d. Proximal inferior vena cava.

    e. Proximal superior vena cava (transesophageal).

    f. Proximal coronary sinus (transesophageal).

  7. Pericardial disease

    a. Effusion.

    b. Tamponade.

    c. Thickening.

  8. Pleural effusion

D. Limitations of study

  1. Physical characteristics of ultrasound

    a. Energy dissipation by bone, cartilage, or air.

    b. Higher-frequency transducers increase resolution of nearby structures, but penetration into distant structures is poorer.

    c. Distance from Doppler probe decreases peak velocity limit detection.

  2. Patient physical characteristics

    a. Barrel chest, emphysema.

    b. Bony deformities of the chest (kyphoscoliosis, pectus excavatum or carinatum).

    c. Marked obesity.

    d. Large pleural effusion, fibrosis, or cardiac malposition.

    e. Patient position and breathing may affect reproducibility of study.

  3. M-mode study

    a. Apex and right-sided structures not well visualized (only 80–85% have optimal LV views).

  4. Two-dimensional study

    a. Tomographic views seen, but three-dimensional reconstruction necessary by evaluation of multiple orthogonal views.

    b. Limited frames for visualization per cardiac cycle (approximately 60 frames per second)

    c. Occasional reverberations which mimic abnormalities.

    d. Apical view frequently limited by endocardial dropout of LV and RV walls.

    e. Frequent echo shadowing distal to prosthetic valves. Valves themselves may be highly echogenic, masking abnormalities in interstices.

    f. Pericardium is quite echogenic, and thickened pericardium may be difficult to differentiate.

    g. Calcified native valves prevent adequate assessment of valve orifices.

  5. Doppler study

    a. Doppler beam has to be within 20° of flow direction to display optimal velocities.

b. Precise quantification of valvular regurgitation or shunt is difficult.

c. Visualization of ascending aorta and transverse thoracic aorta by transesophageal study requires the biplane probe.

d. Misinterpretation of aortic stenosis vs. mitral regurgitation in apical views.

E. Contraindications

1. Transthoracic: virtually none unless thoracic surface "windows" are unavailable.

2. Transesophageal

a. Absolute: active esophageal or oral pharyngeal disease, active peptic ulcer.

b. Relative: history of peptic ulcer, esophageal varices.

c. Infective: Endocarditis prophylaxis should be used only with patients with prosthetic valves who are not undergoing diagnostic evaluation for infective endocarditis. Patient should be NPO, except for oral medications, for at least 3 hr before procedure.

F. Complications

1. Transthoracic

a. Occasional mild bruise if transducer is applied too strenuously.

b. Allergy to ECG electrodes.

2. Transesophageal (rare)

a. Dysrhythmias.

b. Upper gastrointestinal bleeding.

c. Arterial O_2 desaturation.

d. Sinus tachycardia with sodium glycopyrrolate used to dry secretions. Glaucoma and asthma are contraindications for its use.

e. Respiratory arrest after sedation with midazolam—(Versed)—rare.

3. Stress echocardiogram

a. None for echocardiographic part of study.

G. Risks and benefits

1. Risks are negligible.

2. Costs of follow-up study may be reduced to conform to growing considerations of cost/benefit analysis. "Catered echocardiograms" might be considered (e.g., echocardiogram to assess degree of left ventricular hypertrophy alone could be cheaper than standard echocardiogram).

3. It is expected that only 80–85% of usual transthoracic studies are optimal. (> 95% of transesophageal studies).

4. Stress echocardiograms are optimal in > 85% of cases where large studies are performed.

IV. Cardiac Catheterization and Angiography

A. Technical description

1. Insertion of catheter

a. Direct approach through exposure of an artery or vein (brachial).

b. Percutaneous—insertion into femoral artery or vein.

2. Catheterization

a. Needle (cannula is inserted in vessel, with obturator inserted centrally in canula).

b. Obturator is removed and blood flow demonstrated through hub of canula.

c. Guidewire is threaded into canula and vessel, and canula is removed.

d. Catheter is inserted over guidewire into vessel, and guidewire is removed. Catheter is attached externally to an infusion system and the pressure gauge.

e. Catheter tip is positioned in heart or blood vessel for:

(1) recording of pressure.

(2) Hydrogen electrode sampling for shunts.

(3) Angiographic dye injection.

(4) Endomyocardial biopsy

3. Specific procedures

a. Right heart catheterization from peripheral vein to right atrium, right ventricle, pulmonary artery, and for endomyocardial biopsy.

b. Left heart catheterization from peripheral artery to aorta, left ventricle, and for selective coronary artery catheterization.

c. Left atrial (LA) catheterization—usually by transatrial septal approach from right heart catheterization. Rarely performed except for catheter valvulotomy of mitral valve and if catheter cannot be crossed retrograde from aorta to left ventricle in severe aortic stenosis.

B. Indications

1. Cardiac catheterization

a. Valvular heart disease.

b. Congenital heart disease.

c. Evaluation of endomyocardial samples.

d. Interventional cardiology (septostomy, angioplasty, valvulotomy), therapeutic procedures which will not be further described in this chapter.

e. Cardiomyopathy.

2. Coronary arteriography

Involves injection of angiographic dyes selectively into the coronary arteries.

a. Emergency
   (1) Acute myocardial infarction with cardiogenic shock, acute ventricular septal defect, or severe mitral regurgitation.
   (2) Possibly acute myocardial infarction to evaluate vasculature for use of thrombolytic agents or evaluation of results, (selective, not usually necessary with thrombolytic agents).
b. Urgency
   (1) Unstable angina, especially with failure to respond to antianginal medications.
   (2) Markedly abnormal exercise test.
c. Less urgent or elective
   (1) Before cerebrovascular procedures in patients with stable clinical coronary artery disease or after cerebrovascular diagnostic procedure has been performed.
   (2) Before other elective surgical procedures in patients with stable clinical coronary artery disease, especially for peripheral vascular disease operations.
   (3) Rarely, to make a diagnosis of coronary artery disease when noninvasive tests are equivocal.
3. Left ventriculography/angiography
   Injection of angiographic dye into LV or aorta to evaluate left ventricular size and function, aortic size, and presence and degree of aortic or mitral regurgitation. Presence of obstructive cardiomyopathy or proximal aortic dissection.
C. Potential findings
   1. Sequential catheter location—useful in evaluating complex congenital malformations.
   2. Pressure measurement
      a. Specific measures
         (1) Right atrial mean, right ventricular peak and diastolic, pulmonary artery (PA) mean, systole, diastole, pulmonary wedge (reflects LA mean pressure).
         (2) Aortic systolic over diastolic, LV peak and diastolic.
         (3) Special measurements using high-fidelity pressure manometers at the tip of catheter in LV (dp/dt, negative dp/dt, "Tau"—a measure of late systolic LV pressure decrease reflecting end systolic relaxation.

b. Significance
   (1) Left-sided heart disease and pulmonary vein stenosis associated with increased pulmonary wedge pressure (> 12 mmHg). Mitral regurgitation may be associated with large systolic V-wave on phasic measure trace. This is also seen with acute development of ventricular septal defect after myocardial infarction.
   (2) High PA pressure (> 30 mmHg systolic) with normal wedge pressures suggest isolated pulmonary artery hypertension.
   (3) RV systolic/diastolic pressure < 3:1 suggests restrictive cardiomyopathy or constrictive pericarditis. Constrictive pericarditis is also suggested by equalization of LV and RV, diastolic pressures and RA-PC mean pressures which are slightly elevated (10–25 mmHg).
   (4) Left ventricular end-diastolic pressure > 13 mmHg suggests diastolic compliance abnormality, frequently found in LV dysfunction.
3. Blood sampling
   a. For O_2 saturation—determination of location and calculation of shunts.
   b. With air bag collection for systemic cardiac output and calculation of peripheral vascular resistance. Other methods of determining cardiac output:
      (1) Injection of indocyanine green dye and blood sampling.
      (2) Thermodilution catheter in pulmonary artery. Evaluates right-sided cardiac output unless there is a left-to-right shunt at the pulmonary level. With left-to-right shunt at any level or with a right-to-left shunt, this test does not reflect systemic cardiac output.
4. Angiography
   a. General
      (1) Findings: visualization of aorta and LV routine. Visualization of RA, RV, and PA not usually done in adult lab. Rarely, visualization of LA accomplished by right-sided angiography in late (levo) phase.
      (2) Significance: evaluation of LV structure and function; presence of clots, myxomas or masses, aneu-

rysm, obstructive cardiomyopathy; quantification of mitral or aortic regurgitation; demonstration of shunts, aortic root dissections, or aneurysm.

b. Selective catheterization of coronary arteries, left main ostium, left anterior descending coronary artery, left circumflex coronary artery, right coronary artery by specially constructed catheters (Sones, Judkins, Amplatz).

c. Findings

Evaluation of presence and degree of coronary artery obstruction or coronary A-V fistula or ectatic coronary artery.

5. Combination studies (pressure, cardiac output determination)

a. Presence and degree of aortic stenosis using Gorlin formula or modification, determined by:

(1) Pressure gradient.

(2) Filling period.

(3) Stroke volume estimate (cardiac output/heart rate (CO/HR)

b. Study can be accomplished during exercise to determine effect on cardiac function and pressures.

6. Endomyocardial biopsy: evaluation of histopathology and dilated cardiomyopathy and serially after heart transplant.

D. Limitations of technique

1. Invasive approach: discomfort to patient and definite mortality and morbidity.

2. Angiographic data are silhouettes, not tomographic views.

3. May not be able to visualize LV or get LV pressures if significant arterial stenosis exists or if aortic prosthetic valves are in place (transseptal technique is now rarely used).

E. Contraindications

1. Most contraindications are relative and may be reversed.

a. Anticoagulated state.

b. Severe renal insufficiency (because of angiographic contrast.

c. Febrile illness.

d. Severe hypertension.

e. Electrolyte imbalance or digitalis toxicity.

f. Uncontrolled ventricular dysrhythmias.

g. Uncontrolled pulmonary edema.

h. During cerebrovascular accident.

F. Complications

1. Mortality: $< 0.10–1\%$:, depending on patient's age and severity of underlying diseases.

2. High risk

a. Severe three-vessel coronary disease, especially with valvular disease and poor LV function.

b. Severe aortic stenosis.

c. Noncardiac disease: renal, cerebrovascular, marked pulmonary hypertension.

d. Severe LV dysfunction.

e. Marked O_2 desaturation (right-to-left shunts).

f. Infants or elderly patients.

3. Reactions to angiographic dye.

4. Rare: emboli, perforation of the heart or great vessels, cerebrovascular complications from air or emboli.

5. Arterial thrombosis or hematoma at site of catheter insertion.

6. Coronary arteriography: coronary stenosis, clot, dissection, myocardial infarction, dysrhythmias, coronary artery spasm.

G. Risks and benefits

1. Mortality is very low in high-volume laboratories (> 300 cases a year).

2. The gold standard for coronary artery visualization.

3. Still the most direct means of determining intercardiac pressures and of estimating shunts and silhouette. Three-dimensional (compressed into two-dimensional) visualization of cardiac chambers.

V. ECG, Vectorcardiography, and Approach to the Diagnosis of Cardiac Arrhythmias

The approach to these tests is that of further diagnosis after the history and physical examination have suggested cardiovascular disease.

A. The ECG

1. Technical description

a. The surface ECG is accomplished by placing metallic or other conducting electrodes on the wrist and ankles, with special exploring electrodes over six positions on the chest. The exploring electrodes include (1) V_1: fourth interspace to the right of the sternum, (2) V_2: fourth interspace to the left of the sternum, (3) V_3: midway between V_2 and V_4, (4) V_4: fifth interspace of the midclavicular line, (5) V_5: anterior axillary line at the level of V_4, and (6) V_6: midaxillary line at the level of V_4.

b. Additonal electrodes are placed to the right or left of these evaluations of special cardiac geometries with respect to the chest wall. These evaluations include dextrocardia or abnormal positioning of the heart due to chest deformities or intrathoracic deformities such as pleural effusion, and sometimes assessment of RV infarction.

2. Indications
   a. The diagnosis of dysrhythmias and heart blocks.
   b. Anatomic and metabolic abnormalities which affect conduction (e.g., LV hypertrophy, chamber thickening, presence of electrolyte abnormalities, myocardial ischemia or myocardial infarction, and pericarditis).
   c. Specific points that are of value in diagnosis include:
      (1) Electrical alternans suggest pericardial effusion.
      (2) Q-T interval increases with type 1A antiarrhythmic agents (quinidine, procainamide).
      (3) Increased Q-T interval enhances susceptibility to ventricular arrhythmias.
      (4) Exaggerated upright U-wave, especially in the precordial leads suggests hypokalemia.
      (5) Peaked T-waves suggest hyperkalemia.
      (6) Short Q-T interval may be noted in hypercalcemia and prolonged QT interval in hypocalcemia.

B. Vectorcardiography
   1. Technical description
      a. Vectorcardiography uses a triaxial reference system to produce loops which depict atrial and ventricular depolarization and ventricular repolarization.
      b. The direction and appearance of these loops are useful in providing further information which may be obscure on the ECG:
         (1) The presence of inferior wall myocardial infarction where Q wave in leads 2, 3 and AVF on the surface ECG may not be diagnostic.
         (2) The presence of ventricular hypertrophy in association with conduction defects which may be masked in the surface ECG.
         (3) The diagnosis of myocardial infarction in association with bundle branch block patterns.

C. Approach to the diagnosis of cardiac arrhythmias
   1. The ECG is most useful in evaluating arrhythmias already present.
   2. Exercise testing is more sensitive than a standard 12-lead resting ECG in detecting ventricular ectopy but has less prognostic significance than ambulatory ECG (Holter) monitoring. Exercise ECGs, of course, are most useful for the diagnosis of underlying ischemia.
   3. Ambulatory ECG monitoring is useful for diagnosis of the presence, of complex arrhythmia and the correlation of symptoms with ECG abnormalities.
   4. Transtelephonic communication of ECG signals to a recorder-receiver at a central station allows assessment of dysrhythmias when they are relatively infrequent and brief and depend upon the patient's responsibility for activating the unit and transmitting the ECG signal by telephone.
   5. ECG monitoring is also useful in the evaluation of silent ischemia on the basis of ST-segment changes. With new systems which more reliably document ST abnormalities, this may provide additional prognostic and diagnostic information.
   6. With dysrhythmias, especially ventricular extrasystoles, there is considerable spontaneous variation (as much as 85%) from day to day in the number of ventricular premature depolarizations. This must be considered in evaluating the effect of an antiarrhythmic agent.

D. Signal Averaging
   1. Signal averaging is another noninvasive technique which looks at a part of the surface ECG. Because of improvement in the signal-to-noise ratio, it detects cardiac signals of a few microvolts and is applied to late ventricular potentials at the end of the QRS complex.
   2. These abnormal potentials, reflecting delayed conduction in the ventricle, are found in patients with sustained and inducible ventricular tachycardia, especially after myocardial infarction.
   3. The specificity of the test is high, that is, patients with absence of late potentials are much less likely to develop life-threatening arrhythmias.

4. The predictive accuracy for the presence of abnormal late potentials is not high, that is, many patients with abnormal late potentials do not develop life-threatening arrhythmias.

5. The presence of abnormalities must be used in conjunction with other prognostic data, including ambulatory 24-hr ECG recording, stress testing, and the cardiac ejection fraction to provide a comprehensive profile of risk for cardiovascular events.

E. Invasive procedures: technique
1. Multipolar catheter electrodes are inserted into the venous or arterial system and then into various parts of the heart on the basis of passive recording of local electrical signals from conduction in the heart and responses to electrical stimulation from the exploring electrode.

2. The following condition can be diagnosed:
   a. The site of atrioventricular block.
   b. The location of reentry pathways.
   c. The recovery of function of the sinoatrial node.
   d. Pathways for various types of tachycardia, both supraventricular and ventricular.
   e. Effects of ventricular stimulation on the production of sustained ventricular tachycardia. This information may provide prognostic information, as well as information on the efficacy of antiarrhythmic agents in suppressing life-threatening arrhythmias.

F. Esophageal ECG
1. This is accomplished by placing an electrode in the esophagus, which allows recording of atrial and ventricular potentials.

2. This technique may be useful for differentiating supraventricular tachycardia with aberrancy from ventricular tachycardia by allowing atrial activity to be demonstrated. The demonstration of atrioventricular dissociation with a wide QRS tachycardia would more likely suggest ventricular tachycardia than supraventricular tachycardia with aberrancy.

3. This technique could also be useful for differentiating supraventricular tachycardia from atrial flutter with 2:1 atrioventricular conduction when atrial activity cannot be seen on the surface ECG and carotid artery pressure does not increase atrioventricular block, as may be the case in atrial flutter.

G. Complications
1. The risks of noninvasive studies are virtually nil. Appropriate grounding prevents shocks, which may cause burns or arrhythmias.

2. Invasive electrophysiologic studies
   a. Usual complications of intracardiac catheterization including hemorrhage, arterial injury, venous thrombosis, and cardiac perforation.
   b. Risks associated with electrophysiologic stimuli include sustained ventricular tachycardia or ventricular fibrillation. Mortality and morbidity are very low; the mortality rate is approximately 0.05–0.1%.

H. Contraindications
1. There are virtually no contraindications to noninvasive studies with the exception of exercise testing, which should not be performed in patients with unstable angina or within a few days after acute myocardial infarctions.

2. The presence of certain resting ECG abnormalities may obscure the diagnostic impact of the ECG and the exercise test. These abnormal conditions include:
   a. Bundle branch block patterns.
   b. Nonspecific ST- and T-wave abnormalities.
   c. Digitalis effect.
   d. Ventricular preexcitation.
   In these situations, other means of evaluating ischemia, including nuclear imaging and ECG wall motion studies before and after exercise, will be more helpful.

3. Invasive electrophysiologic studies should not be performed in certain unstable conditions such as immediately after acute myocardial infarction or with unstable or resting angina.

I. Costs and benefits
1. The ECG is an excellent screening procedure for underlying cardiac disease in adults over the age of 25. It may be used serially with considerable frequency in patients with dysrhythmia, blocks or during acute myocardial infarction and should be repeated at least annually in patients with underlying heart disease.

2. The vectorcardiogram is useful as an adjunct to the ECG and specific diagnostic situation and is not usually evaluated serially.

3. Signed-averaged ECGs may be useful after myocardial infarction or prognostic profiling and in patients with cardiomyopathy. Otherwise, the use of serial studies using signal averaging requires further evaluation.
4. Exercise stress testing with evaluation of changes in the ECG should be used only under specialized circumstances such as the following:
   a. Men over the age of 35 and women over the age of 40 who plan to participate in an exercise program.
   b. After myocardial infarction to determine the prognosis and to assess rehabilitation procedures.
   c. To assess the effects of exercise on ventricular rate, especially in patients with atrial fibrillation and isolated ventricular ectopic activity in conjunction with agents which increase atrioventricular block with atrial fibrillation or presumably suppressed ventricular ectopic beats.
5. Invasive electrophysiologic studies are probably required in all patients who have undergone a cardiac arrest or have had sustained ventricular tachycardia in order to assess the efficacy of antiarrhythmic agents to characterize the arrhythmia and to provide prognostic information.
   More detailed information is provided in Chapter 17 (Arrhythmias).

VI. **Additional Noninvasive Imaging Techniques**
A. Nuclear techniques
   1. Exercise ^{201}Th imaging
      a. Technical description
         (1) Patient is exercised to the point of maximal stress, at which point ^{201}Th is injected intravenously.
         (2) Scanning is performed within 3–10 min after completion of exercise.
         (3) Ischemic myocardial zones show decreased perfusion immediately after exercise, which reperfuse on scans done several hours after exercise.
         (4) Some centers are using intravenous dobutamine as a pharmacologic stress agent. This agent may be helpful in the study of patients who cannot perform standard treadmill exercise (e.g., those with peripheral vascular disease or musculoskeletal or neurologic disorders). Dobutamine acts to enhance myocardial contractility and oxygen demand. In patients with coronary disease, regions of ischemia will be produced and identified with scanning.
      b. Indications
         (1) Diagnosis of coronary artery disease.
         (2) Demonstration of the physiologic significance of known coronary artery stenosis.
         (3) Evaluation of pharmacologic or surgical therapy.
      c. Potential findings
         (1) Reversible myocardial perfusion defects represent ischemia.
         (2) Fixed perfusion defects seen both with exercise and at rest represent zones of infarction.
      d. Limitations
         (1) Inability to attain maximal levels of exercise.
         (2) Medications that limit the maximal heart rate response.
         (3) Scans may be normal in patients who have significant coronary disease but extensive collateral flow.
      e. Contraindication
         Need to avoid radiopharmaceuticals during pregnancy.
      f. Complications
         (1) IV infiltration.
         (2) Similar to those of regular treadmill testing.
      g. Costs and benefits
         More costly than regular stress testing but more sensitive and specific.
         A new radionuclide agent being used in place of ^{201}Th in some centers is ^{99m}Tc sestamibi. This agent is taken up by myocardial cells proportionately to regional blood flow. The advantages of this agent are better image quality and reduced attenuation artifact. A disadvantage is that this radionuclide washes out of the myocardium very slowly, so patients with abnormal initial scans must return for a resting study 1 to 2 days later.
   2. I.V. dipyridamole with ^{201}Th imaging
      a. Technical description.
         (1) IV dipyridamole causes dilatation of normal coronary arteries by in-

creasing the level of interstitial adenosine. This, in turn, acts on the smooth muscle of coronary arterioles to increase flow through normal coronaries.

(2) There is resultant decreased perfusion to those areas of myocardium supplied by diseased coronary arteries.

(3) After the physiologic effect of the IV dipyridamole is achieved, ^{201}Th is injected and scanning is performed.

(4) Scanning is repeated several hours later to observe for reperfusion.

b. Indications

(1) Useful in patients who are unable to perform standard exercise testing.

(2) May be helpful in patients who have had previous suboptimal standard exercise testing.

c. Potential findings
Similar to those of regular exercise ^{201}Th imaging.

d. Limitation
Cannot be used in patients requiring aminophylline

e. Contraindications

(1) Severe asthma or bronchospastic disease.

(2) Hypotension.

(3) Recent myocardial infarction.

(4) Allergy to dipyridamole.

f. Complications

(1) Angina

(2) Headache

(3) Hypotension

(4) Dyspnea

3. Gated blood pool scanning

a. Principle
Provides accurate assessment of the glocal LV ejection fraction.

b. Technical considerations

(1) Radionuclide is injected IV and attains equilibrium in the blood pool.

(2) Timing with the ECG allows triggering and gating during specific times in the cardiac cycle.

(3) Gating allows comparison of systolic versus diastolic changes in the blood pool volume and calculation of the ejection fraction.

c. Potential findings

(1) Resting ejection fraction.

(2) With supine positioning of patient, the exercise ejection fraction can be obtained.

d. Limitations

(1) Dependent on accurate measurement of background activity.

(2) Care must be taken to isolate the LV from other surrounding structures.

B. Computer tomography (CT)

1. Technical description

a. Cross-sectional x-ray imaging of the heart.

b. Images are reconstructed by computer.

c. Ultrafast CT uses the technique of a scanning electron beam tube to acquire images.

d. ECG-gated CT allows evaluation of LV wall motion.

2. Indications

a. Quantification of the location and extent of myocardial infarction by the use of contrast infusion.

b. Studies of an LV mass.

c. Global measurement of LV function with the use of ECG gating.

d. Evaluation of aortic aneurysms and dissections.

e. Evaluation of congenital heart disease.

f. Evaluation of pericardial disease.

3. Limitations

a. Can image only one tomographic slide at a time with standard scanners.

b. Cardiac motion limitations result in degradation of image quality.

C. Magnetic resonance imaging (MRI)

1. Technical description

a. Nuclear magnetic resonance is exhibited by certain atomic nuclei that have magnetic properties due to their charge and spin.

b. *Nuclear magnetic resonance* refers to the absorption and reemission of an applied radiofrequency electromagnetic energy by certain nuclei found in biological systems. This is observed when these nuclei are placed in a magnetic field.

c. MRI uses the principles of resonance and relaxation in making an image.

d. MRI does not use ionizing radiation.

e. It requires ECG gating to the cardiac cycle to gain optimal images.

2. Indications

a. Myocardial tissue characterization.

   b. Myocardial perfusion imaging.
   c. Analysis of cardiac anatomy.
3. Limitations
   a. More costly than other imaging techniques.
   b. Nonportable technique.
   c. Lengthy imaging time.
4. Contraindications
   a. Patients with pacemakers or intracranial clips or dependent on life support devices.
   b. Patients who are hemodynamically unstable cannot easily be scanned safely.
D. Positron emission tomography (PET)
1. Technical description
   a. A *positron* is a positively charged electron emitted by certain unstable atoms in the process of decay.
   b. Positrons interact with electrons, producing a photon pair that can be detected with radiation detectors and recorded.
   c. PET cameras contain detectors attached to photomultiplier tubes that produce electronic signals, which are then converted to digital information to produce a tomographic image.
   d. A positron radiotracer is injected IV, and cardiac imaging is then obtained.
   e. The positron tracers are analogs of elements present in metabolism.
2. Indications
   a. Evaluation of the physiologic severity of coronary artery disease.
   b. Quantification and location of myocardial infarction.
   c. Determining the presence of myocardial viability.
   d. With the use of ECG gating, parameters of LV function may be studied.
3. Limitations
   a. The glucose analog ^{18}F fluoro-2-deoxyglucose (FDG) used as a radiotracer may not be consistently taken up in normally perfused myocardium of diabetic patients.
   b. There is variability of uptake of FDG in patients fasting at rest.
   c. The procedure is costly.
   d. Anatomic correlations are poorer than those achieved with other imaging techniques.
4. Contraindications.
   a. Situations in which administration of a radiopharmaceutical agent would be contraindicated (e.g., pregnancy).

Bibliography

Bonow RD, Berman DS, Gibbons RJ, et al: Cardiac Position Emission Tomography. *Circulation* 84:447–454, 1991.

Brown KA: Prognostic value of thallium-201 myocardial perfusion imaging: *Circulation* 83:363–381, 1991.

Brundage BH: Comparative Cardiac Imaging, Rockville, Aspen Publishers, Inc. Maryland, 1990.

Hollenberg M, Zoltick JM, Go M, et al: Comparison of a quantitative treadmill exercise score with standard electrocardiographic criteria in screening asymptomatic young men for coronary artery disease. *N Engl J Med* 313:600–606, 1985.

Matsuzaki M, Toma Y, Kusukawa R: Clinical applications of transesophageal echocardiography. *Circulation* 82:709–722, 1990.

Miller DD: Clinical cardiac imaging. McGraw-Hill, New York, N.Y.

Pohost PM: New concepts in cardiac imaging, G.K. Hall Medical Publishers, Boston, 1985.

Popp AL: Echocardiography. *N Engl J Med* 323:101–109, 165–172, 1990.

Sox HC, Jr, Garber AM, Littenburg B: The resting electrocardiogram as a screening test. *Ann Int Med* 111:489–502, 1989.

Stewart RE, Schwaiger M, Molina E, et al: Comparison of Rubidium-82 positron emission tomography and thallium-201 SPECT imaging for detection of coronary artery disease. *Am J Cardiol* 67:1303–1310, 1991.

Tape TG, Mushlin AI: The utility of chest radiographs. *Ann Intern Med* 104:633–670, 1986.

Table 16-1. Diagnostic Cardiac Testing: Commonly Available Tests

Condition	Reason
A. *No Overt Cardiac Disease: History/Physical Exam*	
ECG	Periodically after age 35 (every 2–5 years)
Treadmill stress test	For exercise programs: Men > 35 (every 2 years) Women > 40
B. *Diagnosis of Ischemic (Metabolic) Heart Disease (Plus History)*	
ECG	Serially during infarction, unstable angina.
	At least once annually thereafter.
	Evaluation periodically (every 6 months) during stable angina.
	Evaluation of electrolyte disturbances [K^+, Ca^{2+}, Mg^{2+}]
Vectorcardiogram	Prior inf. MI, MI pattern with bundle branch block
Signal-averaged ECG	Post-MI infarction: prognostic index.
Echocardiogram	Post-MI, wall motion score, clots, aneurysm, prognostic index, mitral regurgitation, VSD.
	For demonstration of ischemia (reversible defects).
Graded exercise test: thallium, echocardiogram, dipyridamole, dobutamine, adenosine	Periodically after MI (limited submaximal maximal). With stable angina. Demonstrates ECG abnormalities, nonperfused areas, wall motion abnormalities (echocardiography).
Ambulatory (24-hr) ECG	For S-T abnormalities: evidence of ischemia (silent or associated with angina).
Gated blood pool scan	Prognostic index after MI.
Coronary arteriogram	Evaluation of coronary artery disease in angina, myocardial infarction.
C. *Diagnosis of Structural/Functional Heart Disease (Plus History or Physical Exam)*	
ECG	LVH, RVH, atrial abnormality, pericarditis.
Vectorcardiogram	Hypertrophy when ECG BBB pattern obscures diagnosis.
Echocardiogram	Chamber structure, LV and RV systolic performance, valvular structure/function, shunts, congenital heart disease, thoracic aortic dissection, tumors, clots in chambers, cardiomyopathy.
Exercise gated blood pool scan versus rest	Ejection fraction (LV)—for decisions about operations in chronic aortic or mitral regurgitation, diastolic LV inflow characteristics (at rest).
CT scan	Aortic dissection, intracardiac masses, pericardial thickening, LV mass (LVH), tomographic representation of chamber structures.
Cardiac catheterization/ angiography	LV volume changes, shunt quantification, estimation of left-sided valvular regurgitation and stenosis, clot in LV. Evaluation of congenital heart disease, cardiomyopathy. Definitive evaluation of LV systolic/diastolic performance, right-sided pressure data.
D. *Electrophysiologic Abnormalities (History of Syncope, Dizziness, Palpitations)*	
ECG	Identification of dysrhythmia, blocks, & pre-excitation pattern.
Ambulatory 24-hr ECG monitoring	Correlation of symptoms with ECG findings: Evaluation of frequency of dysrhythmia/blocks and efficiency of antiarrhythmic agents/devices. Most sensitive determinant of dysrhythmia.
Treadmill stress test	Evaluation of ventricular rate in chronic arterial fibrillation and presence of ventricular arrhythmia with and without antiarrhythmic agents during exercise.

(continued)

Table 16-1. Continued

Condition	Reason
Invasive electrophysiologic study	After sustained ventricular tachycardia, S/P cardiac arrest (especially not associated with MI): to map induced ventricular tachycardia and efficacy of drug suppression. After syncope or evidence for blocks: to evaluate overt or covert block in SAN, AVN, HIS bundle, Purkinje system. Assesses need for pacemaker.
E. *Special Studies Not Usually Available*	
MRI scan	Structural heart abnormalities, including clots, masses, pericardial effusion, evaluation of LVH.
Ultrafast CT scan	Intracardiac and proximal aorta/PA blood flow, heart chamber structure/function.
PET scan	Localization of ischemia and metabolic defects in anginal syndromes, especially in absence of epicardial CAD, and with ambiguous ECG or ^{201}Th stress test findings.

Abbreviations: ECG, electrocardiogram; MI, myocardial infarction; VSD, ventricular septal defect; LVH, left ventricular hypertrophy; RVH, right ventricular hypertrophy; LV, left ventricle; RV, right ventricle; SAN, sinoatrial node; AVN, atrioventricular node; PA, pulmonary artery; CAD, coronary artery disease.

CHAPTER 17

Arrhythmias

Annabelle S. Volgman, M.D.
Thomas A. Buckingham, M.D.

Cardiac Arrhythmias

I. Definition and Introduction

The term *arrhythmia* is actually a misnomer because its Latin roots suggest a meaning of "no rhythm." Nonetheless this term has become established in medicine and is accepted to mean an abnormal cardiac rhythm. This may include tachycardias, bradycardias, or temporary disturbances such as ectopic beats or pauses. Cardiac electrophysiology, the study of the conduction system of the heart, has become a very important field in clinical cardiology. This is due to the advent of new diagnostic procedures and antiarrhythmic therapies (including drugs, ablative therapies, and devices). The fact that antiarrhythmic therapies can occasionally worsen arrhythmias or be *proarrhythmic* has become recognized as a major problem.

II. Etiology

Cardiac arrhythmias can occasionally occur in the absence of heart disease, but serious arrhythmias are usually associated with some cardiac pathology.

A. Congenital heart disease may be associated with a variety of rhythm disturbances. Wolff-Parkinson-White syndrome is caused by abnormal atrioventricular (AV) connections involving muscle tissue formed during embryogenesis of the heart. These abnormal pathways lead to a variety of reentrant rhythms using the accessory pathway and the normal AV node.

B. Diseases causing left ventricular dysfunction are associated with severe ventricular arrhythmias such as sustained ventricular tachycardia or ventricular fibrillation. The most common etiology of these arrhythmias is coronary artery disease, but cardiomyopathy and valvular heart disease may also be associated. The degree of left ventricular dysfunction is associated with the risk of these arrhythmias and with the prognosis in a quantitative fashion (i.e., the lower the ejection fraction, the worse the prognosis).

C. Electrolyte abnormalities, particularly disturbances of potassium, calcium, and magnesium balance, are commonly associated with arrhythmias. Abnormalities of thyroid metabolism also may cause brady- or tachy-arrhythmias.

D. Drugs may be arrhythmogenic by a variety of mechanisms. As already mentioned, antiarrhythmic agents can be proarrhythmic and can cause or worsen cardiac arrhythmias iatrogenically. Other drugs that can cause arrhythmias include those shown in Table 17-1.

III. Pathophysiology of Arrhythmias

A. Normal properties of the cardiac tissues and conduction system include excitability, threshold phenomena, refractoriness, and automaticity. Atrial and ventricular myocardium and the specialized conduction system have action potentials which can be recorded at the cellular membrane level. Depolarization and repolarization of the cells are caused by rapid influx and efflux of ions and are modulated by the autonomic nervous system and other factors. *Excitability* refers to the ability of cardiac tissue to be excited by an electrical stimulus. This stimulus must be of a certain amplitude or *threshold*. Immediately after excitation, the cardiac cell or tissue will not be excitable for a brief period of time known as the *refractory period*. Cardiac cells tend to depolarize slowly and spontaneously until threshold is reached, when the action potential will fire. The rate at which cardiac cells do this is called their *automaticity*. The pacemaker cells of the heart, located in the sinus and AV nodes, have increased automaticity. In healthy cardiac tissue, depolarization and repolarization are rapid and uniform in nature. With

disruption of the myocardium by various types of heart disease, these processes become inhomogeneous and more arrhythmogenic.

B. Mechanisms
   It is important to understand the mechanisms of these arrhythmias in order to understand their treatment. There are three important mechanisms involved in tachyarrhythmias:
   1. Reentry is believed to be the most common cause of clinical tachycardias. It is caused by the electrical impulse traveling around an anatomic circuit with properties of unidirectional block and slowed conduction.
   2. Enhanced automaticity causes tachycardias by increasing the rate of pacemaker cells in various parts of the heart (i.e., sinus tachycardia, junctional tachycardia, accelerated idioventricular rhythm, and parasystole). It can be caused by increased catecholamines or electrolyte imbalances or by disease or injury to local cardiac tissues.
   3. *Triggered activity* refers to the occasional appearance of oscillatory electrical activity during repolarization. This may occur with *torsades de pointes* ("twisting of the axis"), which is a polymorphic form of ventricular tachycardia associated with long QT intervals.

IV. Diagnosis

A. History
   Patients may be asymptomatic or may complain of palpitations, presyncope, or syncope. Patients may also present as resuscitated survivors of cardiac arrest or with documented episodes of sustained ventricular tachycardia.

B. Clinical signs and physical and findings
   Examination of the pulse rate and character should always be performed carefully in patients suspected of having arrhythmias. Both the apical and peripheral pulses should be assessed. An assessment of whether the patient is hemodynamically stable can be made by examination of the blood pressure, mental status, skin color, and temperature. There are a variety of physical findings caused by AV dissociation which suggest a diagnosis of ventricular tachycardia. These include cannon "a"-waves in the neck veins, variable pulse pressure, and a

Table 17-1. Drugs That Cause Tachyarrhythmias

Antiarrhythmic drugs (proarrhythmic response)
   Type 1A*: procainamide, quinidine, disopyramide
   Type 1B: lidocaine, mexiletine, tocainide
   Type 1C: flecainide, encainide, propafenone
   Type 1: ethmozine
   Type 3*: amiodarone, bretylium, sotalol
   Type 4*: bepridil
Digitalis
Phenothiazines*
Tricyclic antidepressants*
Catecholamines
Aminophylline
Antihistamines*: terfenadine, astemizole

*These drugs can prolong the Q-T interval, which can cause torsade de pointes.

variable S1. Carotid sinus massage can be used as a diagnostic or therapeutic maneuver in the presence of tachycardias. This procedure should be done with an electrocardiographic (ECG) recording. The patient is first auscultated for carotid bruits, which if present are a relative contraindication to this procedure. Five seconds or less of moderate pressure and massage is applied first to the right carotid sinus, with close observation of the patient and the ECG. Pressure is stopped immediately if symptoms or slowing occurs. After a brief test, the massage is repeated on the left side. Tachycardias that use the AV node as part of the reentrant circuit will often be terminated by carotid sinus massage. Atrial flutter or atrial tachycardia will show transient slowing on the ventricular rate with visible flutter or p waves. The same effect can be accomplished with the use of adenosine, 6 to 12 mg given rapidly intravenously.

C. Diagnostic Tests.

1. Electrocardiography (ECG) is the most important test of a patient's rhythm status. Whenever possible, a 12-lead ECG should be recorded of any brady- or tachyarrhythmia. Patients at risk should also be connected to continuous ECG telemetry monitoring. It is incumbent upon the physician to review all ECG strips on patients to ensure an accurate diagnosis. Strong efforts should be made to include sufficient samples of the patient's ECG strips in the medical record to document all rhythms observed and related events (medications, etc.).

2. Exercise testing can be undertaken to delineate the patient's underlying heart disease or to determine if the arrhythmia is exercise or stress related. This test is often combined with a nuclear imaging technique such as thallium or cardiolyte scanning.

3. Echocardiography is useful in determining underlying heart disease and the severity of left ventricular dysfunction.

4. Ambulatory 24-hr ECG monitoring (Holter) is useful to diagnose arrhythmias which may occur intermittently. It can be used to quantitate ventricular ectopy and its response to therapy.

5. Event recorders are portable ECG devices that can be carried for long periods

of time by a patient and used to capture the ECG when symptoms occur. The ECG can then be transferred by phone for physician review.

6. Cardiac catheterization is very useful to determine the etiology and severity of underlying cardiac disease.

7. Electrophysiology studies are performed using electrode catheters placed in the heart for stimulation and recording. These studies allow detailed evaluation of the patient's conduction system and rhythm disturbance.

8. Tilt table testing is used in patients with recurrent syncope thought to be due to abnormal vagal reflex responses. Recently, the addition of isoproterenol infusion during tilt table testing has increased the sensitivity of the test and therefore made it more useful.

V. **Classification of Arrhythmias**

The following outline is a summary of the different arrhythmias that are seen clinically. For each arrhythmia, the following will be discussed in detail: (1) definition, (2) causes, (3) diagnosis, (4) differential diagnosis, and (5) treatment.

A. Tachyarrhythmias
   1. Sinus node arrhythmias
      a. Sinus tachycardia
      b. Sinus node reentry
   2. Atrial Arrhythmias
      a. Multifocal atrial tachycardia (chaotic atrial rhythm)
      b. Paroxysmal atrial tachycardia
      c. Atrial flutter
      d. Atrial fibrillation
   3. AV Junctional Rhythms
      a. AV nodal reentry: common and uncommon types
      b. AV reentry related to accessory pathways
         (1) Manifest (WPW syndrome) with antegrade preexcitation
         (2) Concealed accessory pathway
      c. Junctional rhythm
   4. Ventricular tachycardias
      a. Accelerated idioventricular rhythm
      b. Ventricular tachycardia
         (1) Monomorphic
         (2) Polymorphic
      c. Ventricular fibrillation and flutter
B. Bradyarrhythmias
   1. Failure of impulse formation

a. Sick sinus syndrome (sinus pauses, sinus bradycardia)
b. Hypersensitive carotid sinus syndrome
c. Wandering atrial pacemaker
2. Failure of conduction
   a. SA block
   b. AV block
C. Ectopic activity
1. atrial, junctional, and ventricular ectopics
D. Tachyarrhythmias
1. Sinus node arrhythmias
   a. Sinus tachycardia
      (1) *Definition:* a rhythm arising from the sinoatrial (SA) node, $\geq$ 100 bpm.
      (2) *Causes:* usually a normal response to increased adrenergic tone such as physical or emotional stress.
      (3) *Diagnosis:* the p-waves are identical to the normal sinus p-waves, there is a 1:1 ratio of the p-waves to QRS complexes, and the onset and termination are not abrupt.
      (4) *Differential diagnosis:* this cannot be distinguished from sinus node reentry unless the onset or termination is seen.
      (5) *Treatment:* no treatment is usually required unless the tachycardia is chronic and may compromise left ventricular function, such as in patients with severe cardiomyopathy. The treatment to slow down the tachycardia is β-1 selective β-adrenergic antagonists. However, since this is a normal response to stress, treatment of the underlying cause of the stress is the best treatment.
   b. Sinus node reentry
      (1) *Definition:* a rhythm arising from the sinus node with a reentry circuit consisting of two functionally distinct pathways confined to the sinus node.
      (2) *Causes:* usually seen in patients with sick sinus syndrome. This is probably caused by inhomogeneity of the SA node, which causes different conduction velocity and refractory periods, thereby allowing reentry to occur.

(3) *Diagnosis:* sudden onset or termination of tachycardia ($\geq$ 100 bpm), with p-waves identical to the sinus p-waves.
(4) *Differential diagnosis:* this cannot be distinguished from sinus tachycardia unless the onset or termination is seen.
(5) *Treatment:* usually does not require treatment unless the patient is symptomatic. Antiarrhythmic drugs which have a negative chronotropic effect on the sinus node, such as β-adrenergic antagonists and calcium channel blockers, can be used.
2. Atrial Arrhythmias
   a. Multifocal atrial tachycardia (chaotic atrial rhythm)
      (1) *Definition:* a rhythm arising from at least three different ectopic atrial foci
      (2) *Causes:* the exact cause is unknown, but this rhythm is often seen in patients with severe chronic obstructive pulmonary disease. Other diseases associated with this rhythm are cardiac disease, hypertension, and diabetes mellitus.
      (3) *Diagnosis:* three distinct p-waves must be seen in the same lead, in addition to the sinus p-wave and there are variable P-P, R-R, and P-R intervals.
      (4) *Differential diagnosis:* this rhythm can appear similar to atrial fibrillation, since both rhythms are irregularly irregular, especially if the amplitudes of the p-waves are small.
      (5) *Treatment:* if the arrhythmia is persistent and the fast rates cause hemodynamic compromise, β-1, selective antagonists or calcium channel blockers may be effective.
   b. Paroxysmal atrial tachycardia: (ectopic (automatic) atrial tachycardia and reentrant atrial tachycardia)
      (1) *Definition:* a rhythm arising from the atrium.
      (2) *Causes:* ectopic atrial tachycardia is due to increased automaticity in an ectopic focus in the atrium.

Reentrant atrial tachycardia is due to a reentry mechanism arising from different pathways in the atria. Both rhythms are common in patients with dilated atria.

(3) *Diagnosis:* the rate is usually ≥ 100 bpm and < 250 bpm; the p-wave morphology is different from the sinus p-wave morphology.

(4) *Differential diagnosis:* this condition can be distinguished from sinus tachycardia and sinus node reentry by the p-wave morphology. It can be distinguished from atrial flutter by the rate of the atria; the atrial rate is usually 150 to 250 bpm in paroxysmal atrial tachycardia and 250 to 350 bpm in atrial flutter. This can sometimes be difficult to distinguish from AV nodal reentry, AV reentry, and junctional tachycardia.

(5) *Treatment:* usually no treatment is required, since the episodes are usually very transient. If it is necessary to treat, Class Ia, Ic & III drugs can be effective in suppressing the arrhythmia.

c. Atrial flutter

(1) *Definition:* a rapid, regular atrial rhythm, with atrial rates usually ranging from 250 to 350 bpm and variable conduction to the ventricles.

(2) *Causes:* usually found in patients with dilated atria due to other cardiopulmonary disease. The mechanism is thought to be a reentry circuit confined to the atrial tissue.

(3) *Diagnosis:* because of the rapid atrial rates, the p-waves resemble a sawtooth pattern and are called *flutter (F) waves.* There is usually variable conduction ranging from 1:1 to 4:1 or higher. The most common ventricular response rate is 150 bpm in untreated cases. If the conduction is 1:1, the ventricular rates become dangerously high and require immediate electrical cardioversion. If the conduction is ≥ 4:1 in untreated cases, this is usually due to conduction disease of the AV node.

(4) *Differential diagnosis:* it is sometimes difficult to differentiate atrial flutter with 2:1 conduction from paroxysmal atrial tachycardia and supraventricular tachycardia due to AV nodal reentry and AV reentry. A helpful diagnostic method is to block the AV node either by a physiologic maneuver such as carotid sinus massage or with medications such as intravenous adenosine or verapamil. If the ventricular response slows down, the flutter waves become easier to recognize. If the rhythm is terminated, the other supraventricular tachycardias mentioned are more likely.

(5) *Treatment:* If the patient is hemodynamically unstable, the treatment is electrical cardioversion. If the patient is hemodynamically stable, the initial treatment is to block the conduction through the AV node such that the ventricular rate is ≤ 100 bpm. If the atrial flutter persists, chemical cardioversion can be attempted using class Ia, Ic, and III drugs. Since this is a reentry mechanism, overdrive atrial pacing is another mode of terminating this rhythm as long as the atrial rate is less than 340 bpm. If chemical cardioversion fails to convert the rhythm to sinus rhythm, electrical cardioversion can be used.

d. Atrial fibrillation

(1) *Definition:* a chaotic rhythm arising from the atria which prevents effective contraction of the atria.

(2) *Causes:* usually found in patients with dilated atria due to cardiopulmonary diseases or hyperthyroidism. It is also seen in patients with no detectable organic heart disease. The mechanism of atrial fibrillation is unclear, but it may be multiple reentry circuits.

(3) *Diagnosis:* there are no discernible p-waves on any surface ECG lead, and the ventricular complexes are irregularly irregular.

(4) *Differential diagnosis:* this rhythm

can sometimes appear similar to multifocal atrial tachycardia, but it can be differentiated by lack of organized p-waves in all surface ECG leads. When the ventricular response is very rapid, the rhythm can be regular and can appear similar to atrial flutter.

(5) *Treatment:* if the patient is hemodynamically unstable, immediate electrical cardioversion is necessary. If the patient is hemodynamically stable, the ventricular rate should be slowed with AV nodal blockers such as digitalis, calcium channel blockers, or β-adrenergic antagonists. If chemical cardioversion is to be attempted, drugs such as class Ia, Ic & III can be used.

If the QRS complexes are intermittently wide and bizarre, the presence of an accessory bypass tract should be considered. In patients with accessory bypass tract in atrial fibrillation, drugs that slow the AV node can accelerate the conduction through the accessory bypass tract and cause ventricular fibrillation because of the very rapid ventricular rates. This rhythm should be treated with drugs that affect the refractoriness of the accessory bypass tract such as classes Ia, Ic, and III.

In chronic atrial fibrillation (> 48–72 hours in duration), the patient should be anticoagulated prior to an attempt to cardiovert the rhythm chemically or electrically. There are no large studies to demonstrate the optimal duration of anticoagulation prior to cardioversion, but 2–3 weeks is generally appropriate. The duration of drug maintenance is dependent on the underlying cause. If the cause, such as hyperthyroidism, is treated, then chronic therapy is unnecessary. If the underlying cause cannot be cured, chronic therapy with an AV nodal blocker and/or a class Ia, Ic, or III is used to maintain sinus rhythm. A car-

diac echocardiogram should be obtained to assess the atrial size, since large atria (≥ 6.0 cm) rarely stay in sinus rhythm and attempts at cardioversion may be futile.

3. Atrioventricular junctional rhythms
   a. AV nodal reentry
      (1) *Definition:* this rhythm arises from two functionally distinct pathways confined to the AV node. There are two types: common and uncommon. In the common type, the antegrade conduction through the AV node is via the pathway with the slower conduction because the usual pathway (the fast pathway) is still refractory from a previous impulse. The impulse from the slow pathway conducts to the ventricle and also retrograde through the other AV node pathway (the fast pathway), which by then is no longer refractory. This circuit is the mechanism by which reentry can occur in the AV node. The uncommon type utilizes the fast pathway as the antegrade limb and the slow pathway as the retrograde limb.
      (2) *Causes:* no particular disease predisposes patients to having two functionally distinct AV nodal pathways.
      (3) *Diagnosis:* this is a regular rhythm, usually with narrow QRS complexes, identical to the sinus QRS complexes. Occasionally, the complexes may be wide if there is aberrant conduction through the bundle branches. A very good indication that a supraventricular tachycardia (SVT) is due to AV nodal reentry is during the initiation of the SVT. Commonly, a premature atrial complex is conducted with a much longer PR interval, and subsequently the SVT is initiated. In the common type, the retrograde p-waves may be buried in the QRS complex or occur at the final phase of the QRS complex. In the uncommon type, the retrograde p-waves can be seen after the QRS complex.
      (4) *Differential diagnosis:* this SVT can-

not be differentiated from paroxysmal atrial tachycardia or from orthodromic reciprocating tachycardia of the Wolff-Parkinson-White syndrome.

(5) *Treatment:* initial treatment for this rhythm consists of maneuvers to cause AV nodal block, such as the valsalva maneuver or carotid sinus massage (as long as no carotid bruits are auscultated). If maneuvers do not terminate the arrhythmia, intravenous medications that block the AV node can be used. Good initial drugs to use are adenosine or verapamil, since these are both fast acting. For long-term therapy, drugs that block the AV node will cause slowing and blockage in the pathways, such as beta-adrenergic antagonists and calcium channel blockers. Other antiarrhythmic drugs that can be used are drugs that affect the retrograde fast pathway, such as the class 1 and 3 antiarrhythmic agents.

Recently, catheter ablation has been found to be an effective method of treatment. One of the AV nodal pathways is selectively ablated after mapping of the AV node area. The risk of complete heart block exists and requires permanent pacemaker implantation.

b. Atrioventricular reentry
(1) *Definition:* this rhythm occurs in patients with an accessory bypass tract in the AV groove. This bypass tract may have the capacity to (a) conduct antegrade from the atrium to the ventricle; (b) retrograde from the ventricle to the atrium; or (c) both. These bypass tracts have different conduction velocities and refractory periods from the AV node. Premature atrial or ventricular beats can cause a reentry circuit to occur, utilizing the AV node as one pathway and the accessory bypass tract as the other pathway. There are two types of AV reentry: (a) orthodromic reciprocating tachycardia and (b) antidromic reciprocating tachycardia. In orthodromic reciprocating tachycardia, the AV node is the antegrade limb of the reentry circuit and the accessory bypass tract serves as the retrograde limb. In antidromic reciprocating tachycardia, the accessory bypass tract is the antegrade limb and the AV node is the retrograde limb of the reentry circuit.

(2) *Causes:* in patients with Wolff-Parkinson-White syndrome, there is usually no associated cardiac disease, but there is an increased incidence of Ebstein's anomaly. The accessory bypass tract is formed in utero during the separation of the atrial muscle from the ventricular muscle. The accessory bypass tracts are muscle bands that fail to be separated and therefore become direct communications between the atria and the ventricles.

(3) *Diagnosis:* if the bypass tract is capable of conducting impulses antegradely from the atria to the ventricles, this will activate a part of the ventricle prior to the activation of the ventricles from the AV node. This early activation of the portion of the ventricle is manifested by an early deflection of the QRS complex known as the *delta wave.* This early activation or preexcitation causes a short P-R interval, usually ≤ 0.12 sec. If the bypass tract has no antegrade properties but can conduct in a retrograde fashion, there will be no evidence of preexcitation on the surface ECG leads. This is known as a *concealed bypass tract.*

(4) *Differential diagnosis:* orthodromic reciprocating tachycardia, since it is a narrow QRS tachycardia, cannot be differentiated from SVT due to AV nodal reentry or paroxysmal atrial tachycardia unless the existence of an accessory pathway is known. Antidromic reciprocating tachycardia is usually a wide QRS tachycardia which is difficult

to differentiate from SVT with aberrancy or from monomorphic ventricular tachycardia.

(5) *Treatment:* initial treatment for this rhythm consists of maneuvers to cause AV nodal block, such as the valsalva maneuver or carotid sinus massage (as long as no carotid bruits are auscultated). If maneuvers do not terminate the arrhythmia, intravenous medications that block the AV node can be used. A good initial drug to use is adenosine or verapamil, since these are both fast-acting. For long-term therapy, drugs that block the AV node such as β-adrenergic antagonists and calcium channel blockers can be used. Other antiarrhythmic drugs that can be used are drugs that affect the accessory bypass tract such as the class 1 and 3 antiarrhythmic agents.

Recently, catheter ablation has been found to be an effective method of treatment. The accessory bypass tract is selectively ablated after mapping the AV groove.

c. Junctional rhythm
  (1) *Definition:* a rhythm that arises from the AV nodal region. There are two types of junctional rhythm: (a) escape and (b) accelerated.
  (2) *Causes:* The escape junctional rhythm occurs as a result of a decrease in sinus rate, high-degree AV block proximal to the level of the bundle of His, or a long pause following a premature atrial or ventricular complex. The accelerated junctional rhythm is mostly seen in patients with digoxin toxicity.
  (3) *Diagnosis:* this is usually a narrow, complex rhythm unless there is a preexisting bundle branch block which is not preceded by sinus p-waves but can be followed or preceded by retrograde p-waves. The rate of the junctional escape rhythm is 35–60 bpm, and the rate

of the accelerated junctional rhythm is > 60 bpm.
  (4) *Differential diagnosis:* in both types of junctional rhythms, the QRS complexes can be preceded by retrograde p-waves which cannot be differentiated from ectopic atrial tachycardia. Accelerated junctional rhythm can also be difficult to differentiate from AV nodal reentrant tachycardia and orthodromic reciprocating tachycardia in Wolff-Parkinson-White syndrome. The clinical setting is helpful in this differential diagnosis.
  (5) *Treatment:* junctional escape rhythm does not require treatment; it is the underlying cause that requires therapy. If the escape rhythm is insufficient to maintain hemodynamic stability, medications that can accelerate the AV node can be given, such as atropine or isoproterenol. If the rhythm persists, a temporary pacemaker may be necessary. Accelerated junctional rhythm, if caused by digoxin toxicity, only requires removal of the toxin.

4. Ventricular tachycardias
  a. Accelerated idioventricular rhythm
    (1) *Definition:* a rhythm arising from ventricular muscle which occurs when the supraventricular pacemakers have a slower rate than the intrinsic or enhanced rate of the ventricular tissue (i.e., < 100 bpm).
    (2) *Causes:* this rhythm is an escape rhythm due to other rhythm disturbances, or myocardial ischemia/infarction.
    (3) *Diagnosis:* this is a wide QRS complex rhythm. In idioventricular rhythm, the rate is usually 30 to 50 bpm. In accelerated idioventricular rhythm, the rate is usually 60 to 100 bpm.
    (4) *Differential diagnosis:* this rhythm can be difficult to differentiate from junctional rhythms with aberrancy. If the focus of the idioventricular rhythm is near the septum, the QRS complexes may

appear narrow and similar to the junctional beats.

(5) *Treatment:* no treatment is necessary for this rhythm as long as the patient is hemodynamically stable. If the rate is inadequate for hemodynamic stability, a temporary pacemaker may be necessary until the underlying rhythm disturbance is corrected.

b. Ventricular tachycardia

(1) Monomorphic ventricular tachycardia

(a) *Definition:* a rhythm that arises from the ventricular tissues causing a wide QRS tachycardia, with rates > 100 bpm and a single morphology.

(b) *Causes:* the most common cause of monomorphic ventricular tachycardia is a reentry circuit due to an infarcted area of the ventricle as a result of a myocardial infarction. Other causes are (1) bundle branch reentry, seen in some patients with dilated cardiomyopathy; (2) idiopathic ventricular tachycardia which is responsive to verapamil; and (3) right ventricular outflow tract tachycardia seen in patients with right ventricular dysplasia; (4) repetitive monomorphic ventricular tachycardia responsive to beta adrenergic blockers.

(c) *Diagnosis:* a wide QRS complex tachycardia in which the atrial contractions are dissociated from the ventricular contractions unless there is retrograde ventriculoatrial conduction.

(d) *Differential diagnosis:* this can sometimes be difficult to differentiate from SVT with aberrant conduction. If there is evidence of AV dissociation or there are fusion beats, the rhythm would most likely be ventricular tachycardia. If these conditions are not readily evident, another method with a high specificity for ventricular tachycardia is demonstration of the absence of an RS complex in all precordial leads. If an RS complex is present in one or more leads, an RS interval of more than 100 msec is also highly specific for ventricular tachycardia.

(e) *Treatment:* in sustained monomorphic ventricular tachycardia, the patient is at high risk for recurrence and sudden cardiac death. Although studies are still ongoing to define the best method of guiding antiarrhythmic therapy, some studies suggest that invasive electrophysiology testing may be better than noninvasive Holter guided therapy. Treatment includes all classes of antiarrhythmic drugs implantable cardioverter defibrillator devices with or without antitachycardia pacemakers and ablative surgery. Catheter ablation for treatment of monomorphic ventricular tachycardia is still under clinical investigation.

(2) Polymorphic ventricular tachycardia

(a) *Definition:* a rhythm that arises from the ventricular tissues causing a wide QRS tachycardia, with rates > 100 bpm. A single morphology cannot be identified.

(b) *Causes:* some studies suggest that polymorphic ventricular tachycardia may be secondary to ischemia or multiple foci of reentry circuits. Other causes include metabolic abnormalities, as well as all the causes of torsade de pointes, both acquired and congenital. Table 17-2 presents a complete list of the causes of QT prolongation.

(c) *Diagnosis:* this rhythm is usually a wide QRS complex

Table 17-2. Causes of Q-T Prolongation

Acquired

Drug induced: class Ia, Ic, III, IV (Bepridil)
 tricyclic antidepressants and phenothiazines,
 antihistamines (terfenadine astemizole),
 miscellaneous (organophosphate poisons)
Electrolyte abnormalities: hypomagnesemia,
 hypokalemia, and hypocalcemia
Myocardial ischemia and disease
Central nervous system disease
Bradycardia
Mitral valve prolapse
Nutritional states: malnutrition or severe weight loss
Hypothyroidism
Congenital
Jervell Lange-Nielsen syndrome: associated with
 hearing loss, autosomal recessive inheritance
Romano Ward syndrome: no hearing loss,
 autosomal dominant inheritance

tachycardia with a changing bundle branch block pattern or axis. A specific polymorphous ventricular tachycardia that is seen in the presence of a long Q-T interval is called *torsade de pointes*.

(d) *Differential diagnosis:* this rhythm can sometimes be difficult to differentiate from atrial fibrillation in a patient with an accessory bypass tract.

(e) *Treatment:* the patient is usually hemodynamically unstable in sustained polymorphic ventricular tachycardia, and emergent electrocardioversion is necessary. Once the patient is stabilized, the underlying cause needs to be identified and corrected.

c. Ventricular fibrillation and flutter

(1) *Definition:* rhythms that arise from the ventricular tissues and result in sudden death.

(2) *Causes:* these rhythms usually have the same etiologies as monomorphic and polymorphic ventricular tachycardia.

(3) *Diagnosis:* ventricular fibrillation is a chaotic rhythm with no recognizable P-, QRS-, or T-waves.

Ventricular flutter is a rapid ventricular tachycardia with no recognizable ventricular complex component.

(4) *Differential diagnosis:* ventricular fibrillation leads to hemodynamic collapse. Atrial flutter with 1:1 conduction and with aberrancy can appear similar to ventricular flutter.

(5) *Treatment:* since both rhythms lead to sudden cardiac death, immediate electrocardioversion to convert the rhythm must be done.

E. Bradyarrrhythmias

1. Failure of impulse formation

a. Sick sinus syndrome

(1) *Definition:* sinus node dysfunction manifested as lack of impulse formation and slow as well as rapid sinus rhythms.

(2) *Causes:* this syndrome is associated with many cardiac diseases, but the etiology of the sinus node dysfunction is unclear. Its clinical manifestation is due either to lack of impulse formation in the sinus node or to inability of the impulse to be transmitted to the atria.

(3) *Diagnosis:* a 12-lead ECG or a long-term ambulatory ECG reveals one or more of the following: (a) sinus bradycardia, sinus arrest, SA block; (b) junctional escape rhythm, with or without retrograde atrial conduction; (c) atrial arrhythmias, most commonly atrial fibrillation; and (d) sinus bradycardia alternating with sinus tachycardia.

(4) *Differential diagnosis:* all of the above rhythms have differential diagnoses.

(5) *Treatment:* in patients with symptomatic bradycardia, the treatment is usually permanent pacemaker implantation. In patients with tachycardia, treatment consists of antiarrhythmic drugs that slow the sinus node, such as β-adrenergic antagonists and calcium channel blockers. However, these drugs may aggravate the bradycardia, and often these

patients have to be treated with pacemakers and antiarrhythmic drugs.

b. Hypersensitive carotid sinus syndrome

(1) *Definition:* there are two types of this syndrome: (a) cardioinhibitory or vagal and (b) vasodepressor. The cardioinhibitory type is manifested as bradycardia or asystole, with mechanical stimulation of the carotid sinus, and is inhibited by atropine. The vasodepressor type is manifested as vasodilatation and hypotension. It is induced by an abrupt decrease in peripheral resistance and can be inhibited by epinephrine. There can also be a mixture of the two types in a patient.

(2) *Causes:* the exact mechanism of the cardioinhibitory type is unknown, but it is mediated by the parasympathetic nervous system. It is commonly found in elderly men with coronary artery disease and hypertensive heart disease.

(3) *Diagnosis:* the cardioinhibitory type can be diagnosed by carotid sinus massage, which can cause a significant pause (ventricular asystole for > 3 sec). A systolic arterial pressure drop of 30 to 50 mmHg during carotid sinus stimulation can be used to diagnose the vasodepressor type.

(4) *Differential diagnosis:* this syndrome may be part of the sick sinus syndrome.

(5) *Treatment:* in symptomatic patients, a permanent pacemaker is the treatment for the cardioinhibitory type. In patients with the vasodepressor type, treatment is more difficult but patients will usually have a favorable response with supportive leg stockings and volume expanders such as mineralocorticoids. Fludrocortisone acetate have been found to be useful in these patients and can be used in conjunction with the leg stockings.

c. Wandering pacemaker

(1) *Definition:* a rhythm in which the pacemaker shifts from one to another; the pacemaker can be sinus, atrial or junctional. This rhythm is slower than multifocal atrial tachycardia (rate < 100 bpm).

(2) *Causes:* usually any physiologic or pathologic process that enhances the vagal tone.

(3) *Diagnosis:* p-wave morphology is different and P-R intervals change.

(4) *Differential diagnosis:* can appear similar to premature atrial complexes, sinus arrhythmia, junctional beats, and atrial fibrillation.

(5) *Treatment:* the treatment is to correct the underlying cause of the process that enhances the vagal tone.

2. Failure of conduction

a. SA block

(1) *Definition:* impulse formation occurs in the sinus node, but it is not propagated into the atrial conduction system and atrial muscle.

(2) *Causes:* there are physiologic (carotid hypersensitivity), pharmacologic (digitalis and quinidine toxicity, atropine, salicylates), and pathologic (damage to or degenerative disease of the SA node) causes.

(3) *Diagnosis:* there are three types of SA block: first-, second-, and third-degree. Since the sinus node is not represented in the ECG, first-degree SA block cannot be recognized by a surface ECG. Second-degree SA block is further subclassified as type I (Wenckebach) or type II (Mobitz II). In type I, sinus-to-atrial conduction becomes progressively longer until the sinus impulse is blocked. This can be recognized as (a) progressive shortening of the P-P intervals of the cycles preceding a pause; (b) the P-P interval of the cycle that includes the pause is less than twice the length of the P-P interval just prior to the pause; and (c) the P-P interval following

the dropped beat is longer than the P-P interval immediately preceding the pause. In type II the P-P interval that includes the pause is a direct multiple of the P-P interval. Third-degree SA block is indistinguishable from sinus arrest, and escape beats are seen.

(4) *Differential diagnosis:* first-degree SA block may appear similar to sinus arrhythmia.

(5) *Treatment:* patients who are asymptomatic do not need treatment. Patients who are symptomatic are treated with permanent pacemakers.

b. AV block

(1) *Definition:* there is atrial contraction, but also conduction delay through the AV node and His bundle system.

(2) *Causes:* there are three causes: physiologic (vagal stimulation), pharmacologic (digitalis, Class 1A, 2, 3 and 4 antiarrhythmic agents toxicity; antiarrhythmic agents), and pathologic (damage to or degenerative disease of the AV node).

(3) *Diagnosis:* there are three types of AV block: first-, second-, and third-degree. First-degree AV block is P-R prolongation > 0.20 sec. Second-degree AV block is further subclassified as type I (Wenckebach) or type II (Mobitz II). In type I, the P-R interval becomes progressively longer until there is a nonconducted atrial beat. This can be recognized as (a) progressive shortening of the P-R intervals of the cycles preceding a pause; (b) the R-R interval of the cycle that includes the pause is less than twice the length of the R-R interval just prior to the pause; and (c) the R-R interval following the dropped beat is longer than the R-R interval immediately preceding the pause. In type II the R-R interval that includes the pause is a direct multiple of the R-R interval. Third-degree AV

block is complete heart block, and AV dissociation with escape beats is seen.

(4) *Differential diagnosis:* second-degree AV block can sometimes be confused with nonconducted atrial premature beats.

(5) *Treatment:* patients with first- and second-degree AV block type I are usually asymptomatic and do not need treatment. Wenckebach periodicity is present in all patients when the atrial rates exceed the AV node's ability to conduct the impulse. Patients with second-degree AV block type II and third-degree AV block are usually symptomatic and are treated with cardiac pacing. The underlying cause of the block needs to be treated. If the symptomatic AV block persists, permanent pacing is indicated.

F. Ectopic Activity

1. Atrial, junctional, and ventricular ectopics

a. *Definition:* an extra impulse that can arise from any cardiac tissue.

b. *Causes:* most likely, enhanced automaticity due to increased adrenergic tone, reentry, and parasystole. Diseases that cause atrial enlargement usually cause atrial and junctional ectopic beats, while diseases that cause ventricular dysfunction cause ventricular ectopic beats. These ectopic beats are also seen in patients with no apparent structural heart disease.

c. *Diagnosis:* ectopic beats can occur early (premature beat) or late (atrial escape beat) in the cardiac cycle. Atrial ectopic beats usually have a different p-wave morphology from the sinus p-waves. If the atrial ectopic beats occur very early, the atrial beats may not be conducted. Junctional ectopic beats usually are manifested as narrow QRS beats unless there is aberrancy. These beats can be preceded or followed by a retrograde p-wave. Ventricular ectopic beats are usually wide QRS complexes.

d. *Differential diagnosis:* junctional ectopic beats can sometimes resemble atrial ectopic beats if there are retrograde p-waves. Junctional beats that are aberrant can also resemble ventricular ectopic beats.

e. *Treatment:* no treatment is necessary unless the patient is very symptomatic. The underlying cause should be corrected prior to initiation of treatment.

VI. Differential Diagnosis

A. ECG criteria for tachycardias

When the patient is stable and if the ECG of the arrhythmia has been obtained, the rhythm can then be determined by systemically going through three steps:

1. Determine whether the QRS complexes are predominantly narrow or wide.
2. Determine the heart rate.
3. Search for p-waves, which may be hidden in the QRS or the T-waves.

After determining these conditions, the differential diagnosis can be narrowed, as shown in Table 17-3. Ladder diagrams are also quite useful for the analysis of various rhythm disturbances on the ECG. Care should be taken that ECG artifacts are excluded as a potential cause of the ECG abnormality.

VII. Treatment

A. Emergent management of arrhythmias

There are several potentially dangerous arrhythmias that need to be treated quickly. The most important factor in determining whether treatment needs to be administered emergently is how well the rhythm is tolerated hemodynamically. In simple terms, this is assessed by the patient's state of consciousness and blood pressure. If the patient is hemodynamically stable and asymptomatic, one should obtain a 12-lead ECG to allow a more precise diagnosis. However, if the patient is unstable with hypotension, presyncope, or syncope, treatment should be administered immediately. If no pulse is present, cardiopulmonary resuscitation and advanced cardiac life support should be started. These protocols and methods are not covered here. If the patient is bradycardic and hypotensive, give atropine, 1–2 mg IV initially, followed by an infusion of isoproterenol, 1–5 µg/kg/min. If the patient is persistently bradycardic and hypotensive, external or transvenous temporary pacing should be done. The rate at which the pacemaker is set should be determined by hemodynamic parameters.

Both supraventricular and ventricular tachyarrhythmias should be treated emergently when they cause hemodynamic compromise. If the patient has a hemodynamically unstable tachycardia, immediate DC cardioversion is the best therapy. Once the tachyarrhythmia is treated and a safer rhythm is achieved, drug therapy should be initiated to prevent recurrence of the tachyarrhythmia.

B. Cardioversion and defibrillation

DC cardioversion is usually performed for the elective conversion of atrial fibrillation or ventricular tachycardia to sinus rhythm. In this case, 100 to 200 J is delivered, synchronized to the R wave. For ventricular fibrillation, an unsynchronized shock of higher energy levels (usually 300 to 360 J) is used.

C. Drugs

1. Classification system: the modified Vaughn-Williams classification system is useful if its limitations are kept in mind.

D. Devices

1. Pacemakers

a. Pacemakers are used to treat symptomatic, severe bradyarrhythmias such as sick sinus syndrome or complete AV block.

b. A three-letter code is used to describe the mode of pacing. In this code, the first letter refers to the chamber paced, the second to the chamber sensed, and the third to the action the pacemaker takes when it senses. Abbreviations used include A, atrial, V, ventricular, D, dual or both, I, inhibited, and T, triggered. For example, a

Table 17-3. Differential Diagnosis of Tachycardias

QRS Complex	Heart Rate	
	Slow	Fast
Narrow	Sinus, AJR	ST, SVT, MFAT, AF, AFL
Wide	AJRa, AIVR	SVTa, VT, VF, TP

Abbreviations: AJR, accelerated junctional rhythm; AJRa, accelerated junctional rhythm with aberrancy; AF, atrial fibrillation; AFL, atrial flutter; AIVR, accelerated idioventricular rhythm; MFAT, multifocal atrial tachycardia; SVT, supraventricular tachycardia including paroxysmal atrial tachycardia, atrioventricular nodal reentry and atrioventricular reentry; ST, sinus tachycardia; TP, torsades de pointes; VF, ventricular fibrillation; VT, ventricular tachycardia.

VVI pacemaker is a ventricular demand pacemaker.

2. Implantable cardiovertor defibrillators are used to treat patients with malignant ventricular arrhythmias (sustained ventricular tachycardia or ventricular fibrillation) who are refractory to or intolerant of antiarrhythmic therapy. The device works by sensing a malignant rhythm and then defibrillating the patient via electrodes placed around the heart. More advanced versions of the device will be able to convert some rhythms back to normal by pacing techniques and will also be able to treat bradyarrhythmias.

E. Catheter ablation

This relatively new approach is of particular value for many SVTs. In the past, DC current was used to deliver energy through an electrode catheter placed next to an accessory pathway (in Wolff-Parkinson-White syndrome) or an arrhythmia focus in an attempt to cure the condition. More recently, radiofrequency energy has been used with greater safety and success.

F. Surgical approaches

Surgery can be used for arrhythmias refractory to the above approaches. In patients with ventricular tachycardia and a left ventricular aneurysm, aneurysmectomy with electrophysiology-map guided resection of the arrhythmia focus can be performed, with a 10% operative mortality and an 80% overall success rate.

VIII. **Patient Monitoring**

Follow-up can be performed, using the same diagnostic studies described earlier as appropriate.

IX. **Prognosis**

Prognosis is dependent on the presenting arrhythmia and the severity and prognosis of the underlying heart disease. An important predictor of risk in patients with ventricular arrhythmias is the degree of left ventricular dysfunction.

Bibliography

Brugada P, Brugada J, Mont L, et al: A new approach to the differential diagnosis of a regular tachycardia with a wide QRS complex. *Circulation* 83:1649–1659, 1991.

Chou TC: *Electrocardiography in Clinical Practice*, ed 2. Philadelphia, WB Saunders, 1986.

Chung EK: *Principles of Cardiac Arrhythmias*, ed 3. Baltimore, Williams & Wilkins, 1983.

Marriott HJL: *Practical Electrocardiography*, ed 8. Baltimore, Williams & Wilkins, 1988.

CHAPTER 18

Congestive Heart Failure

John T. Barron, M.D., Ph.D.
Joseph E. Parrillo, M.D.

I. **Definition**

Congestive heart failure is a term describing a group of syndromes of myocardial dysfunction, the common feature of which is abnormally elevated left ventricular end-diastolic and pulmonary capillary wedge pressures, resulting in pulmonary edema. Two general categories of cardiac dysfunction can be discerned.

A. Systolic dysfunction, accounting for the majority of cases, is characterized by impaired myocardial contractility and is usually accompanied by a reduced left ventricular ejection fraction ($< 50\%$), although impairment of right ventricular function is frequently also present.

B. Diastolic dysfunction, accounting for 10 to 30% of cases, is characterized by normal or mildly reduced systolic function, but the major abnormalities are impaired diastolic compliance and active relaxation properties of the left ventricle.

The failing myocardium frequently exhibits both systolic and diastolic abnormalities.

II. **Etiology**

A. Systolic dysfunction

1. Ischemia and infarction (i.e., myocardial infarction with attendant scarring and fibrosis of the myocardium) leads to loss of myocardium and of subsequent contractile function.

   a. In the absence of frank infarction, ischemic but viable myocardium may exhibit hypocontractile function. This is referred to as *stunned* or *hibernating* myocardium.

2. States of chronic pressure overload

   a. Chronic hypertension—leads to left ventricular hypertrophy and, if long-standing, may result in dilatation and diminished contractility.

   b. Obstruction to aortic outflow, that is, aortic stenosis.

3. States of chronic volume overload

   a. Valvular heart disease
      (1) Mitral regurgitation
      (2) Aortic regurgitation

   b. Congenital heart disease
      (1) Ventricular septal defects
      (2) Patent ductus arteriosus

4. Cardiomyopathies—diseases affecting cardiac muscle directly

a. Dilated cardiomyopathy
   (1) Infectious processes producing myocarditis: viral (e.g., echo and coxsackie viruses) and parasitic (Chagas disease).
   (2) Chronic inflammatory/immunological processes (e.g., collagen vascular disease).
   (3) Endocrinologic abnormalities (e.g., thyroid disorders).
   (4) Toxins (e.g., ethanol, cobalt).
   (5) Nutritional deficiencies (e.g., selenium, thiamine).
   (6) Idiopathic—no identifiable etiology.

B. Diastolic dysfunction
   1. Chronic pressure overload in hypertension and aortic disease leads to left ventricular hypertrophy and an increase in myocardial mass. Hypertrophied myocardium may have abnormal compliance and relaxation properties.
   2. Restrictive cardiomyopathies
      a. Infiltrative disease processes
         (1) Amyloidosis.
         (2) Granulomatous diseases (sarcoidosis).
         (3) Hemochromatosis.
         (4) Idiopathic fibrosis of myocardium, with and without eosinophilia.
   3. Hypertrophic cardiomyopathies (HCM). Marked myocardial hypertrophy develops in the absence of hypertension or other known causes of hypertrophy. HCM has a genetic component to its etiology; it is autosomal dominant with variable penetrance.
      a. Obstructive type: a gradient can be demonstrated across the left ventricular outflow tract. Usually the septum is thickened to a greater extent than the free wall of left ventricle; this condition is termed *asymmetrical septal hypertrophy (ASH)*. The obstruction is usually caused by apposition of hypertrophied septum with the anterior mitral valve leaflet.
      b. Nonobstructive type: there is no gradient across left ventricular outflow tract. This may be seen with ASH or with concentric hypertrophy.

III. Pathophysiology
A. Systolic dysfunction and acute congestive heart failure

1. Physiologic compensatory mechanisms
   The failing myocardium generates insufficient contractile force, resulting in reduced forward cardiac output and decreased arterial blood pressure. This triggers a series of compensatory neurohumoral reflexes which serve to augment forward cardiac output and maintain normal blood pressure.
   a. Increase in heart rate (cardiac output = heart rate × stroke volume).
   b. Increase in systemic vascular resistance (SVR) (blood pressure = cardiac output × SVR).
   c. Increase in ventricular preload shifts the position of the left ventricle to a higher position on the Frank-Starling curve, resulting in augmented contractile force. Preload is increased by:
      (1) Venoconstriction
      (2) Increased intraventricular volume as a consequence of enhanced salt and water reabsorption by the kidney in response to reduced renal blood flow.
   d. Increase in myocardial contractility
      Attempt to offset the initial impaired contractile performance of the left ventricle. It is mediated by catecholamines (epinephrine and norepinephrine) and possibly by other hormones.
2. Neurohormones in congestive heart failure
   a. Catecholamines
      (1) Norepinephrine—predominantly an α-adrenergic agonist with some β-adrenergic activity.
      (2) Epinephrine—both a β- and an α-adrenergic agonist. Catecholamine secretion mediates arterial and venous vasoconstriction, and increases heart rate and contractility.
   b. Renin-angiotensin-aldosterone system.
      Renin is released from the kidney in response to reduced renal blood flow. Renin promotes conversion of angiotensin I to angiotensin II, which is a potent vasoconstricting agent with inotropic properties. Angiotensin II also results in elaboration of aldosterone, which promotes increased salt and water reabsorption by the kidney.

c. Antidiuretic hormone (vasopressin). It is secreted by the hypothalamus and is involved in volume regulation.

d. Atrial natriuretic factor. Produced in the right and left atria in response to elevated pressures. It has inotropic and vasodilating properties, as well as natriuretic actions. Its precise role in heart failure is presently ill-defined.

B. Systolic dysfunction and chronic congestive heart failure

1. "Overshoot" of compensatory mechanisms. Arterial vasoconstriction, although initially beneficial, is eventually deleterious to the myocardium if extended chronically. Systemic vascular resistance is a major component of left ventricular afterload. Increased afterload impedes left ventricular ejection, leading to further diminution of cardiac output. This results in more intense vasoconstriction and a further increase in afterload. Thus, a vicious circle is initiated.

2. Chronic neurohormonal activation
Catecholamine and angiotensin exert an adverse effect on myocardial cells when present in high concentrations for extended periods. This may account for a further depression of myocardial performance. Furthermore, chronic exposure to catecholamines results in a down-regulation of β-1 receptors in the heart, rendering the heart less responsive to the inotropic effect of β-adrenergic agonists.

3. Biochemical abnormalities of failing myocardium

   a. Abnormal handling of intracellular Ca^{+2}.

   b. Alteration of myosin isoform composition.

   c. Diminution of phosphodiesterase activity.

C. Diastolic dysfunction

1. Compliance and diastolic relaxation abnormality of the ventricles result in elevated left ventricular filling pressure, causing pulmonary edema.

2. Altered Frank-Starling relationship
Although left ventricular filling pressure is elevated, the poorly distensible, noncompliant left ventricle operates on a low position on the Frank-Starling ventricular performance curve. Therefore, con-

tractile force and thus cardiac output may be diminished.

IV. **Diagnosis**

A. History—specific causes of cardiac decompensation should be sought.

B. Signs and symptoms

1. Dyspnea on exertion; if there is severe congestive heart failure, dyspnea may occur at rest. Paroxysmal nocturnal dyspnea, orthopnea, and nocturia may occur as a consequence of mobilization of edema fluid at night in the supine position.

2. Fatigue—manifestation of the low cardiac output state.

3. Peripheral edema.

4. Distended neck veins indicative of elevated right-sided cardiac pressures.

5. Heart failure attributable to congenital or valvular heart disease may have additional specific signs and symptoms.

C. Functional classification of heart failure
The extent and severity of heart failure are important prognostically. The New York Heart Association's functional classification categorizes heart failure into four functional classes:

   • Class I—patients with cardiac disease but with no or minimal limitation of physical activity; prognosis good.

   • Class II—slight limitation of physical activity; ordinary physical activity may produce symptoms; prognosis good with therapy.

   • Class III—marked limitation of physical activity; less than ordinary physical activity produces symptoms; prognosis fair with therapy.

   • Class IV—severe limitation of physical activity, with symptoms present at rest; prognosis poor despite therapy.

D. Physical examination

1. Cardiac examination

   a. Palpation

      (1) Point of maximal impulse (PMI) displaced laterally and inferiorly.

      (2) Precordial lifts or heaves indicative of hypertrophied and/or dilated right or left ventricle.

      (3) Palpable fourth or third heart sounds.

   b. Auscultation

      (1) Irregular rhythm if atrial fibrillation is present; ectopic beats indicative of premature ventricular or atrial contractions are common.

(2) Fourth or third heart sounds.

(3) Systolic murmur indicative of mitral valve incompetence as a consequence of marked dilatation of the left ventricular cavity.

(4) Other auscultative features may be present with specific congenital or valvular causes of heart failure.

2. Lung examination
   a. Pulmonary crackles or rales; diminished breath sounds in bases indicative of the presence of pleural effusion.
   b. Diffuse wheezes and rhonchi may indicate interstitial and/or alveolar pulmonary edema.

3. Neck examination
   a. Jugular venous distension at 45°
   b. Hepatojugular reflux
      Gentle pressure applied on the abdomen in the right upper gradient increases venous return, which is not accommodated in the right heart, where pressure is already elevated. Consequently, jugular venous distension increases or now becomes manifest.

4. Abdomen
   a. In chronic severe heart failure, the liver may be enlarged, tender, and pulsatile (tricuspid regurgitation) as a consequence of elevated right heart pressure. Ascites may also be present.

5. Extremities
   a. Varying degrees and extent of lower extremity edema.
   b. Clubbing may be present in long-standing heart failure.
   c. Cyanosis may be present in congenital heart disease with right-to-left shunting or in states of severely depressed cardiac output.

E. Diagnostic tests
   1. Chest x-ray
      Usually exhibits cardiomegaly, pulmonary vascular redistribution, and interstitial and/or alveolar pulmonary edema. Pleural effusions are often seen. Specific radiologic findings may also suggest specific congenital or valvular diseases. Cardiomegaly may not be present in cases of predominant diastolic dysfunction.
   2. Electrocardiogram
      Nonspecific ST- and T-wave abnormalities are common. Q-waves are usually indicative of prior myocardial infarction. Voltage criteria suggestive of ventricular hypertrophy may also be present.
   3. Echocardiography
      Discerns systolic and diastolic abnormalities, assesses the presence of wall motion abnormalities suggestive or ischemic heart disease, and assesses the presence of congenital or valvular diseases. Also provides a good estimate of the left ventricular ejection fraction.
   4. Gated blood pool nuclear scanning
      Provides a more quantitative measure of the left ventricular ejection fraction.
   5. Cardiac catheterization and coronary angiography
      Diagnostic gold standard. Provides measurement of intracardiac pressures, cardiac output, and pulmonary and systemic resistances and defines the coronary anatomy.

V. **Differential Diagnosis**
   A. Any disease process resulting in dyspnea is included in the differential diagnosis.
      1. Acute and chronic lung processes
      2. Noncardiogenic pulmonary edema
   B. Any disease process producing chronic fatigue should be considered.
   C. Volume overload states
      1. Renal insufficiency
      2. Liver failure

VI. **Treatment**
   Goals of treatment are to achieve hemodynamic stability and to improve symptoms and survival. The underlying cause of heart failure should be corrected if possible.
   A. Systolic dysfunction—acute severe heart failure.
      1. Diuretics
         a. Furosemide, 20 to 120 mg intravenously one to four times daily, depending on the severity of pulmonary edema. K^+ supplementation usually required.
         b. Metalozone, 5 to 15 mg orally once or twice daily, may be added for more brisk diuresis or used in patients refractory to furosemide alone.
      2. Vasodilators
         Used to decrease ventricular afterload, decrease preload, and relieve pulmonary edema.
         a. Acute or severe heart failure

(1) Nitroprusside

Give 0.5 to 10 μg/kg/min titrated to maintain systolic blood pressure of approximately 100 to 110 mmHg. Placement of an arterial catheter for close blood pressure monitoring is usually needed.

(2) Nitroglycerin

Give 20–40 to 400–600 μg/min as needed, titrated to a systolic blood pressure of 100–110 mmHg. Topical nitroglycerin ointment, 1 to 2 in. every 6 hr, may be used in milder forms of heart failure.

Intravenous agents may be weaned as the patient improves and oral vasodilators described below are instituted.

(3) Inotropes

(a) Dobutamine, 5–20 μg/kg/min.

(b) Amrinone: 0.75 mg/kg loading dose over 15 min, then 5–20 μg/kg/min.

(c) Dopamine, 2–20 μg/kg/min. Dopamine is the preferred agent when hypotension complicating heart failure is present. It may also be used in doses of 2–25 μg/kg/min to enhance renal blood flow and promote diuresis.

(d) Digoxin—a modest inotropic agent that is available orally for long-term therapy. It is most useful to control the heart rate in atrial fibrillation. It may be loaded over 24 hr, giving a total dose (in three to four doses) of 1.0 to 1.25 mg, followed by 0.125 to 0.25 mg daily.

(4) Intra-aortic balloon pump (IABP)

For patients with refractory heart failure inadequately responsive to maximal drug therapy described above. The device is inserted in the ascending aorta. The balloon inflates during diastole and deflates during systole, thus reducing ventricular afterload and improving coronary blood flow. It is contraindicated in aortic regurgitation and aortic dissection.

B. Systolic dysfunction—chronic congestive heart failure or mild acute congestive heart failure

The regimen of diuretic and digoxin is standard therapy. Patients who are inadequately controlled or have a left ventricular ejection fraction < 40% should also be treated with a vasodilator.

1. Diuretic

Furosemide, 20 to 80 mg once or twice a day as needed. K^+ supplementation usually required.

2. Digoxin, 0.25 to 0.25 mg orally daily

3. Vasodilator

a. Angiotensin-converting enzyme inhibitors—preferred agents

(1) Captopril: start at 6.25 mg orally three times per day; advance to 50 mg three times per day as tolerated.

(2) Enalapril: start at 5 mg orally twice per day; advance to 20 mg twice per day as tolerated

(3) Lisinopril: start at 5 mg orally daily; advance to 20 mg daily as tolerated

b. Combination of isosorbide dinitrate, 20–40 mg two to three times per day, and hydralazine, 25–75 mg daily as tolerated.

C. Diastolic dysfunction (with normal or near-normal systolic function)

1. Mild diuresis

a. Overdiuresis may decrease left ventricular filling pressures and size to the point where ventricular performance is adversely affected because of the Frank-Starling mechanism

b. Furosemide, 20 to 40 mg orally daily.

2. β-blockade

a. Decreases the heart rate, allowing more time for diastolic filling of the left ventricle. β-blockers are especially effective in hypertrophic obstructive cardiomyopathy because negative inotropic effects help relieve outflow tract obstruction.

b. Agents

(1) Propranolol, 20 to 80 mg four times daily.

(2) Other β-blockers are probably equally effective.

3. Ca^{+2} channel blockade

a. Lusitropic agents improve the diastolic properties of the myocardium, modestly slow the heart rate, and are modestly negative inotropic.

b. Agents
   (1) Verapamil, 80–240 mg three times per day.
   (2) Diltiazem, 30–120 mg two or three times per day.

D. Hypertrophic obstructive cardiomyopathy (see Chapter 22)

1. β-blocker and/or Ca^{+2} channel blocker as above.

2. Disopyramide (because of its negative inotropic properties) in cases refractory to the above agents. The dose is 400–800 mg daily in divided doses.

3. Surgical myotomy or myomectomy of the septum in refractory cases with severe heart failure.

VII. Patient Monitoring

A. Acute

Patients with severe refractory heart failure, especially with hemodynamic instability, should be monitored with a pulmonary artery catheter to help guide therapeutic management. An arterial line is also indicated in patients who are unstable, especially if pressors are required.

B. Chronic

Serial echocardiograms may be performed to gauge noninvasively the improvement or deterioration of ventricular function. A gated nuclear ventriculogram may also be performed to assess quantitatively the changes in ejection fraction.

C. Therapeutic regimen

Adjustments in diuretics and other medicines are frequently needed on an outpatient basis. In patients with severe heart failure (New York Heart Association class IV), intermittent infusions of dobutamine or oral levodopa may provide symptomatic improvement. A subgroup of patients with idiopathic dilated cardiomyopathy may benefit symptomatically from cautious use of low doses of β-blockers, though this therapy is controversial.

VIII. Prognosis

The course of congestive heart failure is variable, depending on the severity of disease on initial presentation and the underlying pathology. Heart failure attributable to valvular lesions, hypertension, or congenital heart disease usually improves substantially with correction of the primary pathology. Idiopathic dilated cardiomyopathy has a bleak prognosis, with 2-year mortality of 30 to 50%. Heart failure due to multiple myocardial infarctions also has a poor long-term prognosis. Suitable candidates who remain severely symptomatic despite maximal medical management should be considered for cardiac transplantation.

Bibliography

Dzau VJ, Creager MA: Progress in angiotensin converting enzyme inhibition in heart failure: Rationale, mechanisms, and clinical response. In Weber KT (ed): *Heart Failure: Current Concepts and Management.* Cardiology Clinics, Series 7/1. Philadelphia, WB Saunders, 1989, pp 87–89.

Parmley WW: Principles in the management of congestive heart failure. In Parmley WW, Chatterjee K (eds): *Cardiology,* Vol 2: *Cardiovascular Disease.* Philadelphia: JB Lippincott, 1989.

Rahimtoola SH: The pharmacologic treatment of chronic congestive heart failure. *Circulation* 80:693–699, 1989.

Stauffer JC, Gaasch WH: Recognition and treatment of left ventricular diastolic dysfunction. *Prog Cardiovasc Dis* 32:319–325, 1990.

Weber KT, Janicki JS: Pathological heart failure. In Weber KT (ed): *Heart Failure: Current Concepts and Management.* Cardiology Clinics, Series 7/1. Philadelphia: WB Saunders, 1989, pp 11–25.

CHAPTER 19

Valvular Heart Disease

Lloyd W. Klein, M.D.
John T. Barron, M.D., Ph.D.

I. Aortic Stenosis (AS)
  A. Etiology
    1. Supraventricular AS
      a. Disease of children; rare in adults
      b. Associated with:
        (1) Hypercalcemia of infancy
        (2) "Elfin" facies
        (3) William syndrome: mental retardation, prominent forehead
        (4) Congenital rubella
      c. Cause of outflow obstruction
        (1) Hourglass deformity of the ascending aorta
        (2) Diaphragm-like stenosis of the ascending aorta.
        (3) Hypoplasia of the ascending aorta
      d. Other associations
        (1) Stenosis of aortic arch branches
        (2) Peripheral pulmonary arterial stenosis (rubella syndrome)
        (3) Myxomatous mitral valve
        (4) Type (1) above associated with coronary artery ostial stenosis
    2. Valvular aortic stenosis
      a. Congenital
        (1) Bicuspid valve—two unequal-sized cups, with a poorly developed raphe extending into the larger cusp.
          (a) Affects 1–2% of the adult population (most common congenital heart defect).
          (b) Usually calcifies and becomes stenotic at ages 40–60.
          (c) Present in 80% of patients with coarctation of the aorta; also associated with patent ductus arteriosus.
          (d) A 4:1 male predominance.
        (2) Unicuspid valve—severe aortic stenosis in infancy/childhood.
      b. Acquired
        (1) Calcific
          (a) Acquired tricuspid valve stenosis of the elderly due to deposition of calcium in the sinuses of Valsalva.
          (b) Calcification and fibrosis prevent normal opening of cusps.
        (2) Rheumatic
          (a) Commonly associated with mi-

tral valve thickening; isolated aortic involvement rare.

   (b) Commissural fusion with fibrous contracture is cause of stenosis.

   (c) The rigid orifice which results frequently is both stenotic and regurgitant.

  (3) Rare causes

   (a) Rheumatoid—nodular thickening of valve cusps.

   (b) Ochronosis.

3. Subvalvular aortic outflow obstruction

  a. Membranous type—a fibrous collar encircles the outflow tract

  b. Idiopathic hypertrophic subaortic stenosis (IHSS)—dynamic outflow obstruction caused by abnormal septal hypertrophy with impingement on outflow tract by anterior mitral valve leaflet. A form of cardiomyopathy but may be confused with aortic stenosis.

B. Hemodynamic determinants

1. Severity of valvular obstruction to left ventricular (LV) outflow.

  a. Aorta: LV systolic mean or peak-to-peak gradient dependent on cardiac output (Gorlin formula: area of cardiac output/(gradient)$^{1/2}$).

  b. Critical AS: gradient > 50 mmHg with normal cardiac output; valve area < 0.7 cm^2.

  c. With exercise, cardiac output does not increase due to increased gradient and arteriolar vasodilation.

2. Adequacy of LV hypertrophy.

  a. Stroke volume (SV) initially maintained by LV hypertrophy; when LV dilation occurs to compensate further, congestive heart failure (CHF) will eventually result.

  b. Elevated left ventricular end-diastolic pressure (LVEDP) is not due to CHF but rather to diminished compliance secondary to hypertrophy; pre-A-wave LV pressure is true reflection of pulmonary venous pressure.

  c. LV hypertrophy counterbalances increased wall stress, but dilation further increases wall stress, with consequent decreased ejection fraction.

3. Preservation of atrial transport

  a. Atrial contraction provides 40% of SV versus 10–30% in normal individuals.

  b. Atrial fibrillation or AV dissociation causes rapid deterioration.

C. Symptoms

1. Hemodynamically significant aortic stenosis can precede symptoms; 3–5% of "asymptomatic" patients experience sudden death.

2. Exertion may cause syncope due to inability to increase cardiac output; blood pressure falls due to arteriolar vasodilation.

3. Angina may occur due to increased myocardial oxygen demand in the context of diminished perfusion and coronary flow reserve. Also, expect coexistent coronary artery disease (CAD) in 50% of patients with angina.

4. LV failure (dyspnea, orthopnea, paroxysmal nocturnal dyspnea, pulmonary edema) is the most serious symptom, with 80% mortality within 4 years of onset.

5. Gastrointestinal hemorrhage due to angiodysplasia of the right side of the colon.

D. Physical signs

1. Diminished pulse pressure ("parvis et tardus" pulse).

  a. Delayed carotid upstroke *not* observed in elderly patients with less compliant vessels.

2. Prominent a-wave in jugular venous pulse.

3. S$_4$ gallop.

4. Length and intensity of systolic ejection murmur and lateness of peaking in systole should correlate with severity. Hypertension or LV failure shorten the murmur, causing underestimation of severity.

5. Murmur radiates to carotid arteries.

6. Valsalva maneuver and standing decrease the murmur; premature ventricular contractions and amyl nitrate increase it.

7. Soft, single-split S$_2$.

8. Aortic ejection sound in young patients.

  a. Gallavardin effect: murmur may be located only at the apex, simulating mitral regurgitation.

E. Noninvasive evaluation

1. Electrocardiogram (ECG) almost invariably shows severe LV hypertrophy.

2. Chest x-ray—shows calcification, dilated aortic root, cardiac silhouette size.

3. Echocardiography/Doppler—above plus relative wall thickness, coexistent regurgitation and other valvular lesions, wall motion, gradient determination.

F. Treatment

1. Medical therapy
   a. Asymptomatic patient: subacute bacterial endocarditis (SBE) prophylaxis, avoidance of strenuous exercise and competitive sports.
   b. onset of symptoms
      (1) Echocardiography/Doppler ultrasound to assess gradient and valve area; if subcritical, catheterization is required.
      (2) Advanced age (i.e., > 70 years) *not* a contraindication to surgery.
      (3) Onset of LV dilation with CHF: digitalis, diuresis, and consideration of surgery.
      (4) Avoid nitrates and marked diuresis, which may prompt preload reduction/dehydration, hypotension, and death.
2. Aortic valve replacement
   a. Results
      (1) There is 4–5% mortality without LV failure; 5–10% mortality with CHF or low ejection fraction (EF).
      (2) If CAD is present, coronary artery bypass graft should be done; however, increased mortality and postoperative infarction.
   b. Early complications (6 weeks postoperatively)
      (1) Staphylococcal and anaerobic endocarditis
      (2) Paravalvular leak
   c. Late complications
      (1) Thromboembolism—prescribe anticoagulants or aspirin, depending on prosthetic valve used.
      (2) Hemolysis—especially common with paravalvular leak.
      (3) Bacterial endocarditis.
      (4) Persistent CHF, dysrhythmia.
3. Balloon valvuloplasty
   a. Possibly beneficial in selected elderly or critically ill patients who are not surgical candidates.
   b. Short-term results show frequent incidence of strokes, procedure-related seizures, hemorrhage, need for surgical arterial repair, and calcium emboli. Fatal LV rupture also described.
   c. Long-term follow-up shows recurrence rate of up to 50%.
   d. Currently, valve replacement suggested except under unusual circumstances, using valvuloplasty as a bridge to surgery.

II. **Aortic Insufficiency (AI)**
   A. Etiology
      1. Valvular
         a. Rheumatic—due to contraction of leaflets; male preponderance.
         b. Infectious endocarditis
         c. Collagen vascular diseases
            (1) Ankylosing spondylitis
            (2) Lupus erythematosus
            (3) Reiter's disease
            (4) Rheumatoid arthritis
            (5) Relapsing polychondritis
            (6) Behcet's syndrome
         d. Sinus of Valsalva aneurysm—congenital or acquired
         e. Aortic cusp fenestration
         f. Congenital bicuspid valve
         g. With large ventricular septal defect, due to inadequate support of noncoronary cusp and herniation into defect (supracristal)
      2. Secondary to aortic root dilation
         a. Hypertension—usually mild AI produced
         b. Marfan's syndrome—cystic medial necrosis
         c. Acute ascending aortic dissection—usually due to long-standing hypertension or Marfan's syndrome or pregnancy
         d. Syphilitic aortitis—marked dilation of ascending aorta with calcification
         e. Uremia
         f. Mycotic aneurysm
         g. Ehlers-Danlos syndrome
         h. Osteogenesis imperfecta
         i. Giant cell aortitis
         j. Takayasu's disease
         k. Traumatic
   B. Hemodynamic determinants
      1. Chronic AI
         a. Regurgitant orifice size
            (1) From 40% to 60% of backflow occurs in the first 0.2 sec in early diastole
         b. Aortic—LVEDP pressure gradient across orifice
            (1) LV volume overload induces LV dilation in an elongated but preserved semiellipsoidal shape to compensate and normalize stroke volume.
            (2) However, LV dilation increases LV wall stress (La Place's law). The ratio

of LV wall thickness to LV cavity radius remains constant.

(3) Initially, the increased left ventricular end-diastolic volume (LVEDV) leads to increased SV, without change in LVEDP. In later stages, increased LVEDV further increases LVEDP, with decreased EF and, ultimately, decreased SV.

(4) In most severe stage, aortic diastolic pressure equals LVEDP; LA and PCWP rise, but not as high as LVEDP, leading to premature mitral valve closure.

   c. Duration of diastole (i.e., diastolic period per minute)

2. Acute AI

   a. Course determined by lack of time to allow LV compensation to develop.

(1) Hence, the regurgitant volume flows into a normal-sized LV, leading immediately to the condition described in Subsection b (4) above. Additionally, cardiac output is low, and the physical signs associated with wide pulse pressure (see below) are absent.

C. Physical examination

1. Wide arterial pulse pressure

   a. Rapid arterial upstroke and collapse due to decreased aortic diastolic pressure.

(1) Corrigan's pulse—marked pulsations over any peripheral artery.

(2) De Musset's sign—rhythmic head bobbing synchronous with heart beat.

(3) Quincke's sign—alternate nail bed reddening and blanching.

(4) Pistol shot sound—characteristic systolic murmur over femoral artery.

(5) Duroziez's sign—biphasic femoral artery bruit detectable by applying mild stethoscope pressure.

2. Auscultation

   a. Decrescendo, early diastolic murmur.

(1) Severity of AI correlates with duration, not loudness, of murmur.

(2) In valvular etiologies, murmur heard best at lower left sternal border and apex.

(3) In aortic root etiologies, murmur heard best along right sternal border.

   b. Systolic ejection murmur may be associated with AS or may be due to turbulence from increased SV.

   c. S_3 gallop and Austin Flint murmur (mid-late diastolic rumble) indicate severe AI.

   d. Valsalva maneuver and squatting increase murmur; amyl nitrate decreases murmur.

   e. In acute AI, findings are those of tachycardia, peripheral vasoconstriction, and pulmonary congestion.

3. Noninvasive evaluation

   a. ECG—LV hypertrophy

   b. Chest x-ray—LV dilation, mild ascending aorta dilation except in aortic dissection, Marfan's syndrome, and syphilis.

   c. Echocardiogram

(1) Fine fluttering of mitral valve

(2) Increased LV volume and aortic root size

(3) vegetation, premature mitral closure if present.

(4) Doppler ultrasound—to assess severity.

4. Aortography—to assess degree of contrast reflux

D. Treatment

1. Medical therapy

   a. SBE prophylaxis

   b. Antistreptococcal prophylaxis, if origin is rheumatic, up to age 35.

   c. Screening and penicillin therapy for syphilis.

2. Aortic valve replacement

   a. Acute AI

(1) First sign of CHF or hemodynamic instability.

(2) Premature mitral closure.

(3) Endocarditis—emboli, refractory CHF

     (a) Probably for staphylococcal and fungal infections.

     (b) Possibly for very large vegetations.

(4) Aortic dissection with acute AI—urgent surgery required.

   b. Chronic AI

(1) Symptomatic AI requiring medical therapy.

(2) Known enlarging cardiac silhouette by chest x-ray or when EF has recently become < 50%.

(3) Asymptomatic—controversial indications include:

(a) Fall in EF by radionuclide angiography with exercise.
(b) LV systolic dimension > 55 mm or echo.
(c) Based on inability to perform normal amount of exercise.

   c. Operative Outcome
      (a) Perioperative mortality 5%
      (b) EF often decreases by 5% or more, so EF < 20% preoperatively is the informal limit for surgical candidacy.

III. Mitral Stenosis

A. Etiology
1. Rhematic (only common cause)
2. Left arterial tumor (myxoma, thrombus)
3. Calcified mitral annulus (in presence of *massive* calcification)
4. Congenital

B. Hemodynamic determinants
1. Severity of valvular obstruction to LV inflow
   a. Critical valve area < 1.0 cm^2, or assuming normal LVEDP and cardiac output, an LV-LA pressure gradient of 10–15 mmHg, and a pulmonary capillary wedge pressure (PCWP) of 25 mmHg (with onset of CHF).
2. Rate of transmittal blood flow (determined by cardiac output and heart rate).
   a. Since one defense against CHF is to diminish volume with sodium restriction or diuretics, which also decreases cardiac output, calculation of valve area is particularly crucial (Gorlin formula).
   b. Atrial fibrillation, which is associated with a rapid ventricular rate and a shortened diastolic filling period, thus tends to raise PCWP and to increase the chances of CHF, especially due to loss of atrial transport.
3. Pulmonary vascular resistance
   a. With chronic pulmonary venous hypertension, pulmonary artery pressure increase pari passu.
   b. In many patients, the rise in pulmonary resistance is disproportionate to the elevation of LA/PCWP; thus, pulmonary vascular disease may cause symptoms and may not reverse completely (or even substantially) with medical or surgical treatment.
   c. When pulmonary hypertension attains systemic pressure, the patient is no longer operable.

C. Symptoms
1. Exertional dyspnea—usually the first symptom.
2. Fatigue and weakness.
3. Orthopnea and paroxysmal nocturnal dyspnea in later stages.
4. Hemoptysis (rupture of bronchopulmonary varices).
5. Syncope—uncommon in rheumatic disease but highly suggestive of myxoma or thrombus.
6. Emboli and palpitations in setting of chronic and/or paroxysmal atrial fibrillation.

D. Physical Findings
1. Palpation and inspection
   a. The LV size is normal in uncomplicated MS; thus, an abnormal heave and/or a displaced point of maximal impulse (PMI) suggests superimposed conditions.
   b. With pulmonary hypertension, a right ventricular (RV) heave, prominent jugular venous a-wave, and signs of chronic right heart failure are expected.
2. Auscultation
   a. Low-pitched, mid-late diastolic rumble heard best at the apex in the left lateral decubitus position.
   b. Neither the intensity of the murmur nor its length is reflective of its severity. In pulmonary hypertension, the murmur is often quite soft.
   c. In patients with sinus rhythm, there is presystolic accentuation of the murmur.
   d. An opening snap is commonly heard at the apex; it should be distinguished from second heart sound splitting by lack of variance with respiration.
   e. The first heart sound is accentuated.
   f. The pulmonary component of the second heart sound is accentuated if pulmonary hypertension is present.

E. Noninvasive evaluation
1. Electrocardiogram
   a. Atrial fibrillation is found in about one-third of patients.
   b. When sinus rhythm is present, left atrial enlargement is seen, evidenced by a broad, notched P-wave in the inferior leads and a wide negative deflection in V$_1$ (*P mitrale*).
   c. In uncomplicated MS, there is no LV hypertrophy.

d. As MS advances and pulmonary hypertension appears, the axis shifts rightward and RV hypertrophy develops.

2. Chest x-ray—left atrial (LA) dilation, calcified mitral valve, RV hypertrophy, pulmonary artery dilation, pulmonary venous congestion.

3. Echocardiogram/Doppler ultrasound—decreased diastolic slope of the anterior leaflet is diagnostic; thickened leaflets and calcification visible.

F. Therapy
1. Medical
a. Digoxin to control ventricular rate in atrial fibrillation; β-blockers useful if sinus rhythm is present.
b. Diuretics for symptomatic relief.
c. Asymptomatic patients may limit exertion severely, with major lifestyle changes, yet claim no symptoms.
d. Anticoagulation to prevent emboli.
e. SBE prophylaxis.
f. Rheumatic fever prophylaxis if age < 35.

2. Surgery
a. Valve replacement indicated when:
(1) Right heart failure becomes manifest.
(2) Dyspnea affects lifestyle.
b. Commissurotomy possible when there is no or minimal calcification and mitral regurgitation.
c. Pulmonary vascular resistance calculation before surgery to assess operative risk.

3. Valvuloplasty
a. Reasonable short- and long-term results in very experienced hands at a few centers.
b. Requires transseptal approach.
c. Very dilated LA, severe calcification, and presence of MR or LV dilation have poorer prognosis.

IV. Mitral Insufficiency
A. Etiology
1. Organic valvular diseases
a. Acquired
(1) Infectious endocarditis—perforation of leaflet, vegetation on valve, ruptured chordae.
(2) Rheumatic.
(3) Trauma.
(4) Rare causes—lupus erythematosus, Marfan's syndrome, carcinoid, scleroderma, Takayasu's aortitis, endocardial fibroelastosis.
b. Congenital
(1) Mitral valve prolapse—myxomatous degeneration, redundant leaflet tissue.
(2) Anomalous chordal insertion.
(3) Associated with common AV canal or ostium primum atrial septal defect, and corrected transposition of the great vessels.

2. Papillary muscle causes
a. Dysfunction or infarction due to coronary artery disease
b. Dysfunction due to infiltrative diseases—amyloid, sarcoid.

3. Chordal rupture
a. Endocarditis.
b. Myxomatous degeneration.
c. Ischemia/infarction.

4. Annular dilation
a. Produced by marked LV dilation—cardiomyopathy, hypertension, or with multiple myocardial infarctions.
b. Mitral annular calcification.

B. Hemodynamic determinants
1. Size of regurgitant orifice
a. Leakage occurs during ventricular systole from an actively contractile LV to an isometrically relaxed LA; thus, the leak is pansystolic.
b. As 50% of LV stroke volume may be ejected into the LA rather than into the aorta, cardiac output is diminished.
c. The LV dilates in a globular fashion to compensate and maintain SV and cardiac output. Eventually, EF decreases and LVEDP increases.

2. Systolic LV-LA pressure gradient
a. As LV dilates, LA dilates to keep LA and LVEDP normal.

3. LA compliance
a. When LA dilation is no longer an effective compensatory mechanism, LVEDP increases and pulmonary venous congestion results.
b. In acute MR, neither chamber has the time to dilate, and an acute volume overload is superimposed on the LA and pulmonary venous circulation, leading to acute CHF.

C. Physical Findings
1. Auscultation

a. Parasystolic murmur of blowing quality radiating to left axilla heard best at the apex.

b. When posterior leaflet or papillary muscle is dysfunctional, the murmur may radiate to the base of the heart and to the neck, mimicking AS.

c. Severity of MR correlates with intensity of murmur *except* in acute MR, when *no* murmur may be audible due to low cardiac output (c.o.)

2. Signs of right-sided failure, depending on pulmonary artery hypertension and RV dilation.

D. Noninvasive evaluation

1. ECG—may be normal, or suggestive of left atrial enlargement, left ventricular hypertrophy, or pulmonary hypertension, if present.

2. Echocardiography/Doppler—diagnostic of both severity and cause.

E. Cardiac catheterization

1. Pulmonary artery wedge pressure (PAWP) will show large v-waves when the LA is noncompliant, i.e., in acute MR or with severe chronic MR and massive LV and LA dilation.

2. Pulmonary hypertension, if present.

3. LV angiography—to assess degree of insufficiency.

F. Treatment

1. Medical therapy

a. Arteriolar vasodilation with no or minimal symptoms (i.e., New York Heart Association class I).

b. Six-month to yearly follow-up with noninvasive tests to plan surgery prior to marked LV dilation.

2. Surgical therapy

a. Repair of valve possible for annular dilation, redundant leaflet, and some cases of ruptured chordae.

b. Replacement required for most cases of organic vulvular and papillary muscle etiologies.

c. EF will usually decrease 5–10%. Thus, patients with EF < 20–25% are not usually considered surgical candidates.

d. Valve surgery indications

(1) Before LVEF < 55%.

(2) Before LV end-systolic volume > 50 ml/sq m.

(3) Before pulmonary artery

(4) New York Heart Association class III or significant class II symptoms.

V. Mitral Valve Prolapse (MVP)

A. Definition

Displacement or billowing superiorly of one or both mitral leaflets beyond the plane of the mitral valve annulus during systole.

B. Etiology

1. Idiopathic in most individuals with syndrome

a. Prevalence of 5–10% in general population

b. Strong hereditary component; transmitted as an autosomal dominant trait

2. Connective tissue disorder

a. Marfan's syndrome

b. Ehlers-Danlos syndrome

c. Osteogenesis imperfecta

d. Holt-Oram syndrome

3. Congenital malformation and other heart diseases

a. Primum and secundum atrial septal defects

b. Ebstein's anomaly

c. Hypertrophic obstructive cardiomyopathy

d. Wolf-Parkinson-White syndrome

e. Tricuspid valve prolapse frequently coexists

4. Acquired

a. Rheumatic

b. Papillary muscle dysfunction from any cause (e.g., coronary artery disease)

c. Rupture of chordae tendinae

C. Pathophysiology

1. Myxomatous proliferation and/or degeneration of mitral leaflets, resulting in billowing of leaflets into left atrium. May be associated with mitral insufficiency. MVP most common cause of mitral regurgitation requiring valve replacement.

2. Papillary muscle dysfunction leads to incorrect coaptation of mitral leaflets, resulting in prolapse with varying degrees of mitral insufficiency.

3. Other than the consequences of mitral regurgitation, the pathophysiology of the syndrome complex (i.e., palpitations, chest discomfort, dyspnea) is largely unknown.

D. History, signs, and symptoms

1. Features of idiopathic (acquired) form

a. Occurs predominantly in young women but can appear in both sexes and at all ages.

b. Asthenic habitus common.

c. Other associations:

(1) Pectus excavatum
(2) Straight back
(3) Shallow chest
d. Associated with thyroid disorders
e. Association with anxiety neurosis has been proposed
2. Symptoms and signs
a. Common—variable and evanescent
(1) Palpitations—especially during periods of psychological stress or upon exposure to stimulants such as caffeine or nicotine.
(2) Chest discomfort—non exertional and atypical.
(3) Dyspnea—may occur at rest or upon exertion. Dyspnea may be prominent if mitral regurgitation is significant.
b. Rare
(1) Cerebral embolic events—thought to be due to platelet thrombi arising from mitral valve.
(2) Syncope and sudden death—attributable to malignant ventricular arrhythmias.
(3) Other forms of MVP
History and features determined predominantly by associated cardiac pathology
E. Cardiac examination
1. Midsystolic click
a. Heard at left lower sternal border and apex.
b. Maneuvers which decrease volume of LV cavity (e.g., standing, straining phase of Valsalva maneuver) move click closer to the first heart sound.
c. Maneuvers which increase volume of LV cavity (e.g., raising thre legs in prone position, squatting) move click closer to the second heart sound.
2. Mid-late systolic murmur
a. May or may not be present.
b. Occasional early systolic murmur heard.
c. Maneuvers which affect movement of click usually affect murmur similarly; maneuvers may also result in murmur if this is not heard in the supine position.
3. Rhythm—may reveal frequent extrasystoles. Both click and murmur can be variable and evanescent.
F. Diagnosis
1. Physical examination
Midsystolic click (with or without murmur) that moves with maneuvers.

2. Noninvasive tests
a. Two-dimensional echocardiography and Doppler ultrasound
(1) Systolic displacement of one or both mitral leaflets at least 1 mm beyond mitral annulus.
(2) Doppler ultrasound may detect and assess the magnitude of coexisting mitral regurgitation.
3. Any co-existing cardiac pathology may also be assessed.
a. Electrocardiography
(1) Usually normal ECG, but T wave inversion in inferior leads may be seen. QT prolongation also reported. Atrial and ventricular extrasystoles not uncommon. Supraventricular and ventricular tachycardia also may occur.
(2) Ambulatory 24 hour Holter monitoring.
(a) Indicated to assess type and extent of symptomatic arrhythmias.
(3) Invasive tests—Left ventriculography
(a) Prolapse of mitral valve into left atrium
(b) Magnitude and severity of mitral regurgitation may be assessed.
(c) Any co-existing cardiac pathology may be assessed.
Note: Test rarely indicated; no advantage over echocardiography.
G. Differential diagnosis
1. Any cardiac or noncardiac cause of chest discomfort.
2. Other cardiac causes of ectopic beats.
3. Pulmonary and other cardiac causes of dyspnea.
H. Treatment
1. Asymptomatic or minimally symptomatic patients.
a. Reassurance of patient.
b. Avoidance of caffeine or nicotine.
2. Symptomatic patients
a. Chest discomfort and palpitations (severely symptomatic).
(1) β-blocker therapy: propranolol, 80–240 mg/day.
(2) Ca^{+2} channel blocker for patients intolerant of β-blocker: verapamil, 120–240 mg/day in divided doses.

b. Cerebral embolic events
   (1) Aspirin, 324 mg daily.
c. Syncope and sudden death
   (1) Electrophysiological studies to guide antiarrhythmic therapy.
d. Severe mitral valve regurgitation
   (1) Medical therapy for mitral regurgitation as outlined above.
   (2) Mitral valve replacement surgery when clinically indicated.
   (3) MVP patients with murmur
       (a) Antibiotic prophylaxis for dental and other surgical procedures.

I. Prognosis

In absence of malignant ventricular arrhythmias and severe mitral regurgitation, life expectancy similar to that of general population.

II. Tricuspid Stenosis and Insufficiency

A. Stenosis
   1. Etiology
      a. Rheumatic
         Isolated rheumatic tricuspid stenosis rare; almost always accompanied by rheumatic mitral valve disease.
   2. Hemodynamic determinants
      Significant stenosis: mean diastolic gradient $\geq$ 2 mmHg; a gradient of 5 mmHg is usually required to produce systemic venous congestion.
   3. Signs and symptoms
      a. Fatigue indicative of low cardiac output state.
      b. Marked peripheral edema due to venous congestion.
      c. Hepatomegaly; liver may be tender and pulsatile. Hepatic congestion may cause jaundice.
      d. Ascites.
   4. Pathophysiology
      a. Obstruction to flow across tricuspid valve leads to elevated RA pressure, resulting in systemic venous congestive.
   5. Physical findings
      a. Palpation and inspection
         (1) Distended jugular veins.
         (2) Prominent jugular venous a-wave.
         (3) Marked hepatomegaly with hepatic pulsation.
         (4) Ascites and marked pitting edema.
      b. Auscultation
         (1) Tricuspid opening snap may be audible at left lower sternal border.

The presence of an opening snap suggests a pliable but stenotic valve.
   (2) Medium-pitched diastolic murmur heard at left lower sternal border, accentuated by inspiration.
   (3) Presystolic murmur corresponding to atrial systole in normal sinus rhythm diminishes before the first heart sound.
   6. Diagnosis
      a. Noninvasive tests
         (1) Echocardiography and Doppler ultrasonography.
         (2) Electrocardiography: prominent p-waves indicative of RA enlargement.
   7. Treatment
      a. Medical
         (1) Mild diuresis to relieve systemic congestion.
         (2) Digoxin to control ventricular rate in atrial fibrillation.
      b. Surgical
         (1) Valve replacement should be undertaken with a gradient $\geq$ 5 mmHg (corresponding valve orifice area of approximately 2.0 cm^3).
         (2) Surgery should be performed at time of surgery for mitral valve. As an alternative to valve replacement, open commissurotomy should be considered.
B. Tricuspid valve insufficiency (TI)
   1. Etiology
      a. Anatomically normal valve, i.e., functional TI. Secondary to elevated PAWP or to dilatation of tricuspid annulus from elevated right ventricular end-diastolic pressure (RVEDP). Mild TI is a common finding on Doppler echocardiography of normal hearts.
      b. Organic anatomically abnormal valve
         (1) Rheumatic
         (2) Endocarditis
         (3) Tricuspid valve prolapse—myoxomatous change
         (4) Traumatic—chest trauma in auto accident, for example
         (5) Papillary muscle dysfunction—ischemia or trauma
         (6) Ebstein's anomaly
         (7) Connective tissue disorder
         (8) Radiation
   2. Hemodynamic determinants

a. Pulmonary artery (and RV systolic) pressures > 60 mmHg suggest that TI is functional. Significant TI with these pressures < 40 mmHg suggests at least a component of valve pathology.

3. Signs and symptoms
   a. If TI is functional, features of primary cardiac pathology predominant.
   b. Signs of right-sided failure
      (1) Massive edema
      (2) Hepatomegaly and hepatic tenderness
      (3) Ascites
      (4) Jugular venous distension
      (5) Symptoms of reduced cardiac output

4. Physical findings
   a. Palpation and inspection
      (1) Distended jugular vein with prominent v-wave.
      (2) Hepatomegaly with hepatic pulsation
      (3) Ascites and peripheral edema
      (4) RV lift
   b. Auscultation
      (1) Right-sided S_3 (heard at left lower sternal border and accentuated by inspiration).
      (2) With pulmonary hypertension present, P_2 may be accentuated.
      (3) Presystolic ejection murmur heard at left lower sternal border or in subxiphoid region. Murmur accentuated with inspiration.

5. Diagnosis
   a. Noninvasive
      (1) Echocardiography and Doppler ultrasound
      (2) Electrocardiography
         (a) Features of underlying cardiac pathology prevail

(b) Right bundle branch block may be present with RV volume or pressure overload.

6. Treatment
   a. Functional—treat underlying pathology
      (1) Diuresis to relieve systemic venous congestion.
      (2) Consider surgical tricuspid valvuloplasty or tricuspid annuloplasty with Carpentier ring in cases with severe TI producing refractory systemic congestion.
   b. Organic
      (1) Endocarditis
         (a) Appropriate intravenous antibiotics.
         (b) Valvulotomy in recurrent endocarditis (e.g., drug addicts); surgically replace valve in future after complete sterilization with antibiotics.
      (2) Other organic processes
         (a) Medical management with diuretics or digoxin as necessary.
         (b) Refractory, severe systemic congestion requires surgical replacement of valve with prosthesis.

Bibliography

Barron JT: Severe aortic or mitral regurgitation. In Parrillo JE (ed): *Current Therapy in Critical Care Medicine*, ed 2. Philadelphia, BC Decker, 1990, pp 142–147.

Braunwald E: Valvular heart disease. In Braunwald E (ed): *Heart Disease*. Philadelphia, WB Saunders, 1988, pp 1023–1092.

Ross J: Left ventricular function and the timing of surgical treatment in valvular heart disease. *Am Heart J* 94:498–504, 1981.

CHAPTER 20

Coronary Artery Disease

Gary L. Schaer, M.D.
Edward L. Passen, M.D.

I. Angina Pectoris
   A. Definition
   Angina pectoris is chest discomfort due to myocardial ischemia.
   B. Pathophysiology
   Angina pectoris is caused by myocardial ischemia resulting from an imbalance between myocardial oxygen supply and demand. Because the myocardium normally extracts close to the maximum quantity of oxygen from blood, increased oxygen demand can only be met by increasing coronary blood flow and oxygen supply.
   1. Reduced myocardial oxygen supply
      a. Atherosclerosis. Atherosclerotic plaques (composed of lipid, fibrous tissue, and sometimes calcium) grow within the intima of the coronary artery and become significant when the luminal diameter is narrowed $\geq 70\%$.
      b. Thrombosis. Rupture of an atherosclerotic plaque may lead to platelet aggregation and thrombus formation within the coronary artery. This may substantially reduce the myocardial oxygen supply, producing unstable angina or acute myocardial infarction (see below).
      c. Coronary vasospasm (see below). Severe coronary vasoconstriction in the presence of a fixed coronary obstruction (or occasionally with normal coronary arteries) may severely reduce the myocardial oxygen supply and produce angina in the absence of an increase in myocardial oxygen demand.
      d. Reduced oxygen-carrying capacity. Severe anemia, hypoxemia, carbon monoxide exposure.
   2. Increased myocardial oxygen demand
   In the presence of a significant coronary stenosis, the following may precipitate angina: physical exertion, emotional stress, severe hypertension, severe left ventricular (LV) hypertrophy, tachyarrhythmias, exposure to cold.
   3. Risk factors
   Cigarette smoking, hypercholesterolemia, hypertension, diabetes mellitus, a family history of premature coronary disease, age, sex, and obesity.
   C. Diagnosis
   1. History
      a. Typical angina

Patients usually describe a retrosternal constriction, burning, pressure, or heaviness that may radiate down the medial aspect of the left arm or into the neck or jaw. Patients are more likely to describe chest "discomfort" rather than "pain," which is crescendo-decrescendo and usually lasts for 1–5 min. It is typically precipitated by exertion (or emotional stress) and relieved by rest, although it may also occur at rest (see the discussion of unstable angina and variant angina in Section II).

b. Atypical (nonischemic) chest pain
Nonexertional sharp, fleeting chest pains (< 30 sec) or very prolonged dull aches localized over the left chest are rarely due to myocardial ischemia. Chest pains worsened by movement of the arms, shoulders, or torso are also atypical of myocardial ischemia and suggest a musculoskeletal etiology.

2. Physical findings
Physical examination is frequently normal. A careful search for signs of vascular disease should be performed, including a fundoscopic examination as well as palpation and auscultation of the carotid and peripheral arteries. Cardiac examination should include auscultation for murmurs suggesting aortic stenosis, papillary muscle dysfunction, or hypertrophic cardiomyopathy. Examination during an anginal episode may reveal a transient S_3 or S_4 gallop, murmur of mitral regurgitation (papillary muscle dysfunction), or signs of LV failure.

3. Diagnostic tests
a. Electrocardiogram (ECG)
Although the resting ECG may appear normal despite significant coronary artery disease, the presence of Q-waves (confirming a prior myocardial infarction), ST-segment depression, or T-wave inversion, suggest the diagnosis. Obtaining a stat ECG during an episode of angina (before giving nitroglycerin, if possible) can be extremely helpful. The ECG with pain should be carefully compared with prior ECGs to detect new ST-segment depression or more subtle T-wave changes indicating myocardial ischemia.

b. Exercise stress tests
These tests utilize a graded increase in exercise (usually on a treadmill) to provoke myocardial ischemia, which can then be detected on the ECG. To increase sensitivity and specificity in patients with a resting ECG abnormality (or in those more likely to have a false-positive or false-negative test), the stress test can be combined with an imaging modality such as thallium, echocardiography, or radionuclide ventriculography. It is important to note that any type of stress testing is *contraindicated* in patients with unstable angina pectoris or acute myocardial infarction until the condition has clearly stabilized.

(1) Exercise ECG
ECG, symptoms, and blood pressure are continuously monitored during incremental increases in workload. Exercise is increased until the target heart rate is reached (85% of the predicted maximum) or the patient develops angina, severe shortness of breath, a fall in blood pressure, ventricular tachyarrhythmias or marked ST-segment depression (> 2 mm). A positive (abnormal) test is defined by a > 1 mm horizontal or downsloping depression of the ST segment. If the patient is unable to achieve the target heart rate despite the absence of ECG abnormalities or chest pain, the test is considered nondiagnostic. The incidence of a false-positive test is about 15%, but this is increased in the presence of an abnormal resting ECG (especially left ventricular hypertrophy), in patients on cardiac drugs (e.g., digoxin), and in women. False-negative tests are even more common (25–30%), especially if the coronary stenosis involves a more electrically silent region (e.g., the posterior wall).

(2) Exercise thallium imaging
Regional myocardial perfusion can be assessed by injecting the radioisotope thallium[201] immediately after exercise. Patients are scanned immediately after exercise and again 2–4 hr later. Myocardial ischemia is suggested by the presence of a reversible perfusion defect (a "cold spot" on the scan immediately after exercise which "redistributes" or fills in on the

later scan). A perfusion defect that persists on the late scan suggests a prior myocardial infarction. ^{99m}Tc sestamibi (Cardiolite) is a newer, technetium-labeled compound that may produce image resolution superior to that of thallium, particularly in very overweight patients.

(3) Exercise radionuclide ventriculography (multigated angiogram, MUGA). This technique combines ^{99m}Tc labeling of red blood cells with exercise (bicycle ergometry). An ECG-gated nuclear ventriculogram is obtained at rest to assess global LV function (ejection fraction) and regional contractility. When the scan is repeated at maximal exercise, myocardial ischemia will be identified by the appearance of a new wall motion abnormality (hypokinesis or akinesis) and a transient depression of the global ejection fraction.

(4) Exercise echocardiography
This modality is similar to an exercise radionuclide ventriculography, except that two-dimensional echocardiography is used to image the heart in multiple planes to identify exercise-induced regional wall motion abnormalities.

c. Pharmacologic cardiac stress imaging permits the noninvasive detection of myocardial ischemia in patients unable to exercise sufficiently to reach their target heart rate.

(1) Dipyridamole thallium scanning
Dipyridamole (Persantine) administered IV is a coronary vasodilator which provokes myocardial ischemia by shunting coronary blood flow away from the myocardium supplied by a significantly obstructed coronary artery. This creates a transient cold spot which is detected by thallium imaging. Repeat scanning several hours later provides evidence of redistribution after the effects of dipyridamole have worn off.

(2) Adenosine thallium scanning
This newer technique is based on the same principle as dipyridamole testing. Adenosine is a shorter-acting and more potent agent.

(3) Dobutamine thallium scanning and dobutamine echocardiography
These tests utilize the β-agonist dobutamine to augment myocardial contractility and heart rate to provoke myocardial ischemia.

d. Coronary angiography
This invasive test remains the gold standard for diagnosis of coronary artery disease, permitting quantitation of the degree and extent of coronary artery obstruction. Left ventriculography (to define regional and global LV function) and hemodynamic measurements are usually performed at the same time. It should be considered in (1) patients with anginal symptoms and a positive exercise test in whom a revascularization procedure percutaneous transluminal coronary angioplasty (PTCA), or coronary artery bypass graft (CABG) is contemplated; (2) in asymptomatic patients with an exercise test demonstrating severe ischemia (markedly positive exercise ECG or evidence of a large or multiple thallium defects); and (3) in patients with severe anginal symptoms (typical or atypical) in whom the diagnosis is in doubt because of an indeterminate stress test. The risks of a serious complication (death, myocardial infarction, stroke) from coronary angiography is 0.1–0.2%.

D. Treatment
1. Modify cardiac risk factors: correct hypercholesterolemia; discontinuation of cigarette smoking; treat hypertension and diabetes; advise weight reduction and regular aerobic exercise.
2. Correct exacerbating medical conditions, such as hypertension, thyrotoxicosis, chronic obstructive pulmonary disease (COPD), anemia, heart failure, and cardiac arrhythmias.
3. Medical therapy
Agents are chosen because of their ability to improve the myocardial oxygen supply or reduce the demand. Always consider potential adverse effects before commencing therapy.
a. Therapeutic goals
(1) Prevention or relief of anginal episodes
(2) Prevention of myocardial infarction
(3) Improvement in survival

b. Nitrates. These agents are beneficial because they reduce myocardial oxygen demand (by vasodilating capacitance vessels and reducing LV wall stress) and increase the myocardial oxygen supply (by coronary artery vasodilation and increasing collateral blood flow).

(1) Acute anginal attack is best treated with sublingual nitroglycerin (0.4–0.6 mg) and may be repeated twice if the pain is not relieved within 5 min. Caution patients to take the drug while seated or supine and to seek medical attention immediately if symptoms persist.

(2) For prevention of anginal attacks, nitrates are administered orally or transcutaneously (paste or patch).

(3) Tachyphylaxis will occur with all nitrate preparations and reduce their effectiveness unless an 8- to 12-hr "nitrate-free" interval is permitted daily.

c. β-adrenergic blockers. These agents are very useful because they reduce the myocardial oxygen demand by decreasing heart rate and blood pressure. They also prevent the chronotropic and inotropic response to physical exertion or emotional stress. The dose should be titrated in each patient to reduce the resting heart rate to 55–60 bpm and prevent an exercise-induced increase in heart rate above 100 bpm.

(1) Choice of β-blocker. β_1-selective agents (metoprolol, atenolol) are less likely to worsen symptoms of COPD or peripheral vascular disease. Lipid-insoluble agents (e.g. atenolol, nadolol) are less likely to be associated with central nervous system (CNS) side effects.

(2) Potential adverse effects

(a) Worsening of heart failure (due to negative inotropic effects).

(b) Exacerbation of COPD or asthma.

(c) Worsening of symptoms of peripheral vascular disease.

(d) CNS effects (depression, fatigue).

(e) Masking of hypoglycemia in diabetic patients.

(f) Abrupt withdrawal may precipitate angina and myocardial infarction.

d. Calcium channel antagonists. These agents are potent coronary vasodilators, thereby increasing the myocardial oxygen supply. They also reduce the myocardial oxygen demand by reducing afterload and lowering the heart rate (verapamil and diltiazem).

(1) Nifedipine is a potent arteriolar vasodilator with minimal negative inotropic properties. A sustained-release preparation (Procardia XL) can be given once a day and avoids the disadvantage of shorter-acting preparations which reflexively increase the heart rate (and thus the myocardial oxygen demand). Nifedipine is the calcium antagonist of choice in patients with depressed LV function, bradycardia, or heart block. Amlodipine is a newer calcium blocker similar to nifedipine, that has the additional benefit of proven safety in patients with concomitent LV dysfunction.

(2) Verapamil is also a potent coronary vasodilator but has important negative inotropic and chronotropic properties. It may exacerbate heart failure in patients with LV dysfunction or in those concurrently on β-blockers. It is contraindicated in patients with advanced heart block.

(3) Diltiazem shares the beneficial antihypertensive and coronary vasodilating effects of the other calcium blockers, but it also possesses negative inotropic and chronotropic properties somewhat milder than those of verapamil. Like verapamil, it should be used with caution (if at all) in patients with signs of congestive heart failure, bradycardia, or advanced heart block.

4. Percutaneous transluminal coronary angioplasty (PTCA)

This nonsurgical revascularization technique is accomplished by inflating a balloon-tipped catheter across a significant coronary stenosis. Patients with a coronary stenosis ($\geq 70\%$ luminal diameter) which involves one or more vessels are candidates, provided that they (a) have evidence of inducible ischemia on stress testing; (b) are candidates for CABG if PTCA is unsuccessful;

and (c) do not have a significant left main stenosis. Although PTCA is usually successful (> 90% of cases), significant complications include urgent CABG (1.5–4%), myocardial infarction (0.5–5%), and death (0.1–0.5%). Restenosis (significant renarrowing of a previously successfully dilated artery in 1–3 months) occurs in 25–40% of initially successful dilatations and can usually be treated by repeat PTCA. No pharmacologic therapy has yet been proven to reduce the incidence of restenosis.

5. New interventional devices
   a. Excimer laser coronary angioplasty utilizes a fiberoptic catheter to deliver focused quantities of laser energy directly to the atherosclerotic plaque. This new technique is demonstrating a high success rate and a low complication rate for some lesions not ideally suited for PTCA.
   b. Directional coronary atherectomy utilizes a catheter-mounted rotating blade which "shaves" the atherosclerotic plaque and removes it from the body. It has also been shown to successfully treat some coronary lesions not ideally suited for PTCA.
   c. Rotational atherectomy (Rotablator). This device grinds atherosclerotic plaque into fine particles using a high-speed rotating diamond-encrusted stainless steel burr, mounted on the tip of a flexible catheter. This approach is especially useful in calcified and fibrotic coronary stenoses not optimally treated with PTCA.
   d. Coronary stents are miniature coils of stainless steel mesh which can be inserted into a coronary artery to scaffold the treated vessel. Stents are useful for severe coronary dissections caused by PTCA reducing the need for urgent bypass surgery. Because a stent is a foreign body prone to thrombosis, patients must be aggressively anticoagulated following stent placement.

6. Coronary artery bypass grafting (CABG) Bypass surgery is also an effective revascularization strategy and is indicated for significant left main disease (> 50% diameter narrowing), as well as in most patients with severe multivessel disease, particularly when accompanied by LV dysfunction. Surgical revascularization is also indicated for symptomatic patients with less extensive coronary disease when lesions are unsuitable for coronary angioplasty. The risks of CABG include a 1–2% operative mortality rate and a 5–10% risk of perioperative myocardial infarction. In addition, 15–25% of saphenous vein grafts close within the first year of CABG. The internal mammary arteries (both left and right) are more long-lasting conduits than saphenous vein grafts.

II. Unstable Angina Pectoris
A. Definition

Unstable angina is a clinical syndrome characterized by chest pain which is of new onset or has worsened in severity, duration or frequency and is not associated with enzyme or electrocardiographic (ECG) evidence of myocardial infarction. It is part of a spectrum of acute coronary syndromes which also includes non-Q and Q-wave myocardial infarction.

B. Etiology and pathophysiology

Rupture of a coronary atherosclerotic plaque is the most important pathophysiologic event in unstable angina. The consequences of plaque rupture include platelet aggregation, thrombus formation, and coronary vasoconstriction (due in part to release of platelet-derived vasoconstrictors). These events substantially narrow the coronary artery lumen, reduce coronary blood flow, and diminish the myocardial oxygen supply. Myocardial ischemia may therefore result despite a stable myocardial oxygen demand. If the thrombotic obstruction to coronary blood flow progresses to complete occlusion, myocardial infarction results.

C. Diagnosis
1. History

Patients with unstable angina typically present with severe angina of recent onset, a marked worsening in the pattern of their previous symptoms (crescendo angina), or angina at rest. Anginal symptoms soon after myocardial infarction (postinfarction angina) also fall under this diagnosis.

2. Diagnostic tests
   a. Stress tests are *contraindicated* in the acute phase of unstable angina and should only be considered once the patient has stabilized on medical therapy.
   b. Electrocardiography (ECG). During an episode of chest pain, transient ST-segment depression (occasionally elevation) and T-wave inversions are often seen.

These changes may occasionally persist despite lack of enzyme evidence of infarction.

   c. **Coronary angiography.** Most patients should undergo coronary angiography after they have stabilized medically.

     (1) Indications

       (a) Recurrent chest pain despite medical therapy

       (b) ECG evidence of a large area of myocardium at risk

       (c) Stress-induced ischemia after medical stabilization

     (2) Goals. Coronary angiography is used to determine the lesion responsible for the unstable syndrome (the "culprit" lesion) and to clarify the extent of disease in the remainder of the coronary vasculature.

     (3) Angiographic findings. Evidence for intracoronary thrombus (filling defect, hazy or smudged appearance) is often seen. In the 10–15% of patients found to have insignificant coronary artery disease, coronary artery spasm or a noncardiac (e.g., gastrointestinal) cause of chest pain should be strongly considered. In the 85–90% of patients with significant coronary obstructions, PTCA or CABG can be considered.

D. Treatment

  1. **Initial approach.** All patients with unstable angina should be admitted to the hospital, and therapy should be instituted promptly.

    a. Perform ECG (during angina if possible).

    b. Obtain IV access and place the patient on a cardiac monitor.

    c. Administer nitroglycerin, 0.4 mg sl (which may be repeated provided that the systolic blood pressure is > 100 mmHg).

    d. Give aspirin (non-enteric coated), 160–325 mg orally or chewed (see Subsection 2 (a) below).

    e. Treat anxiety with benzodiazepines; analgesics should be used sparingly (if at all) in an attempt to monitor the response of angina to specific anti-ischemic therapy.

    f. Treat factors which could exacerbate myocardial ischemia (by augmenting myocardial oxygen demand), including anemia, hypertension, supraventricular arrhythmias, congestive heart failure, and thyrotoxicosis.

  2. **Medical therapy.** Goals include (a) relief of myocardial ischemia; (b) prevention of further ischemic episodes; and (c) stabilization and initial healing of the ruptured atherosclerotic plaque.

    a. **Aspirin**

    The presence of a fresh, partially obstructing intracoronary thrombus has been demonstrated by coronary angioscopy and pathologic studies. Antiplatelet treatment with aspirin (160–325 mg chewed or orally) should begin promptly after the diagnosis is considered and continued daily. The major adverse effect is an increased risk of bleeding, but this is outweighed by the benefits of reducing episodes of ischemia and infarction.

    b. **Heparin**

    Systemic anticoagulation should be added to aspirin in patients with unstable angina who also demonstrate ischemic ECG changes, as well as in patients with recurrent angina despite medical therapy. Because the risk of bleeding is increased in patients receiving both aspirin and heparin, close observation is essential. Administer heparin as an IV bolus of 5,000 units, followed by 1,000 units/hr by constant infusion. The dose should be titrated to achieve a partial thromboplastin time of 1.5–2 times control.

    c. **Nitrates**

    These agents are particularly useful in unstable angina because they increase the myocardial oxygen supply (by coronary vasodilation and increased collateral blood flow) and reduce the demand (by decreased preload and afterload). IV nitroglycerin is best administered in the critical care unit and is superior to topical or oral nitrates because of its immediate onset, short duration, and precise titration. The drip should be started at 5 to 10 μg/min and can be increased as needed to completely eliminate angina. Systolic arterial pressure should be reduced by 10–20 mmHg but should not be lower than 100 mmHg. Doses as high as 200–400 μg/min may be needed in some cases. Frequent blood pressure monitoring is important, as an occasional patient will become hypotensive during even low-dose infusions. Nitrate-induced hypotension is usually due to vasodilation and can therefore be rapidly corrected by transient dose reduction, and IV boluses of normal saline (100–200 ml). In patients with marked or persistent hemodynamic instability, especially in the presence of signs of heart failure (e.g., pulmonary rales), direct measurement of the pulmonary capillary wedge pressure and cardiac output is recommended. Continue IV nitroglycerin for 1–2 days after the last bout of angina to permit stabilization of the involved coronary artery. IV nitroglycerin can then be discontinued and oral or topical nitrates (Nitropaste) begun.

d. Calcium channel antagonists

These agents are beneficial because they are potent coronary vasodilators capable of preventing periodic coronary vasoconstriction resulting from platelet-derived products (e.g., thromboxane A_2, serotonin) released at the site of the ruptured atherosclerotic plaque. Calcium antagonists also reduce the myocardial oxygen demand by lowering afterload, preload, and heart rate (diltiazem, verapamil). For many patients with unstable angina, diltiazem is a useful agent. It may be started along with IV nitroglycerin at a dose of 30–60 mg orally every 6–8 hr. Because diltiazem possesses negative inotropic properties, it should be used with caution (if at all) in patients with signs of congestive heart failure. Amlodipine (5–10 mg po qd) or a long-acting nifedipine preparation (e.g., Procardia XL 30–60 mg po qd) are excellent alternatives.

e. β-adrenergic blockers

These agents are beneficial because they reduce the myocardial oxygen demand by decreasing the heart rate and arterial pressure and are indicated in patients with anginal symptoms inadequately controlled by aspirin, IV nitroglycerin, and a calcium channel antagonist. β-blockers are particularly beneficial in those patients with a persistently rapid heart rate not due to volume depletion or reduced cardiac output. β-blocker therapy may be instituted with the short-acting agent propranolol, 20 mg orally every 6 hr, and then titrated to a resting heart rate of 55–60 bpm. An alternative oral β-blocker is the β_1-selective agent metoprolol, which can be started at 25 mg orally every 6 hr and increased to up to 100 mg orally twice per day. In patients in whom more rapid β-blockade is desired, metoprolol can be given IV at a dose of 5 mg every 5 min for three doses, followed by the above oral starting dose. Because of their negative inotropic effects, β-blockers should generally not be administered to patients with signs of congestive heart failure or with moderate to severe depression of left ventricular function. Caution should also be exercised in patients with a resting bradycardia (< 50 bpm) and in those with a history of obstructive lung disease or asthma.

f. Thrombolytic therapy

Despite the evidence that intracoronary thrombus is important in the pathophysiology of unstable angina, a recent randomized trial (TIMI-3) failed to show a beneficial effect of thrombolytic therapy.

g. Angina refractory to maximal medical therapy

Because these patients are at very high risk of infarction, they should undergo immediate coronary angiography followed by a revascularization procedure (PTCA or CABG). Placement of an intra-aortic balloon pump in the catheterization laboratory may be needed to stabilize these patients prior to angiography.

3. PTCA

Coronary angioplasty has been shown to be a safe and effective treatment for many patients with unstable angina. Although reported success rates range from 85 to 94%, several studies have documented a higher complication rate than with elective angioplasty. This is probably due to the presence of intracoronary thrombus. The procedure is indicated for those patients with single- or double-vessel disease in whom the lesion responsible for the unstable syndrome (the *culprit* lesion) is amenable to balloon dilatation. Patients with more extensive multivessel disease, left main disease, or significantly depressed left ventricular function may be better candidates for bypass surgery (see

Subsection 4 below). If possible, coronary angioplasty should be delayed until systemic heparin (in addition to aspirin, nitrates, and calcium blockers) has been given for 3–5 days. This may encourage resolution of associated coronary thrombus and permit initial healing of the ruptured atherosclerotic plaque. This approach appears to reduce the incidence of angioplasty-associated acute complications (abrupt closure, distal embolization, myocardial infarction and the need for emergency bypass surgery), particularly in those patients in whom intracoronary thrombus had been identified on the initial coronary angiogram. As in patients with stable angina, an important long term disadvantage of coronary angioplasty is the risk of restenosis, which ranges from 25 to 40%, depending on the site of balloon dilatation.

4. CABG

Bypass surgery is also an effective revascularization strategy for patients with unstable angina and is indicated for significant left main disease and in most patients with severe triple-vessel coronary disease. Preoperative placement of an intra-aortic balloon pump is very helpful in stabilizing these patients by augmenting coronary blood flow and reducing myocardial oxygen demand. Surgical revascularization is also indicated for patients with less extensive coronary disease when lesions are unsuitable for coronary angioplasty.

Bibliography

Baim DS: Interventional catheterization techniques: percutaneous transluminal balloon angioplasty, valvuloplasty and related procedures. In Braunwald E, (ed): *Heart Disease.* W.B. Saunders, 1992; Chap 41, pp 1365–1381.

Beller GA et al: Sensitivity, specificity and prognostic significance of noninvasive testing for occult or known coronary disease. Prog Cardiovasc Dis 29:241–270, 1987.

Fuster V, Badiman I, Cohen M, et al: Insights into the pathogenesis of acute ischemic syndromes. Circulation 77:1213–1220, 1988.

Rutherford JD, Braunwald E: Chronic ischemic heart disease. In Braunwald E, (ed): *Heart Disease.* W.B. Saunders, 1992; Chap 40, pp 1292–1364.

Sherman CT, Litvack F, Grundfest W, et al: Coronary angioscopy in patients with unstable angina pectoris. *N Engl J Med* 315:913–919, 1986.

Theroux P, Ouimet H, McCans J, et al: Aspirin, heparin or both to treat acute unstable angina. *N Engl J Med* 319:1105–1111, 1988.

CHAPTER 21

Acute Myocardial Infarction

Lloyd W. Klein, M.D.
Gary L. Schaer, M.D.
Edward L. Passen, M.D.

Myocardial infarction is a medical emergency requiring prompt evaluation and treatment. In recent years, treatment has changed from a passive supportive role to an active interventional approach aimed at restoring blood flow to the previously occluded coronary artery.

I. Diagnosis
  A. History
    1. Chest pain due to myocardial infarction usually resembles angina but is more severe and prolonged (see Chapter 20).
    2. Some patients, particularly diabetics, hypertensives, and the elderly, may have either no chest pain at all or unusual anginal equivalents (e.g., shortness of breath).
    3. The characteristics of the chest discomfort, along with the patient's past medical history and risk factors for coronary artery disease, should suggest the diagnosis of myocardial infarction.
    4. Noting the time of onset of chest pain is important because it permits estimation of the likelihood of myocardial salvage with reperfusion therapy.
  B. Physical examination

1. The physical examination in patients with myocardial infarction may be normal, may provide clues to underlying atherosclerosis (e.g., peripheral vascular disease), or may reveal coronary risk factors (e.g., hypertension).
2. Obtain accurate baseline vital signs, identify potential complications of infarction (cardiogenic shock, right ventricular infarction, congestive heart failure).
3. Exclude other cardiac problems (aortic stenosis, other valvular disease, hypertrophic cardiomyopathy, pericarditis).
4. Exclude other noncardiac ailments that may cause chest pain (aortic dissection, pulmonary embolism, pneumothorax, peptic ulcer disease).
  C. Electrocardiogram (ECG)
    1. Should be obtained immediately.
    2. Initial ECG changes depend on the time the ECG is first recorded in relation to the onset of symptoms.
    3. Acute myocardial infarction should not be excluded on the basis of an initially normal ECG, since changes may be delayed or intermittent.

4. Repeating the ECG one or more times increases the diagnostic yield and should be considered particularly when the diagnosis is in doubt. Minor ST-segment or T-wave changes should not be overlooked.

5. ST-segment elevation is most suggestive of acute myocardial infarction and frequently identifies the location of myocardial injury (i.e., anterior, inferior, lateral).

6. Other causes of ST-segment elevation should be considered, especially Prinzmetal's angina, ventricular aneurysm, pericarditis, and early repolarization.

7. Although the development of Q-waves usually suggests a completed infarct, if significant chest pain and ST-segment elevation persist, the infarct may still be evolving and may be amenable to myocardial salvage with reperfusion.

8. In Q-wave infarctions the ECG demonstrates an evolving decrease in R-wave voltage, return of the ST-segment to baseline, symmetric inversion of the T-waves, and pathologic Q-waves.

9. In non-Q-wave infarctions (caused by subtotal or intermittent coronary occlusion by thrombus and/or spasm) the ECG usually demonstrates an evolving ST-segment depression and/or T-wave inversions in the area overlying the infarction.

D. Cardiac enzymes
  1. Irreversibly injured myocardial tissue releases creatine kinase (CK) into the blood.
  2. The MB isoenzyme of CK is most specific for myocardial necrosis and should be obtained immediately and serially for 24–36 hr.
  3. Lack of elevation of CK or its MB fraction excludes infarction.
  4. Plasma CK usually exceeds normal levels 4–6 hr after the onset of infarction, peaks at 2–10 times normal levels within 24 hr, and returns to baseline in 4 days.
  5. When thrombolytic therapy successfully opens the occluded coronary artery, the rate of enzyme release is altered, usually resulting in a high and rapid CK peak.

II. Management
  A. General care
    1. The patient should be transferred to the coronary care unit as soon as possible.
    2. Complete bed rest is mandatory in the acute period.
    3. ECG monitoring for arrhythmias should begin immediately.

4. Intravenous access should be obtained.
5. The patient should be NPO until medically stable.
6. Intramuscular injections are to be avoided to prevent hematoma formation if thrombolytic therapy or anticoagulation is utilized, and to prevent confusion from muscle CK release.
7. Supplemental oxygen should be administered by nasal prongs (2–4 l/min).

B. Analgesia and sedation
  1. Morphine sulfate (1–4 mg IV) is the analgesic of choice because it is potent, rapidly acting, and has favorable hemodynamic effects (venodilation). In addition, if adverse effects occur (i.e., hypotension, respiratory depression), the effects of morphine can be rapidly reversed by Narcan.
  2. Sedation with benzodiazepines may also be useful to reduce myocardial oxygen demand in anxious patients.
  3. Analgesics and sedatives should be carefully titrated to avoid respiratory depression and hemodynamic instability.

C. Conventional medical therapy
  1. Aspirin
    a. Early administration of aspirin to patients with acute myocardial infarction has become standard practice. Unless contraindicated by an allergic history, aspirin (160–325 mg chewable or orally) should be given promptly to the patient with presumed infarction.
    b. The mechanism of aspirin's beneficial effect is platelet inhibition. Aspirin irreversibly inactivates platelet cyclooxygenase, thereby impairing platelet aggregation and reducing the release of platelet-derived vasoconstrictors (thromboxane A_2, serotonin).
    c. The main toxicity of aspirin is dose-related gastrointestinal symptoms.
    d. Aspirin alone has been shown to be an effective reperfusion agent, even when thrombolytic agents are contraindicated.
  2. Nitrates
    a. Nitrates should be instituted immediately.
    b. Unless contraindicated by hypotension (systolic blood pressure < 90 mmHg), therapy should begin with a sublingual nitroglycerin.
    c. Although this dose may be repeated

again in 5–10 min, it is best to continue therapy with IV nitroglycerin. This therapy may be started at 5–10 μg/min and increased in increments of 5–10 μg/min every 5 min.

d. Titration to pain resolution may not be practical or possible. A 10–20% reduction in systolic blood pressure is a reasonable target for titration, but the systolic blood pressure should not be permitted to fall to < 100 mmHg.

e. Nitrates have several beneficial effects in acute myocardial infarction.

   (1) Nitrates reduce myocardial ischemia in patients with vasospastic etiology.

   (2) With thrombotic occlusion of a coronary artery, nitrates are beneficial because they reduce myocardial oxygen demand by decreasing venodilation and preload.

   (3) Nitrates may also increase the myocardial oxygen supply by increasing collateral blood flow to the ischemic region.

f. The major adverse effect of nitrates is hypotension, which is more likely to occur in patients who are volume depleted or who have right ventricular infarction (see Subsection). Nitrate-induced hypotension may also be associated with a reflex tachycardia that further worsens myocardial ischemia by increasing myocardial oxygen demand.

3. Heparin

a. Although routine systemic anticoagulation with heparin has not been shown to improve survival independently in the emergent treatment of acute myocardial infarction; its utility in unstable angina has led to its routine use in infarction treated without thrombolysis. Its major value is as an adjunct to thrombolytic therapy to diminish reocclusion following successful reperfusion (see Subsection 3,b).

b. Systemic heparin has been shown to reduce the incidence of left ventricular mural thrombi and systemic embolism in patients with a large anterior myocardial infarction.

4. β-blockers

a. Early use of β-blockers in acute myocardial infarction has been shown to re-

duce ischemic pain, nonfatal reinfarction, cardiac arrest, and death.

b. Their mechanism of action involves a dose-dependent competitive binding to β_1-receptors in the heart, which cause an increase in heart rate and myocardial contractility when stimulated. By inhibiting cardiac β-adrenergic receptors, β-blockers cause a reduction in heart rate, blood pressure, and contractility, all of which reduce the myocardial oxygen demand.

c. Left ventricular wall stress is also reduced.

d. The threshold for ventricular fibrillation is raised.

e. β-blockers should be avoided in patients with signs of heart failure, bradycardia, severe first-degree atrioventricular (AV) block, and second- or third-degree AV block. Caution is also advised for those with obstructive lung disease and peripheral vascular disease.

f. For patients with acute myocardial infarction in whom no contraindications exist, β-blockers should initially be administered IV to achieve immediate β-blockade, followed by oral administration.

5. Antiarrhythmic therapy

a. Some authors recommend prophylactic lidocaine for all patients with proven or suspected acute myocardial infarction; others await documented frequent or complex ventricular ectopy.

b. The bolus dose and infusion rate should be reduced by one-half in elderly patients and in those with severe heart failure, hypotension, or liver disease.

c. Toxic manifestations primarily involve the central nervous system (lethargy, confusion) and should prompt reduction or discontinuation of the drug.

D. Thrombolytic therapy

1. Indications and contraindications

a. Thrombolytic therapy should be considered promptly in all patients presenting with acute myocardial infarction. It is essential that treatment be instituted as soon as possible, preferably within 4 hr of symptom onset, because the longer the delay to reperfusion, the lower the potential for myocardial salvage.

b. A candidate for thrombolytic therapy presents with chest pain persisting for > 30 min but < 6 hr, associated with ST-segment elevation of at least 1 mm (0.1 mV) in at least two contiguous leads. In addition, there should be no contraindications to thrombolytic therapy (see Subsection 1,d).

c. Patients with intermittent chest pain for > 6 hr should also be considered for thrombolytic therapy, provided ST-segment elevation persists.

d. Thrombolytic therapy has not been shown to be beneficial when the ECG demonstrates other than ST-segment elevation or left bundle branch blocks (LBBB) (i.e., ST-segment depression, T-wave abnormalities).

e. Before administering a thrombolytic agent, the clinician should weigh the potential benefits (estimated by the duration of ischemia and the amount of myocardium in jeopardy) versus the risks (estimated by age, the presence of other medical problems, and potential bleeding complications). Although the elderly seem to derive the most benefit from thrombolytic therapy, they are also more likely to have complications.

f. Absolute contraindications to thrombolytic therapy include active internal bleeding; known bleeding diathesis; a history of cerebrovascular accident, intracranial neoplasm, arteriovenous malformation, or aneurysm; recent intracranial or intraspinal surgery or trauma; recent major surgery; or severe uncontrolled hypertension.

g. Relative contraindications include prolonged cardiopulmonary resuscitation, recent invasive procedures, poorly controlled hypertension, hemorrhagic ophthalmic conditions (i.e., diabetic proliferative retinopathy), and postpartum condition or menstruation. A history of a prior allergic reaction or treatment with streptokinase should not preclude the use of another thrombolytic agent.

h. About one-third of patients presenting with an acute myocardial infarction are eligible for thrombolytic therapy using the above guidelines.

2. Choice of a thrombolytic agent

a. The IV route is preferred because it facilitates rapid treatment, thereby accelerating the time to reperfusion. The intracoronary route is less often used because of the intrinsic delay in performing emergency catheterization and because appropriate invasive facilities may not be routinely available.

b. Thrombolytic agents may be generally classified as fibrin-selective or nonselective.

   (1) Fibrin-selective agents (e.g., tissue plasminogen activator) locally activate the plasminogen-fibrin complex, cause less systemic fibrinogen breakdown, and achieve a higher 90-min patency rate.

   (2) Nonselective agents (e.g., streptokinase, urokinase, APSAC) cause systemic fibrinolysis and a systemic lytic state. The resulting elevation in fibrin split products produces platelet inhibition, which may be beneficial by reducing the incidence of reocclusion following successful reperfusion.

   (3) Despite the systemic lytic state produced by the nonselective agents, the incidence of bleeding complications does not appear to be significantly different from that observed with the fibrin-selective agents.

c. Tissue plasminogen activator (t-PA)

   (1) t-PA or alteplase is a serine protease enzyme produced by vascular endothelial cells and is commercially produced by recombinant DNA technology. It is a fibrin-selective agent with a marked affinity for the plasminogen-fibrin complex.

   (2) Multicenter clinical trials have demonstrated that t-PA is the most effective thrombolytic agent in achieving prompt reperfusion of the occluded coronary artery. The patency rate at 90 min is 70–75%, whereas streptokinase (see Subsection 2,d) achieves a 90-min patency rate of 40–50%.

   (3) Clinical trials have also demonstrated that t-PA reduces mortality and improves left ventricular function.

(4) "Front loaded" dosing, as used in the GUSTO trial, produced 80% patency at 90 minutes and a 1% improvement in mortality vs. streptokinase.

d. Streptokinase

(1) Streptokinase is a non-fibrin-selective thrombolytic agent which is a product of β-hemolytic streptococci.

(2) Multicenter clinical trials have demonstrated 90-min infarct-related artery patency rates of 40–50%, which is considerably lower than those achieved with t-PA. However, the patency rate at 24 hr increases to 85%, which is comparable to that of t-PA.

(3) This agent has also been clearly shown to reduce mortality and improve left ventricular (LV) function in patients with myocardial infarction. Although both GISSI-II and ISIS-III demonstrated that streptokinase produced the same reduction in mortality as t-PA, GUSTO revealed a 1% mortality advantage among patients using t-PA.

e. APSAC

(1) APSAC is an anisoylated derivative of streptokinase which results in greater persistence of fibrinogenolytic activity and improved thrombolytic potency compared with an equivalent dose of streptokinase.

(2) Although APSAC also produces a systemic fibrinolytic state, it may be somewhat more fibrin-selective than streptokinase.

(3) Clinical trials which have demonstrated a mean 90-min patency rate of 60–70%.

(4) APSAC has also been shown to reduce mortality and improve LV function. ISIS-III showed that APSAC has an impact on mortality rates equivalent to those of t-PA and streptokinase.

f. Urokinase

(1) Although urokinase is approved by the Food and Drug Administration for intracoronary use, it is not presently approved for IV adminis-

tration in acute myocardial infarction.

(2) However, recent clinical trials have shown that IV urokinase (2–3-million-unit bolus) is an effective therapy, with 90-min patency rates of 60–67%.

3. Adjunctive medical therapy

a. Aspirin is probably the most important agent to use in combination with thrombolytic therapy because it has been demonstrated to reduce mortality further and to decrease the rate of reinfarction following successful thrombolysis (ISIS-II). Aspirin (160–325 mg orally daily) should probably be continued indefinitely following myocardial infarction.

b. The precise role of heparin as an adjunct to thrombolytic therapy has not yet been completely defined. At the present time, heparin (5,000-unit bolus, then 1,000 units/hr by continuous infusion) should be administered 1 hr after beginning thrombolytic therapy. It should be continued for 1–3 days, maintaining the partial thromboplasin time at 1.5–2 times control. The major purpose of heparin is to prevent reocclusion of the newly reperfused coronary artery.

c. β-blockers should be administered early and IV in all patients receiving thrombolytic therapy, provided that there are no contraindications. Immediate β-blockade has been shown to decrease significantly the incidence of recurrent ischemia and reinfarction in this patient population (TIMI-II).

E. Indications for invasive procedures after thrombolysis

1. Patients with persistent (or intermittent) chest pain and continued ST-segment elevation despite the administration of thrombolytic therapy should be considered for emergency cardiac catheterization within 1–2 hr.

2. Many of these patients should be considered for "rescue" coronary angioplasty, aimed at reperfusing the occluded infarct–related vessel by mechanical means.

3. If coronary angiography demonstrates significant left main or triple-vessel disease, or if the anatomy is otherwise unsuitable for coronary angioplasty, patients should be considered for emergency bypass surgery.

4. Whether or not to perform diagnostic cardiac catheterization prior to hospital discharge is currently a matter of debate. Cardiac catheterization is usually performed in those patients who spontaneously develop rest or exertional angina (postinfarction angina); and in those patients in whom angina is provoked by a submaximal exercise test.

5. In addition, diagnostic cardiac catheterization is often recommended for patients at high risk for ischemic complications postdischarge, such as those with significant left ventricular dysfunction, extensive infarct territory (particularly anterior infarction), and complex ventricular arrhythmias. It is also recommended in younger patients (age < 55).

F. Primary coronary angioplasty: Reperfusion without thrombolysis
1. When acute infarction patients present with absolute or relative contraindications to thrombolytic therapy, an invasive approach should be strongly considered.
2. Emergent diagnostic catheterization is done to define the infarct-related vessel.
3. Primary (or direct) angioplasty of the infarct-related vessel should then be performed to restore coronary blood flow.
4. This invasive approach is also valuable in patients in whom the diagnosis is in doubt, such as those with typical ischemic chest pain without ST-segment elevation or those with atypical symptoms.
5. Increasingly, the use of direct angioplasty in patients with cardiogenic shock is being recommended after diagnosis and stabilization.
6. The precise role of direct percutaneous transluminal coronary angioplasty in routine myocardial infarction management remains controversial. Recent studies suggest an improved outcome with regard to decreased recurrent ischemia and non-fatal infarction with angioplasty compared to thrombolytic therapy.

III. **Coronary Morphology and Acute Coronary Syndromes: Pathophysiologic Hypothesis**
   A. Introduction
      In recent years, new observations based on improved technology have changed our concepts of coronary pathogenesis. Thrombus formation secondary to plaque fissuring or rupture appears to be the common link in these syndromes.

B. Platelets and thrombosis
   1. Platelet adhesion and vessel wall injury
      a. The loss of integrity of the endothelial lining in a normal blood vessel by superficial injury results in attachment of a layer of adherent platelets to the underlying subendothelium.
      b. Platelets attach to exposed subendothelium, a process dependent on platelet membrane receptors, adhesive macromolecules that circulate in the blood or are released by platelet granules, and exposure of activating sites in the subendothelium.
      c. These receptors are recognized by fibrinogen molecules which bind to them and form links between platelets, constituting the essential process in aggregation.
      d. Platelet activation occurs via three pathways: (1) direct stimulation by thrombin and collagen, (2) adenosine diphosphate released from platelet granules, and (3) arachidonic acid converted to thromboxane A_2 by cyclooxygenase and thromboxane synthetase in the platelet.
      e. In addition, the clotting mechanism may be activated by exposure of blood to the damaged endothelial surface (intrinsic system) and to released tissue factor (extrinsic system). Thrombin is then generated, further promoting platelet aggregation.

C. Coronary morphology in acute ischemic syndromes
   Occurrence of thrombosis superimposed on deep arterial wall injury or a ruptured plaque is the mechanism of coronary arterial occlusion in myocardial infarction and unstable angina.
   1. Unstable angina
      a. Patients with progressive symptoms but without rest angina have a ruptured plaque without thrombosis.
      b. Because such plaque rupture is often found in an area of a relatively minor preexisting lesion, the increase in exertional symptoms is ascribed to a decrease in coronary blood flow due to rupture of a relatively small, soft, "fatty" plaque, which acutely increases the degree of stenosis.
      c. There is increasing evidence that unsta-

ble angina at rest may be produced mainly by the occurrence of intermittent thrombosis superimposed on the lesion.

    d. Vasoconstriction or spasm may also contribute to exertional angina at decreased workloads (*mixed angina*), as well as to episodes of rest pain in patients with unstable angina.

    e. Abnormalities of coronary tone have been demonstrated in unstable patients with coronary stenoses by coronary arteriography following intracoronary injection of acetylcholine and ergonovine.

2. Non-Q-wave infarction

    a. About one-fourth of patients with non-Q-wave infarctions have completely occluded infarct-related vessels, the distal territory usually being well supplied by collaterals.

    b. In most other patients, a transient complete occlusion which resolves within the first 1 or 2 hr (*spontaneous thrombolysis*) is responsible for the ischemic event.

    c. Most often, nontotal obstructions with some preserved antegrade flow are found. These obstructions may close totally and reopen intermittently (*stuttering* infarction).

    d. In yet other cases, transient hypotension may be the initiating factor.

    e. The angiographic morphology of the infarct-related stenosis has been shown to be the same as described for unstable angina, confirming the role of plaque rupture as the initiating factor in the majority of cases.

3. Q-wave infarction

    a. The patient who develops a Q-wave infarction almost always exhibits an occlusive thrombus overlying an area of plaque rupture at angiography.

    b. One may hypothesize that in Q-wave infarction the thrombus is more fixed, lasting for at least several hours due to a greater extent of vessel wall damage or ulcer than in other coronary syndromes.

    c. The incidence of total occlusions diminishes with time over the first 24 hr after the event, suggesting spontaneous thrombolysis after the infarction has occurred. The opposite pattern has been described with non-Q-wave infarction.

IV. Complications of Acute Myocardial Infarction

A. Introduction

The consequences of myocardial infarction are many. They include (1) development of ventricular fibrillation and sudden cardiac death, most commonly in the first few minutes, (2) development of various cardiac arrhythmias and heart block, (3) cardiogenic shock, (4) congestive heart failure, (5) ventricular aneurysm, (6) clot in the LV, (7) rupture of the intraventricular septum or LV free wall, (8) rupture or dysfunction of the papillary muscles of the mitral valve, (9) venous thrombosis and pulmonary embolism, and (10) pericarditis.

B. Systolic ventricular performance

1. In myocardial infarction, various focal LV contraction abnormalities may occur, including (a) hypokinesis, (b) akinesis, (c) dyskinesis, and (d) aneurysm formation. *Hypokinesis* is decreased contraction, *akinesis* is absence of contraction, and *dyskinesis* is paradoxic expansion or systolic bulging. *Paradoxic systolic expansion* decreases the forward blood flow or stroke volume of the LV.

2. The hemodynamic consequences of increasing amounts of infarcted myocardium on systolic performance are determined by the Frank-Starling curve: a progressive decrease in systolic performance (stroke work) despite increasing LV filling pressure.

3. Increasing diastolic stiffness in the infarcted zone of the myocardium may actually improve global LV systolic function since it tends to minimize systolic paradoxic wall motion.

4. Clinical heart failure accompanies a combined area of abnormal contraction exceeding 25%, and cardiogenic shock accompanies loss of more than 35% of the LV myocardium. Cardiogenic shock is fatal in 80–90% of patients.

5. Reversible ischemia has been hypothesized to cause diminution or absence of segmental ventricular contraction for extended periods (up to several days), called *stunned myocardium*. It is possible that with reperfusion this myocardium can renew its contractile properties, an issue of great controversy today.

6. Patients with myocardial infarction can occasionally have reduced contractile func-

tion in noninfarcted zones of the myocardium. This may occur because the coronary artery supplying the noninfarcted region of the ventricle is obstructed, and previously was perfused from collaterals from the infarcted vessel, a condition termed *ischemia at a distance*.

C. Diastolic ventricular function

1. The major characteristic of diastolic performance after myocardial infarction is decreased LV compliance. This increases diastolic pressure for any given volume. Thus the left ventricular end-diastolic pressure is frequently between 12 and 18 mmHg.

2. The Frank-Starling law determines that it is helpful to have an increased filling pressure to support systolic function when systolic performance is reduced.

D. Complications of myocardial infarction

1. Rupture of the free wall of the left ventricle.

   a. More frequent in the elderly and in women, and more common in hypertensive than normotensive individuals.

   b. Usually occurs 3 to 5 days following an infarct.

   c. Preceded by infarct expansion, that is, a thinning and disproportionate dilatation within the softened necrotic zone.

   d. Rupture usually results in electromechanical dissociation and death unless the diagnosis is made and drainage of pericardial blood is performed promptly.

   e. Rarely, complete rupture may be contained by a fibrotic pericardium, producing an LV diverticulum or a large false aneurysm or pseudoaneurysm which maintains communication with the cavity of the LV but does not cause immediate death of the patient.

2. Rupture of the interventricular septum

   a. Occurs with either anteroseptal infarcts, involving the apex, or inferior wall infarcts, involving the posterior-basal part of the intraventricular septum.

   b. This produces a left-to-right shunt of blood, resulting in hypotension with shock.

3. Rupture of the papillary muscle

   a. Produces severe congestive heart failure associated with acute severe mitral regurgitation.

   b. Caused by complete necrosis of the full thickness of the papillary muscle.

4. Ventricular aneurysm

   a. A circumscribed, noncontractile outpouching of the LV occurring in 12–15% of patients surviving a myocardial infarction.

   b. The wall of the aneurysm is thin compared to the rest of the LV. The wall bulges with systole, thus decreasing stroke volume.

   c. Aneurysm associated with clot formation usually develops in the apex of the LV.

   d. Occasionally systolic emboli occur from these clots.

   e. A true LV aneurysm rarely ruptures.

5. Right ventricular (RV) infarction

   a. More frequent than many clinicians realize.

   b. Generally associated with obstructive lesions of the right coronary artery.

   c. It is less common than LV infarcts because of the lower oxygen demands of the RV.

   d. RV infarcts occur more commonly with conditions associated with increased RV oxygen needs, such as cor pulmonale.

   e. A shock-like syndrome may occur with an RV infarct, primarily because of the markedly decreased output of the RV to the pulmonary circulation and the subsequent decrease in LV filling.

6. Ventricular arrhythmias

   a. Usually occurs during the acute phase.

   b. Ventricular tachycardia, which frequently leads to ventricular fibrillation and cardiac arrest, is usually due to acute ischemia.

   c. When arrhythmias occur unassociated with acute ischemia, an aneurysm may be the electrical substrate. Electrophysiologic testing is mandatory in these cases.

7. AV block

   a. After anterior infarcts, blocks below the bundle of His may produce second- and third-degree AV blocks, as well as various bundle branch blocks, which are associated with a very high mortality.

   b. AV block associated with anterior infarction generally requires pacemaker therapy.

   c. With inferior infarction, blocks above

the bundle of His may occur, also producing second- and third-degree AV block. These AV blocks are usually reversible and are not associated with high mortality.

   d. Various arrhythmias are associated with a poor prognosis after infarction, including the development of supraventricular tachycardia and bundle branch blocks.

E. Long-term prognosis after infarction

  1. Certain findings are associated with increased mortality. These include:

    a. Persistent diffuse ST depression of the ECG.

    b. Complex ventricular arrhythmias.

    c. Recurrent supraventricular arrhythmias.

    d. Decreased LV ejection fraction, especially < 40% (normal, 55–70%).

    e. The development of ischemic changes on ECG during low-intensity treadmill stress testing.

    f. Recurrent angina.

  2. In addition, the classical risk factors of smoking, hypercholesterolemia, and elevated blood pressure become even more significant predictors of recurrent coronary events and cardiovascular mortality.

  3. Currently, there are a limited number of pharmacologic interventions which may affect long-term mortality. These include:

    a. β-blockers (for 2–3 years).

    b. Possibly aspirin.

    c. Angiotensin-converting enzyme inhibitors (in post-myocardial infarction patients with severe congestive heart failure or diminished ejection fraction (<40%).

    d. Calcium antagonists after non-Q-wave infarcts (but not after Q-wave infarcts).

Bibliography

Modern Management of Acute Myocardial Infarction in the Community Hospital. Jeffrey Anderson, editor. Marcel Dekker, New York, 1991.

Pasternak RC, Braunwald E, Sobel BE, "Acute Myocardial Infarction" in Braunwald E (ed) *Heart Disease: A Textbook of Cardiovascular Medicine,* 3rd edition. Chapter 39, pp 1200–1291. WB Saunders, Philadelphia, 1992.

Clinical Strategies in Ischemic Heart Disease E. Corday and HJC Swan, editors. Williams and Wilkins, Baltimore, 1979.

Topol E, "Mechanical Interventions For Acute Myocardial Infarction" in Topol E (editor), *Textbook of Interventional Cardiology.* Chapter 14, pp 269–299. WB Saunders, Philadelphia, 1990.

Topol E, "Thrombolytic Intervention" in Topol E (editor) op. cit.

CHAPTER 22

Cardiomyopathy and Myocarditis

Lloyd W. Klein, M.D.
Joseph E. Parrillo, M.D.

Cardiomyopathy

I. Definition

A. A disease, often of unknown etiology, in which the basic pathophysiologic and dominant clinical feature is myocardial dysfunction. The diagnosis of cardiomyopathy implies the exclusion of ischemic, hypertensive, congenital, valvular, and pericardial diseases.

B. Classification

   1. May be based on functional presentation
      a. Hypertrophic—inappropriate left ventricular (LV) hypertrophy, often with asymmetrical septal involvement and preserved or increased contractility.
      b. Dilated—characterized by LV dilation, contractile dysfunction, and symptoms of congestive heart failure (CHF).
      c. Restrictive—an LV endocardial abnormality (e.g., scarring) causing impaired diastolic filling.
   2. Another useful classification system is based on etiology:
      a. Primary—the cause of the heart disease is unknown and is not part of a systemic disorder.
      b. Secondary—the cause may be known (e.g., alcohol) or is a manifestation of a systemic illness (e.g., amyloid).

C. Often, these two classification systems are combined to describe a given patient.

II. Hypertrophic Cardiomyopathy (HCM)

A. Definition of terminology and subtypes
   Hypertrophy can occur in any part of the ventricular wall, but certain patterns are most typical:

   1. Idiopathic hypertrophic subaortic stenosis (IHSS)—a form of HCM in which a dynamic subaortic outflow obstruction is present or inducible. Septal hypertrophy is a cardinal manifestation.
   2. Nonobstructive HCM—no rest or provokable gradient; asymmetric septal hypertrophy is present.
   3. Apical HCM
      a. Yamaguchi's HCM: spade-like configuration on two-dimensional echocardiogram and/or left ventriculogram; electrocardiography (ECG) demonstrates giant inverted T-waves in the precordial leads; there is no outflow gradient.

b. Maron described an atypical form with a small, poorly contractile apical segment and a markedly narrowed midventricular channel. A pressure gradient may be found, and the T-waves are not deeply inverted.

4. Genetically transmitted forms
   a. Autosomal dominant transmission with partial penetrance is the probable cause in the majority of patients with HCM.
   b. May be human leukocyte antigen (HLA) related or linked to Friedrich's ataxia, Pompe's disease, Duchenne's muscular dystrophy, or Fabry's disease
   c. May have concentric LV hypertrophy.

5. Asymmetric septal hypertrophy may be associated with lentiginosis, acromegaly, hyper- or hypothyroidism, and hyperparathyroidism.

6. Athletes may demonstrate any of these patterns, which may be associated with sudden death.

7. HCM may occur in the elderly (> 70 years old) in any morphologic type. When concentric LV hypertrophy occurs, it is difficult to separate HCM from hypertensive heart disease.

B. Morphology
   1. Anatomy
      a. Hypertrophic LV with normal or increased function and small or normal-sized LV chamber (at least in the early stages).
      b. The hypertrophy is often asymmetric, with a predilection for the basal septum, but may be concentric or localized to other segments.
      c. Systolic anterior motion of the anterior mitral valve leaflet occurs in the obstructive forms (i.e., IHSS).
      d. Endocardial plaque found at the point of mitral-septal contact.
      e. Dilated left atrium.
   2. Histology
      a. Myocardial fiber disarray
         (1) Five percent or more of myocardium in 80% of HCM
         (2) gross disorganization, with a characteristic "whorled" pattern.
         (3) Prominent fibrosis.
         (4) *Not* pathognomonic though highly suggestive of HCM.
      b. Medial hypertrophy of intramural coronary arteries.

(1) Reduced luminal area.
(2) Occurs mostly in the septum.
(3) May be responsible for myocardial ischemia.

C. Pathophysiology
   1. Impaired outflow during systole caused by the narrowing of the outflow tract due to asymmetric hypertrophy *plus* abnormal mitral valve motion.
      a. Obstructive types (IHSS): dynamic obstruction worsened by:
         (1) Increased contractility (catecholamines, inotropes).
         (2) Decreased preload (volume loss, venous pooling, induced by standing or use of nitrates).
      b. Dynamic obstruction decreased by:
         (1) Increased afterload (arteriolar vasoconstriction).
         (2) Negative inotropes (calcium antagonists, β-blockers).
   2. Impaired diastolic filling
      a. Impaired relaxation due to LV hypertrophy.
      b. Disproportionate contribution of atrial transport to LV filling.
   3. One-third of patients have mitral regurgitation.
   4. Myocardial ischemia/scarring
      a. Reduced coronary flow reserve.
      b. Small vessel disease (see Subsection B, 2 above).
      c. Septal perforator "squeeze" during systole.
   5. Associated with arrhythmias
      a. Ventricular arrhythmias and sudden death—most common cause of mortality in IHSS.
      b. Supraventricular tachycardia, especially atrial fibrillation; potential for further diminished LV filling and for systemic embolization.
      c. Occasional association with atrioventricular bypass tracts.
   6. Increased incidence of infectious endocarditis
      a. Septal endocardial plaque
      b. Outflow tract
      c. Mitral regurgitation

D. Clinical findings
   1. Symptoms
      a. Dizziness, syncope
      b. Dyspnea and fatigue
      c. Palpitations

d. Chest pain, typical and atypical
e. Sudden death–2–3% incidence per year

2. Physical exam
   a. Blood pressure usually normal; with severe pressure gradient may be low; in elderly HCM, may be associated with hypertension.
   b. Arterial pulse—brisk upstroke, bifid systolic contour, prolonged ejection time (in IHSS).
   c. Jugular venous pulse—prominent a-wave.
   d. Apical impulse—sustained LV heave, palpable S_4 gallop.
   e. Auscultation
      (1) Systolic ejection murmur at lower left sternal border augmented by maneuvers which decrease LV size (e.g., Valsalva maneuver); murmur decreased by increasing afterload with squatting.
      (2) S_4 gallop.
      (3) Paradoxically split S_2.
      (4) Mitral regurgitation in one-third of patients.

E. Diagnostic evaluation
   1. Echocardiography/Doppler Ultrasound
      a. Thickened (hypertrophied) LV wall: basal septum most frequent; also apex, generalized hypertrophy, free wall hypertrophy.
      b. LV hypercontractility and small chamber size.
      c. LA dilation.
      d. LV outflow tract obstruction.
         (1) Systolic anterior motion of the anterior mitral valve leaflet.
         (2) Prolonged mitral-septal contact with resting obstruction.
         (3) Aortic valve closure during mid- or early systole.
      e. Doppler ultrasound can quantitate the pressure gradient and demonstrate midsystolic obstruction, mitral regurgitation, and abnormal LV filling.
   2. Cardiac catheterization
      a. Normal to hyperdynamic LV systolic function.
      b. LV outflow obstruction.
         (1) Resting gradient.
         (2) Provokable gradient—Valsalva response to premature ventricular contractions; (PVCs), amyl nitrite, isoproterenol; decreased gradient with phenylephrine.

      (3) Assess mitral regurgitation.
      (4) Quantitate LV filling pressure.
      (5) Assess coronary arteries.

F. Prognosis
   1. Recurrent syncope—usually responsive to negative inotropes which decrease the pressure gradient.
   2. Congestive heart failure
      a. Also responsive to medications which decrease the pressure gradient and enhance diastolic relaxation.
      b. When mitral regurgitation becomes more severe and/or LV dilation ensues in the later stages, *judicious* doses of nitrates, diuretics, and digoxin may be useful. Such agents are contraindicated in any patient with resting or provokable outflow tract obstruction.
   3. Sudden death—usually due to ventricular arrhythmias, but may also occur with heavy exercise (athletes) or with marked subaortic obstruction.
   4. High-risk profile
      a. Age of 10–30 years
      b. Family history of sudden death
      c. Marked LV hypertrophy
      d. Marked resting or provokable gradient
      e. Presence of ventricular tachycardia (8% mortality per year) or frequent PVCs on ambulatory monitoring

G. Treatment
   1. Negative inotropes which decrease the pressure gradient and enhance LV diastolic filling.
      a. β-blockers—30–50% response rate.
      b. Calcium channel blockers, especially verapamil—60% response rate
      c. Combined propranolol-verapamil therapy—anecdotally effective in refractory cases, but increased incidence of sinoatrial (SA) and atrioventricular (AV) blocks reported.
      d. May actually worsen the condition in patients with elevated pulmonary venous pressures, LV dilation, and/or mitral regurgitation.
   2. Digitalis, diuretics—as noted, usually considered contraindicated but may have a role in selected cases with severe mitral regurgitation and LV dilation
   3. Antiarrhythmics
      a. Disopyramide—also a negative inotrope which may be synergistic in reducing the subaortic gradient.

b. Amiodarone—conflicting reports in the literature at this time.

4. Surgery—myotomy/myectomy, with or without mitral valve replacement.

    a. Indicated in patients with medically refractory symptoms, a significant subaortic gradient (> 50 mmHg), and/or mitral regurgitation.

    b. Operative mortality of 5–8% plus possibility of ventricular septal defect and conduction blocks, occasionally requiring AV sequential pacing.

    c. Among operative survivors, 95% experience a reduced gradient and improved symptoms.

III. Dilated Cardiomyopathy (CM)

A. Characterization

1. Demonstrably diminished LV systolic function.
2. Four-chamber cardiac enlargement.
3. Symptoms result primarily from LV dysfunction.
4. LV hypertrophy not prominent for degree of LV dilation.
5. Mitral regurgitation may occur due to LV dilation.
6. Histology shows interstitial and perivascular fibrosis, cellular infiltrates, and myocyte hypertrophy and degeneration.

B. Etiologies (Common)

1. Idiopathy—most common
       a. May be related to an autoimmune response to a previous viral myocarditis.
       b. Enterovirus RNA has been found in many patients with end-stage dilated CM.
2. Metabolic
       a. Nutritional
           (1) Beri-beri (high output)
           (2) Selenium deficiency
       b. Endocrine
           (1) Acromegaly
           (2) Hypothyroidism
           (3) Diabetes
       c. Electrolyte
           (1) Hypophosphatemia
           (2) Hypocalcemia
3. Toxic/drug-related
       a. Alcohol
       b. Adriamycin, cyclophosphamide
       c. Catecholamines
       d. Cocaine
4. Hematologic—may be nonspecific response to any chronic anemia

    a. Sickle cell anemia
    b. Polycythemia vera

5. Systemic diseases
    a. Sarcoid
    b. Uremia
    c. Scleroderma
    d. Peripartum

C. Clinical manifestations

1. Symptoms—those of LV failure
       a. Diminished cardiac output—fatigue, weakness.
       b. Elevated pulmonary venous pressure—dyspnea, paroxysmal nocturnal dyspnea, orthopnea.
       c. Right-sided failure—late and ominous sign (i.e., peripheral edema, abdominal distension).
       d. Chest pain—may suggest concomitant ischemic disease.
       e. Cardiac cachexia—late stage.
       f. Systemic emboli—(i.e., cerebrovascular accidents and pulmonary emboli).

2. Physical examination
       a. Arterial pulse—low systolic pressure, narrow pulse pressure; pulsus alternans with severe LV failure.
       b. Neck vein distension—frequent; prominent a-wave; prominent v-wave suggests superimposed tricuspid regurgitation.
       c. Engorged liver, edema, and ascites with right heart failure
       d. Cardiac exam
           (1) LV and perhaps RV heaves with laterally displaced apical impulse.
           (2) Gallop rhythms.
           (3) Mitral and/or tricuspid regurgitation murmurs.

D. Diagnostic Evaluation

1. Chest x-ray—enlarged chambers, pulmonary venous congestion, pleural effusions.
2. ECG—dysrhythmias, conduction defects, abnormal Q-waves and ST changes, ventricular and atrial enlargement.
3. Echocardiogram—four-chamber enlargement, excludes other causes of heart failure; LV thrombus.
4. Coronary angiography—excludes ischemic origin.
5. Transvenous endomyocardial biopsy
       a. May diagnose uncommon specific causes (e.g., hemochromatosis, radiation fibrosis, anthracycline toxicity, myocarditis, sarcoidosis).

b. Most likely to show lymphocytic and/or fibroblastic infiltration in patients with a presumed preceding viral illness and a short duration of cardiac symptoms.

c. The incidence of myocarditis proved by biopsy dilated CM patients is low, usually 3–10%.

d. The interobserver variability in interpreting biopsy specimens for myocarditis is high.

e. In patients with cellular infiltrates, prednisone therapy may produce a modest improvement in ventricular performance; however, its long-term benefit is minimal and the side effect profile is significant.

E. Prognosis

1. Usually, progressive deterioration over several years, but with a substantial early mortality soon after presentation.

2. Mortality of 75% within 5 years; a minority (10–20%) of patients improve and achieve long-term survival.

3. Most therapies are symptomatic and do not seem to alter the prognosis; however, vasodilators (isordil and hydralazine) and angiotensin converting enzyme (ACE) inhibitors have shown modest improvement in survival in heart failure patients, including those with dilated CM.

F. Treatment

1. Digitalis, diuretics, venodilators (nitrates).

2. ACE inhibitors or hydralazine-isordil combination.

3. Intravenous inotropes

a. β-adrenergic agonists—dobutamine.

b. Phosphodiesterase inhibitors—amrinone; oral form (milrinone) recently shown to improve symptoms but worsen the prognosis.

4. β-blocker therapy in very low doses has been associated with improved exercise tolerance and ventricular performance in some dilated cardiomyopathy (DCM) patients. However, it is difficult to identify prospectively the subgroup that responds. Benefit may be due to β-receptor up-regulation.

5. Levodopa—may improve LV function in a subgroup of patients.

6. Anticoagulants—prevent pulmonary and systemic emboli.

7. Antiarrhythmic therapy—controversial: Is the therapeutic benefit of PVC control greater than the risk of proarrhythmia?

8. Cardiac transplantation in end-stage, refractory cases.

IV. **Restrictive Cardiomyopathy**

A. Clinical characteristics

1. Defined by normal LV chamber size, normal or mildly abnormal systolic function, increased LV thickness, and the sine qua non, abnormal diastolic function with restrictive hemodynamics.

2. Myocardial infiltration, fibrosis, or hypertrophy due to an underlying disease process is responsible for diastolic dysfunction.

3. Differentiation from constrictive pericarditis is typically a fundamental clinical problem and is mandatory, as the latter is surgically remediable.

4. No specific therapy exists. The prognosis is that of the underlying disease.

B. Etiology

1. Amyloidosis—most common cause in United States. May be associated with systemic amyloidosis or limited to the heart. May be secondary to immune dyscrasias, chronic infectious or inflammatory conditions, or familial. Cardiovascular amyloid may also present with a syndrome of orthostatic hypotension, arrhythmias, conduction disturbances, and/or dysautonomia.

2. Hemochromatosis—may present as a dilated or restrictive CM. Suspected especially in diabetics with characteristic bronze skin coloration. May also occur with chronic liver disease, defects in hemoglobin synthesis, or excessive iron intake or abnormal iron metabolism. Therapy with repeated phlebotomy or iron chelation with desferoxamine may provide substantial benefit.

3. Sarcoid—may present as a dilated or restrictive CM. Primary cardiac involvement in this chronic granulomatous disorder with multisystem involvement is difficult to recognize, especially since cor pulmonale due to pulmonary disease is much more common. Conduction defects, AV block, LV failure, and ventricular arrhythmias should raise the suspicion of this disease.

4. Hypereosinophilic syndrome—frequently associated with Loeffler's endocarditis, an endomyocardial fibrosis frequently associated with overlying thrombus that produces profound restriction to ventricular filling. Treatment with antieosinophil therapy has been associated with improved survival.

5. Endocardial fibroelastosis—usually seen in young children

C. Clinical manifestations
   1. Symptoms
      a. Exercise intolerance—inability to increase cardiac output by tachycardia without decreasing the filling time.
      b. Weakness and dyspnea (heart failure).
   2. Physical Exam
      a. Signs of right-sided heart failure may be more prominent than those of left-sided heart failure—neck vein distension, peripheral edema, enlarged liver, ascites.
      b. S_3 and/or S_4 gallops.
      c. Kussmaul's sign—inspiratory increase in venous pressure.

D. Diagnostic Evaluation
   1. Noninvasive tests
      a. ECG: low voltage despite demonstration of thickened LV on echocardiogram.
      b. Chest x-ray—pericardial calcification, if present, is helpful in making a differential diagnosis in favor of constrictive pericarditis.
      c. Computed tomography (CT) scanning, magnetic resonance imaging (MRI)—distinguish between pericardial and myocardial thickening.
   2. Invasive tests
      a. Hemodynamics—equalization of diastolic pressures with prominent "y" descent in atrial chambers, "dip and plateau" pattern in ventricular chambers. To distinguish from constriction, one must show some separation of LV from RV diastolic pressure (e.g., Valsalva maneuver, PVCs, volume loading). The crucial point is to prove a differential effect i.e. LV > RV. Otherwise, one cannot exclude either diagnosis.
      b. Endomyocardial biopsy—definitive diagnosis if the endocardium is thick or infiltration with amyloid, iron, or granuloma (sarcoid) can be clearly demonstrated.

E. Treatment
   1. Therapy aimed at the underlying disease if possible.
   2. Diuretics can produce some symptomatic improvement if used judiciously.

Infectious Myocarditis

I. **Pathophysiology**
   A. Inflammatory process caused by an infectious agent
      1. May be acute or chronic.
      2. Involves the myocardium, interstitium, and/or vascular structures.
      3. The process may be diffuse or focal and is randomly distributed.
      4. The histologic findings are nonspecific and do not aid in identifying a particular agent.
   B. Damage caused by several mechanisms
      1. Production of toxin (i.e., diphtheria).
      2. Invasion of myocardium.
      3. Immunologically mediated.
   C. Myocardial involvement is frequently subclinical. It has been hypothesized that idiopathic dilated cardiomyopathy may be the culmination of virus-initiated, immunologically mediated damage
   D. Clinical consequences dependent on the size, extent, and location of infective foci.

II. **Clinical Manifestations**
   A. Clinical expression may range from subclinical, due to focal inflammation alone, to acute and fulminant CHF with diffuse involvement.
   B. Usual presenting findings include heart failure, dysrhythmias, chest pain, and/or ECG changes.
   C. Nonspecific symptoms include fatigue, dyspnea, and palpitations.
   D. Physical findings
      1. Fever
      2. Tachycardia
      3. S_3 gallop
      4. Normal-sized or dilated LV with hypocontractility
      5. Pulmonary and/or systemic emboli
   E. ECG changes
      1. ST-segment and T-wave abnormalities
      2. PVCs
      3. AV block and intraventricular conduction defect (complete AV block may cause death).

III. **Diagnostic Evaluation**
   Diagnostic evaluation is mainly dependent on identification of the associated systemic illness (see Section V below) and/or viral titers or other serologic testing.
   A. Serum myocardial enzyme elevation (creatine kinase, serum glutamic-oxaloacetic transaminase), though frequently not present.
   B. Echocardiogram—diffuse LV wall motion abnormalities.
   C. Radionuclide scanning—with ^{67}Ga or ^{99m}Tc pyrophosphate to identify abnormal myocardial uptake.

D. Transvenous endomyocardial biopsy—pathologic findings to diagnose myocarditis positively. Isolation of virus very unlikely. A small group of patients have negative biopsy despite all other signs of myocarditis.

IV. Treatment

A. Usual supportive measures directed toward symptoms and signs (e.g., heart failure, dysrhythmias).

B. Immunosuppressive agents—some patients respond to prednisone and azathioprine, but their unequivocal value has not been established by a controlled trial. Such therapy is *not* indicated in patients without histologic evidence of inflammation (lymphocytes, fibroblasts), or in those with a positive gallium scan or a consistently elevated erythrocyte sedimentation rate without another evident cause.

V. Common or Important Etiologic Agents

A. Viral

1. Coxsackie: Both A and B viruses cause myocarditis, but coxsackie B is the more frequent cause of viral myocarditis. Clinical symptoms are those suggesting acute viral infection (i.e., pleurodynia, myalgia, upper respiratory infection, arthralgia, fever); chest pain, palpitations, and dyspnea are suspicious symptoms.

2. Echovirus—similar to coxsackie in terms of presentation.

3. Influenza virus.

4. Poliomyelitis—myocarditis is a frequent finding with this rare illness.

5. Human immunodeficiency virus (HIV)—acquired immunodeficiency virus (AIDS)

   a. Myocarditis is common but not usually clinically manifest.

   b. CHF, LV dysfunction, ventricular arrhythmias, and ECG charges in AIDS patients should raise suspicions, especially late in the course of the illness.

   c. Infectious myocarditis in AIDS patients may also be due to any number of other opportunistic agents.

6. Cytomegalovirus.

7. Mycoplasma pneumonia.

8. Psittacosis.

B. Rickettsial

1. Scrub typhus.

2. Rocky Mountain spotted fever.

C. Bacterial

1. Diphtheria—myocarditis is the most common cause of death and occurs in 25% of cases. Damage is caused by a toxin which inhibits protein synthesis. Signs appear after 1 week of illness. Cardiomegaly, CHF, and elevated serum CK are common. Cardiovascular collapse may ensue. Urgent treatment with antitoxin is called for; antibiotics are less important. Steroids are of no value, but carnitine may be a useful adjunct.

2. Streptococcal—rheumatic fever and its sequelae are forms of immune myocarditis, with or without valvulitis.

D. Spirochetal

1. Syphilis—aortitis is the more usual manifestation of chronic luetic disease, but in congenital syphilis, myocarditis is a severe manifestation.

2. Lyme disease—carditis occurs in 5–10% of cases about 3–6 weeks after the initial illness. It is manifest as a transient myocarditis, with varying degrees of AV block. Ceftriaxone, penicillin, or tetracycline therapy usually brings resolution; serologic confirmation should be sought.

E. Protozoal

1. Chagas' disease (*Trypanosoma cruzi*)—most frequent cause of CHF and sudden death in South and Central America.

   a. Acute phase—transmission by bite of reduviid bug, classically dropping (*vinchuga*) from the ceiling at night, biting around the eyes (eyelid swelling: Romana's sign) or through the skin (chagoma). Fever, myalgia, diaphoresis, and CHF ensue; most patients recover. Young children most often develop clinical, acute phase disease. Immune myocytolysis by antibody and cell-mediated immunity directed against *T. cruzi*-infected cells is the pathogenesis of the acute myocarditis.

   b. Latent phase—*no* clinical sequelae for 10–30 years!

   c. Chronic chagas' disease—occurs in 30% of infected individuals; manifestations range from simple seropositivity to isolated ECG changes, CHF, dysrhythmia, emboli, right bundle branch block, left anterior hemiblock, posterior-apical aneurysms, and sudden death. A dilated, four-chamber CM is usual, but RV dilation may be most prominent. An autoimmune mechanism is suggested by increased levels of IgG directed against myocyte sarcolemma, an anti-*T. cruzi* membrane antibody which cross-reacts with the myocyte sarcoplasmic reticulum, and an IgG anti-idiotype, antisarcolemma antibody. The complement fixation test and the enzyme-linked immunosorbent assay (ELISA) are useful diagnostically.

Bibliography

Anderson DW, Virmani R, Reilly JM, et al: Prevalent myocarditis at necropsy in the acquired immunodeficiency syndrome. *J Am Coll Cardiol* 140:2023–2031, 1988.

McIntosh CL, Maron BJ: Current operative treatment of obstructive hypertrophic cardiomyopathy. *Circulation* 78:487–495, 1988.

Maron BJ, Bonow RO, Cannon RO, et al: Hypertrophic cardiomyopathy. *N Engl J Med* 316:780–788, 844–852, 1987.

Parrilo JE, Aretz T, Palacios I, et al: The results of transvenous endomyocardial biopsy can frequently be used to diagnose myocardial diseases in patients with idiopathic heart failure. Endomyocardial biopsies in 100 consecutive patients reveal a substantial incidence of myocarditis. *Circulation* 69:93–101, 1984.

Parrillo JE, Cunnion RE, Epstein SE, et al: A prospective, randomized, controlled trial of prednisone for dilated cardiomyopathy. *N Engl J Med* 321:1061–1068, 1989.

Popma JJ, Cigarroa RG, Busa LM, et al: Diagnostic and prognostic utility of right sided catheterization and endomyocardial biopsy in idiopathic dilated cardiomyopathy. *Am J Cardiol* 63:955–958, 1989.

Sadigursky M, Von Kreuter BF, Ling PY, et al: Association of elevated anti-sarcolemma, anti-idiotype antibody levels with the clinical and pathologic expression of chronic Chagas myocarditis. *Circulation* 80:1269–1276, 1989.

CHAPTER 23

Diseases of the Aorta

William Piccione, Jr., M.D.
Hassan Najafi, M.D.

The aorta originates at the aortic valve and contributes all major arterial branches (coronaries, brachiocephalics, renal, visceral) before terminating at its bifurcation into the iliacs. Pathologic processes affecting the aorta include trauma, atherosclerosis, aneurysmal disease, dissection, infection and degenerative processes such as cystic medial necrosis.

I. Trauma (Nonpenetrating)

  A. Etiology

    Blunt traumatic injury to the aorta is generally associated with a rapid deceleration injury.

  B. Pathophysiology

    Rapid deceleration applies a shearing force secondary to differential rates of deceleration within the aorta.

    1. Most common site of injury is the junction of the fixed aortic arch with the relatively mobile descending aorta, that is, just distal to the left subclavian.

    2. Less common sites are the root of the aorta and the origin of the innominate artery.

    3. Blunt trauma as a cause of abdominal aortic rupture is rare.

  C. Diagnosis

    1. History

      a. History of major trauma, usually a motor vehicle accident or fall, is obtainable.

      b. Patients usually present with multisystem injuries.

      c. Mean age is 26–31 years.

    2. Clinical signs and findings

      a. Associated trauma including orthopedic and neurologic injuries common.

      b. Clinical triad of increased blood pressure in upper extremities, decreased pressure in lower extremities, and widened mediastinum on chest x-ray (CXR) are diagnostic but not always present.

    3. Diagnostic tests

      a. CXR findings of widened mediastinum, left pleural effusion, deviation of trachea or nasogastric tube, "blurring" of aortic knob.

      b. Aortogram is the study of choice to identify acute aortic disruption.

      c. Computed tomography (CT) scan is helpful to evaluate untreated survivors who develop a late false aneurysm.

    4. Treatment

      a. Surgical repair is the treatment of choice.

5. Prognosis
   a. Traumatic aortic disruption usually fatal, with a small percentage (< 20%) of patients surviving to receive medical care.
   b. Only 5% of untreated survivors will live long enough to develop false aneurysms.
   c. Results of surgical repair are excellent.
      (1) Patients may succumb to associated injuries.
      (2) Paraplegia occurs in 5% of patients undergoing surgical repair secondary to temporary or permanent disruption of blood supply to the spinal cord.

II. Aneurysmal Disease

A. Etiology
   1. Degenerative process (atherosclerosis or cystic medial necrosis) is the most common etiology (> 90%) (Table 23-1).
      a. Aneurysms may be single or multiple and occur at any level. The fusiform variety is more common than the saccular form.
      b. Terminal aorta is affected most frequently, followed by the descending aorta and the ascending aorta.
   2. Syphilis, once common, is now rarely seen as an etiology.
      a. Syphilitic aneurysms exhibit a predilection for the thoracic aorta, particularly the ascending aorta; often they are saccular.

Table 23-1 Etiologic Classification of Aortic Aneurysms

Degenerative
  Atherosclerosis
  Medial necrosis
  Pregnancy related
Inflammatory
  Infectious (bacterial, syphilitic, mycobacterial, etc.)
  Noninfectious (autoimmune, Takayasu's
    syndrome, polyarteritis, Kawasaki disease, etc.)
Structural
  Postcoarctation
  Traumatic
  Postsurgical (anastomotic, graft degeneration)
Congenital
  Marfan's syndrome
  Ehlers-Danlos syndrome

Source: Adapted from Rutherford RD (ed): *Vascular Surgery.* Philadelphia, WB Saunders, 1984, p 746

3. Mycotic aneurysms occur secondary to infection weakening the aortic wall.
   a. Clinical course may be complicated by systemic sepsis and/or rupture.
   b. Aortic involvement may result from lodging of septic emboli in bacterial endocarditis, embolization to the vasa vasorum, or direct extension from adjacent septic foci.
   c. Current series demonstrate an increasing incidence of gram-negative and anaerobic species.
   d. Immunodeficient hosts may exhibit virtually any pathogen, including mycobacteria fungi, and *Campylobacter.*
   e. *Salmonella* is particularly virulent and currently accounts for half of all cases.
      (1) *Salmonella* infection of the arterial wall may cause rupture without prior aneurysm formation.
4. Takayasu's aortitis is an inflammatory disorder of the aorta and its branches that may cause both occlusive and aneurysmal lesions.
   a. Etiology unclear; possible autoimmune disorder.
   b. Generally affects young persons (< 30 years) and women, who account for 90% of cases.
   c. Hypertension is a common finding, either from stenotic lesions of the suprarenal aorta or from renal artery stenosis.
   d. Death is commonly due to congestive heart failure or myocardial infarction.
5. Marfan's syndrome and other connective tissue disorders such as Ehlers-Danlos syndrome (see Section IV).

B. Pathophysiology of atherosclerotic aneurysm
   1. Poorly understood process whereby atherosclerotic degeneration weakens the aortic wall.
      a. Virtually all aneurysms expand with time and many eventually rupture.
      b. Larger-diameter aneurysms generally expand more rapidly than smaller ones (LaPlace's law)
   2. Risk factors same as those for atherosclerotic occlusive disease (see Subsection III, A).

C. Diagnosis
   1. Thoracic aortic aneurysms may be asymptomatic until they become large or rupture.
      a. May cause dull, aching pain.

b. Often found incidentally on CXR.

c. Symptoms may develop from compression of local structures.

   (1) Hoarseness with recurrent laryngeal nerve involvement.

   (2) Dysphagia with esophageal compression.

2. Abdominal aortic aneurysms may be detected by the patient or physician as a pulsatile mass. More commonly, they are discovered incidentally on x-rays of the spine, on abdominal ultrasound scans, or on abdominal exploration for other conditions.

a. Tenderness implies impending rupture.

b. Distal pulses are intact unless there is concurrent occlusive disease.

c. Overwhelming majority of aneurysms contain laminated clots.

3. Ruptured aortic aneurysms are usually fatal.

a. Ascending aneurysms rupture into the pericardial sac and cause tamponade.

b. Descending aortic aneurysms rupture into the left hemithorax.

c. Abdominal aortic aneurysms may rupture into one of four cavities:

   (1) Intra-abdominal; usually fatal.

   (2) Retroperitoneal; may locally tamponade long enough for the patient to seek medical care.

   (3) Into adjacent bowel, with the patient presenting with gastrointestinal hemorrhage.

   (4) Into the inferior vena cava (rare); patients present in congestive heart failure with a continuous abdominal bruit.

4. Diagnostic tests

a. CT scan with contrast is usually adequate.

b. Magnetic resonance imaging (MRI) may replace CT scan as modality of choice. Negates the need for contrast material.

c. Small, asymptomatic aneurysms may be followed by ultrasound.

d. Transesophageal ultrasound helpful in evaluating thoracic aneurysms.

e. Aortogram is often necessary to confirm the diagnosis and to delineate the extent of the lesion and its relationship to major arterial branches.

5. Differential diagnosis

a. CT scan or MRI can usually differentiate aneurysmal disease from nonvascular masses.

6. Treatment

a. Surgical resection and placement of interposition graft is treatment of choice, with excellent results.

b. Small (< 4 cm diameter), asymptomatic aneurysms may be followed by noninvasive means and resected if they continue to expand.

7. Prognosis

a. A 30–40% chance of death by eventual rupture if untreated.

b. Excellent prognosis with surgical resection.

c. Resection of descending aortic aneurysms carry the risk of paraplegia secondary to interruption of the spinal cord blood supply.

III. **Atherosclerotic occlusive disease**

A. Etiology

1. Atherosclerosis is a generalized disorder of the arterial system. Known risk factors include genetic predisposition, dietary factors, diabetes, hyperlipidemias, tobacco abuse, and hypertension.

B. Pathophysiology

1. Accumulation of atherosclerotic plaque reduces effective intraluminal diameter.

2. Blood flow generally unaffected until lumen is reduced by 50%.

3. Symptoms attributable to insufficient blood flow to organs and/or extremities.

C. Diagnosis

1. Supported by presence of known risk factors.

2. Symptoms dependent on branch arteries compromised.

a. Coronaries—angina, myocardial infarction.

b. Brachiocephalic—neurologic, transient ischemic attacks.

c. Renals—hypertension, renal insufficiency.

d. Visceral—"intestinal angina," weight loss.

e. Iliacs—claudication.

3. "Leriche syndrome"

a. Thrombotic occlusion of infrarenal aorta.

b. Increasing hypertension implies renal artery encroachment by ascending thrombus.

c. Impotence occurs secondary to internal iliac artery compromise.
d. Bilateral claudication.
e. Weak or absent femoral pulses.
D. Diagnostic tests
1. Aortography essential to assess the location, severity, and extent of lesion.
2. Possible future role for intravascular ultrasound.
E. Treatment
1. Surgical reconstruction is mainstay of therapy.
a. Long-term results of aortic reconstruction are generally good; thrombosis of aortic grafts is rare.
b. Associated coronary atherosclerotic disease is major cause of perioperative morbidity/mortality.
c. Elderly or symptomatic patients should have thorough preoperative evaluation for possible concurrent coronary or carotid artery disease.
2. Increasing role of transluminal angioplasty in treatment of aortic branch vessel stenosis, (e.g., renal, iliac, visceral arteries).
a. Currently limited role for angioplasty of the aorta itself or for carotid arteries.

IV. Dissection
A. Definition
Disruption of the aortic intima, which allows the arterial media to separate, forming a "false lumen" that may then propagate throughout the enter aorta and its branches.
1. Term *aneurysme dissequant* introduced by Laennec in 1819 is a misnomer, since the aorta is not acutely aneurysmal.
2. *Aortic dissection* is a more appropriate term.
B. Pathophysiology
Initial event is a tear in the aortic intima allowing blood under systemic pressure to separate (*dissect*) the layer of media.
1. Result is a *double-barrel* aorta with both a true lumen and a false lumen, with the outer wall of the false lumen consisting of an adventitial layer and some media.
2. The septum or "flap" between the true and false lumens consists of an intimal layer and some media.
3. Most common point of origin is in the ascending aorta just above the aortic valve.
4. Second most common site is just distal to the takeoff of the left subclavian.
5. Rupture of false lumen is most common cause of death.

a. Ascending aortic dissection ruptures into pericardial cavity.
b. Descending aortic dissection ruptures into left hemithorax.
6. Morbidity and death also result from compromise of aortic branch vessels, including the coronary arteries.
a. Aortic valve incompetence will result if the valvular apparatus becomes involved.
C. Classification
1. Based on area of aorta involved.
2. Original classification by DeBakey (types I, II, III).
a. Types I and II originate in ascending aorta, with type I extending into the descending aorta. Type II is confined to the ascending aorta.
b. Type III involves the descending aorta.
3. Classification of Najafi
a. Anterior, involving the ascending aorta.
b. Posterior, involving the descending aorta.
4. Acute dissections are < 2 weeks old.
D. Diagnosis
1. Predisposing factors
a. Hypertension present in 70–90% patients.
b. Male:female ratio 3:1.
c. Association with pregnancy.
d. Association with Marfan's syndrome.
(1) Inheritable connective tissue disorder with transmission to offspring of approximately 50%.
(2) Associated ocular findings, tall stature, highly arched palate, joint hyperextensibility.
2. Clinical signs and physical findings
a. Severe "tearing" pain present in most patients.
(1) Pain in ascending aorta usually referred to anterior chest.
(2) Pain in descending aorta usually referred to interscapular area and back.
b. Cardiac manifestations include acute aortic valve incompetence and/or myocardial infarction if coronaries are compromised.
(1) Right coronary artery more frequently involved.
(2) Cardiac tamponade with rupture into pericardial space.
c. Neurologic manifestations.

(1) Cerebrovascular accident with carotid compromise.

(2) Paraparesis or paraplegia due to impairment of blood supply to the spinal cord.

(3) Peripheral neuropathy in instances of frankly ischemic limbs.

d. Renal dysfunction.

e. Acute abdomen with intestinal ischemia if visceral arteries compromised.

f. Physical Findings

(1) Patients often appear to be vasoconstricted and "shocky."

(2) Blood pressure may be elevated.

(a) Hypotension usually signifies cardiac compromise or aortic rupture.

(3) Absence or diminution of pulses depends on location of dissection.

3. Diagnostic tests

Routine CXR may provide valuable information such as widened mediastinum, double aortic density representing superimposition of true and false lumens, and separation of calcium within the aortic wall.

a. Aortic angiography remains the diagnostic test of choice to define the location and extent of dissection, as well as the relationship of major branch vessels.

b. Ultrasound helpful to identify the intimal flap and to assess the aortic valve.

c. CT and MRI are valuable adjuncts but have not replaced aortography.

d. Future role of transesophageal and intravascular ultrasound.

e. Routine serum chemistries usually not helpful in diagnosis.

4. Differential diagnosis

Pain associated with dissection is usually severe and pathognomonic.

a. Anterior chest pain with ascending dissection may be confused with acute myocardial infarction.

5. Treatment

Dissection of the ascending aorta should be treated surgically, with placement of interposition graft.

a. Aortic valve replacement may be necessary.

b. Composite replacement of ascending aorta and aortic valve with reimplantation of coronary arteries usually required in patients with Marfan's syndrome due to diffuse nature of degenerative changes.

c. Uncomplicated dissections of the descending aorta may be managed medically with strict blood pressure control and β-blockade to reduce the shearing force (dp/dt).

(1) Aneurysmal degeneration of the false channel or compromise of major branch vessels warrants surgical correction of descending dissections.

6. Prognosis

a. Perioperative mortality significantly higher in patients with ruptured aneurysms.

b. Operative mortality for ascending dissections is 10–20% at most centers.

c. Ten-year actuarial survival for patients leaving the hospital is approximately 60%.

Bibliography

Akins CW, Buckley MJ, Daggett W, et al: Acute traumatic disruption of the thoracic aorta: A ten-year experience. *Ann Thorac Surg* 31(4):305–308, 1981.

Crawford ES: Marfan's syndrome. *Ann Surg* 198(4):488–505, 1983.

DeSanctis RW, Doroghaze RM, Austen WG, et al: Aortic dissection. *N Engl J Med* 317(17):1060–1067, 1987.

Najafi H, Javid H, Hunter JA, et al: An update on treatment of aneurysms of the descending thoracic aorta. *World J Surg* 4:553–561, 1986.

Piccione W Jr, DeLaria GA, Najafi H: Descending thoracic aneurysms. In Bergan JJ, Yao JST (eds): *Aortic Surgery.* Philadelphia, WB Saunders, 1989, pp 247–266.

Roberts WC: Aortic dissection: Anatomy, consequences and causes. *Am Heart J* 101(2):195–213, 1981.

CHAPTER 24

Lipid Disorders and Lipoprotein Metabolism

Robert S. Rosenson, M.D.

I. Definition

Lipid disorders encompass a variety of metabolic disorders classified as either as primary, resulting from a presumed genetic etiology, or secondary to other metabolic derangements or systemic diseases.

A. Hypercholesterolemia has been categorized into three strata by the Adult Treatment Panel of the National Cholesterol Education Program.

	Total Cholesterol (mg/dl)	Low Density Lipoprotein (LDL) Cholesterol (mg/dl)
Desirable	< 200	< 130
Borderline	200–239	130–159
High	< 240	< 160

B. Hypertriglyceridemia
   1. The classification of hypertriglyceridemia is evolving to include lower levels. The Triglyceride Consensus Conference sponsored by the National Institutes of Health met in 1983 and defined triglyceride elevations according to the following schema:
   Desirable   < 250 mg/dl
   Borderline   250–500 mg/dl
   Elevated   < 500 mg/dl
   Recently, the importance of triglyceride elevations in coronary heart disease (CHD) has attained greater significance. A more appropriate classification is to categorize triglyceride levels according to the Lipid Research Clinics population distributions by comparing with age- and sex-matched controls.
   2. Disorders manifest as hypertriglyceridemia result from:
      a. Accumulation of very low density lipoprotein (VLDL) (type IV hyperlipoproteinemia, or HLP).
      b. Impaired clearance of chylomicron and VLDL remnants (type III HLP) or familial dysbetalipoproteinemia.
      c. Hyperchyolomicronemia or exogenous hypertriglyceridemia resulting from accumulation of chylomicrons alone (type I HLP) or with VLDL (type V HLP).

C. Hypoalphalipoproteinemia [low high density lipoprotein cholesterol (HDL-C) levels]

1. Abnormalities in reverse cholesterol transport, as measured by reduced cholesterol content of HDL enhances the risk of the development of CHD.
2. Classification of HDL-C levels based upon CHD risk is a practical tool in the assessment and management of dyslipidemias. In the Framingham Heart Study, the median HDL-C level for men was 45 mg/dl and for women it was 55 mg/dl. According to the "risk multiplier" for HDL-C, the relative risk for CHD increases by approximately 25% for every 5 mg/dl decrement in HDL-C and falls about 12.5% for every 5 mg/dl increase in HDL-C.
3. Genetic disorders of HDL metabolism are defined by HDL levels below the tenth percentile compared with age- and sex-matched controls.

II. Lipoprotein Disorders

Hyperlipidemias result from overproduction and/or impaired clearance of lipoproteins. Abnormalities in lipoprotein removal may be due to defects in the lipoprotein receptor or ligand for the receptor. A classification of lipoprotein disorders is presented in Table 24-1.

A. Familial hypercholesterolemia (FH)
1. Cardinal features
   a. Selective elevation of LDL-C level.
   b. Deposition of LDL-derived cholesterol in tissue sites, especially in the skin (xanthomata) and arteries (atheroma).
2. Genetics
   a. Autosomal dominant inheritance with a gene-dosing effect. Homozygotes are more adversely affected than heterozygotes.
   b. Homozygous familial hypercholesterolemia
      (1) Genetics: phenotypic frequency of 1/1,000,000.
      (2) History
         (a) CHD often occurs prior to age 10 years and as early as 18 months of life.
         (b) Total cholesterol levels most often exceed 600 mg/dl.
      (3) Physical findings
         (a) Tendon xanthomas [see Subsection A,2,c(4)(a)], arcus corneus, and xanthelasma are common.
         (b) Planar cutaneous xanthomas are raised, yellowish plaques that develop at sites of cutaneous trauma such as elbows, knees, and buttocks.
   c. Heterozygous FH
      (1) Genetics
         (a) The phenotypic frequency is about 1/500.
         (b) Familial history of premature CHD (event prior to age 55 years) in a parent, sibling, or first-degree relative with documented LDL-C levels exceeding 190 mg/dl.
      (2) CHD begins in the third decade. By the age of 60 years, approximately 50% of individuals have experienced a myocardial infarction.
      (3) Elevations in lipoprotein (a) [Lp(a)], a modified form of LDL, increases the susceptibility to CHD in these subjects.
      (4) Physical findings
         (a) Xanthomas of the tendons are diagnostic of FH. Tendon xanthomas may involve the Achilles tendon, knee, elbow, or dorsum of the hand. They increase with age and become manifest in 75% of heterozygotes.
         (b) Arcus corneus and xanthelasma are frequent but not pathognomonic for FH.

B. Familial defective apoprotein B-100
1. History
   a. Cause of moderate hypercholesterolemia in which the apo B-100 ligand has a base substitution in the binding domain, resulting in defective binding to the LDL receptor.
2. Laboratory tests
   a. This disorder can be identified only with molecular biology techniques.
3. Therapy
   a. 3-hydroxy-3-methylglutaryl coenzyme A (HMG-CoA) reductase inhibitors may be ineffective in reducing LDL-C levels.

C. Polygenic hypercholesterolemia
1. History
   a. Genetics are poorly understood. Familial aggregation of hypercholesterolemia with premature onset of CHD is common.
   b. Accounts for about 85% of all cases of hypercholesterolemia.

Table 24-1. Classification of Dyslipidemias

Disorders of Cholesterol Metabolism	**Combined Hyperlipidemia (LDL + VLDL)**

Disorders of Cholesterol Metabolism

Primary
   Familial hypercholesterolemia (LDL receptor
      defects)
   Familial defective apoprotein B-100
   Polygenic (includes exogenous
      hypercholesterolemia)
Secondary
   Renal disease
   Nephrotic syndrome
   Hypothyroidism
   Cushing's syndrome
   Dysglobulinemias
   Acute intermittent porphyria
   Cholestatic liver diseases

Disorders of Triglyceride Metabolism

Primary
   Exogenous hyperlipidemia
         (hyperchylomicronemia syndrome)
      Familial hypertriglyceridemia
      Sporadic
      Multiple defect hyperlipidemia
      Familial lipoprotein lipase deficiency
      Apoprotein C-II deficiency
      Apoprotein C-III inhibitor
Secondary
   Exogenous (chylomicron) hyperlipidemia
      Dysglobulinemias
      Systemic lupus erythematosus
   Endogenous (VLDL) hyperlipidemia
      Diabetic hyperlipidemia
      Dysglobulinemias
      Uremia
      Hypothyroidism
      Nephrotic syndrome
      Glycogenosis, type I
      Lipodystrophies
      Chronic renal failure
      Uremia
   Exogenous
      Estrogen use
      Glucocorticoid use
      Chronicle ethanol use
      Stress-induced

Combined Hyperlipidemia (LDL + VLDL)

Primary
   Familial combined hyperlipidemia (familial
      multiple type hyperlipidemia)
Secondary
   Nephrotic syndrome
   Hypothyroidism
   Dysglobulinemias
   Cushing's syndrome
   Glucocorticoid use
   Sress-induced

Hypoalphalipoproteinemia

Primary
   Familial hypoalphalipoproteinemia
   Apo A-I deficiency
   Apo A-I/C III deficiency
   Apo A-I structural variants
   Fish eye disease
   Tangier disease
   Lecithin cholesterol: Acyl transferase deficiency
Secondary
   Exogenous androgens
   Associated disorders of triglyceride metabolism

Source: Havel RJ: Approach to the patient with hyperlipidemia. *Med Clin North Am* 66(2): 319–333. Table 2 reprinted with permission.

c. Consumption of high saturated fat diet,
   with its effect on down-regulation of the
   LDL receptor, may account for the high
   prevalence of this disorder in industrialized countries.

2. Laboratory tests
   a. Enrichment of the LDL particle with
      apoprotein B confers greater atheroge-
      nicity.
   b. Lp(a) is a modified LDL particle with

two apoprotein (a) ligands attached to the apoprotein B moiety. Lp(a) is found in the LDL density range and is a component of the estimated LDL-C fraction. Apoprotein(a) bears homology to plasminogen and serves to interfere with endogenous fibrinolysis. An elevated Lp(a) level is an independent risk factor for coronary, cerebral, and femoral atherosclerosis. A high content of Lp(a) increases atherogenicity of the LDL fraction.

D. Familial combined hyperlipidemia (familial multiple-type hyperlipoproteinemia)
  1. Genetics
     a. Autosomal dominant due to an overproduction of hepatogenously derived apo B-100.
     b. Hyperlipidemia develops in puberty or early adulthood. Only 10–20% of children express hyperlipidemia.
     c. Manifest as one of three phenotypes: increased VLDL as a triglyceride (TG) elevation, LDL as a total cholesterol (TC) elevation, or combined elevations of VLDL and LDL.
     d. Most frequent familial lipoprotein disorder with a prevalence of 1% in the North American population.
     e. Most common genetic disorder associated with premature CAD.
  2. Physical findings
     a. Rarely associated with oxygen.
  3. Laboratory findings
     a. Characterized by elevations in apo B-100.
     b. Elevations in TG, TC, or both are observed.

E. Familial hypertriglyceridemia (type IV lipoprotein pattern)
  1. Genetics
     a. Autosomal dominant
     b. Manifest by moderate TG elevations in the range of 200–500 mg/dl, with an onset late in puberty or early in adulthood.
  2. History
     a. Often accompanied by obesity, hyperglycemia, hyperinsulinemia, hypertension, and hyperuricemia.
     b. Exacerbated by ethanol consumption, worsening of the glycemic state, exogenous estrogen use, and hypothyroidism.

  3. Diagnosis
     a. Due to an elevation in VLDL.
     b. Occurs in 5% of patients with premature CAD. Risk of CHD increases greatly when accompanied by reduced HDL-C level. Familial hypertriglyceridemia with hypoalphalipoproteinemia is the most common disorder in patients undergoing coronary arteriography prior to age 55 years, with a prevalence of 17% in one series.

F. Exogenous hypertriglyceridemia
  1. Genetics
     a. The underlying causes result from inactivity of lipoprotein lipase (LPL). Apo C-II, the cofactor for LPL, is an enzyme localized to the endothelium and serves to hydrolyze triglyceride from the core of chylomicrons and VLDL, thereby generating remnant particles.
     b. The frequency of familial LPL deficiency is 1/1,000,000.
  2. History
     a. Frequent episodes of abdominal pain and pancreatitis.
     b. Often associated with secondary conditions of diabetes mellitus (poorly controlled), pancreatitis, and dysglobulinemia.
  3. Physical findings
     a. Lipemia retinalis, eruptive xanthomas, and hepatosplenomegaly.
  4. Laboratory tests
     a. Marked hypertriglyceridemia with normal or slightly elevated total cholesterol.
     b. Fasting plasma refrigerated overnight results in a creamy supernatant and a clear infranatant.

G. Mixed hypertriglyceridemia (type V HLP)
  1. Genetics
     a. Results from overproduction of VLDL and chylomicrons and VLDL remnants.
     b. Familial forms result in part from low levels of LPL. Glucose intolerance and hyperuremia are frequent accompaniments.
  2. History
     a. TG elevations exceeding 1,000 mg/dl are associated with pancreatitis.
     b. Hypertriglyceridemia is worsened by secondary disorders of TG metabolism (see Subsection E,2,b).
  3. Physical findings

a. Marked hypertriglyceridemia with TG levels above 2,000 mg/dl are associated with lipemia retinalis, eruptive xanthoma, and hepatosplenomegaly.

b. Polyneuropathy with symptoms of tingling and numbness of the extremities can occur.

4. Laboratory findings

a. Marked elevation in TG. TC is increased due to increased VLDL-C; LDL-C is reduced.

b. Fasting plasma refrigerated overnight is characterized by a creamy supernatant composed of chylomicrons and a turbid, VLDL-rich infranatant.

H. Familial dysbetalipoproteinemia (Type III HLP)

1. Genetics

a. Autosomal dominant inheritance.

b. Manifestation of this disorder requires the presence of two Apo E2 alleles and a metabolic abnormality such as diabetes mellitus, hypothyroidism, obesity, and/or ethanol consumption. Apo E2 has a low affinity for the LDL receptor; therefore, VLDL remnants which bear apo E on their surface are not cleared from the plasma efficiently. A dense VLDL particle known as β-VLDL is formed. Chylomicron remnants also possess apo E and therefore accumulate in this disorder.

2. History

a. Premature coronary artery and especially peripheral vascular disease is common.

3. Physical findings

a. Tuberoeruptive xanthomas and xanthomas of the palmar creases (xanthomata striata palmaris).

b. Evidence of coronary and peripheral atherosclerotic vascular disease.

4. Laboratory findings

a. Plasma cholesterol and triglyceride levels are increased.

b. β-VLDL is present on agarose gel electrophoresis.

I. Familial hypoalphalipoproteinemia

1. Genetics

a. Autosomal dominant

b. Frequency: 4% of individuals with premature coronary atherosclerosis.

2. Laboratory findings

a. HDL-C below the 10th percentile compared with age- and sex-matched controls.

III. **Major Secondary Disorders of Lipoproteinemia Metabolism**

A. Non-insulin-dependent diabetes mellitus (NIDDM)

1. Insulin resistance causes hypertriglyceridemia due to enhanced synthesis and decreased lipolysis of VLDL-TG. Glucose and free fatty acids serve as a substrate for TG synthesis. Insulin stimulates lipoprotein and hepatic triglyceride lipase. Therefore, insulin resistance or relative insulin deficiency is associated with an impairment in the catabolism of TG-containing lipoproteins and lower HDL-C levels.

B. Cholestatic liver diseases

1. History

a. Primary biliary cirrhosis and similar disorders are accompanied by hypercholesterolemia reportedly as high as 2,000 mg/dl. The hypercholesterolemia results from an accumulation of lipoprotein-X (LP-X), a phospholipid micelle that forms around a core of albumin. The clinical sequelae of hypercholesterolemia have been associated with the hyperviscosity syndrome, but no clear association with CHD has been established.

2. Physical findings

a. Xanthomata striae palmare occur when the cholesterol level approaches 1400 mg/dl. These lesions are also present in familial dysbetalipoproteinemia.

b. Xanthomas occur at peripheral sites such as legs and arms.

3. Laboratory findings

a. LP-X migrates to the cathode on agarose gel electrophoresis, in contrast to other lipoproteins that travel to the anode. The cathodally migrating band is extracted, and the phosphorus content is measured. LP-X is reported as the concentration of LP-X phospholipid.

C. Chronic renal failure

1. Characterized by hypertriglyceridemia due to delayed catabolism of VLDL. This results from impairment in lipoprotein and hepatic triglyceride lipases.

D. Nephrotic syndrome

1. Hypercholesterolemia is the most common lipid abnormality observed. As the nephrotic syndrome progresses, impairment in lipolysis of triglyceride-containing lipoproteins produces an associated hypertriglyceridemia.

E. Hypothyroidism
   1. Associated with increased LDL-C. Thyroxine has important regulatory functions in the metabolism of LDL by (a) stimulating the α-hydroxylase reaction, the rate-limiting step in the conversion of cholesterol to bile acids, and (b) increasing the synthesis of the high-affinity LDL receptors.

IV. **Treatment** (see Table 24-2)

After excluding secondary disorders affecting lipoprotein metabolism, a management strategy designed to attain target goals is initiated. Nonpharmacologic lifestyle changes are the first step in management and must be continued when drugs are employed.

A. Dietary modification
   1. Dietary cholesterol and saturated fats raise plasma cholesterol, with saturated fats having a much greater impact.
   2. Foods containing high quantities of cholesterol include egg yolks, as well as animal fats including milk, milk products, and meats.
   3. The major sources of high saturated fats include meats, dairy products, and baked goods.
B. Caloric restriction
   1. A decrease in body leanness, or overweightedness, raises the TC, or LDL-C,

TG, and reduces HDL-C; therefore efforts to maintain or attain lean body weight play a central role in the management of the dyslipidemic patient.

C. Aerobic exercise
   1. Exercise lowers heart rate and blood pressure, improves glycemic control, lowers TG, and raises HDL-C.
   2. For individuals without manifestations of CHD, an aerobic exercise program is designed to raise the heart rate to 70% of the maximum. Exercise involves "warm-up" and "cool down" phases. Exercise is increased by 5-min increments until 30 min of continual exercise is attained for a minimum of three times weekly. Subjects with stable angina pectoris have exercise prescriptions based on 70% of the heart rate at which ischemic ST-segment changes appear.

D. Hypolipidemic agents
   1. Bile acid sequestrants
      a. Agents: Cholestyramine and colestipol.
      b. Mechanism: Binding of the bile acids in the intestine interrupting the enterohepatic circulation. Hepatic cholesterol is reduced, thereby stimulating synthesis of LDL receptors.
      c. Dosing
         (1) Cholestyramine, 8–24 g daily
         (2) Colestipol, 10–30 g daily
         (3) Administration: The agents should be ingested within 30 min of a meal for cholestyramine as 4 g twice daily or for colestipol as 5 g twice daily. Another regimen includes a double dose at bedtime (e.g., cholestyramine, 8 g nightly, or colestipol, 10 g daily). Based upon the response and tolerability of the agents, the doses can be increased.
      d. Anticipated results
         (1) LDL-C is lowered by 10–30%, depending on the dosage.
         (2) HDL-C may rise by 5–8%.
         (3) TG can increase.
      e. Adverse effects
         (1) Impairs the absorption of fat-soluble vitamins, digoxin, warfarin, thiazide diuretics, β-adrenergic antagonists, thyroxine, and phenobarbital.
         (2) Nausea, bloating, cramping, and constipation.
         (3) Raises hepatic transaminase and alkaline phosphatase levels.

Table 24-2. Management of Dyslipidemias

↑TC	↑TC and TG	↑TG	↓HDL
EXCLUDE SECONDARY DISORDERS OF LIPOPROTEIN METABOLISM			
ATTAIN BODY LEANESS			
REDUCE TOTAL CALORIES			
REDUCE TOTAL & SATURATED FATS REDUCE DIETARY CHOLESTEROL	REDUCE CONCENTRATED SUGARS		
	AEROBIC EXERCISE		
HMG-CoA REDUCTASE INHIBITORS			
	GEMFIBROZIL		
BILE ACID SEQUESTRANTS	(+TG LOWERING AGENT)		
NICOTINIC ACID			
EXOGENOUS ESTROGENS (POSTMENOPAUSAL WOMEN ONLY)			
PLASMA EXCHANGE			

2. Nicotinic acid or niacin
   a. Mechanism: Inhibits the hepatic pro-
      duction of VLDL and its metabolites,
      intermediate density lipoprotein (IDL)
      and LDL. VLDL triglyceride is lowered.
      Nicotinic acid impairs the catabolism of
      HDL, which contributes to its HDL-
      raising effects of 30–40%.
   b. Dosing
      (1) Dosage, 1–12 g daily. The HDL-
          raising properties are observed with
          a 1-g total daily dose, whereas the
          VLDL-lowering properties are not
          usually noted until the dosage is
          increased to 3 g or more.
      (2) Administration
          (a) Ingest on food-filled stomach.
          (b) Pretreat with aspirin 30 min
              prior to dosing for 7–10 days in
              order to minimize prostaglan-
              din-mediated side effects.
          (c) Initiate dosing with 100 mg
              three times daily and gradually
              increase to targeted dosage as
              tolerated.
          (d) Crystalline niacin is preferred
              to sustained-release prepara-
              tions due to the greater inci-
              dence of hepatotoxicity with the
              latter agents.
   c. Adverse effects
      (1) Cutaneous: Prostaglandin-medi-
          ated side effects include cutaneous
          flushing, warm sensation ("hot
          flashes"), and pruritus. Other der-
          matologic reactions are hyperpig-
          mentation, acanthosis nigricans,
          and dry skin.
      (2) Gastrointestinal: nausea, vomiting,
          dyspnea, and diarrhea.
      (3) Hepatic: elevation of hepatocellular
          enzymes with jaundice and fulmi-
          nant hepatitis.
      (4) Metabolic
          (a) Hyperglycemia, unmasking of
              diabetes mellitus in susceptible
              patients, and worsening of the
              glycemic state in those treated
              medically for diabetes mellitus.
      (5) Hyperuricemia with acute gouty ar-
          thritis.
3. HMG-CoA reductase inhibitors
   a. Agents: lovastatin, pravastatin, and sim-
      vastatin.

   b. Mechanism: specific competitive inhibi-
      tor of hydroxy-methyl glutaryl-CoA re-
      ductase, the rate-limiting step in choles-
      terol biosynthesis. Reduction in
      intrahepatic cholesterol level stimulates
      the synthesis of LDL receptors by the
      liver, thereby facilitating clearance of
      LDL and VLDL remnant particles.
   c. Dosing
      (1) Lovastatin: 20 mg with the evening
          meal; can be increased to 20 mg
          twice per day, which is more effica-
          cious than 40 mg with the evening
          meal. The maximum dose is 80 mg
          daily.
      (2) Pravastatin: dosage is 10–40 mg
          daily.
      (3) Simvastatin: Dosage 10–40 mg daily.
   d. Anticipated results
      (1) With lovastatin, LDL lowering
          ranges from 20 to 40% over the
          dosage range of 10–80 mg daily;
          TG falls by 25% and HDL-C rises by
          10–13%.
   e. Adverse effects
      (1) General: headache, fatigue, sleep
          disturbance with lovastatin.
      (2) Gastrointestinal: nausea, diarrhea,
          constipation, abdominal cramps,
          and flatulence.
      (3) Incidence of myalgia/myositis is
          0.5% with lovastatin but increases
          with concomitant administration of
          gemfibrozil, nicotinic acid, cyclos-
          porine, and erythromycin. Com-
          pared with the other reductase in-
          hibitors, pravastatin has a lower
          incidence of myopathy, especially in
          combination with gemfibrozil and
          nicotinic acid.
4. Gemfibrozil
   a. Mechanism
      (1) VLDL production is decreased and
          catabolism is increased. TG level is
          lowered dramatically.
      (2) HDL level is increased through its
          effects on
          (a) stimulating apo A-I synthesis
              and
          (b) activating lipoprotein lipase,
              which reduces the residence
              time of VLDL, thereby reduc-
              ing the transfer of cholesterol in
              HDL to VLDL.

    b. Dosing
      (1) Dosage: 600 mg twice per day.
      (2) Administration: prior to meals on an empty stomach.
    c. Anticipated results: total cholesterol is lowered by 11%.
    d. Adverse effects
      (1) Gastrointestinal: nausea, cramping, bloating, flatulence, frequent loose stools.
      (2) Hepatic: transaminitis; promotes cholesterol gallstone formation.
    e. Drug interactions: displaces coumadin from albumin-binding sites, thereby potentiating the anticoagulant effect.
  5. Probucol
    a. Mechanism: reduces oxidative modification of LDL, which may reduce its atherogenicity; however, the agent has not been evaluated in clinical trials of atherosclerotic vascular disease.
    b. Dosing: 500 mg twice per day.
    c. Anticipated results: lowers LDL-C by 10%, with an accompanying fall in HDL-C of 10–30%.
    d. Adverse effects
      (1) Gastrointestinal: loose stools, diarrhea,
      (2) Hematologic: eosinophilia.
      (3) Cardiac: prolongation of QT interval.
      (4) Miscellaneous: angioneurotic edema.

Bibliography

Arad Y, Ramakrishman R, Ginsberg HN: Lovastatin therapy reduces low density lipoprotein apoB levels in subjects with combined hyperlipidemia by reducing the production of apoB-containing lipoproteins: implications for the pathophysiology of apoB production. *J Lipid Res* 31:567–582, 1990.

Atmeh RF, Stewart JM, Boag DE, et al: The hypolipidemia action of probucol: A study of its effect on high and low density lipoproteins. *J Lipid Res* 24:585–595, 1983.

Austin MA, King MC, Vranizan KM, et al: Atherogenic lipoprotein phenotype: A proposed genetic marker for coronary heart disease risk. *Circulation* 82:495–506, 1990.

Austin MA: Plasma triglyceride and coronary heart disease. *Arteriosclerosis Thromb* 11:2–14, 1991.

Brown M, Goldstein JL: Drugs used in the treatment of hyperlipoproteinemias. In Gilman AG, Rall TW, Nies AS, et al (eds): *Goodman and Gilman's, The Pharmacological Basis of Therapeutics*, ed 8. New York, Pergamon Press, 1990, pp 874–886.

Brown MS, Goldstein JL: A receptor-mediated pathway for cholesterol homeostasis. *Science* 232:34–47, 1986.

Brunzell JD: Familial lipoprotein lipase deficiency and other causes of the chylomicronemia syndrome. Scriver CR, Beaudet AL, Sly WS, Valle D. In *The Metabolic Basis of Inherited Diseases*. ed 4. New York, McGraw-Hill, 1989, pp 1165–1180.

Castelli WP, Anderson K: A population at risk: Prevalence of high cholesterol levels in hypertensive patients in the Framingham Study. *Am J Med* 80(Suppl 2A):23–32, 1986.

Chait A, Bierman EL, Albers JJ: Regulatory role of triiodothyronine in the degradation of low density lipoprotein by cultured human skin fibroblasts. *J Clin Endicrinol Metab* 48:887–889, 1979.

Chan MK, Varghese Z, Moorhead JF: Lipid abnormalities in uremia, dialysis, and transplantation. *Kidney Int* 19:625–637, 1981.

Consini A, Mazzotti M, Fumagalli R, et al: Poor response to simvastatin in familial defective apo-B-100. *Lancet* 337:305, 1991.

Etchason JA, Miller TD, Squires RW, et al: Niacin-induced hepatitis: A potential side effect with low-dose time-release niacin. *Mayo Clin Proc* 66:23–28, 1991.

Goldstein JL, Brown MS: Familial hypercholesterolemia. In *The Metabolic Basis of Inherited Diseases*, ed 4. New York, McGraw-Hill, pp 1215–1250, 1989.

Gordon T, Castelli WP, Hjortland MC, et al: High-density lipoprotein as a protective factor against coronary heart disease. The Framingham Study. *Am J Med* 62:707–714, 1977.

Grundy SM, Vega GL: Fibric acids: Effects on lipids and lipoprotein metabolism. *Am J Med* 83(suppl. 5B):9–20, 1987.

Havel RJ: Approach to the patient with hyperlipidemia. *Med Clin North Am* 66:319–333, 1982.

Hay RV, Rosenson RS: Pathophysiology and management of hypercholesterolemia. *Compr Ther* 15:45–53, 1989.

Innerarity TL, Mahley RW, Weisgraber KG, et al: Familial defective apolipoprotein B that causes hypercholesterolemia. *J Lipid Res* 1337–1349, 1990.

Joven J, Villabona C, Vilella E, et al: Abnormalities of lipoprotein metabolism in patients with the nephrotic syndrome. *N Engl J Med* 323:579–548, 1990.

Luria MH: Effect of low-dose niacin on high-density lipoprotein cholesterol and total cholesterol/high-density lipoprotein cholesterol ratio. *Arch Intern Med* 148:2493–2495, 1988.

Mahley RW, Rall SC Jr: Type III hyperlipoproteinemia (dysbetalipoproteinemia): The role of apolipoprotein E in normal and abnormal lipoprotein metabolism. Scriver CR, Beaudet AL, Sly WS, Valle D. In *The Metabolic Basis of Inherited Diseases*, ed 4. New York, McGraw-Hill, pp 1195–1214, 1989.

National Institutes of Health Consensus Conference on the Treatment of Hypertriglyceridemia. *JAMA* 251:9–15, 1984.

Report of the National Cholesterol Education Program Expert Panel on Detection, Evaluation, and Treatment of High Blood Cholesterol in Adults. *Arch Intern Med* 148:36–69, 1988.

Rifkind BM, Segal P: Lipid Research Clinics Program reference values for hyperlipidemia and hypolipidemia. *JAMA* 250:1869–1872, 1983.

Rosenson RS, Baker AL, Chow M, et al: Hyperviscosity syndrome in a hypercholesterolemic patient with pulmonary biliary cirrhosis. *Gastroenterology* 98:1351–1357, 1990.

Scanu AM, Fless GM: Lipoprotein(a) heterogeneity and biological relevance. *J Clin Invest* 85:1709–1715, 1990.

Schaefer EJ: Clinical, biochemical and genetic features in familial disorders of high density lipoprotein deficiency. *Arteriosclerosis* 4:303–322, 1984.

Schaefer EJ, McNamara JR, Genest J Jr, et al: Clinical significance of hypertriglyceridemia. *Semin Thromb Hemos* 14:143–148, 1988.

Seed M, Happichler F, Reaveley D, et al: Relation of serum lipoprotein(a) concentration and apolipoprotein(a) phenotype to coronary heart disease in patients with hypercholesterolemia. Scriver CR, Beaudet AL, Sly WS et al. (eds) *N Engl J Med* 322:1494–1505, 1990.

Stalder M, Pometta D, Suenram A: Relationship between plasma insulin levels and high density lipoprotein cholesterol levels in healthy men. *Diabetologia* 21:544–548, 1981.

Steinberg D, Parthasarathy S, Carew TE, et al: Beyond cholesterol: modifications of low-density lipoprotein that increase its atherogenicity. *N Engl J Med* 320:915, 924, 1989.

Thompson GR, Soutar AK, Spengel FA, et al: Defects of receptor-mediated low density lipoprotein catabolism in homozygous familial hypercholesterolemia and hypothyroidism in vivo. *Proc Natl Acad USA* 78:2591–2595, 1981.

Vergani C, Betale G: Familial hypo-alpha-lipoproteinemia. *Clin Chem Acta* 114:45–52, 1981.

Wiklund O, Angelin B, Bergman M, et al. Pravastatin and gemfibrozil alone and in combination for the treatment of hypercholesterolemia. Am J Med 94:13–20, 1993.

Zavaroni I, Dall'Aglia E, Alpi O, et al: Evidence for an independent relationship between plasma insulin and concentration of high density lipoprotein cholesterol and triglyceride. *Atherosclerosis* 55:259–266, 1985.

CHAPTER 25

Hypertension: Pathogenesis and Patient Management

Philip R. Liebson, M.D.

I. Pathogenesis
  A. Introduction
    1. Age, Race, and Gender
      a. Children of hypertensive parents tend to have higher blood pressures than children of nonhypertensive parents.
      b. Women appear to be more protected against target organ damage for a given blood pressure than men.
      c. Blacks are more likely to have target organ damage for a given blood pressure than whites.
    2. Hemodynamics
    All patients with essential hypertension have a peripheral vascular resistance which appears increased above the appropriate range, even though cardiac output may be normal or, especially in younger individuals, increased.
  B. Specific pathogenetic mechanisms
    1. Heredity
    Essential (primary) hypertension is considered to be polygenic and may be affected by such factors as salt sensitivity, catecholamine levels, renin-angiotensin-aldosterone activity, possible localized membrane defects, and disorders which tend to cause retention of sodium and water. This, in turn, leads to increased intracellular calcium, which may result in increased peripheral arterial resistance, followed by an elevation in blood pressure.
      a. Cellular membrane defects
        (1) Sodium-potassium-ATPase system
        Abnormalities in the activity of this system may lead to an increase in intracellular sodium and, in turn, to an increase in intracellular calcium, increasing vascular reactivity and peripheral vascular resistance.
        (2) Increased calcium in cells
        Primary increase in intracellular calcium ions may be associated with an intrinsic membrane defect, possibly independent of the sodium-potassium-ATPase system.
      b. Sympathetic nervous system
        (1) In some hypertensive patients, catecholamine levels may be increased.
        (2) Increased angiotensin also tends to sensitize norepinephrine receptors, as does corticosteroids.

c. Renin-angiotensin-aldosterone system
Approximately 10% of hypertensives have increased plasma renin activity, 60% have normal plasma renin activity, and 30% have decreased plasma renin activity.

2. Environmental
   a. Increased sodium intake
      (1) Cross-sectional epidemiologic studies demonstrate that hypertension in the general population appears to be directly correlated with average sodium intake and inversely correlated with potassium intake.
      (2) There is evidence that 35% of patients with essential hypertension appear to be sensitive to sodium.
   b. Obesity
      (1) Blood pressure correlates directly with body mass index.
      (2) Obesity is associated with increased blood volume and cardiac output and with increased insulin resistance. It is possible that insulin resistance may be associated with increased sodium retention by the renal tubules.
   c. Alcohol
      Increase in alcohol consumption is associated directly with increased blood pressure.
   d. Diet
      (1) Licorice contains glycyrrhizinic acid, which is associated with sodium retention and increased blood pressure.
      (2) Certain foods, such as cheeses, contain tyramine, which may profoundly increase blood pressure, especially when the patient is taking a monoamine oxidase (MAO) inhibitor.

3. Congenital/endocrine/structural abnormalities and secondary hypertension. A more detailed discussion in Chapter 87 (Orlowski, J: Hypertension)
   a. Pregnancy
      In certain women, especially those with previous hypertension, young primigravidas, diabetics, and grand multiparas, blood pressure may increase considerably, with preeclampsia or eclampsia.
   b. Coarctation of the aorta
      In this condition, blood pressure in the upper extremities is increased. Blood pressure in the lower extremities may be normal.
   c. Increased cardiac output
      Disorders which lead to increased cardiac output may be associated with systolic hypertension. These include:
      (1) Hyperthyroidism
      (2) Patent ductus arteriosus
      (3) Beriberi (vitamin B_1 deficiency)
      (4) Aortic regurgitation
      (5) Arteriovenous fistulas
   d. Renal and renovascular disease
      (To be covered in the renal section)

C. Pathogenic mechanisms of accelerated/malignant hypertension Table 25-1.
   1. Although accelerated hypertension can be attributed to specially defined endocrine abnormalities such as pheochromocytoma, aldosteroma, or excess adrenocorticoids, it is commonly independent of specific endocrine causation.
   2. Specific disease entities may be associated with reflex catecholamine activity, which leads to marked increases in blood pressure over a short period of time. Examples include:
      a. Head trauma
      b. Preeclampsia or eclampsia
      c. Cerebral hemorrhage
      d. Aortic dissection
      e. Burns
      f. Postoperative effects

D. Associated abnormalities in hypertension
   There is increasing evidence that hypertension is related to other metabolic abnormalities which, in turn, may be independent risk factors for cardiovascular disease. These include the following:
   1. Dyslipidemia
   2. Diabetes mellitus
   3. Increased uric acid
   4. Polycythemia

Table 25-1. Possible Pathogenic Mechanisms of Primary Hypertension

Sodium intake
Catecholamine sensitivity
Increased renin-angiotensin-aldosterone activity
Renal tubular defect in sodium reabsorption
Increased smooth muscle permeability to calcium ion
Polygenic factors

5. Smoking
E. Consequences of hypertension
1. Cardiac
    a. Pressure overload
        (1) Hypertensive individuals have a relative or absolute increase in peripheral vascular resistance, which in turn causes an increased systolic load on the left ventricular wall.
        (2) Chronic compensation leads to left ventricular hypertrophy.
        (3) Increased stress per unit area of myocardium may lead to ischemia because of increased myocardial oxygen needs, especially with underlying coronary artery disease.
    b. Diastolic compliance
        In hypertensive individuals even with normal-appearing left ventricles, echocardiographic and gated blood pool radioisotope studies demonstrate a decrease in early inflow from the left atrium to the left ventricle.
    c. Left ventricular hypertrophy/congestive heart failure
        Left ventricular hypertrophy (LVH) is found in a substantial percentage of individuals with hypertension. As many as 50% of hypertensive individuals may have LVH on the basis of echocardiographic evaluation. Electrocardiography demonstrates LVH in only 10% of individuals.
    d. Dysrhythmia/sudden cardiac death.
    e. Coronary artery disease/myocardial infarction. Hypertension is a significant risk factor for coronary artery disease.

2. Arterial
    a. Aortic dissection
        Tears of the thoracic aorta are frequently associated with hypertension.
    b. Aortic aneurysm
        Abdominal as well as thoracic aorta aneurysms are more common in hypertension, especially in cigarette smokers.
    c. Cerebrovascular accident
    d. Nephrosclerosis

II. **Cardiovascular Risk and Patient Management: Epidemologic Studies and Clinical Trials** Table 25-2.
A. Evidence of increased cardiovascular risk with hypertension
    1. The 30-year Framingham Study and the Multiple Risk Factor Intervention Trial (MRFIT) observation study of 360,000 men have determined conclusively that elevated blood pressure is associated with increased risk of cardiovascular death, coronary heart disease, fatal myocardial infarction, stroke, renal disease, and congestive heart failure. The risk increases with blood pressures above 110/70 mmHg.
    2. There is also some evidence that, especially in patients with clinical coronary heart disease, lowering blood pressures to below 135/85 mmHg may be associated with increased cardiovascular events.
B. Evidence of the association of cardiovascular risks
    1. Lipids
        a. Aside from the increased association of dyslipidemia with hypertension, the combined risk of elevated cholesterol and increasing blood pressure is multi-

Table 25-2. Selected Hypertensive Emergencies and Urgencies: Flow Diagram (Blood Pressure > 200 Systolic)

CVA Coma	Malignant hypertension	Congestive heart failure	Aortic dissections	Catecholamine excess
Lower BP No more than 20–30% in first 24 hr	Lower SP to < 160 mmHg initially	Lower SP to < 160 mmHg initially	Lower SP to < 100 mmHg	SP to < 160 mmHg initially
Nitroprusside Labetalol	Nitroprusside Labetalol	Nitroprusside Nitroglycerine Hydralazine	Nitroprusside β-blockers Labetalol	Phentolamine or Phenoxybenzamine, then β-blocker

SP = systolic pressure.

plicative in respect to cardiovascular disease.
2. Smoking
Smoking in conjunction with elevated blood pressure increases the risk of coronary heart disease and is a strong multiple risk factor in cerebrovascular accidents and aortic aneurysm.
3. Diabetes/insulin resistance
Approximately 60% of diabetics have hypertension. There is also increasing evidence of an association between increased insulin resistance in general and elevated blood pressure.
4. Viscosity
Hypertensives appear to have increased blood viscosity. Increased viscosity may play a role in the development of LVH.
C. Evidence of effectiveness of risk reduction
1. Malignant hypertension
The five year survival rate from malignant hypertension has increased gradually from 0% in the untreated state to over 75%. There is overwhelming evidence for the benefits of treatment in patients with this condition.
2. Moderate-severe hypertension
Nonmalignant hypertension produces more morbidity and mortality than malignant hypertension based upon the large number of patients with nonmalignant forms. There is clear-cut evidence for reduction of hypertension-induced cardiovascular morbidity and mortality in relation to the initial diastolic pressure.
3. Mild hypertension
Even mild hypertension (diastolic pressures of 90–95 mmHg) has been associated with demonstrated benefits, although benefits at lower levels of blood pressure have been modest.
4. Systolic hypertension in the elderly
A recent report from the Systolic Hypertension in the Elderly Study (SHEP) indicated that the treatment of this condition (found in 6–18% of elderly patients above 60 years of age) decreased the incidence of stroke by 35% over 5 years. Major cardiovascular events were reduced.

III. Management: Principles and Practice
A. Blood pressure control
1. In general, the aim of blood pressure reduction is to achieve a diastolic blood pressure below 140 mmHg and a diastolic blood pressure below 90 mmHg.
2. Because of the variability and stress of blood pressure, measurement of pressure should be accomplished in at least two readings which are no more than 5 mmHg apart.
3. Multiple sets of readings are encouraged especially by nonphysician personnel and away from the office setting by the patient.
4. Drug therapy is generally used for patients with systolic blood pressure above 160 mmHg and diastolic blood pressure above 95 mmHg.
5. Blood pressure should not be lowered excessively because of the possibility of decreasing perfusion to vital organs, especially in patients with preexisting coronary disease.
6. Elderly patients with systolic hypertension have been shown to benefit from systolic pressure reduction below 160 mmHg with the use of modest doses of thiazide diuretics.
B. Organ system damage: Prevention and reversal
1. Heart
a. There is no evidence that lowering blood pressure reverses the pathology of coronary artery disease.
b. On the other hand, decreased blood pressure under these circumstances tends to decrease myocardial oxygen needs and therefore may be beneficial.
c. In congestive heart failure with hypertension, antihypertensive agents are particularly important in improving cardiac performance.
2. Arterial disease
a. In patients with aortic aneurysms, antihypertensive agents are beneficial in decreasing stress on the aneurysmal wall.
b. Both reduction in blood pressure and the rate of rise of left ventricular pressure (dp/dt) are important.
C. Therapeutic Interventions
1. Nonpharmacologic
a. Sodium reduction
Limitation of sodium intake to less than 2 g/day is effective in producing a modest decrease in blood pressure, especially in patients with relative volume load hypertension.
b. Weight reduction
In patients with body mass indices about 15% above ideal weight, a decrease in

weight may be associated with a blood pressure decrease of 5–10 mmHg.

c. Activity status

In patients who are sedentary, modest activity such as daily walking for 1–2 hr or a program of submaximal exercise for 30 min three times a week may be associated with a decrease in blood pressure.

d. Limitation of alcohol

Those who drink should do so in moderation, that is, no more than 1 oz of ethanol daily. This is equivalent to 2 oz of 100-proof whiskey, 8 oz of wine, or 24 oz of beer.

2. Pharmacologic

a. General principles

(1) Blood pressure considerations

(a) In patients with diastolic blood pressure above 104 mmHg, there is considerable evidence that reduction of blood pressure with drugs decreases cardiovascular mortality and morbidity.

(b) In patients with milder hypertension in the diastolic range of 90–104 mmHg, there is clearcut protection against congestive heart failure, stroke, progression to more severe levels of hypertension, and cardiovascular mortality.

(c) On the other hand, protection against the complications of coronary artery disease using antihypertensive drugs has not been convincingly demonstrated.

(d) It is recommended that patients whose diastolic blood pressure is 90–94 mmHg and who are otherwise at low risk for developing cardiovascular disease should be treated initially with nonpharmacologic approaches.

(e) The 1993 report of the Joint National Committee on Hypertension recommends that diuretics and beta-blockers are recommended as first choice agents unless contraindicated because of their evaluation in long-term control clinical trials demonstrating reduction of morbidity and mortality, or be-

Table 25-3 Selected Use of Antihypertensive Agents

Category	Initial Class Suggested
Young patients	β-blockers, ACE inhibitors
Elderly patients	Calcium channel blockers, diuretics
Blacks	Calcium channel blockers, diuretics
Diabetics	Diuretics, ACE inhibitors
Myocardial infarction, ischemia	β-blockers, calcium channel blockers
Tachyarrhythmias	Calcium channel blockers (verapamil)
Congestive heart failure	Diuretics, ACE inhibitors
Systolic hypertension in the elderly	Diuretic (chlorthalidone), possibly with β₁-blocker (atenolol)

cause other agents may be specially indicated. Other agents suitable for initial monotherapy include calcium antagonists, angiotensin converting enzyme inhibitors, alpha-1-receptor blockers and alpha-beta-blocker (labetalol).

D. Specific classes of agents

1. Diuretics

a. Most effective diuretics include thiazides, potassium-sparing agents, and loop diuretics. The last should be reserved for renal insufficiency.

b. Diuretics increase urinary sodium excretion and reduce plasma volume and cardiac output. After 6 to 8 weeks, although plasma volume gradually re-

Table 25-4 Precautions with Antihypertension Agents

Condition	Medications to Avoid
Congestive heart failure	Calcium channel blockers, β-blockers
Myocardial infarction	Hydralazine, direct vasodilators
Diabetics	Diuretics, β-blockers
Bronchospastic disease	β-blockers
Volume depletion	ACE inhibitors
Bilateral renovascular hypertension	ACE inhibitors
Postural hypotension	α-blockers
Lipid abnormalities	Thiazides, loop diuretics, β-blockers

turns to normal, as does cardiac output, there appears to be a fall in peripheral vascular resistance.

c. Continuous diuretic therapy is associated with a blood pressure decrease of approximately 10 mmHg.

d. Diuretics are especially useful with other agents which may cause sodium retention.

e. More recent studies suggest that lower doses of diuretics are reasonable, such as 25 mm hydrochlorothiazide.

f. With renal insufficiency manifested by a serum creatinine level above 2.5 mm/dl, thiazides are usually not effective and therapy with furosemide or metolazone may be needed.

g. Side effects of diuretics include hypokalemia, hypomagnesemia, hyperuricemia, hyperlipidemia, and hyperglycemia.

h. Nonsteroidal anti-inflammatory drugs may inhibit the effects of thiazides and loop diuretics.

2. β-blockers

a. These agents are unique among antihypertensives in that peripheral vascular resistance may increase early in their administration.

b. Cardiac output falls by 15–20%, probably due to decreased heart rate and contractility, and there is a decrease in renin release of about 60%.

c. The initial increased peripheral vascular resistance may reverse so that eventually peripheral vascular resistance is close to normal.

d. Some β-blockers have intrinsic sympathomimetic activity (ISA), such as pindolol and acebutolol, which produce an agonist response. These drugs may be useful in patients with a relatively slow heart rate. ISA agents also blunt the adverse effects on lipid metabolism seen with non-ISA β-blockers.

e. β-blockers are especially suitable in younger patients and whites.

f. Clinical conditions in which β-blockers could be used as monotherapy include those with:
(1) Hyperkinetic hypertension.
(2) Marked anxiety and coexisting ischemic heart disease.

g. β-blockers may increase peripheral vascular disease, leading to bronchospasm and congestive heart failure in those with underlying disease.

h. Non-ISA β-blockers induce modest lipoprotein changes, especially an increase in triglycerides and a decrease in high density lipoprotein (HDL) cholesterol.

i. β-blockers used in patients with pheochromocytoma may produce unimposed α-adrenergic action, leading to hypertensive crisis.

j. Intravenous labetalol has been used successfully to treat hypertensive emergencies, especially with catecholamine excess.

3. Central sympathetic agents

a. Central α-agonists include methyldopa (Aldomet), clonidine (Catapres), and guanabenz (Wytensin)

b. These agents act centrally to stimulate α-2 receptors, which in turn decrease sympathetic outflow from the central nervous system, leading to a decrease in peripheral resistance with little effect on cardiac output.

c. Renal blood flow is usually well maintained, and postural hypotension is unusual.

d. Methyldopa may be given in doses ranging from 250 to 3,000 mg/day in a twice daily dosage. Side effects include sedation, orthostatic hypotension, autoimmune phenomena including a positive antinuclear antibody test in 10% of patients, and, rarely, clinically apparent hemolytic anemia or hepatitis.

e. Clonidine can be used as often as once an hour. Usual doses are 0.1 to 1 mg/day. It may be given transdermally, which may allow smoother blood pressure control for as long as 7 days; skin rashes occasionally occur. Clonidine withdrawal hypertension has been noted because of rapid rebound. This may be treated by reinstitution of clonidine or the use of an α-adrenergic antagonist.

f. Both methyldopa and clonidine are associated with fluid retention; guanabenz is not.

g. Guanabenz has also been shown to reduce serum cholesterol levels in some studies.

4. Peripheral sympatholytic agents (α-1 blockers)

a. These include prazosin and doxazosin. These agents block α-mediated vasoconstriction at the postsynaptic receptor.

b. Prazosin is associated with a first-dose hypotension. Thus, it is advisable to give the initial dose to a patient in the recumbent position.

c. The favorable hemodynamic changes include a fall in peripheral vascular resistance, with maintenance of cardiac output and heart rate.

d. These agents may be especially suitable in patients with asthma or peripheral vascular disease or in those with lipid abnormalities. They are frequently used with a diuretic.

5. ACE inhibitors

a. These agents inhibit converting enzyme, thus preventing the formation of angiotensin II and decreasing the effect of the renin-angiotensin-aldosterone system.

b. Agents include captopril, enalapril, lisinopril, fosinopril, and quinapril.

c. Captopril is usually given three times a day, enalapril twice a day, lisinopril and fosinopril once a day.

d. The main effect is the decrease in peripheral vascular resistance, with little effect on heart rate, cardiac output, or fluid volume.

e. Other effects of these agents may include an increase in the concentration of vasodepressor hormone by inhibition of the breakdown of bradykinin and an increase in the levels of vasodilatory prostaglandins.

f. These agents are less effective in blacks, possibly because of lower renin levels.

g. The effect on hypertension may not be seen for 1 to 2 weeks, so the initial doses should be moderated slowly.

h. It is best to initiate therapy twice a day with captopril and once a day with enalapril because of a possibly dramatic drop in blood pressure early in therapy. Sometimes an initial dose of captopril as little as 6.5 mg should be given.

i. Hypotension may occur especially if the sodium concentration in the plasma is less than 140 mEq/l.

j. These agents, along with β-blockers, are associated with potassium retention, and hyperkalemia can result.

k. Side effects are relatively uncommon and include dysgeusia (with captopril), hypersensitivity reaction, or persistent cough.

l. There are no central nervous system side effects, no reduction in cardiac output, and no effect on sympathetic activity, lipids, glucose, or uric acid.

m. In patients with bilateral renal vascular hypertension, therapy may be associated with marked fall in renal perfusion. This is also the case for solitary kidneys.

n. These agents are especially useful in patients with diabetic neuropathy because they reduce efferent arterial or resistance secondary to a reduction in angiotensin II.

6. Calcium channel blockers

a. These agents include verapamil, nifedipine, nicardipine, amlodipine, diltiazem, and isradipine. They are a diverse group of agents even though they are considered as members of one class.

b. The dihydropyridine derivatives, including nifedipine, nicardipine, amlodipine, and isradipine, have the greatest peripheral vasodilatory action, with little effect on cardiac conduction. The other two agents diltiazem and verapamil are also effective antihypertensives.

c. These agents are associated with renal vasodilatation leading to sodium loss.

d. On the other hand, unlike other antihypertensive agents, their effectiveness may be reduced by dietary sodium restriction.

e. They are especially useful in elderly and black hypertensives.

f. They are usually contraindicated in patients with congestive heart failure.

7. Pure vasodilators

a. These include hydralazine and minoxidil. They are effective in producing marked vasodilation and are usually second- or third-line agents.

b. They produce a significant reflex sympathetic effect and fluid retention, and thus should be used with diuretics and possibly sympatholytic agents.

c. Side effects of hydralazine include a lupus-like syndrome, seen in 10–20% of patients, which is dose dependent, especially in doses over 200 mg/day.

d. About 3% of patients given minoxidil develop pericardial effusions, usually those with renal insufficiency.

e. Pure vasodilators produce dilatation of arteries but not of veins.

f. Intravenous vasodilators include nitroprusside and diazoxide, which are usually used for hypertensive crises.

E. Patient characteristics suggesting the initial drug

1. Age, race, and sex

a. Younger individuals and whites usually respond better to β-blockers and ACE inhibitors; blacks and older patients respond better to diuretics and calcium antagonists.

b. There is no effect of gender on the significant response to drugs.

c. There is evidence that hypertension in blacks is more severe than that in whites, with more frequent strokes, end-stage renal disease, congestive heart failure, and LVH.

d. There are no recognized differences in responses to nonpharmacologic therapy between whites and blacks.

e. Older patients may be more sensitive to volume depletion and sympathetic inhibition than younger patients. Thus, antihypertensive therapy should be initiated at smaller doses in the elderly.

f. Drugs which may cause orthostatic hypotension include α-1 blockers, labetalol, and guanethidine.

2. Coronary artery disease

a. Effort should be made to avoid rapid reductions in blood pressure.

b. β-blockers and calcium entry blockers are especially useful in patients with anginal pectoris. β-blockers reduce postinfarct secondary events and mortality.

c. Aggressive measures to control hyperlipidemia and eliminate cigarette smoking should also be instituted in these patients.

3. Congestive heart failure
ACE inhibitors and diuretics are especially useful in these patients. With regard to LVH, agents which have been shown to cause regression of hypertrophy include β-adrenergic blockers, ACE inhibitors, and calcium antagonists. Diuretics and direct-acting vasodilators appear to be less effective.

4. Peripheral vascular disease
β-adrenergic antagonists are contraindicated. ACE inhibitors and calcium antagonists may be beneficial in patients with severe peripheral vascular disease, especially Raynaud's disease or collagen vascular diseases.

5. Diabetes mellitus

a. β-blocking agents should be avoided.

b. Diabetic nephropathy may be associated with hypoaldosteronism, with resulting hyperkalemia. Therefore, potassium-sparing diuretics, ACE inhibitors, and β-blockers which may aggravate hyperkalemia should be used cautiously. Most antihypertensive therapies are effective in diabetic patients, however.

c. In patients who have neuropathic complications of diabetes, orthostatic hypotension may occur. Therefore, drugs which aggravate orthostatic hypertension should be used with caution.

6. Obstructive lung disease or asthma
β-blockers should be avoided.

7. Renal Disease (See Chapter 87)

8. Aortic dissection

a. Agents which increase left ventricular dp/dt should be used cautiously unless β-blockers are also used.

b. Agents which tend to increase dp/dt despite a decrease in blood pressure include trimethaphan and diazoxide.

c. Usually effective agents include nitroprusside and labetalol.

d. β-blockers in conjunction with vasodilators are particularly effective because of their modification of left ventricular dp/dt.

9. Cerebrovascular disease
Systolic blood pressure should not be decreased below 160 mmHg especially in acute situations. In the period when an acute ischemic cerebral infarction or transient ischemic attack occurs, antihypertensive therapy may be withheld temporarily unless systolic blood pressure is very high, that is, above 220 mmHg.

10. Pregnancy

a. With preeclampsia, modified bed rest and a normal sodium diet may be effective. Volume reduction is detrimental.

b. Methyldopa and hydralazine are effective in reducing blood pressure.

c. β-blocking agents may also be effective.

d. ACE inhibitors are contraindicated because of their possible effects on the fetus.

e. Calcium channel blockers may produce a decrease in uterine contractions during labor and should be avoided in late pregnancy.

11. Hypertensive crises or emergencies (Table 2).

a. Vasodilators include sodium nitroprusside, nitroglycerin, diazoxide, and hydralazine.

b. The dose of nitroprusside is 0.5–10 μg/kg/min as an IV infusion.

c. Nitroglycerin can be given as 5–100 μg/min as an IV infusion.

d. Diazoxide is given as a 50- to 150-mg bolus, which may be repeated, but hypotension can be produced. This drug should be given cautiously.

e. Hydralazine can be given as 10–20 mg IV, but its initial effect begins in 10–30 min. It may cause tachycardia and aggravation of anginal pectoris.

f. Effective adrenergic inhibitors include labetalol, a 20- to 80-mg IV bolus every 10 min or a 2 mg/min IV infusion.

g. Oral agents for hypertensive emergencies should be given with caution. Standard drugs which have been given include:

(1) Captopril, 25 mg.

(2) Clonidine, 0.1–0.2 mg, repeated every hour.

(3) Minoxidil, 2.5–5 mg, repeated every 2–3 hr.

(4) Nifedipine, 10 mg, repeated every 30 min.

Bibliography

Bakris GL, Frohlich ED: The evolution of antihypertensive therapy: An overview of four decades of experience. *J Am Coll Cardiol* 14:1595–1608, 1989.

Farnett L, Mulrow CD, Linn WD, et al: The J-curve phenomenon and the treatment of hypertension. Is there a point beyond which pressure reduction is dangerous? *JAMA* 265:489–495, 1991.

The fifth report of the Joint National Committee on detection evaluation, and treatment of high blood pressure. (JNCV). *Ann Int Med* 53:154–183, 1993.

Littenberg B, Garber AM, Sox HC Jr: Screening for hypertension. *Ann Intern Med* 112:192–202, 1990.

SHEP Cooperative Research Group: Prevention of stroke by antihypertensive drug treatment in older persons with isolated systolic hypertension. Final results of the Systolic Hypertension in the Elderly Program (SHEP). *JAMA* 265:3255–3264, 1991.

CHAPTER 26

Drugs Used in Cardiac Disease

Catherine M. MacLeod, M.D., F.R.C.P.(C), F.A.C.P., F.C.P.

Therapeutic Classification

I. **Drugs Used to Treat Arrhythmias**
   A. Class I: sodium channel blocking drugs
   B. Class II: beta-adrenergic receptor blockers
   C. Class III: potassium channel modulating agents
   D. Class IV: calcium channel blockers
   E. Class V: other drugs used to treat arrhythmias
      1. Purine receptor antagonists—adenosine
      2. Anticholinergic agents—Atropine
      3. Cardiac glycosides—Digoxin

II. **Drugs Used in Congestive Heart Failure**
   A. Cardiac stimulants
      1. Sympathomimetic drugs
      2. Cardiac glycosides
      3. Bipyridines
      4. Glucagon
   B. Preload reducers
      1. Diuretics
      2. Nitrates
   C. Afterload reducers
      1. Angiotensin-converting enzyme inhibitors
      2. Nitrates (high doses)

III. **Drugs Used in Coronary Artery Disease**
   A. Drugs to increase coronary artery perfusion
      1. Nitrates
      2. Calcium channel blockers
   B. Drugs to decrease the myocardial workload
      1. Beta-adrenergic receptor blockers
      2. Calcium channel blockers (prominent myocardial activity)
      3. Nitrates
   C. Drugs used to alter thrombus formation
      1. Antiplatelet drugs
      2. Thrombolytic agents
      3. Parenteral anticoagulants

IV. **Drugs Used in Hypertension**
   A. Drugs affecting the sympathetic nervous system
      1. Alpha-adrenergic receptor blockers
      2. Beta-adrenergic receptor blockers
      3. Sympatholytic agents
   B. Drugs affecting vascular smooth muscle directly
      1. Calcium channel blockers
      2. Direct-acting vasodilators
   C. Drugs with other actions
      1. Angiotensin-converting enzyme inhibitors
      2. Diuretics

Antiarrhythmic Drugs

I. Classification

A. Class I: Sodium channel blocking drugs
   1. Class IA: Procainamide (Pronestyl)
      Quinidine (many trade names)
      Disopyramide (Norpace)
   2. Class IB: Lidocaine (Xylocaine)
      Phenytoin (Dilantin)
      Mexiletine (Mexitil)
      Tocainide (Tonogard)
   3. Class IC: Encainide (Enkaid)
      Flecainide (Tambocor)
   4. Class I: Other
      a. Moricizine (Ethmozine)
      b. Propafenone (Rythmol)

B. Class II: Beta-adrenergic receptor blockers
   1. Esmolol (Brevibloc)
   2. Metoprolol (Lopressor)
      Propranolol (Inderal)
   3. Sotalol (Sotacor)—also Class III

C. Class III: potassium channel modulators
   1. Amiodarone (Cordarone)
   2. Bretylium (Bretylol)
   3. Sotalol (Sotacor)

D. Class IV: calcium channel blockers
   1. Verapamil (Isoptin, Calan)
   2. Diltiazem (Cardizem)

E. Class V: other agents
   1. Purine receptor agonist—Adenosine (Adenogard)
   2. Cardiac glycoside—Digoxin (Lanoxin)
   3. Anticholinergic—Atropine

II. Mechanism of Action

A. *Class I* agents affect myocardial conduction by blocking sodium channels. They are subdivided based on rate of onset and offset of drug binding, state of the sodium channel for drug binding, and additional effects on the action potential (AP). The *Class IA* drugs bind to open sodium channels, with an intermediate rate of both binding and release. By affecting potassium channels, they prolong repolarization. They are vagolytic (antimuscarinic) to varying extents: disopyramide has the greatest and procainamide the least vagolytic action. Quinidine has alpha-adrenergic blocking properties which cause peripheral vasodilation, and procainamide has weak ganglion-blocking action. Disopyramide has direct effects on the myocardium to decrease contractility. At high concentrations they increase the QRS interval.

B. *Class IB* drugs rapidly bind to and release from partially depolarized, ischemic myocardial cells of the ventricles, binding to inactivated sodium channels. There are no additional effects on the cardiovascular system. The effects of these drugs are quite predictable, with no effect on the P-R, QRS, or J-T intervals. The AP is shortened.

C. *Class IC* drugs have the most marked effect on sodium channels, with slow binding and release. They prolong the QRS interval at therapeutic concentrations but do not affect the J-T interval.

D. *Moricizine*, a phenothiazine, is most similar to class IC agents, but the AP is shortened and it is vagolytic. It also has antihistaminic action. *Propafenone* acts like class IC drugs, but it shares with class IA drugs the prolongation of the AP at low concentrations by restricting the outward potassium current. The AP is shortened at high concentrations.

E. *Class II* antiarrhythmic agents are β-adrenergic receptor blockers which inhibit catecholamine-induced arrhythmias, as well as slowing conduction through the atrioventricular (AV) node. At high concentrations, propranolol inhibits sodium channels as do class I agents. With prolonged therapy, the class II drugs prolong the repolarization duration, similar to the action of class III drugs. Esmolol is a very-short-acting β-blocker with rapid onset of prominent antiarrhythmic effects.

F. The chemically diverse *Class III* antiarrhythmic agents affect K$^+$ channels to prolong repolarization. In addition, amiodarone is a noncompetitive α- and β-adrenergic receptor blocker, as well as a calcium channel blocker. Bretylium causes initial release of norepinephrine from sympathetic nerve endings and then depletes the nerve of norepinephrine, causing hypotension, decreased myocardial conduction, and decreased contractility. Sotalol is a nonselective β-adrenergic receptor blocker.

G. *Class IV* drugs are the calcium channel blockers verapamil and diltiazem. They inhibit calcium channels of the AV node and, to a lesser extent, of the sinoatriol (SA) node.

H. *Class V* drugs affect the SA and/or AV nodes. Adenosine stimulates supraventricular purine receptors to increase potassium conductance, hyperpolarize cell membranes, and decrease calcium channel activity. It is also sympatholytic. Digoxin has prominent vagal stimulating activity, slowing the SA rate of depolarization and the AV rate of conduction while improving atrial conduction. Atropine reverses the vagal-mediated depression of AV conduction and SA node activity by means of its anticholinergic (antimuscarinic) action.

III. **Indications**
   A. Class IA
      1. Prophylaxis/treatment of supraventricular and ventricular tachyarrhythmias
   B. Class IB
      1. Prophylaxis/treatment of ventricular arrhythmias, particularly those occurring in association with myocardial ischemia or infarction, heart surgery, or digoxin toxicity
   C. Class IC
      1. Prophylaxis/treatment of tachyarrhythmias not associated with myocardial infarction or ischemia
   D. Class I Other: probably the same as for class IC drugs
   E. Class II
      1. Prophylaxis/treatment of supraventricular tachyarrhythmias
      2. Prophylaxis/treatment of ventricular arrhythmias associated with excess catecholamine stimulation
      3. Prophylaxis in the post–myocardial infarct period
   F. Class III
      1. Prophylaxis/treatment of life-threatening ventricular arrhythmias
   G. Class IV
      1. Prophylaxis/treatment of supraventricular tachyarrhythmias
   H. Class V
      1. Digoxin: treatment of supraventricular tachyarrhythmias and/or control of the ventricular response to intractable supraventricular tachyarrhythmias
      2. Adenosine: emergency treatment of severe supraventricular tachyarrhythmias
      3. Atropine: emergency treatment of hemodynamically unstable bradyarrhythmias secondary to enhanced vagal activity; AV block, asystole

IV. **Significant Drug Interactions**

Drug	Interacting Drug	Effect	Mechanism
Procainamide	H$_2$ blockers	↑ procainamide	↓ metabolism ± excretion
	Neuromuscular blockers	↑ neuromuscular blockade	additive
Quinidine	Digoxin	↑ digoxin	↓ excretion/binding
	Neuromuscular blockers	↑ neuromuscular blockade	additive
Lidocaine	Drugs ↓ metabolism	↑ lidocaine	↓ metabolism
	Cotrimoxazole	methemoglobinemia	additive
Flecainide	Drugs ↓ heart contractility	CHF	additive
Moricizine	Theophylline	theophylline	↑ clearance
Propafenone	Cimetidine	propafenone	↓ metabolism
	Quinidine		
Amiodarone	Anesthetics	cardiac toxicity	unknown
	Anticoagulants (oral)	anticoagulation	↓ metabolism
	Digoxin	arrhythmias	additive
	Quinidine	quinidine effect	unknown
Adenosine	Carbamazepine	heart blockade	additive
	Dipyridamole	adenosine effect	↓ removal
	Theophylline	adenosine efect	antagonism

V. Complications

Drug	CNS	CV	GI	Hematology	Other
Procainamide	+	+ +	±	+ +	SLE*
Quinidine	+	+ +	+ +	+ +	—
Disopyramide	+	+ +	+	+	anticholinergic
Lidocaine	+ +	−	+	−	—
Phenytoin	+ + +	+	+ +	+ + +	immune syndrome
Mexiletine	+ +	+	+	+ +	—
Tocainide	+	+	+	+ +	pneumonitis
Encainide	+ +	+ +	+	−	—
Flecainide	+	+ +	+ +		—
Moricizine	+	+ +	+	−	—
Propafenone	+	+	±	+	?SLE
β-blockers	+	+	±	−	—
Amiodarone	+ +	+ +	+ +	−	lung fibrosis thyroid changes blue-gray skin photosensitivity
Bretylium	−	+ +	+	−	neuromuscular blockade
Ca^{+2} blockers	−	+	+	−	—
Adenosine	±	+ +	±	−	Dyspnea, cough
Digoxin	+	+ + +	+ +	−	—
Atropine	+	+ +	±	−	—

*SLE, systemic lupus erythematosus.

A. Central nervous system (CNS)
1. Mainly confusion
2. Excitation, seizures with some Class IB and IC drugs
3. Ataxia with phenytoin
4. Extrapyramidal reactions with amiodarone
B. Cardiovascular (CV)
1. Proarrhythmias with Class I drugs
2. Congestive heart failure with disopyramide, flecainide, amiodarone, and possibly calcium channel blockers
C. Gastrointestinal (GI)
1. Mainly nonspecific upset
2. Cholestasis with disopyramide, and phenytoin
3. Hepatitis with phenytoin, flecainide, and amiodarone
D. Hematology
1. Neutropenia or agranulocytosis with procainamide, disopyramide, phenytoin, mexiletine, tocainide, and propafenone
2. Thrombocytopenia with quinidine, phenytoin, mexiletine, and tocainide

VI. Contraindications
A. Patients with congestive heart failure should not receive, or should receive with caution, the following drugs: disopyramide, flecainide, propafenone, β-blockers, amiodarone, verapamil or diltiazem, and possibly procainamide.
B. In patients with ventricular ectopic activity or ventricular conducting defects, atropine should be avoided or used with extreme caution. In the presence of AV or SA dysfunction, all drugs should be used with caution, and β-blockers, amiodarone, verapamil, diltiazem, adenosine, and digoxin should be avoided.
C. Patients with asthma or bronchoconstrictive disease should not receive β-blockers or adenosine.
D. Hypersensitivity to a given drug or chemical class of drug obviates the use of the drug or of chemically similar agents when there is evidence of cross-sensitivity.

Cardiotonic Agents
I. Classification
A. Sympathomimetic agents
1. Dobutamine (Dobutrex)
2. Dopamine (Intropin)
3. Norepinephrine (Levophed)
B. Digoxin (Lanoxin)
C. Amrinone (Inocor)
D. Milrinone (Corotrope)
E. Glucagon

Table 26-1. Dose and Handling of Drugs

Class	Drug/Dose	Bioavailability	Onset of Action	Elimination	Elimination t½ Normal	Elimination t½ Renal Dysfunction	Duration of Action
IA	*Disopyramide*						
	PO—initially 300mg Maintenance: 100–200 mg q 6h (extended release: 200–400 mg q 12h)	100%	0.5–3.5 hr	50% metabolism to active metabolite 50% renal excretion	4–10 hr	8–18 hr	1.5–8.5 hr
	Procainamide						
	PO—initially 1.25 g, then 0.75 g in 1 hr, then 0.5–1g q 2–3h Maintenance: 0.5–1 g q 4–6h (extended release: 1 g q 6h)	75–95%	1 hr	40–50% metabolism to active aceainide (NAPA)—class III 50–60% renal excretion	2.5–4.5 hr 6 hr	11–20 hr	4–6 hr
	IV—load 100 mg over 2 min, repeated q 5 min to desired effect, toxicity or ≦ 1 g Maintenance: 2–6 mg/min	—	< 1 min	As above	As above	As above	As above
	Quinidine						
	PO—initially 200–600 mg q 2–3 h to desired effect Maintenance: 200–300 mg tid/qid (extended release: 300–600 mg q 8–12h)	90%	< 1 hr	50–90% metabolism (some metabolites active) 10–50% renal excretion	6 hr	↑	6–8 hrs.
		90%	2–3 hr	as above		As above	12 hr
	IV—800 mg at 20 mg/min, up to 5 g/day	—	< 5 min	As above		As above	6–8 hr

(continued)

199

Table 26-1. Continued

Class	Drug/Dose	Bioavailability	Onset of Action	Elimination	Elimination t½		Duration of Action
					Normal	Renal Dysfunction	
IB	*Lidocaine* IV—load 1–1.5 mg/kg over 1 min, repeat 0.5–1 mg/kg q 5 min PRN to total dose of 225–250 mg infusion 1–4 mg/min	—	< 1 min	90% metabolism to active and toxic metabolites 10% renal excretion	1–2 hr but dose dependent		10–20 min. with initial doses (distribution effect)
	Mexiletine PO—load 400 mg; initially 200 mg q 8h Maintenance: up to 400 mg q 8h	80–90%	0.5–2 hr	85% metabolism 10% renal excretion	10–12 hr (in severe congestive heart failure up to 25 hr)	↕	8–12 hr
	Phenytoin IV—50–100 mg at 50 mg/min q 10–15 min to desired or 15 mg/kg	—	< 1 min	Metabolism	10–15 hr	↕	8–10 hr
	Tocainide PO—initially 400 mg q 8h Maintenance: 400–600 mg q 8h	100%	0.5–2 hr	60% metabolism 40% renal excretion	15 hr	↕	8 hr
IC	*Encainide* PO—initially 25 mg q 8h Maintenance: 50–75 mg q 6–12h	100%	1–3 hr	Metabolism to two active metabolites (genetic enzyme deficiency results in renal excretion)	1–2 hr 3–12 hr 6–11 hr	↕↕ ↑	6–8 hr 8–12 hr
	Flecainide PO—initially 100 mg q 12h Maintenance: 150–200 mg q 12h	100%	1–3 hr	70% metabolism 30% renal excretion	20 hr	Slight	12–18 hr

I Not classified

	%	Onset	Metabolism/Excretion	Half-life		Duration
Moricizine PO—initially 150 mg q 8h Maintenance: 200–400 mg q 8h	30%	up to 24 hr	Metabolism to two active metabolites (over 30 inactive metabolites) Enterohepatic cycling	7–13 hr	↕	8 hr
Propafenone PO—initially 150 mg q 8h Maintenance: up to 300 mg q 8h	4–12%	3–4 hr	60–80% metabolism to two active metabolites 20–40% renal excretion (increased renal excretion with genetic enzyme deficiency)	2–10 hr 10–32 hr	↕ ←	12 hr

II

	%	Onset	Metabolism/Excretion	Half-life		Duration
Esmolol IV—load 0.5 mg/kg over 1 min Maintenance: 0.1 mg/kg/min × 4 min	—	5 min	Red blood cell (RBC) hydrolysis	9 min	↕	10–20 min

(For other agents see the section on β-adrenergic blocking drugs)

III

	%	Onset	Metabolism/Excretion	Half-life		Duration
Amiodarone PO—load 0.8–1.6 g qd × 1–3 weeks Maintenance: 400 mg qd	200–55%	2–3 days (up to 2–3 months)	Metabolism to active metabolite	2.5–107 days 61 days	↕	Weeks to months
IV—300–600 mg over 20–120 min, then 600 mg over 24 hr	—	Delayed	As above	As above		As above
Bretylium IV—initially 5 mg/kg rapid injection, then 10 mg/kg q 15–30 min to 30 mg/kg Maintenance: 1–2 mg/min continuous infusion	—	5–15 min	90% renal excretion	5–10 hr		6–24 hr

(continued)

Table 26-1. Continued

Class	Drug/Dose	Bioavailability	Onset of Action	Elimination	Elimination t½ Normal	Elimination t½ Renal Dysfunction	Duration of Action
	Sotalol PO—80–320 mg bid IV—1–1.5 mg/kg over 5–10 min	70% —	2–3 hr < 15 min	75% renal excretion 25% metabolism	17 hr	↑	12–20 hr
IV	*Diltiazem* IV—0.25 mg/kg over 2 min; 0.35 mg/kg in 15 min if needed; 10–15 mg/hr infusion × 24 hr	—	1–5 min	Metabolism	3–4 hr	↕	0.5–4 hr
	Verapamil IV—5–10 mg over 2 min, then 10 mg in 30 min if needed	—	1–5 min	Metabolism	2–5 hr	↕	0.3—2 hr
V	*Adenosine* IV—6 mg rapid injection—if no effect, 12 mg repeated q 2–5 min	—	Immediate	Metabolism by RBC and vascular endothelium	< 10 sec	↕	< 1 min
	Atropine IV—0.5–1 mg, repeated in 10 min to maximum of 2 mg	—	< 1 min	50–70% metabolism 30–50% renal excretion	2.5 hr	↕	< 30 min
	Digoxin Load 0.4–0.6 mg, then 0.1–0.3 mg to desired effect Maintenance: 0.125–0.75 mg qd	—	5–30 min	50–70% excretion variable metabolism	30–40 hr	60–100 hr	6 days with repeated doses

II. Mechanism of Action

A. *Dobutamine* stimulates myocardial contractility, with little change in heart rate, by binding to and stimulating β_1 receptors on myocardial cell membranes, which increases cyclic adenosine monophosphate (cAMP) and enhances myosin–actin interaction. It is also a mild vasodilator. *Dopamine* stimulates D_1 receptors at low doses to increase renal blood flow, β_1 receptors at higher doses to stimulate myocardial contractility and heart rate, and α_1 receptors at high doses to increase peripheral vascular resistance (PVR). *Norepinephrine* has marked α_1-stimulating properties and thus increases peripheral vascular resistance, with a reflex decrease in heart rate. It may also increase myocardial contractility directly through β_1 and α stimulation.

B. *Digoxin* binds to and inhibits membrane-bound Na^+-K^+ ATPase, an enzyme involved in the active transport of sodium out of cells in exchange for potassium. Binding is potassium dependent: increased K^+ decreases digoxin binding and hypokalemia increases the binding. Intracellular Na^+ increases, activates the Na^+-Ca^{+2} electrogenic exchange mechanism, and thus increases intracellular Ca^{+2}, which produces an increase in the force and rate of muscle contraction. In patients with congestive heart failure whose sympathetic tone is high, the improved hemodynamics decreases the sympathetic tone, decreasing PVR and the renin-angiotensin system. Digoxin stimulates parasympathetic outflow directly and indirectly, causing slowing of the SA node's rate of discharge, improved atrial conduction, and slowing of conduction through the AV node.

At toxic doses, digoxin stimulates the central sympathetic outflow while directly affecting the resting membrane potential of Purkinje cells via loss of intracellular K^+. There is increased automaticity and slower conduction velocity, which, in conjunction with the increased intracellular Ca^{+2}, cause oscillatory electrical activity called *afterdepolarizations*.

C. *Milrinone* and *amrinone* inhibit the phosphodiesterase (PDE) enzyme relatively specific to myocardial and vascular smooth muscle cells—(PDE III). This inhibition causes accumulation of cAMP; increased cAMP results in enhanced contractility without changing heart rate or myocardial oxygen demands in the myocardium and causes peripheral vasodilation in vascular smooth muscle. Milrinone and amrinone also improve left ventricular diastolic relaxation, which increases the time for coronary artery perfusion.

D. *Glucagon* stimulates myocardial adenylyl cyclase activity to increase cAMP, enhancing calcium ion utilization and contractility. This agent is also a direct vasodilator and an opioid antagonist.

III. Indications

A. *Sympathomimetics* are used to maintain adequate cardiac output and blood pressure in severe congestive heart failure and/or hypotension.

B. *Digoxin* is indicated, either alone or in conjunction with diuretics and/or vasodilators, in the treatment of congestive heart failure. It is used to treat and/or prevent recurrent atrial arrhythmias, particularly atrial fibrillation, atrial flutter, and paroxysmal atrial tachycardia.

C. *Amrinone* is used to support myocardial function acutely in severe congestive heart failure, either alone or in combination with other cardiotonic or load-reducing agents. *Milrinone* is used orally and parenterally in congestive heart failure, often in combination with diuretics, other cardiotonic drugs, and/or vasodilators.

D. *Glucagon* has been used to support cardiac function in patients who are in the postoperative recovery phase after open-heart surgery.

IV. Significant Drug Interactions

Drug	Interacting Drug	Effect	Mechanism
Sympatho-mimetics	Theophylline	arrhythmias	additive
		?cardiac necrosis	unknown
Digoxin	Drugs causing decreased K^+	↑ digoxin toxicity	↑ binding
	Antacids, Kaopectate	↓ digoxin levels	↓ absorption
	Bile sequestrants		
	Quinidine/quinine	↑ digoxin levels	↓ excretion/distribute
Amrinone	Glucose IV solution	↓ amrinone effect	chemical interaction
	Furosemide	↓ effect of each drug	precipitation

V. Complications

A. Sympathomimetics
   1. CNS: excitation
   2. CV: arrhythmias, tachycardia (not with norepinephrine), myocardial ischemia
   3. GI: nausea, vomiting
   4. Hematology: platelet function changes—increased with norepinephrine decreased with dopamine and dobutamine
   5. Other: tissue necrosis with extravasation, mainly with norepinephrine but also with dopamine

B. Digoxin
   1. CNS: drowsiness, neuralgic pain of the lower face, confusion, aphasia, delirium, hallucinations, rarely seizures, visual changes such as blurring with a halo effect, altered color perception
   2. CV: AV block, sinus bradycardia, SA block, premature atrial complexes, accelerated AV junctional rhythms from delayed after-depolarizations, premature ventricular complexes, bigeminy, trigeminy, ventricular tachycardia, ventricular fibrillation
   3. GI: vomiting or nausea from central stimulation of the chemoreceptor trigger zone, diarrhea
   4. Other: gynecomastia

C. Milrinone
   1. CV: arrhythmias with increased risk in patients with some severe congestive heart failure

D. Amrinone
   1. CV: hypotension, angina, rarely cardiac arrhythmias
   2. GI: nausea, vomiting, rarely hepatotoxicity
   3. Immune: acute pleuropericarditis with effusions, vasculitis with or without pulmonary infiltrates, acute myositis
   4. Other: thrombocytopenia, nephrogenic diabetes insipidus, hyperuricemia

E. Glucagon
   1. GI: nausea, vomiting
   2. Metabolic: hypokalemia, hyperglycemia
   3. Immune: allergic reactions, particularly dizziness, rash, shortness of breath

VI. Contraindications

A. *Dobutamine* should be avoided in hypertrophic cardiomyopathy and uncorrected hypovolemia. *Dopamine* is not used in pheochromocytoma, tachyarrhythmias, or ventricular ectopy. *Norepinephrine* is of concern in peripheral vascular disease and Raynaud's phenomenon.

B. *Digoxin* should be avoided in patients with ventricular ectopic activity, uncorrected hypokalemia, or ongoing digoxin toxicity. Digoxin toxicity can be treated with digoxin-specific antibody fragment therapy (digoxin FAB). Digoxin should be used with caution in patients with AV block or sick sinus syndrome. It may be detrimental in patients with certain types of Wolff-Parkinson-White syndrome or hypertrophic cardiomyopathy. Acidosis, hypoxia, and excess catecholamines, either endogenous or exogenous, increase digoxin toxicity.

C. *Amrinone* and *milrinone* should be avoided in patients with hypertrophic cardiomyopathy, aortic or pulmonary valvular disease, and hypersensitivity to the bipyridines. With parenteral therapy, a history of anaphylaxis to bisulfites contraindicates the use of amrinone.

D. *Glucagon* should not be used in patients with pheochromocytoma, insulinoma, moderate to severe diabetes mellitus, or known hypersensitivity.

Diuretic Agents

I. Classification

A. "High-ceiling" loop diuretics
   1. Bumetanide (Bumex)
   2. Ethacrynic acid (Edecrin)
   3. Furosemide (Lasix)
B. Thiazide diuretics
   1. Chlorthalidone (Hygroton)
   2. Hydrochlorthiazide (Hydrodiuril)
C. Potassium-sparing diuretics
   1. Amiloride (Midamor)
   2. Spironolactone (Aldactone)

II. Mechanism of Action

A. *High-ceiling loop* diuretics act on the thick ascending loop of Henle of the nephron to compete with chloride at its receptor site on the tubular cell Na^+-K^+-Cl^- cotransporter protein. They prevent reabsorption of all three ions, resulting in an increase in Na^+ excretion of about 25%. Additional actions include an initial increase in venous capacitance and renal blood flow and an increase in calcium excretion. Bumetanide and furosemide, both sulfonamide derivatives, are carbonic anhydrase inhibitors and therefore act in the proximal tubule as well.

B. *Thiazide-type* diuretics act on the Na^+-Cl^- cotransport system of the distal convoluted tubule of the nephron to inhibit Na^+ reab-

Table 26-2. Dose and Handling of Drugs

Drug/Dose	Bioavailability	Onset of Action	Elimination	Elimination t½ Normal	Elimination t½ Renal Dysfunction	Duration of Action
Dobutamine IV—2.5–15 µg/kg/min	—	1–2 min	Metabolism	2 min	—	< 5 min
Dopamine IV—0.5–2 µg/kg/min (low dose) 2–<20 µg/kg/min (moderate dose) 20–50 µg/kg/min (high dose)	—	< 5 min	Metabolism	2 min	—	< 10 min
Norepinephrine IV—2–12 µg/kg/min	—	Rapid	Metabolism	1 min	—	1–2 min
Digoxin PO—load 0.25–0.5 mg, then 0.1–0.3 mg q 6–8 h *or* 0.125–0.5 mg bid or qd to desired effect (≦ 1.5 mg) Maintenance: 0.05–0.35 mg qd	60–80%	1–2 h	50–70% renal excretion, variable metabolism (GI inactivation)	30–40 hr	60–100 hr	6 days
IV—load 0.4–0.6 mg, then 0.1–0.3 mg to desired effect Maintenance: 0.125–0.75 mg qd	—	5–30 min	As above	As above	As above	As above

(continued)

Table 26-2. Continued.

Drug/Dose	Bioavailability	Onset of Action	Elimination	Elimination t½		Duration of Action
				Normal	**Renal Dysfunction**	
Amrinone						
IV—load 0.75 mg/kg over 2–3 min, repeat in 30 min prn	—	< 10 min	Acetylation with genetic distribution	3–6 hr	6–12 hr	3–6 hr
Maintenance: 5–10 µg/kg/min						
Milrinone						
PO—10–15 mg tid	92%		Renal excretion	1.5–2.5 hr	3.8	6–8 hr
IV—load 50 µg/kg over 10 min	—					
Maintenance: 0.375–0.75 µg/kg/min up to 1.13 mg/kg/day						
Glucagon						
IV—load 2–3 mg, repeated prn	—	1–2 min	Metabolism	3–6 min		3–6 min
Maintenance: 1–10 hr						

sorption. Like other sulfonamide diuretics, these drugs are inhibitors of carbonic anhydrase. Thiazides decrease calcium excretion and reduce urinary volume in patients with diabetes insipidus. With long-term administration, thiazides cause decreased peripheral vascular resistance, probably because of decreased activity of the Na^+-Ca^{+2} transport pump across vascular smooth muscle cells, with a decrease in intracellular Ca^{+2}.

C. *Amiloride* acts on the distal convoluted tubule and the collecting tubule of the nephron to block the sodium-reabsorbing channels in a noncompetitive manner. K^+ and H^+ secretion are diminished. The drug is a weak natriuretic agent.

D. Aldosterone binds to specific receptors on the capillary side of the very distal part of the nephron, interacts with the cell nucleus to alter protein synthesis, and causes an increase in Na^+ transport from the lumen of the tubule into the cell. *Spironolactone* competitively binds to the aldosterone receptor to prevent aldosterone-receptor complex formation, and Na^+ reabsorption at this site.

E. All diuretic agents except spironolactone are filtered at the glomerulus and act directly on the renal tubule via the lumen. Most gain access to the tubular cells at their site of action from the lumen of the tubule by active transport.

III. Indications

A. *High ceiling loop* diuretics are the most effective drugs to treat the Na^+ and water overload associated with congestive heart failure, hepatic cirrhosis, and renal insufficiency. They are usually used alone but may be combined with a thiazide or K^+-sparing diuretic to enhance sodium and water excretion in refractory edema. They lower plasma calcium levels in symptomatic hypercalcemia.

B. *Thiazide-type* diuretics are the drugs of choice in the long-term management of mild to moderate edema in patients with cardiac, hepatic, and renal insufficiency. They are the diuretics of choice in the treatment of essential hypertension, either alone or in combination with other antihypertensive agents. Other uses include the treatment of diabetes insipidus and the treatment of hypercalciuria in patients with recurrent calcium salt renal stones.

C. *Potassium-sparing* diuretics are used primarily in conjunction with loop or thiazide diuretics to further increase Na^+ excretion and to reduce the K^+ loss. When used as single agents, their natriuretic action is generally too weak to be effective.

D. *Spironolactone* has been used in the treatment of edema, particularly that associated with hepatic cirrhosis where aldosterone levels may be high. It has also been used in congestive heart failure, mainly in those patients at risk for excessive K^+ loss. A combination of thiazide-type diuretics and spironolactone is frequently employed to increase Na^+ and water excretion and to decrease K^+ loss. Spironolactone has been used in the treatment of hypertension in patients susceptible to hypokalemia and in the diagnosis of primary hyperaldosteronism.

IV. Significant Drug Interactions

Drug	Interacting Drug	Effect	Mechanism
Loop diuretics	Drugs K^+	Severe hypokalemia	additive
	Drugs causing ototoxicity	↑ risk of ototoxicity	additive
	Lithium	↑ lithium levels	↓ renal excretion
	Neuromuscular blockers	↑ block	↓ K^+
	Oral anticoagulants	↑ anticoagulation	↓ protein binding
Thiazides	Drugs K^+	Severe hypokalemia	additive
	Allopurinol	↑ toxicity	↓ oxipurinol excretion
	Amantadine	↑ amantadine levels	↓ excretion
	Calcium antacids	↑ risk Ca^{+2}	↓ renal excretion
Amiloride	ACE* inhibitors	↑ K^+	additive
Spironolactone	ACE inhibitors	↑ K^+	additive
	Cholestyramine	hyperchloremic acidosis	↓ renal clearance Cl^-

*ACE, angiotensin converting enzyme.

V. Complications

A. High ceiling loop diuretics

The major complications result from electrolyte imbalances, such as hyponatremia, hypokalemia, and hypochloremic alkalosis, which occur in up to 10–15% of patients. Other adverse events include the following:

1. CNS: ototoxicity when large doses are given to patients with renal function impairment or confusion
2. CV: chest pain with bumetanide, orthostatic hypotension
3. GI: bleeding with ethacrynic acid, pancreatitis, jaundice
4. GU: hematuria with ethacrynic acid
5. Hematology: leukopenia/agranulocytosis, thrombocytopenia
6. Immune: activation of systemic lupus erythematosus
7. Other: gout, hyperglycemia, photosensitivity, IV irritation

B. Thiazide-type diuretics

The electrolyte imbalances mentioned above are seen but are less severe and less frequent than those caused by the high ceiling loop diuretics. Other adverse effects include the following:

1. CV: orthostatic hypotension
2. GI: cholestatic hepatitis, cholecystitis, pancreatitis, aggravation of hepatic insufficiency
3. GU: worsening of renal insufficiency
4. Hematology: agranulocytosis, thrombocytopenia
5. Immune: allergic skin reactions or urticaria
6. Other: hyperuricemia with or without gout, hyperglycemia, photosensitivity

C. Potassium-sparing diuretics

The most frequent abnormality is hyperkalemia, occurring in 10–15% of patients. Other adverse effects include the following:

1. CNS: dizziness, ataxia
2. GI: nonspecific upset
3. GU: nephrolithiasis, decreased sexual ability
4. Immune: allergic skin reactions, anaphylaxis
5. Other: photosensitivity, muscle cramps

D. Spironolactone

Hyperkalemia is most common; other side effects include the following:

1. CNS: headache, dizziness
2. GI: nausea or vomiting, abdominal cramps, diarrhea
3. GU: decreased sexual ability
4. Hematology: agranulocytosis
5. Immune: rashes, anaphylaxis

6. Endocrine: gynecomastia, hypertrichosis, abnormal menses

VI. Contraindications

A. All sulfonamide-derived diuretics (thiazides, bumetanide, and furosemide) should be avoided in patients with significant sulfonamide hypersensitivity. Diuretics should be avoided in anuric patients or those with severe renal function impairment. Patients with systemic lupus erythematosus should be treated with high ceiling loop diuretics and thiazide diuretics with caution, as these agents exacerbate or activate lupus erythematosus. All high ceiling loop diuretics can aggravate pancreatitis and should therefore be avoided, if possible, in patients with a history of or active pancreatitis.

B. Potassium-sparing diuretics should not be used in patients with hyperkalemia.

Nitrates

I. Classification

A. Rapidly acting formulations

1. Nitroglycerin
   a. Parenteral (Nitrostat, Nitrobid, and others)
   b. Sublingual (Nitrostat)
   c. Lingual aerosol (Nitrolingual)
   d. Buccal (Nitrogard)
2. Isosorbide Dinitrate
   a. Sublingual (Isordil)
   b. Chewable tablets (Sorbitrate)

B. Long-acting formulations

1. Nitroglycerin
   a. Oral extended-release capsules and tablets (Nitrobid, Nitrospan)
   b. Ointment (Nitrobid, Nitrol)
   c. Transdermal systems (Nitrodur, Transder-nitro)
   d. Extended-release buccal tablets (Nitrogard)
2. Isosorbide dinitrate
   a. Extended-release capsules and tablets (Isordil, Isorbid)
   b. Oral tablets (Isordil, Isorbid)

II. Mechanisms of Action

A. The nitrates are metabolized by smooth muscle to release nitric oxide, which acts via cyclic guanosine monophosphate (cGMP) to alter enzyme activation; these changes result in dephosphorylation of the light chain of myosin, decreasing its interaction with actin. The result is relaxation of smooth muscle.

B. Venous smooth muscle is most affected at low doses, but as the dose is increased, arterial and

Table 26-3. Dose and Handling of Drugs

Drug/Dose	Bioavailability	Onset of Action	Elimination	Elimination t½ Normal	Elimination t½ Renal Dysfunction	Duration of Action
Bumetanide						
PO—initially 0.5–2 mg qd Maintenance: up to 10 qd	90%	30–60 min*	45–50% renal excretion 40% metabolism 2.5% biliary excretion	1–1.5 hr	↔	4–6 hr*
IV—0.5–1 mg q 2–3h (up to 10 mg/day)	—	5 min	As above	As above		As above*
Ethacrynic acid						
PO—initially 50–100 mg qd Maintenance: up to 400 mg qd	75%	30 min*	70% metabolism 20% renal excretion	1–2 hr	↔	6–8 hrs*
IV—0.5–1 mg/kg q 2–4h	—	5 min*	as above	as above	as above	
Furosemide						
PO—initially 20–80 mg qd Maintenance: up to 600 mg qd	60–70%	30–60 min*	100% metabolism	1–2 hr	1.5–2.5 hr	6–8 hr*
IV—20–40 mg q 2h up to 100–200 mg q 2h	—	5 min*	As above	As above		2 hr*
Chlorthalidone						
PO—25–100 mg qd or 100–200 mg qod	> 90%	2 hr*	~100% renal excretion	35–50 hr	↑	48–72 hr*
Hydrochlorthiazide						
PO—25–100 mg qd or qod	> 90%	2 hr*	~100% renal excretion	15 hr	↑	6–12 hr*
Amiloride						
PO—5–10 mg qd	15–20%	< 2 hr*	20–50% renal excretion 40% fecal excretion	6–9 hr	↔	24 hr*
Spironolactone						
PO—25–200 mg qd to qid	> 90%	Inactive prodrug	Metabolism to active canrenone which has renal excretion	13–24 hrs	↔	2–3 days*

*Onset and duration of antihypertensive action prolonged—onset in 3–4 days and duration for 1 week after discontinuation.

then arteriolar smooth muscle are relaxed. Smooth muscle cells of the bronchial, biliary, and GI systems are also relaxed.

    C. Tolerance to the effects of nitrates is seen, particularly when the dose is high. It has been reported with intravenous administration of nitroglycerin after 48 hr, and with continuous use of transdermal patches. Depletion of cellular components required for the generation of nitric oxide (NO), or a reduced effect of NO on activation of cGMP, may be responsible.

After long-term exposure to nitrates, abrupt withdrawal of the agent may cause intense vasospasm, producing myocardial ischemia and vascular insufficiency.

III. Indications

Nitrates are used in the treatment and prophylaxis of acute or chronic angina pectoris, acute hypertension associated with myocardial ischemia or infarction, and as adjunctive therapy in congestive heart failure (decreased preload and afterload).

IV. Significant Drug Interactions

Drug	Interacting Drug	Effect	Mechanism
All nitrates	Opioids	↑ risk of hypotension	additive
IV nitroglycerin	Heparin	↓ anticoagulation	? antagonism
	Norepinephrine	↓ effect of each drug	antagonism

V. Complications

    A. CNS: headache from vasodilation
    B. CV: hypotension (mainly postural), palpitations
    C. GI: nausea, vomiting
    D. Hematology: methemoglobinemia, significant in severe anemia
    E. Skin: rash from topical preparations
    F. Immune: allergic skin reactions
    G. Other: tolerance phenomenon, withdrawal syndrome

VI. Contraindications

The nitrates should be avoided in severe anemia or severe hepatic dysfunction; cerebral hemorrhage or head trauma; hypertrophic cardiomyopathy; glaucoma; hyperthyroidism; significant hypotension; and pericardial tamponade or constrictive pericarditis.

Angiotensin-Converting Enzyme Inhibitors

I. Classification

    A. Captopril (Capoten)
    B. Benazepril (Lotensin)
    C. Enalapril (Vasotec)
    D. Enalaprilat (Vasotec)

    E. Fosinopril (Monopril)
    F. Lisinopril (Prinivil)

II. Mechanism of Action

These drugs, or their active metabolites, competitively inhibit kininase II (angiotensin-converting enzyme, ACE), a nonspecific dipeptidyl carboxypeptidase responsible for the conversion of inactive angiotensin I to active angiotensin II and for the conversion of active bradykinin to inactive metabolites. The ACE inactivation prevents formation of the vasoconstricting angiotensin II and allows accumulation of the vasodilating bradykinin. ACE inhibitors may increase the production of prostaglandin E_2 and prostacyclin in tissues through the enhancing effect of bradykinin on the synthesis of vasodilating prostaglandin. Local platelet aggregation is diminished.

III. Indications

These drugs have been used successfully in the treatment of hypertension and congestive heart failure. With the latter condition, they have usually been given in association with digoxin and/or diuretics.

IV. Significant Drug Interactions

Drug	Interacting Drug	Effect	Mechanism
All ACE inhibitors	Anesthetics (inhaled)	↑ risk of severe hypotension	additive
	K^+-sparing diuretic	hyperkalemia	additive
	Lithium	↑ lithium toxicity	↓ renal excretion
Captopril	Allopurinol	↑ skin reactions	unknown
	Cimetidine	↑ severe neuropathy	? additive

Table 26-4. Dose and Handling of Drugs

Drug/Dose	Onset of Action	Elimination	Elimination t½ Normal	Elimination t½ Renal Dysfunction	Duration of Action
Nitroglcerin		Metabolism to less active dinitrates, then to inactive metabolites			
PO—extended-release tablets 1.3–6.5 mg q 8–12h	15–30 min		1–4 min	—	8–12 hr
Sublingual—0.3–0.6 mg q 3–5 min to maximum of 4 tablets	1–3 min		40 min	—	30–60 min
Lingual aerosol—0.4 mg	2–4 min			—	30–60 min
Topical—ointment 15–30 mg q 6–8h; transdermal patch 0.1–0.6 mg/hr for 12–14 hr q 24h	< 30 min				4–8 hr
	< 30 min				8–24 hr
IV—initially 10–20 µg/min titration up to 200 µg/mn	< 1 min				5–20 min
Isosorbide dinitrate		Metabolism to active mononitrate metabolites, then conjugation			
PO—5–40 mg q 6h (extended-release tablets, 20–80 mg q 8–12h)	15–40 min		45 min	—	4–6 hr
	30 min		2–5 hr		12 hr
Sublingual—2.5–5 mg q 2–3 2–3 hr prn	2–5 min				1–2 hr

V. Complications
A. CNS: fatigue
B. CV: excessive hypotension with or without angina
C. GI: diarrhea, loss of taste, nausea
D. GU: proteinuria, renal failure in renal artery stenosis
E. Hematology: neutropenia, agranulocytosis
F. Immune: angioedema, rash often associated with fever, joint pain and positive antinuclear antibodies (ANA)
G. Other: dry cough, hyperkalemia

VI. Contraindications
Patients should not receive ACE inhibitors in the presence of untreated hyperkalemia or bilateral renal artery stenosis, or with a history of angioedema or anaphylaxis with prior ACE inhibitors. ACE inhibitors should be used with caution in patients with autoimmune disease involving the kidney.

β-Adrenergic Blocking Drugs

I. Classification
A. Nonselective, no intrinsic sympathomimetic activity (ISA)
   1. Lipid-soluble—propranolol (Inderal)
   2. Water-soluble—nadolol (Corgard)
B. Nonselective with ISA: lipid-soluble—pindolol (Visken)
C. Selective, no ISA
   1. Lipid-soluble—metoprolol (Lopressor)
   2. Water-soluble—esmolol (Brevibloc)
D. Selective with ISA: water-soluble—acebutolol (Sectral)
E. Nonselective + α_1-blocker: water-soluble—labetalol (Normodyne, Trandate)

II. Mechanism of Action
A. The β-adrenergic receptor blocking drugs (β-blockers) competitively inhibit catecholamine binding at β-adrenergic receptors. As sympathetic activity increases, the effect of these drugs becomes more evident. β-blockers result in blunting of myocardial responses to catecholamines from sympathetic nerves or from the adrenal medulla. There is a decrease in maximal heart rate and blood pressure response to stress. The workload of the heart is decreased and, with ischemia, less myocardium is at risk of necrosis. Because catecholamines can be a cause of cardiac arrhythmias, the β-blockers can decrease the risk of catecholamine-induced arrhythmias.

B. The blood pressure effects of the β-blockers are complex. The initial response is lowering of blood pressure from decreased cardiac output, particularly during stress. With acute administration, the nonselective β-blockers increase the PVR. Over a period of days to weeks, the PVR decreases and the blood pressure, both systolic and diastolic, decreases. This change is most apparent in hypertensive individuals. Possible explanations for the gradual decrease in PVR include:
   1. Decreased renin production
   2. Decreased central sympathetic outflow
   3. Decreased NE release from peripheral neurons
   4. Resetting baroreceptors
   5. Enhanced production/effect of vasodilating prostaglandins.
C. β-blockers can be relatively specific for myocardial β_1-receptors or can block both β_1- and β_2-receptors, the latter located on smooth muscle cells of bronchi and arterioles supplying skeletal muscles and parts of the mesenteric circulation. At high doses, the specificity is lost. Some β-blockers demonstrate partial agonist activity (ISA) when resting sympathetic tone is low but blunt the response to catecholamines when sympathetic activity is high; this effect may decrease the up-regulation of β-receptors and thus decrease the withdrawal rebound phenomenon. Lipid solubility affects pharmacokinetic properties such as the first-pass effect, hepatic metabolism, renal excretion, and elimination half-life. It also affects CNS penetration. Additional effects seen include α-adrenergic receptor blockade (labetalol), class III antiarrhythmic properties (sotalol), and membrane-stabilizing effects (propranolol).

III. Indications
A. All β-blockers except esmolol are indicated for hypertension and for prophylaxis of chest pain in stable classical angina. Drugs such as propranolol, metoprolol, esmolol, and sotalol are used to treat tachyarrhythmias. Esmolol gives rapid, short-term control of the ventricular response in atrial fibrillation or atrial flutter and controls the rate of sinus tachycardia in patients who are hemodynamically unstable.
B. Other uses (of propranolol in particular) include thyrotoxicosis, migraine prophylaxis,

Table 26-5. Dose and Handling of Drugs

Drug/Dose	Bioavailability	Onset of Action	Elimination	Elimination t½ Normal	Elimination t½ Renal Dysfunction	Duration of Action
Captopril PO—Initially 25 mg bid or tid Maintenance: up to 150 mg bid or tid	75% (fasting)	0.25–1 hr	50% metabolism 50% renal excretion	3 hr	3.5–32 hr	6–12 hr
Benazepril PO—initially 10 mg Maintenance: 20–40 mg qd or bid	> 37%	Prodrug	80–90% metabolism to active benazeprilat, then 90% renal excretion, 10% biliary excretion	0.6–1.1 hr ~11 hr	— ↑	24 hr
Enalapril PO—initially 5 mg qd Maintenance: up to 40 mg qd	60%	Prodrug	80% metabolism to active enalaprilat, then renal excretion	11 hr	↑	24 hr
Enalaprilat IV—1.25 mg over 5 min q 6h	—	15 min	100% renal excretion	11		6 hr
Fosinopril PO—initially 10 mg Maintenance: 20–40 mg qd or bid	32–36%	Prodrug	Metabolism to active fosinoprilat, then 50% renal excretion, 50% biliary excretion	— ~12 hr	— ↕	24 hr
Lisinopril PO—initially 10 mg qd Maintenance: up to 80 mg qd	25%	1 hr	100% renal excretion	12 hr	↑	24 hr

hypertrophic cardiomyopathy, prophylaxis for myocardial reinfarction/postinfarct cardiovascular adverse events, essential tremor,

tachycardia and tremor of anxiety, mitral valve prolapse syndrome and, as an optic solution, open-angle glaucoma.

IV. Significant Drug Interactions

Drug	Interacting Drug	Effect	Mechanism
All β-blockers	Antacids	↓ β-blockade	↓ absorption
	Cimetidine	↑ β-blockade	↓ metabolism/excretion
	Hypoglycemics	severe hypoglycemia	↓ symptoms/response
	Neuromuscular blockers	↑ extent/duration of neuromuscular blockade	potentiation
	Theophylline	↑ theophylline level	↓ clearance

V. Complications
A. CNS: nightmares, vivid dreams, or insomnia (more prevalent with lipid-soluble β-blockers)
B. CV: congestive heart failure (less with ISA β-blockers); bradycardia, SA or AV node conduction block; exacerbation of peripheral vascular disease or Raynaud's phenomenon (with nonselective, non-ISA β-blockers); withdrawal syndrome with severe hypertension and tachycardia (less with ISA β-blockers)
C. GI: constipation
D. Metabolism: blunting of clinical manifestations of hypoglycemia, delay in recovery from insulin-induced hypoglycemia
E. Respiration: precipitation of bronchospasm in patients with asthma or bronchoconstrictive disease who receive nonselective β-blockers with no ISA or a high dose of any β-blocker
F. Immune: positive ANA, rarely with arthralgias or myalgias
   Esmolol, with a very short half-life, has fewer complications. It can cause short-lived bradyarrhythmias, SA or AV node dysfunction and bronchospasm, and/or dyspnea. The incidence of CNS adverse effects is increased, and local phlebitis at the injection site has been reported.

VI. Contraindications
A. Nonselective β-blockers should not be used in patients with congestive heart failure, AV block, asthma, bronchoconstrictive lung disease, peripheral vascular disease, Raynaud's disease, or brittle insulin-dependent diabetes mellitus.
B. Selective β₁-receptor blocking agents should not be used in high doses in the patient populations mentioned above and are still restricted in patients with congestive heart failure.

C. β-blockers with ISA should be used with caution in the patient population outlined for exclusion from nonselective β-blockers.

Calcium Channel Blockers
I. Classification
A. Major myocardial effects: Verapamil (Calan, Isoptin, Verelan)
B. Major vascular effects: Nifedepine (Procardia, Adalat)
   Felodipine (Plendil, Renedil)
   Isradipine (DynaCirc)
   Nimodipine (Nimotop)
   Nicardepine (Cardene)
C. Equal myocardial/vascular effects: Diltiazem (Cardizem)

II. Mechanism of Action
A. These chemically diverse drugs bind to and competitively inhibit voltage-sensitive "L" calcium channels in cardiac and smooth muscle cells. The resulting decreased calcium channel responsiveness to membrane depolarization decreases intracellular free calcium ions and thus diminishes the actin–myosin interaction.
B. Because of differing binding characteristics to the calcium channel, the drugs produce different blocking effects. Verapamil (a diphenylalkylamine) delays recovery of the channel from its inactive state to its resting stage and thus has the greatest effect on cardiac tissue. Conduction through the SA and AV nodes is slowed and contractility is attenuated; arteriolar smooth muscle is also relaxed. Dihydropyridines do not affect the recovery time of the channels, and thus have only a slight effect on the myocardium but a greater effect on arteriolar smooth muscle. The decreased PVR

Table 26-6. Dose and Handling of Drugs

Drug/Dose	Bioavailability	Onset of Action	Elimination	Elimination t½ Normal	Elimination t½ Renal Dysfunction	Duration of Action
Propranolol						
PO—40–640 mg/day bid or tid (sustained release 60–160 mg qd)	30% (first-pass effect)	1–1.5 hr	Metabolism to active 4-hydroxy metabolite plus inactive metabolites	3–5 hr / >12 hr	—	>12 hr / 24 hr
IV—1–10 mg at 1 mg/min, repeated in 2 min and then in 4 hr	—	10 min	Less 4-hydroxy metabolite formed	3–5 hr		<12 hr
Metoprolol						
PO—10–200 mg bid (extended release 100–400 mg qd)	50%	1–2 hr	Metabolism (3–10% renal excretion)	3–4 hr	—	>12 hr
IV—5 mg q 2 min × 3 doses	—	20 min	As above		As above	As above
Atenolol						
PO—50–200 mg qd	40%	2–4 hr	85–100% renal excretion	6–7 hr	16–144 hr	~24 hr
IV—5 mg over 5 min, repeated in 10 min	—	10–20 min	As above		As above	As above
Pindolol						
PO—5–30 mg bid	90%	1–2 hr	Metabolism	3–4 hr	—	>12 hr
Labetalol						
PO—100–600 mg bid	20–33%	2–4 hr	Metabolism	4–8 hr	—	12 hr
IV—20 mg over 2 min, then 40–80 mg q 10 min to total of 300 mg	—	5 min	As above		As above	4–6 hr

causes reflex stimulation of sympathetic outflow, producing an increased myocardial conduction rate and increased contractility. Diltiazem (a benzothiazepine) has prominent activity on conduction through the SA and AV nodes, little effect on myocardial contractility, and a strong relaxation effect on arteriolar smooth muscle.

III. Indications
A. All agents are useful in the treatment of hypertension and angina pectoris. By decreasing myocardial oxygen demand, verapamil is used to treat hypertrophic cardiomyopathy.
B. Verapamil and diltiazem are used to treat supraventricular tachyarrhythmias.
C. Nimodepine is used to treat subarachnoid hemorrhage-associated neurologic deficits if used within 96 hours of the hemorrhage.

IV. Significant Drug Interactions

Drug	Interacting Drug	Effect	Mechanism
All Ca^{+2} blockers	Carbamazepine	↑ neurotoxicity	↑ metabolism
	Theophylline	↑ toxicity	unknown
	Valproic acid	↑ valproate effect	↓ metabolism
Verapamil and diltiazem	Cimetidine	↑ Ca^{+2} blockade	↓ metabolism
	Disopyramide and flecainide	congestive heart failure	additive
Nifedipine	Phenytoin	↑ phenytoin toxicity	unknown

V. Complications
A. CNS: headache, dizziness, angina (with the dihydropyridines)
B. CV: flushing, pedal edema, hypotension (with the dihydropyridines), bradycardia, AV block (with verapamil and diltiazem)
C. GI: constipation, nausea (with verapamil)
D. Other
  1. Arthritis (with nifedipine)
  2. Allergic skin reactions, including erythema multiforme and Stevens-Johnson syndrome (with verapamil or diltiazem)

VI. Contraindications
A. These drugs should be avoided in severe hypotension, aortic stenosis, bradycardia, or congestive heart failure; acute myocardial infarction; and significant hypersensitivity to a given chemical family.
B. Verapamil and diltiazem are not advised in patients with significant AV block or SA node dysfunction.

Antiplatelet Drugs
I. Classification
A. Aspirin
B. Dipyridamole (Persantin)
C. Ticlopidine (Ticlid)
II. Mechanism of Action
A. Aspirin (ASA) has unique activity as an antiplatelet agent. At *low* doses, it irreversibly inhibits platelet cyclooxygenase by acetylation of its active site, decreasing production of prostaglandins, including thromboxane A_2. The latter compound is a powerful stimulus for platelet aggregation and vasoconstriction. The inhibitory effect of aspirin on platelet aggregation lasts for the life span of the platelet, which cannot synthesize new enzyme. Although aspirin also inhibits endothelial cell production of prostacyclin, which has vasodilating and antiplatelet aggregation properties, this effect is short, as endothelial cells can synthesize new cyclooxygenase. When aspirin is given in *high doses*, the main metabolite of aspirin, salicyclic acid accumulates and is a reversible inhibitor of cyclooxygenase, like other nonsteroidal anti-inflammatory drugs (NSAIDs). It affects endothelium and platelets equally, so platelets can regain normal function when the drug is no longer present.
B. Dipyridamole inhibits the uptake of adenosine; it thus enhances the local effect of adenosine as a vasodilator in arterioles. In platelets, it increases cAMP by inhibiting cyclic nucleotide phosphodiesterase or by blocking uptake of adenosine, which stimulates A_2 receptors to increase adenylyl cyclase. The increased cAMP decreases platelet reactivity. There may be synergy between dipyridamole and aspirin.

Table 26-7. Dose and Handling of Drugs

Drug/Dose	Bioavailability	Onset of Action	Elimination	Elimination t½ Normal	Elimination t½ Renal Dysfunction	Duration of Action
Diltiazem						
PO—initially 30 mg tid or qid; Maintenance: up to 120 mg tid (extended release initially 60–120 mg bid)	40%	0.5–1 hr	Metabolism to active metabolite desacetyldiltiazem, then further metabolism	5–8 hr	↔	4–8 hr
Maintenance: up to 180 mg bid; IV—0.25 mg/kg over 2 min, then 0.35 mg/kg over 2 min in 15 min if needed; Maintenance: 10–15 mg/hr infusion ×24 hr	—	1–5 min	As above	3.4 hr	↔	0.5–4 hr
Felodipine						
PO—initially 5 mg qd; Maintenance: 5–10 mg qd	20%	2–5 hr	Metabolism	11–16 hr	↔	24 hr
Isradipine						
PO—initially 2.5 mg bid; Maintenance: 2.5–10 mg bid	15–24%	2–3 hr	Metabolism	8 hr	↕	> 12 hr
Nicardipine						
PO—initially 20 mg tid; Maintenance: 20–40 mg tid	35%	30 min	Metabolism	8.6 hr	↔	6–8 hr
Nifedipine						
PO—initially 20 mg tid; Maintenance: up to 60 mg tid (extended release initially 30–60 mg qd); Maintenance: up to 120 mg qd	35%	20 min	Metabolism	5 hr	↕	4–8 hr / 12–24 hr
Nimodipine						
PO—60 mg q4h × 21 days	13%	1–2 hr	Metabolism	8–9 hr	↔	4–6 hr
Verapamil						
PO—initially 80–120 mg tid; Maintenance: up to 160 mg tid or 240 mg bid (extended release initially 120–240 mg qd); Maintenance: up to 480 mg qd	20–35%	1–2 hr	Metabolism to active metabolite norverapamil, then to inactive metabolites	4.5–12 hr / 10 hr	↕↕	8–12 hr / 24 hr
IV—5–10 mg over 2 min, then 10 mg in 30 min if needed	—	1–5 min	As above	2–5 hr	↔	20 min–2 hr

C. Ticlopidine, or more likely an active metabolite of this drug, interacts with platelet glycoprotein IIb/IIIa to inhibit binding of fibrinogen to activated platelets. This inhibition prevents platelet aggregation and clot retraction. There is no effect on the production of thromboxane A_2 or other prostaglandins.

III. Indications

A. These drugs are adjuncts in patients with coronary artery disease, particularly following myocardial infarction, when platelet aggregation is enhanced. Aspirin at low daily doses decreases the incidence of acute cardiovascular illnesses.

B. The drugs are used, alone or as adjunctive agents, as prophylaxis against thrombus formation in the heart or valves and against embolic phenomena in patients with prosthetic valves.

IV. Significant Drug Interactions

Drug	Interacting Drug	Effect	Mechanism
Aspirin	Drugs with GI cytotoxicity	↑ risk of GI bleeding	additive
	Drugs ↓ hemostasis	↑ risk of bleeding	additive
	Zidovudine (AZT)	↑ AZT toxicity	↓ glucuronidation
Dipyridamole	Drugs ↓ hemostasis	↑ risk of bleeding	additive

V. Complications

A. All antiplatelet drugs
   1. GI: gastric erosions, ulceration and bleeding, nausea, vomiting
B. Aspirin
   1. CNS: salicylism with tinnitus, decreased hearing, confusion, headache, dizziness, drowsiness, visual disturbances
      a. With a toxic dose, hallucinations and seizures
   2. Hematology: anemia from GI bleeding, hemolytic anemia in patients with glucose-6-phosphate dehydrogenase deficiency
   3. Respiratory: bronchospasm in patients with asthma, nasal polyps, and allergies
   4. Immune: anaphylactoid reactions, rashes, hives, urticaria, fever
C. Dipyridamole
   1. CNS: dizziness, headache
   2. CV: "coronary steal" phenomenon in patients with coronary artery disease (at onset of therapy or with rapid IV administration)
   3. Immune: rashes
   4. Other: flushing
D. Ticlopidine
   1. GI: diarrhea
   2. Hematology: severe neutropenia

VI. Contraindications

A. Patients with bleeding gastrointestinal ulcers, hemophilia, active sites of bleeding or disorders of coagulation or platelet function should not receive these medications.

B. Aspirin should not be used in patients with thrombocytopenia, asthma plus nasal polyps, or a history of anaphylaxis or severe sensitivity reactions to aspirin or other NSAIDs.

C. Patients with unstable angina or sensitivity to dipyridamole should not be given this medication.

Thrombolytic Agents

I. Classification

A. Indirect plasminogen activators
   1. Streptokinase (Streptase)
   2. Anistreplase (Eminase)
B. Direct plasminogen activators
   1. Urokinase (Abbokinase)
   2. Prourokinase (Saruplase—investigational)
   3. Alteplase (Activasert-PA)

II. Mechanism of Action

Either directly or indirectly, all the thrombolytic agents cause activation of circulating plasminogen to plasmin, an active, nonspecific protease. The active protease degrades fibrin, fibrinogen, and coagulation factors V and VIII, as well as α_2-antiplasmin, which binds to plasmin to inactivate its effect. Plasminogen may be activated in the circulation or at the site of fibrin clots by streptokinase or urokinase. More preferential activation at the site of fibrin deposition is demonstrated with prourokinase, anistreplase, and alteplase. The end result is the lysis of fibrin clots at all sites of formation.

Table 26-8. Dose and Handling of Drugs

Drug/Dose	Onset of Action	Elimination	Elimination t½ Normal	Elimination t½ Renal Dysfunction	Duration of Action
Aspirin (ASA) PO—80–325 mg qd	30–60 min	Metabolism to salicylate (also active NSAID), then metabolism to inactive metabolites	15–20 min 2–20 hr	↔	7–10 days (antiplatelet action)
Dipyridamole PO—75–100 mg qid (usually with aspirin)	1–2 hr	Metabolism; biliary excretion with enterohepatic cycling	1–12 hr	↔	6 hr
Ticlopidine PO—250 mg bid	Prodrug	Metabolism to active metabolite	No data	No data	> 4 days

III. Indications

These agents are used to treat deep vein thrombosis, pulmonary embolus, acute coronary artery occlusion (in conjunction with heparin and aspirin), and acute arterial thromboembolism.

IV. Significant Drug Interactions

Drug	Interacting Drug	Effect	Mechanism
All	Drugs ↓ hemostasis	↑ risk of hemorrhage	additive
Streptokinase	Antihypertensives	↑ risk of severe hypotension	unknown

V. Complications

All agents have the potential to cause hemorrhage, particularly at sites of vascular access. Embolic phenomena have been described with their use. Reperfusion arrhythmias may occur after acute coronary occlusion treated with thrombolytic agents. Other adverse effects include the following:

A. Streptokinase: fever
B. Anistreplase: allergic reactions including anaphylaxis

VI. Contraindications

All agents: dissecting aneurysm; intracranial AV malformation; brain tumor; active bleeding; cerebrovascular accident; acute severe, uncontrolled hypertension

Parenteral Anticoagulants

I. Classification

A. Regular heparin
B. Low molecular weight heparin

II. Mechanism of Action

A. Regular heparin serves as a catalyst by binding both activated thrombin and antithrombin III in a conformation that enhances their interaction 100-fold. This interaction dramatically increases the effect of antithrombin III to inhibit activated thrombin, a protease that changes fibrinogen to fibrin. The binding of antithrombin III to heparin also causes exposure of the reactive site of antithrombin III for binding to and subsequent inhibition of activated factors X, IX, XI, and XII and kallikrein.

B. Low molecular weight heparin cannot bind both antithrombin III and thrombin, but it increases exposure of the antithrombin III reactive site to activated coagulation factors, mainly factor X_a.

III. Indications

A. Heparin
  1. Adjunct to thrombolytic therapy and aspirin in acute coronary artery thrombosis
  2. Treatment/prophylaxis of deep vein thrombosis and pulmonary embolus
  3. Prophylaxis for thromboembolism during cardioversion
  4. Prevention of blood clotting in extracorporeal circulation

B. Low molecular weight heparin: prevention of deep vein thrombosis and pulmonary embolism in certain surgical procedures.

IV. Significant Drug Interactions

Drug	Interacting Drug	Effect	Mechanism
Heparin	Drugs ↓ hemostasis	↑ risk of hemorrhage	additive
	ACE inhibitors	↑ K^+	both ↓ aldosterone
	Nitroglycerin IV	↓ anticoagulation	? antagonism
	K^+-sparing diuretic	↑ K^+	additive

V. Complications

A. The major adverse effect is bleeding, and the risk increases with age, liver disease, and renal disease. In some patients with inherited or acquired antithrombin III deficiency, resistance to heparin is seen.

B. Other adverse effects include thrombocytopenia, which is mild in 2–5% of patients and occurs within 2–15 days of onset of therapy. In < 1% of patients, a severe form of thrombocytopenia is seen, usually 7–14 days after starting therapy.

Table 26-9. Dose and Handling of Drugs

Drug/Dose	Onset of Action	Elimination	Elimination t½ Normal	Elimination t½ Renal Dysfunction	Duration of Action
Streptokinase IV—250,000 IU over 30 min, then 100,000 IU/hr *or* 1,500,000 IU over 1 hr	Clot dissolves in 45 ± 15 min	? Metabolism	25–35 min	—	≤ 24 hr
Anistreplase IV—30 U over 3–5 min	Clot dissolves in ~45 min	Metabolism	70–120 min	—	≤ 24 hr
Urokinase IV—load 1000–4500 IU/kg Maintenance: 4400 IU/kg/hr	Clot dissolves in ~45 min	Metabolism	20 min	—	≤ 24 hr
Alteplase IV—load 10-mg bolus, then 50 mg/hr × 1 hr, then 20 mg/hr × 2 hr	Clot dissolves in ~45 min	? Metabolism	35 min	—	≤ 24 hr

221

C. Abnormal liver function tests and osteoporosis may occur with therapy given over 3 months. Hyperkalemia from aldosterone synthesis inhibition is seen, and skin necrosis from thrombosis associated with severe thrombocytopenia rarely occurs.

VI. **Contraindications**

These drugs should be avoided in patients with hypersensitivity to pork or beef proteins, threatened abortion, dissecting or cerebral aneurysm, cerebrovascular hemorrhage, active uncontrolled hemorrhage, severe uncontrolled hypertension, or previous severe heparin-induced thrombocytopenia.

α-Adrenergic Receptor Blocking Agents

I. **Classification**
   A. Nonselective (α_1 and α_2 blockade)
      1. Phenoxybenzamine (Dibenzyline)
      2. Phentolamine (Regitine)
   B. Selective (α_1 blockade only)
      1. Prazosin (Minipress)
   C. Selective with other actions
      1. Labetalol (Normodyne, Trandate)—β-blockade
      2. Ketanserin (Sufrexal)—serotonin/histamine antagonism

II. **Mechanism of Action**
   A. α-Adrenergic receptor blockers (α-blockers) are chemically diverse, with different binding characteristics. Phenoxybenzamine irreversibly binds to α_1 and α_2 receptors to prevent catecholamine stimulation, causing vasodilation of both arterioles and veins. Reflex sympathetic output produces tachycardia and increased myocardial contractility. Phentolamine and tolazoline act in a similar manner but are competitive inhibitors. Tolerance to the vasodilating action of these drugs may occur.

Prazosin competitively inhibits α_1 receptors selectively. This inhibition relaxes smooth muscle of arterioles and veins, and also relaxes the smooth muscle of the urinary bladder trigone and sphincter. No tolerance is seen with this α_1-specific blocker.
   B. Other agents which demonstrate α_1 competitive inhibition, such as labetalol and ketanserin, have multiple sites of action, but all decrease peripheral vascular resistance by α_1-receptor antagonism.

III. **Indications**
   A. *Phenoxybenzamine* may be used in pheochromocytoma to control hypertension and diaphoresis preoperatively, as well as for chronic management in patients who are unable to undergo surgery or who have malignant pheochromocytoma. It has been used in the treatment of benign prostatic hypertrophy. *Phentolamine* has been used for the short-term management and prevention of paroxysmal hypertension in patients prior to and during surgery for pheochromocytoma, and to prevent skin necrosis and dermal sloughing secondary to extravasation of norepinephrine.
   B. *Prazosin* is useful in patients with essential hypertension and with concurrent elevations of low density lipoprotein (LDL)-cholesterol and/or triglycerides. Prazosin tends to lower LDL-cholesterol and triglycerides while elevating high-density (HDL) lipoprotein-cholesterol.
   C. *Labetalol* has been useful in managing severe or malignant hypertension and may be of value in treating hypertension in patients with classic angina secondary to coronary artery disease. The exact role of *ketanserin* in the management of hypertension has yet to be determined.

IV. **Significant Drug Interactions**

Drug	Interacting Drug	Effect	Mechanism
Prazosin	β-blockers	↟ first-dose effect	additive

V. **Complications**
   A. Phenoxybenzamine
      1. CNS: miosis, confusion
      2. CV: postural hypotension, reflex tachycardia
      3. GI: dry mouth
      4. GU: inability to ejaculate
      5. Other: nasal congestion
   B. Phentolamine and Tolazoline
      1. CV: postural hypotension, tachycardia, myocardial infarction
      2. GI: nonspecific upset
      3. Other: nasal congestion, flushing or redness of face

Table 26-10. Dose and Handling of Drugs

Drug/Dose	Onset of Action	Elimination	Elimination t½		Duration of Action
			Normal	Renal Dysfunction	
Heparin IV—load 5000–10,000 U Maintenance: 700–2000 U/hr	Immediate	Reticuloendothelial uptake Metabolism	1 hr (100 u/kg) 2.5 hr (400 u/kg) 5 hr (800 u/kg) Varies also with disease	—	1–5 hr (use of protamine sulfate decreases the duration of action)
Low molecular weight heparin SC—5000 U qd	20–60 min	As above	3 hr		Up to 24 hr

C. Prazosin
   1. CNS: numbness or tingling of extremities, drowsiness
   2. CV: first-dose phenomenon with orthostatic hypotensive reaction, bradyarrhythmias, edema, withdrawal rebound hypertension
   3. GI: nonspecific upset
D. Labetalol
   1. CNS: sleep disturbances, anxiety, fatigue, sedation
   2. CV: hypotension, bradycardia, congestive heart failure, angina with abrupt withdrawal
   3. GI: constipation
E. Ketanserin
   1. CV: postural hypotension, Torsades de Pointes when used with diuretic
   2. GI: constipation or diarrhea, dry mouth
   3. Other: nasal congestion

VI. Contraindications
The α-adrenergic blocking agents should not be used in patients with hypotension or cardiogenic shock.

Sympatholytic Agents
I. Classification
A. Central action
   1. Clonidine (Catapres)
   2. Methyldopa (Aldomet)
B. Autonomic ganglia: trimethaphan (Arfonad)
C. Sympathetic nerve endings: guanethidine (Ismelin)

II. Mechanism of Action
A. These drugs act at different levels within the sympathetic division of the autonomic nervous system (SANS) to decrease the effect of the SANS on the cardiovascular system.

B. Clonidine and methyldopa penetrate the (CNS) to stimulate the α_2 receptors of the SANS within the CNS in or around the nucleus tractus solitarius. A negative feedback signal to decrease central SANS outflow is produced. Clonidine is an active drug; methyldopa is a prodrug which is metabolized by CNS neurons to the active methylnorepinephrine and methylepinephrine.
C. Trimethaphan competitively inhibits acetyl choline activity in autonomic ganglia, blocking both sympathetic and parasympathetic efferent pathways.
D. Guanethidine is actively taken up by peripheral sympathetic neurons by the NE reuptake mechanism. It binds to NE storage vesicles, releases NE acutely, and then depletes the vesicle of NE, which cannot reaccumulate. It uncouples the neuronal action potential from release of NE.

III. Indications
A. Clonidine and methyldopa are used to treat essential hypertension when other antihypertensive agents cannot be used. Clonidine is useful in treating and preventing migraine headaches, dysmenorrhea, menopausal flushing, and opioid withdrawal.
B. Trimethaphan is used primarily in surgery to produce controlled hypotension, but it has also been used to treat pulmonary edema in patients with combined pulmonary and systemic hypertension and in hypertensive emergencies associated with acute dissecting aortic aneurysms.
C. Guanethidine is a third-line drug in the treatment of severe, poorly controlled hypertension.

IV. Significant Drug Interactions

Drug	Interacting Drug	Effect	Mechanism
Clonidine	Antidepressants (tricyclics)	↓ hypotensive action	antagonism
	β-blockers	↑ BP on withdrawal of β-blocker	unknown
	Naloxone	↓ clonidine effect	antagonism
Methyldopa	Bromocriptine	↓ bromocriptine effect	antagonism
	Haloperidol	↑ mental confusion	additive
	Levodopa	↑ risk psychosis ↓ effect levodopa	unknown
	Monoamine oxidase inhibitors	↑ CNS excitation	unknown
Guanethidine	Antidepressants (tricyclics)	↓ hypotensive effects	↓ neuronal uptake guanethidine

Table 26-11. Dose and Handling of Drugs

Drug/Dose	Bioavailability	Onset of Action	Elimination	Elimination t½ Normal	Elimination t½ Renal Dysfunction	Duration of Action
Phenoxybenzamine PO—initially 10 mg bid Maintenance: 20–40 mg bid or tid	20–30%	Several hours	Metabolism	< 24 hr		> 3–4 days
Phentolamine IV—5 mg 1–2 hr prior to surgery for pheochromocytoma *or* 0.5 mg/kg/min infusion	—	Rapid	13% renal excretion	19 min		20 min
Prazosin PO—initially 1 mg at bedtime Maintenance: 3–5 mg bid or tid	70%	< 2 hr	Metabolism	3 hr		4–6 hr

V. **Complications**
   A. Central α-2 agonists (clonidine and methyl-dopa)
      1. CNS
         a. Sedation, depression, vivid dreams or nightmares
         b. With toxic levels, pinpoint pupils
      2. CV:
         a. Edema; bradycardia; rebound hypertension in sudden withdrawal associated with anxicty, chcst pain, palpitations, headache, increased salivation, nausea, vomiting, abdominal cramps
         b. Raynaud's phenomenon
      3. GI: nonspecific upset, dry mouth
      4. GU: decreased sexual ability
      5. Other
         a. With clonidine patch, itching, red skin, irritation
         b. Dry, itching, or burning eyes, nasal congestion
   B. Methyldopa (in addition to the above)
      1. GI: colitis, cholestasis, or hepatitis
      2. Hematology: Coombs'-positive test (< 5% developing hemolytic anemia), granulocytopenia, thrombocytopenia
      3. Immune: drug fever, systemic lupus erythematosus syndrome
      4. Other: hyperprolactinemia
   C. Peripheral sympatholytic agents (guanethidine)
      1. CV: edema, orthostatic hypotension, bradycardia, angina, pulmonary edema
      2. GI: diarrhea, dry mouth, nausea, vomiting
      3. GU: difficulty in ejaculation, nighttime urination
      4. Other: muscle pain or tremors, nasal congestion, blurred vision, alopecia, skin rash

VI. **Contraindications**
   A. The central α₂ agonists (clonidine and methyldopa) should be used with caution in patients with AV node dysfunction, cerebrovascular accidents, or significant mental depression.
   B. Methyldopa should not be used in patients with active hepatic disease or pheochromocytoma.
   C. Guanethidine is not recommended in patients with cerebrovascular insufficiency or pheochromocytoma.

Direct-Acting Vasodilators
I. **Classification**
   A. Oral: arteriolar action—hydralazine (Apresoline) minoxidil (Loniten)
   B. Parenteral
      1. Arteriolar action—Hydralazine (Apresoline) Diazoxide (Hyperstat)
      2. Arteriolar and venous—Nitroprusside (Nipride)

II. **Mechanism of Action**
   A. Hydralazine, minoxidil, and diazoxide act on arteriolar smooth muscle with little, if any, effect on the venous circulation, whereas nitroglycerin acts preferentially on venous smooth muscle at low doses but will affect both venous and arteriolar smooth muscle at high doses. (see Nitrates) Nitroprusside affects both arteriolar and venous smooth muscle at therapeutic doses.
   B. These drugs may interact with endothelial cells to cause release of endothelium-derived relaxing factor (EDRF), which is NO or produces NO, or the drugs may form NO in or near the vascular smooth muscle. NO, through an increase in cGMP, causes enzymatic changes resulting in dephosphorylation of the light chain of myosin. This process decreases the myosin–actin interaction and thus causes vasodilation.
   C. Other vasodilating effects of hydralazine include hyperpolarization and interference with mobilization of ionized calcium in arteriolar smooth muscle cells. Minoxidil may also cause hyperpolarization via its active metabolite, minoxidil-NO-sulfate.
   D. Hydralazine, minoxidil, and diazoxide cause reflex sympathetic outflow with increased heart rate and myocardial contractility. There is a sympathetic-stimulated increase in renin production, causing fluid and water retention by the kidney. The result is attenuation of the blood pressure-lowering effect of these drugs over time. The addition of diuretics and/or β-blockers decreases this tolerance by blunting the reflex effect.
   E. Nitroprusside causes little reflex sympathetic activation. Nitroglycerin has dose-dependent effects on the systemic vasculature but has only a slight to moderate ability to increase sympathetic outflow.

III. **Indications**
   A. *Hydralazine* is used to treat hypertension, usually in combination with other agents such as diuretics and α-blockers or cardiac-active calcium channel blockers. It is not a drug of first choice. It has been used in the acute management of congestive heart failure. Parenterally, it has been given as an adjunct in the treatment of malignant or accelerated hypertension.

Table 26-12. Dose and Handling of Drugs

Drug/Dose	Bioavailability	Onset of Action	Elimination	Elimination t½ Normal	Elimination t½ Renal Dysfunction	Duration of Action
Clonidine						
PO—initially 0.1 mg bid Maintenance: 0.2–1.2 mg bid	100%	30–60 min	50% metabolism 40% renal excretion 10% enterohepatic cycling	12–16 hr	41 hr	~ 12 hr
Transdermal—initially 0.1 mg/day × 1 week Maintenance: up to 0.3 mg/day	Varies with site of placement	2–3 days		7 days per transdermal system 8 hr after removing system		
Methyldopa						
PO—initially 250 mg bid to tid Maintenance: up to 1.5 g bid	50%	2–4 hr	30% CNS metabolism 40% hepatic metabolism 30% renal excretion	2 hr	4–6 hr	24–48 hr
Methyldopate						
IV—0.25–0.5 g over 30–60 min q 6h up to 1 g q 6–12h	—	0.5–2 hr	As above	As above		10–16 hr
Trimethophan						
IV—1–4 mg/min, increased prn to desired effect	—	Immediate	Renal excretion	No data	—	10–15 min
Guanethidine						
PO—initially 10–12.5 mg qd Maintenance: up to 100 mg qd	3–30%	2–6 hr	50–75% metabolism 25–50% renal excretion	4–8 days		1–3 weeks

B. *Minoxidil* is an alternative drug to treat severe hypertension uncontrolled by other medications. It is used in conjunction with diuretics. It may be valuable in the treatment of severe hypertension in patients with renal insufficiency.

C. *Diazoxide* and *nitroprusside* are useful in the

management of hypertensive emergencies. Nitroprusside has been used to reduce pre- and afterload in acute myocardial dysfunction, such as severe congestive heart failure, acute myocardial infarction with hypertension, and open heart surgery.

IV. Significant Drug Interactions

Drug	Interacting Drug	Effect	Mechanism
Hydralazine	β-blockers	↑ β-blockade	unknown
Minoxodil	Diazoxide	severe hypotension	additive

V. Complications
A. Hydralazine
   1. CNS: headache, peripheral neuritis from relative pyridoxine deficiency
   2. CV: angina, hypotension, palpitations, arrhythmias, edema, pulmonary congestion, flushing of the face
   3. GI: nonspecific upset
   4. Immune: fever, positive ANA, systemic lupus erythematosus-like syndrome, usually seen after > 6 months of therapy at doses > 200 mg/day (more common in slow acetylators and in patients with renal insufficiency)
   5. Other: nasal congestion, watering or irritated eyes
B. Minoxidil
   1. CNS: paresthesias, peripheral neuritis, headache
   2. CV: angina, arrhythmias, palpitations, hypotension, severe edema, flushing of the skin, pericarditis or pericardial effusion, electrocardiographic T-wave changes, pulmonary hypertension (with long-term use)
   3. Immune: skin rashes including Stevens-Johnson syndrome
   4. Other: hypertrichosis
C. Nitroprusside
   1. CV: rebound hypertension on discontinuing therapy
   2. Metabolism
      a. Thiocyanate toxicity in patients with decreased renal function after long-term therapy, with CNS dysfunction (ataxia, blurred vision, dizziness, headache,

confusion, agitation, tinnitus, disorientation, restlessness, tremors with progression to seizures and coma), abdominal pain, nausea, vomiting, hypothyroidism, weakness, shortness of breath
      b. Cyanide toxicity with high-dose therapy in patients with reduced stores of sulfur-containing compounds (CNS toxicity with agitation, confusion, lethargy, convulsions and coma associated with loss of reflexes and widely dilated pupils, tachypnea, tachycardia with hypotension, arrhythmias)—prevented with concurrent administration of sodium thiosulfate in susceptible patients
D. Diazoxide
   1. CV: excess hypotension
   2. Metabolism: hyperglycemia

VI. Contraindications
A. Hydralazine should not be used in aortic aneurysm, cerebrovascular accidents, or significant coronary artery disease. It should be used with caution in patients with renal insufficiency because of the increased incidence of systemic lupus erythematosus-like syndrome.
B. Minoxidil should be avoided if possible in patients with cerebrovascular accidents, coronary insufficiency, myocardial infarction, and pericardial effusions.
C. Nitroprusside should not be used in patients with compensatory hypertension, such as AV shunt or coarctation of the aorta, hypothyroidism, or encephalopathy unrelated to hypertension.

Table 26-13. Dose and Handling of Drugs

Drug/Dose	Bioavailability	Onset of Action	Elimination	Elimination t½ Normal	Elimination t½ Renal Dysfunction	Duration of Action
Hydralazine						
PO—initially 20 mg bid Maintenance: up to 100 mg bid	15–30% (fast acetylators) 35–50% (slow acetylators)	45 min	GI and hepatic acetylation Metabolism in blood 2–4% renal excretion	2–4 hr	↔	3–8 hr
IV—10–40 mg, repeated prn to desired effects	—	10–20 min	11–14% renal excretion Metabolism in blood Hepatic metabolism	2–4 hr	↔	as above
Minoxidil						
PO—initially 5 mg qd Maintenance: up to 100 mg qd	90%	30 min	> 90% hepatic metabolism to active and inactive metabolites	4.2 hr	↔	24–48 hr
Sodium nitroprusside						
IV—initially 0.5 μg/kg/min, with increase to desired effect up to 10 μg/kg/min Maintenance: ≤3 μg/kg/min	—	30 sec	RBC conversion to NO and cyanide Cyanide metabolized in liver to thiocyanate Thiocyanate excreted via kidney	< 3 min 7 days	↔ ↑	3 min
Diazoxide						
IV—1–3 mg/kg, repeated q 5–15 min to desired effect up to 1.2 g/day	—	1 min	50% renal excretion	21–36 hr	20–53 hr	2–12 hr

229

Bibliography

Antonaccio MJ (ed): Cardiovascular Pharmacology, ed 3. New York, Raven Press, 1990.

Drug Information for the Health Care Professional, ed 13. Rockville, MD, The United States Pharmacopeial Convention, Inc, 1993.

Dukes MNG (ed): Meyer's Side Effects of Drugs. Amsterdam, Elsevier, 1988.

Frishman WH, Charlap S (guest eds): Cardiovascular Pharmacotherapy III. *Medical Clinics of North America* 73(2), 1988.

Frishman WH, Michelson, EL (guest eds): Cardiovascular Pharmacotherapy II. Antiarrhythmic and Antihypertensive Drugs. *Medical Clinics of North America* 72(2), 1988.

Frishman WH, Weiner DA (guest eds): Cardiovascular Pharmacotherapy I. Anti-Ischemic Drugs. *Medical Clinics of North America* 72(1), 1988.

Gilman AG, Rall TW, Nies AS, et al (eds): Goodman and Gilman's The Pharmacological Basis of Therapeutics. Elmsford, NY, Pergamon Press, 1990.

Messerli FH (ed): Cardiovascular Drug Therapy. Philadelphia, WB Saunders, 1990.

Rizack MA (ed): Handbook of Adverse Drug Interactions. New Rochelle, NY, Medical Letter, 1987.

Vaughan Williams MJ (ed): Antiarrhythmic Drugs. Handbook of Experimental Pharmacology, vol 89. Berlin, Springer-Verlag, 1989.

SECTION 4

Pulmonary Medicine

Approach to the Patient with Pulmonary Problems: Cough, Dyspnea, Hemoptysis, Solitary Pulmonary Nodule

Yousef N. Nawas, M.D.

Cough

I. Definition

Cough is the sudden explosive release of air following forceful expiration against a closed glottis.

II. Pathophysiology

A. Cough is an important physiologic mechanism that clears the central airways of foreign material and excess secretions; additionally, it may occasionally be the only sign of serious disease.

B. The cough receptors are found mainly in the larynx, trachea, and bronchi; other sites are the tympanic membrane and the pleura. Thus, in rare instances, cough can occur due to irritation of the tympanic membrane by a hair.

III. Differential Diagnosis

A. The most common cause of acute self-limiting cough is viral upper respiratory tract infection. Other causes are pneumonias and foreign body aspiration.

B. The most common cause of chronic cough is smoking. "Smoker's cough" is related to chronic bronchitis but is usually ignored by smokers.

C. Differential diagnosis of chronic cough
   1. Postnasal drip from chronic rhinosinusitis

   2. Bronchial asthma
   3. Gastroesophageal reflux
   4. Chronic bronchitis
   5. Bronchiectasis
   6. Aspiration: neuromuscular disease
   7. Angiotensin-converting enzyme (ACE) inhibitors
   8. Pulmonary congestion: heart failure
   9. Interstitial lung disease

D. A new cough or changing pattern of a cough in a smoker should raise the suspicion of bronchogenic carcinoma.

E. Differential diagnosis of nocturnal cough:
   1. Bronchial asthma
   2. Postnasal drip
   3. Gastroesophageal reflux
   4. Pulmonary congestion

IV. History and Physical Examination

A. A correct diagnosis can be reached in 70–80% of cases by the history and physical examination alone. The specific diagnostic tests are included in Table 27-1.

B. The sputum may be of diagnostic significance if the cough is productive.
   1. Large amounts of expectorated sputum are usually seen in bronchiectasis.

Table 27-1. Diagnosis of Cough

Disease	History	Physical Exam	Diagnostic Test
Chronic bronchitis	Smoker Chronic cough Smoking cessation reduces cough	Early inspiratory crackles Prolonged expiratory phase	Irreversible airway obstruction by spirometry after inhaled bronchodilators
Asthma	Recurrent attacks of cough, shortness of breath (SOB), and wheezing	Wheezes Prolonged expiratory phase May be normal	Reversible airway obstruction by spirometry
Postviral hyperreactive airway disease	Persistent cough following upper respiratory infection Induced by cold air and respiratory irritants	May be normal	Positive methacholine challenge test
Gastroesophageal reflux	Heartburn Nocturnal cough	May be normal	Upper GI series may show hiatus hernia Low pH on esophageal pH monitoring
Aspiration	Cough on swallowing Neuromuscular disease Elderly persons with swallowing difficulties	Crackles at lung bases	Cine-esophagogram may demonstrate aspiration
Postnasal drip	Chronic sinusitis Nasal congestion	Sinus tenderness	Sinus x-rays
Bronchogenic carcinoma	Smoker Change in cough pattern Hemoptysis	May show signs of postobstructive pneumonia or a mass	Abnormal chest x-ray Sputum cytology Bronchoscopy may show endobronchial mass
Pulmonary congestion	Dyspnea on exertion Orthopnea and Paroxysmal Nocturnal Dyspnea	S3 gallop Crackles in bases	Chest x-ray may show cardiomegaly and signs of pulmonary edema MUGA (Multigated Cardiac Scan) scan and echocardiogram show reduced ejection fraction

2. Purulent sputum with rust-colored blood is seen in pneumococcal pneumonia.
3. "Currant-jelly" sputum is seen in Friedlander's pneumonia.
4. Foul-smelling sputum indicates anaerobic infection, as in lung abscess and bronchiectasis.
5. Pinkish, frothy sputum indicates pulmonary edema.

V. Treatment
  A. Specific therapy should be directed at the cause of the cough:
    1. Chronic bronchitis
      a. Discontinue smoking
      b. Bronchodilators may be helpful
      c. Anti-inflammatory topical steroids
    2. Bronchial asthma
      a. Bronchodilators
      b. Anti-inflammatory topical steroids
    3. Postnasal drip
      a. Decongestants
      b. Antibiotics
    4. Gastroesophageal reflux
      a. Elevation of the head of the bed
      b. Antacids or H2 blockers
      c. Metaclopramide may be helpful
      d. Avoidance of chocolate, caffeine. Alcohol and their agents that decrease LES-tone (lower esophageal sphincter)
    5. Bronchogenic carcinoma

a. Surgical removal if possible
6. Pulmonary congestion
   a. Preload and afterload reducers
B. Nonspecific therapy
1. Codeine
2. Dextromethorphan

VI. Complications of Cough
A. Spread of airborne infection
B. Cough syncope
C. Rib fractures
D. Inguinal hernias
E. Stress incontinence

Dyspnea
I. Definition
A. Dyspnea is the sensation of difficult, labored, and uncomfortable breathing.
B. It may occur with exertion or at rest.
C. It may be influenced by position.
1. Orthopnea: dyspnea in the recumbent position that is relieved after sitting up. It may occur with either heart or lung disorders.
2. Platypnea: dyspnea in the erect position. It occurs mainly in chronic liver disease.
3. Paroxysmal nocturnal dyspnea: sudden dyspnea that awakens the patient from sleep. This is more indicative of heart disorders.

II. Mechanisms
A. Cortical influences: anxiety, fear.
B. Increased ventilatory drive: acidemia, hypercarbia, hypoxemia.
C. Increased work of breathing: airway obstruction, restrictive lung disease.
D. Abnormality of the ventilatory apparatus: neuromuscular diseases.

III. Differential Diagnosis
A. Acute dyspnea
1. Anxiety/hyperventilation
2. Bronchial asthma
3. Pulmonary edema
4. Pulmonary embolism
5. Pneumothorax
   a. Spontaneous
   b. Traumatic
B. Chronic dyspnea
1. Respiratory disorders:
   a. Airway disease: bronchial asthma, chronic obstructive pulmonary disease (COPD)
   b. Parenchymal lung disease: interstitial lung disease, pneumonia, malignancy
   c. Pulmonary vascular disease: primary and secondary pulmonary hypertension

   d. Pleural disease: pleural effusion
   e. Chest wall deformity: kyphoscoliosis
2. Neuromuscular disease
   a. Phrenic nerve dysfunction
   b. Myasthenia gravis
   c. Amyotrophic lateral sclerosis
3. Cardiovascular diseases
   a. Congestive heart failure
   b. Right-to-left shunts
4. Anemia
5. Deconditioning

IV. History and Physical Examination (Table 27-2)
A comprehensive history is essential to evaluate dyspnea. The following points should be clarified: the onset, duration, timing, intensity, frequency, initiating factors, aggravating and relieving factors, and associated symptoms (e.g., cough, wheezing, and chest pain).

V. Diagnosis
A. History and physical examination
B. Complete blood count (CBC): exclude anemia
C. Arterial blood gases
1. Metabolic acidosis
2. Increased (A-a) O_2 difference (Alveolar-arterial oxygen difference)
D. Chest x-ray
1. Pneumothorax
2. Hyperinflation: emphysema
3. Small lung volumes: interstitial lung disease
4. Consolidation: pneumonia
5. Cardiomegaly and pulmonary edema
6. Prominent central pulmonary vessels: pulmonary hypertension
7. Raised hemidiaphragm, small pleural effusion: Pulmonary embolism
E. Pulmonary function tests
1. Obstructive lung disease: forced expiratory volume in 1 sec/forced vital capacity (FEV_1/FVC) < 70%
2. Restrictive lung disease: total lung capacity (TLC) < 80%
3. Reduced diffusing capacity of the lungs for carbon monoxide (DL_{CO}): pulmonary embolism, emphysema, interstitial lung disease, pneumonia
4. Increased DLCO: pulmonary hemorrhage, asthma, mild heart failure
F. Maximum inspiratory and expiratory pressures: decreased in neuromuscular diseases and chest wall deformity.
G. Methacholine challenge test: if dyspnea is episodic and pulmonary function tests are normal, with no other evidence of cardiopulmonary disease

Table 27-2. History and Physical Examination

Disease	History	Physical Examination				
		Inspection	Palpation	Percussion	Auscultation
Anxiety	"I can't take a deep breath"	Irregular breathing and frequent sighs	Normal	Normal	Normal
Asthma	Recurrent attacks of dyspnea, cough, and wheezes	Apprehensive Uses accessory respiratory muscles Wheezes may be heard	Normal	Normal or hyperresonant	Prolonged expiratory phase Wheezes
COPD	Smoking history Baseline coughing and dyspnea	Uses accessory respiratory muscles Purse-lipped breathing Increased anteroposterior diameter of the chest	Normal to decreased tactile vocal fremitus (TVF)	Loss of cardiac dullness Normal to large lung volumes	Prolonged expiratory phase Wheezes Early inspiratory crackles
Interstitial lung disease	Progressive SOB associated with cough No wheezes	Rapid, shallow breathing	Small lung volumes	Normal	Late inspiratory crackles in lung bases
Spontaneous pneumothorax	Sudden, acute pleuritic chest pain and dyspnea	Frequently tall and thin Rapid, shallow breathing	Mediastinum may be shifted away from affected side Reduced TVF	Hyperresonance of side affected	Decreased breath sounds on affected side
Pleural effusion	SOB	Rapid, shallow breathing	Mediastinum may be shifted Reduced TVF	Dullness to percussion	Reduced breath sounds
Pneumonia	Fever, chills and rigors Cough Pleuritic chest pain	Rapid breathing	Increased TVF (Tactile Vocal Fremitus)	Dullness to percussion	Bronchial breathing E to A change Egophony Whispering pectiroloquy Crackles
Pulmonary edema	Myocardial dysfunction Orthopnea and Paroxysmal nocturnal dyspnea	Rapid breathing	Laterally displaced apical impulse	Increased cardiac dullness	Bilateral basal crackles S3

H. Echocardiogram:
  1. Wall motion abnormalities
  2. Signs of pulmonary hypertension
VI. Treatment (Underlying Cause)
A. Obstructive lung disease: bronchodilators
B. Interstitial lung disease: depends on the etiology
C. Pulmonary embolism: anticoagulation
D. Pneumothorax: chest tube
E. Pneumonia: antibiotics
F. Pulmonary edema: diuretics, preload and afterload reducers

Hemoptysis
I. Definition
Hemoptysis is the coughing up of blood that originates in the respiratory tract below the larynx.
II. Classification
A. Hemoptysis ranges from blood streaks to massive bleeding.
  1. Mild hemoptysis: < 20 ml per 24 hr.
  2. Moderate hemoptysis: 20–200 ml per 24 hr.
  3. Severe hemoptysis: 200–1000 ml per 24 hr; 600 ml per 24 hr is the usually quoted number in massive hemoptysis.
B. The rate of bleeding is related to morbidity and mortality.
III. Pathophysiology
A. The lung receives blood from two sources:
  1. The pulmonary arteries, which are a low-pressure system.
  2. The bronchial arteries, which are a high-pressure system.
B. Bleeding may occur from either system but is more common from the bronchial arterial circulation.
C. Hemorrhage can occur due to several mechanisms:
  1. Inflammation of well-vascularized mucosa, as in tracheobronchitis.
  2. Proliferation of bronchial circulation, as in bronchiectasis.
  3. Necrosis of tumor tissue or rupture of a vessel, as in ulcerating bronchial tumor.
  4. Rupture of Rasmussen's aneurysm in the wall of a tuberculous cavity.
  5. Severe inflammation of lung parenchyma, as in pneumonia.
  6. Rupture of distended pulmonary venules and capillaries, as in heart failure.
  7. Pulmonary infarction, as in pulmonary embolism and pulmonary vasculitis.

IV. Differential Diagnosis
A. Tracheobronchitis
B. Bronchiectasis
C. Bronchogenic carcinoma
D. Tuberculosis
E. Bacterial pneumonia
F. Fungal infections
G. Lung abscess
H. Pulmonary infarction
I. Mitral stenosis
J. Heart failure
K. Goodpasture's syndrome
L. Bronchial adenoma
M. Idiopathic pulmonary hemosiderosis
N. Arteriovenous fistulas
O. Coagulopathy
P. Trauma
  The first four causes constitute more than two-thirds of the cases of hemoptysis.
V. History
A. It is very important to differentiate hemoptysis from hematemesis (gastrointestinal bleeding) and epistaxis (nasopharyngeal bleeding).

Hemoptysis	Hematemesis
Coughing up blood	Vomiting blood
Bright red blood	Brownish in color
Frothy	No froth
Alkaline reaction	Acidic reaction

B. It is important to know:
  1. The duration and quantity of the bleeding and whether there were previous episodes.
  2. Smoking history.
  3. The underlying cardiopulmonary diseases.
  4. Bleeding disorders.
VI. Physical examination
This may be normal. If there are findings, they may suggest the cause and site of bleeding. The following are helpful:
A. General condition and vital signs.
B. Head and neck exam, which may show an extrapulmonary source of bleeding.
C. Cervical lymphadenopathy, which may be due to malignancy.
D. Signs of lung consolidation suggestive of pneumonia.
E. Wheezes and early inspiratory crackles suggestive of COPD.
F. Localized wheeze suggestive of partial endobronchial obstruction due to a mass or an aspirated foreign body.
G. S3 sound suggestive of heart failure.

VII. Diagnostic Workup

    A. History and physical examination.

    B. CBC with differential.

    C. Platelet count, prothrombin time, and partial thromboplastin time.

    D. Arterial blood gases.

    E. Sputum examination for cytology, Gram stain, acid-fast stain, and culture.

    F. Chest x-ray.

    G. Bronchoscopy: the most important diagnostic test for determining the site of bleeding.

    H. Conventional tomography of the chest.

    I. Computed tomography (CT) scan of the chest.

    J. Angiography.

        The first six diagnostic tools are needed for all patients with hemoptysis. The other procedures are considered in various circumstances.

VIII. Management

    A. Management depends upon the rate of bleeding, as well as the age, smoking history, and general condition of the patient.

    B. Goals of therapy

       1. Airway stabilization

       2. Localization of bleeding

       3. Control of bleeding

       4. Treatment of underlying disease

    C. Mild hemoptysis

       1. Reassurance

       2. Cough suppressants

       3. Supplemental oxygen if needed

       4. Treat the underlying cause

    D. Moderate and severe hemoptysis

       1. Bed rest

       2. Airway protection, including proper suctioning and postural drainage

       3. Lateral decubitus position, with the bleeding side down

       4. Cough suppression with codeine; avoid oversedation

       5. Early localization of the bleeding site, preferably using bronchoscopy

       6. If bleeding persists, consider:

          a. Tamponading the bleeding segment, using a Fogarty catheter through a bronchoscope

          b. Cold bronchoalveolar lavage

          c. Pitressin injection

          d. Topical thrombin

          e. Bronchial arterial embolization

       7. Treatment of underlying disease

Solitary Pulmonary Nodule (SPN)

I. Definition

    A. SPN is a round or oval density, 1–3 cm in diameter, seen on a chest x-ray surrounded by air-containing lung, with no evidence of other pulmonary disease.

    B. A single nodule larger than 3 cm in diameter is called a *solitary pulmonary mass*.

    C. The following facts are helpful in understanding the importance of reliably diagnosing SPN:

       1. About 30% of newly diagnosed lung cancers present as a solitary nodule or mass on the initial chest x-ray.

       2. Forty-four percent of all SPNs are malignant lesions, and most of them are bronchogenic carcinomas.

       3. There is convincing evidence of improved survival after resection of early stage tumors.

       4. Confirming the benignity of the SPN noninvasively can help the patient avoid the small but real risk of morbidity and mortality of thoractomy.

II. Differential Diagnosis

    A. Malignant tumors

       1. Bronchogenic carcinoma

       2. Single metastatic tumor

       3. Carcinoid

    B. Benign tumors

       1. Hamartoma

    C. Granulomas

       1. Histoplasmosis

       2. Tuberculosis

       3. Blastomycosis

       4. Aspergillosis

       5. Coccidioidomycosis

    D. Others

       1. Hydatid cyst

       2. Bronchial cyst

       3. Pseudotumor (loculated fluid in a fissure)

       4. Rheumatoid nodule

       5. Rounded atelectasis

       6. Arteriovenous malformation

III. History and Physical Examination

    A. SPN is a radiological entity. It is usually found accidentally on a routine chest x-ray. The patient is usually asymptomatic, and the physical exam is usually normal unless the patient has a preexisting lung disease.

    B. Factors that are likely to differentiate malignant from benign lesions:

       1. Age of the patient

          a. In patients less than 35 years of age, less than 1% of SPNs are malignant.

          b. Sixty-five percent of noncalcified SPNs are malignant in patients 65 years of age or older.

2. A smoking history increases the risk of malignancy.
3. Size of the nodule:
   a. The larger the nodule, the higher the risk of malignancy.
   b. About 5% of benign SPNs are > 3 cm.
4. Calcification
   a. Fewer than 1% of pulmonary malignancies appear calcified on chest radiographs.
   b. The following patterns of calcification in an SPN are reliable signs of benignity: diffuse, laminated, popcorn, speckled, and central.
   c. Eccentric calcification, on the other hand, may prove to be scar carcinoma.
5. Properties of the nodule
   a. Lobulation and shagginess of the borders of an SPN are suggestive of malignancy.
6. Rate of growth
   a. *Doubling time* refers to the time required for the nodule to double in volume (not in diameter).
   b. A lesion that doubles in size in < 20 days or in > 465 days is most unlikely to be malignant.
   c. A single malignant cell has to undergo about 30 doubling times to become visible on a routine chest x-ray.

IV. Diagnostic tests
A. Radiologic tests to show a pattern of calcification consistent with benignity:
   1. Routine chest x-ray
   2. Low-kilovolt chest x-ray and fluoroscopy
   3. Digital radiography
   4. CT scan of the chest with densitometry
B. Sputum cytology
   1. About 10–20% of lung cancers have positive sputum cytology.
C. Fiberoptic bronchoscopy with washings, brushings, and biopsies may be helpful, especially in large, centrally located nodules.
D. Transthoracic needle aspirate biopsy (TNBA)
   In experienced hands, most malignant SPNs can be identified using TNBA. Benign lesions are harder to diagnose for two reasons:
   1. They are harder to penetrate.
   2. Fragments of tissue are needed for diagnosis.
E. Thoracotomy with excision of SPN.

V. Diagnostic Workup

A. From 10% to 20% of small or subtle lesions interpreted as SPN are not real. A repeat chest x-ray, oblique views, or nipple markers may be helpful to confirm the presence of an SPN.
B. Comparison with old radiographs showing the same lesion unchanged in size over 2 years is a sure sign of benignity.
C. CT scan of the chest to determine:
   1. The number of nodules: if multiple, proceed with workup to rule out metastasis.
   2. Calcification using densitometry if the SPN was not noted on the chest x-ray.
D. The above-mentioned workup will determine whether the nodule is intraparenchymal and will stop further workup of an SPN of confirmed benignity, either through the presence of calcification or the doubling time.
E. Workup of noncalcified SPN depends upon:
   1. The age of the patient.
   2. The size of the nodule.
F. In patients who are < 30 years of age and have a nodule < 2 cm:
   1. Obtain a chest x-ray every 3 months for 1 year. If there is no change in size, stop further workup.
G. In patients who are > 30 years of age and have a nodule of any size, there are two main approaches:
   1. Histologic diagnosis using bronchoscopy and transthoracic needle aspiration biopsy (TNAB). If malignancy is demonstrated, surgery is done immediately. If it is not demonstrated, repeat the chest x-ray every 3 months. If malignancy is suggested by the doubling time, surgery should be done immediately.
   2. Immediate surgery: warranted in cases where there is a high suspicion of malignancy.

Bibliography

Cough

Braman SS, Corrao WM. Cough: Differential diagnosis and treatment. *Clin Chest Med* 8(2):177–188, 1987.

Fuller RW, Jackson DM. Physiology and treatment of cough (editorial). *Thorax* 45(6):425–430, 1990.

Irwin RS, Curley FJ. The treatment of cough: A comprehensive review. *Chest* 99(6):1477–1484, 1991.

McCool FD, Leith DE. Pathophysiology of cough. *Clin Chest Med* 8(2):189–195, 1987.

Dyspnea

Cherniack NS, Altose MD. Mechanisms of dyspnea. *Clin Chest Med* 8(2):207–214, 1987.

Killian KJ, Jones NL. Respiratory muscles and dyspnea. *Clin Chest Med* 9(2):237–248, 1988.

Mahler DA. Dyspnea: Diagnosis and management. *Clin Chest Med* 8(2):215–230, 1987.

Tobin MJ. Dyspnea: Pathophysiologicv basis, clinical presentation, and management. *Arch Intern Med* 150:1604–1613, 1990.

Hemoptysis

Conlan AA. Massive hemoptysis: Diagnostic and therapeutic implications. *Surg. Annu.* 17:337–354, 1985.

Israel RH, Poe RH. Hemoptysis. *Clin Chest Med* 8(2):197–205, 1987.

Johnston H, Reisz G. Changing spectrum of hemoptysis. Underlying causes in 148 patients undergoing diagnostic flexible fiberoptic bronchoscopy. *Arch Intern Med* 149:1666–1668, 1989.

Naidich DP, Funt S, Ettenger NA, et al. Hemoptysis: CT-bronchoscopic correlations in 58 cases. *Radiology* 177(2): 357–362, 1990.

Solitary Pulmonary Nodule

Caskey CI, Templeton PA, Zerhouni EA. Current evaluation of the solitary pulmonary nodule. *Radiol Clin North Am* 28(3):511–520, 1990.

Cummings SR, Lillington GA, Richard RJ, et al. Managing solitary pulmonary nodules: The choice of strategy is a "close call." *Am Rev Respir Dis* 134:453–460, 1986.

Khouri NF, Mejiane MA, Zerhouni EA. The solitary pulmonary nodule: Assessment, diagnosis, and management. *Chest* 91(1):128–133, 1987.

Swensen SJ, Jett JR, Payne WS, et al. An integrated approach to evaluation of the solitary pulmonary nodule. *Mayo Clin Proc* 65:173–186, 1990.

CHAPTER 28

Diagnostic Methods

Michael R. Silver, M.D.

I. Imaging Techniques
  A. Computed tomography (CT) has largely replaced conventional tomography for imaging thoracic lesions. For localization of metallic foreign bodies, tomograms are more cost effective than CT, but CT allows three-dimensional localization better than tomograms. Infusion allows differentiation of blood from other fluids and tissues. Calcium (bone), fat, and air also have different appearances. Housefield numbers may be useful in differentiating malignant and benign lesions in some situations and are able to discern fluid from blood (when infusion is used) and from tissue.

    1. Procedure
      a. An x-ray beam of variable width (1–12 mm) is rotated 360° around the body in 1° increments.
      b. High-resolution (1-mm)-width or standard (10-mm)-width beams usually employ images reconstructed using sophisticated computer algorithms.
    2. Indications and potential findings
      a. Images can be reconstructed for frontal, sagittal, or coronal orientation.
      b. Images can be re-created to demonstrate subtle differences in bone or tissue densities.
      c. Useful for localizing and identifying:
        (1) Vascular abnormalities (e.g., dissecting aortic aneurysm).
        (2) Chest wall abnormalities (invasion/destruction of ribs from a primary neoplasm or extension of an intrathoracic process).
        (3) Pleural processes (loculated effusion, mesothelioma).
        (4) Mediastinal abnormalities
          (a) Excels at identifying tissues based on density.
          (b) Best method to visualize the mediastinum noninvasively.
          (c) Allows differentiation of fat from tissue and from fluid.
        (5) Pulmonary parenchymal abnormalities (small nodules, presence of calcium, bronchiectesis).
    3. Limitations of the study
      a. Patients must be able to lie still for the procedure.
      b. Weight and size limitations for CT scanners.

c. Without contrast, it is difficult to differentiate tissue from vessels.
4. Contraindications
   a. No absolute contraindications to CT without contrast; pregnancy is a relative contraindication.
   b. Allergic reaction to contrast agents is a relative contraindication; however, new agents may be used in patients with allergies to older dyes.
5. Complications
   a. Allergic reactions to contrast.
   b. Acute tubular necrosis (ATN) from dye.
6. Risks and benefits
   a. Aside from radiation exposure, there are no risks without contrast related to this procedure.
   b. Patients with intravascular volume depletion, renal insufficiency, and/or diabetes mellitus are at increased risk for ATN from contrast.
   c. The procedure is expensive.
B. Ventilation-perfusion scanning is useful for determining the presence of abnormalities in ventilation and/or perfusion of the lung. The test usually includes six views of lung perfusion, although when done at the bedside, only two views are usually obtained.
1. Procedure
   a. Perfusion scanning
      (1) Usually uses macroaggregates of human serum albumin radiolabeled with ^{99m}Tc (half-life, 6 hr).
      (2) Particle size should be 10 to 50 μm in diameter (smaller particles pass through capillaries; larger particles may simulate pulmonary embolism).
      (3) To avoid false positives (nonvisualization), there should be at least 60,000 particles, and ideally 100,000.
   b. Ventilation scanning
      (1) Detected by the patient inhaling radioactive gas, usually ^{133}Xe.
      (2) Identifies areas of normal ventilation, reduced ventilation, and delayed washout of inspired gas.
2. Indications
   a. Detection of acute or chronic pulmonary thromboembolism.
   b. Sequential scans sometimes used to monitor the response to treatment.
   c. Perfusion scanning may demonstrate intracardiac or intrapulmonary right-to-left shunting.

d. Quantitate ventilation and perfusion to each lung in patients with reduced pulmonary function who are being considered for a lobectomy or pneumonectomy.
3. Potential findings
   a. Abnormal ventilation/perfusion ($\dot{V}/\dot{Q}$) scans occur when ventilation is seen in an area that did not trap radiolabeled albumin, usually caused by vascular occlusion (thromboembolism) and/or vasoconstriction (chronic obstructive pulmonary disease, COPD).
   b. Defects are categorized anatomically as subsegmental, segmental, or lobar and can be single or multiple.
   c. When an abnormal chest radiograph in the area with a $\dot{V}/\dot{Q}$ abnormality occurs, the perfusion defect may be described as larger, smaller, or the same size as the radiographic abnormality.
   d. A recent approach to investigation of pulmonary embolism has integrated the clinical index of suspicion with imaging studies.
      (1) Normal chest radiograph, a high clinical index of suspicion, absence of obstructive lung disease, and a lobar or multisegmental abnormality (high-probability scan) strongly suggest thromboembolism.
      (2) Normal chest radiograph, an intermediate or low clinical index of suspicion, a high-probability scans can be falsely positive (see Chapter 32)
4. Limitations of the study
   a. Only two views of perfusion increase the false-positive rate.
   b. Patients with COPD have a higher false-positive rate.
   c. A $\dot{V}/\dot{Q}$ mismatch does not indicate whether a defect is acute or chronic.
   d. An old $\dot{V}/\dot{Q}$ defect may resolve over time.
5. Contraindications
   None
6. Complications
   a. When appropriate-size particles are used, side effects or allergic reactions are rare.
7. Risks and benefits
   a. Although the risk/benefit ratio suggests that everyone with unexplained dyspnea should undergo a $\dot{V}/\dot{Q}$ scan, it is

important to consider how the information will be used to make clinical decisions *before* ordering the scan.

C. Thoracoscopy is a surgical procedure in which the visceral and parietal pleura and the lung are directly inspected and may be sampled, usually utilizing fiberoptic or rigid instrumentation.

1. Procedure
   a. In some European countries, the procedure is routinely performed under local anesthesia.
   b. In the United States, it is often performed under general anesthesia
   c. A pneumothorax is induced and a thoracoscope is inserted through an incision in an intercostal space.
   d. Abnormalities in the lung, or in the visceral and parietal pleura, are directly visualized and can be biopsied.

2. Indications
   a. Unexplained exudative pleural effusion.
   b. Increasingly used in the performance of open lung biopsy.

3. Potential Findings
   a. Malignancy, tuberculosis, adhesions, etiology of interstitial lung disease, diagnosis of lung and pleural space disease.

4. Limitations of the study
   a. Increased costs.
   b. Special training of operators.

5. Contraindications.
   a. Bleeding diathesis.
   b. Inability to tolerate pneumothorax.
   c. Inability to tolerate general anesthesia.

6. Complications
   a. Bleeding, persistent pneumothorax, bronchopleurocutaneous fistuala, hypotension (rarely), death (rarely).

7. Risks and benefits
   a. Higher yield than pleural biopsy but higher morbidity.
   b. Invasive procedure to diagnosis disease (metastatic cancer) which may have a poor prognosis and limited treatment options.

II. Fiberoptic Bronchoscopy

A. Procedure
   1. Usually performed under local anesthesia.
      a. Bronchoscope is most often inserted through nares; it can also be inserted orally.
      b. Topical anesthesia is applied to upper airways before procedure and to lower airways during procedure.
   2. Usually consists of:
      a. Direct inspection of upper airways, vocal cords, and tracheobronchial tree to at least the fourth-order bronchi seventh-order bronchi can be visualized with pediatric bronchoscopes).
      b. Bronchoalveolar lavage in which 100–200 ml of sterile saline in 20- to 50-ml aliquots are instilled through the bronchoscope into a segment of lung in which the bronchoscope has been "wedged" and then aspirated. This allows sampling of terminal bronchioles and alveoli.
      c. Bronchial brushing, in which small brushes (often 7 mm) are passed through the bronchoscope and rubbed vigorously over abnormal mucosal lesions or passed into abnormal segments and rubbed.
   3. Other procedures which may be performed at the time of bronchoscopy:
      a. Endobronchial biopsy, in which 1- to 3-mm^3 pieces of tissue are obtained by biopsying directly visualized areas.
      b. Transbronchial biopsy, in which 1- to 3-mm^3 pieces of tissue, usually containing alveoli, are obtained from an abnormal area of lung not directly visualized. Fluoroscopic guidance may be used to localize the lesion during the procedure.
      c. Protected catheter/brush cultures, in which distal airway secretions are sampled and quantitative aerobic microbiologic cultures are performed.
      d. Transbronchial needle aspiration, in which a needle (18- to 23-gauge, 3–11 mm) is passed, under direct vision, through the bronchial wall to sample lymph nodes or peribronchial masses.

B. Indications
   1. Suspected endobronchial lesion (usually from volume loss on chest x-ray or localized wheezing.
   2. Hemoptysis.
   3. Unknown pulmonary parenchymal lesions (e.g., chronic pneumonia).
   4. Unexplained cough or hypoxemia, especially in immunocompromised hosts.
   5. Aspiration of retained secretions.

6. Research evaluation of lung disease (using BAL bronchoalveolar lavage).
7. Evaluation of persistent cough.

C. Potential findings
   1. Endobronchial obstruction
      a. Foreign body, secretions, malignancy, or extrinsic compression which may result from middle lobe syndrome (e.g., hilar adenopathy in tuberculosis, histoplasmosis, or malignancy).
   2. Inflammation
      a. Bronchitis, endobronchial granulomatous disease, malignancy without obstruction.
   3. Parenchymal abnormalities with normal airways.
      a. Malignancy, sarcoid, fibrosis.
   4. Recovery of viral, mycobacterial, fungal, parasitic, or protozoan pathogens.
   5. Alveolar hemorrhage.
   6. Tracheo- or bronchoesophageal fistula.
   7. Perforated bronchus.

D. Limitations of the study
   1. Some lesions may be too distal in the tracheobronchial tree to visualize.
   2. Removal of foreign bodies more difficult than with rigid bronchoscopy.
   3. Control of hemorrhage more difficult than with rigid bronchoscopy.
   4. Small biopsy pieces may preclude identification of the etiology of interstitial lung diseases (except sarcoid).
   5. Insufficient tissue to diagnose invasive fungal infections (can document the presence of fungal elements).

E. Contraindications
   1. Inability to oxygenate or ventilate the patient.
   2. Severe asthma attack is a relative contraindication.
   3. Coagulopathy or bleeding diathesis is a contraindication to biopsy and brushing but not to bronchoalveolar lavage or diagnostic bronchoscopy.
   4. Inability of the patient to cooperate may necessatite utilization of general anesthesia if the procedure is truly necessary.

F. Complications
   1. From biopsy—bleeding, fever, pneumothorax, death.
   2. From brushing—bleeding, pneumothorax.
   3. From lavage—transient hypoxemia, fever, pneumothorax.
   4. From anesthetic—drug reactions, anaphylaxis, death.
   5. From procedure—epistaxis, hoarsness, fever.

G. Risks and benefits
   1. Much less morbidity than open lung biopsy (gold standard).
   2. Bronchoscopy with lavage is safe in patients with thrombocytopenia or acute respiratory failure
   3. BAL has high predictive value for diagnosing nonbacterial infections such as *Pneumocystis carinii*, mycobacterial disease, and fungal disease.
   4. Addition of biopsy improves the yield for tuberculosis, sarcoid, and malignancy but increases the risk.
   5. Biopsy has a low yield for diagnosing interstital lung disease (except sarcodiosis).

III. Mediastinoscopy

A. Procedure
   1. Performed under general anesthesia.
   2. Incision above the suprasternal notch.
   3. Exploration of scalene nodes, superior and anterior mediastinum to the level of the subcarinal nodes.

B. Indications
   1. Superior or anterior adenopathy without a clinical diagnosis.
   2. Superior or anterior adenopathy in high-risk patients with lung cancer being considered for thoracotomy and resection of lung.
   3. Staging of patients with lung cancer.

C. Potential findings
   1. Location of benign or malignant adenopathy.
   2. Lymphoma.
   3. Sarcodiosis.

D. Limitations of the study
   1. Cannot visulize hilar structures (anterior mediastinotomy is needed).
   2. More difficult in patients with prior surgery or radiation treatment.
   3. Depending on the location of positive nodes, the patient may still be operable and resectable (controversial).

E. Contraindications
   1. Inability to tolerate general anesthesia.
   2. Bleeding diathesis.

F. Complications
   1. Hemorrhage (3–4%), recurrent laryngeal nerve injury (< 4%), pneumothorax (< 1%), wound infection (< 1%), death.

G. Risks and benefits
  1. Largest benefit is the reduction of the number of thoracotomies for unresectable lung cancer.
  2. Clinical controversy concerns what CT findings are so suggestive of mediastinal spread of cancer that they allow the patient to be correctly labeled as unresectable and to avoid mediastinoscopy and/or thoracotomy.

IV. **Pulmonary Function Tests**
Pulmonary function testing generally has four components:
  1. Spirometery (with or without bronchodilators).
  2. Assessment of lung volumes.
  3. Assessment of diffusion capacity.
  4. Arterial blood gas sampling.
  A. Procedure
    1. Spirometery performed in seated patients at rest.
    2. Lung volumes measured by helium dilution or body plethysmography.
  B. Indications
    1. Unexplained dyspnea.
    2. Assessment of airway reactivity (with or without provocation).
    3. Quantitation of degree of pulmonary impairment.
    4. Demonstration of improvement with bronchodilator therapy.
    5. Diagnosis of lung hemorrhage (diffusion capacity).
    6. Reduced exercise tolerance of unknown etiology.
    7. Complete pulmonary functional assessment.
  C. Potential findings
    1. Obstructive and/or restrictive lung disease.
    2. Alteration in acid-base status.
    3. Abnormalities in oxygenation.
    4. Changes in blood-alveolar surface area.
  D. Limitations of the study
    1. Spirometry requires patient's cooperation.
    2. Underestimation of lung volumes in patients with obstructive lung disease.
    3. Underestimation of function in patients recovering from acute illness.
  E. Contraindications
    1. Unstable angina.
    2. Recent myocardial infarction.
    3. Stable angina (relative contraindication).
  F. Complications
    1. Rare; usually those associated with sampling of arterial blood.

G. Risks and benefits
  1. Low-risk procedure, useful for quantifying patient's function.
  2. Only significant drawback is the cost of testing.

V. **Exercise Testing**
The exercise in exercise testing may consist of running, walking, bicycling, or isolated arm or leg exercises. The testing involves measurement of heart rate and rhythm, blood pressure, respiratory rate, oxygen saturation, expired oxygen and carbon dioxide concentration, tidal volume, minute ventilation, and sometimes continuous sampling of arterial oxygen and carbon dioxide tensions and pH. Testing also involves calculation of oxygen consumption, carbon dioxide production, dead space ventilation, sometimes cardiac output, and shunt fraction.
  A. Procedure
    1. In pulmonary patients, the bicycle ergometer is used and work is increased continuously until the patient is unable to exercise further, target values are reached, or a cardiopulmonary event occurs.
  B. Indications
    1. Reduced exercise tolerance of unknown etiology.
    2. Determination of anaerobic threshold for athletic training.
    3. Determination of disability.
  C. Potential findings
    1. Patient has ventilatory limitation of exercise.
    2. Patient has cardiac limitation of exercise.
    3. Indeterminte study if patient was unable to exercise sufficiently.
    4. Results suggesting pulmonary hypertension, malingering, congestive heart failure, or lung disease.
  D. Limitations of the study
    1. Patients may be deconditioned, which limits the study.
    2. Without arterial blood gas sampling, cardiac output and dead space are not measurable.
    3. Patients with neuromuscular diseases may have difficulty with exercise.
    4. Patients with untreated hypertension may appear to be cardiac limited.
  E. Contraindications
    1. Unstable angina.
    2. Recent myocardial infarction.
    3. Stable angina (relative contraindication).
    4. Exercise-induced asthma (relative contraindication).
    5. Pulmonary hypertension.

F. Complications
   1. Musculoskeletal injury, cardiac arrhythmia, angina, myocardial infarction, complications from arterial line placement, death.
G. Risks and benefits
   1. In patients without cardiovascular disease, risks are relatively low.
   2. In deconditioned patients (the majority tested), the etiology of exercise-induced dyspnea may not be identified; however, certain etiologies may be excluded.
   3. In patients with severe heart or lung disease, testing may confirm the clinical impression without providing additional useful information.

VI. **Bronchial Provocation Techniques**
   A. Procedure
      1. Patients with suspected reactive airway disease are exposed to a nonspecific stimulant (histamine, methacholine) or a specific stimulant (exercise, cotton dust, tolvere diisocyanates) and monitored for the development of airflow obstruction.
   B. Indications
      1. Unexplained cough.
      2. Suspected asthma with normal spirometry.
      3. Document reactivity to an occupational or household antigen.
      4. Patients considered for lung resection.
   C. Potential findings
      1. No evidence of increased sensitivity to specific or nonspecific stimulants.
      2. Hyperresponsive airways with reduced forced expiratory volume in 1 sec/forced vital capacity (FEV_1/FVC) to specific or nonspecific antigens.
   D. Limitations of the study
      1. Patients with only a late-phase reaction (4–12 hr after testing) will be initially negative.
      2. Positive results are consistent with the diagnosis but do not establish the cause and effect.
      3. Difficult to do occupational testing in patients with preexisting obstructive airway disease.
   E. Contraindications
      1. For nonspecific stimulus:
         a. Known asthma.
         b. Obstructive airway disease by spirometry.
      2. For antigen specific testing
         a. Known asthma (relative contraindication).
         b. Obstructive airway disease by spirometry (relative contraindication).
   F. Complications
      1. Precipitation of asthmatic attack or status asthmaticus, death.
   G. Risks and benefits
      1. As many as one-third of patients with normal spirometry and cough may have abnormal provocation testing, suggesting reactive airway disease as the etiology for cough.
      2. Patients with obstructive airway disease or severe cardiac disease are at increased risk for adverse events.
      3. Some patients demonstrate reactivity; interpretation of the clinical significance of this finding is difficult.

Bibliography

American Thoracic Society: Clinical role of bronchoalveolar lavage in adults with pulmonary disease. *Am Rev Respir Dis* 142:481–486, 1990.

Anders GT, Johnson JE, Bush BA, et al: Transbronchial lung biopsy without fluoroscopy: A seven-year perspective. *Chest* 94:557–560, 1988.

Dramer El, Divgi CR: Pulmonary applications of nuclear medicine. *Clin Chest Med* 12:55–75, 1991.

Fedullo PF, Shure D: Pulmonary vascular imaging. *Chest* 8:53–64, 1987.

Khouri NF, Meziane MA, Zerhouni EA, et al: The solitary pulmonary nodule: Assessment, diagnosis, and management. *Chest* 91:128–133, 1987.

Mahler DA, Horowitz MB: Pulmonary function testing. In: Pulmonary and Critical Care Medicine. RC Bone ed. Mosby Year Book 1992.

Newell JD: Evaluation of pulmonary and mediastinal masses. *Med Clin N Amer* 68:1463–1480, 1984.

Prakash UB. Bronchoscopy: In: Pulmonary and Critical Care Medicine. RC Bone ed. Mosby Year Book 1992.

Value of the ventilation/perfusion scan in acute pulmonary embolism. Results of the prospective investigation of pulmonary embolism diagnosis (PIOPED). The PIOPED Investigators. *JAMA* 263(20):2753–9, 1990.

Wiedermann HP, MA Meziane: Diagnostic imaging of the chest. In: Pulmonary and Critical Care Medicine. RC Bone ed. Mosby Year Book 1992.

CHAPTER 29

Pleural Disease

Larry Casey, M.D., Ph.D.

Pneumothorax

I. Definition

Pneumothorax is defined as air in the pleural space.

II. Etiology

Any process that causes a tear or perforation of the visceral pleura can produce a pneumothorax.

A. Spontaneous
1. Peak incidence between ages 20 and 30 years.
2. A 4:1 male predominance.
3. Predilection for tall, thin individuals.
4. Smoking may be a risk factor.
5. Majority of cases occur during sedentary activity, but 20% may be associated with strenuous activity and 5% occur after a forceful cough or sneeze.
6. If it occurs in an atypical patient, one should look for other underlying lung disease.
   a. Eosinophilic granuloma
   b. Sarcoidosis
   c. Usual interstitial pneumonia
   d. Desquamative interstitial pneumonia
   e. Pneumoconioses
   f. Emphysema
   g. Pneumonia
   h. Tuberculosis
B. Iatrogenic
1. Thoracentesis
2. Subclavian or internal jugular vein catheterization
3. Transbronchial or percutaneous lung biopsy
4. Liver biopsy
5. Positive-pressure ventilation
6. Nerve block
C. Traumatic
1. Penetrating chest trauma
2. Rib fracture
3. Deceleration injury with bronchial rupture
4. Abdominal trauma with transdiaphragmatic injury

III. Pathophysiology

A. Direct perforation of the visceral pleura
B. Rupture of a subpleural bleb or bulae
C. Necrotizing parenchymal process that erodes through its visceral pleura
D. Partial endobronchial obstruction, producing a "check-valve" leading to progressive hyperinflation

E. Tension pneumothorax: continued pumping of air into the pleural space, raising pleural pressure and thus causing total collapse of the lung and a shift of the mediastinum, which can impair cardiac output, causing hypotension, shock, and death.

IV. Diagnosis
A. History
1. Symptoms depend on the clinical context
   a. Dyspnea
   b. Chest pain, usually pleuritic and of sudden onset
   c. History of trauma or invasive procedures
2. Clinical signs and physical findings
   a. Tachypnea
   b. Tympanic percussion on the side of the pneumothorax
   c. Decreased fremitus
   d. Decreased breath sounds
   e. Subcutaneous emphysema
   f. Signs of tension pneumothorax
      (i) Shift of the trachea away from the involved side
      (ii) Increasing tympany on the involved side
      (iii) Tachycardia
      (iv) Hypotension
B. Diagnostic tests
1. Chest roentgenogram is diagnostic.
   a. Small pneumothorax may be missed; inspiratory and expiratory films should be ordered
   b. Sometimes difficult to determine if the x-ray represents a pneumothorax or a large bullus in patients with emphysema

V. Differential Diagnosis
The differential diagnosis is usually limited but may include worsening of preexisting pulmonary or cardiac disease or a pulmonary embolus.

VI. Treatment
Treatment of a pneumothorax is dependent upon the underlying etiology and the size of the pneumothorax.
A. Small pneumothorax (less than 10%)
1. Observation if caused by spontaneous pneumothorax without underlying lung disease and sometimes if caused by lung biopsy.
B. Large pneumothorax, traumatic pneumothorax, or pneumothorax in a patient on a ventilator.
1. Insertion of a chest tube with closed drainage

VII. Patient Monitoring
A. Patients being observed for small pneumothorax must have frequent assessment of vital signs and a physical examination.
B. If the chest tube becomes nonfunctional or if the air leak is very large with a stiff lung, the patient can still develop tension pneumothorax despite the presence of a chest tube.
C. In patients on ventilators who become hemodynamically unstabled and in whom a clinical diagnosis of pneumothorax is made, do not wait for x-ray confirmation before inserting the chest tube.

VIII. Prognosis
The insertion of a chest tube into a patient with a tension pneumothorax is a lifesaving procedure resulting in rapid, dramatic improvement in hemodynamics and gas exchange.
A. Persistent air leaks (> 7 days) usually require surgery.
B. Patients with spontaneous pneumothorax have a high incidence of recurrence. If more than two episodes occur, the patient should have surgery or chemical pluerodesis.

Pleural Effusions
I. Definition
A pleural effusion is defined as an abnormal accumulation of fluid within the pleural space.
II. Etiology
A. Transudate: increased hydrostatic pressure or decreased oncotic pressure results in fluid filtration across the pleural surface. Examples include:
1. Congestive heart failure
2. Cirrhosis
3. Nephrotic syndrome
4. Volume overload
5. Peritoneal dialysis
6. Myxedema
7. Superior vena caval obstruction
B. Exudate: inflammation or other disease processes affecting the pleural surface itself. Examples include:
1. Malignancies (primary or metastatic)
2. Infectious
   a. Bacterial (empyema or parapneumonic)
   b. Tuberculosis
   c. Fungal
3. Immunologic diseases
   a. Rheumatoid arthritis
   b. Systemic lupus erythematosus

    c. Post–cardiac injury syndrome
    d. Sarcoidosis
  4. Drug-induced effusions
    a. Nitrofurantoin
    b. Dantrolene
    c. Methysergide
    d. Bromocriptine
    e. Methotrexate
  5. Miscellaneous
    a. Pulmonary infarction
    b. Pancreatitis
    c. Intra-abdominal infections
    d. Asbestos exposure
    e. Chylous or pseudochylous effusion
    f. Trauma

III. Pathophysiology

Fluid flux across a membrane is governed by the Starling equation, which balances hydrostatic and oncotic forces across the membrane, and by two coefficients that represent the membrane permeability to fluid or protein.

IV. Diagnosis

A. History—overshadowed by the underlying disease. If the effusion is large, the patient will complain of shortness of breath.

B. Clinical signs and physical examination
  1. Tachypnea
  2. Dullness to percussion
  3. Diminished breath sounds
  4. Decreased tactile and vocal fremitus
  5. Bulging intercostal margins
  6. Mediastinal shift
  7. Egophony and bronchial breath sounds caused by lung compression

C. Diagnostic tests
  1. Chest x-ray
  2. Lateral decubitus x-ray if the effusion is small or to determine if the fluid is free-flowing
  3. Thoracic ultrasound if the effusion is very small or loculated.
  4. Thoracentesis
    a. Culture
    b. Protein
    c. Lactic dehydrogenase (LDH)
    d. Cell count

    e. Cytology
  5. Pleural biopsy
    a. Tuberculosis
    b. Malignancy

V. Differential Diagnosis

The principal differential is between transudates and exudates.

A. Transudate
  1. Clear or straw-colored
  2. Total protein < 3 g
  3. Protein/serum protein < 0.5
  4. LDH/serum LDH < 0.6
  5. Total LDH < 200

B. Exudate
  1. Amber-colored, blood-tinged, or milky
  2. Total protein > 3 g
  3. Protein/serum protein > 0.5
  4. LDH/serum LDH > 0.6
  5. Total LDH > 200

VI. Treatment

If patient is not symptomatic, treatment is directed at the underlying etiology

A. Chest tube insertion
  1. Symptomatic malignant effusions
    a. May require sclerosis
  2. Traumatic effusions
  3. Bacterial infection in the pleural space (empyema)

B. Surgery
  1. Open pleural biopsy when workup is negative and etiology is unknown
  2. Pleurectomy for some cases of refractory malignant effusion
  3. Loculated empyema or complicated parapneumonic effusion
  4. Thoracoscopy

VII. Prognosis

A. Prognosis is dependent upon the underlying condition

Bibliography

Light R. (ed) Pleural Disease. In Clinics in Chest Medicine. WB Saunders, 1985.

Upper Airway Obstruction

Robert L. Rosen, M.D.

I. **Definition**
The upper airway is defined as the region between the mouth and carina. Although obstruction is infrequent, it is a serious management problem.

II. **Etiology**
Obstruction can result from both structural and functional abnormalities. Foreign body aspiration is the most common cause.
   A. Blunt trauma to the neck may occur from sports injuries or auto accidents and should prompt evaluation for an associated cervical spine injury.
   B. Infectious causes include Ludwig's angina (hypopharyngeal or laryngeal abscess); bacterial epiglottis, usually due to hemophilus influenza B; viral croup; bacterial tracheitis; and squamous papilloma.
   C. Structural abnormalities include laryngomalacia, vocal cord polyps, subglottic stenosis, laryngeal webs, laryngeal saccular cysts, subglottic hemangiomas, and benign and malignant neoplasms.
   D. Abnormal laryngeal function due to paradoxical vocal cord motion, unilateral and bilateral vocal cord paralysis, spastic dysphonia, or laryngospasm.
   E. Laryngeal edema related to systemic anaphylaxis, asthma, or Cl' esterase inhibitor deficiency.

III. **Pathophysiology**
Physiologic abnormalities depend on whether the site of obstruction is extrathoracic or intrathoracic and on whether it is fixed or variable.
   A. The extrathoracic upper airway, surrounded by atmospheric pressure, tends to collapse during inspiration, while the intrathoracic upper airway, surrounded by pleural pressure, normally opens.
   B. Stiff, nonpliable lesions are not affected by changes in the phase of respiration, and the resulting obstruction is independent of the level of obstruction.
   C. The effect of variable, pliable lesions is dependent on the level of obstruction. Variable extrathoracic lesions are worsened on inspiration as the airway collapses, while intrathoracic lesions may be compensated for by the normal inspiratory airway enlargement.

IV. **Diagnosis**

    A. Exertional dyspnea is a major complaint. Cough or a change in voice also frequently occurs.

    B. Isolated inspiratory stridor or wheezing should alert one to the possibility of upper airway obstruction. The finding is most prominent over the trachea.

    C. Flow-volume curves often point to the diagnosis, which can then be confirmed by soft-tissue radiographs and direct visualization of the larynx and trachea.

        1. A variable obstructing lesion above the suprasternal notch (extrathoracic) will cause a flattening of the inspiratory loop of the flow-volume curve.

        2. A variable lesion between the suprasternal notch and the carina will result in airflow limitation during expiration.

        3. A fixed obstruction, either intra- or extrathoracic, causes flattening of both the inspiratory and expiratory loops of the flow-volume curve.

V. **Differential Diagnosis**

Upper airway obstruction is commonly confused with obstructive lung disease, mainly asthma.

VI. **Treatment**

Acute upper airway obstruction is usually an acute medical emergency. Treatment is directed at ensuring an adequate airway while the underlying cause is determined and managed.

    A. Nebulized epinephrine is useful in reducing localized edema.

    B. Inhalation of a helium/oxygen mixture, which has a lower density than room air, can help overcome the density-dependent increased resistance seen in upper airway obstruction.

Bibliography

Acres JC, Kryger MH. Clinical significance of laryngeal function tests: Upper airway obstruction. *Chest* 80:207–211, 1981.

Jacobson S. Upper airway obstruction. *Emerg Med Clin North Am* 7:205–217, 1989.

Proctor DF. The upper airways: The larynx and trachea. *Am Rev Respir Dis* 115:315–341, 1977.

CHAPTER 30-B

Asthma

Robert L. Rosen, M.D.

I. **Definition**
Asthma is a reversible obstructive lung disease associated with inflammation and increased airway responsiveness to a variety of stimuli.

II. **Etiology**
Asthma affects 5–10% of the population, with prevalence rates showing an increase over the last 10 years.
   A. The etiology of asthma is currently unclear, but it appears that genetic factors interact with various environmental factors.
      1. Air pollution, both environmental and occupational, as well as childhood cigarette exposure, may sensitize the airways.
      2. Repeated allergen exposure may play a role in the development of asthma.
      3. Viral respiratory infections related to adenovirus, coronavirus, respiratory syncytial virus, parainfluenza virus, and influenza viruses have all been implicated as etiologic agents.
   B. Asthma is associated with increased bronchial sensitivity to histamine and methacholine, cold air, osmolarity of inhaled solutions, irritants such as sulfur dioxide and cigarette smoke, climatic conditions, and exercise.

III. **Pathophysiology**
Asthma results from complex interactions between inflammatory cells, mediators, and the cells and tissues of the airways.
   A. Histologic findings in the airways include mucosal edema, infiltration of the bronchial mucosa or submucosa with inflammatory cells, contraction and hypertrophy of airway smooth muscle, and obstruction of the distal airways with mucus, desquamative epithelial debris, and eosinophils.
   B. Mechanisms of airway hyperresponsiveness include airway inflammation, abnormalities in bronchial epithelial integrity, alterations in autonomic neural control of airways, and changes in intrinsic bronchial smooth muscle function.
      1. An initial trigger may be the release from bronchial mast cells, macrophages, and epithelial cells of inflammatory mediators including histamine, chemotactic factors for neutrophils, eosinophils, and basophils, platelet activating factor, and leukotrienes and prostaglandins, resulting in directed migration and activation of inflammatory cells.

2. Inflammatory damage of airway epithelium leads to increased permeability to inhaled allergens, irritants, and inflammatory mediators and to the loss of production of epithelial-derived protective endopeptidases and relaxant factors.

3. Alterations in parasympathetic control of airway tone is suggested by increased responsiveness to cholinergic substances.

4. Increased airway smooth muscle responsiveness and bronchial smooth muscle hypertrophy lead to further airway narrowing and increased resistance to airflow.

C. An allergen-induced asthmatic response is often biphasic.

1. An early phase is associated with mast cell degranulation, and mediator release occurs within minutes of allergen inhalation and resolves within 1–3 hr.

2. A late-phase response is associated with cellular infiltration and subsequent inflammation 2–6 hr after allergen exposure, and may last for 48 hr.

D. Airflow obstruction is determined by the internal diameter of the airway lumen, with exacerbations characterized by decreases in expiratory airflow.

1. Morphologic mechanisms include bronchial wall edema, mucus production, smooth muscle contraction, and hypertrophy.

2. Peak flow rates decrease and the work of breathing increases.

E. Exacerbations lead to alterations in lung mechanics, gas exchange, and hemodynamics.

1. Residual volume increases secondary to air trapping and functional residual capacity rises, so that respiration occurs closer to total lung capacity, thus aiding in maintaining airway patency.

2. During respiration, use of accessory respiratory muscles (the sternocleidomastoid muscles) help maintain the lungs in a hyperinflated state.

3. Hypoxemia results from the mismatching of ventilation and perfusion.

4. Alveolar ventilation is often maintained with hypocapnia until more severe airflow obstruction causes the flow rates to fall below 25% of predicted, at which time arterial CO_2 increases and ventilatory failure may ensue.

5. Hypoxia-induced increases in pulmonary vascular resistance may lead to a right ventricular strain pattern on an electrocardiogram.

6. Pulsus paradoxus related to increased negative pleural pressure correlates with severe airway obstruction.

IV. **Diagnosis**

The diagnosis of asthma is based on a consistent history associated with physical findings of intermittent airway obstruction.

A. Symptoms, precipitating/aggravating factors, age of onset, and the impact of disease may vary from patient to patient, as well as within the individual patient over time.

1. Cough, wheezing, shortness of breath, chest tightness, and sputum production may be continuous or associated with seasonal variations. Symptoms may vary throughout the day and may worsen at night.

2. Precipitating and/or aggravating factors include viral respiratory infections, inhalational exposure to environmental or occupational allergens or chemicals, nonspecific changes in weather (especially cold air), emotional factors, exercise, drugs (aspirin, nonsteroidal anti-inflammatory drugs, β-blockers), and certain food additives (sulfites).

3. Asthma can present initially in every age group from infancy to old age.

4. Associated conditions include a history of allergic rhinitis, sinusitis, nasal polyps, or atopic dermatitis.

B. Physical findings are primarily limited to the upper respiratory tract, chest, and skin.

1. Nasal polyps, nasal discharge, and postnasal drip are often associated with asthma and may result in exacerbations.

2. Wheezing is the classic breath sound of asthma, but it is not a reliable indicator of severity because the intensity of breath sounds may be reduced in severe airway narrowing. Prolonged expiration is typical of airflow obstruction.

3. Rashes or flexural eczema may reflect an atopic disposition.

C. Spirometry documenting reversible airway obstruction is the key diagnostic study; however, the study may be normal between acute exacerbations. Other studies are useful both diagnostically and in the search for etiologic factors during acute exacerbations.

1. The chest x-ray will typically show hyperinflation, but localized areas of atelectasis may be related to mucus plugging.
2. White blood cell analysis will typically show a moderate elevation in number related to acute demargination of neutrophils, as well as an eosinophilia if the exacerbation is allergen related.
3. Sputum and nasal secretions contain eosinophils.
4. Serum IgE levels are moderately elevated, and skin testing may reveal atopy.

V. Differential Diagnosis

A wide variety of situations associated with recurrent cough and wheezing are often confused with asthma.

A. In infants and children, possibilities include foreign body aspiration, airway compression related to enlarged lymph nodes or tumor, congenital stenosis of the airways, bronchopulmonary dysplasia, cystic fibrosis, and swallowing dysfunction leading to recurrent aspiration.
B. In adults, asthma is often confused with mechanical airway obstruction due to tumor or foreign bodies, laryngeal dysfunction, chronic obstructive lung disease, congestive heart failure, pulmonary embolism, cough secondary to drugs (β-blockers and angiotensin-converting enzyme inhibitors).

VI. Treatment

The therapeutic goal is to control bronchospasm, as well as to reduce chronic airway inflammation.

A. Bronchodilator agents are the cornerstone of therapy for acute asthma. Although they do not affect the underlying inflammation, they give the fastest relief.
   1. β-Adrenergic agonists are the most potent bronchodilators.
      a. When administered by the inhalational route, these agents have rapid onset of action and few side effects.
      b. Although effective when delivered orally or parenterally, these routes are associated with increased incidence of systemic side effects such as palpitations and tremor.
      c. Primary effect is smooth muscle relaxation, but mucociliary function is also improved.
      d. The presumed action is the stimulation of cyclic adenosine monophosphate (cyclic AMP), leading to smooth muscle relaxation.
   2. Inhaled anticholinergic agents act as primary bronchodilators by blocking the production of cyclic guanosine monophosphate (cyclic GMP).
      a. They are usually less effective then β-adrenergic agents.
      b. They have a slower onset of action than β-agonists but may have a more prolonged duration of action.
   3. The role of methylxanthines, primarily theophylline, is currently being reevaluated.
      a. Their mechanism of action is thought to be as an antagonist of adenosine, although inhibition of phosphodiesterase activity in bronchial smooth muscle has been considered in the past.
      b. These drugs have a narrow therapeutic window with many side effects.
B. Anti-inflammatory agents block the development of bronchial inflammation and have preventive activity.
   1. Corticosteroids are the most effective anti-inflammatory agents.
      a. They interfere with arachidonic acid metabolism and the synthesis of leukotrienes and prostaglandins, increase β-receptor responsiveness, and prevent the release of platelet activating factor and the directed migration and activation of inflammatory cells.
      b. They can be administered parenterally, orally, or by inhalation. The inhalational route is preferred when they are used prophylactically in order to avoid systemic side effects.
   2. Cromolyn sodium can be administered by inhalation as a prophylactic agent.
      a. It inhibits both early- and late-phase, allergen-related bronchospasm.
      b. It may act by stabilizing mast cells and preventing mediator release.
   3. Other anti-inflammatory drugs under investigation include nedocromil sodium, methotrexate, and newer antihistamines.
C. Nonpharmacologic interventions include patient education and avoidance of situations that precipitate bronchospasm.
   1. Patients and families must be able to identify bronchospasm, define its severity, and respond to exacerbations.

2. Avoidance of triggers including allergens, inhalational irritants such as cigarette smoke, precipitating emotional stresses, and respiratory viruses is important.

3. Although not as useful as avoidance of allergens, immunotherapy may be helpful in selected patients.

VII. Patient Monitoring

Although many patients with asthma are able to perceive acute exacerbations, some cannot always recognize when an episode is developing.

A. Peak flow meters can be used at home to quantitate early exacerbations.

B. Patients should be closely observed during pollen and flu seasons. Yearly flu vaccination should be done to prevent severe upper respiratory infections.

VIII. Prognosis

Despite advances in the understanding of the pathophysiology of asthma and improvements in pharmacologic interventions, the morbidity and mortality of asthma have been increasing over the last decade.

A. Possible explanations for the increase in deaths include increasing environmental factors, side effects from the medications used in treatment, inadequate therapy during an acute exacerbation with hesitancy among physicians to use corticosteroids, psychosocial problems including denial of the severity of the disease, and lack of access to appropriate care.

B. An increased risk of death from asthma is found in black Americans compared to whites, in patients hospitalized for asthma within the previous year, and in patients who have required intubation in the past for status asthmaticus.

C. Chronic asthma can result in irreversible changes in pulmonary status, presumably from uncontrolled inflammation.

Bibliography

Djukanovic R, Roche WR, Wilson JW, et al. Mucosal inflammation in asthma. *Am Rev Respir Dis* 142:434–457, 1990.

Hargreaves FE, Dolorich J, Newhouse MT. The assessment and treatment of asthma: A conference report. *J Allergy Clin Immunol* 85:1098–1111, 1990.

McFadden ER, Gilbert IA: Asthma. *New Engl J Med* 327:1928–1937, 1992.

National Asthma Education Program. *Guidelines for the Diagnosis and Management of Asthma.* Pub No. 91-3042. Bethesda, MD, U.S. Department of Health and Human Services, August 1991.

Chronic Obstructive Pulmonary Disease

Robert L. Rosen, M.D.

I. Definition

The term *chronic obstructive pulmonary disease (COPD)* encompasses a group of lung disorders that have long-standing obstruction to airflow as a common abnormality. Although COPD can be subdivided into various types, most patients display overlapping presentations and strict definitions are often not useful clinically.

A. Chronic bronchitis, defined clinically by the long-standing presence of excessive bronchial secretions with accompanying productive cough. Cough productive of sputum on most days for 3 consecutive months for 2 consecutive years.

B. Emphysema, defined by anatomic changes; destruction of alveolar walls, with resultant permanent abnormal enlargement of air spaces distal to terminal nonrespiratory bronchioles.

C. Asthmatic bronchitis, similar to chronic bronchitis, but with more eosinophilic secretions that are more responsive to bronchodilator and anti-inflammatory therapy.

II. Epidemiology

Inhalational exposure to a variety of agents, as well as a history of atopy, have been implicated in the cause of COPD.

A. Approximately 30 million Americans have COPD, with a resultant 75,000 deaths per year.

B. Cigarette smoking is a contributing factor in 90% of cases, although only 15% of smokers acquire COPD.

1. The degree of physiologic and pathologic lung change is quantitatively related to the number of "pack-years" of smoking. Individuals with > 40 pack years usually have demonstrable physiologic, though not necessarily clinically significant, abnormalities.

2. Airway/alveolar injury results from oxidants and an imbalance of elastase/antielastase. These effects are modulated by α_1-antitrypsin.

3. The oxidant effect of cigarette smoke stimulates the release of white blood cell elastases and depresses α_1-antitrypsin activity.

4. Cigarette smoke depresses alveolar macrophage function, impairs tissue repair

by inhibiting the synthesis of new elastin, and slows mucus transport.

C. Occupational exposure to dusts and fumes, including grain dusts, cotton, coal, and isocyanate, contributes to the development of COPD in some individuals.

D. Childhood respiratory problems, including poor pulmonary function at birth and recurrent lower respiratory infections in infancy, have been implicated as etiologic factors.

E. Atopy (increased IgE or skin test responsiveness) and/or nonspecific bronchial hyperresponsiveness may constitute risk factor(s) for the development of COPD.

F. Hereditary and/or environmental impairment of antioxidant defense mechanisms in blood cells or lung tissue predisposes patients to COPD.

1. α_1-Antitrypsin deficiency is the only well-recognized genetic factor associated with emphysematous changes, especially in smokers.

2. Deficiencies in other protease inhibitors may lead to similar changes.

III. Pathophysiology

The pathologic changes of COPD reflect abnormalities in bronchi, bronchioles, and lung parenchyma.

A. Bronchi show submucosal gland enlargement, mucosal edema, smooth muscle hypertrophy, and infiltration with neutrophils and lymphocytes, as well as eosinophils in the case of asthmatic bronchitis.

B. Bronchioles contain a mix of inflammation, luminal mucus, goblet cell metaplasia, and distortion due to peribronchiolar fibrosis and loss of alveolar attachments.

C. Changes of emphysema consist of alveolar as well as noncartilaginous bronchiolar destruction.

1. Centrilobular emphysema, originating at the center of a lobule, results in destruction of respiratory bronchioles.

   a. It is commonly associated with cigarette smoking and often involves upper lung fields.

   b. Loss of radial traction leads to premature collapse of small airways during expiration.

2. Panlobular emphysema develops from dilated alveolar ducts at the periphery of lobules and is associated with α_1-antitrypsin deficiency.

D. Physiologic changes of COPD result from airway narrowing leading to increased airway resistance.

1. Increased airway resistance leads to increased work of breathing.

2. Increased thoracic volumes resulting from air trapping and increased lung compliance of emphysema lead to alterations in lung mechanics. This places the diaphragm and other respiratory muscles at a mechanical disadvantage.

3. Hypoxemia results from ventilation/perfusion ($\dot{V}/\dot{Q}$) mismatching, with a preferential reduction in ventilation.

4. Hypoxemia is seen less commonly in emphysema than in bronchitis, since in emphysema both respiratory tissue and the vascular bed are destroyed, thus preserving $\dot{V}/\dot{Q}$ relationships better than in bronchitis.

5. Hypercarbia is a consequence of the increased work of breathing.

6. Hypoxic pulmonary vasoconstriction, as well as emphysematous destruction of alveolar capillaries, results in pulmonary hypertension and cor pulmonale.

7. Polycythemia compensates for chronic hypoxemia.

IV. Diagnosis

COPD may be suspected on the basis of the patient's history and physical examination, with laboratory data used to confirm the diagnosis.

A. Dyspnea, frequently associated with chronic cough, sputum production, and recurrent respiratory infections, is the hallmark of COPD.

1. COPD typically affects middle-aged and older persons.

2. Dyspnea is frequently worsened with exercise.

3. Sputum of chronic bronchitis is typically thick and white/yellow in color and worse in the morning, while sputum of asthmatic bronchitis is clear but "sticky," and flares are often related to environmental factors.

B. Physical findings depend on the severity of the obstructive process.

1. Early findings include hyperinflation of the chest with increased resonance to percussion, prolonged expiration, poor diaphragmatic excursion, and expiratory rhonchi or wheezes.

2. With disease progression, patients may use accessory muscles of respiration and develop signs of dyspnea at rest.

3. Severe disease is associated with findings of pulmonary hypertension, including a palpable and auscultatory prominent P2, right-sided cardiac prominence with a heave or gallop, and signs of right-sided heart failure, as demonstrated by jugular venous distention and peripheral edema.

4. Patients with hypoxemia may have cyanosis, but clubbing is not seen in uncomplicated COPD.

C. Pulmonary function tests (PFTs), chest roentgenograms, and arterial blood gas analysis are important in defining obstructive lung disease and quantifying the degree of impairment.

1. Spirometric evaluation shows reduction in forced expiratory volume in 1 sec (FEV_1), forced expiratory volume in 1 sec/forced vital capacity percentage ($FEV_1/FVC\%$), and forced expiratory flow (FEF_{25-75}).

2. Reversibility of obstruction following bronchodilator inhalation is seen in asthmatic bronchitis.

3. Total lung capacity, functional residual capacity, and residual volume are typically increased due to air trapping and increased lung compliance.

4. A reduction in diffusion capacity is associated with emphysema.

5. Arterial blood gas analysis can detect impairments in oxygen uptake or carbon dioxide elimination.

6. Chest roentgenography may show hyperinflation, diaphragmatic flattening in the lateral projection, and vascular attenuation. Bullae are pathognomonic for emphysema.

7. Sputum examination distinguishes eosinophilic from neutrophilic secretions and is useful in determining the asthmatic bronchitis component.

V. Differential Diagnosis

COPD can be confused with any disease that has dyspnea as a major manifestation.

A. Acute lung processes including acute bacterial or viral upper respiratory disease, pneumonia, acute exposure to inhaled fumes or toxins, or allergic asthma.

B. Chronic lung processes including bronchiectasis, mycobacterial or fungal processes, interstitial lung disease, noninfectious granulomatous disease, or fibrosing alveolitis.

C. Cardiac dysfunction including congestive heart failure and valvular heart disease.

VI. Treatment

Management of COPD is directed at decreasing airway resistance and reversing its physiologic consequences.

A. Based on pulmonary function tests (PFTs), only 15–20% of COPD patients appear to respond to bronchodilators, but many patients show clinical improvement after appropriate bronchodilator therapy.

1. Inhaled β-adrenergic agonists are well tolerated, have few systemic side effects, and may improve mucociliary function.

2. Inhaled anticholinergic agents have been found to be effective, either alone or in conjunction with β-adrenergics (as bronchodilating agents).

3. Theophyllines are currently used less often as initial therapy because of their potential side effects but remain part of the therapeutic regimen due to their ease of administration and long action.

B. Anti-inflammatory agents help reduce airway secretions and edema.

1. Corticosteroid therapy benefits certain patients with COPD, especially those with an asthmatic bronchitis component. Low-dose oral regimens (5–10 mg/day) or inhaled preparations can reduce the inflammatory response.

2. Inhaled cromolyn may have benefit in patients with an allergic component.

C. Antibiotics are often useful during acute bronchitic flares, but their benefit has never been firmly established.

D. Prevention of acute attacks includes yearly influenza immunization.

E. Recently there has been renewed interest in expectorants, but their overall impact on disease is probably small. Mucolytic agents should be used cautiously due to the risk of paradoxically increasing mucous production or producing bronchospasm.

F. The survival of hypoxemic COPD patients is improved by long-term oxygen therapy.

1. Appropriate candidates are clinically stable patients who are chronically hypoxemic, with a resting arterial $PO_2 < 55$

torr, or who have a PO_2 of 55–59 torr but evidence of polycythemia or right heart failure.

2. Patients should receive supplemental oxygen for at least 12 hr/day, with close to 24 hr/day being optimal.

3. Patients with intermittent hypoxemia, either nocturnal or exercise related, may benefit from supplemental oxygen, but few data exist to confirm this conclusion.

VII. Patient Monitoring

Patients with COPD need to be observed for symptomatic deterioration or signs of impending right heart failure.

A. Routine PFTs add little to the management of these patients.

B. When nonacute decompensation occurs, arterial blood gas analysis should be done to determine whether the patient is a candidate for supplemental oxygen.

VIII. Prognosis

The course of COPD is dependent on the predominant type of pathology and the degree of disease present when the patient seeks medical intervention.

A. Most patients are relatively asymptomatic until FEV_1 decreases below 1.0 liters. At $FEV_1 < 0.8$ liters, most patients become severely limited.

B. Once significant COPD is present, the yearly decline in FEV_1 is approximately 50–75 ml/year, compared to a normal decline of 25–40 ml/year (although the standard deviation is large).

C. Patients with asthmatic bronchitis may fare better than those with a more emphysematous form of COPD. Ten-year mortality is 60% in emphysema and 15% in asthmatic bronchitis.

D. The initial value for FEV_1 is the single best predictor of survival, with age being the only other relevant predictor.

1. The 5-year survival rate for patients with FEV_1 of 1.0 liter is 50%, whereas for those with an FEV_1 of 0.75 liter it is approximately 25%.

2. Increasing age is associated with an increased risk of death.

3. Diffusion capacity, cor pulmonale, and resting heart rate have minimal predictive power after adjustment for FEV_1 and age.

Bibliography

Dosman JA, Cockroft DW (eds). Obstructive lung disease. *Med Clin North Am* 74(3):547–850, 1990.

Murray JF (ed). Chronic airways disease—Distribution and determinants, prevention and control. *Chest* 96(3):301S–378S, 1989.

Petty TL (ed). Diagnosis and treatment of chronic obstructive pulmonary disease. *Chest* 97(2):1S–33S, 1990.

Snider GL. Emphysema: The First Two Centuries—and Beyond. *Am Rev Respir Dis* 146:1334–44, 1615–22, 1992.

Standards for the diagnosis and care of patients with chronic obstructive pulmonary disease and asthma. *Am Rev Respir Dis* 136:225–243, 1987.

Bronchiectasis

Robert L. Rosen, M.D.

I. Definition

Bronchiectasis is defined pathologically as an abnormal and permanent dilation of the subsegmental airways.

II. Etiology

Once a common problem (prior to the widespread availability of antibiotics), bronchiectasis remains a complication of suppurative lung processes.

A. Focal bronchiectasis is localized to a segment or lobe.

1. Foreign body aspiration associated with unchewed food or dental elements often leads to localized disease on the right and in the lower lobe or posterior segments of the upper lobe.

2. A bacterial pneumonia or lung abscess may resolve, with structural changes localized to a single lobe.

3. Adenopathy, broncholiths, or benign lung tumors may lead to partial airway obstruction and subsequent bronchiectatic changes.

B. Diffuse disease is often a consequence of a widespread pulmonary process or systemic disease.

1. Aspiration of gastric contents or corrosive chemicals, as well as inhalation of noxious gases such as anhydrous ammonia or sulfur dioxide, may result in acute inflammation and long-term airway damage.

2. Tuberculosis, necrotizing bacterial pneumonia, and viral pneumonia related to measles, whooping cough, pertussis, or adenovirus may all resolve with parenchymal destruction and fibrosis

3. Humoral immunodeficiency, especially panhypogammaglobulinemia, is associated with recurrent suppurative pulmonary processes leading to bronchiectatic changes.

4. Ciliary dyskinesia syndromes result in repeated pulmonary infections and airway abnormalities.

5. Allergic bronchopulmonary aspergillosis involves an immunologically mediated reaction leading to mucosal inflammation and bronchiectatic changes classically involving central bronchi.

6. The recurrent infections of cystic fibrosis result in the structural changes of bronchiectasis.

III. Pathophysiology

The defining structural abnormalities lead directly to the classic clinical finding of copious secretions.

A. Affected airways are tortuous, dilated, and partially obstructed by thick, purulent secretions.

B. Distal bronchioles and alveoli are destroyed and replaced by fibrotic strands.

C. Histologic abnormalities include inflammation, mucosal ulceration, bronchomalacia, muscular hypertrophy, and neovascularization.

D. Peripheral airways become inflamed and filled with secretions, leading to a cycle of recurrent inflammation with even more secretions.

IV. Diagnosis

Bronchiectasis should be suspected in patients with the clinical syndrome of recurrent cough productive of copious amounts of secretions.

A. Patients typically have a chronic intermittent cough which is worse upon awakening and is associated with excessive purulent secretions.

1. Historical factors such as previous sinus/pulmonary infections or recurrent aspiration are often present.

2. The sputum is typically described as being cupful in amount and assuming a characteristic three-layer appearance.

3. Blood-streaked sputum is frequently seen.

B. Physical findings are not specific.

1. Crackles or wheezes are heard over the involved areas.

2. Clubbing and hypertrophic osteoarthropathy are commonly seen in long-standing disease and distinguish bronchiectasis from bronchitis.

3. Sinus involvement and nasal polyps may be seen.

C. The diagnosis is made by the finding of areas of dilated airways by thin-section computed tomography or bronchography.

1. Blood counts may show anemia of chronic infection, erythrocytosis related to hypoxemia, or leukocytosis related to chronic infection.

2. Sputum cultures often show normal upper airway flora.

3. Serum protein electrophoresis and immunoglobulin quantitation may show a polyclonal increase in IgG levels related to chronic infection or deficiencies if causative.

4. PFTs often show evidence of obstruction but may also have a restrictive pattern.

5. If focal disease is suspected, bronchoscopy should be performed, looking for an obstructing lesion.

V. Differential Diagnosis

Bronchiectasis must be considered in patients with chronic cough or atypical presentations of bronchitis or asthma.

VI. Treatment

Since bronchiectasis is a permanent structural abnormality, cure is not possible. Therapy is directed at preventing disease progression and complications.

A. Intermittent infectious flares usually respond to broad-spectrum antibiotics such as trimethoprim-sulfamethoxazole, ampicillin, or tetracycline given on a prolonged or rotating schedule.

B. Bronchodilator therapy and bronchial hygiene techniques benefit many patients.

C. Surgical resection of focal disease is sometimes appropriate but is not suitable for diffuse disease unless localized bleeding complications develop.

D. Gamma globulin therapy for hypogammaglobulinemia or prednisone for allergic bronchopulmonary aspergillosis is helpful if these conditions are causes of disease.

VII. Prognosis

Since the advent of antibiotics, the prognosis of bronchiectasis has markedly improved. Complications can lead to cor pulmonale or massive hemoptysis, but death is usually due to other causes.

Bibliography

Barker AF, Bardana EJ Jr. Bronchiectasis: Update of an orphan disease. *Am Rev Respir Dis* 137:969–978, 1988.

Grenier P, Maurice F, Musset D, et al. Bronchiectasis: Assessment by thin-section CT. *Radiology* 161:95–99, 1986.

leRoux BT, Mohlala ML, Odell JA, et al. Suppurative diseases of the lung and pleural space: Bronchiectasis. *Curr Probl Surg* 23:97–158, 1986.

Chapter 30-E

Cystic Fibrosis

Robert L. Rosen, M.D.

I. **Definition**

Cystic fibrosis (CF) is the most commonly occurring lethal inherited disease of white Americans. It is a syndrome consisting of chronic suppurative lung disease and/or exocrine pancreatic insufficiency in association with an elevated sweat chloride concentration.

II. **Epidemiology**

In the United States, there are about 30,000 individuals with CF and approximately 12 million who carry the CF gene.

A. Inherited in an autosomal recessive pattern, its incidence approximates 1:2,000 in white populations, 1:17,000 in black Americans, and 1:90,000 in Polynesians.

B. The most common genetic defect, found in 68% of patients, is a deletion of three base pairs at the F508 locus on chromosome 7, which codes for a single amino acid (phenylalanine) and results in an abnormal protein termed *cystic fibrosis transmembrane regulator (CFTR)*.

C. No clinical or biochemical abnormalities are noted in heterozygotes for the CF gene.

III. **Pathophysiology**

The major clinical manifestations of CF are suppurative lung disease and exocrine pancreatic insufficiency. The consequences of CF are related to a defect in the regulation of the chloride ion channel in epithelial cells.

A. Abnormal CFTR blocks epithelial chloride channels, resulting in impaired chloride ion transport across epithelial cells.

1. Chloride ions trapped within CF cells lead to excess sodium ion reabsorption, an abnormal mucosal transmembrane potential difference, and increased water drawn into epithelial cells, resulting in thick, sticky, dehydrated mucus in airways and abnormal pancreatic secretions.

2. The apical membrane of airway epithelial cells, as well as nasal epithelium, sweat glands, and pancreatic tissue, are the sites most often affected.

B. The precise mechanisms leading to suppurative lung disease remain unclear.

1. Bacterial adherence and colonization, especially by *Pseudomonas aeruginosa*, may result from impaired mucociliary clearance; abnormalities of cellular and humoral immunity such as an increase in nonopsonic IgG subclasses, particularly

of IgG2, which impairs opsonin-mediated bacterial clearance; and enhanced bacterial binding to respiratory epithelium related to poor nutritional status.

2. Bacterial colonization results in the copious production of alginate by the mucoid phenotype of *P. aeruginosa.*
   a. The alginate forms a polysaccharide matrix around the microorganisms, inhibiting macrophage and neutrophil ingestion.
   b. Alginate also reduces the efficacy of mucociliary and cough mechanisms, and its volume may obstruct small airways.
3. A type III immune complex response, induced by antigen related to either *P. aeruginosa* or *Aspergillus* which colonizes the airways, may activate a proteolytic process which results in the degradation of connective tissue.

C. Structural alteration results from the progressive damage to airway wall structures.
   1. Chronic bronchitis, bronchiolitis, and mucopurulent airway plugging are obstructive changes found in all age groups.
   2. Bronchiectasis, the predominant pathologic finding, increases with disease progression.
   3. Bronchiolar stenosis, scarring, and pneumonia are found in advanced disease stages.

D. Altered function results from altered structure.
   1. Obstructive lesions beginning in small peripheral airways lead to increased airflow resistance, hyperinflation, and impaired ventilation-perfusion relationships.
   2. Airway hyperreactivity frequently contributes to the obstructive abnormality.
   3. Bronchiectatic changes lead to airway wall instability.
      a. Distention occurs during deep inspiration due to abnormally compliant structures and leads to increased dead space volume.
      b. Increased compressibility by positive transthoracic pressure adds a dynamic component to airway obstruction.

E. The respiratory flora in CF are varied.
   1. *Pseudomonas aeruginosa* is the most commonly isolated organism.

2. *Staphylococcus aureus* and *Hemophilus influenzae* may be the initial infecting organisms.
3. Other species of the gram-negative, nonfermenting group, as well as anaerobes, have been isolated.
4. Recently, an increasing frequency of *P. cepacia* colonization has been associated with shortened survival in some patients.

IV. **Diagnosis**
CF is generally diagnosed during childhood because of recurrent pulmonary and gastrointestinal problems.

A. The history is dominated by recurrent respiratory infections and gastrointestinal complaints.
   1. Pulmonary exacerbations characterized by cough productive of purulent, blood-streaked sputum, fever, weight loss, and anorexia.
   2. Asthma, nasal polyps, and chronic sinusitis are common.
   3. Gastrointestinal symptoms in children include failure to thrive, frequent bulky, greasy stools, fatty food intolerance, excessive flatus, and crampy abdominal pain.
   4. Older patients have fewer gastrointestinal symptoms, but recurrent episodes of pancreatitis may occur.
   5. Reproductive problems are common.
      a. Azoospermia, present in 95% of men, results from blockage of the vas deferens with viscid material.
      b. Women with CF have reduced fertility related to abnormal cervical mucus, which acts as a barrier to sperm penetration.
      c. Menstrual irregularities and secondary amenorrhea related to pulmonary infections are common.

B. Physical findings are not diagnostic of CF but are a reflection of the underlying pathophysiologic abnormalities.
   1. Nutritional status is generally poor, related to malabsorption and the chronic suppurative process in the lungs.
   2. Nasal polyps are common, occurring in 41% of adult CF patients compared with 10% of children.
   3. Sinusitis occurs in more than 90% of CF patients.
   4. Pulmonary hyperinflation, rhonchi, and wheezes are commonly present.

5. Evidence of cor pulmonale may develop in long-standing disease.
6. Hypertrophic pulmonary osteoarthropathy increases in prevalence with advancing age.

C. Diagnostic tests
1. Elevated sweat chloride concentration, combined with either chronic pulmonary disease or pancreatic insufficiency, is the key diagnostic criterion for CF.
   a. Ninety-eight percent of patients with CF have sweat chloride concentrations > 60 mEq/liter.
   b. In children, sweat chloride testing separates patients with and without CF, with almost no overlap.
   c. Healthy adults have sweat chloride values ≤ 70 mEq/liter, so that higher levels are necessary for a diagnosis.
   d. Diagnosis in adults is more difficult because of the belief that CF is a pediatric disease.
2. In the future, DNA analysis or the use of nasal potential differences may replace the sweat chloride test.
3. Chest x-ray may show interstitial and reticular markings related to bronchiectasis. Air trapping, hilar adenopathy, and solitary nodules due to inspissated mucus are also seen.
4. Although exocrine pancreatic insufficiency can be inferred by elevated fat excretion in a 72-hr stool collection, definitive diagnosis requires intubation of the duodenum, with direct measurement of the basal and secretin-stimulated output of bicarbonate, trypsin, chymotrypsin, amylase, and lipase.

V. Differential Diagnosis
A. CF should be part of the differential diagnosis of obstructive lung disease in children and young adults.
1. Bronchiectasis in relation to immunoglobulin deficiency syndromes or immotile cilia syndrome can resemble CF.
2. Chronic infections, such as tuberculosis or fungal infection, allergic bronchopulmonary aspergillosis, and sarcoidosis can mimic the findings in CF.
B. Gastrointestinal diseases, which mimic CF, include pancreatitis and inflammatory bowel disease.

VI. Treatment
A. Antimicrobial chemotherapy is the mainstay of therapy.
1. Antibiotic intervention affects bacterial colonizers such as *Pseudomonas*, resulting in a decreased antigenic supply for the immunologic cascade, leading to lung damage.
2. Except in acute exacerbations, there is a greater effect on the long-term course of the disease.
3. Antimicrobial chemoprophylaxis risks the development of resistent microorganisms.
B. Chest physiotherapy is a standard mechanical treatment.
1. It reduces the consequences of obstructing secretions, such as atelectasis and hyperinflation.
2. It clears purulent secretions, reducing the antigenic supply and proteolytic activity.
C. Nutritional supplementation may benefit younger patients in the phase of airway growth.
D. Bronchodilators have a beneficial effect in patients in whom bronchospasm contributes to airway obstruction.
1. Bronchodilators must be tailored to the patient.
2. Paradoxical effects have been noted in cases where increased bronchial smooth muscle tone compensates mechanically for structural damage.
E. Mucolytic agents reduce sputum viscosity in vitro, but there is no evidence of a beneficial long-term effect. In addition, these agents may increase bronchial reactivity and reduce ciliary activity.
F. Experimental therapies include antipseudomonal vaccines, selective sodium transport blockers, inhibitors of alginate biosynthesis, anti-inflammatory agents, and synthetic inhibitors of neutrophil-derived elastase.
G. Heart-lung and double lung transplantation have resulted in improved lung function and no recurrence of the disease in the transplanted lung.

VII. Patient Monitoring
The complications of the suppurative lung process and the pancreatic dysfunction must be part of patient monitoring in patients with CF.

A. Pneumothorax may result when subpleural blebs rupture through a pleura weakened by degenerative changes.
   1. Rarely, it occurs in children younger than 10 years; it also occurs in about 20% of older CF patients.
   2. The frequency of recurrence is > 50%, with an associated mortality rate of up to 19%.
   3. Pleurodesis should be undertaken even after the first episode.
B. Hemoptysis, while rare in children under 10 years of age, occurs in > 50% of older patients.
   1. Massive hemoptysis occurs in 8% of adult CF patients and is associated with frequent recurrence.
   2. Therapy for massive hemoptysis includes resection or bronchial artery embolization.
C. Intestinal obstruction increases with age and is present in 17% of adult patients.
   1. Meconium ileus equivalent occurs in 10% of patients and usually in these older than 10 years.
   2. Intussusception or high fecal impaction at the ileocecal junction results from abnormal fecal consistency.
      a. Incomplete digestion, abnormal intestinal gland secretions, or abnormal intestinal fluid and electrolyte transport makes the fecal stream semisolid instead of liquid.
      b. Inspissated feces adhering to the bowel wall may act as lead points for intussusception.
D. Cholelithiasis, due to abnormal enterohepatic circulation of bile acids, occurs in 40–50% of patients with CF and is more common in adults than in children.

E. Abnormal liver function is present in one-third of these patients.
   1. Biliary cirrhosis, in association with pancreatic insufficiency, has been found in 25% of CF patients at autopsy.
   2. Fatty infiltration occurs in 30% of patients but progresses to frank cirrhosis in < 5%.
   3. Hepatic failure with gastrointestinal hemorrhage is uncommon but accounts for nearly all nonpulmonary deaths in CF patients who survive beyond infancy.
F. Exocrine pancreatic insufficiency, with greatly reduced or absent release of digestive enzymes, results in malabsorption syndromes and occurs in 80–90% of children and 95% of adults.
G. Glucose intolerance occurs in 40–60% of patients, but only 8% require insulin.

VIII. Prognosis
The prognosis of CF has improved markedly with the advent of improved antibiotic therapy.
A. Median age at death has risen from less than 2 years in the 1940s to 28 years today.
B. One-third of CF patient are older adolescents and adults.
C. Mortality is related to pulmonary complications in 90% of cases.

Bibliography

Riordan JR, Rommens JM, Kerem B-S, et al. Identification of the cystic fibrosis gene: Cloning and characterization of complementary DNA. *Science* 245:1066–1072, 1989.

diSant'Agnese PA, Davis PB. Cystic fibrosis in adults. *Am J Med* 66:121–132, 1979.

Wood RE, Boat TF, Doershuk CF: Cystic fibrosis. *Am Rev Respir Dis* 113:833–870, 1976.

Zach MS: Lung disease in cystic fibrosis—an updated concept. *Ped Pulmonol* 8:188–202, 1990.

CHAPTER 31

Interstitial Lung Disease

Michael W. Heniff, M.D.
David B. Rubin, M.D.

Idiopathic Pulmonary Fibrosis (IPF)

I. Definition

IPF is a progressive interstitial fibrotic lung disease of unknown etiology.

II. Pathophysiology

The proposed chronologic sequence of events is as follows:

A. An unknown factor(s) incites the accumulation of mononuclear and polymorphonuclear leukocytes within the alveoli.

B. Alveolitis results in epithelial and endothelial cell damage, which may activate fibroblasts to migrate, proliferate, and produce abundant extracellular matrix.

C. Pulmonary parenchyma is eventually replaced with fibrous tissue in association with cystic changes and distortion of small airways.

D. Destruction of lung parenchyma and hypoxia results in pulmonary hypertension and cor pulmonale.

III. Diagnosis

A. Diagnosis of exclusion: no evidence of exposure to known pneumotoxins (e.g., radiation or Cytoxan), collagen vascular disease, infection, occupational exposure (e.g., asbestos), hypersensitivity pneumonitis, sarcoidosis, aspiration, or cardiac-related lung disease.

B. Clinical presentation

1. Symptoms: cough and progressive exertional dyspnea

2. Signs: inspiratory crackles and clubbing (in 60% of cases of advanced disease)

3. Chest x-ray: increased linear and reticular radiopacities (interstitial) and associated changes; 10% of patients have a normal chest x-ray.

4. Pulmonary function: restrictive pattern, lowered diffusing capacity of the lungs for carbon monoxide ($D_{L_{CO}}$) and widened alveolar-arterial oxygen pressure (PA_{O_2}–Pa_{O_2}) difference.

IV. Natural History and Prognosis

A. Cough and exertional dyspnea months to years prior to diagnosis.

B. Rare spontaneous regression; a progressive disease with survival for 2–10 years after diagnosis; 30–50% of patients die within 5 years of diagnosis.

C. Rapidity of progression is variable: weeks to months with Hamman-Rich syndrome; up to 20 years in some patients with IPF.

D. A familial form of IPF has been identified.

V. **Differential Diagnosis** (See Section III, A)

VI. **Diagnostic Evaluation**

Guidelines for patient evaluation are depicted in the decision tree (Figure 31-1). Open lung biopsy that includes histological analysis of collagen deposition is the definitive test.

VII. **Indices of IPF Activity and Severity**

A. No one test consistently correlates with disease activity.

B. Routine monitoring every 2 to 3 months may be useful in management.
  1. Pulmonary function tests (PFTs): especially the ventilatory capacitory (VC), total lung capacity (TLC), $D_{L_{CO}}$ and PA_{O_2}–Pa_{O_2} difference.
  2. Exercise PFT: determine oxygen desaturation.
  3. Chest x-ray: changes do not always parallel the fibrotic process; especially helpful in assessing for pneumonia or pulmonary edema.

C. Less routine: computed tomography (CT) and magnetic resonance imaging (MRI) estimate the extent of disease better than chest x-ray but are not necessarily more helpful in monitoring fibrotic activity.

D. Controversial or experimental: bronchoalveolar lavage and gallium scan. Would not use in routine clinical settings.

VIII. **Therapy**

Therapeutic guidelines are presented in Figure 31-2. The mainstay of treatment until recently involved the use of steroids, oxygen, antibiotics, fluid management, and routine measures for respiratory hygiene and rehabilitation. Lung transplantation is becoming the ultimate therapeutic option.

Radiation-induced Lung Injury

I. **Definition**

Inflammation and edema progressing to varying degrees of fibrosis following lung irradiation; referred to as *radiation pneumonitis, pleurapneumonitis,* or *pneumopathy.*

II. **Etiology**

A. The true incidence of lung disease caused by radiation therapy is unknown. The best estimate of clinically significant disease is 10%, but all patients develop some degree of pneumonitis/fibrosis.

B. Pneumonitis can occur at doses as low as 2 Gy but are more likely to occur with higher radiation exposure. Standard radiation therapy for lung cancer is 2 Gy/day, for a total of 40 to 60 Gy administered over 4 to 6 weeks. Pneumonitis/fibrosis not uncommonly occurs after mediastinal radiation therapy for lymphoma.

C. The longer the interval between radiation doses, the lower the incidence of clinically significant pneumonitis/fibrosis; in general, normal tissue tolerance to radiation is improved with lower radiation dose rates.

D. The greater the irradiated lung volume, the more likely that radiation lung disease will be manifested clinically.

E. Oxygen and chemotherapy can potentiate radiation pneumotoxicity; bleomycin is the classic example, but in the susceptible individual, many different drugs and possibly oxygen therapy and malnutrition can enhance the likelihood of radiation lung disease.

III. **Pathophysiology**

A. Acute changes (hours to weeks): increased leukocyte adhesion to endothelium, increased perivascular edema, discharge of surfactant from type II cells; sparse destruction and swelling of endothelial and epithelial cells; suspected enhanced intravascular procoagulant state.

B. Intermediate (weeks to months): inflammatory cell infiltration, destruction and increased proliferation of endothelial and type II epithelial cells. These events may promote fibroblast proliferation and increased synthesis of extracellular matrix proteins.

C. Late (months to years): loss of vessels and alveolar epithelial structure; interstitial fibrosis.

D. Diminished host defenses increase the possibility of a complicating infection.

IV. **Diagnosis**

A. History of radiation exposure to the lungs.

B. Chest x-ray: pneumonitis is evident 2 weeks to 6 months after treatment: typical radiodensity (interstitial and/or alveolar) is demarcated by the field of radiation exposure; fibrosis is evident 6 months to years after treatment, and loss of lung volume is demonstrated.

V. **Differential Diagnosis**

Usually the diagnosis is easy, but it can be confounded by the presence of underlying lung disease: malignancy, infection, drug pneumotoxicity, or graft-versus-host disease.

VI. **Clinical Presentation and Natural History**

A. Most cases are subclinical.

B. Pneumonitis
  1. Initial presentation occurs 1 to 3 months

after irradiation; often resolves spontaneously within days of symptom onset
but can evolve to fibrosis.

2. Symptoms can range from a mild, nonproductive cough to severe dyspnea and
fever.

3. Signs include auscultation that reflects
consolidation, pleural effusion or pleural
rub; tachypnea, cyanosis, and adult respiratory distress syndrome in the most severe cases.

4. Laboratory tests: hypoxemia, restrictive
pattern, lowered $D_{L_{CO}}$; leukocytosis and
elevated erythrocyte sedimentation rate
are less helpful.

5. Chest X-ray: radiation density delineation per exposure field; CT scan determines infiltrates at earlier times and is
more accurate in estimating the extent of
lung involvement.

C. Fibrosis

1. Occurs 2 months to 2 years after therapy,
usually preceded by evidence of pneumonitis.

2. Chest x-ray: contraction of lung volume
in relation to exposure field.

3. PFT: progression of restrictive pattern,
hypoxemia, and loss of $D_{L_{CO}}$.

4. Perfusion lung scan: reduced pulmonary
blood flow to affected areas.

5. Progression of symptoms and signs noted
for pneumonitis.

D. Prognosis

1. Depends on amount of irradiated lung.

2. Pneumonitis: varies from spontaneous
recovery to rapid respiratory failure.

3. Fibrosis: can progress for up to 2 years
after exposure.

VII. Treatment

A. Supportive care, possibly including oxygen
and antibiotics when specified.

B. Corticosteroid, 60–100 mg/day for 3–4
weeks; effective for pneumonitis but not for
fibrosis.

C. Experimental: penicillamine, antioxidants.

D. Underlying systemic disease limits the option of lung transplant, but this may be
considered for a cancer patient with a long
life expectancy.

Interstitial Pneumonia

I. Definition

A group of lung diseases characterized by a
diffuse infiltrate on chest x-ray and histologically by destruction of the gas exchange components in the lung and associated with inflammatory cells.

II. Etiology

Interstitial lung disease can be secondary to
more than 150 specific causes, but over 80% of
these fall into three general groups:

1. Pneumonoconiosis
2. Drug-induced
3. Hypersensitivity pneumonitis

III. Pathophysiology

The pathophysiology of injury to the lung by a
variety of causes is made easier to detect by the
fact that the lung is very limited in the way it
responds to injury. The usual sequence of
events is as follows:

A. Alveolitis associated with epithelial and endothelial cell damage that may progress to
the next stage.

B. Alveolar wall destruction, with increased
collagen deposition and scar formation leading to fibrosis.

IV. Diagnosis

The diagnosis of a specific disease in a patient
who presents with interstitial pneumonia depends upon obtaining a careful history, observing clinical signs, and performing diagnostic
tests.

A. History, with particular attention to:

1. Duration and type of symptoms: most of
the disorders have a subacute to chronic
presentation. A more acute presentation
may be more closely associated with an
infectious cause (pneumocystis carinii
pneumonia, viral, mycoplasma) discussed elsewhere.

2. Occupational history, with particular attention to asbestos, silica, mold, soil, dust,
birds, animals, and plants.

3. Complete drug history—both prescribed
and illicit drugs taken in the past.

4. Family history of collagen vascular disease, pulmonary fibrosis, or vasculitis.

5. Review of systems with attention to
cough, hemoptysis, shortness of breath,
dyspnea on exertion, and signs of systemic disease such as weight loss, rash,
fever, myalgia, arthritis, or hematuria.

B. Clinical Signs

1. Cyanosis or clubbing.

2. Rash, alopecia, erythema nodosum, lymphadenopathy, rheumatoid nodules,
muscle or joint tenderness.

3. Cardiac exam for an increased P_2 or
right-sided S_3 heart sound.

4. Lungs: frequently these disorders will produce diffuse crackles on lung exam.
5. Edema.

C. Diagnostic tests. The use of these tests will be guided by the clinical picture and may vary from a comparable history and characteristic chest x-ray, as in the pneumoconioses, to open lung biopsy, as may be required in pulmonary fibrosis.

Helpful diagnostic tests include:

1. Chest x-ray, arterial blood gases, and pulmonary function tests to document the disease and possibly to follow its progression.
2. Routine blood work such as a complete blood count can be helpful to identify anemia or polycythemia secondary to hypoxia. Urinalysis and biochemistry screen are useful in identifying coexistent renal disease, as seen in collagen vascular disease, Wegener's granulomatosis, or Goodpasture's syndrome.
3. Bronchoscopy with bronchoalveolar lavage (BAL) and biopsy—not required in every case, but helpful in ruling out infection and may give adequate tissue for diagnosis without open lung biopsy. At some centers, the number and type of inflammatory cells in the BAL are used to aid in diagnosis and management, but this is not routine.
4. Exercise testing may be helpful.
5. Precipitin testing for antibodies when hypersensitivity pneumonitis is suspected.
6. Autoimmune profile.
7. Antineutrophilic cytoplasmic antibodies can be useful in Wegener's granulomatosis and vasculitis.
8. CT or MRI.
9. Biopsy of the lung is sometimes required.

V. Differential Diagnosis
A. Infection (viral, mycoplasma, PCP)
B. Pneumoconiosis
C. Pulmonary fibrosis
D. Sarcoidosis
E. Bronchiolitis obliterans
F. Pulmonary alveolar proteinosis
G. Hypersensitivity pneumonitis
H. Histiocytosis X
I. Collagen vascular disease
   1. Rheumatoid arthritis
   2. Systemic lupus erythematosus
   3. Polymyocytis-dermatomyocytis
   4. Mixed connective tissue disease
   5. Scleroderma
J. Ankylosing spondylitis
K. Vasculitides
   1. Wegener's granulomatosis
   2. Churig-Straus syndrome
L. Lymphomatoid granulomatosis
M. Chronic eosinophilic pneumonia
N. Goodpasture's syndrome
O. Drug-induced e.g., chemotherapy antibiotics, narcotics
P. Neoplastic (lymphoma, breast, bronchoalveolar cell carcinoma)
Q. Amyloidosis
R. Pulmonary hemosiderosis
S. Graft-versus-host disease
T. Lymphangioleiomyomatosis

VI. Treatment, Prognosis, and Patient Monitoring
These depend on the specific etiology identified as the cause.

Hypersensitivity Pneumonitis
I. Definition
Immunologic lung disease characterized by lymphocytic and granulomatous interstitial and alveolar filling caused by intense or prolonged exposure to inhaled organic dust in a susceptible host.

II. Etiology
A. Inhalation of almost any organic dust particles of the proper size can cause hypersensitivity pneumonitis, but the following agents are well described:
   1. Mold, hay, or grass
   2. Sugar cane
   3. Compost
   4. Cork
   5. Grain
   6. Wood
   7. Contaminated water from a sauna, air conditioner, or humidifier
   8. Fertilizer
   9. Detergent
   10. Cheese
   11. Animal droppings, feathers, or hair
   12. Snuff
   13. Toluene, isocyanates, epoxy resins
B. Common to all of these particles are the following:
   1. Particle size enabling them to come to rest in the lung
   2. Commonly, these are organic proteins.
   3. Thermophilic actinomycetes are often found along with the organic material.

III. Pathophysiology
The inhalation of an antigen by a susceptible host initiates the following sequence of events:

A. Initially, an increase in polymorphonuclear leukocytes is seen in the alveoli and small airways.

B. Later, mononuclear cells follow, with granuloma formation.

C. If the exposure to the initiating agents continues, scarring and fibrosis can occur.

IV. **Diagnosis**

A. History—obtaining a complete history is important, with attention to the following:

1. Occupational history with exposures.

2. Hobbies (gardening, woodworking, raising birds).

3. Other symptoms associated with collagen vascular disease or other causes of interstitial lung disease.

4. Drug history.

B. Typical symptoms depend on whether the disease is acute, subacute, or chronic.

1. Acute—typically 6–8 hr postexposure. The patient complains of dyspnea, fever, and cough, with or without interstitial infiltrates on chest x-ray.

2. Subacute—appears insidiously over weeks with cough, dyspnea, and cyanosis. This form may also occur following the acute form.

3. Chronic—more gradual onset of cough and increasing dyspnea over months to years more commonly seen with prolonged low-dose exposure to the antigen.

C. Diagnostic tests

1. Routine tests can be helpful to exclude other causes and to follow the disease.

a. Complete blood count, SMA-6, autoimmune profile, arterial blood gases.

b. Chest x-ray can be normal, but usually in the acute phase, patchy interstitial or reticulonodular infiltrates are seen. Later, changes of chronic fibrosis may be seen.

c. PFTs may be useful in the more chronic forms. Typically, they demonstrate a restrictive pattern and a decreased $D_{L_{CO}}$.

d. Serum precipitant test against suspected antigens should always be done, but it must be interpreted with caution. An elevated titer may simply indicate exposure and may be unrelated to the lung disease; conversely, the lack of an elevated titer may be due to the fact that the offending antigen is not represented in the test battery.

e. Bronchoscopy with transbronchial biopsy and BAL may be required to exclude other causes. It is used at some centers to aid diagnosis and guide treatment, but it is not routinely used. BAL that indicates an inflammatory reaction may be amenable to steroid therapy.

f. Open lung biopsy is occasionally needed.

V. **Differential Diagnosis**

Please see the Differential Diagnosis of interstitial pneumonias for a complete list.

VI. **Treatment**

The key to all forms of treatment is avoidance of the offending agent.

A. Acute form—usually the patient will recover without treatment if the offending antigen is not encountered again. However, fulminant cases or cases which progress to the subacute form should be treated as below.

B. Subacute—prednisone, 1 mg/kg/day or its equivalent for 7–14 days, followed by a 2- to 6-week taper guided by the patient's clinical status.

C. Chronic—prednisone, 1 mg/kg/day for 2–4 weeks, followed by a taper to the lowest dose released. If there is no observed improvement, the steroids can be tapered to zero. In the future, cyclosporine or possibly desensitization may be used, as some animal studies have shown promise.

VII. **Monitoring**

Emphasizing avoidance of further exposure is key in follow-up. The use of chest x-ray, arterial blood gas analysis, and PFTs may be helpful in guiding steroid therapy. Repeated BAL and gallum scans are not usually indicated except for experimental protocols.

VIII. **Prognosis**

A. Acute—usually self-limited but can progress to the subacute or, rarely, to the fulminant form.

B. Subacute—if treated early, prior to the development of fibrosis, progression of disease may be minimized.

C. Chronic—although steroids are given to limit any ongoing inflammation, once fibrosis occurs it is generally irreversible.

Collagen Vascular Disease (CVD)

Lung involvement in CVD can manifest in many forms. An outline of lung disease in CVD follows.

Scleroderma

I. Definition

A generalized connective tissue disease characterized by inflammatory, fibrotic, and degenerative changes in the skin and internal organs.

II. Etiology and Pathophysiology

Unknown, but there are three possible explanations:

A. Primary abnormality of the vasculature

B. Immunologic abnormalities

C. Abnormal inflammatory process

D. May also be related to chronic aspiration from achalasia.

III. Diagnosis

The diagnosis of lung disease due to scleroderma is usually made on clinical grounds in a patient with the typical cutaneous manifestations and an infiltrate on chest x-ray.

A. History

1. Pulmonary complaints are the presenting symptom in 1% of patients.

2. Sixty percent of patients with pulmonary involvement present with dyspnea.

3. Seventeen percent present with pleuritic chest pain.

4. Ten percent present with cough, usually nonproductive.

B. Physical exam—in addition to classic cutaneous manifestations, the lung exam reveals rales in 40% of patients and a pleural rub in 13%. Pulmonary hypertension is rare in pure scleroderma but is more common in the CREST syndrome. With pulmonary hypertension, the following may be heard on a cardiac exam:

1. Fixed split S_2, $_s2\geqslant$, at the apex.

2. Pulmonic or tricuspid regurgitation.

3. A right ventricular heave may be palpable.

C. Tests

1. Rheumatoid factor is found in 25–35% of patients, antinuclear antibody is positive in 40–80%, and an elevated erythrocyte sedimentation rate is common.

2. The chest x-ray typically shows interstitial lung disease or fibrosis.

3. PFTs usually show a restrictive pattern, with or without some obstruction and a low $D_{L_{CO}}$.

4. Lung biopsy is usually not needed for the diagnosis but may be required to rule out other disease or to exclude infection in a rapidly deteriorating patient.

IV. Differential Diagnosis

Usually the diagnosis is relatively easy in the patient with typical clinical and chest x-ray findings. However, in the patient who presents with pulmonary disease first, the differential diagnosis is the same as for IPF.

V. Treatment

No consistently effective treatment presently exists, but the following have been used:

A. Steroids.

B. Vasodilators for pulmonary hypertension.

C. D-Penicillamine—presently the most promising treatment, but more study is needed.

VI. Prognosis

The patient who develops lung disease generally has a worse prognosis. However, this is not because of worsening PFTs but because of frequent pneumonias. Patients who develop pulmonary hypertension have the worst prognosis.

Polymyositis-Dermatomyositis (PM-DM)

I. Definition

Inflammatory disease of the skin and muscle characterized by:

A. Weakness of the limb girdles, neck, and pharynx.

B. Bimodal age peaks at ages 12 and 50.

C. Male:female ratio of 2:1.

II. Diagnosis

A. The diagnosis of PM-DM depends upon fulfilling four of the following diagnostic criteria:

1. Symmetrical proximal muscle weakness.

2. Increased serum muscle enzymes.

3. Typical electromyographic pattern.

4. Biopsy.

5. The rash of dermatomyositis.

B. Pulmonary disease occurs in 5% of patients as cough or dyspnea. The diagnosis of pulmonary disease due to PM-DM depends on the diagnosis for PM-DM as above coupled with the following:

1. A diffuse interstitial infiltrate on chest x-ray.

2. A restrictive pattern on PFTs.

3. Impaired oxygenation.

a. Bronchoscopy should be done to rule out infection.

III. Differential Diagnosis

The differential diagnosis of an interstitial pattern on chest x-ray is the same as that of interstitial pneumonia, but special attention should be given to ruling out infection or drug-induced disease.

IV. Treatment

Prednisone, 1 mg/kg/day for 1 month, followed by a taper has been the mainstay of treatment, with varying results. Other potentially helpful drugs include:

A. Azathioprine

B. Cyclosporine

C. Cyclophosphamide

   1. However, these drugs are not routinely recommended.

V. Prognosis

Variable. Important prognostic factors include the following:

A. Pulmonary fibrosis occurs with increased frequency in patients with the anti-Jo-1 antibody.

B. An underlying malignancy is found in up to 10% of patients, commonly of the breast, ovary, or stomach, and will obviously affect the prognosis.

Systemic Lupus Erythematosus (SLE)

I. Definition

A chronic systemic inflammatory disease of multiple organ systems with frequent involvement of the lung. Common lung syndromes in SLE include the following:

A. Pleurisy in 40%

B. Effusions in 24%

C. Pneumonitis in 30%

D. Pneumonia

E. Pulmonary hemorrhage

F. In contrast to the other cardiovascular diseases, fibrosis is rare; 50% of SLE patients will develop lung disease.

II. Diagnosis

The diagnostic criteria for SLE are presented elsewhere. Lung disease in an SLE patient may present with any of the above complaints, along with fever, tachypnea, and hypoxia and chest x-ray findings of interstitial or alveolar infiltrates. Pleural effusion on chest x-ray is also common.

A. Pleural effusions—exudative LE cells are diagnostic. Thoracentesis may be used to rule out infection (i.e., tuberculosis or empyema).

B. Pneumonitis—bronchoscopy is needed to rule out infection or hemorrhage.

C. PFTs in SLE may show a mild restrictive pattern and small airway disease. In cases of pulmonary hemorrhage the $D_{L_{CO}}$ may be increased.

III. Differential Diagnosis of Pulmonary Disease in SLE

A. Pulmonary embolism, especially in patient with the lupus anticoagulant

B. Infection

C. Vasculitis

D. Pulmonary hemorrhage from other causes

E. Drug-induced pulmonary disease

IV. Treatment

The pulmonary complications found in SLE are typically treated, with varying success, as follows:

A. Prednisone, 1 mg/kg/day.

B. If the patient fails to respond to the above regimen, azothioprine or cyclophosphamide can be added.

V. Prognosis

Extremely variable, ranging from resolution to rapid progression and death in severe cases of pneumonitis or hemorrhage.

Mixed Connective Tissue Disease (MCTD)

I. Definition

A syndrome with overlapping features of scleroderma, SLE, rheumatoid arthritis, and PM-DM.

II. Diagnosis

Pulmonary dysfunction occurs in 80% of patients with MCTD; however, most cases are asymptomatic.

A. Patients who have a clinical picture of MCTD and serologic evidence of the disease (positive antinuclear antibody, ribonucleoprotein, coupled with radiographic or physiologic (PFTs) evidence of interstitial lung disease do not need a biopsy.

B. Bronchoscopy may be needed to rule out infection in some patients.

C. Chest x-ray typically shows fine reticular infiltrates in the middle and low lung fields in 33% of patients.

III. Differential Diagnosis

Differentiating MCTD from the other forms of connective tissue disease is important, as is exclusion of infection.

Rheumatoid Arthritis

I. Definition

A systemic disorder of unknown etiology characterized by the following:

A. Subacute to chronic inflammation of peripheral joints in a symmetric distribution.

B. Multiple possible lung manifestations.

   1. Pleural effusion with characteristic low glucose level

   2. Pulmonary nodules

   3. Pneumoconiosis

4. Pulmonary vasculitis
5. Interstitial fibrosis
6. Bronchiolitis obliterans
C. Lung disease can precede joint symptoms, although it may also be related to drug/therapy (i.e., methotrexate) especially in men.

II. Diagnosis
A. In a patient with known rheumatoid arthritis and diffuse pulmonary infiltrates, a clinical diagnosis of rheumatoid lung can be made without biopsy if the patient presents with typical slowly progressive disease. Progression of disease over days to weeks requires bronchoscopy to rule out other causes.
B. The pleural effusion is exudative, with a low glucose level, and typically resolves spontaneously over time, although not always.

III. Treatment
A. Rheumatoid lung disease is generally poorly responsive to any treatment, and asymptomatic patients should not be treated.
B. If the patient becomes dyspneic with routine activity, the following treatment is tried:
   1. Prednisone, 1 mg/kg/day for 1 month, followed by a taper.
   2. After 1 month, PFTs are used to assess the response to therapy. A positive response is considered to be one of the following, although less than 5% of all patients respond well.
      a. A 10% increase in forced vital capacity.
      b. A 20% increase in $D_{L_{CO}}$.
      c. A 5-mm Hg decrease in the A-a difference.
   3. Cytotoxic agents have not shown to be helpful in rheumatoid lung.

IV. Monitoring
Asymptomatic patients should not be monitored for disease, as they would not be treated, and no evidence shows that detecting and treating lung disease earlier changes the outcome.

V. Prognosis
Typically rheumatoid lung progresses over years, but very few patients die of respiratory failure.
A. Pleural effusions tend to wax and wane.
B. Nodules may resolve, persist, or cavitate.
C. Caplan's syndrome (in coal miners) and bronchiolitis obliterans are also variable in course.

Sjogren's syndrome
I. Definition
A. Can be associated with lung disease
   1. Interstitial infiltrates
   2. Obstruction
   3. Bronchiectasis
   4. Pleural effusion
   5. Fibrosis
B. What distinguishes Sjogren's syndrome from the other diseases is that a lymphocytic interstitial pneumonitis thought to be a low-grade lymphoma can occur.

II. Diagnosis
A. Dry eyes and mouth
B. Parotid and lacrimal swelling or pain
C. Aspirin-sensitive hepatitis
D. Biopsy and siccant syndrome establish diagnosis

III. Monitoring—as in other connective tissue diseases

IV. Treatment—as in other connective tissue diseases. Attention must be paid to keeping cornea and mouth moist

V. Prognosis—guarded, depending on pulmonary and gastrointestinal involvement

Bibliography

Carrington CB, Gaensler EA. Clinical-Pathologic Approach to Diffuse Infiltrative Lung Disease. In W.M. Thurlbeck (ed.) *The Lung: Structure, Function, and Disease.* Baltimore: Williams & Wilkins, 1978.

Fraser RG, Pare JA. P. *Diagnosis of Diseases of the Chest.* Philadelphia: Saunders, Vol. 1, pp. 423–435; Vol. 3, pp. 1690–1707, 1977.

Fulmer JD, Crystal RG. Interstitial Lung Disease. In D.E. Simmons (ed.) *Current Pulmonology.* Boston: Houghton Mifflin, 1979. Vol. 1.

Gross NJ. Pulmonary effects of radiation therapy. *Ann Intern Med* 86:81–89, 1977.

Interstitial Lung Disease. Ed 2. Schwarz MI, King TE Jr. (Eds.) Mosby Year Book, St. Louis, MO. 1993.

Liebow AA. Definition and classification of interstitial pneumonia in human pathology. *Prog Resp Res* 8:1–33, 1975.

Lourenco RV, Turino GM, Davidson LAG, et al: The regulation of ventilation in diffuse pulmonary fibrosis. *Am J Med* 38:199–216, 1965.

Wiedemann HP, Matthay RA. Pulmonary Manifestations of Collagen Vascular Diseases. *Clinics in Chest Medicine* 10:677–691, 1989.

CHAPTER 32

Diseases of the Pulmonary Circulation

J. Peter Szidon, M.D.

Thromboembolism

I. Definition

Spontaneous clotting within the lumen of one or more systemic veins (venous thrombosis), with or without dislodgement of the clot and subsequent obstruction of one or more pulmonary arteries (pulmonary embolism).

II. Etiology

A. Spontaneous venous thrombosis is caused by:
1. Stasis.
2. Injury to the intima.
3. Alterations in clotting (antithrombin III, protein S or C deficiencies).

B. The following clinical factors predispose to venous thrombosis and pulmonary embolism:
1. Previous episode of venous thrombosis
2. Prolonged immobility
3. Surgery
4. Congestive heart failure
5. Advanced age
6. Cancer
7. Obesity
8. Use of estrogen-containing contraceptives

III. Pathophysiology

A. Venous thrombosis usually begins in the calf veins. There may be no external manifestations.

B. Progression of the thrombus to thigh veins (deep vein thrombosis) can also be clinically silent, or there may be signs of inflammation (pain and edema).

C. Embolization to the lungs may be clinically inapparent or may elicit a range of manifestations.

D. Dyspnea and tachypnea are related to the stimulation of juxta-alveolar vagal afferents.

E. Pulmonary infiltrates on chest X-rays, pleuritic chest pain, pleural effusions, and hemoptysis can be attributed to atelectasis and/or infarction of the lung downstream from the site of embolization.

F. Hypoxemia is caused by ventilation/perfusion mismatch and by decreased mixed venous oxygen tension.

G. Hypotension, shock, and signs of acute cor pulmonale are caused by massive embolization, with obstruction of more than 75% of the vascular bed.

H. Pulmonary hypertension above 40 torr does not occur in acute pulmonary embolism unless there is preexisting cardiovascular disease.

IV. **Diagnosis**
   A. History
      1. Sudden dyspnea, pleuritic pain, hemoptysis.
   B. Physical findings
      1. Tachycardia, tachypnea, signs of acute cor pulmonale (see below), signs of pleural effusion.
      2. The clinical clues are not in themselves diagnostic. In combination with predisposing factors, they suggest the diagnosis and establish the need to obtain confirmatory evidence.
   C. Diagnostic tests
      1. Impedance plethysmography (IPG) of the lower extremities has high sensitivity/specificity for deep vein thrombosis.
      2. Real-time B-mode ultrasonography of the groin is an alternative test.
      3. A normal ventilation-perfusion scan in most instances rules out pulmonary embolism.
      4. Unmatched segmental defects in the presence of normal chest x-rays in patients suspected of having pulmonary embolism are sufficient to recommend anticoagulation.
      5. Other defects or a low index of suspicion for pulmonary embolism make these findings nondiagnostic.
      6. Pulmonary angiography is indicated in patients who either have negative IPG and nondiagnostic scans or a contraindication to anticoagulants.

V. **Differential Diagnosis**
   A. Pulmonary infarcts should be differentiated from infectious causes of lung infiltrates (pneumonias) and causes of pleuritic chest pain/effusion.
   B. Acute cor pulmonale should be distinguished from pericardial tamponade, pneumothorax with tension, acute obstruction of the superior vena cava, and right-sided myocardial infarction. Electrocardiogram (ECG), echocardiogram, and chest X-rays are used for this purpose.

VI. **Treatment**
   A. Alternatives for prophylaxis
      1. Low dose subcutaneous heparin: 5000 U every 8 or 12 hr.
      2. Warfarin to prolong the prothrombin time (PT) by 1.2 to 1.3 times the control value.
      3. Intermittent mechanical compression of the lower limbs with cuffs.
   B. Recommended treatment
      1. Intravenous heparin: loading dose is a 5000-U bolus, followed by continuous infusion at the rate of 1000 U/hr.
      2. Add warfarin after 7–10 days.
      3. Discontinue heparin after 5 days of overlap with warfarin.
      4. Greenfield filter: recommended when recurrence of embolism is presumed to carry a high mortality risk or when anticoagulants are absolutely contraindicated.
      5. Thrombolytic agents (tissue plasminogen activator, streptokinase) are recommended in massive embolism.

VII. **Patient Monitoring**
   A. Patients should be monitored by ECG for arrhythmias, clinically for circulatory stability (heart rate, blood pressure), and for signs of bleeding as a complication of anticoagulation.
   B. The Activated Partial Thromboplastin Time (APTT) should be used to monitor the efficacy of heparinization and to lessen the risk of bleeding: the desired clinical level of APTT is 1.5 to 2.5 times control level using the continuous infusion method.
   C. The PT should be monitored for warfarin use: the desired clinical level of PT is 1.5 times control.

VIII. **Prognosis**
   The mortality of pulmonary embolization can be reduced from 30% to 8% by appropriate anticoagulation. Deep vein thrombosis can result in chronic venous insufficiency (postphlebitic syndrome), which may be prevented by the use of thrombolytic agents.

Bibliography

Hull RD, Raskob GE, Hirsh J. The diagnosis of clinically suspected pulmonary embolism. *Chest* 89:417S–425S, 1986.
   Moser KM. Venous thromboembolism. *Am Rev Respir Dis* 141:235–249, 1980.

Cor Pulmonale
I. **Definition**
   Right ventricular enlargement secondary to respiratory disease (pulmonary vascular, parenchymal, chest wall, or abnormal ventilatory

drive) producing pulmonary hypertension. Cor pulmonale can be acute or chronic. The definition does not include etiologies of pulmonary hypertension related to left heart or congenital heart disorders.

II. **Etiology**

A number of disease processes can lead to chronic cor pulmonale. Acute cor pulmonale is usually caused by massive pulmonary embolism or acute exacerbation of chronic obstructive pulmonary disease (COPD).

A. Pulmonary vascular disorders
   1. Chronic thromboembolic occlusion
   2. Scleroderma, calcinosis, Raynaud's, sclerodactily, teleaugiectasia, polymyositis, lupus erythematosus
   3. Cirrhosis
   4. Veno-occlusive disease
   5. Fibrosing mediastinitis
   6. Chronic mountain sickness
   7. Familial pulmonary hypertension
   8. Primary pulmonary hypertension
B. Parenchymal disorders
   1. COPD (emphysema, cystic fibrosis, bronchiectasis)
   2. Interstitial lung diseases (usual interstitial pneumonitis, sarcoidosis, pneumoconiosis)
   3. Extensive surgical loss of lung tissue
C. Chest wall disorders
   1. Obesity
   2. Kyphoscoliosis
   3. Neuromuscular disorders (Duchenne's muscular dystrophy, amyotrophic lateral sclerosis)
D. Abnormal ventilatory drive
   1. Central nervous system (CNS) lesions (Arnold-Chiari syndrome, atlantoaxial dislocation, tumors)
   2. Congenital central hypoventilation

III. **Pathophysiology**

A. Pulmonary hypertension leads to increased afterload of the right ventricle, which induces dilation and/or hypertrophy. Subsequently, right-sided heart failure may ensue.
B. Pulmonary hypertension can be caused by factors which reduce the vascular cross-sectional area: emphysematous destruction, surgical excision, embolization, or vasoconstriction.
C. Chronic hypoxia induces hypertrophy of vascular smooth muscle in small pulmonary arterioles.

IV. **Diagnosis**

A. History
   1. Patients should have a history consistent with one of the etiologies listed above.
   2. Dyspnea and fatigue on exertion are common complaints.
   3. Exertional syncope or angina-like pain can occur in severe pulmonary hypertension.
   4. Hemoptysis may be present.
B. Physical findings
   1. The physical findings of right ventricular hypertrophy include left parasternal lift, loud P_2 sound, right-sided third and fourth heart sounds, and murmurs of tricuspid and/or pulmonic regurgitation.
   2. Right ventricular failure is associated with distended jugular veins, hepatomegaly, and edema.
   3. Other physical findings are related to the underlying conditions.
C. Diagnostic tests
   1. ECG and echocardiograms can be used to document right ventricular enlargement. ECG evidence correlates well with the degree of pulmonary hypertension.
   2. Radionuclide evaluation of left ventricular function is helpful to confirm the absence of dysfunction.
   3. Cardiac catheterization is used to establish the severity of pulmonary hypertension and the absence of left heart dysfunction.
   4. Pulmonary function tests are important to characterize parenchymal and chest wall etiologies.
   5. Arterial blood gas analyses are useful to diagnose hypercapnia.
   6. Ventilation-perfusion scans and angiography are often necessary to establish the etiology of pulmonary vascular disorders.

V. **Treatment**

A. Treatment of chronic cor pulmonale is dependent on the underlying cause.
B. Endarterectomy can reverse pulmonary hypertension associated with chronic thromboembolic occlusion.
C. The use of pulmonary vasodilators (hydralazine, nifedipine) is controversial.
D. Lung transplantation is an option in primary pulmonary hypertension.
E. Hypoxic pulmonary hypertension associated with parenchymal diseases (PO_2 less

than 55 torr) can be improved with 18 hr or more of daily oxygen use. This leads to increased survival.

F. Digitalis is not effective.

G. Diuretics should be used judiciously.

H. Nocturnal ventilation using a nasal mask and a portable ventilator is useful in preventing hypoventilation during sleep in neuromuscular disorders.

Bibliography

Fishman AP. Chronic cor pulmonale. *Am Rev Respir Dis* 114:775–787, 1976.

Primary Pulmonary Hypertension

I. Definition

A rare disease of unknown etiology causing obliteration of medium-sized and small pulmonary vessels, pulmonary hypertension, and cor pulmonale. According to its predominant pathologic feature, it has been classified into three subgroups: primary plexogenic arteriopathy, recurrent thromboembolism (microemboli), and veno-occlusive disease. It affects women twice as often as men. The median age at diagnosis is approximately 35 years.

II. Etiology

The cause of primary pulmonary hypertension is unknown. An abnormal vasoconstrictive stimulus, a disorder of endothelial-mediated coagulation, and a disorder of vascular smooth muscle growth have been postulated.

III. Pathophysiology

A. Proliferation of the intima and media of small vessels leads to narrowing and occlusion.

B. Progressive pulmonary hypertension causes cor pulmonale and right ventricular failure.

C. Syncope and sudden death are ascribed to fixed, reduced cardiac output.

D. Plexiform lesions consist of a bundle of small vessels that fill the lumen of a dilated, thin-walled artery. They can rupture and cause hemoptysis.

E. Severe hypoxemia can occur if the atrial septum secundum is not fused to the foramen ovale (20%), resulting in right-to-left shunting.

IV. Diagnosis

A. History

The onset can be insidious, with exertional dyspnea, fatigue, and syncope being the most common symptoms. Raynaud's disease, angina-like chest pain, and arthralgias are less common.

B. Physical findings

The findings on physical exam are those of right ventricular hypertrophy, pulmonary hypertension, and right ventricular failure discussed above for cor pulmonale.

C. Diagnostic tests

The diagnosis requires the exclusion of the conditions listed below under Differential Diagnosis. The following tests are useful:

1. Echocardiogram to diagnose left heart diseases.

2. Pulmonary function tests to exclude parenchymal lung diseases and hypoventilation.

3. Cardiac catheterization to determine the magnitude of pulmonary hypertension and the presence of left heart disease.

4. Cardiopulmonary exercise testing to demonstrate specific patterns of response which suggest the need for further testing in patients presenting with unexplained dyspnea.

5. Angiography is necessary if ventilation-perfusion ($\dot{V}/\dot{Q}$) scans suggest chronic thromboembolic occlusion.

6. Lung biopsy is not necessary.

7. Transbronchial biopsy is contraindicated.

V. Differential Diagnosis

A. Left heart disease (mitral valve disease, left atrial myxoma).

B. Intracardiac shunts (atrial septal defect, ventricular septal defect, patent ductus arteriosus).

C. Chronic thromboembolic occlusion.

D. Pulmonary vascular obstruction (mediastinitis, tumor emboli, filariasis, schistosomiasis).

E. Parenchymal lung disease (obstructive, restrictive).

F. Alveolar hypoventilation (neuromuscular disorders, central).

VI. Treatment

A. Oral anticoagulants can be used to slow the progression of microembolization.

B. Vasodilators have been disappointing; most patients fail to respond.

C. Demonstration of responsiveness to hydralazine, nifedipine, or prostacyclin should be done in the cardiac catheterization laboratory before instituting therapy.

D. Lung or heart-lung transplantation is effective. Early results are encouraging.

VII. Prognosis

In the absence of lung transplantation or with a lack of substantial response to vasodilators, the disease is uniformly fatal within 2–5 years of the diagnosis. Occasional patients survive for more prolonged periods.

Bibliography

Rich S. Primary pulmonary hypertension. *Progr Cardiovasc Dis* 31:205–238, 1988.

Pulmonary Vasculitides

I. Definition

A group of disorders characterized pathologically by acute or chronic inflammation of pulmonary vessels. Pulmonary vasculitis is usually part of multiorgan involvement. The following entities are considered:

1. Wegener's granulomatosis
2. Allergic granulomatosis and angiitis (Churg-Strauss syndrome)
3. Necrotizing sarcoid-like granulomatosis
4. Lymphomatoid granulomatosis
5. Benign lymphocytic angiitis and granulomatosis
6. Takayasu's disease
7. Hypersensitivity vasculitis (Henoch-Schonlein purpura, collagen diseases, mixed cryoglobulinemia)
8. Behcet's syndrome

II. Etiology

A variety of mechanisms have been implicated, including reactions to the deposition of immune complexes, cell-mediated immunity, and direct antibody attack. The exact mechanisms of inflammation are not known.

III. Diagnosis

A. Clinical findings
1. There is no typical presentation. The symptom complex at presentation is variable and can range from the incidental finding of an abnormal x-ray in an asymptomatic patient to a severe systemic illness with fever, weight loss, anemia, and evidence of involvement of one or more organs: kidney, skin, peripheral nerves, CNS, heart, and lung.
2. Patterns of involvement can be those of specific disorders.
3. Churg-Strauss patients have a history of asthma.

B. Diagnostic tests
1. Patients with Wegener's granulomatosis and Churg-Strauss have circulating antineutrophil cytoplasmic antibodies.
2. Patients with Churg-Strauss syndrome can have eosinophilia and elevated IgE levels.
3. Chest x-rays can reveal nodules or patchy infiltrates with cavities.
4. Bronchoscopy may show endobronchial involvement in Wegener's granulomatosis.
5. Histologic confirmation is necessary for diagnosis.
6. Nasal septum or kidney are useful biopsy sites for Wegener's granulomatosis.
7. Transbronchial biopsy has a low yield.
8. Open lung biopsy is required for diagnosis in the majority of pulmonary vasculitis.

IV. Differential Diagnosis

Pulmonary infections, particularly granulomatous ones (tuberculosis, fungi), should be ruled out by appropriate cultures.

V. Treatment

A. Immunosuppressive agents (cyclophosphamide, azathioprine) are used alone or in conjunction with glucocorticosteroids.
B. Renal failure in Wegener's granulomatosis is treated with hemodialysis or transplantation.

VI. Prognosis

The prognosis is variable, and depends on the specific disorder and the severity of the disease.

Bibliography

Leavitt RY, Fauci AS. Pulmonary vasculitis. *Am Rev Respir Dis* 134:149–166, 1986.

Hemorrhagic Lung Syndromes

I. Definition

A syndrome consisting of acute or chronic diffuse hemorrhage into the interstitial spaces of the lung.

II. Etiology

Diffuse pulmonary hemorrhage can occur during the course of the following disorders:

1. Antiglomerular basement membrane disease (Goodpasture's syndrome)
2. Collagen vascular disease (lupus, rheumatoid arthritis, scleroderma)
3. Wegener's granulomatosis
4. Subacute bacterial endocarditis
5. Cryoglobulinemia

6. Inhalation of trimellitic anhydride
7. Idiopathic pulmonary hemosiderosis
8. Severe thrombocytopenia

III. Pathophysiology
A. Diffuse hemorrhage can cause hemoptysis.
B. If hemorrhage is severe or recurrent, iron deficiency and microcytic anemia may ensue.
C. Infiltration of air spaces causes hypoxemia, rapid shallow breathing, and respiratory distress.
D. With repeated episodes of hemorrhage, progressive pulmonary fibrosis with restrictive lung disease and eventually cor pulmonale can develop.

IV. Diagnosis
A. History
Rapid, progressive dyspnea, cough, and hemoptysis.
B. Physical findings
Diffuse end-expiratory inspiratory crackles.
C. Diagnostic tests
1. Chest x-rays show diffuse air space consolidation.
2. The diffusing capacity for carbon monoxide (DL_{CO}) is elevated.
3. Circulating antiglomerular basement membrane antibodies are present in Goodpasture's syndrome and antineutrophil cytoplasmic antibodies in Wegener's granulomatosis.
4. Hematuria and proteinuria with granular or red cells casts occur in both diseases.
5. Bronchoalveolar lavage shows hemosiderin-laden macrophages and persistently blood-stained lavage fluid.
6. Renal biopsy may be necessary to diagnose Goodpasture's syndrome, Wegener's granulomatosis, or lupus.
7. Open lung biopsy is used in idiopathic hemosiderosis.

V. Differential Diagnosis
The triad of hemoptysis, anemia, and diffuse lung infiltrates can be present in infections (cytomegalovirus, herpes, fungal dissemination in immunocompromised hosts), hemorrhagic diathesis (excessive anticoagulation, leukemias), or some vascular malignancies (Kaposi's sarcoma in AIDS).

VI. Treatment
A. Corticosteroids and cyclophosphamide are effective in Goodpasture's syndrome and Wegener's granulomatosis. Plasmapheresis is recommended in the former.
B. Long-term dialysis and transplantation are used to manage renal failure.
C. In the remaining disorders, treatment is symptomatic and supportive.

VII. Patient Monitoring
Recurrent lung hemorrhage is detected by monitoring serial chest X-rays and measuring the diffusing capacity for carbon monoxide.

VIII. Prognosis
The prognosis depends on the underlying condition.

Bibliography

Matthay RA, Bromberg SI, Putnam CE. Pulmonary renal syndromes: A review. *Yale J Biol Med* 53:497–523, 1980.

Congenital Malformations

I. Definition
A group of diverse disorders in which an embryologic abnormality leads to malformation of portions of the lung vasculature. The following disorders will be considered:
1. Pulmonary sequestration
2. Scimitar syndrome
3. Arteriovenous malformation

II. Etiology
Numerous theories have been proposed: vascular traction, vascular insufficiency, and accessory budding.

III. Pathophysiology
A. Intrapulmonary sequestrations (90%) are left-sided, do not communicate with normal airways, and receive an aberrant systemic blood supply from the aorta.
B. Cysts can become infected and rupture into neighboring lung tissue.
C. The scimitar syndrome includes a wide range of congenital anomalies: a hypoplastic right lung, an aberrant systemic supply to the right lung, and a characteristic pattern of anomalous venous drainage of a major portion of the right lung which, on chest x-rays, resembles a Turkish scimitar.
D. Arteriovenous malformations are single or multiple and cause systemic venous blood to shunt past the alveoli. Severe hypoxemia and secondary polycythemia can result.
E. Paradoxical embolization of septic material can cause cerebral abscesses.

IV. Diagnosis
A. History
Patients with sequestration can be asymptomatic or can present with cough, sputum

production, and fever. The severe form of scimitar syndrome is seen in pediatric patients. The mild form is seen in adults and is usually asymptomatic. Patients with arteriovenous malformations have exertional dyspnea and, rarely, hemoptysis.

B. Physical findings
Patients with arteriovenous malformations have cyanosis, clubbing, and, at times, a bruit over the site of the malformation, the loudness of which increases with inspiration. Telangiectasias can be seen around the mouth.

C. Diagnostic tests
1. Patients with sequestration can be diagnosed by demonstrating the aberrant systemic vessel with an aortic angiogram.
2. The scimitar syndrome has a characteristic appearance on chest x-rays.
3. Arteriovenous malformations can be diagnosed by pulmonary angiography.

V. Differential Diagnosis
A. Sequestration can be confused with cavitary infections and bronchiectasis.
B. The scimitar syndrome is easily diagnosed by its appearance on chest x-rays.
C. Arteriovenous malformations should be distinguished from other causes of hypoxemia polycythemia (i.e., intracardiac shunts and chronic lung diseases).

VI. Treatment
A. The scimitar syndrome requires no treatment.
B. Sequestrations can be excised surgically if there is bleeding or recurrent infection.
C. Arteriovenous malformations can be obstructed with detachable balloons or coils inserted via catheters. Surgical excision is an option with single lesions.

VII. Prognosis
A. Prognosis of the mild form of scimitar syndrome is excellent.
B. Sequestrations can cause recurrent pulmonary infections and severe bleeding.
C. Arteriovenous malformations can also cause disability due to their effect on exercise tolerance and their propensity for systemic embolization.

Bibliography

Clements BS, Warner JO, Shinebourne EA. Congenital bronchopulmonary vascular malformations: Clinical application of a simple anatomical approach in 25 cases. *Thorax* 42:409–416, 1987.

Cigarette Smoking

Vidysagar Chodimella, M.D.
Christopher G. Murlas, M.D.

I. Problem

Experimental, epidemiological, and clinical evidence accumulated over the past two decades indicates that cigarette smoking is a major risk factor in several diseases, including chronic obstructive airway disease and lung cancer. Certain conclusions concerning the health consequences of smoking made in the U.S. Surgeon General's Report of 1989 are important to reiterate here.

A. Smoking-related health problems

"1. The Surgeon General's Report of 1964 concluded that cigarette smoking increases overall mortality in men, causes lung and laryngeal cancer in men, and causes chronic bronchitis. The Report also found significant associations between smoking and numerous other diseases.

2. Reports of the Surgeon General since 1964 have concluded that smoking increases mortality and morbidity in both men and women. Disease associations identified as causal since 1964 include coronary heart disease, arteriosclerotic peripheral vascular disease, lung and laryngeal cancer in women, oral cancer, esophageal cancer, chronic obstructive pulmonary disease, intrauterine growth retardation, and low-birthweight babies.

3. Cigarette smoking is now considered to be a probable cause of unsuccessful pregnancies, increased infant mortality, and peptic ulcer disease; to be a contributing factor for cancer of the bladder, pancreas, and kidney; and to be associated with cancer of the stomach.

4. Accumulating research has elucidated the interactive effects of cigarette smoking with certain occupational exposures to increase the risk of cancer, with alcohol ingestion to increase the risk of cancer, and with selected medications to produced adverse effects.

5. A decade ago, the 1979 Report of the Surgeon General found smokeless tobacco to be associated with oral cancer. In 1986, the Surgeon General concluded that smokeless tobacco was a cause of this disease.

6. Research in the present decade has established that involuntary smoking is a cause of disease, including lung cancer, in healthy nonsmokers, and that the children

of parents who smoke have an increased frequency of respiratory infections and symptoms.

7. In 1964, tobacco was considered habituating. A substantial body of evidence accumulated since then, and summarized in the 1988 Surgeon General's Report, has established that cigarettes and other forms of tobacco are addicting. Given the prevalence of smoking, tobacco use is the nation's most widespread form of drug dependency.

8. Studies dating from the 1950s have consistently documented the benefits of smoking cessation for smokers of all age groups.

9. Recent evidence, including that presented in this . . . Report, documents that cigarette smoking is a cause of cerebrovascular disease (stroke) and is associated with cancer of the uterine cervix."

II. Physiochemistry and Toxicology of Tobacco

A. The estimated number of compounds in tobacco smoke exceeds 4,000, including many that are pharmacologically active, toxic, mutagenic, and carcinogenic.

B. Forty-three carcinogens have been identified in tobacco smoke.

C. Carcinogenic tobacco-specific nitrosamines are found in high concentrations in smokeless tobacco.

D. Cigarette smoke contains tarry particles of respirable size suspended in a mixture of organic and inorganic gases. Smoke-induced lung injury is mediated by two classes of free radicals:

1. Free radicals in the gas phase
   a. Short-lived, with a half-life of about 5 min.
   b. Inorganic and organic radicals.
   c. Inactive α_1-protease inhibitor affecting the elastase-antielastase balance in the lung.

2. Tar radicals
   a. Are stable indefinitely.
   b. A major tar radical has been identified as a quinone-hydroquinone complex.
   c. Act by reducing molecular oxygen to superoxide, eventually leading to the formation of H_2O_2 and hydoxyl radicals.
   d. Tar radicals are associated with lower carcinogenicity but larger oxidant stress.
   e. Chelate metals that catalyze the decomposition of H_2O_2 and cleave DNA.

III. Pathogenesis of Lung Injury

Lung injury is modulated by several factors, including age at smoking, smoke dilution, smoking habits, tar, nicotine content, and quantity of activated charcoal in the filters.

A. Lung injury is preceded by retention and activation of smoke constituents to protoxins in the lung.

1. Major activating systems in the lung are P-450 and flavin-dependent monooxygenase and arachidonic acid-dependent monooxygenase systems.

2. Aromatic hydrocarbons and nitrosamines bind to DNA. Their subsequent activation results in DNA damage, which may be responsible for carcinogenicity or cocarcinogenicity associated with smoking.

3. Nicotine, an important alkaloid found in tobacco, is responsible for several organic changes in the lungs and behavioral patterns of smokers. Nicotine's action is mediated by inhibition of histamine catabolism and enhanced neutrophil responsiveness to chemotactic agents.

4. Cadmium compounds found in tobacco smoke are associated with increased chemotaxis, enhanced neutrophil recruitment, and increased epithelial permeability.

B. Pulmonary response to cigarette smoke

1. Effect on lung development
   a. Increased incidence of respiratory infections in the newborn infants of smoking mothers.
   b. Associated with abnormal lung growth in utero.
   c. Significant decrease in both disaturated phosphotidylcholine and phosphotidyl glycerol.

2. Inflammatory response of the lung
   a. Neutrophil-mediated response: cigarette smoking is associated with increased numbers of neutrophils in bronchoalveolar lavage (BAL) fluid, increased release of neutrophil elastase, and increased release of leukotriene B_4, with enhanced recruitment of neutrophils to the site of inflammation.
   b. Complement mediation: activation of C3 and alternative pathways of complement activation.
   c. Macrophage-mediated response characterized by increased numbers of pulmonary macrophages in BAL fluid,

increased oxidative metabolism of alveolar macrophages, and induction of changes in the membrane protein composition of macrophages.

3. Airway response: varies with nicotine content of smoke and is characterized by:
   a. Bronchoconstriction and hypercapnea.
   b. Increased epithelial permeability related to oxidant-induced changes in cell morphology.
   c. Diminished mucociliary clearance related to the ciliotoxic effect of smoke and abnormal epithelial chloride secretion.

4. Repair mechanisms of the lung are affected via:
   a. Inhibition of lysyl oxidase, a major repair enzyme in the lung.
   b. Increased macrophage and neutrophil elastase burden on the lung.
   c. Inactivation of transglutaminase, an enzyme necessary for cross-linking structural protein molecules in the repair process.

IV. Smoking Prevention and Cessation Activities

Observations made in the U.S. Surgeon General's Report of 1989 are again worth quoting:

A. Smoking prevention activities

"1. Diverse program approaches to the prevention of smoking among youth grew out of antismoking education efforts in the 1960s. These approaches include media-based programs and resources; smoking prevention as a part of multicomponent school health education; psychosocial prevention curricula; and a variety of other resources developed and sponsored by professional and voluntary health organizations, Federal and State agencies, and schools and community groups.

2. Psychosocial curricula addressing youths' motivations for smoking and the skills they need to resist influences to smoke have emerged as the program approach with the most positive outcomes. Evolution in program content has been accompanied by a shift since the 1960s in prevention program focus from youths in high school and college to adolescents in grade 6 through 8.

3. Existing prevention programs vary greatly in the extent to which they have been evaluated and used. Psychosocial prevention curricula have been intensively developed over the last decade and have been the most thoroughly evaluated and best documented; however, they are generally not part of a dissemination system. More widely disseminated smoking prevention materials and programs, such as those using mass media and brochures, have not always been as thoroughly evaluated; however, they have achieved wider use in the field.

4. The model of stages of smoking behavior acquisition underlies current smoking prevention programs and suggests new intervention opportunities, ranging from prevention activities aimed at youth children to cessation programs for adolescent smokers.

5. There has been and continues to be a lack of smoking prevention programs that target youth at higher risk for smoking, such as those from lower socioeconomic backgrounds or school dropouts."

B. Smoking education and cessation activities

"1. During the past 25 years, National voluntary health agencies, especially the American Cancer Society, the American Heart Association, and the American Lung Association, have played a significant role in educating the public about the hazards of tobacco use.

2. Individual and group smoking cessation programs evolved from an emphasis on conditioning-based approaches in the 1960s, to the cognitively based self-management procedures of the 1970s, to the relapse prevention and pharmacologically based components of the 1980s.

3. There has recently been an increased emphasis on targeting specific groups of smokers for cessation activities (e.g., pregnant women, Hispanics, blacks).

4. Packaging and marketing of self-help smoking cessation materials have become more sophisticated and there is more of an emphasis on relapse prevention, while much of the content has changed relatively little over the years.

5. Mass-mediated quit-smoking programs have become an increasingly popular strategy for influencing the smoking behavior of a large number of smokers."

C. Smoking control

1. Policies pertaining to information and education

   "a. The Federal Government's efforts to

reduce the health consequences of cigarette smoking have consisted primarily
of providing the public with information and education about the hazards of
tobacco use. Two of the most well-
known mechanisms are the publication
of the Surgeon General's Reports and
the requirement of warning labels on
cigarette packages. A system of rotating
health warning labels is now required
for all cigarette and smokeless tobacco
packaging and advertisements.

b. Current laws do not require health
warning labels on all tobacco products
and do not require monitoring of the
communications effectiveness of the
warnings. Furthermore, existing laws
do not provide administrative mechanisms to update the contents of labels to
prevent the overexposure of current
messages or to reflect advances in scientific knowledge, such as new information about the addictive nature of tobacco use.

c. There is insufficient evidence to determine the independent effect of cigarette warning labels, particularly the rotating warning labels required since
1985, on public knowledge about the
health effects of smoking or on smoking
behavior.

d. Information about tar and nicotine
yields appears on all cigarette advertisements but not on all cigarette packages.
Levels of other hazardous constituents
of tobacco smoke, such as carbon monoxide, hydrogen cyanide, and ammonia, are not disclosed on packages or
advertisements. Little information is
available to the public about the identity

or health consequences of the additives
in tobacco products."

2. Economic incentives
"a. Cigarette excise taxes are imposed by
the Federal Government (16 cents per
pack), all State governments, and nearly
400 cities and counties. On average,
Federal and State excise taxes add 34
cents per pack to the price of cigarettes.
Cigarette excise tax rates have fallen
since 1964 in real terms because the rate
and magnitude of periodic tax increases
have not kept pace with inflation.

b. Studies demonstrate that increases in
the price of cigarettes decrease smoking
particularly by adolescents. It has been
estimated that an additional 100,000 or
more persons will live to age 65 as a
result of the price increases induced by
the 1983 doubling of the Federal excise
tax on cigarettes.

c. In 1964, smoking status was not considered in the determination of insurance
premiums. Currently, nearly all life insurers but only a few health, disability,
and property and casualty insurers offer premium discounts for nonsmokers.
Few health insurers reimburse for the
costs of smoking cessation programs or
treatment."

Bibliography

NHLBI workshop summary. Effects of tobacco smoke
components on cellular and biochemical processes in the
lung. *Am Rev Resp Dis* 136:1058–1064, 1987.

*Reducing Health Consequences of Smoking—25 Years of
Progress.* A Report of the Surgeon General. 1989. U.S. Gov't
Public, 3426, Washington D.C.

Silicosis

Vidyasagar Chodimella, M.D.
Christopher G. Murlas, M.D.

I. **Definition**
Silicosis is lung disease due to prolonged inhalation of crystalline silicon dioxide.

II. **Etiology**
  A. Occupational exposure to SiO_2 occurs whenever the earth's crust is broken and silicon-containing rock and sand is gathered, processed, or used (e.g., mining, tunneling, and excavating; quarrying granite and sandstone; foundries of ferrous metals, abrasives, and ceramics).
  B. The severity of disease depends on the period and intensity of exposure to silicon dioxide

III. **Pathogenesis**
The basic process of silicotic fibrogenesis is as follows:
  A. Ingestion of silica particles by alveolar macrophages, with damage to lysosomal membranes leading to autolysis of alveolar macrophages and release of silica particles.
  B. The sequence of events is repeated by freshly recruited alveolar macrophages.
  C. Hyperplasa of type II pneumonocytes, which secrete lipid factors that modify the tissue's reaction to silica.

  D. Disruption of type I alveolar epithelial cells, exposing the fibroblasts to macrophage-secreted fibrogenic factors.
  E. Cell matrix interactions, with deposition of collagen in the area of lung injury.
  F. Hyalinization of collagen related to deposition of material derived from immunoglobulins.

IV. **Pathology**
Pathology is dependent on chronicity, incubation time, and exposure level. Silicosis may present in the
  A. Chronic, or classic, form
    1. Occurs after prolonged exposure to silica dust containing less than 30% quartz. This disorder is more common in the upper lobes.
    2. Characterized by a nodule composed of an acellular center with concentric collagen fibers.
    3. Other features, though less common, include interstitial fibrosis, pleural plaques, and regional lymphadenopathy with peripheral calcification.
  B. Accelerated form
    1. Occurs following shorter and heavier exposure to silica dust.

2. Histologic features are similar to those of the chronic form but also include granulomas, more diffuse interstitial fibrosis, hyperplasia of type II pneumonocytes, and pleural plaques.

C. Acute form
   1. Occurs following intense exposure to fine silica dust for shorter periods.
   2. Characterized by features similar to those of pulmonary alveolar proteinosis and interstitial pneumonitis.
   3. Presence of silica particles in the proteinaceous fluid obtained from bronchoalveolar lavage.

V. Other Manifestations
A. Rhematoid silicotic nodules with central necrosis and calcification.
B. Complicating tuberculosis characterized by caseous granulomas.
C. Associated bronchitis or emphysema in silicotic smokers.
D. Extrathoracic manifestations: silicotic nodules and lymph nodes of the neck, abdomen, liver spleen, and bone marrow.

VI. Diagnosis
A. History and clinical feature
   1. History of occupational exposure to silica. Evolution of symptoms depends on intensity of exposure.
   2. Chronic silicotics may have no symptoms or signs except possibly abnormal chest films. Dyspnea on exertion indicates complicating features like progressive massive fibrosis, pulmonary tuberculosis, and/or obstructive airway disease.
   3. Cough in silicosis usually develops during advanced stages. It is typically dry and intractable but may be productive if bronchial infections are coincident. Hemoptysis may indicate coincident tuberculosis.
   4. Chest pain, fever, and weight loss are uncommon. Their presence should warn of the possibility of coincident tuberculosis.
   5. Clubbing is not a feature of complicated silicosis.
B. Radiologic picture
   1. Classic pattern
      a. Long exposure period (10–20 years) before appearance of radiologic abnormalities.
      b. Multinodular opacities 1–10 mm in diameter, fairly well circumscribed and calcified.
      c. Nodular pattern preceded by or associated with a reticular pattern.
      d. Enlarged hilar lymph nodes.
   2. Silicosis secondary to diatomaceous earth exposure
      a. Absent nodularity.
      b. Linear or reticular pattern.
      c. Upper zone predominance.
   3. Complicated silicosis
      a. Homogeneous area of consolidation of nonsegmental distribution, usually affecting the upper lobes.
      b. Opacities are irregular and ill-defined, with multiple "pseudopodia" extending into the surrounding parenchyma.
      c. More common in mid-lung zones at the periphery and tend to progress toward the hilum.
      d. Gradual incorporation of nodular lesions into massive consolidation in the upper zones, with frequent cavitation.
      e. Enlargement of the bronchial artery, with neovascularization and peripheral bronchopulmonary shunts.
      f. Enlarged hilar lymph nodes with peripheral calcification ("eggshell" calcification) is a pathognomonic feature.
      g. Unilateral diaphragmatic paralysis due to compression of the phrenic nerve may occur.
      h. Caplan's syndrome: manifestation of rheumatoid lung and characterized by the presence of large necrobiotic nodules superimposed on a background of simple silicosis.

VII. Pulmonary Function Tests
A. May be normal in early stages of the disease.
B. Dyspnea associated with restrictive and/or obstructive patterns.
C. Decreased diffusing capacity.
D. Evidence of arterial hypoxemia in patients with progressive massive fibrosis (PMF). Late stages of this disease are associated with CO_2 retention.

VIII. Management
A. Chronic silicosis
   1. Care directed to preventing progression, as well as surveillance for and treatment of complications such as tuberculosis.
   2. D-Penicillamine has been suggested by some authors, but its beneficial effects have not been proven.

B. Acute silicosis
   1. Bronchoalveolar lavage may be useful if and when silicosis manifests as alveolar proteinosis.
   2. Vigorous treatment of complicating mycobacterial infection.

IX. Prognosis

Prognosis depends on:
A. Extent of the parenchymal response to silica.
B. Presence and progression of interstitial fibrosis.
C. Progression of clinical disability.
D. Presence of complicating mycobacterial infection, obstructive airway disease, and/or cor pulmonale.

Bibliography

Banks DE, Morring KL, Bochleke BA, et al. Silicosis in silica flour workers. *Am Rev Respir Dis* 124:445–450, 1981.

Becklake MR. Silicosis, in Dunn CDR, Garnett HM, Jacobs P (eds): *Environmental Pollution and Man.* Monograph No. 3. Newburgh, IN, Immunology and Hematology Research Foundation, 1984, pp 85–93.

Dickie HA. Asbestos and silica: Their multiple effects on the lung. *Disease-a-Month* 28(12):1–79, 1982.

Morgan WKC, Seaton A. *Occupational Lung Diseases,* ed 2. Philadelphia, WB Saunders, 1984.

CHAPTER 33-C

Coal Worker's Pneumoconiosis (CWP)

Vidyasagar Chodimella, M.D.
Christopher G. Murlas, M.D.

I. **Definition**
CWP is an occupational lung disease resulting from prolonged exposure to coal dust.

II. **Etiology**
A. Occupations where the risk is high include coal mining and trimming; mining and milling of graphite in carbon plants; manufacturing or extensive use of carbon electrodes or carbon black.
B. Predisposing factors include cigarette smoking, chronic bronchitis, and emphysema. These conditions interfere with the pulmonary clearance mechanisms of inhaled dust particles.

III. **Pathogenesis**
A. Simple CWP results from accumulation of considerable amounts of inert coal dust with minimal tissue reaction.
1. Inhalation of coal particles less than 1 μm in diameter which are deposited in the alveoli.
2. Inert coal particles engulfed by alveolar macrophages move toward the bronchioles, to be expectorated in the sputum.
3. In the face of an overwhelming dust load, failure of the clearance mechanism with retention of dust in the alveoli and engagement of lymphatics.
4. Tissue reaction to inert coal dust includes small, pigmented lesions (coal macules) in the upper lobes (consisting initially of aggregates of dust-laden macrophages which may progress to fibrosis). Enlarged coal macules impinge on and weaken adjacent airways to create centrilobular emphysema. Other features include subpleural dust deposits, enlargement of hilar and mediastinal lymph nodes, and pigmentation of parietal pleural lymphatics.
B. Progressive massive fibrosis (PMF)
1. Factors predisposing to the development of PMF are unclear at present. PMF appears to be associated with:
a. Amorphous accumulation of protein, mineral dust, and calcium phosphate.
b. Mycobacterial infection.
c. Autoimmune reaction characterized by rheumatoid antinuclear and antilung antibodies.
2. Lesions are usually found in the posterior segment of the upper lobes or the apical segment of the lower lobes.

3. Histologic picture is similar to that of the coal nodule of simple CWP. Additional features include coarse hyalinized collagen, central calcification due to ischemia or complicating tuberculosis, vasculitis, and cardiac hypertrophy.

C. Caplan's syndrome or rheumatoid pneumoconiosis
   1. Lesions are larger than coal nodules and often unpigmented.
   2. Microscopically similar to the rheumatoid silicotic lesion and characterized by central necrosis, cavitation, perivascular plasma cell infiltration, and vasculitis.

IV. Diagnosis

Diagnosis is usually based on chest film findings and a history of occupational exposure.

A. Clinical manifestations are variable.
   1. Patients with simple pneumoconiosis suffer little clinical disability, and their disease shows little progress if they are removed from the dust-ridden environment.
   2. Those with PMF may present with exertional dyspnea, cough with mucoid expectoration or hemoptysis, and attacks of acute purulent bronchitis/bronchiolitis. Occasionally patients may expectorate black sputum (melanoptysis) resulting from the rupture of cavitating PMF lesions into the airways.
   3. Signs and symptoms of complicating obstructive airway disease and cor pulmonale may occur.
   4. Presence of rheumatoid arthritis or subcutaneous rheumatoid nodules should raise the possibility of Caplan's syndrome.

B. Radiological features
   1. Simple pneumoconiosis: early stages characterized by the presence of small, round, nodular opacities 1–5 mm in diameter. Associated with no calcification or central, punctate calcification.
   2. Complicated pneumoconiosis
      a. Large opacities 1 cm in diameter in the upper lung zones on a background pattern of simple pneumoconiosis.
      b. PMF typically starts near the periphery of the lung and presents as a mass with a smooth, well-defined lateral border which parallels the rib cage. The medial margin often is ill-defined.
      c. Homogeneous consolidation with or without cavitation.
      d. Presence of calcification and compensatory emphysema of parenchyma surounding the PMF lesion.
   3. Caplan's syndrome
      a. Pulmonary nodules are more regular in contour and more peripherally located than the masses of PMF.
      b. Nodules range from 0.5 to 5.0 cm in size.

V. Pulmonary Function Tests

A. Usually minimal disturbance of lung function unless complicated by PMF.

B. Lung function deficits in simple CWP include:
   1. Increased residual volume; reduction in vital capacity may be minimal.
   2. Occasional abnormality of the dead space/tidal volume ratio and/or frequency dependence of compliance.
   3. Reduced carbon monoxide diffusing capacity.
   4. Decreased elastic recoil.

C. PMF is characterized by more frequent and more marked abnormalities than simple CWP, as well as by eventual development of substantial airflow limitation and pulmonary hypertension.

VI. Differential Diagnosis

A. Complicated CWP
   1. Bronchial carcinoma
   2. Pulmonary tuberculosis

B. Simple CWP
   1. Other dust diseases like silicosis

C. Complications
   1. Mycobacterial infection
   2. Caplan's syndrome
   3. Scleroderma
   4. Chronic obstructive pulmonary disease
   5. Cor pulmonale with right heart failure

VII. Treatment

No effective treatment (other than general supportive care) has been established.

VIII. Prevention

A. Effective dust suppression.

B. Early recognition of dust retention by routine radiography.

C. Close surveillance and prompt management of complicating mycobacterial infections, including tuberculosis.

Bibliography

Kleinerman J. Pathology standards for coalworker' pneumoconiosis. Report of the Pneumoconiosis Committee of the College of American Pathologists. *Arch Pathol Lab Med* 103:375–385, 1979.

Rom WN (ed). *Environmental and Occupational Medicine.* Boston, Little-Brown, 1983.

Asbestos-Related Lung Diseases

Christopher G. Murlas, M.D.
Vidyasagar Chodimella, M.D.

I. **Definition**
   Asbestos-related lung diseases are forms of pneumoconiosis due to the inhalation of asbestos.

II. **Etiology**
   A. The etiologic agent is asbestos, which occurs naturally in fiber forms.
   B. Exposure to asbestos commonly occurs in several settings.
      1. Occupational: as in mining, milling, transporting, manufacturing, applying, and using the raw fiber or manufactured product.
      2. Indirect occupational or environmental: as results from working in the vicinity of a workplace or of an individual whose job involves direct handling of the material (e.g., carpenters or welders in ship building or ship repair); or domestic exposure, as may occur, for example, when handling fiber-laden work clothes.
   C. The different types of asbestos minerals and fibers, and the settings in which they are used, are summarized in Table 33D-1.

III. **Pathophysiology**
   A. Important determinants of potential disease are the dose delivered to the lung; dimensions of the fiber (longer and thinner fibers appear to be more oncogenic); the fiber type; and the biologic durability of the fiber.
   B. Long asbestos fibers (50 μm) tend to follow the axial bronchi to the lower lobes, where they are deposited. Some may penetrate the lung or diaphragm to reach the pleural space or peritoneum, respectively.
   C. Summary of events leading to asbestosis:
      1. Activation of macrophages by fibers, leading to the release of various enzymes and mediators.
      2. Alveolar epithelial injury and alveolitis due, in part, to the fiber burden, as well as to enzyme and mediator effects.
      3. Extension of the process to the interstitium, eventually leading to fibrosis.
   D. In general, asbestos-related lung diseases can be classified into two forms:
      1. Parenchymal disease, including parenchymal fibrosis and bronchial carcinoma.
      2. Pleural:
         a. Benign reactions, including pleural plaques, pleural thickening, and/or benign pleural reaction.
         b. Mesothelioma.

Table 33D-1.   Asbestos Minerals and Their Uses

Mineral: Type of Group and Form	Main Commercial Uses and/or Other Human Exposures
Cummington-grunerite	No current commercial uses
Tremolite	Has rural domestic uses (e.g., stucco); may or may not be removed in processing
Serpentine	
Chrysotile (white asbestos)	Friction materials; paper products; textiles; asbestos cement products (pipes, gutters, tiles, roofing sheets); insulation, fireproofing
Amphibole	
Crocidolite (blue asbestos)	Used in combination mostly in cement
Anthophyllite	Filler in plastics and rubber
Amosite (brown)	Used generally in combination and for many of the applications listed above

Source: Adapted from Rom WN (ed.) *Environmental and Occupational Medicine* Boston, Little-Brown, 1983.

    E. The Stanton hypothesis may help explain the between-fiber differences in carcinogenic potential. Stanton emphasized the importance of fiber size: carcinogenic potential increases directly with fiber length and inversely with fiber diameter (under approximately 1.5 μm). The variable persistence of different fibers in lung tissue may help to explain the biologic gradient in human mesothelioma production related to the major asbestos fiber types. Fiber absorption of cigarette carcinogens also appears to be important toxicologically.

IV. Diagnosis
  A. Clinical features
    1. History of asbestos exposure.
    2. Symptoms
      a. Symptoms are insidious in onset and may slow the progression to total disability.
      b. Exertional dyspnea: dyspnea out of proportion to physical and radiologic signs may be indicative of asbestosis.
      c. Cough is usually nonproductive.
      d. Sputum may be purulent in smokers, suggesting purulent bronchitis or bronchiectasis. Hemoptysis, if present, should prompt the exclusion of malignancy.
      e. Chest pain is uncharacteristic and should prompt consideration of a possible superimposed process, especially malignancy.
    3. Physical signs are usually nonspecific unless complications or extensive disease are present.
      a. Central cyanosis, usually precipitated by effort, may be severe if chronic airflow obstruction complicates the picture.
      b. Clubbing of fingers and toes often indicates pulmonary fibrosis with hypoxemia.
      c. Hypertrophic osteoarthropathy suggests the possibility of a complicating bronchial carcinoma.
      d. If interstitial fibrosis is present, high-pitched crackles, occurring during inspiration and persisting after coughing, are usually present; thickening and secretions in the small airways are thought to be responsible for these findings.
  B. Radiologic features
    1. Pulmonary fibrosis
      a. Signs of interstitial fibrosis
        (1) Lower lobe predominance.
        (2) Gradual progression toward mid-lung zones.
      b. Complicating airspace disease
        (1) Evidence of bronchiectasis with multiple cavities may be present.
        (2) Parenchymal lesions or mediastinal widening suggests the possibility of bronchial carcinoma.
    2. Pleural fibrosis and plaques
      a. Pleural fibrosis usually typified by homogeneous opacification in the lower and mid-lung zones, involving lateral and posterior costophrenic sulci.
      b. This disorder may be associated with pleural effusion, which may be minimal and detectable on lateral decubitus views only. Large volumes of fluid, reaccumulating rapidly after aspiration, suggest the possibility of malignancy.
      c. Pleural plaques

(1) Usually bilateral and tend to follow rib lines. Oblique chest films may be useful in identifying them. Involvement of lung spaces is uncharacteristic.

(2) Involvement of lateral parietal and diaphragmatic pleura is pathognomonic of asbestosis.

(3) Plaque calcification suggests that plaques are benign.

3. Pulmonary function abnormalities

a. A restrictive ventilatory disorder associated with a decreased carbon monoxide diffusing capacity and an increased (A-a) oxygen difference are usually evidence of interstitial fibrosis.

b. An obstructive pattern may also occur, especially in smokers.

4. Other investigations

a. Biopsy of lesions present.

b. Bronchoalveolar lavage to identify fibers if present.

c. Gallium scan to assess the activity of a possible alveolitis.

5. Differential diagnosis: includes sarcoidosis, diffuse interstitial fibrosis, emphysema, bronchiectasis, honeycomb lung, and collagen vascular diseases.

V. Management

A. In the early stages of asbestosis, corticosteroid therapy has been suggested by some authors, although its efficacy has not been established. Serial chest films and pulmonary function tests, including measurement of carbon monoxide diffusing capacity, may be useful in monitoring the response to steroid therapy.

B. Tuberculosis complicating the disorder is common, especially in advanced cases. Consequently, the surveillance for and treatment of complicating tuberculosis are important. Asbestosis-related neoplasia of the lung, pleura, ovary, and gastrointestinal tract usually represents a very difficult management problem, and few generalizations can be made.

VI. Prognosis

A. Although the extent and progression of disease are often related to the intensity of exposure, asbestosis, once acquired, usually progresses slowly and relentlessly even after removal of the patient from further exposure. Pulmonary function deficits correlate more closely with morbidity and mortality in asbestosis than do the radiologic features.

B. The prognosis of complicating lung cancer is usually worse than that in the general population. Few cases, however, are resectable due to impaired ventilatory function, pulmonary and pleural fibrosis.

C. Pleural mesothelioma associated with asbestosis runs an inexorable course.

VII. Prevention and Control

The following measures should be used to protect workers from occupational exposure

A. Asbestos fibers should be shipped in dust-proof bags. Crocidolite, which is responsible for malignant mesothelioma, should be handled mechanically.

B. Maneuvers at work that can give rise to asbestos dust should be carried out under proper exhausts, and with respiratory and body protection.

C. Notification of processes involving crocidolite should be sent to the appropriate regulatory authorities.

D. Measures to prevent accidental exposures, including signs indicating asbestos-containing materials, are important precautions.

E. Medical surveillance of asbestos workers

1. Full occupational history at the time of hiring, along with physical examination, chest films, and lung function parameters, is appropriate.

2. Symptoms suggestive of asbestosis should be investigated immediately.

3. Periodic examination of the workers at risk may be important to assess the efficacy of precautions, although these measures have not been shown to be associated with decreased morbidity and mortality due to asbestosis.

Bibliography

Becklake MR. Asbestos-related diseases of the lungs and other organs: Their epidemiology and implications for clinical practice. *Am Rev Respir Dis* 114:187–227, 1976.

Becklake MR. Asbestos-related diseases of the lungs and pleura: Current clinical issues. *Am Rev Respir Dis* 126:187–194, 1982.

Craighead JE, Mossman BT. The pathogenesis of asbestos-associated diseases. *N Engl J Med* 306:1446–1455, 1982.

Morgan WKC, Seaton A. *Occupational Lung Diseases*, ed 2. Philadelphia, WB Saunders, 1984.

Other Pneumoconioses

Vidyasagar Chodimella, M.D.
Christopher G. Murlas, M.D.

Beryllium Disease

I. Definition

Occupational lung disease resulting from exposure to beryllium.

II. Etiology

Exposure to beryllium occurs in:

A. Fluorescent light industry.

B. Industries manufacturing alloys, ceramics, and x-ray and vacuum tubes.

C. All industries that producing airborne beryllium, including melting, casting, grinding, drilling, and machining.

III. Pathophysiology

A. Beryllium enters the body via the lungs, although the manifestations are systemic.

B. Acute berylliosis is a dose-related, toxic lung injury characterized by acute irritation damage to the upper airways, bronchiolitis, pulmonary edema, and chemical pneumonitis.

C. Chronic beryllium disease is the result of delayed hypersensitivity reaction to beryllium compounds which act as haptens and trigger cellular immune reactions. Chronic beryllium lesions are characterized by:

1. Mononuclear infiltrate of the alveolar walls.

2. Coalescence of cellular infiltrates into granulomas containing epithelioid cells, giant cells, and macrophages in various stages of activation.

3. Variable amount of fibroblastic activity that progresses to interstitial fibrosis.

4. Granulomas found in several organs, including thoracic and abdominal lymph nodes, spleen, and liver.

5. Cutaneous lesions, if present, are considered to be the result of direct contact.

IV. Diagnosis

A. Diagnostic criteria for beryllium disease

1. History of exposure.

2. Objective evidence of lower respiratory disease and a clinical course consistent with berylliosis.

3. Radiologic evidence of interstitial fibronodular disease.

4. Impaired pulmonary function.

5. Histopathologic changes in the lung and lymph nodes.

Table 33E-1.   Other Common Pneumoconioses

Disease	Cause	Source of Dust	Pathological Effect
Baritosis	Barium sulphate	Mining of barium salts	Chest film changes only
Siderosis	Iron oxide	Welding	Chest film changes only
Stannosis	Tin oxide	Smelting	Chest film changes
Kaolinosis	Hydrated Al silicate	China clay	Simple pneumoconiosis
Aluminosis	Stamped Al	Explosives and paints	Nodular fibrosis, emphysema, bulla, pneumothorax
Talcosis	Hydrated Mg silicate	Rubber industry	Pulmonary fibrosis

Source: Adapted from Crofton and Douglas (1983).

6. Demonstration of the presence of beryllium in biologic material (e.g., lung, lymph nodes, urine).

B. Acute berylliosis: clinical and radiologic features are similar to those of chemical pneumonitis.
  1. Clinical features include dyspnea, cough, chest pain, hemoptysis, rales, and cyanosis.
  2. The radiologic picture suggests patchy airspace consolidation.

C. Chronic berylliosis
  1. Multisystem disorder in which granulomas develop throughout the body, including the lungs.
  2. Usually develops without preceding acute berylliosis.
  3. Symptoms precipitated by stress (e.g., pregnancy, surgery).
  4. Clinical features include dyspnea and progressive, unremitting cough.
  5. Physical signs are consistent with pulmonary fibrosis.
  6. Radiologic features are neither specific nor diagnostic.
    a. Diffuse, finely granular haziness of mid-lung zones.
    b. Bilateral diffuse nodular opacities.
    c. Presence of regional lymph nodal enlargement, with or without calcification.
    d. Advanced cases show a reticular pattern with conglomeration of nodular shadows.
    e. Ten percent of cases may present as spontaneous pneumothorax.

7. Pulmonary function tests may reveal restrictive, obstructive or mixed patterns.

V. **Differential Diagnosis** (Table 1)
Beryllium disease is differentiated from other noncaseating granulomatomas diseases (such as sarcoidosis) by:
  A. Absence of uveal tract, tonsil, parotid gland, and bone involvement.
  B. No change in tuberculin reactivity unless the patient is receiving steroid treatment.

VI. **Treatment**
  A. Prolonged therapy with steroids has been advocated.
  B. Specific measures for incidental infection, cor pulmonale, or spontaneous pneumothorax.

VII. **Preventive Measures**
Preventive measures should be directed toward controlling atmospheric beryllium to less than 2 $\mu g/m^3$.

Bibliography

Becklake MR. Chronic airflow limitation and its relationship to dusty occupations. *Chest* 88:608–617, 1985.

Crofton JR, Douglas A. *Respiratory Diseases*, ed 3. London, Blackwell, 1983.

Cullen MR. Respiratory diseases from hard metal exposure: A continuing enigma. *Chest* 86:513–514, 1984.

Pruess OP, van Orstrand HS. Beryllium disease: Update and review, in *VIth International Pneumonconiosis Conference 1983.* (W. Rom, ed.) Bochum, Bergbau-Berfsgenossenschaft, 1984, pp 1159–1167.

Rom WN (ed). *Environmental and Occupational Medicine.* Boston, Little, Brown, 1983.

Occupational Asthma

Christopher G. Murlas, M.D.

I. **Definition**
  A. The term *occupational asthma* refers to asthma that is of new onset and is caused by environmental or workplace exposures. Common agents causing this disorder include animal danders and secretions, insects and crustaceans, vegetable gums, and enzymes from plants or bacteria. Small molecular weight substances such as acid anhydrides, platinum, and resins fall into this group.
  B. Some authors have also described as occupational asthma those cases of preexisting asthma that are worsened by such exposures. However, these environmental exposures are not causal. Asthmatics are commonly irritated by a wide variety of chemical, physical, and pharmacologic stimuli, and thus their bronchial hyperreactivity is nonspecific. This disorder has become a major health issue because:
    1. It is a very common disease.
    2. Many patients with disease are often clinically asymptomatic until aggravated by exposure to one or more agents which have no effect on nonasthmatics.
    3. Exacerbations of preexisting asthma in the workplace cause significant morbidity and mortality worldwide.

II. **Etiology**
Agents thought to cause occupational asthma can be divided into two broad categories (Table 33F-1):
  A. Low molecular weight compounds. These are usually inorganic chemicals with a molecular weight below 1,000. The prevalence of asthmatic reactions to these chemicals is low. A history of atopy is uncommon, but IgE antibody production may occur, along with peripheral eosinophilia.
  B. High molecular weight substances. These are often organic materials. Reaction to high molecular weight compounds is thought to be IgE dependent; specific IgE antibodies can be demonstrated, and skin tests with the putative agent are often positive.

III. **Pathophysiology**
  A. Although the pathophysiology by which certain low molecular weight chemical agents may cause occupational asthma has been characterized, the mechanisms of most

Table 33F-1. Common Agents Associated with Occupational Asthma

High Molecular Weight Substances		Inorganic and Organic Agents of Low Molecular Weight	
Substance	Representative Occupation or Industry	Substance	Representative Occupation or Industry
Animal proteins		Anhydrides	
Laboratory animals	Animal breeders, laboratory workers	Phthalic, trimellitic, hexahydrophthalic, tetrachlorophthalic	Plastics industry, epoxy resins
Domestic animals	Farmers, poultry breeders, veterinarians, meat workers	Dyes	
		Azo, anthraquinone	Cloth dyeing
Birds	Bird breeders, poultry processors	Fluxes	
Sea squirts	Osyter workers, wood pulp workers	Colophony	Electronics industry
		Aminoethylethanolamine	Aluminum soldering
Prawns	Prawn workers	Diisocyanates	
Grain weevils/mites	Granary workers, farmers, dock workers	Toluene diisocyanate (TDI)	Automobiles, paints, TDI manufacture
Enzymes (aminal)		Diphenylmethane diisocyanate	Foundry core workers, polyurethane foam
Subtilisin	Detergent manufacturers	Hexamethylene diisocyanate	Paints
Trypsin, pancreatin	Pharmaceutical industry		
Enzymes (plant)		Metallic salts	
Papain, bromelain, pectinase, diastase	Food industry, pharmaceutical industry	Nickel	Metal plating
		Chromium	Cement, tanning, metal plating
Plant proteins			
Cereal grains	Farmers, granary workers, millers, dock workers, bakers	Aluminum	Aluminum fluoride and sulfate workers
		Platinum slats	Platinum refining
Legumes (coffee, soy and castor beans)	Farmers, dock workers, food processors, fertilizer workers		
Seeds (cotton, flax, linseed)	Bakers, fertilizer workers, flax workers, oil producers		
Vegetable gums			
Karaya, tragacanth, acacia, arabic, quillaja	Food industry, printers, manufacturers		

Source: Adapted from Moller et al. (1986).

causes of asthma remain poorly understood at present.

B. Immunologic mechanisms, especially IgE-mediated hypersensitivity responses, are important in some cases. Low molecular weight compounds are usually incomplete allergens (i.e., haptenic) and must react first with a protein carrier before they are capable of causing an immunologic response. It is believed that industrial chemicals, such as isocyanates and anhydrides, act in this manner, probably by combining with respiratory tract proteins. Mast cells and basophils play a central role in these allergic reactions. Perturbation of cell surface membranes by cross-linking IgE antibodies stimulates the synthesis of several bronchoactive mediators, including the sulfidopeptide leukotrienes, prostaglandins, and platelet activating factor.

C. Certain low molecular weight chemicals may cause nonimmunoglobulin-mediated mast cell stimulation by activation, via either the classic or alternative complement pathway.

D. An agent may produce a pharmacologic response and may act directly on bronchial smooth muscle to cause bronchospasm. Toluene diisocyanate, for example, has been reported to act as a partial β-adrenergic antagonist. The organophosphate pesticides may cause bronchospasm and increased airway secretions by inhibiting acetylcholinesterase and allowing the accumulation of acetylcholine at cholinergic receptor sites on bronchial smooth muscle and secretory glands.

E. Most low molecular weight chemicals are irritants and stimulate rapidly adapting irritant receptors located in close proximity to the airway epithelium. Activation of both types of sensory fibers results in vagally mediated cough, laryngeal constriction, mucous secretion, and changes in airway diameter.

F. Another response mechanism of the lung is bronchoconstriction due to airway injury. Transient increases in nonspecific airway reactivity are associated with reversible airway epithelial damage such as that occurring after ozone exposure. The observed increase in airway reactivity may also relate to increased sensitivity of vagal irritant reflexes or an increase in airway permeability.

G. Bronchial hyperreactivity is a characteristic feature of occupational asthma and is nonspecific. The increased responsiveness of the airways occurs to a variety of provocative stimuli.

1. Mucosal damage itself may produce acute bronchial hyperreactivity because airway epithelial cells are known to elaborate products that result in smooth muscle spasm.

2. The airway inflammation that ensues after epithelial cell injury may or may not augment the acute hyperreactivity that occurs. The mechanisms explaining the chronic, persistent airway hyperreactivity found in chronic asthma, whether occupationally associated or not, are entirely unknown.

   a. It is possible that airway inflammatory and immunologic mechanisms interact to cause persistent asthma.

   b. In addition to causing acute bronchial hyperreactivity, the initial environmental exposure and tissue injury may lead to a chronic inflammatory state, with or without an associated production of antigen(s) consisting of altered tissue proteins with or without the putative agent itself. Subsequent exposure to the same agent could then perpetuate the inflammatory response, including persistent airway epithelial and vascular permeability.

IV. **Diagnosis**

A. History and symptoms

1. Often the key in diagnosing occupational asthma is a thorough occupational history. The association between environmental exposure(s) and the onset of asthma is often overlooked because de novo asthma in adults is so common. A detailed list of materials encountered in the workplace and home environments may identify a known etiology.

2. Work-related asthma is typically manifested by dyspnea, cough, wheezing, and/or chest tightness. Late-occurring asthmatic responses are common. In many cases, cough may be the predominant or only symptom. The cough tends to occur during the day but may be especially troublesome at night, sometimes interrupting sleep. Symptoms usually occur, or are most severe, during or shortly after the workday and improve during weekends and vacations. However, in some cases, particularly those related to isocyanate or western red cedar, symptoms may persist for months or years after termination of exposure.

3. There are several common variations to the usual presentation:

   a. Immediately after exposure, symptoms of bronchospasm may be minor or absent.

   b. If these symptoms are absent, they may manifest 4–12 hr later (the so-called late asthmatic response or late-phase reaction). Late and dual asthmatic responses occur more commonly than simple immediate responses in some forms of work-induced asthma.

   c. Early on, many patients complain primarily or solely of a cough, which may or may not be productive.

   d. As in nonoccupational asthma, rhinitis may precede the onset of asthma by months to years.

B. Physical findings
1. Wheezing, if present, may be the only physical finding.
2. Confirming the diagnosis is sometimes difficult and may require special diagnostic procedures. It is useful to document work-related declines in expiratory airflow over a day or week, using a peak flow meter or spirometer. However, such monitoring does not exclude the diagnosis because cases in which there is persistent or nominal obstruction may be overlooked.
3. Serial pulmonary function tests over a longer period of time may detect more gradual declines in ventilatory function.
   a. Spirometry carried out before and after a work shift can be diagnostic, but is insensitive and may yield normal results in over one-half of affected workers if done only once.
   b. Measurement of peak expiratory flow with a portable peak flow meter, preferably at regular intervals during workdays and on weekends for 2 weeks, can be quite helpful. A recurring repeated difference of more than 20% between a day's maximal and minimal values, and the temporal relationship between symptoms and the workplace or putative environment, are helpful in confirming the diagnosis.
C. Diagnostic tests
1. Determining bronchial reactivity to methacholine, histamine, or cold air challenge may be extremely helpful in the evaluation of patients with suspected occupational asthma. However, a positive challenge test to methacholine, histamine, or cold air, although sensitive, is nonspecific. The causative agent is not identified, nor is a definitive diagnosis made, by such testing. The agent may be suspected if bronchial reactivity increases after a period of work (presumably due to a late-occurring asthmatic response). Normal airway responsiveness, however, does not rule out the presence of work-related asthma.
2. When work-related asthma is mediated, in part, by immunologic mechanisms, prick or intradermal skin testing for immediate hypersensitivity may help to identify the specific cause. This technique is suitable for many plant and animal proteins and for a few chemicals such as phthalic anhydride and platinum salts. Generally, most industrial chemicals are unreliable when used directly for skin testing. The radioallergosorbent test (RAST) may be also be useful but does not replace skin testing.
3. Many cases of occupational asthma can be confirmed only by specific bronchial inhalation challenge testing. Exposure to suspected agents should be preformed in a clinical laboratory under close observation by a physician in case severe reactions occur. The method of inhalation exposure differs according to the form of the reagent (i.e., fume, vapor, dust) to be investigated.
V. **Differential Diagnosis**
A. Asthmatic reactions to high or low molecular weight compounds must be differentiated from hypersensitivity pneumonitis, a disease caused by similar compounds and having some overlapping features. Shortness of breath and cough, as well as similar timing of symptom onset, tend to blur these two diagnoses. Hypersensitivity pneumonitis generally presents with a dry cough, rales rather than wheezes, fever, interstitial infiltrates on the chest radiograph, and a decreased carbon monoxide diffusing capacity on pulmonary function tests. The disease represents an irritant response occurring at the alveolar-capillary level, as opposed to the bronchial level, and is usually caused by a type III (IgE) response. It can have a permanent effect and may be fatal if not diagnosed quickly.
B. Brief, intense exposure to high levels of inhaled irritants can cause asthma, or reactive airways dysfunction syndrome (RADS), or toxic inhalation. RADS must be differentiated from toxic inhalation. Toxic inhalation is an alveolar-capillary response to inhaled irritants, whereas RADS is a bronchial response. Toxic inhalations are caused by substances that are caustic to the lower airways, such as chlorine gas and sulfur dioxide. Depending on the nature of the inhaled substance, the concentration, and the duration of exposure, toxic inhalation can cause respiratory distress, noncardiogenic pulmonary edema, and death. RADS and toxic

inhalation share certain manifestations. For example, hypoxemia often immediately follows RADS exposure, and varying durations of airway obstruction may be seen following toxic exposure.

VI. Treatment

A. Prevention: The major objective in management is prevention. To benefit all workers at risk, the offending agent should be identified as soon as possible.

   1. Until the afflicted worker can be transformed from his or her usual workplace, a properly fitting respiratory device can be used on a short-term basis.

   2. If exposure is avoided, symptoms of occupational asthma usually resolve. Several studies have documented that bronchial hyperreactivity, measured by histamine or methacholine challenge, can also improve after removal from the workplace. However, there are some cases that do not respond so favorably.

B. Medications

   1. Drug treatment of individuals with occupational asthma is predicated on the same principles that apply to naturally occurring asthma. Patients usually respond to conventional therapy.

   2. Exacerbating factors such as various physical conditions, aeroallergens, and chemical irritants need to be identified and avoided.

   3. The choice of medications depends on the severity of asthma, as judged clinically, and the results of pulmonary function testing.

   4. For certain mild or moderate cases, β-adrenergic agonists and cromolyn sodium usually suffice to control symptoms.

   5. For more difficult cases, systemic corticosteroids may be required. Steroids are particularly helpful and may be necessary to control late asthmatic responses, which are common in occupational asthma. Whenever possible, systemic corticosteroids should only be used as a burst regimen for a short period of time.

   6. In certain situations, such as laboratory animal handler's asthma and exercise-induced bronchospasm, cromolyn sodium is extremely useful in reducing or preventing clinical symptoms when used before an unavoidable exposure to offending agents. However, the effects of cromolyn may not be long-lasting, and it usually proves ineffective with continued or heavy occupational exposures.

C. Immunotherapy

At present, there is limited and mixed experience concerning immunotherapy in the management of occupational asthma. There are reports of success with this form of treatment, especially in baker's asthma and laboratory animal handler's asthma, but additional critically evaluated trials are needed to confirm its utility.

VII. Patient Monitoring

A. If workers are exposed to an agent known to cause occupational asthma, periodic medical surveillance is mandatory. Serial measurement of nonspecific airway responsiveness can be quite useful in monitoring the progress of patients with occupational asthma. Exposure to the etiologic agent often causes an acute increase in nonspecific airway responsiveness that can persist for days to weeks.

B. In helping to develop control measures to prevent occupational asthma in the workplace, the chest physician and allied health workers may be faced with the difficult situation in which even the maintenance of threshold limit values may not protect some persons at risk. Changes instituted in the cotton industry, which included the washing and steaming of cotton before its processing, exemplify how alterations in the manufacturing process can reduce or prevent disease.

VIII. Prognosis

The natural history of occupational asthma is uncertain. Recent evidence suggests that asthma initially caused by workplace exposure may persist for many years after exposure ceases and that the likelihood of persistent asthma increases with the duration of symptoms. With avoidance of an identified occupational asthma-causing agent, many workers report resolution of their symptoms. Several studies have documented that bronchial hyperreactivity, as measured by histamine or methacholine challenge, may also improve following removal from the workplace. However, there are reports (including those of western red cedar workers) suggesting that not all workers may have such an optimistic prognosis.

Bibliography

Moller DR, Murlas CG, Baughman RP, et al. New directions in occupational asthma to small molecular weight compounds. *Semin Respir Med* 7:225–240, 1986.

Murlas CG, Brooks SM. Treatment of occupational asthma, in Cherniack RM (ed): *Current Therapy of Respiratory Disease*. Philadelphia, BC Decker, 1987, pp 110–112.

Chapter 33-G

Pulmonary Disease Secondary to Drugs

Christopher G. Murlas, M.D.

I. Classification of Drug Reactions

A. Respiratory disorders related to therapeutic drug use cause significant morbidity and mortality each year. As many as 1% of all hospital deaths annually may be related to the use (not abuse) of one or more medications.

B. Approximately 100 drugs have been reported to cause respiratory disease. Although in most cases it is not known how certain drugs cause disease, several mechanisms have been identified. In general, these can be summarized as follows:

1. Drug reactions that occur in any person
   a. Overdosage. The reaction is directly related to the amount of overdosage. This reaction can also result from drug accumulation due to organ failure, preventing catabolism or normal excretion.
   b. Side effects. These are unavoidable pharmacologic effects of the drug (e.g., sedation caused by antihistamines). Most drugs cause one or more side effects, and some are particularly serious.
   c. Secondary effects. These effects are indirect but not necessarily inevitable results of the drug's primary action (e.g., immunosuppression by corticosteroids).
   d. Drug interaction. One or more drugs may inhibit, enhance, or otherwise alter the biotransformation of another drug.

2. Reactions that occur only in susceptible persons, based, in some situations, on genetic predisposition
   a. Intolerance. A qualitatively normal but quantitatively enhanced pharmacologic drug effect (e.g., digitalis-induced atrial-ventricular block occurring with therapeutic doses).
   b. Idiosyncracy. A qualitatively abnormal drug effect, that is, one that does not correspond to the usual pharmacologic actions of the drug (e.g., hemolytic anemia in patients with glucose-6-phosphate dehydrogenase deficiency).
   c. Allergy or hypersensitivity. An immune response associated with the formation of specific antibodies or sensitized lymphocytes.

3. "Toxic" reactions due to metabolites (but that do not occur in all persons)

$$O_2 \xrightarrow{e^-} O_2^{-} \xrightarrow{e^- + 2H^+} H_2O_2 \xrightarrow{e^- + H^+} H_2O + OH\cdot \xrightarrow{e^- + H^+} H_2O$$

$$2O_2^{-} + 2H^+ \xrightarrow{\text{superoxide dismutases}} O_2 + H_2O_2$$

$$2H_2O_2 \xrightarrow{\text{catalases}} O_2 + 2H_2O$$

$$H_2O_2 + 2\ GSH \xrightarrow{\text{glutathione peroxidase}} 2H_2O + GSSG$$

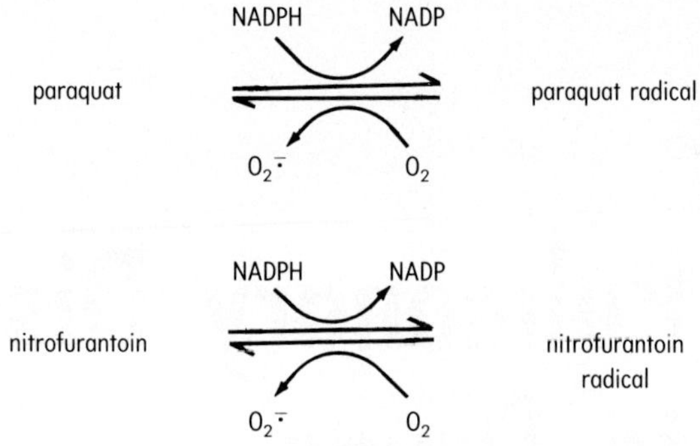

FIGURE 33G-1. Common reactions leading to the generation of free radicals of oxygen.

a. Arylating and alkylating intermediates that covalently bind to tissue, producing epithelial necrosis and tissue edema (postulated but not yet proven in humans).

b. Production of free radical intermediates of oxygen, namely, the superoxide anion radical (O_2^-), hydrogen peroxide (H_2O_2), and the hydroxy radical (OH^-). These oxygen radicals generate singlet electron transfers and disrupt critical cell functions (Figure 33G-1). Some drugs (e.g., nitrofurantoin) may produce pulmonary fibrosis by stimulating oxygen radical generation within certain lung cells. This overwhelms the normal antioxidant protective mechanisms available to scavenge such radi-

Table 33G-1. Chemotherapeutic Agents Inducing Pulmonary Disease

Cytotoxic Reaction
Produces cellular atypia, especially type II pneumocytes
Frequently irreversible
Subacute
No eosinophilia
Fever common
Examples include busulfan, bleomycin, nitrosoureas, chlorambucil, mitomycin, hydroxyurea, melphalan, and cyclophosphamide.
Procarbazine; uracil mustard, and 6-mercaptopurine may also produce such reactions.

Noncytotoxic reaction
No cellular atypia
? Hypersensitivity reaction
Usually acute
Eosinophilia common
Fever common
Examples include cyclophosphamide, methotrexate, procarbazine, bleomycin, and cytosine arabinoside.

Source: Adapted from Rosenow (1980).

Table 33G-2. Drugs That May Induce SLE

Antiarrhythmic drugs	Antituberculous drugs
Practotol	Isoniazid*
Procainamide*	Para-aminosalicyclic acid
Quinidine	Streptomycin
Antibiotics	Phenothiazines
Griseofulvin	Chlorpromazine
Nitrofurantoin	Levomepromazine
Penicillin	Perazine
Sulfonamides	Perphenazin
Tetracycline	Promethazine
Anticonvulsant drugs	Thioridazin
Carbamazepine	Miscellaneous
Diphenylhydantoin*	Amoproxan
Ethosuximide	Anthiomaline
Mephenytoin	D-Penicillamine
Phenylethylacetylurea	Methysergide
Promidone	Methylthiouracil
Trimethadione	Oral contraceptives
Antihypertensive drugs	Oxyphenisatin
Hydralazine*	Phenylbutazone
Methyldopa	Prophylthiouracil
	Tolazamide

*Drugs that elicit ANA in a large percentage of individuals taking the drug even without clinical symptoms. These drugs account for >90% of the cases, with the exception of chlorpromazine.

Table 33G-3. Respiratory Disorders Associated with Certain Drugs In Which the Pathophysiology Is Either Not Well Understood Or Is Unknown

Interstitial pneumonitis/fibrosis
  All chemotherapeutic agents
  Nitrofurantoin (both acute and chronic reactions)
  Drug-induced SLE
  Oxygen
  Gold
  Aspirated oil
  D-Penicillamine
  Talc
  Sulfasalazine
  Drug-inducing PIE reactions
  Methysergide
Pleural effusion
  Nitrofurantoin (acute)
  Methysergide (chronic)
  Drug-induced SLE (acute and chronic)
  Chemotherapeutic agents
  Dantrolene
Hilar/mediastinal adenopathy or widening
  Methotrexate
  Corticosteroids
  Dilantin
Drug-induced acute noncardiac pulmonary edema
  Heroin, methadone, propoxyphene
  Aspirin (very low $PaCO_2$)*
  Hydrochlorthiazide
  Chlordiazepoxide*
  Ethylchlorvynol*
  Blood (leukoagglutinin)
  Dextran
Drug-induced pulmonary infiltrate(s) with
  eosinophilia
  Nitrofurantoin
  Mexthotrexate
  Sulfonamides
  Sulphasalazine
  Penicillin
  Isoniazid, para-aminosalicylic acid
  Procarbazine
  Salicylates
  Carbamazepine
  Imipramine
  Cromolyn sodium
  Ritalin

Bronchospasm
  β-blockers
  Nitrofurantoin
  Aspirin ibuprofen, indomethacin, fenoprofen
  Drug-inducing pulmonary infiltrates with
    eosinophilia
  Many nebulized medications
  15-Methyl-prostaglandin-F2-α
  Isoproterenol
Drug-induced pulmonary granulomas
  Mineral oil
  Talc
  Methotrexate
  Bacille Calmette-Guérin (BCG)
  Cromolyn sodium
Pulmonary hypertension (vasospasm and/or emboli)
  Oral contraceptives
  Aminorex
  15-Methyl-prostaglandin-F2-α
Drug-induced pulmonary disease that may be on
  immunologic basis
  Drug-induced SLE
  Chemotherapeutic agents
  Many narcotics
  Leukoagglutinins
  Penicillamine
  Talc
  BCG
  Drugs inducing PIE
Respiratory paralysis secondary to antibiotics
  Neomycin
  Streptomycin
  Kanamycin
  Polymyxin B
  Colistin
  Gentamicin

*Ibuprofen and other anti-inflammatory agents can produced a subacute, non-cardiac pulmonary edema due to sodium retention.
Note: Clubbing rarely occurs in drug-induced pulmonary disease, and when it does, it has no diagnostic significance.
Source: Adapted from Rosenow (1980).

cals and incites an inflammatory reaction, which may subsequently become fibrotic.

c. Chemotherapeutic drug injury may cause either cytotoxic or noncytoxic reactions (Table 33G-1 on p. 306). The mechanisms producing disease from many drugs of this class are perhaps best known. Considerable research has been done concerning bleomycin in particular. This is because initial protocols required close monitoring, as well as the fact that animal studies closely correlated with observations in humans. Reactions to bleomycin are common if more than 450 U is used, and these reactions are potentiated if hemithoracic radiation therapy, oxygen supplementation, or nitrosoureas are also administered. Not all chemotherapeutic drugs are as clearly dose-related as bleomycin.

d. Pulmonary phospholipidosis. More than 20 cationic amphiphilic drugs (e.g., amiodarone) are known to induce a phospholipid storage disorder in many cells of the body, including the lungs. It is not known, however, whether this phospholipidosis is a secondary effect or the primary cause of the interstitial pneumonitis that occurs.

e. Drug-induced systemic lupus erythematosus (SLE) (Table 33G-2 on p. 306). Two groups of drugs are associated with drug-induced SLE. In the first group, aninuclear anibody (ANA) formation is common, but only a small percentage of these lead to the development of clinical symptoms of SLE. The second group includes a large number of drugs that have been (though rarely) reported to induced SLE. ANA formation in this group is not common. A multitude of drugs have been reported, but each may only rarely induce SLE. Exactly how drugs incite anibodies to nuclear protein is unclear at present becausc these agents are in themselves nonimmunogenic. In drug-induced SLE, the antibodies are primarily against histones, in contrast to the idiopathic onset of SLE, in which the ANA are more heterogeneous. Drug-induced SLE produces pleuropulmonary symptoms or chest roentgenogram abnormalities in approximately 50% of cases. In contrast to de novo SLE, complement is normal in drug-induced SLE and renal involvement is rare. ANA (single-stranded) is positive, whereas native (double-stranded) ANA is negative in this syndrome.

II. Associated Respiratory Disorders

Respiratory disorders are associated with certain drugs in which the pathophysiology is either not well understood or is unknown. Various drugs associated with some common disorders are summarized in Table 33G-3 on p. 307.

Bibliography

Cooper JAD Jr, White DA, Matthay RA. Drug-induced pulmonary disease: Part 1: Cytotoxic drugs. *Am Rev Respir Dis* 133:321–340, 1986. Part 2: Noncytotoxic drugs. 133:488–505, 1986.

Rosenow EC III (ed). Drug-induced pulmonary disease. *Semin Respir Med* 2:45–96, 1980.

CHAPTER 34

Miscellaneous Lung Diseases

Larry Casey, M.D., Ph.D.

Alveolar Proteinosis

I. Definition
A rare disease characterized by the deposition of an amorphous proteinaceous material rich in lipids within alveoli.

II. Etiology
Unknown. May be a response to chemical irritants. Possible associations:

A. Acute silicosis

B. Inhalation of inert dusts of extremely fine particulate matter

C. Human immunodeficiency virus–positive patients

D. Possible autosomal recessive inheritance

E. Lymphoid and hematologic malignancies

III. Pathophysiology
A. Chemical analysis

  1. The intra-alveolar material is similar in composition to surfactant; however, it has no surface-active properties.

B. Microscopic analysis

  1. Alveoli filled with granular, acidophilic, periodic acid-Schiff (PAS)–positive material.

  2. Electron microscopy shows many lamellar bodies similar to surfactant.

  3. Alveolar septae are generally normal or have minimal thickening from fibrosis or inflammation.

C. Abnormal macrophage function

  1. The alveolar material impairs macrophage function, leading to an increased incidence of fungal, tuberculous, and bacterial infections.

IV. Diagnosis
A. History

Usually presents insidiously. An abrupt onset suggests infection. Common clinical complaints include:

  1. Dyspnea.

  2. Cough.

  3. Sputum production, sometimes described as containing "tissue."

  4. Weight loss.

B. Clinical signs and physical exam

  1. Frequently, there are no abnormal physical findings.

  2. Rales.

  3. Cyanosis.

  4. Clubbing.

  5. Peak incidence is between 30 and 50 years of age, the disease occurs in all age groups.

6. A 3:1 male:female ratio.
C. Diagnostic tests
   1. Diagnostic test is the demonstration of PAS-positive material in alveoli or sputum. Lung biopsy may be either transbronchial or open.
   2. Hypoxemia.
   3. Pulmonary function tests show a restrictive pattern, with decreased carbon monoxide diffusing capacity.
   4. Chest x-ray shows diffuse bilateral perihilar infiltrates similar to those of congestive heart failure. Other patterns:
      a. Lobar consolidation.
      b. Miliary or interstitial infiltrates.
      c. Hilar adenopathy, pleural effusion, or cavities suggest infection.
   5. Lactic dehydrogenase may be elevated.
   6. Secondary polycythemia.

V. Differential Diagnosis
Any disease producing a diffuse alveolar-filling pattern on chest x-ray.
A. Pulmonary edema
   1. Cardiogenic
   2. Noncardiogenic
B. *Pneumocystis carini*
C. Intrapulmonary hemorrhage
D. Acute toxic inhalation
E. Atypical pneumonias

VI. Treatment
For moderate or severe disease, the treatment is bilateral whole lung lavage done under general anesthesia and lavaging one lung at a time.
A. Placement of a Carlens or double-lumen endotracheal tube for differential ventilation of the lungs.
B. Inhalation of 100% FIO_2.
C. Instillation of warmed normal saline into one lung followed by gravity-dependent drainage.
D. Total volume of saline is generally between 10 and 20 liters or until the turbidity of the lavage fluid clears.

VII. Patient Monitoring
A. Arterial blood gases
B. Chest x-ray
C. Pulmonary function tests
D. Watch for infection, including:
   1. Nocardia
   2. Cryptococcosis
   3. Aspergillosis
   4. Tuberculosis
   5. Bacterial infections

VIII. Prognosis
A. The overall prognosis is variable; approximately 30% of patients may have spontaneous resolution of symptoms, and 30% will die from the disease or from an infection.
B. Bilateral whole lung lavage can result in dramatic improvement and resolution of the disease over several months after the lavage.

Bibliography

Davidson J and MacLeod W. Pulmonary alveolar proteinosis. *Br J Dis Chest* 63:13, 1969.

Rosen S, Castleman B, and Liebow A. Pulmonary alveolar proteinosis. *N Engl J Med* 258:1123, 1958.

Eosinophilic Granuloma
I. Definition
Eosinophilic granuloma is a chronic proliferative disorder characterized by aggregates of atypical lymphocytes and granulomatous infiltration of the lung and bones. It is classified as part of histiocytosis X, along with Letterer-Siwe disease and Hand-Schuller-Christian disease.

II. Etiology
There is no known etiology. The disorder occurs at 20 to 40 years of age, with a slight male predominance. It is not hereditary.

III. Pathophysiology
The diagnostic features on histologic examination is the presence of atypical histiocytes (Langerhans histiocytes) containing characteristic organelles seen on electron microscopy, called *Birbeck granules*, that have the shape of tennis rackets. The Langerhans histiocytes are present with an admixture of eosinophils, lymphocytes, plasma cells, and multinucleated giant cells.
A. Upper lobe predominance. Destruction of alveolar septa results in cyst formation and honeycombing.
B. Other organ involvement includes:
   1. Bone—the disorder was originally described as a bone disease
   2. Skin
   3. Hypothalamus—diabetes insipidus is common
   4. Lymph nodes

IV. Diagnosis
A. History (20% of patients are asymptomatic)
   1. Cough
   2. Dyspnea
   3. Chest pain

4. Pneumothorax, especially in young men
5. Polyuria-polydipisia of diabetes insipidus
6. Weight loss
7. Fever

B. Clinical signs and physical findings
   Physical examination is usually unremarkable, although there may be wheezes or rales.

C. Diagnostic tests
   Laboratory tests are nonspecific.
   1. Pulmonary function tests show restrictive lung disease, but with an elevated residual volume (if there is extreme honeycombing).
   2. The diffusing capacity for carbon monoxide is typically reduced.
   3. There may or may not be evidence of airway obstruction.
   4. Arterial hypoxemia is usually present, either at rest or with exercise.
   5. Chest x-ray
      a. Upper lobe infiltrate, with relative sparing of the lung bases.
         (1) Indistinct nodules.
         (2) Coarse linear densities.
         (3) Bullae.
         (4) Honeycombing.
         (5) Some enlargement of the hilum may occur, but not like that which occurs in sarcoidosis.
   6. Definitive diagnosis requires biopsy
      a. Electron microscopic demonstration of Langerhans histiocytes in either lung biopsy or bronchoalveolar lavage fluid

V. **Differential Diagnosis**
   A. Sarcoidosis
   B. Tuberculosis
   C. Fungal infections
      1. Histoplasmosis
      2. Cryptococcosis
      3. Bastomycosis
      4. Aspergillosis
   D. Silicosis/pneumoconiosis
   E. Idiopathic interstitial pneumonia (usual interstitial pneumonia, desquamative interstitial pneumonia), lymphocytic interstitial pneumonia
   F. Vasculitis

VI. **Treatment**
   A. Self-limited in most patients.
   B. Steroids will improve systemic symptoms and speed resolution of nodular infiltrates.
   C. Radiation is used to treat progressive bone lesions and diabetes insipidus.

VII. **Patient Monitoring**
   A. Arterial blood gases.
   B. Chest X-ray.
   C. Pulmonary function tests.
   D. Watch for pneumothorax.
      1. From 10% to 20% of patients develop spontaneous pneumothorax.
      2. Watch for diabetes insipidus.

VIII. **Prognosis**
   A. Most patients recover with minimal residual symptoms.
   B. A small percentage develop progressive pulmonary fibrosis with cor pulmonale.

Bibliography

Friedman PJ, Liebow AA and Sokoloff J. Eosinophilic granuloma of lung. *Medicine* 60:385, 1981.

Sarcoidosis

I. **Definition**
   Systemic granulomatous disease of unknown etiology.

II. **Etiology**
   Unknown.

III. **Pathophysiology**
   A. Noncaseating granulomas.
   B. Bonchealveolar lavage shows increased numbers of T lymphocytes.
   C. Cutaneaus anergy.

IV. **Diagnosis**
   A. History
      1. Thirty percent of patients are asymptomatic and present with an abnormal chest x-ray taken for other reasons.
      2. Symptoms depend on organ involvement.
         a. The most commonly affected organ is the lung. Symptoms:
            (1) Cough
            (2) Dyspnea
            (3) Chest pain
            (4) Hemoptysis
            (5) Sputum production
   B. Clinical signs and physical findings
      The physical findings are usually limited to the effects of granuloma formation within the involved organs.
      1. Skin
         a. Lupus pernio—smooth, chilblain-like swelling of the face and digits of the hands and feet that becomes firm and indurated.

b. Erythema nodosum—may occur early in the disease and is associated with a favorable outcome.

c. Plaques and nodular lesions.

2. Lymph nodes
   a. Cervical and supraclavicular lymphadenopathy.

3. Lacrimal or salivary gland involvement

4. Eyes
   a. Anterior uveitis
   b. Keratoconjunctivitis
   c. Chorioretinitis

5. Arthralgia is not usually associated with redness, swelling, or heat and is most prominent in the wrists, elbows, ankles, and knees.

6. Fatigability and malaise

7. Fever

8. Lung
   a. Frequently no findings
   b. Wheezing from endobronchial sarcoid
   c. Rales with extensive pulmonary involvement

9. Hepatosplenomegaly

C. Diagnostic tests

There is no single diagnostic test, but routine laboratory tests may help support the diagnosis.

1. Hypergammaglobulinemia

2. Hypercalcemia and hypercalciuria

3. Elevated alkaline phosphatase

4. Chest radiographic classification at presentation
   a. Stage 0—normal (5–16%)
   b. Stage I—bilateral hilar adenopathy (25–40%)
   c. Stage II—bilateral hilar adenopathy with pulmonary infiltrates (24–49%)
   d. Stage III—pulmonary infiltrate without hilar adenopathy (6–15%)

5. Usual biopsy sites
   a. Lung (transbronchial biopsy or open lung)
   b. Lymph node (supraclavicular or mediastinal)
   c. Skin
   d. Subconjunctival
   e. Parotid

6. Angiotensin converting enzyme (ACE) may be elevated in patients with sarcoidosis, but this is not specific.
   a. Other diseases with elevated ACE
      (1) Gaucher's disease
      (2) Tuberculosis
      (3) Granulomatous colitis
      (4) Leprosy
      (5) Lymphangiomyomatosis
      (6) Diabetic retinopathy
      (7) Alcoholic cirrhosis
      (8) Hyperthyroidism
      (9) Bacterial pneumonia
      (10) Acute respiratory distress syndrome

7. Gallium scan
   ^{67}Ga lung scan may show increased uptake in the lung parenchyma, hilar lymph nodes, and parotid and salivary glands.
   a. Gallium uptake is nonspecific, as other infectious or noninfectious diseases can also cause increased gallium uptake in the lung.
   b. The combination of uptake in the lung, lymph nodes, and salivary glands in the appropriate clinical setting is strongly suggestive of sarcoidosis but is not diagnostic.
   c. Gallium scanning has no role in following the course of sarcoidosis (except in research protocols).

8. Kveim test is positive in 70–90% of patients with sarcoidosis.
   a. Limitations
      (1) Available in only a few centers.
      (2) Takes 4–6 weeks.
      (3) Requires a skin biopsy and an experienced pathologist.

9. Bronchoalveolar lavage showing increased numbers of T lymphocytes.

V. Differential Diagnosis

A. Tuberculosis

B. Fungal infection

C. Lymphoma

D. Diseases associated with biopsies showing noncasceating granulomas
   1. Tuberculosis
   2. Fungal diseases
   3. Beryllium disease
   4. Drug reactions

VI. Treatment

The majority of patients with sarcoidosis do not require treatment.

A. Many patients improve spontaneously.

B. Steroid treatment is reserved for patients with symptomatic organ involvement.

C. Steroids may decrease the inflammatory component, but there is no evidence that they prevent fibrosis or improve survival.

VII. Patient Monitoring

A. Follow the patient's symptoms as a guideline to the indication for therapy and the effectiveness of therapy.

B. Chest x-ray.

C. Pulmonary function tests.

D. Watch for the development of infections (particularily tuberculosis and fungal infections), especially if the patient becomes febrile.

E. Hemoptysis in a patient with cavities suggests an aspergillus fungus ball.

F. Watch for the numerous side effects of steroid therapy.

VIII. Prognosis

A. Many patients improve spontaneously.

B. Patients with Löffgrens syndrome (asymptomatic hilar adenopathy, erythema nodosum, and polyarticular arthalgias) have a better prognosis. Treatment requires only nonsteroidal anti-inflammatory drugs.

C. Patients presenting with fibrosis have a worse prognosis.

Bibliography

Siltzbach LE and Jones DG. Course and prognosis of sarcoidosis around the world. *Am J Med* 57:847, 1974.

Winterbauer R, Belve N, and Mooses KD. A clinical interpretation of bilateral hilar adenopathy. *Ann Intern Med* 78:65, 1973.

Mitchell DN and Scodding JG. Sarcoidosis: State of the art. *Am Rev Resp Dis* 110:774, 1974.

Lymphangiomyomatosis

I. Definition

Lymphangiomyomatosis is characterized by hamartomatous proliferation of smooth muscle within the lungs.

II. Etiology

The etiology is unknown. However, the high incidence of this disorder in young women, the occasional exacerbation during pregnancy, and the therapeutic benefit of hysterectomy or progesterone therapy suggest an important role of hormones in its pathogenesis.

III. Pathophysiology

Pathologically, there are nodular masses of smooth muscle cells that may occur in the pleura and alveolar walls, as well as around lymphatics, venules, and bronchioles.

A. Bronchiolar obstruction leads to alveolar obstruction and formation of cysts.

B. Venous obstruction causes venous distention and rupture, resulting in hemosiderosis.

C. Lymphatic obstruction causes lymphatic rupture and the formation of a chylothorax.

IV. Diagnosis

A. History

1. Major symptom is progressive dyspnea.

2. Patients may have a slightly productive cough.

B. Clinical signs and physical examination

1. Classic triad

a. Chylous pleural effusion

b. Hemoptysis

c. Spontaneous pneumothorax

2. Physical examination

a. Rales and/or rhonchi

b. Signs of a pleural effusion

C. Diagnostic tests

The diagnosis is established by biopsy.

1. Chest x-ray: reticulonodular infiltrate with cysts, blebs, or honeycombing at the bases. Despite the interstitial infiltrate, the lungs appear to be hyperinflated.

2. Pulmonary function tests

a. Both obstructive and restrictive patterns

b. Reduced diffusion capacity

c. Progressive increase in total lung capacity

d. Hypoxemia

3. Laboratory tests

These tests are nonspecific, except for the presence of a chylous pleural effusion.

V. Differential Diagnosis

A. All causes of interstitial lung disease

B. Sarcoidosis

C. Eosinophilic granuloma

D. Pulmonary hemosiderosis

VI. Treatment

A. Progesterone therapy or hysterectomy can prevent the progression of the disease if instituted early.

B. β-Agonists can be given for the treatment of bronchospasm.

C. Oxygen can be given if the patient is hypoxemic.

D. Surgical or chemical obliteration of the pleural space is performed for large, recurrent effusions or pneumothorax.

VII. Patient Monitoring

A. Watch for the development of spontaneous pneumothorax.

B. Watch for enlargement of the pleural effusion.

C. Follow arterial oxygenation, pulmonary function tests, and chest x-rays.

VIII. Prognosis

A. Early treatment with progesterone or hysterectomy may prevent progression of the destructive lung disease.

B. Patients presenting with extensive cystic changes and hyperinflation may live for only 3–10 years.

Bibliography

Carrington CB et al;. Lymphangiomyomatosis. Physiologic-pathologic-radiologic correlations. *Am Rev Resp Dis* 116:977, 1977.

McCarty KS et al. Pulmonay lymphangiomyomatosis responsive to progesterone. *N Engl J Med* 303:1461, 1980.

Pulmonary Idiopathic Hemosiderosis

I. Definition

Chronic recurrent intrapulmonary hemorrhage with hemosiderin-laden macrophages.

II. Etiology and Pathogenesis

The etiology and pathogenesis are unknown. Possible etiologic agents include:

A. Early manifestations of systemic lupus erythematosus (SLE).

B. Exposure to insecticides, hydrocarbons, or other toxins

C. Genetic predisposition

III. Diagnosis

The diagnosis is established by demonstrating the presence of intrapulmonary hemorrhage and/or hemosiderin-laden macrophages in the absence of:

A. No focal cause of bleeding.

B. No pulmonary venous hypertension (congestive heart failure, mitral stenosis).

C. No systemic vasculitis or immunologic disease.

D. Wegener's granulomatosis and Goodpasture's syndrome.

E. The diagnosis may have to be revised over time with the subsequent development of an autoimmune disease.

   1. History

     a. May or may not have hemoptysis

     b. Fatigue

     c. Dyspnea

   2. Clinical signs and physical examination

     a. Pallor

     b. Rales

   3. Laboratory tests

     a. Hemosideren-laden macrophages.

     b. Iron deficiency anemia.

     c. Chest x-ray—bilateral alveolar infiltration, especially prominent in the hilum and lower lobes, which clears over 2–3 days, forming a reticular pattern that becomes normal in about 2 weeks.

     d. Pulmonary function tests show a normal to mildly restrictive defect with a markedly elevated diffusing capacity at the time of intrapulmonary hemorrhage.

IV. Differential Diagnosis

A. Wegener's granulomatosis

B. Goodpasture's syndrome

C. Mitral stenosis

D. Congestive heart failure

E. Systemic vasculitis

F. Any focal site of bleeding

V. Treatment

A. High-dose steroids may help during the acute intrapulmonary bleed, but no controlled trials have been done.

B. Long-term steroids probably do not alter the course of the disease.

C. The role of immunosuppressants such as azathioprine is unclear.

D. Supportive therapy with oxygen, mechanical ventilation if necessary, and blood transfusions can be provided.

VI. Patient Monitoring

A. Follow autoimmune profiles, as many patients will subsequently develop an autoimmune disease, most commonly SLE.

B. Sequential pulmonary function tests, particularly the diffusing capacity test and the diffusing/alveolar ventilation test, are helpful.

C. Hemoglobin.

VII. Prognosis

Prognosis is highly variable. Death may occur from massive intrapulmonary hemorrhage. The variability in outcome makes the interpretation of the results of therapy difficult.

Bibliography

Fuleiban FJD, Abboud RJ and Hubayter R. Idiopathic pulmonary hemosiderosis. *Am Rev Resp Dis* 98:93, 1968.

Soergel KH and Sommers SC. Idiopathic pulmonary hemosiderosis and related syndromes. *Am J Med* 32:499, 1962.

CHAPTER 35

Drug-Induced Lung Disease

Michael R. Silver, M.D.

ABBREVIATIONS

A = Patterns of injury

B = Rapidity of onset

C = Frequency

D = Radiographic appearance

E = Clinical

F = Risk factors

G = Dosage

H = Steroids

 I = Mortality

BOOP bronchiolitis obliterans with organizing pneumonia

Acetylsalicylic acid (aspirin) I

A noncardiogenic pulmonary edema
B 1–2 days
C common[1]
D diffuse alveolar infiltrates
E cough, dyspnea

F increased age, chronic ingestion, smoking
G overdose
H ineffective
I low

Acetylsalicylic acid II

A pseudosepsis
B weeks to months
C rare
D diffuse alveolar infiltrates
E fever, leukocytosis, hypotension, multisystem organ failure
F
G
H
I high

Amiodarone

A chronic pneumonitis, fibrosis, BOOP, noncardiogenic pulmonary edema[7]

---

[1]Only after overdose.

[7]When combined with oxygen therapy.

B   1–180 days
C   1–6%
D   reticular, acinar, reticulonodular, pleural effusions,[2] diffuse alveolar infiltrates[7]
E   dyspnea, nonproductive cough, fever, weight loss
F   greater than 400 mg/day, decreasing diffusion capacity (DL_{co}), oxygen therapy
G   maintenance
H   probably effective
I   high

Amphotericin

A   noncardiogenic pulmonary edema
B   1–2 days
C   occasional
D   diffuse alveolar infiltrates
E   dyspnea
F   leukocyte transfusion
G   idosyncratic
H
I   low

Ampicillin

A   hypersensitivity pneumonitis
B   days
C   occasional
D   diffuse alveolar infiltrates
E   dyspnea, fever, eosinophilia
F
G   idiosyncratic
H
I   low

Angiotensin-converting enzyme inhibitors

A   none
B
C   common
D   normal
E   cough
F   more common in women
G
H
I   none

Azathioprine

A   chronic pneumonitis, fibrosis
B   weeks
C   rare
D   reticulonodular
E   cough, dyspnea
F
G
H
I

Bleomycin I

A   chronic pneumonitis, BOOP
B   days to weeks
C   common
D   reticulonodular, nobular, pneumothorax[2]
E   cough, dyspnea
F   greater than 450–500 U/cumulative, supplemental oxygen therapy,[3] increased age, radiotherapy,[4,5] concurrent cyclophosphamide, ?renal failure
G   cumulative
H   equivocal
I   low

Bleomycin II

A   hypersensitivity pneumonitis
B   days
C   occasional
D   acinar, diffuse alveolar infiltrates,[3] pleural effusion[2]
E   dyspnea, eosinophilia, fever
F
G   idiosyncratic, ?cumulative
H   effective
I   low

Bleomycin III

A   acute pleritic/pericardial pain[9]
B   1–2 days
C
D   normal
E   chest pain, dyspnea
F   does not reoccur with subsequent administration

---

[2]Uncommon.
[3]As little as 30% FIO_2 may increase the risk of toxicity.
[4]Sequence of radiotherapy unimportant.
[5]Less than 3,300 rads of pulmonary radiation may be safe.
[9]Only one study reported.

---

[2]Uncommon.
[7]When combined with oxygen therapy.

G first or second dose only
H
I low

Bromocriptine

A chronic pleural effusions
B months to years
C occasional
D pleural effusions
E lymphocytic pleural effusions, elevated sedimentation rate
F
G symptoms resolve when drug discontinued
H
I low

Busulfan

A chronic pneumonitis, alveolar proteinosis
B 6 weeks to 10 years, average 3 years
C common
D acinar, reticular, reticulonodular
E nonproductive cough, dyspnea, weight loss, fever
F < 500 mg probably safe, 2,900 mg average for patients with disease, probably radiotherapy
G cumulative
H
I high (mean survival, 5 months)

Carbamazepine

A hypersensitivity
B days
C rare
D acinar
E dyspnea, fever, eosinophilia
F
G
H effective
I low

Carmustine

A chronic pneumonitis
B months to years
C common
D reticular, pneumothorax[2]
E dyspnea, nonproductive cough

F younger patients, no drug threshold
G cumulative[9]
H
I high

Chlorambucil

A chronic pneumonitis
B 6–36 months
C rare
D reticular
E cough, dyspnea, fever, anorexia
F
G
H probably ineffective
I high (50%)

Chlordiazepoxide

A noncardiogenic pulmonary edema
B 1–2 days
C rare
D diffuse alveolar infiltrates
E dyspnea
F
G
H
I low

Chlorpropamide

A noncardiogenic pulmonary edema
B 1–2 days
C rare
D diffuse alveolar infiltrates
E dyspnea
F
G
H
I low

Chlorpromazine[14]

Cocaine

A noncardiogenic pulmonary edema, BOOP, pulmonary hemorrhage, fibrosis[13]
B 1–2 days

---

[2]Uncommon.

[9]Only one study reported.
[14]Suggested to cause drug-induced SLE.
[13]Rare.

C   rare
D   diffuse alveolar infiltrates, acinar infiltrates, retic-
    ular[13]
E   dyspnea
F
G
H
I   low

Colchicine

A   noncardiac pulomonary edema
B   1–2 days
C   rare
D   diffuse alveolar infiltrates
E   dyspnea
F   overdose
G   overdose
H
I   low

Cromolyn

A   noncardiogenic pulmonary edema
B   1–2 days
C   rare
D   diffuse alveolar infiltrates
E   dyspnea
F
G
H
I   low

Cyclophosphamide

A   hypersensitivity pneumonitis, BOOP
B   2 weeks–13 years, usually weeks
C   occasional
D   acinar
E   cough, dyspnea, fever, eosinophilia
F   ?oxygen therapy, ?concurrent vincristine
G   idiosyncratic
H   effective
I   high

Cytosine Arabinoside

A   noncardiogenic pulmonary edema

B
C   common
D   diffuse alveolar infiltrates
E   dyspnea, hemoptysis[2]
F
G
H
I   high

Dantrolene

A   noncardiogenic pulmonary edema
B   1–2 days
C   rare
D   diffuse alveolar infiltrates
E   dyspnea
F
G
H
I   low

Dipyridamole[9]

A   acute airflow obstruction
B   minutes to hours
C   rare
D   normal
E   dyspnea, wheezing
F
G
H
I   low

Diphenylhydantoin[14]

A   hypersensitivity pneumonitis
B   3–6 weeks
C   rare
D   acinar, diffuse alveolar infiltrates, hilar and medi-
    astinal adenopathy
E   dyspnea, fever, eosinophilia
F
G
H   effective
I   low

---

[13]Rare.

[2]Uncommon.
[9]Only one study reported.
[14]Suggested to cause drug-induced SLE.

Esophageal Variceal Sclerotherapy

A   pleural effusions, noncardiogenic pulmonary edema[13]
B   1–2 days
C   common
D   mediastinal widening, pleural effusions, atelectasis, infiltrates, diffuse alveolar infiltrates[13]
E   fever, chest pain, dyspnea
F
G
H
I   low

Ethchlorvynol

A   noncardiogenic pulmonary edema
B   1–2 days
C   rare
D   diffuse alveolar infiltrates
E   dyspnea
F   only after overdose
G
H
I   low

Fludarabine monophosphate

A   chronic pneumonitis, fibrosis
B   1–2 days
C   rare
D   reticulonodular
E   fever, dyspnea, cough
F
G   idiosyncratic
H   +
I   low

Gold salts

A   chronic pneumonitis, fibrosis, BOOP, hypersensitivity penumonitis[2]
B   1–180 days (usually < 3 months)
C   occasional
D   reticulonodular
E   dyspnea, eosinophilia, cough, fever, dermatitis, wheezing[2]
F

---
[13]Rare.
[2]Uncommon.

G
H   equivocal
I   low

Haloperidol

A   noncardiogenic pulmonary edema
B   1–2 days
C   rare
D   diffuse alveolar infiltrates
E   dyspnea
F
G   only after overdose
H
I   low

Heroin

A   Noncardiogenic pulmonary edema
B   1–2 days
C   occasional
D   diffuse alveolar infiltrates
E   dyspnea
F
G   only after overdose
H
I   low

Hyskon (Low Molecular Weight Dextran)

A   noncardiogenic pulmonary edema
B   hours
C   uncommon
D   diffuse alveolar infiltrates
E   dyspnea, coagulopathy
F   procedure lasts for more than 45 min, inflamed endometrial surfaces
G   more than 500 ml used
H
I   low

Hydrochlorothiazide

A   noncardiogenic pulmonary edema
B   20 min to 2 days
C   rare
D   diffuse alveolar infiltrates
E   dyspnea, cough, fever, altered blood pressure
F   almost exclusively in women, intermittent, not daily therapy
G   idiosyncratic, occurs with rechallenge

H   equivocal
I   low

Hydralazine[12]

A   hypersensitivity penumonitis
B   days
C   rare
D   acinar, diffuse alveolar infiltrates
E   dyspnea, fever, eosinophilia
F
G
H
I   low

Imipramine

A   Hypersensitivity pneumonitis
B   days
C   rare
D   acinar, diffuse alveolar infiltrates
E   dyspnea, fever, eosinophilia
F
G
H
I   low

Interleukin-2

A   noncardiogenic pulmonary edema, acute airflow
     obstruction
B   1–2 days
C   common
D   diffuse alveolar infiltrates, pleural effusions
E   dyspnea
F
G   idiosyncratic
H
I   low

Isoniazid[12]

A   hypersensitivity pneumonitis
B   days
C   rare
D   acinar, diffuse alveolar infiltrates
E   dyspnea, fever, eosinophilia
F

G
H
I   low

Lidocaine

A   noncardiogenic pulmonary edema
B   1–2 days
C   rare
D   diffuse alveolar infiltrates
E   dyspnea
F   parenteral, oral, or topical
G   idiosyncratic
H
I   low

Lomostine (CCNU)[9]

Same as carmustine

Mecamylamine

A   hypersensitivity pneumonitis
B   days
C   rare
D   acinar, diffuse alveolar infiltrates
E   dyspnea, fever, eosinophilia
F
G
H
I   low

Melphalan

A   chronic pneumonitis
B   1–4 months
C   rare
D   reticular, reticulonodular, acinar
E   cough, dyspnea, malaise
F
G
H
I   high

Mephenesin caramate

A   hypersensitivity pneumonitis
B   days

---

[12]Known to cause drug-induced systemic lupus erythematosus (SLE).

[9]Only one study reported.

C   rare
D   acinar, diffuse alveolar infiltrates
E   dyspnea, fever, eosinophilia
F
G
H
I   low

Methadone

A   noncardiogenic pulmonary edema
B   1–2 days
C   rare
D   diffuse alveolar infiltrates
E   dyspnea
F
G   only after overdose
H
I   low

Methotrexate I

A   hypersensitivity pneumonitis, BOOP
B   days (weeks[10])
C   occasional (common[10])
D   acinar, diffuse alveolar infiltrates, pleural effusions[2]
E   dyspnea, fever, eosinophilia, pleuritic chest pain, dermopathy,[2] dough[10]
F   ?concurrent nitrofurantoin, ?concurrent cyclo-phosphamide
G   frequency of administration (daily, weekly vs. monthly), not cumulative dose
H
I   low

Methotrexate II

A   noncardiogenic pulmonary edema
B   1–2 days
C   occasional
D   diffuse alveolar infiltrates
E   dyspnea
F   ?concurrent cyclophosphamide
G   idiosyncratic, discontinuation not required, may not occur with reinstitution of therapy, can occur after intrathecal administration
H
I   low

Methylphenidate

A   hypersensitivity pneumonitis
B   days
C   rare
D   acinar, diffuse alveolar infiltrates, emphysema
E   chest pain, wheezing, dyspnea, hemoptysis
F
G
H
I   low

Mitomycin

A   chronic pneumonitis, BOOP
B   days to months
C   occasional
D   reticular, reticulonodular, pleural effusions, hilar adenopathy[13]
E   cough, dyspnea, bronchospasm[6]
F   radiation, oxygen, concurrent vinblastine therapy
G
H
I

Naloxone

A   noncardiogenic pulmonary edema
B   1–2 days
C   rare
D   diffuse alveolar infiltrates
E   dyspnea
F
G
H
I   low

Nebulized Medications (Pentamidine, Beclomethasone, Airway Propellents)

A   acute airway obstruction
B   minutes to hours
C   rare
D   normal
E   dyspnea, wheezing, cough
F

---

[10]With chronic low-dose administration.
[2]Uncommon.

[13]Rare.
[6]When combined with vinblastine.

G
H
I   low

Nitrofurantoin I

A   noncardiogenic pulmonary edema
B   1–180 days, 90% within 1 month
C   common
D   reticular, reticulonodular, nodular
E   dyspnea, fever, rash, fatigue, arthralgia, pleuritis,
     effusions, cyanosis,[2] wheezing[13]
F   inversely related to number of prior exposures
G
H
I   low

Nitrofurantoin II

A
B   2–60 months of continuous therapy
C   occasional
D   acinar, pleural effusions
E   cough, dyspnea, eosinophilia
F
G
H   not effective
I   high

Nitrosoureas[8]

Para-aminosalicylic Acid

A   hypersensitivity pneumonitis
B   days
C   rare
D   acinar, diffuse alveolar infiltrates
E   dyspnea, fever, eosinophilia, lymphadeonpathy,
     dermatitis, angioneurotic edema
F
G
H
I   low

Penicillin[14]

A   hypersensitivity pneumonitis
B   days
C   rare
D   acinar, diffuse alveolar infiltrates
E   dyspnea, fever, eosinophilia
F
G
H
I   low

Penicillamine[14] I

A   BOOP
B   early or late
C   rare
D   normal
E   cough, fever[2]
F
G
H
I   high

Penicillamine II

A   chronic pneumonitis,[13] fibrosis[13]
B   1–180 days
C   rare
D   reticular, reticulonodular
E   cough, dyspnea, fever[2]
F
G
H
I   low

Penicillamine III

A   pulmonary hemorrhage
B   early or late
C   rare
D   acinar, diffuse alveolar infiltrates
E   cough, hemoptysis
F   ?cumulative
G
H
I   high

---

[2]Uncommon.
[13]Rare.
[8]Produces a clinical picture similar to that of sarcoidosis.

---

[14]Suggested to cause drug-induced SLE.
[2]Uncommon.
[13]Rare.

Procainamide

Cause of drug-induced SLE

Procarbazine

A   hypersensitivity pneumonitis, chronic pneumo-
   nitis[13]
B   days
C   rare
D   acinar, diffuse alveolar infiltrates
E   dyspnea, fever, eosinophilia, rash
F
G
H
I   low

Propoxphene

A   noncardiogenic pulmonary edema
B   1–2 days
C   rare
D   diffuse alveolar infiltrates
E   dyspnea
F
G   only with overdose
H
I   low

Protamine[9]

A   acute airflow obstruction
B   minutes to hours
C   rare
D   normal
E   dyspnea
F
G
H
I   low

Ritodrine

See Tocolytics

Semustine[9]

See Carmustine

Sulfonamide[14]

A   hypersensitivity pneumonitis
B   days
C   rare
D   acinar, diffuse alveolar infiltrates
E   dyspnea, fever, eosinophilia
F
G
H
I   low

Sulfasalazine

A   hypersensitivity pneumonitis, acute broncho-
   spasm, BOOP[13]
B   days
C   rare
D   acinar
E   fever, cough, dyspnea, eosinophilia
F
G   idiosyncratic
H   effective
I   low

Sulfadimethoxine

A   hypersensitivity pneumonitis
B   days
C   rare
D   acinar, diffuse alveolar infiltrates
E   dyspnea, fever, eosinophilia
F
G
H
I   low

Talc

A   Fibrosis, progressive massive fibrosis
B   months to years
C   uncommon
D   upper lobe nodules, retraction, pneumothorax
E   dyspnea, cough
F
G   progresses even after drugs discontinued
H
I   high

---

[13]Rare.
[9]Only one study reported.

[14]Suggested to cause drug-induced SLE.
[13]Rare.

Terbutaline

See Tocolytics

Thiazide

See Hydrochlorothiazide

Tocainide

A   chronic pneumonitis, fibrosis
B   1–180 days
C   rare
D   reticular, reticulonodular
E   cough, dyspnea, fever[2]
F
G
H   equivocal
I   low

Tocolytics (Ritodrine, Terbutaline)

A   noncardiogenic pulmonary edema
B   1–2 days
C   occasional
D   diffuse alveolar infiltrates
E   dyspnea
F   use of steroids, anemia, fluid overload, twin gestation, multiparous
G   idiosyncratic
H   not effective
I   low

Tumor Necrosis Factor

A   noncardiogenic pulmonary edema
B   1–2 days
C   rare
D   diffuse alveolar infiltrates
E   reduced $D_{L_{CO2}}$ weeks after administration,[9] dyspnea
F
G
H
I   low

Vinblastine

A   interstitial pneumonitis, noncardiogenic pulmonary edema[2]

B   days
C   rare
D   reticular, diffuse alveolar infiltrates
E   bronchospasm, dyspnea
F   concurrent mitomycin-C administration increases risk to 5%
G
H
I

Vindesine

A   acute bronchospasm
B   days
C   occasional
D   normal, acinar
E   dyspnea, wheezing
F   concurrent mitomycin therapy
G
H
I   high[11]

VM-26

A   noncardiogenic pulmonary edema
B   days
C   rare
D   diffuse alveolar infiltrates
E   dyspnea
F
G
H
I

Bibliography

Cooper JAD Jr, DA White, RA Matthay. Drug-induced pulmonary disease: part 1. cytotoxic drugs. *Am Rev Respir Dis* 133:321–340. 1986.

Cooper JAD Jr, DA White, RA Matthay. Drug-induced pulmonary disease: part 2. noncytotoxic drugs. *Am Rev Respir Dis* 133:488–505. 1986.

EC Rosenow III, JL Myers, SJ Swensen, and RJ Pisani. Drug-induced pulmonary disease: an update. *Chest* 102: 239–250. 1992.

Vogelzang PJ, SM Bloom, JW Mier, MB Atkins. Chest roentgenographic abnormalities in IL-2 recipients. *Chest* 101:746–752. 1992.

---

[2]Uncommon.
[9]Only one study reported.

[11]If chest radiograph is abnormal.

SECTION 5

Critical Care and Emergency Medicine

CHAPTER 36

Cardiopulmonary Resuscitation (CPR)

Paul K. Hanashiro, M.D.
Jerrold B. Leikin, M.D.

I. General Considerations

A. Cardiopulmonary arrest is still the leading cause of death in the United States (approximately 400,000 deaths per year).

B. CPR in the treatment of cardiopulmonary arrest is effective, but only if performed early.

C. The therapeutic window for CPR is extremely short (4–6 min to initiate treatment).

D. The percentage of long-term survivors have been disappointingly low (2%–26% in large series).

E. Early response times, immediate defibrillation, with endotracheal intubation and combined cardiopulmonary support are keys to a successful outcome.

F. Bystander CPR prior to definitive CPR seems to widen the therapeutic window, thereby increasing the rate of successful outcomes.

G. External cardiac compression provides, at best, 25% of normal circulatory flow and is inadequate to provide long-term circulatory support.

H. Major issues that need to be resolved:

1. Provide means of enhancing early response and treatment times.

2. Provide early defibrillation.

3. Improve artificial circulation during resuscitation.

4. Protect brain function during resuscitation.

II. Objectives of CPR

A. Provide emergent temporary cardiopulmonary support for patients who suffer abrupt cessation of cardiopulmonary function.

B. Restore spontaneous cardiopulmonary function as rapidly as possible.

III. Clinical Situations of Sudden Cardiopulmonary Arrest

Sudden collapse with unresponsiveness, apnea, and pulselessness (indications for CPR).

A. Cardiac arrest

1. Tachyarrhythmias

a. Ventricular fibrillation.

b. Ventricular tachycardia with hemodynamic instability.

c. Supraventricular tachycardia with hemodynamic instability.

2. Bradyarrhythmias

a. Asystole.

b. Complete heart block with inadequate ventricular response.

3. Electromechanical dissociation

a. Hypoxia
   (1) Intubation of the esophagus or of the left or right mainstem bronchus.
   (2) Tension pneumothorax
   (3) Pulmonary edema/hemorrhage
   (4) Upper airway obstruction
b. Pericardial tamponade
c. Massive pulmonary embolus
d. Myocardial or aortic rupture
e. Shock—cardiogenic, septic, anaphylactic, hemorrhagic, adrenal
f. Exsanguination
g. Severe acidosis

B. Respiratory arrest
   1. Acute upper airway obstruction
   2. Primary apnea
      a. Chemical or drug-induced
      b. Fatigue
      c. Central nervous system (CNS) dysfunction

IV. Techniques of CPR

A. Defibrillation—most urgent need in the presence of ventricular fibrillation.
   1. Best results obtained when performed within 6 min of ventricular fibrillation.
   2. Success rate for defibrillation rapidly decreases with increasing interval from the onset of ventricular fibrillation to the time of defibrillation
   3. Should be the first therapeutic maneuver when ventricular fibrillation is first identified.
      a. Single precordial thump can be tried initially in witnessed arrest, with or without identification of ventricular fibrillation.
      b. Electrical defibrillation is the definitive treatment for ventricular fibrillation.
         (1) Consecutive attempts at 200, 300, and 360 J prior to other CPR maneuvers.
         (2) Follow ventricular fibrillation drug protocol in refractory ventricular fibrillation (Table 36-1).
   4. Automatic external defibrillators—simplify training and use, thereby allowing trained laypeople to apply early defibrillation

B. "ABCs" of CPR
   1. A—Airway control
   2. B—Breathing
      a. Airway control and breathing are best accomplished simultaneously by endotracheal intubation.

Table 36-1. Drug Therapy in Refractory Ventricular Fibrillation

Epinephrine—5- to 10-ml 1:10,00 IV bolus or through endotracheal tube if IV access is not available; repeat every 5 min.

Lidocaine—75 mg or 1.5 mg/kg IV bolus; repeat with 50 mg every 10 min × 3; start infusion at 2 mg/min.

Bretylium—500 mg or 5 mg/kg IV; repeat with 10 mg/kg every 5 min × 2.

Procainamide—100 mg in 5 min or 20 mg/min up to 1.0 g; start infusion at 1–2 mg/min.

Consider $MgSO_4$, propranolol, amiodarone

Note: Defibrillation attempts should be made after each additional drug administration while CPR is being maintained.

b. Intubation should take less than 15 sec per attempt. Ventilation should be interposed with cardiac compression.
c. Tracheal intubation allows additional access for drugs such as epinephrine, atropine, naloxone, and lidocaine when venous access is not available. The dose should be 2–2.5 times the IV dose.

3. C—Circulation
   a. External chest compression is effective in providing artificial circulation for only a short period, since it provides only 25% of normal circulation.
      (1) Mechanism of flow generation is in debate (whether due to direct compression of the heart or to increasing intrathoracic pressure).
      (2) Several methods to increase flow have been tested experimentally using thoracic vests, mast suits, and interposed thoracic and abdominal compression, with varying results. However, their clinical superiority has not been established.
      (3) Current American Heart Association guidelines recommend a compression:relaxation ratio of 1:1 and a compression rate of 80–100/min. Compressions should be 2–2.5 in. in depth in the adult patient.
   b. Open cardiac massage
      (1) Cardiac output is double that obtained by external chest compressions.
      (2) Effective in specific settings, such as the operating room or catherization laboratory when conventional CPR is unsuccessful.

(3) Impractical in the field or in open wards.

c. Cardiopulmonary assist devices in appropriate settings such as operating rooms, catheterization laboratories, and emergency departments may be effective; they can also be used in hypothermia cases as warming devices.

C. Venous access

Venous access should be established as soon as possible for the administration of medications and fluids.

1. A peripheral vein, including the femoral vein, is the simplest approach, although transit time is delayed by about 90 sec.
2. Placement of a central line should be attempted after intubation for more rapid delivery of fluids and medication.
    a. Internal jugular approach—any of the three following approaches is preferred over the subclavian approach:
       (1) Anterior
       (2) Central
       (3) Posterior
    b. Subclavian vein approach—increases risk of pneumothorax.
    c. Venous cutdowns are rarely indicated for the adult victim.

D. Medications

1. Epinephrine—the most important drug in CPR.
    a. Effective in ventricular fibrillation, asystole, and electromechanical dissociation due to its chronotropic, inotropic, and vasoconstrictive effects.
    b. Increases coronary and cerebral flow.
    c. Converts fine ventricular fibrillation to coarse ventricular fibrillation, making defibrillation more effective.
    d. Dosage: A 1.0-mg bolus is given early in CPR, either IV or into an endotracheal tube; it may be repeated at 3- to 5-min intervals. Recent reports suggest higher concentrations (2–10 mg), particularly in refractory cases, but its clinical use is not clearly established.
2. Dopamine—used in high doses to maximize the α-adrenergic effects of raising the blood pressure. Dosage: 10–40 μ/kg/min IV.
3. Atropine—used in asystole or bradycardia. Dosage: 0.5-mg IV bolus every 5 min up to 2 mg or 1-mg bolus into an endotracheal tube.
4. Sodium bicarbonate—no longer recommended as a first-line drug in CPR; listed only for severe acidosis and hyperkalemia. Dosage: 1 mEq/kg followed by 0.5 mEq/kg at 10-min intervals, preferably guided by arterial pH determinations.
5. Lidocaine—used in refractory ventricular fibrillation or tachycardia. No longer used as prophylaxis for preventing primary ventricular fibrillation in routine acute myocardial infarction.
    a. Early distribution half-life is 8 min; therefore, multiple loading doses must be given.
    b. Dosage: 75 mg or 1.5 mg/kg IV bolus; repeat with 50 mg at 8- to 10-min intervals up to a total of 225 mg or 3 mg/kg. Start concomitant infusion at 2 mg/min.
6. Bretylium—used in refractory ventricular fibrillation after lidocaine.
    a. Works synergistically with lidocaine.
    b. May cause hypotension.
    c. Dosage: 5 mg/kg IV bolus; repeat in 5 min with 10 mg/kg.
7. Calcium—no longer used in routine CPR.
    a. Clinical studies show no benefit.
    b. Potential deleterious effect.
       (1) Reperfusion injury
       (2) CNS dysfunction
    c. Consider use in:
       (1) Patients receiving calcium channel blocker therapy or experiencing toxicity.
       (2) Suspected hyperkalemia (renal failure) or hypocalcemia.
    d. Dosage: 10% $CaCl_2$—5 ml every 10 min × 4.
8. Magnesium—may be used in refractory ventricular dysrhythmias or torsade de pointes. Dosage: 1- to 2-g IV bolus in 1–2 minutes; repeat in 5–10 min; concomitant infusion 2–20 mg/min.

E. Adjunctive therapy

1. Pacemaker therapy
    a. Must be used early in CPR to be effective.
    b. Indications
       (1) Witnessed asystole with intermittent, spontaneous response to conventional CPR.
       (2) Postresuscitation bradycardia <50 beats/min unresponsive to medications (atropine, 1–2 mg IV, or isoproterenol infusion, 2–10 μg/min).

(3) Second- or third-degree heart block after resuscitation.

(4) Unstable spontaneous rhythm after resuscitation.

(5) Recurrent or incessant ventricular tachycardia refractory to drugs.

c. Nonindication

(1) Ventricular fibrillation.

(2) Electromechanical dissociation with heart rate >50 beats/min.

(3) Unwitnessed asystole unresponsive to conventional CPR.

(4) Terminal asystole after prolonged CPR.

2. Brain resuscitation

a. The brain is most sensitive to anoxic injury, leading to:

(1) Postresuscitation hypoperfusion.

(2) Cascade of toxic metabolic events causing further brain injury.

(3) Major determinant of ultimate survival.

b. Many experimental studies show promise, such as barbiturate anesthesia, calcium entry blockers, desferoxamine, short-term hypothermia, hyperbaric oxygenation, carotid perfusion, and hemodilution.

c. Clinical investigations thus far have been disappointing.

3. End-tidal CO_2 and arteriovenous CO_2, pH gradients.

a. Reflect tissue acidosis and flow.

b. May be used to assess effectiveness in CPR.

c. May have prognostic value.

V. CPR—Practical Considerations

A. General

1. American Heart Association (AHA) Standards and Guidelines for Basic Life Support (BLS) and Advanced Cardiac Life Support (ACLS) are still the cornerstones for CPR.

2. Updated AHA Guidelines

a. BLS

(1) Call 911 or other source of help.

(2) Open airway with head tilt and chin lift.

(3) Two slow breaths initially instead of four quick breaths

(4) Increase compression rate to 80–100/min.

(5) Clear foreign bodies from the airway with the Heimlich maneuver instead of the back slap.

b. ACLS

(1) Defibrillation—three consecutive shocks initially in ventricular fibrillation prior to CPR.

(2) Sodium bicarbonate is no longer a first-line drug.

(3) Calcium is no longer recommended in routine CPR.

(4) Lidocaine is the first-line drug treatment in refractory ventricular fibrillation

3. The setting of CPR is often chaotic, with rapid changes occurring in cardiopulmonary arrest from moment to moment, requiring multiple interventions almost simultaneously.

a. A team leader must be assigned to coordinate activities.

b. A set of priorities must be established and pursued in a simple, systematic fashion.

B. Therapeutic priorities

Table 36-2 summarizes the priorities for CPR. The therapeutic maneuvers are best accomplished by a team, with each member assigned to a specific therapeutic maneuver. When this is not possible, the AHA, BLS, and ACLS guidelines are instituted until additional help arrives.

1. Ventricular fibrillation—best outcome achieved if defibrillation is performed early.

a. Witnessed arrest with no monitors or defibrillator—use single precordial thump, then CPR.

b. Identified ventricular fibrillation/ventricular tachycardia

(1) Defibrillate immediately with 200 J; if no response occurs, repeat in rapid sequence at 300 J and at 360 J.

(2) In refractory ventricular fibrillation, initiate conventional CPR and use drug treatment protocol for ventricular fibrillation.

2. Asystole—poor outcome; may be the end stage of prolonged ventricular fibrillation.

a. Initiate CPR.

b. Epinephrine—give 1 mg early via endotracheal or IV access; repeat doses every 5 min.

c. Atropine—give 1-mg IV bolus; repeat in 3–5 min up to a total of 0.04 mg/kg.

d. Consider bicarbonate, 1 mEq/kg IV bolus, preferably with pH monitoring.

Table 36-2. CPR Priorities

Defibrillate

As soon as ventricular fibrillation is identified, defibrillate starting at 200 J and repeating with 300 J and 360 J consecutively if no response is noted.

ABCs of CPR

A—Establish and clear airway

B—Ventilate

Mouth-to-mouth resuscitation

Bag-valve-mask preferred in emergency room setting

Mechanical ventilation

Note: A and B accomplished simultaneously by tracheal intubation; this provides an additional route for certain drugs; intubation attempt must take less than 15 sec per attempt.

Ventilation should be interposed.

C—Chest compression: use 1:1 compression: relaxation ratio; 2–2.5 in. 80–100 beats/min.

Establish venous access

Medications in CPR: tracheal route—epinephrine, atropine, lidocaine, naloxone

Intravenous route—epinephrine is the key drug.

Pacemaker Insertion—effective if used early.

Assess underlying cause of cardiac arrest and institute treatment.

e. Consider defibrillation or check alternative leads for ventricular fibrillation.

f. Consider pacing only if intermittent, spontaneous, organized cardiac rhythm is noted.

3. Electromechanical dissociation—poor outcome if treatable causes are not detected and corrected.

a. Correctable causes

(1) Hypoxia

(a) Airway obstruction

(b) Pneumothorax

(c) Pulmonary edema

(2) Hypovolemia

(3) Cardiac tamponade

(4) Acidosis

(5) Shock

(6) Pulmonary embolus

b. Unlikely correctable cause

(1) Myocardial or aortic rupture

(2) Massive myocardial damage

(3) Prolonged ischemia

c. Epinephrine in combination with a high concentration of dopamine infusion should be used to secure hemodynamic stability, along with volume challenges in hypovolemic states.

d. Bicarbonate therapy should be used to correct severe metabolic acidosis.

e. Repeated efforts should be made to identify and correct the cause of the electromechanical dissociation.

4. Respiratory arrest

a. Clear airway

(1) With signs of acute obstruction

(a) Foreign body—apply Heimlich maneuver or remove manually.

(b) No foreign body

i) Puncture cricothyroid membrane with 10- to 14-gauge angioneedle catheter and ventilate with intermittent jet.

ii) Cricothyrotomy.

b. Naloxone—at least 2 mg IV if there is no sign of obstruction.

c. Tracheal intubation and mechanical ventilation.

5. Assessment and treatment of underlying cause of cardiac arrest

a. Definitive corrective measures

(1) Cardiac tamponade—pericardiocentesis

(2) Pneumothorax—thorocentesis and tube insertion

(3) Hypovolemia—volume repletion

(4) Acute ischemic syndromes—revascularization

(5) Pulmonary embolus—possible thrombolytic therapy

(6) Acidosis—bicarbonate therapy

6. Terminating CPR

a. Terminate if no spontaneous response of organized cardiac activity is noted within 10–15 min of advanced life support.

b. Continue CPR in the following situations:
   (1) Hypothermia
   (2) Drug-induced arrest
   (3) Electrocution
   (4) Refractory ventricular fibrillation—when CPR is initiated within 6 min and is being maintained adequately, by evidence of spontaneous movements of the victim, adequate oxygenation, and absence of acidosis by blood gas measurements. (Thoracotomy and open cardiac massage might be an option.)
7. Survival unlikely if CPR extends beyond 30 min.
   a. Linear regression model predicting out-of-hospital cardiac arrest survival rate equals 67% − 2.3% per minute of CPR − 1.1% per minute to defibrillation − 2.1% per minute to A.C.L.S. therapy. Without any treatment, the decline in survival rate is 5.5% per minute
   b. Patients with asystole or electromechanical dissociation at the scene usually have poor outcome.
8. Postarrest care
   a. Maintain cardiopulmonary support until patient is stable.
   b. Monitor CNS function meticulously, especially for signs of increased intracranial pressure and hypoxemia.
   c. Pursue definitive treatment of the underlying problem, such as coronary revascularization procedures, surgery, etc.
   d. Monitor for multiorgan dysfunction.
9. Future considerations in CPR
   a. Increased use of automatic external defibrillators.
      (1) Use by first responders, including All emergency medical technicians, police, fireman, family members of high-risk cardiacs, personnel in aid stations in public gatherings.
   b. Simplify and increase training in BLS—bystander CPR shown to increase successful outcomes.
   c. Improve techniques in external cardiac massage to increase flow—extensive experimental investigations show limited clinical utility.
   d. Improve brain resuscitation with techniques instituted during arrest and pos-

tarrest periods—probably a combination effort—to protect the metabolic functions of the brain while restoring perfusion to the brain.
   e. Use of interposed abdominal-aortic counterpulsation (IAC-CPR) to improve survival in cardiac arrest.
      (1) Open hands over umbilicus, with 100 mm pressure at a rate equal to chest compression.
      (2) Abdominal compression coordinates with early relaxation phase.
      (3) In-hospital cardiac arrest survival rates (including that of neurologically intact patients) improved with use of IAC-CPR.
      (4) Continuous abdominal compression may be effective.
   f. Use of cough—CPR may be effective in ventricular fibrillation for up to 93 sec.
      (1) Instruct patient to cough hard at 1- to 3-sec intervals.
      (2) A cough can generate up to 25 J.
      (3) It can cardiovert ventricular tachycardia.
   g. Use of active chest compression-decompression devices (ACD-CPR).

Bibliography

Abramson SA. Randomized clinical study of thiopental loading in comatose survivors of cardiac arrest: Brain resuscitation clinical trail 1 study group. *N Engl J Med* 314:397–403, 1986.

American Heart Association. *Textbook of Advanced Cardiac Life Support.* Dallas, TX, American Heart Association, 1987. Emergency Cardiac Care Committee and Subcommittees, American Heart Association. Guidelines for cardiopulmonary resuscitation and emergency cardiac care, 1:introduction. *JAMA* 268:2172–2183, 1992.

Barton C, Callaham M. High-dose epinephrine improves the return of spontaneous circulation rates in human victims of cardiac arrest. *Ann Emerg Med* 20:722–725, 1991.

Becker LB, Ostrander MP, Barrett J, et al. Outcome of CPR in a large metropolitan area—where are the survivors?. *Ann Emerg Med* 20:355–361, 1991.

Beless DJ, Otsuki JA, Davis WE. Neurologically intact survivor of prolonged ventricular fibrillation: A case for intermediate dose epinephrine and postresuscitation infusion. *Am J Emerg Med* 10:133–135, 1992.

Bleske BE, Chow MS, Zhao H, et al. Effect of different dosages and modes of sodium bicarbonate administration during cardiopulmonary resuscitation. *Am J Emerg Med* 10:525–532, 1992.

Brown CG, Martin DR, Pepe PE, et al. A comparison of

standard-dose and high-dose epinephrine in cardiac arrest outside the hospital. *N Engl J Med* 327:1051–1055, 1992.

Callaham M, Madsen CD, Barton CW, et al. A randomized clinical trial of high-dose epinephrine and norepinephrine vs. standard-dose epinephrine in prehospital cardiac arrest. *JAMA* 268:2667–2672, 1992.

Christenson JM, Hamilton DR, Scott-Douglas NW, et al. Abdominal compressions during CPR: Hemodynamic effects of altering timing and force. *J Emerg Med* 10:257–266, 1992.

Cohen TJ, Tucker KJ, Lurie KG, et al. Active compression-decompression. A new method of cardiopulmonary resuscitation. *JAMA* 267:2923, 1992.

Cummins RO, Eisenberg MS, Bergner L, et al. Automatic external defibrillation: Evaluations of its role in the home and in emergency medical services. *Ann Emerg Med* 13:798–801, 1984.

Del Guercio L, Feins N, Cohn J, et al. Comparison of blood flow during external and internal cardiac massage in man. *Circulation* 31(suppl 1):171–180, 1965.

Eisenberg MS, Horwood BT, Cummins RO, et al. Cardiac arrest and resuscitation: A tale of 29 cities. *Ann Emerg Med* 19:179–186, 1990.

Eitel DR, Walton SL, Guerci AD, et al. Out-of-hospital cardiac arrest: A six-year experience in a suburban-rural system. *Ann Emerg Med* 17:808–812, 1988.

Goetting MG, Paradis NA. High-dose epinephrine in refractory pediatric arrest. *Crit Care Med* 17:1258–1262, 1989.

Grundler W, Weil MH, Rackow EC. Laboratory investigation, cardiac arrest: Arteriovenous carbon dioxide and pH gradients during cardiac arrest. *Circulation* 74:1071–1074, 1986.

Halperin HR, Weisfeldt MC. New approaches to CPR: Four hands, a plunger or a vest. *JAMA* 267:2940–2941, 1992.

Hanashiro PK, Wilson JR. Cardiopulmonary resuscitation: A current perspective. *Med Clin North Am* 70:729–747, 1986.

Hargarten KM, Stueven HA, Waite EM, et al. Prehospital experience with defibrillation of coarse ventricular fibrillation: A ten-year review. *Ann Emerg Med* 19:157–162, 1990.

Haynes BE, Mendoza A, McNeil M, et al. A statewide early defibrillation initiative including laypersons and outcome reporting. *JAMA* 266:545–547, 1991.

Hillis M, Sinclair D, Butler G, et al. Prehospital cardiac arrest suvival and neurologic recovery. *J Emerg Med* 11:245–252, 1993.

Holliman CJ, Bates MA. Review of all studies of cardiopulmonary resuscitation in animal models reported in the Emergency Medicine literature for the past ten years. *Am J Emerg Med* 10:347–353, 1992.

Joslyn SA, Pomrehn PR, Brown DD. Survival from out-of-hospital cardiac arrest: Effects of patient age and presence of 911 Emergency Medical Services phone access 1993. *Am J Emerg Med* 11:200–206, 1993.

Kouwenhoven WB, Jude JR, Knickerbocker GG. Closed chest cardiac massage. *JAMA* 173:1064–1067, 1960.

Larsen MP, Eisenberg MS, Cummins RO, et al: Predicting survial from out-of-hospital cardiac arrest: A graphic model. *Ann Emerg Med* 22(11):1652–1658, 1993.

Levine RL, Pepe PE, Fromm RE, et al. Prospective evidence of a circadian rhythm for out-of-hopsital cardiac arrests. *JAMA* 267:2935–2937, 1992.

McGrath RB. In-house cardiopulmonary resuscitation—after a quarter of a century. *Ann Emerg Med* 16:1365–1368, 1987.

Martin DR, Olson DW, Aprahamian C, et al. Prehospital bicarbonate use in cardiac arrest: A 3-year experience. *Am J Emerg Med* 10:4–7, 1993.

Martin GB, Gentile NT, Paradis NA, et al. Effect of epinephrine on endtidal carbon dioxide monitoring during CPR. *Ann Emerg Med* 19:396–398, 1990.

Neumar RW, Bircher NG, Sim KM, et al. Postresuscitation metabolic acidosis after high-dose epinephrine administered during cardiopulmonary resuscitation (abstract). *Circulation* 86(Suppl I):I-546, 1992.

Ornato JP, Levine RL, Young DS, et al. The effect of applied chest compression force on systemic arterial pressure and end-tidal carbon dioxide concentration during CPR in human beings. *Ann Emerg Med* 18:732–737, 1989.

Prehospital cardiac arrest treated by urban first-responders: Profile of patient response and prediction of outcome by ventricular fibrillation waveform. *Ann Emerg Med* 22(11): 1664–1667, 1993

Polin K, Leikin JB. High-dose epinephrine in cardiopulmonary resuscitation. *JAMA* 269:1383, 1993.

Redding JS, Pearson JW: Evaluation of drugs for cardiac resuscitation. *Anesthesiology* 24:203–207, 1963.

Reich H, Angelos M, Safar P, et al. Cardiac resuscitability with cardiopulmonary bypass after increasing ventricular fibrillation times in dogs. *Ann Emerg Med* 19:887–890, 1990.

Richless LK, Schrading WA, Polana J, et al. Early defibrillation program: Problems encountered in a rural/suburban EMS system. *J Emerg Med* 11:127–134, 1993.

Rieser MJ. The use of cough—CPR in patients with acute myocardial infarction. *J Emerg Med* 10:291–293, 1992.

Sack JB, Kesselbrenner MB, Bregman D, et al. Survival from in-hospital cardiac arrest with interposed abdominal counterpulsation during cardiopulmonary resuscitation. *JAMA* 267:379–385, 1992.

Safar P. Cerebral resuscitation after cardiac arrest: A review. *Circulation* 74:138–153, 1986.

Sanders AB, Kern KB, Otto C, et al. End-tidal carbon dioxide monitoring during cardiopulmonary resuscitation. *JAMA* 262:1347–1351, 1989.

Sterz F, Safar P, Tisherman S, et al. Mild hypothermic cardiopulmonary resuscitation improves outcome after prolonged cardiac arrest in dogs. *Crit Care Med* 19:379–389, 1991.

Stiell IG, Hebert PC, Weitzman BN, et al. High dose epinephrine in adult cardiac arrest. *N Engl J Med* 327:1045–1050, 1992.

Valenzuela TD, Spaite DW, Meislin HW, et al: Emergency vehicle intervals versus collapse-to-CPR and collapse-to-defibrillation intervals: Monitoring emergency medical services system performance in sudden cardiac arrest. *Ann Emerg Med* 22(11):1678–1683, 1993.

Valenzuela TD, Spaite DW, Meislin HW. Case and survival definitions in out-of-hospital cardiac arrest: Effect on survival rate circulation. *JAMA* 267:272–274, 1992.

van der Hoeven JG, Waanders H, Comier EA, et al: Prolonged resuscitation efforts for cardiac arrest patients who cannot be resuscitated at the scene: Who is likely to benefit? *Ann Emerg Med* 22(11):1659–1663, 1993.

Van Hoeyweghen RJ, Bossaert LL, Mullie A, et al. Survival after out-of-hospital cardiac arrest in elderly patients. *Ann Emerg Med* 21:1179–1184, 1992.

Weaver WD, Hill D, Fahrenbrugh CE, et al. Use of the automatic external defibrillator in the management of out-of-hospital cardiac arrest. *N Engl J Med* 319:661–666, 1988.

Weisfeldt ML, Chandra N, Tsitlik J. Increased intrathoracic pressure—not direct heart compression—causes the rise in intrathoracic vascular pressures during CPR in dogs and pigs. *Crit Care Med* 9:377–378, 1981.

White BC, Aust SD, Arfors KE, et al. Brain injury by ischemic anoxia: Hypothesis extension—a tale of two ions? *Ann Emerg Med* 13:862–867, 1984.

Yakaitis RW, Otto CW, Blitt CD. Relative importance of alpha and beta adrenergic receptors during resuscitation. *Crit Care Med* 7:292–296, 1979.

CHAPTER 37

Endotracheal Intubation and Mechanical Ventilation

Eric Gluck, M.D.

Positive-pressure ventilation is given to reduce the work of breathing to a level commensurate with adequate oxygen loading (PaO_2) and adequate ventilation, as demonstrated by the partial pressure of carbon dioxide (PCO_2) and the pH of the blood. It is indicated for intrinsic diseases of the lung, as well as extrinsic alterations in the mechanical properties of the chest wall or neural drive

I. **Types**
   A. Volume limited
      1. Most commonly used.
      2. Preset volume delivered at a preset rate and flow, regardless of the pressure required. Alarms can be set to prevent excessive intrapulmonary pressure. Guarantees a given minute ventilation.
   B. Pressure limited
      1. Gas is delivered to the patient at preset flow rate and respiratory frequency until a given airway pressure is achieved, regardless of the volume delivered. This prevents excessive intrapulmonary pressure. Minute ventilation will vary if the resistance of the airways or the compliance of the lung changes significantly. Alarms can

be set to warn of falling (Ve) minute ventilation or (Vt) tidal volume.
   C. High Frequency
      1. Small volumes of high-flow gas delivered at frequencies greater than 60 beats per minute. Reduces peak airway pressure. Can support ventilation for prolonged periods of time. No randomized study showed improved survival. A nonrandomized study with ventilator frequencies of 300 beats per minute showed improved gas exchange.

II. **Indications**
   A. Respiratory failure—hypoxia or hypoxemia.
   B. Ventilatory failure—inability to remove adequate quantities of CO_2.
   C. Reduction in the work of breathing to allow for better performance of the other organs.

III. **Modes**
   A. Assist control
      1. Ventilator delivers preset volume, at preset flow and minimum respiratory rate.
      2. Patient can trigger the ventilator to deliver additional ventilator breaths as nec-

essary, with only a trivial increase in the work of breathing. Thus additional ventilations are completely supported.

3. Work of breathing is near zero if the patient is not triggering the machine for additional breaths.

4. No restriction on the amount of ventilation the patient can generate.

5. Excellent initial mode of ventilation for the patient in acute respiratory failure.

B. Synchronized intermittent mandatory ventilation (IMV)

1. Ventilator delivers a preset volume at a preset rate and flow.

2. Any additional breaths desired by patient are not supported.

3. Work used to breathe through the endotracheal tube (ET) and the ventilator circuit increases the work of breathing for spontaneous breaths.

4. As the number of IMV breaths decreases the patient's work of breathing gradually increases, making this mode a useful tool for weaning.

5. IMV rates of 4 or less probably result in excessive work to breathe and should be avoided.

C. Pressure support ventilation

1. Ventilator delivers a preset pressure in response to the patient's demand for a breath

2. At levels of pressure support sufficient to overcome all the resistive and elastic forces of the lung, the work of breathing approaches zero and the mode is similar to that of assisted control

3. Requires the patient to have an active medullary center for respiration (pharmacologic paralysis is contraindication)

4. As the pressure support is reduced, the patient must supply the additional pressure to support an adequate tidal volume and minute ventilation.

5. Work of breathing per breath gradually increases as the pressure support is reduced, making this technique useful for weaning.

6. Pressure support ventilation is distinguished from IMV and assisted control in that there are no preset ventilator breaths.

7. Pressure support levels less than 5 are associated with excessive work of breathing in most patients.

8. Can be combined with IMV to support the spontaneous ventilations in difficult-to-wean patients.

D. Continuous positive airway pressure

1. Provides positive airway pressure above atmospheric pressure during inspiration and exhalation.

2. Positive end-expiratory pressure (PEEP) used for spontaneously breathing patients.

3. Can be delivered to patients who are intubated or breathing spontaneously through a mask.

4. Used for patients with mildly unstable alveoli, as in congestive heart failure or resolving adult respiratory distress syndrome (ARDS).

IV. Settings

A. Tidal volume

1. Recommendation: 7–10 cc/kg.

2. Smaller tidal volumes should be accompanied by sighs to prevent atelectasis.

3. Recent animal experiments suggest that larger volumes may enhance lung injury and may be edemagenic.

B. Respiratory rate

1. In the (A/C) assist control mode, the patient is free to choose his or her own rate if medullary centers are still functional.

2. Tendency to underestimate necessary minute ventilation (RR X Vt) respiratory rate time tidal volume

a. Chronic obstructive pulmonary disease (COPD)—range, 5–10 liters/min.

b. ARDS—range, 10–20 liters/min.

c. Trauma, sepsis, burns—15–30 liters/min.

3. Check adequacy of minute ventilation by arterial blood gas determination of $PaCO_2$.

C. Inspiratory Flow

1. Sets inspiratory:expiratory (I:E) ratio by establishing the time it takes for inspiration to be completed.

2. Crucial in establishing a comfortable ventilatory regimen for the patient.

a. Flows which are too high lead to coughing and bucking of the ventilator.

b. Flows which are too low lead to air hunger and increased inspiratory work.

3. Longer I:E for patients with obstructive airways disease (1:4 or greater), shorter I:E for patients with restrictive diseases (1:1 or 1:2).

4. Increasing the flow will increase the peak airway pressure, which some think may be responsible for barotrauma.

D. FiO2
   1. Usually best to start with fractional inspired oxygen (FiO_2) of 0.95 unless one is reasonably certain how good oxygen loading will be. An FiO_2 of 1.0 has been associated with absorptive atelectasis.
   2. Using a lower FiO_2 to start could subject the patient to hypoxia for an unnecessary length of time.
   3. Titrate down the oxygen concentration, using oximetry and arterial blood gases.
   4. Object—to achieve arterial saturation of >90 with an FiO_2 of 0.5 or less.

E. Waveform
   1. Ventilators generally supply three waveforms, i.e., the pattern of gas flow once the mechanical breath is activated.
      a. Square wave
         (1) Supplies tidal volume at a constant flow rate.
         (2) Allows for the shortest inspiratory time.
         (3) Associated with the highest peak airway pressures.
         (4) Dissimilar to the normal spontaneous flow pattern.
         (5) Useful in patients with high minute ventilation demands.
      b. Descending ramp
         (1) Inspiratory flow increases very rapidly and then declines slowly.
         (2) Most similar to normal inspiratory flow patterns.
         (3) End-inspiratory flow pattern may improve the distribution of ventilation within the lung.
         (4) Most commonly used pattern of gas flow.
         (5) Lower peak airway pressures than with square waves but requires longer inspiratory time to deliver tidal volume.
         (6) Used commonly in patients with obstructive lung diseases such as COPD and asthma, since it is a good compromise between peak pressure and inspiratory time.
      c. Sine wave
         (1) Least often used waveform.
         (2) Associated with the longest inspiratory times and the lowest peak airway pressure.
         (3) Reported to achieve better gas mixing within the lung, but little data are available to substantiate this conclusion.
         (4) Has found some utility in patients with patchy obstructive lung disease.
      d. Inspiratory pause
         (1) Not really a waveform. Prevents the onset of exhalation for preset length of time (0.1–1 sec).
         (2) Suggested that this may result in more uniform gas mixing within the lung, but little clinical data are available to support its use.

F. Positive end-expiratory pressure
   1. Raises mean airway pressure, increasing the surface area for oxygen transfer.
   2. Establishes an end-expiratory pressure which prevents alveolar collapse and small airway closure at the end of expiration.
   3. Most useful in conditions with increased elastic recoil of the lung, such as ARDS and cardiogenic pulmonary edema.
   4. Titrated to give an acceptable level of oxygen saturation in the arterial blood at a safe FiO_2 (0.5 or less).
   5. Useful range: 5–25 cm H_2O.
   6. High levels are associated with cardiac depression due to poor ventricular filling.
   7. May falsely elevate pulmonary capillary wedge (pcw) pressure measurements.
   8. Does not reduce lung water but may decrease further lung water accumulation.

G. Sighs
   1. Sigh volume: 2–3 × Vt
   2. 2–8 per hour.
   3. Prevents atelectasis associated with small tidal volumes (5–7 cc/kg).
   4. May be useful in secretion removal.
   5. Not required when larger tidal volumes are used.
   6. Peak airway pressure must be monitored closely.

V. Monitoring
   A. Physical exam
      1. Vital signs should be monitored frequently.
      2. Patients should be assessed several times

each day, paying attention to evenness of air entry and peripheral perfusion.

3. Check synchrony of chest and abdomen during spontaneous respirations.
4. Check adventitial sounds
5. Lower intercostal retraction suggestive of hyperinflation.

B. Airway pressure
   1. Peak airway pressure necessary to overcome the elastic and resistive forces.
      a. May correlate best with presence of barotrauma.
   2. Plateau pressure generated by the elastic forces of the lung.
   3. Peak-plateau difference proportional to airway resistance and inspiratory flow and inversely proportional to ET tube size.
   4. Mean airway pressure correlates best with impairment of cardiac function.

C. Arterial blood gas and oximetry
   1. $PaCO_2$ assesses adequacy of ventilation, but the endpoint should be an appropriate arterial pH.
   2. PaO_2—assesses efficiency of oxygen loading.
      a. Goal: PaO_2 above 60 torr, FiO_2 below 0.5.
   3. Saturation closely approximates total amount of oxygen carried by the blood.
   4. Oximetry can be used to tirate FiO_2
      a. Poor correlations may be associated with dark races and shift of the oxyhemoglobin dissociation curve.
      b. May not measure saturation in patients with poor peripheral perfusion.

D. Capnography
   1. Measures exhaled PCO_2 continuously.
   2. Inaccurate in patients with obstructive lung disease and in those with rapid respiratory rates.
      a. Trends may be more useful than actual correlation with arterial blood gas sample.
   3. Limited utility in intensive care units, though reviewed favorably in operating rooms.

E. Compliance
   1. Dynamic compliance (peak inspiratory pressure–PEEP)/tidal volume
      a. Measures resistive and elastic components of the work of breathing.
      b. Normal range: 35–50 cc/cm H_2O.
   2. Static compliance (Static Pressure–PEEP)/tidal volume

a. Measures the elastic component of the work of breathing.
b. Normal range: 50–75 cc/cm H_2O.
c. Plateau inspiratory pressure is obtained by trapping the gas within the lung at the end of exhalation and allowing the pressure to equilibrate. The difference between dynamic and static compliance is the resistive component. This falls to zero when the flow is zero.

F. Airway resistance
   1. Most ventilators now incorporate the software necessary to perform measurements.
   2. Most useful in patients with obstructive airway disease.
   3. Major component of measurement is the resistance of the ET tube.
   4. Can be used to assess weanability and the patient's response to bronchodilator therapy.
   5. Normal range: < 2.5 cm H_2O/liter/sec.

G. Minute ventilation
   1. Measures dead space ventilation and alveolar ventilation.
   2. Measures the demand for ventilation.
   3. Increases with a high respiratory quotient (RQ), increased CO_2 production, or increased dead space (such as with pulmonary embolism).
   4. Should be < 12 liters/min at the time of extubation.

H. Chest x-ray
   1. Should be obtained daily to evaluate position of ET tube.
   2. Useful monitor for barotrauma, infection, and lung water.

I. Useful formulas: see Table 37-1.

VI. Weaning
   A. Transfer of the work of breathing back from the machine to the patient.
      1. Try not to exceed the work of breathing that the patient will be called upon to do after extubation; otherwise, the patient may remain on the mechanical ventilator for an unnecessary length of time.
   B. Methods of Weaning. No study has shown one of the following methods to be superior to the others.
      1. T piece
         a. Intermittently switched from assist control to T piece.
         b. Patient breathes spontaneously with-

Table 37-1. Monitoring Mechanical Ventilation: Common Formulas

$$\dot{V}E = V_T \times \text{Rate}$$

$$\dot{V}E = \dot{V}A + \dot{V}D$$

$$\text{desired rate} = \text{initial rate} \times \frac{\text{initial PaCO}_2}{\text{desired PaCO}_2}$$

$$\frac{\dot{V}D}{V_T} = \frac{\text{PaCO}_2 - \text{PECO}_2}{\text{PaCO}_2}$$

$$D(A - a)O_2 = PAO_2 - PaO_2$$

$$PAO_2 = PIO_2 - \frac{PaCO_2}{R}$$

$$PIO_2 = (P_B - P_{H_2O}) \times FIO_2$$

$$PAO_2 = PIO_2 - PaCO_2 \left[FIO_2 + \frac{1 - FIO_2}{R} \right]$$

The normal value of the $D(A\text{-}a)O_2 < \frac{\text{age}}{4} + 12$

$$\frac{PaO_2}{PAO_2} > 0.75$$

$$\frac{PaO_2 i}{PAO_2 i} = \frac{PaO_2 f}{PAO_2 f}$$

$$CaO_2 = SaO_2 \times Hgb \times 1.34 + PaO_2 \times 0.003$$

$$\frac{\dot{Q}s}{\dot{Q}_T} = \frac{CIO_2 - CaO_2}{CIO_2 - C\bar{v}O_2}$$

out ventilator support while on T piece.

c. Gradually increased time and number of trials per day until each trial lasts for 30 min and about 15 trials are done per day.

d. Evaluate for extubation (see below).

e. Advantages
(1) Does not require additional equipment.
(2) Easy to perform and to monitor the patient.
(3) Does not require sophisticated ventilators.

f. Disadvantages
(1) Patient receives total support from the ventilator and then during the trial has to perform excessive work due to the work associated with the ventilator circuit and the ET tube.
(2) Does not appear to be very physiologic.

2. Synchronized intermittent mandatory ventilation SIMV
a. Gradually reduce number of mandatory breaths until patient is receiving only four.
b. Continuous positive airway pressure (CPAP) trial then usually done for about 30 min.
c. Then evaluate for extubation (see below)
d. Advantages
(1) Most ventilators have this mode of ventilation.
(2) Does not require additional equipment.
(3) More gradual assumption of the work of breathing than in the T-piece mode.
e. Disadvantages
(1) Spontaneous breaths are usually not supported (see discussion of pressure support); thus, work of breathing through the ET tube and ventilator may be excessive.
(2) Difficult to predict at what level the patient is actually performing more work on the ventilator than would occur after extubation.

3. Pressure support
a. Pressure support is gradually reduced until the patient is receiving 5–8 cm H_2O with a size 8 ET tube or 8–10 cm H_2O with a size 7 tube.
b. Patient is then evaluated for extubation.
c. Advantages
(1) Patient receives a proportionate amount of support per breath.
(2) Work of breathing never exceeds the work the patient would have to do after extubation.
(3) Appears to be more physiologic.
d. Disadvantages
(1) Patient may not get large inflations, leading to atelectasis.
(2) If the patient receives excess sedation, backup ventilation is produced by the ventilator and may not be adequate.

C. Indices predicting successful extubation
1. Evaluate the demands on the respiratory system, the work of breathing, and the power output of the respiratory muscles
a. Demand

(1) Minute ventilation: should be < 12 liters/min.

(2) CO_2 production may now be directly measured, using metabolic carts.

(3) Carbon dioxide output (VCO_2) > 300 ml, make weaning unlikely.

b. Work

  (1) Elastic

    (a) Static compliance − tidal volume/plateau pressure.

    (b) Values > 30 cc/cm H_2O are usually associated with success.

  (2) Resistive

    (a) Most ventilators allow calculation of resistance.

    (b) Limited by the fact that the ET tube accounts for the majority of the resistance measured.

    (c) Values < 12 cm H_2O/liters/min are usually associated with success.

    (d) If unavailable, peak minus plateau pressure < 10 cm H_2O is usually associated with low airway resistance.

c. Power

  (1) Maximum inspiratory force (MIF)

    (a) Values ≤35 cm H_2O are usually acceptable.

    (b) Not a very reproducible measurement.

    (c) Strongly dependent on patient effort and level of consciousness.

d. Rapid shallow breathing (RSB) index

  (1) Respiratory rate/tidal volume (liters)

    (a) Recently shown to be highly predictive of failure to wean (if > 100).

    (b) Less reliable in predicting success (80% with value < 100).

e. CROP-acronym for a combination of the above measurements

  (1) Dynamic compliance × arterial PO_2/alveolar PO_2 × maximum inspiratory force /respiratory rate

    (a) values >14 are associated with success

f. FiO_2 should be ≤ 0.50.

g. PCO_2 should result in normalized pH.

h. Secretions should be under reasonable control.

i. Good mental status is helpful but not mandatory.

j. In marginal cases, consider the clinical course if improvement is likely; wait.

D. Point of extubation

1. Once the above measurements are achieved, the patient should be tried on CPAP with minimal ventilator support for a short period of time.

2. If patient can maintain a tidal volume > 300 cc and a respiratory rate < 35, extubation should be attempted.

3. Prior to removing the ET tube, the cuff should be deflated and the patient should be observed for air leakage around the tube.

4. Lack of airflow around the tube suggests tracheal or laryngeal edema and could result in an acute upper airway obstruction after extubation.

E. Failure to wean

1. Causes

a. Work of breathing remains too great.

  (1) Airway resistance cannot be reduced further (e.g., in end-stage COPD, bronchitis).

  (2) Lung or thoracic compliance remains too low, increasing the elastic work of breathing (e.g., pulmonary edema or fibrosis; chest wall abnormalities; obesity; intra-abdominal distention from stool, air, feces, or fluid).

b. Metabolic demand is too high (CO_2 production exceeds ability to ventilate as a result of sepsis or hyperalimentation with glucose-rich fluids and resultant increased RQ).

c. Neuromuscular output is insufficient to ventilate the patient adequately. This can be seen with malnutrition, residual sedation, electrolyte disturbances involving potassium, chloride, sodium, phosphorus, magnesium, calcium, bicarbonate, primary myopathies, intracerebral catastrophes.

VII. Complications

A. Pulmonary

1. Barotrauma—usually attributed to high airway pressure or large tidal volumes. May be more closely related to the underlying lung condition.

2. ET tube–associated problems—kinking,

colonization, self-extubation, tracheal edema, scarring.
3. Ventilator failure.
4. Respiratory muscle atrophy.
B. Cardiac
1. Hemodynamic compromise—appears to be most closely related to mean airway pressure.
   a. Results from inability of the left ventricle to expand fully due to surrounding pressure. May also be affected by the state of the intravascular volume.
2. Hypotension
C. Gastrointestinal
1. Stress ulceration: ≥70% of all intensive care unit patients will develop abnormal gastric mucosae.
   a. All patients on ventilators should receive prophylaxis against ulceration.
2. Gastric distention.
3. Ileus.
D. Renal
1. Renal failure—may be related to redistribution of renal blood flow due to positive intrathoracic pressure or may be humorally mediated.
2. Hyponatremia.
3. Increase in total body water.
E. Infectious disease
1. Nosocomial pneumonia.
2. Sepsis.
F. Nutritional depletion

VIII. **Newer Modes**
A. Inverse I:E ratio ventilation
1. Inspiratory time greater than expiratory time.
2. Increases mean airway pressure without increasing peak inspiratory pressure.
3. Recommended in refractory hypoxia unresponsive to PEEP.
4. Associated with increases in barotrauma and hemodynamic embarrassment.
B. Airway pressure release ventilation
1. Inspiration last > 95 of respiratory cycle.
2. Positive airway pressure maintains lung volume over functional residual capacity until exhalation.
3. Release of pressure allows deflation and removal of CO_2.
4. Lung repressurized to previous pressure.
5. Advantages
   a. Peak inspiratory pressure effectively becomes the PEEP level.

b. Barotrauma should be reduced.
6. Disadvantages
   a. Patient must be paralyzed during ventilation.
   b. Unstable alveoli will not be recruited during inflation.
   c. No controlled studies have been done to demonstrate efficacy in humans with significant lung injury.

IX. **Negative-Pressure Ventilation**
A. Creates a negative pressure around the chest, causing negative intrathoracic pressure to develop, resulting in air being sucked into the lungs.
1. Most closely simulates the normal respiratory physiology.
2. Unable to generate strongly negative pressures or rapid respiratory rates, which limits its utility in patients with high demands or stiff lungs.
3. Iron lungs were the prototype, but their use was limited due to the above problems, as well as poor patient access once inside the ventilator.
4. Other, more modern methods of producing negative pressure are available but are not very useful clinically.

X. **Mechanical ventilation without ET Tubes**
A. Transnasal ventilation without ET tubes is currently being tested, with encouraging results.
B. Will probably be limited to ventilatory assistance rather than providing ventilatory support.
C. May be useful for nighttime support or support of patients with COPD who are not candidates for intubation.

Bibliography

Bone RC, Eubanks D: A clinicians guide to ventilators. How they work and why they fail. *J Crit Illness*, Vol 7(3) March 1992 pg 379.

Bone RC, Eubanks D: Second and third generation ventilators; sorting through the available options. *J Crit Illness*, Vol 7(3) March 1992; pg 399.

Gluck EH, Bone RC, Eubanks D: The technique of instituting mechanical ventilation. *J Crit Illness*, Vol 8(2) August 1992.

Haake et al.: Barotrauma, pathophysiology, risk factors and prevention. *Chest* 1987 91:608–613.

Craven DE, Kunkes LM, Kilinsky V, et al.: Risk factors for pneumonia and fatality in patients receiving continuous mechanical ventilation. *ARRD* 1986: 133: 792–796.

CHAPTER 38

Hemodynamic Monitoring

James E. Calvin, M.D.
Jeffrey R. Snell, M.D.

I. Procedure

A. Description

1. Hemodynamic and electrocardiographic monitoring represent major activities in a critical care unit.

2. Hemodynamic monitoring is achieved using a flow-directed, balloon-tipped catheter which is easily manipulated through the right heart chambers and into the pulmonary artery. Besides enabling passage of the catheter into the pulmonary artery, inflation of the balloon inside the pulmonary artery allows the measurement of pressure within the distal pulmonary artery when there is no antegrade flow, the so-called pulmonary capillary wedge pressure (PCWP), which reflects left atrial and left ventricular diastolic pressures (i.e., left ventricular filling pressures).

3. A thermistor attached to the tip of the catheter allows measurement of cardiac output (CO) using a thermodilution technique.

B. Historical perspective

1. Popularized by the Cedars-Sinai group in the mid-1970s to characterize the severity of acute myocardial infarction and to direct therapy.

2. Rapidly adopted by physicians caring for other critically ill patients and anesthetists looking after high-risk surgical patients.

II. Current Indications

A. In general, RHC with hemodynamic monitoring is used to facilitate a specific management decision and is used when physicians are committed to act on the data.

B. Common indications are listed in Table 38-1.

III. Information Derived from Right Heart Catheterization (RHC)

A. As shown in Table 38-2, right heart catheterization (RHC) allows direct measurement of CO, PCWP, right atrial pressure (RAP) and pulmonary artery pressure (PAP).

B. Figure 38-1 shows typical waveform recordings from the right atrium, right ventricle, pulmonary artery, and pulmonary capillary wedge positions (PCWP).

C. RHC also allows the determination of systemic and pulmonary vascular resistances, right and

Table 38-1. Common Indications for Hemodynamic Monitoring

To establish a specific diagnosis of:
  Ventricular septal defect (VSD)
  Mitral regurgitation
  Right ventricular infarction
  Cardiogenic shock
  Noncardiogenic pulmonary edema
  Cardiac pulmonary edema
  Hypovolemia
  Cardiac tamponade
  Myocardial ischemia in the presence of an
    uninterpretable electrocardiogram
To assist in the managment of:
  Acute myocardial infarction complicated by:
    hypovolemia unresponsive to volume challenge
    hypotension requiring vasoactive agents or
      ventricular assist devices
  Severe congestive heart failure associated with
    hypotension
  Severe pulmonary hypertension requiring
    vasodilator therapy
  Acute pulmonary embolism
To assist in the management of cricitally ill patients
  with:
  Gastrointestinal hemorrhage where volume status
    is uncertain
  Sepsis to optimize preload and oxygen delivery
  Respiratory failure
  Renal failure   } to aid in judicious
  Pancreatitis   } fluid management
  Drug overdose
To assist in the management of cardiac surgical
  patients having:
  Valve replacement (multiple, in the elderly)
  Coronary bypass grafting
  Ventricular aneurysm resection
  Associated high-risk factors
To assist in the management of vascular surgical
  patients having:
  Dissecting aneurysm repair
  Abdominal aortic aneurysm repair
To assist in the management of other surgical
  patients who are at high risk of morbidity and
  mortality:
  Patients having recent myocardial infarction
    (<6 months)
  Patients having a high Goldman classification
  Patients suspected of having serious myocardial
    ischemia or serious left ventricular
    dysfunction

Table 38-2. Information Derived from RHC

Directly measured variables of major therapeutic use:
  CO
  RAP
  PCWP
  PAP
Derived variable of potential therapeutic use:
  Oxygen delivery
  Systemic vascular resistance
  Pulmonary vascular resistance
Derived variables of uncertain significance:
  Left ventricular stroke work index
  Right ventricular stroke work index
  Right ventricular ejection fraction*
  Right ventricular end-diastolic volume*
  Systemic vascular oxygenation†

  *Right ventricular ejection fraction and end-diastolic volume can be measured by a specialized right heart catheter with a fast frequency response.
  †Systemic vascular oxygenation can be measured by specialized right heart catheters that are now commercially available.

left ventricular stroke works, and oxygen delivery (Table 38-3).
  D. Table 38-4 indicates how knowledge of PCWP, the cardiac index, and blood pressure can guide therapy in acute myocardial infarction.
IV. **Limitations of Measurements**
  A. Cardiac output
    1. Derived by a special formula using a dye dilution principle whereby temperature is the indicator.
    2. Error rate: ± 5%.
    3. Error rate is increased by:
      a. Performing repeated measurements at different phases of the respiratory cycle.
      b. Rapid infusion of other IV lines.
      c. Inadvertent warming of the injectate.
      d. Inaccurate measurement of the volume of injectate.
      e. Electrocautery.
      f. Pathological conditions such as tricuspid regurgitation.
    4. Ensure accurate cardiac output by:
      a. Injecting only at the end of expiration.
      b. Inspecting the cardiac output tracing to rule out poor mixing, poor injections, and the presence of recirculation (i.e., VSD).

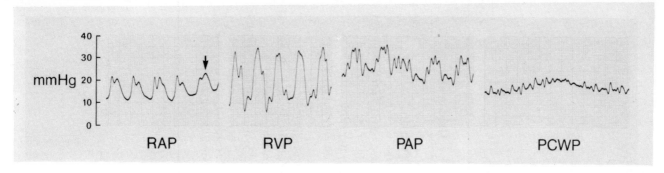

Figure 38-1. Representative pressure tracings from the right atrium, right ventricular, pulmonary artery, and pulmonary capillary wedge pressure positions. Note the venous waveforms in both the right atrial and pulmonary capillary wedge pressure tracings and the step-up in systolic pressure in the right ventricle. As the catheter is passed from the right ventricle into the pulmonary artery, a stepup in the diastolic pressure is seen. In this example, a prominent V wave is noted in the RAP tracing suggestive of tricuspid regurgitation (arrow).

 c. Checking for tricuspid regurgitation (large V-wave on RAP tracing, Figure 38-1).
 d. Double-checking injectate volumes and temperatures and programmable constants.
B. Pulmonary capillary wedge pressure
 1. Does not necessarily measure left ventricular (LV) preload

2. May be influenced by:
 a. Changes in intrathoracic pressure if the tip is not lying in a dependent portion of the lung (West's Zone III, Figure 38-2).
 b. LV inflow tract obstruction (such as by mitral stenosis, which raises left atrial [LA] pressure).
 c. Juxtacardiac pressure such as right ventricular (RV) diastolic pressure, pericar-

Table 38-3. Information Gained from RHC and Arterial Blood Pressure Monitoring

Variable	Formula	Normal Values
Direct measurements		
Cardiac output (CO,L/min)		
Cardiac index (CI,L/min/m^2)	CO/body surface area (BSA)	3.2 ± 0.2 liters/min/km^2
Right atrial pressure (RAP,mmHg)		0–5 mmHg
Pulmonary capillary wedge pressure (PCWP,mmHg)		5–12 mmHg
Mean pulmonary artery pressure (PAP,mmHg)		9–18 mmHg
Mean arterial blood pressure (MAP,mmHg)		90 mmHg
Derived measurements		
LVSW (g − m/m^2)	Stroke volume $\times$ (MAP − PCWP) $\times$ 0.0136/BSA	56 ± 6
RVSW (g − m/m^2)	Stroke volume $\times$ (PAP − RAP) $\times$ 0.0136/BSA	8.8 ± 0.9
PVR (dynes $\cdot$ sec $\cdot$ cm^{-5}/m^2)	$\dfrac{(PAP - PCWP) \times 80}{CO}$	270 ± 15
SVR (dynes $\cdot$ sec $\cdot$ cm^{-5}/m^2)	$\dfrac{(MAP - RAP) \times 80}{CO}$	2180 ± 120
Oxygen delivery (D0$_2$, ml/min/m^2)	CI $\times$ 10 $\times$ Ca0$_2$*	580–600 ml/min $\cdot$ m^2

*CA0$_2$ = arterial oxygen content (ml/dl) = (Hb $\times$ 1.34 $\times$ percent saturation) + (oxygen tension $\times$ 0.0031).
Abbreviations: MAP, mean arterial pressure; CI, cardiac index.

Table 38–4. Hemodynamic Classification and Therapeutic Strategy of Patients with Acute Myocardial Infarction

Subset	Clinical situation	Arterial BP (mmHg)	PCWP (mmHg)	CI (liters/m/m²)	Management
1	Normal	>100	<14	>2.2	Expectant; Observe for arrhythmia; Treat pain; Noninvasive testing for long-term prognosis
2	Hypovolemia (clinically low output)	<100	<14	<2.2	Volume expansion
3	Pulmonary congestion (pulmonary edema)	>100	>18	>2.2	Diuretics/nitroglycerin
4a	Low output and pulmonary edema	>100	>18	<2.2	Arterial vasodilators
4b	Low output and pulmonary edema	<100	>18	<2.2	Inotropic agents, vasodilators, and circulatory assistance
5	RV infarct	<100	<14 (CVP > 10)	<2.2	Optimize PCWP; consider dobutamine early
6	Mitral regurgitation	Variable	>18 (V wave)	usually <2.2	As in 4: consider early surgery
7	Ventricular septal defect	Variable	Usually high	Variable; O_2 step-up in RV	As in 4: consider early surgery

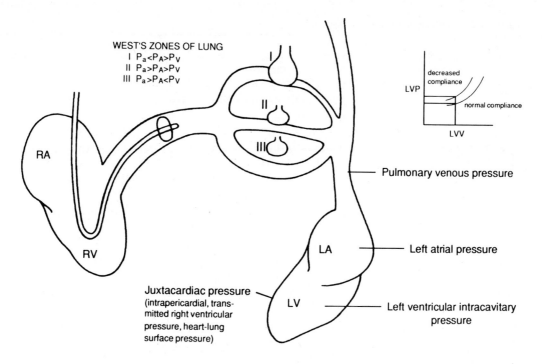

WEST'S ZONES OF LUNG
I $P_a < P_A > P_V$
II $P_a > P_A > P_V$
III $P_a > P_A < P_V$

LVP
decreased compliance
normal compliance
LVV

RA

RV

Pulmonary venous pressure

LA

Left atrial pressure

Juxtacardiac pressure
(intrapericardial, transmitted right ventricular pressure, heart-lung surface pressure)

LV

Left ventricular intracavitary pressure

Figure 38-2. Various influences to be considered when measuring PCWP. The PCWP is measured from the distal lumen of the right heart catheter, with the balloon inflated in such a manner as to obstruct antegrade flow. For this pressure to accurately reflect left atrial and left ventricular diastolic pressure, the catheter tip must be residing in West Zone III, where the pressure gradient for flow is the difference between the pulmonary artery and pulmonary venous pressures (which both exceed the alveolar pressure). Catheter tips that lie in either Zone 1 or Zone 2 may reflect alveolar pressure. Assuming that the PCWP is accurately reflecting left atrial pressure does not necessarily ensure that it is tracking left ventricular preload or left ventricular end-diastolic volume (LVV). Compliance of the left ventricle can markedly influence this relationship, as shown by the insert at the top right. Decreased compliance of the left ventricle can result in a higher left ventricular filling pressure being measured at a given left ventricular end-diastolic

Table 38-5. Complications of RHC

Complication	Incidence (%)
Related to insertion	
Hematoma	0–2.8
Pneumothorax	0.07–1.5
Hemthorax/hemomediastinum	Unpublished
Puncture of lymphatic duct	Unpublished
Air embolism	0.1
Injury to carotid artery	0–13
Injury to trachea, vagus, or phrenic nerve	Unpublished
Ventricular arrhythmia (transient)	19–50
Ventricular arrhythmia (requiring treatment)	0–2
Complete heart block	0–2.6
Guidewire embolism	Unpublished
Knotting	Unpublished
Cardiac or vascular perforation	Unpublished
Failure of catheterization	1.7
Related to long-term maintenance	
Infection	<5
Pulmonary infarction	0.3
Pulmonary artery rupture	0.2
Catheter shredding and embolism	Unpublished

dial pressure, and heart-lung surface pressure, which reduce LV distensibility by either contact pressure or ventricular interaction (Figure 38-2).

   d. Changes in LV diastolic function such as ischemia, hypertrophy, or cardiomyopathy (Figure 38-2).

3. Ensure accurate PCWP measurement by:

   a. Determining that the tip of the catheter is beneath the atria on the cross-table lateral chest x-ray (ensures that the tip is lying in West's Zone III and that there is a continuous column of blood between the catheter tip and the left atrium).

   b. Aspirating oxygenated blood from the distal port when wedged.

   c. Determining that pulmonary artery diastolic pressure (PADP) is greater than PCWP.

   d. Ensuring venous waveform appearance.

Table 38-6. Summary of Cost/Benefit Analysis of RHC

Utility	Accepted Findings
	Diagnosis
Low cardiac output	RHC more reliable than clinical assessment
Low PCWP	RHC more reliable than clinical assessment
High PCWP	RHC more reliable than clinical assessment
VSD	O_2 step-up in RV is an accepted means of diagnosis
Mitral regurgitation (MR)	Giant V-wave in PCWP tracing is strongly suggestive of MR
Pulmonary hypertension	Gold standard for diagnosis
RV infarction	RAP: PCWP >0.80 strongly suggestive of RV involvement
	Prognosis
Hemodynamic subsets in MI	Confers prognostic information and suggests therapeutic options
LVSW	Useful for prognosis in MI (<20 g-m has poor 1-year prognosis)
Pulmonary hypertension	Mortality related to RVSP and RAP
Sepsis	Prognosis better with supranormal cardiac index or oxygen transport Therapy
Changes in therapy	Information from RHC changes therapy 34 to 48% of time
Improved outcome	Few randomized controls
	Survivorship in high-risk surgical patients improved using protocol based on RHC

    e. Avoiding air in the pressure measurement system (tubes and transducer).

    f. Being wary when large pressure swings corresponding to intrathoracic pressure changes are observed.

V. Complications

  A. It is to be expected that RHC has some risk.

  B. Common complications and observed incidence rates are noted in Table 38-5.

VI. Risks and Benefits

  A. Few randomized clinical trials have been performed.

  B. Benefits in the diagnosis of certain low cardiac output states and certain cardiac conditions are noted in Table 38-6.

  C. Some information has good prognostic value.

  D. Improved outcomes have been difficult to demonstrate.

Bibliography

Calvin JE, Technology Subcommittee of the Working Group on Critical Care, Ontario Ministry of Health. Hemodynamic monitoring. A technology assessment. *Can Med Assoc J* 145(2):114–121, 1991.

Forrester JS, Diamond G, Chatterjee K, et al. Medical therapy of acute myocardial infarction by application of hemodynamic subsets. *N Engl J Med* 295:1356–1362, 1404–1413, 1976.

Friesinger GC II, Williams SV, Achord JL, et al. Clinical competence in hemodynamic monitoring—a statement for physicians from the ACP/ACC/AHA task force on clinical privileges in cardiology. *JACC* 15(7):1460–1464, 1990.

Putterman C. The Swan-Ganz catheter: A decade of hemodynamic monitoring. *J Crit Care* 4(7):127–146, 1989.

The ACP/AAC/AHA Task Force on Clinical Privileges in Cardiology. Clinical competence in hemodynamic monitoring. *J Am Cell Cardiol* 15:1460, 1990.

Tuman KJ, Carroll GC, Ivankovich AD. Pitfalls in interpretation of pulmonary artery catheter data. *J Cardiothorac Anesth* 4(5):625–641, 1989.

CHAPTER 39

Shock

Andrew C. Dixon, M.D.
Joseph E. Parrillo, M.D.

I. **Definition**

Shock is a syndrome best defined as a systemic disorder that results in inadequate delivery of oxygen and other nutrients to meet the needs of the tissues. While at the cellular level hypoperfusion always exists, this may not be true at the macrovascular level, where maldistribution of adequate or elevated cardiac output can still result in shock. The development of shock, regardless of its etiology, is clinically heralded by organ dysfunction. It is the recognition of this organ dysfunction that is most often used to diagnose and determine the severity of shock. The low output state is defined as one form of shock which is characterized both clinically and hemodynamically by a reduction in cardiac output.

II. **Etiologies of Shock**

Shock can be broadly classified into five etiologic categories: cardiogenic, extracardiac obstructive, oligemic, distributive, and mixed (see Table 39-1). When classifying shock, it is helpful to understand its effect on cardiovascular physiology—specifically, whether cardiac output is low or high. The first three forms of shock discussed below result in low output, while the latter two may have low, normal, or high cardiac output.

A. Cardiogenic shock

This type of shock results from a failure of forward flow, and includes shock caused by impaired systolic performance, impaired diastolic filling, valvular dysfunction, or a combination of these conditions.

1. Myopathic forms of cardiogenic shock result in reduced forward flow caused by an impairment of systolic contractile performance. When due to an acute myocardial infarction, the most common cause of cardiogenic shock, a loss of 40% or more of the myocardium must occur prior to the development of shock. In this situation, efforts to control ischemic myocardium can result in rapid improvements in cardiac output and resolution of shock. Most forms of dilated cardiomyopathy can also result in the development of shock once the usual compensatory mechanisms have failed in the late stages of this disease.

Table 39-1. Classification of Shock States

1. Cardiogenic Shock
   A. Failure of systolic performance (myopathic)
      Acute myocardial infarction or ischemia
      Cardiomyopathy
      Myocarditis
      Acidosis
      Drugs (e.g., doxorubicin, β-blockers, anesthetics)
   B. Valvular or subvalvular diseases
      Acute mitral regurgitation
      Aortic stenosis or insufficiency
      Mechanical valve failure
      Hypertrophic cardiomyopathy with obstruction
   C. Arrhythmias
      Bradyarrhythmias
      Tachyarrhythmias (e.g., supraventricular tachycardia, ventricular tachycardia)
2. Extracardiac obstructive
   Pericardial tamponade
   Constrictive pericarditis
   Massive pulmonary embolism
   Severe pulmonary hypertension
   Coarctation of the aorta
   Tension pneumothorax
   Positive-pressure ventilation
3. Oligemic
   A. Hemorrhagic
      Trauma
      Gastrointestinal bleeding
      Internal bleeding
         Hemothorax
         Hemoperitoneum
         Ruptured aortic aneurysm
         Fractures
   B. Nonhemorrhagic
      Gastrointestinal Losses
         Vomiting
         Diarrhea
      Renal Losses
      Osmotic diuresis (e.g., diabetic ketoacidosis)
         Diabetes insipidus
         Diuretic-induced losses
         High-output renal failure
      Burns
      Peritonitis
      Pancreatitis
4. Distributive
   A. Drug-induced
      Anesthetics
      Vasodilators
   B. Neuropathic
      Spinal cord injury
      Severe dysautonomia
      Diffuse cerebral injury
   C. Toxic
      Sepsis
      Anaphylaxis
   D. Endocrinologic
      Adrenal insufficiency
      Thyroid disorders
5. Mixed
   Sepsis
   Anaphylaxis
   Pancreatitis
   Burns
   Trauma

2. Numerous valvular lesions, both acute and chronic, can result in shock. Acute mitral insufficiency commonly precipitates shock, usually from a rupture of the cordea tendineae or infarction of the papillary muscle. Impedance to left ventricular outflow, as occurs in aortic stenosis or conditions where hypertrophic tissue exists below the aortic valve (idiopathic hypertrophic subaortic stenosis, asymmetrical septal hypertrophy), can also result in shock, though most commonly after a prolonged period of time with symptomatic disease. Aneurysms of the left ventricle can result in severe ventricular dysfunction and the shock syndrome.

3. Dysrythmias, both ventricular and supraventricular, may also result in shock, due either to inadequate ventricular filling or to a failure of contractile performance.

B. Extracardiac obstructive shock
   In this form of shock, an impairment of venous return to the right or left heart exists, leading to the development of reduced cardiac output.
   1. The prototypic example of this form of shock is pericardial tamponade, in which pericardial fluid under pressure com-

presses the right atrium and ventricle and impedes the return of venous blood to the right side of the heart.

2. Another common example of this form of shock is massive pulmonary embolus, in which obstruction to right ventricular emptying occurs, resulting in failure to fill the left ventricle adequately.

C. Oligemic shock

Oligemic shock is best categorized into hemorrhagic and nonhemorrhagic forms. Regardless of the type of shock, at least 25% of the intravascular volume is usually lost before compensatory mechanisms fail and the development of shock occurs. In addition to the amount of fluid lost; the rate at which it is lost is important in the development of shock; compensatory mechanisms fail earlier when volume loss occurs acutely. Advanced age or the coexistence of other disease processes can also modify the success of compensatory mechanisms in patients with oligemic shock.

1. Hemorrhagic shock occurs as a result of blood loss from any site. It precipitates tissue ischemia not only due to the loss of oxygen-carrying capacity, but also because of the reduction in ventricular preload, which causes diminished cardiac output.

2. Nonhemorrhagic forms of oligemic shock imply a loss of circulating plasma volume, usually from renal or gastrointestinal processes but also occasionally from sequestration within the body (i.e., pancreatitis or severe hypoproteinemia). In this category, shock results from the failure or ventricular filling (preload), with a reduction in cardiac output.

D. Distributive shock

As the name implies, distributive shock occurs when there is a maldistribution of blood flow away from vital organs to the venous capacitance bed. Thus, despite a sufficient circulating blood volume and cardiac output, tissue hypoperfusion exists from inadequate flow and/or delivery of oxygen and other nutrients at the capillary level.

1. Septic shock has characteristically been used as an example of distributive shock. However, in sepsis, depression of myocardial contractility also frequently occurs, leading to a combination of distributive and cardiogenic shock. A better example of pure distributive shock is that which occurs with spinal cord injury, in which peripheral vasodilation is the predominant feature.

E. Mixed forms of shock

These forms of shock are more complex and result from the coexistence of two or more of the types of shock discussed above.

1. Septic shock is the best example of this form because of the coexistence of arterial vasodilation, increased venous capacitance from venodilation (a distributive phenomenon), and reduction in the compliance and contractility of both ventricles (a cardiogenic form of shock).

III. Pathophysiology of the Shock State

Because hypoperfusion, at least at the tissue level, exists in all forms of shock, characteristic metabolic responses occur and can often be used to define both the severity and the prognosis of shock.

A. Systemic Responses

The most important systemic markers of shock are hypotension and metabolic acidosis.

1. Systemic hypotension, when present, is a clear indication that shock exists or is rapidly developing. As noted previously, however, blood pressure is a poor marker of specific organ perfusion. Therefore, the reduction in blood pressure that is necessary before shock develops varies greatly among individuals.

2. Lactic acidosis occurs commonly in shock and reflects the development of anaerobic metabolism due to inadequate delivery of oxygen and other metabolic substrates at the cellular level. While the absolute level of lactate in the circulation varies widely and correlates poorly with either the outcome or the severity of shock, the response of serial lactate levels to treatment can be a useful sign of the adequacy of therapy chosen, that is, if the lactate level falls as a specific treatment is initiated, one can be relatively certain that this treatment has been beneficial.

B. Organ responses

The brain, heart, gut, kidneys, and lungs are the organs most commonly involved in shock, because these organs are most dependent upon adequate perfusion to maintain metabolic function.

1. Cerebral perfusion remains relatively constant over a broad range of blood

pressures because of its complex autoregulatory mechanisms. Once the mean arterial blood pressure (MAP) falls below 60 to 70 mmHg, however, a fall in cerebral perfusion occurs, usually resulting in a deterioration of mental status. As the perfusion pressure falls further, frank coma and eventually irreversible ischemic brain damage occur.

2. The heart is the principal organ involved in the compensatory mechanisms that are employed in early shock, one of the most important being the development of sinus tachycardia. Once these compensatory mechanisms fail, however, coronary perfusion may fall as systemic hypotension progresses, leading to the subsequent development of myocardial ischemia. This can be manifested either by chest pain or by a worsening of systolic pump function, the latter of which tends to aggravate the underlying shock state.

3. The gut is a strongly perfusion-dependent organ, and in the setting of hypoperfusion, mucosal breakdown tends to develop rapidly. This may then precipitate gastrointestinal bleeding and/or intra-abdominal fluid sequestration, as well as enabling translocation of enteric organisms or their cellular components (e.g., endotoxin) across the previously intact mucosal barrier.

4. The kidney, like the brain and heart, displays complex autoregulation over a broad range of perfusion pressures. As perfusion falls, blood is initially redistributed to the renal medulla from the cortex; as it falls further, a significant decrease in glomerular filtration is manifested clinically by a reduction in urine volume and eventually by anuria. The development of oliguria in any patient should be sufficient to prompt a thorough investigation into the cardiovascular and volume status of that individual.

5. Hepatic dysfunction is common in patients with shock and is related to hypoperfusion of the liver. The most common abnormality is elevation of the hepatic transaminases; however, coagulopathy and overt hepatic necrosis may also occur if the duration or extent of hypoperfusion is prolonged or severe. In some forms of shock (e.g., septic shock) the liver has been implicated as a major producer of cytokines. This cascade of inflammatory mediators is thought to be initiated by the liver's role in filtering organisms or endotoxins that have originated from the bowel.

6. While the lung has a dual blood supply and thus is not as dependent on perfusion as are other organs, respiratory failure is very common in shock. This is manifested by diffuse lung infiltrates, impaired oxygenation, and increased work of breathing. Both cardiogenic and noncardiogenic pulmonary edema occur, and must be differentiated by clinical and often invasive diagnostic means. The mechanisms of noncardiogenic pulmonary edema are poorly understood, but may be related to the production of large quantities of cytokines and other inflammatory mediators produced by the hypoperfused liver.

C. Other subcellular responses to shock
A number of other responses occur in shock, all prompted by an effort to maintain perfusion by either stimulating cardiac output, increasing blood pressure, or increasing the effective circulating blood volume.

1. Circulating catecholamine levels rise dramatically in shock, and in doing so cause both α- and β-receptor stimulation. This leads to both cardiac stimulation and peripheral vascular constriction.

2. Numerous hormonal responses occur in shock, including a rise in cortisol, adrenocorticotropic hormone (ACTH), and antidiuretic hormone (ADH), all of which serve to retain salt and water in order to expand the circulating blood volume.

3. Lastly, in response to the metabolic acidosis, a shift in the oxyhemoglobin dissociation curve to the right occurs, allowing more efficient unloading of oxygen at the cellular interface.

IV. Diagnosis
A. Clinical recognition
Because shock is defined as a systemic disorder in which tissue hypoperfusion occurs, it is usually recognized clinically by the development of systemic hypotension or organ dysfunction. As described above, it is the most perfusion-dependent organs that first fail in shock—namely, the brain, kidneys,

Table 39-2. Characteristic Clinical and Laboratory Findings in Shock

Organ System	Clinical Findings	Laboratory/Radiographic Findings
Cardiovascular	Hypotension	Electrocardiographic changes
	Cool, clammy skin	Lactic acidosis
	Tachycardia	Cardiomegaly
	Dysrhythmias	
Renal	Reduced urine output	Increased blood urea nitrogen, creatinine
Central nervous system	Mental status changes	
Hepatic	Peripheral edema	Hypoalbuminemia
	Excessive bleeding	Coagulopathy/disseminated intravascular coagulopathy
		Increased transaminases
		Hyperbilirubinemia
Pulmonary	Tachypnea	Respiratory alkalosis
	Cyanosis	Increased A-a gradient
	Rales	Pulmonary edema
Hematologic	Petechiae	Thrombocytopenia
		Anemia
		Increased white blood cell count
Gastrointestinal	Gastrointestinal bleeding	Mucosal ulcerations
	Abdominal pain	Infarcted bowel
Others	Fever, hypothermia	

and cardiovascular system. Therefore the presence of characteristic abnormalities in the function of these organs usually first alert the physician to the presence of shock (see Table 39-2). Thus the classic triad of oliguria, mental status changes, and poor systemic perfusion (as manifested by poor capillary refill, cool extremities, and often hypotension) should immediately alert the physician to the presence of a shock state, and in order to prevent further end-organ dysfunction, therapy must begin immediately, even before a specific diagnosis is established.

B. Initial assessment

A brief organ-specific assessment should initially be performed in all patients thought to be in shock, with the goal of identifying the underlying cause of shock. Because of the low specificity of the physical examination in determining the cause of shock, invasive hemodynamic monitoring is often needed to diagnose and manage these conditions more reliably.

1. Volume status

It is of the utmost importance to identify the specific volume status of any patient in shock, initially by using clinical criteria

and often by subsequently applying invasive monitoring devices. Clinical signs of volume contraction are nonspecific and difficult to distinguish from those of reduced cardiac output; they include reduced pulse pressure, postural hypotension, tachycardia, oliguria, cool dry skin, and reduced jugular venous pressure. Volume overload, meanwhile, is associated with distended neck veins, peripheral edema, rales, and an S3 gallop on auscultation of the heart. The chest radiograph in patients with hypervolemia often demonstrates the presence of cardiomegaly, pulmonary edema, and/or pleural effusions.

2. Cardiac output

As with volume status, the physical examination is often unreliable in determining cardiac output. Nonspecific findings of oliguria, reduced pulse pressure, delayed capillary refill, cool clammy skin, tachycardia, and mental status changes may all be found in patients with depressed cardiac output, but they are also present in other forms of shock as well. Hyperdynamic forms of shock are usually accompanied by warm skin, a bounding pulse,

Table 39-3.   Characteristic Hemodynamic Findings in Shock

	CO	SVR	PAOP	CVP	Da-vO$_2$
Cardiogenic shock	↓	↑	↑	↔	↑
Acute MI (LV)	↓	↑	↑	↑	↑
Acute MI (RV)	↓	↑	↑	↑	↑
Cardiomyopathy	↓	↑	↑	↑	↑
Acute mitral regurgitation	↓	↑	↑	↑	↑
Aortic stenosis					
Extracardiac obstructive					
Pericardial tamponade	↓	↑	↑	↑	↑
Massive Pulm. Embolus	↓	↑	↔	↑	↑
Oligemic	↓	↑	↓	↓	↑
Distributive					
Vasodilator	↔	↓	↓	↓	0,↓
Spinal cord injury	↑	↓	↓	↓	0,↓
Mixed					
Septic shock (early)	↓	↑	0,↓	↔	↑
After volume resuscitation	0,↑	↓	↔	↔	↓
Premorbid	↔	↑	↔	↔	↑

Abbreviations: CO, cardiac output; SVR, systemic vascular resistance; PAOP, pulmonary artery occlusion pressure; CVP, central venous pressure; Da-vO$_2$, the difference between arterial and venous oxygen contents.

Symbols: 0, no effect; ↔ variable effect; ↑, increase; ↓, decrease.

and tachycardia. Again, hemodynamic monitoring is warranted for those patients without a clear etiology for their shock on physical exam (see Table 39-3).

3. Adequacy of oxygenation
Although peripheral cyanosis is strongly associated with hypoxemia, serial arterial blood gases are needed to manage properly any patient in shock. Supplemental oxygen should be administered to all patients immediately while awaiting the results. The presence of hypoxemia should alert the physician to the likely coexistence of either acute or chronic lung disease. Therapeutically, an arterial saturation of 95% or higher is recommended for all of these patients.

4. Adequacy of tissue perfusion
Clinically, determination of the adequacy of tissue perfusion is made using the criteria cited above, including capillary refill, rate of urine production, warmth of skin, and laboratory determinants of either systemic perfusion or specific organ function (e.g., blood lactate, pH, creatinine, bilirubin, creatine phosphokinase, lipase).

C. Use of hemodynamic monitoring
The use of invasive hemodynamic monitor-

ing has revolutionized the care of patients in shock. Not only can an accurate assessment of volume status and cardiac output be made, but the response to therapy can be rapidly determined.

1. Arterial catheters
Indwelling arterial catheters are relatively safe and easy to place, and provide an immediate and continuous recording of both systolic and mean arterial blood pressures. Although blood pressure correlates poorly with blood flow, the use of these catheters can rapidly alert critical care staff to acute changes in physiology that affect the blood pressure.

2. Pulmonary artery catheters
   a. The pulmonary capillary wedge pressure (PCWP), provides a reasonable assessment of left ventricular preload in patients without severe mitral valvular, ventricular compliance, or pulmonary venous diseases. Patients with a significant elevation of their PCWP (greater than 18 mmHg) will usually be found to have a cardiogenic form of shock, while those with a low PCWP can safely be thought of as having a noncardiogenic form of shock. Equalization of end-diastolic pressures

Table 39-4.   Therapeutic Goals in the Management of Shock

1. Improve oxygen delivery to a level where metabolic needs are met:
    MAP > 65 mm Hg
    Normalize blood lactate level
    Maintain hemoglobin > 10 g%
    Maintain oxygen saturation > 95%
    Maintain cardiac index > 2.2 liters l/min/m^2 in cardiogenic shock and > 4.0 liters/min/m^2 in septic shock*
    Maintain Da-vO$_2$ = arterial − mixed venous oxygen difference < 5.0
    Reverse and/or normalize organ dysfunction
        Renal—blood urea nitrogen, creatinine, urine output
        Hepatic—bilirubin
        Pulmonary—(A-a) gradient
        Central nervous system—mental status
2. Treatment or correction of the underlying cause of shock—for example:
    Ischemia—maximize coronary perfusion with coronary vasodilators or revascularization
                (angioplasty or coronary bypass surgery)
            —Minimize myocardial oxygen consumption
    Oligemic—Volume replacement with appropriate volume expander (e.g., blood, crystalloids, albumin)
    Septic   —antibiotics, surgical drainage of abscess, etc.

*In selected forms of shock (e.g., septic shock) there may be indications for maintaining a considerably higher cardiac index.

(PCWP, pulmonary arterial, right ventricular, and right atrial) is highly suggestive of pericardial tamponade.

   b. Cardiac output, as determind by thermodilution, is also an invaluable tool in managing patients with shock. As described above, low cardiac output can be seen in any form of shock, whereas normal or high cardiac output is seen only in distributive or mixed forms of shock. The characteristic hemodynamic patterns of the various forms of shock are shown in Table 39-3.

   3. Noninvasive determinations of filling pressures and cardiac output
    A number of techniques to determine the cardiac output and filling pressures noninvasively have been described. To date the only one receiving widespread use is the echocardiographic/Doppler assessment of end-diastolic volumes, myocardial contractility, and pulmonary artery pressures.

V. Goals in the Management of Shock
    Specific therapeutic goals must be decided when managing patients in shock. These can be divided into goals associated with the initial resuscitation of the patient in shock and those that require more sophisticated clinical and lab-oratory data, and are therefore necessarily difficult to define and achieve during the initial resuscitation (see Table 39-4).

A. Immediate resuscitative goals
    These are goals that require only a brief physical examination and minimal laboratory evaluation to define and monitor.
    1. Because the determination of adequate perfusion to all tissue beds is difficult, findings suggestive of improving tissue perfusion are initially used to identify the response to therapy. These include the normalization of MAP, development of adequate urine output (> 30 ml/hr), improvement in mental status, resolution of chest pain when present, and resolution of peripheral cyanosis and poor capillary refill.

B. Subsequent therapeutic goals
    These goals require a more thorough evaluation of clinical, laboratory, and hemodynamic parameters but provide much more information about the adequacy of blood flow to individual tissue beds.
    1. As a measure of the adequacy of systemic oxygen delivery, the normalization of a metabolic acidosis, or the return toward normal of a previously elevated serum lactate level, is highly suggestive of a reduction in anaerobic metabolism, with

Table 39-5. Specific Management Strategies in Shock States

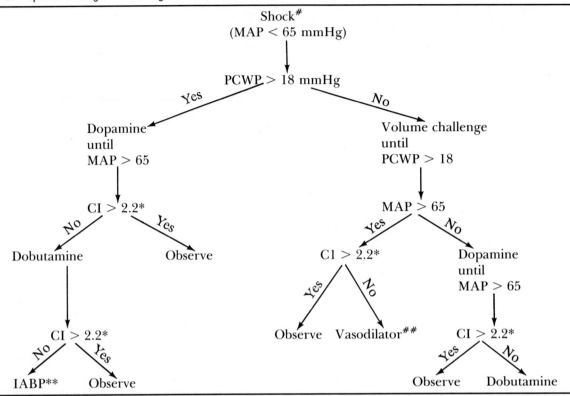

#This is a management strategy for shock associated with hypotension. In nonhypotensive patients in shock, efforts to maximize oxygen delivery using inotropic agents, blood transfusions when necessary, and supplemental oxygen should be performed.

*In septic shock we use a CI > 4.0 because of experimental data suggesting an improved outcome in those patients with a high cardiac output and oxygen delivery.

**Rarely would an intra-aortic balloon pump (IABP) be used in patients with septic shock.

##Vasodilators would rarely be efficacious in situations where vasodilation is often present (e.g., septic shock). In these patients, a dobutamine infusion would be substituted for the vasodilator.

a resultant shift toward aerobic metabolism. This is why it is most useful to determine the lactate level serially rather than on only one occasion.

2. When invasive hemodynamic monitoring is used, the normalization of cardiac output, when reduced, is an appropriate goal in most patients. The specific target cardiac output must be individualized, however, depending on the metabolic stress affecting each patient, as well as the previous cardiovascular function and the adequacy of compensatory reserve. As an example, an elderly patient with a chronically dilated cardiomyopathy will usually not require as high a cardiac index (CI) (cardiac output normalized for body surface area) as a younger individual with an acute myocardial infarction. As a rule of thumb, a CI > 2.2 liters/

min · m^2 is usually adequate in patients with either cardiogenic or extracardiac obstructive forms of shock. Patients with other forms of shock, in particular septic shock, usually benefit from a significantly higher CI (> 4.0 liters/min · m^2), because these patients also have concomitant abnormalities in unloading oxygen at the tissue level.

When available, knowledge of the hemodynamic physiology of the patient prior to the development of shock provides invaluable information that can help determine individual goals.

3. Clear reversal of organ dysfunction, or preferably prevention of organ dysfunction, is a primary goal in managing patients in shock. Metabolic markers of individual organ function (e.g., creatinine, bilirubin) should be followed on a serial

basis to help determine the adequacy of blood flow to these organs (see Table 39-4).

VI. Managing the Patient in Shock

Shock is a medical emergency and requires the immediate institution of therapy in order to correct the underlying physiologic problem, as well as to prevent the development or worsening of organ dysfunction. While the appropriate management of a patient in shock requires a thorough knowledge of the etiology of the shock, initial resuscitative efforts should begin concomitantly with attempts to establish a diagnosis. Following the initial resuscitation, and after invasive monitoring devices have been placed, specific diagnosis and physiology-based management can proceed.

A. Initial resuscitation

While the initial resuscitation occurs in the absence of a complete physiologic database, it should not obviate or delay efforts to establish the etiology of shock. In addition to a brief physical examination with specific attention to volume status and adequacy of systemic perfusion (see Table 39-2), the acquisition of several laboratory tests, including arterial blood gases, a chest radiograph, and an electrocardiogram, should occur during this phase of resuscitation. Clearly, the identification of a reversible form of shock mandates therapy directed to that etiology (i.e., a tension pneumothorax).

1. Restoration of circulating volume

The rapid delivery of intravenous fluids is the initial resuscitative measure in all patients with hypotension and/or shock of unknown etiology. The choice of fluid to be administered is dependent on one's clinical assessment of the type of shock. In patients with obvious hemorrhage, packed red blood cells should be employed; in those with chronic malnourishment or other processes that predispose to hypoalbuminemia (e.g., nephrotic syndrome, cirrhosis), albumin is the fluid of choice. While controversy about the use of crystalloids versus colloids persists, our practice is to use normal saline or lactated Ringer's solution in the remainder of these patients. When given in adequate volumes, these solutions are equally effective in raising the preload at a fraction of the cost of colloids.

Fluid therapy is continued until either the blood pressure normalizes or a better indicator of intravascular volume status (i.e., a pulmonary artery catheter) suggests that the intravascular compartment is adequately expanded.

2. Restoration of blood pressure

Fluid therapy alone is insufficient to normalize blood pressure in many patients in shock, and so must be accompanied by other means while awaiting a diagnosis and physiologically directed therapy. Dopamine is the initial vasopressor we use in patients with hypotension that has not responded to 1–2 liters of crystalloid solution. This agent, given in low doses, improves cardiac performance and augments renal and mesenteric perfusion, while at higher doses it exerts both inotropic (and chronotropic) and vasopressor effects. It can thus be titrated upward until an adequate blood pressure (MAP > 65 mmHg) has been achieved. If an excessively tachycardic response to dopamine occurs, neosynephrine can be substituted, providing the necessary α-agonist activity (raising the blood pressure) without causing unwanted β-stimulatory effects (tachycardia).

3. Placement of intravascular catheters

We employ both indwelling radial artery and pulmonary artery catheters in all patients who do not respond readily to volume therapy. These catheters should be placed during the initial resuscitative efforts by individuals skilled in both the techniques of placement and interpretation of the data derived from these catheters.

B. Subsequent diagnosis and physiology-directed therapy

Once the etiology of shock has been determined and/or invasive monitoring has been employed, a diagnosis is made and physiology-directed therapy is initiated. Because of the broad range of physiologic patterns that are seen in shock, treatment varies considerably among etiologic categories. Below is a general approach to patients within each broad category of shock.

1. Cardiogenic shock

a. Cardiogenic shock results predominantly from pump failure, but it can also be complicated by abnormalities in preload and afterload. In an effort to improve systolic performance, the Starling principle is applied, suggesting that an adequate preload must be maintained. In the absence of pulmonary edema we characteristically push volume therapy until the PCWP reaches 18 mmHg, although some patients will display a further improvement in cardiac output above this level. If this approach fails to raise the CI above 2.2 liters/min/m^2, then either dobutamine or amrinone is added for its additional potent inotropic effects. If high doses of these potent inotropes fail to raise the CI sufficiently and the patient remains in shock, then placement of an intra-aortic balloon pump should be considered. These devices work by maximizing coronary perfusion while reducing afterload during rapid deflation.

b. Patients with cardiogenic shock who have a high afterload (systemic vascular resistance, SVR) respond well to other forms of afterload reduction with agents such as nitroprusside, which provides both arterial and venous vasodilation. Caution must be employed when using these agents because the vasodilatory effect can cause a further fall in blood pressure and in ventricular filling pressures. This effect can often be minimized by ensuring adequate volume replacement (preload) prior to initiating this therapy.

c. In patients with ischemic causes of cardiogenic shock (either acute myocardial infarction or active myocardial ischemia), a primary goal must be to reduce myocardial oxygen consumption and to maximize coronary blood flow (discussed in Chapter 21). Therefore coronary vasodilators, intravenous nitroglycerin, and occasionally β-blockade should be considered in these patients. The early application of emergent coronary angiography will identify those patients best suited for percutaneous transluminal coronary angioplasty or operative revascularization in order to abate and reverse the myocardial injury that is manifested as cardiogenic shock.

2. Extracardiac obstructive shock
This form of shock is almost always amenable to specific therapeutic interventions (e.g., pericardiocentesis in pericardial tamponade or thrombolytic therapy in massive pulmonary embolus), and it is this intervention that will cause a reversal of shock. While performing appropriate diagnostic tests or awaiting definitive therapy, these patients can often be supported temporarily by the use of volume expansion and inotropic therapy with dobutamine or dopamine.

3. Oligemic shock
Oligemic shock, by definition, occurs solely due to a reduction in preload to the left ventricle. The management of these patients therefore consists of rapidly replacing intravascular volume with the appropriate fluid (see the discussion above). Vasopressors or inotropic agents are rarely indicated in this form of shock.

4. Distributive/mixed shock
a. The management of these patients must be carefully individualized, using frequent determinations of cardiac filling pressures, cardiac outputs, and oxygen transport variables. An example of how complex some conditions may be is seen in sepsis, where patients are usually seen initially at a point where they are relatively volume depleted and vasodilated. After adequate volume replacement (we use a pulmonary capillary wedge pressure, PCWP, of > 14 mmHg), these patients usually become hyperdynamic, with elevated cardiac output, reduced SVR, and evidence of a modest reduction in cardiac performance (decreased ejection fraction). In a small number of patients, a late or premorbid phase of septic shock develops, with a severe reduction in myocardial performance (related to myocardial depression) and a SVR that may be either low, normal, or high. These latter patients require high doses of inotropic agents in order to maintain adequate cardiac output.

b. As a rule of thumb, we push the PCWP in all patients with septic shock to 16 mmHg or greater in order to maximize myocardial contractility and oxygen delivery. If patients are persistently hypotensive, a dopamine infusion is begun, titrating the dose to maintain a MAP of > 65 mmHg. If this still fails to raise the MAP adequately, we begin an infusion of norepinephrine (a more potent α- and β-agonist) and reduce the dopamine infusion to the renal vasodilating range (< 5 μg/kg/min). Inotropic therapy is occasionally needed and should be guided by either an inadequate CI (< 4.0 liters/min/m^2) or persistent evidence of tissue hypoxia (manifested by a lactic acidosis or widened arterial-mixed venous oxygen difference). The inotropic agent of choice in this situation is usually dobutamine.

VII. Prognosis

A. The prognosis for a patient who develops shock depends upon a number of factors, including age, presence of preexisting illness or organ dysfunction, severity and etiology of shock, and the rapidity and completeness of response to therapy. While most of these factors cannot be altered once shock has developed, the early recognition of shock and/or organ dysfunction and the rapid institution of treatment can be expected to improve the outcome substantially.

B. Once end organ failure develops, the prognosis worsens significantly. In fact, the presence of three or more failed organs for at least 5 days has been associated with a fatal outcome. Thus early attention to support of the circulation and maintenance of oxygen delivery, as well as efforts to reverse organ dysfunction when it occurs, are vital to improving the outcome of shock.

VIII. Conclusions

Shock is a common disorder of diverse etiologies that is clinically manifested by organ dysfunction resulting from a reduction in oxygen delivery at the micro- or macrovascular level. The mortality of the syndrome is high if treatment is withheld or delayed, but it can be significantly reduced by appropriate management of the process underlying the development of shock, as well as the institution of aggressive measures to restore adequate delivery of oxygen and other nutrients at the cellular level.

Bibliography

Parrillo JE. *Current Therapy in Critical Care Medicine,* ed 2, Philadelphia, BC Decker, 1991, pp 1–350.

Parrillo JE, Parker MM, Natanson C, et al. Septic shock in humans: Advances in the understanding of pathogenesis, cardiovascular dysfunction, and therapy. *Ann Intern Med* 113:227–242, 1990.

Schuster DP, Lefrak SS. Shock, in Civetta JM, Taylor RW, Kirby RR (eds), *Critical Care.* Philadelphia, JB Lippincott, 1988, p 891.

Shoemaker WC. Shock states: Pathophysiology, monitoring, outcome prediction, and therapy, in Shoemaker WC, Ayres S, Grenvik A, et al. *Textbook of Critical Care,* ed 2, Philadelphia, WB Saunders, 1989, p 977.

CHAPTER 40

Acute Respiratory Failure

Robert A. Balk, M.D.
Roger C. Bone, M.D.

I. **Definition**
   A. Respiratory failure is the inability of the respiratory system to meet adequately the oxygenation and/or ventilation demands of the body.
      1. Depending on the duration of the failure and the degree of metabolic compensation, respiratory failure may be described as acute, subacute, or chronic.
      2. The major functions of the respiratory system include:
         a. The oxygenation of blood as it circulates through the capillaries of the lung.
         b. The excretion of carbon dioxide that has been produced through the metabolic processes of the various organ systems.
         c. The lung is also involved in the metabolism of various substances that are either produced in the lung or altered as they pass through the lung.
   B. There are two major types of respiratory failure that are classified according to carbon dioxide elimination.
      1. Type I respiratory failure
         a. Also termed *Hypoxemic respiratory failure*.
         b. Manifested by hypoxemia with a normal or low partial pressure of carbon dioxide ($PaCO_2$).
      2. Type II respiratory failure
         a. Also termed *hypoxemic-hypercapnic respiratory failure*.
         b. Manifested by both hypoxemia and hypercapnia.
   C. Definition of hypoxemia
      1. Hypoxemia refers to inadequate or low levels of oxygen in the arterial blood.

II. **Etiology and Risk Factors for the Development of Respiratory Failure**
   A. The development of acute respiratory failure can be viewed as involving a chain that includes the brain, spinal cord, neuromuscular system, thorax and pleura, upper airway, cardiovascular system, and lower airway. Each of these components is important in maintaining the integrity of the chain. Breaks anywhere along this chain may lead to the subsequent development of acute respiratory failure (Figure 40-1).

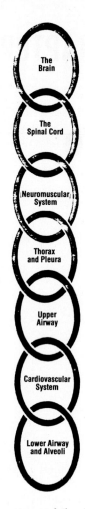

The Brain

The Spinal Cord

Neuromuscular System

Thorax and Pleura

Upper Airway

Cardiovascular System

Lower Airway and Alveoli

Figure 40-1. Chain of respiratory failure/function.

B. Examples of disorders that may involve the components of this chain are as follows.
   1. The brain may be altered by a variety of clinical disorders, including:
      a. Cerebrovascular accidents
      b. Bulbar poliomyelitis
      c. Drug overdose
      d. Central alveolar hypoventilation syndrome
      e. Trauma
      f. Myxedema
      g. Postoperative anesthetic depression
   2. The spinal cord may be affected by:
      a. Guillain-Barré syndrome
      b. Spinal cord trauma
      c. Poliomyelitis
      d. Amyotrophic lateral sclerosis
   3. Examples of neuromuscular disorders include:
      a. Myasthenia gravis
      b. Those due to Curariform drugs
      c. Those due to neuromuscular blocking antibiotics
      d. Those due to organophosphate insecticides
      e. Multiple sclerosis
      f. Hypophosphatemia
      g. Tetanus
      h. Botulism
      i. Myxedema
      j. Peripheral neuritis
      k. Hypokalemic paralysis
      l. Hypomagnesemia
   4. The upper airway may be responsible for the development of acute respiratory failure associated with:
      a. Obstructive sleep apnea
      b. Tracheal obstruction
      c. Postintubation laryngeal edema
      d. Large tonsils and adenoids
      e. Vocal cord paralysis
      f. Epiglottitis
      g. Laryngotracheitis
   5. Abnormalities of the thorax and pleura that may contribute to respiratory failure include:
      a. Muscular dystrophy
      b. Kyphoscoliosis
      c. Rheumatoid spondylitis
      d. Pleural effusion
      e. Massive obesity
      f. Trauma/flail chest
      g. Pneumothorax
   6. Cardiovascular alterations that may lead to respiratory failure include:
      a. Cardiogenic pulmonary edema
      b. Pulmonary embolism
      c. Fat embolism
      d. Venomous snake bite
      e. Uremia
   7. The lower airway and alveoli may be altered by a variety of clinical conditions that in some instances will result in the development of acute respiratory failure. A partial list of some of these disorders includes:
      a. The aspiration of gastric acid or bile
      b. Smoke inhalation
      c. Exacerbations of chronic obstructive pulmonary disease
      d. Cystic fibrosis
      e. Interstitial lung disease
      f. Massive bilateral pneumonia
      g. Near drowning

h. Radiation
i. Septic shock
j. Bronchiolitis
k. Acute exacerbations of asthma
l. Adult respiratory distress syndrome (ARDS)
m. Atelectasis
n. Bronchiectasis
o. Pulmonary contusion
p. Pancreatitis

C. Respiratory muscle depression or dysfunction may predispose the patient to the development of acute respiratory failure. Included in the factors that may potentiate respiratory muscle depression are:

1. The existence of renal failure, which may lead to drug accumulation, hypocalcemia, and electrolyte disorders.
2. The use of anesthetic agents or muscle relaxants.
3. Preexisting neuromuscular disease.
4. Overdose of medications, especially sedatives and narcotics.
5. Hypothermia.
6. The presence of respiratory acidosis.
7. Hypermagnesemia.
8. The use of certain antibiotics, especially in close relationship to the use of various neuromuscular blocking drugs, may be associated with the development of acute respiratory failure.
   a. Aminoglycosides
      (1) Gentamicin
      (2) Tobramycin
      (3) Amakacin
      (4) Streptomycin
      (5) Kanamycin
      (6) Neomycin
   b. Polymyxins
      (1) Colistin
      (2) Polymyxin B
   c. Other
      (1) Viomycin

D. Additional risk factors that may contribute to the subsequent development of acute respiratory failure include:

1. Increased hydrostatic pressure
   a. Congestive heart failure
   b. Fluid overload
2. Recumbency
3. The excessive use of sedatives and/or narcotics.
4. The presence of an ileus, upper abdominal surgery, or gross abdominal distention.

5. Chronic lung disease.
6. Advanced age.
7. Recent history of cigarette use.

III. **Pathophysiology**

A. There are four basic pathophysiologic mechanisms of hypoxemia.

1. Inadequate partial pressure of alveolar oxygen tension (PAO_2).
   a. Hypoventilation
   b. Lowered fraction of oxygen in the inspired air (FiO_2)
2. Mismatching of ventilation and perfusion relationships.
3. Increased shunt fraction.
4. Diffusion abnormalities.

B. Hypercapnia results from a variety of causes, including:

1. Increased CO_2 production ($\dot{V}_{CO_2}$) is seen with:
   a. Fever
   b. Pain
   c. Stress
   d. Increased carbohydrate load
   e. Increased work of breathing
2. Decreased CO_2 excretion, as seen in patients with;
   a. Airway obstruction and/or increased airway resistance
   b. Neuromuscular weakness leading to hypoventilation.
   c. Hypoventilation related to oversedation or central nervous system disorders.
3. The $PaCO_2$ is inversely proportional to the alveolar ventilation (V_A). This relationship is expressed by the equation $PACO_2 = 0.863 \times \dot{V}_{CO_2}/V_A$.
   a. The normal $\dot{V}_{CO_2}$ is approximately 200 ml/min. This number will vary with the metabolic activity.
   b. The $PaCO_2$ is normally maintained under fairly tight control, despite changes in $\dot{V}_{CO_2}$. This is normally the consequence of changes in the Minute Ventilation (Respiratory Rate X Tidal Volume) ($\dot{V}_E$) regulated by peripheral and central chemoreceptors and their feedback to the brain stem.
   c. Even with complete apnea, the $PaCO_2$ increases at a rate of only 6–8 mmHg/min.

IV. **Diagnosis**

A. History

1. Acute respiratory failure exists when the

pulmonary system is unable to meet the oxygenation, ventilation, or metabolic demands of the body. Typically, the patient is acutely dyspneic and manifests a $PaO_2 <$ 50 mmHg, $PaCO_2 > 50$ mmHg, or a decreased arterial pH. As Figure 40-1 illustrates, a wide variety of clinical entities may be associated with or lead to the development of acute respiratory failure.

2. Acute respiratory failure is often a complication or a worsening of a preexisting disorder.

3. The development of the respiratory failure may be acute or acute superimposed upon a more chronic process.

B. Clinical signs and physical findings

1. The clinical signs and physical manifestations of respiratory insufficiency and acute respiratory failure include visual, tactile, and auditory signs.

   a. The visual signs of respiratory distress may include:

     (1) Abnormal rate of respiration or abnormal breathing pattern.

     (2) Gasping respirations or the use of the accessory muscles of respiration.

     (3) Retraction of the thoracic rib cage.

     (4) The presence of foreign matter in the mouth.

     (5) Visible cyanosis or pale, sweaty skin. The patient may also appear apprehensive or in distress.

   b. The tactile signs of respiratory distress may include:

     (1) An increased, decreased, or irregular pulse. A pulsus paradox may be measured or palpable.

     (2) The skin may feel cold and clammy or may be very diaphoretic. Patients with febrile processes may have warm skin.

   c. The auditory and auscultatory signs of respiratory distress may include:

     (1) A silent examination, with little audible air movement.

     (2) Snoring or gurgling respiratory sounds.

     (3) High-pitched, musical stridor or upper airway noises.

     (4) Localized or diffuse wheezing. This may be accompanied by a prolongation of the expiratory phase of respiration.

     (5) The presence of crackles, rales, or rhonchi.

2. The clinical manifestations of acute hypercapnia may include:

   a. A decreased level of consciousness.

   b. The presence of a headache.

   c. Warm skin or a feeling of being flushed.

   d. Hypertension and/or tachycardia.

   e. The subjective complaint of dyspnea, which may or may not be present.

   f. Congested conjunctiva or papilledema of the eyes.

   g. Asterixis on examination.

3. The clinical manifestations of acute hypoxemia may include:

   a. Altered mental status or altered level of mental function.

   b. Usually no sensation of distress. Restlessness or agitation.

   c. The vital signs may reflect tachypnea, tachycardia, or hypertension.

   d. Mild peripheral vasoconstriction.

4. Unfortunately, hypoxemia and hypercapnia are difficult to diagnose from the clinical examination. Laboratory assessment of oxygenation and ventilation abnormalities is imperative in the assessment of these patients.

C. Diagnostic tests

1. Laboratory tests

   a. The hallmark laboratory evaluation for the diagnosis of acute respiratory failure is the arterial blood gas (ABG) test.

   b. In the absence of ABG availability, the use of noninvasive determinants of oxygenation and ventilation status may be used.

   c. Additional laboratory tests as appropriate for diagnosis and/or management of the underlying condition may be useful.

     (1) These tests may include determination of the serum electrolytes, magnesium, calcium, phosphate, and the acid/base status.

2. Roentgenographic studies

   a. Radiologic studies as appropriate for the diagnosis and management of the underlying disorder may give some clues to the etiology of the respiratory failure.

   b. The chest x-ray is typically obtained in this circumstance and may provide evidence of:

(1) Pneumonia and pulmonary infiltrates.

(2) Congestive heart failure.

(3) Pneumothorax.

(4) Trauma.

(5) Pleural effusions.

(6) Atelectasis.

3. Other tests

a. Pulmonary function tests can be used to assess the degree of respiratory compromise. These tests include:

(1) Simple spirometry (forced vital capacity [FVC], forced expiratory volume in 1 sec [FEV_1], FEV_1/FVC)

(2) Maximum inspiratory and expiratory pressures.

(3) Tidal volume, respiratory rate, and minute ventilation.

(4) Determination of pulmonary compliance (static and dynamic components), work of breathing, and airway resistance.

b. Physiologic assessments may be measured or calculated to assist with the diagnosis of acute respiratory failure.

(1) Calculation of the alveolar-arterial oxygen gradient.

(2) PaO_2/PAO_2 ratio.

(3) PaO_2/FiO_2 ratio.

(4) Venous admixture or shunt fraction.

(5) Arterial oxygen content, arteriovenous oxygen difference, tissue oxygen delivery.

(6) Dead space ventilation.

V. Differential Diagnosis

A. The differential diagnosis of acute respiratory failure is primarily related to the differential diagnosis of the underlying predisposing or complicating medical condition(s). In most cases, the onset of acute respiratory failure can be viewed as a later stage or a complication of the underlying injury process. Often there is no arbitrary change that denotes the sudden development of acute respiratory failure. Instead there is a continuum of progressive worsening, with the end result being the onset of failure.

B. In some circumstances, it is important to recognize the specific differential diagnostic possibilities that manifest as acute respiratory failure, since the subsequent approach to patient care and the allocation of resources and efforts may be altered, depending upon the specific conditions that are present. In patients with hopeless or futile conditions, aggressive mechanical ventilatory support may not be appropriate.

C. In other circumstances, the diagnosis of respiratory failure will be based on purely clinical grounds, and there will be no initial supporting laboratory work or confirmatory studies.

VI. Basic Principles of Treatment and Patient Monitoring

A. The basic principles of treatment and management of the patient with acute respiratory failure are the same for most etiologies. The cornerstone of management is specific treatment directed at the underlying disorder that led to the development of the acute respiratory failure.

1. Obviously this necessitates identification of the predisposing disorder or break in the chain (see Figure 40-1) and the institution of specific therapy.

2. This therapy is typically administered in a special care unit or an intensive care unit, utilizing the resources of these specialized units.

a. Included in these resources are trained, experienced staff (nurses, respiratory therapists, and other ancillary personnel).

b. The special care areas may also contain various patient monitors that can assist in ther management of these patients.

(1) Electrocardiography and the ability to use hemodynamic monitors.

(2) Patients on mechanical ventilatory support may be monitored by some of the monitors built into the ventilator.

(3) Monitors of oxygenation

(a) Pulse oximetry is a noninvasive method used to monitor the oxygen saturation of patients with acute respiratory failure. It has been demonstrated to be very reliable and easy to use in the majority of patients.

(b) Transcutaneous measurement of oxygen tension has been shown to be useful in neonates and small children but is not reliable in adults, especially those with poor perfusion and thick skin.

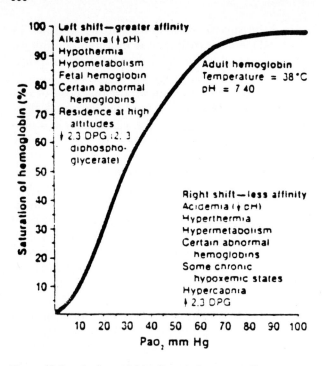

Figure 40-2. Oxyhemoglobin dissociation curve. Factors associated with rightward and leftward shifts of the curve. Right shifts have less affinity for oxygen and a greater release of oxygen to the tissues. Left shifts have greater oxygen affinity and less release of oxygen to the tissues.

(c) Conjunctival measurement of oxygen tension is another method used to monitor oxygenation status, but it is difficult and not as well accepted.

(d) Some of the noninvasive monitors of oxygenation related to changes in oxygen saturation. The relationship of oxygen saturation to PaO_2 is depicted by the oxyhemoglobin dissociation curve, the position of which can be influenced by a number of factors (Figure 40-2).

(4) Monitors of ventilation

(a) Mass spectrometers have been used to analyze the expired gases on a breath-by-breath basis.

(b) End-tidal CO_2 monitors can measure the carbon dioxide concentration of the expired air and seem to work reasonably well in patients without lung disease. Unfortunately, in patients with lung disease, there is so much mismatching of ventilation and perfusion that the value does not adequately reflect the $PaCO_2$.

(c) The transcutaneous CO_2 measurement appears to be a reliable, noninvasive measurement of the $PaCO_2$. The value of this technique in patients with poor perfusion remains to be established.

(5) Other monitors used in the basic management and evaluation of patients with acute respiratory failure may include:

(a) Electrocardiographic monitoring.

(b) Noninvasive blood pressure monitoring.

(c) Invasive hemodynamic monitoring with arterial and pulmonary artery catheters.

(d) Respiratory inductive plethysmography.

B. Oxygenation and/or ventilatory support are frequently necessary to manage these patients and can take many forms. In some circumstances, mechanical ventilation with endotracheal intubation has been avoided by the use of mask or nasal positive-pressure ventilation or other respiratory support devices.

1. Adequate oxygenation should be ensured by the use of supplemental oxygen in patients who are hypoxemic. In circumstances of CO_2 retention, some advocate controlled administration of oxygen using Venturi masks.

a. The Venturi mask allows controlled administration of oxygen from 24% to 50% FiO_2.

b. Nasal canula oxygen can be administered up to approximately 6 liters/min based on the patient's tolerance. However, with this method of oxygen delivery, it is almost impossible to know the exact FiO_2 that is being delivered.

c. Face masks, face shields, and high-humidity/high-flow face masks can be utilized to administer FiO_2 up to 100% in some patients.

2. In patients who do not achieve adequate

oxygenation with the use of supplemental oxygen and who have diffuse lung disease, the use of masked continuous positive airway pressure (CPAP) or, if on mechanical ventilatory support, positive end-expiratory pressure (PEEP) may be of benefit in improving the PaO_2 on a given FiO_2.

    a. PEEP works by decreasing the shunt fraction, increasing the functional residual capacity (FRC), and recruiting more functional lung units.

  3. Mechanical ventilatory support

    a. Positive-pressure ventilation.

      (1) Conventional positive-pressure ventilation.

      (2) Nonconventional positive-pressure ventilation.

        (a) Masked positive-pressure ventilation.

        (b) Nasal positive-pressure ventilation.

        (c) High-frequency ventilation.

        (d) Permissive hypercapnia.

        (e) Low-frequency, positive-pressure ventilation with extracorporeal CO_2 removal.

        (f) Inverse ratio ventilation.

      (3) Negative-pressure ventilation.

      (4) Respiratory assist devices.

        (a) Pneumobelt

        (b) Cuirass

        (c) Poncho or shell

        (d) Rocking bed

        (e) Phrenic nerve pacing

C. Bronchodilator medications are frequently utilized to treat increased airway resistance and/or bronchospasm when present. The bronchodilators may include:

  1. β-Adrenergic agonists.

  2. Corticosteroids.

  3. Theophylline.

  4. Anticholinergic agents.

  5. In some cases, there may even be a role for cromolyn sodium, calcium channel blockers, magnesium, α-adrenergic blockers, and even general inhalational anesthetic agents.

D. Infection is commonly present in patients with acute respiratory failure. The infection may be a cause of the progression to respiratory failure or a complication.

  1. Studies should be performed to determine the etiology of the infection, when present, and culture and sensitivity studies should direct the subsequent antibiotic decisions.

  2. Nosocomial infections, especially nosocomial pneumonia, are well-recognized complications in patients with acute respiratory failure.

    a. Nosocomial pneumonia may be very difficult to diagnose. It may also be difficult to separate the exact etiologic organisms from airway contaminants and colonizers.

    b. Even with positive cultures directing the therapy of nosocomial pneumonia, the morbidity and mortality of the condition remain high.

E. Nutritional support

  1. It is becoming more apparent that critically ill patients may benefit from nutritional support. This is particularly true with enteral nutrition, which has been demonstrated to maintain the mucosal barrier function of the gastrointestinal tract.

    a. Maintaining the intestinal mucosal barrier function may be necessary to avoid the translocation of intestinal bacteria and endotoxins.

    b. Bacterial and endotoxin translocation may be involved in the production of multiple system organ failure (MSOF). MSOF is a frequent complication in the critically ill and is associated with an increased mortality rate.

  2. Proper nutrition may also be important in the maintenance of respiratory muscle function.

    a. Atrophy of the diaphragm and accessory respiratory muscles has been demonstrated in the presence of malnutrition.

    b. In conditions of limited respiratory function, overfeeding and increased carbohydrate loads have been associated with elevated $PaCO_2$ and with respiratory acidosis.

F. Measures to improve the function of the respiratory muscles have been employed to assist in the management of some patients with acute respiratory failure. Some of the techniques used for this purpose include:

  1. Resting the muscles with controlled ventilation.

  2. Proper nutrition.

3. Correction of electrolyte abnormalities.
4. Theophylline, digoxin, and dopamine have been thought to improve respiratory muscle function in some patients.
5. Plasmapheresis has been helpful in some patients with various neuromuscular disorders.

G. Selected patients with either acute or impending respiratory failure have been treated with respiratory muscle stimulants in an attempt to reverse the process.
   1. Respiratory stimulants include:
      a. Doxapram.
      b. Almitrine.
      c. Progesterone (it usually takes weeks to achieve the full beneficial effect).
   2. Respiratory stimulants are often of little benefit, since the patient is typically under maximal stimulus to improve respiratory function.

H. Patients with acute respiratory failure are critically ill and need to be managed with the same care that other critically ill patients require. This involves anticipation and prevention of the complications that may develop in these critically ill patients. Included in these potentially preventable complications are:
   1. Stress ulcer of the gastrointestinal tract.
   2. Deep venous thrombosis and pulmonary emboli.
   3. Nosocomial infections.

VII. Prognosis

A. The prognosis of acute respiratory failure depends to a great extent on the etiology of the respiratory failure and the course of the patient during the subsequent treatment.

B. The prognosis of respiratory failure due to chronic obstructive pulmonary disease has improved over the past several decades. This is probably related to an increased understanding of the pathophysiologic process and the use of home oxygen, bronchodilator therapy, and prudent use of antibiotics.

C. The prognosis associated with the development of ARDS continues to be rather poor, with an overall mortality rate of approximately 50%.
   1. This high mortality rate is somewhat misleading in that there has been a decrease in the number of early deaths related to the inability to achieve adequate oxygenation and/or ventilation.
   2. There is also a wide discrepancy in mortality rate between patients with ARDS of various etiologies.
      a. Patients with ARDS from sepsis continue to have one of the highest mortality rates, reportedly ranging as high as 85–90% in patients with ARDS from gram-negative sepsis.
      b. Patients with ARDS from fat embolism or post–cardiopulmonary bypass have some of the lowest mortality rates when the disorder is properly diagnosed and supportive care is given.
      c. The major causes of death in patients with ARDS at the present time include recurrent sepsis and the development of multisystem organ failure.

D. The prognosis associated with acute respiratory failure from neuromuscular disorders and central nervous system disorders depends to a great extent on the response of the underlying lesion to therapy or its ultimate degree of reversibility.

Bibliography

MacNee W. Treatment of respiratory failure: A review. *J R Soc Med* 78:61–71, 1985.

Marini JJ. Monitoring during mechanical ventilation. *Clin Chest Med* 9:73–100, 1988.

Martin L. Respiratory failure. *Med Clin North Am* 61:1369–1396, 1977.

Pingleton SK. Complications of acute respiratory failure. *Am Rev Respir Dis* 137:1463–1493, 1988.

Pontpoppidan H, Geffin B, Lowenstein E. Acute respiratory failure in the adult. Parts 1, 2, 3. *N Engl J Med* 287:690–698, 743–752, 799–806, 1972.

CHAPTER 41

Multiple System Organ Failure

Robert A. Balk, M.D.
Roger C. Bone, M.D.

I. Introduction

  A. Definition

    1. The definition of the multiple system organ failure (MSOF) syndrome is somewhat controversial at this time.

    2. Most agree that the syndrome is present when there is dysfunction or overt failure of more than two organ systems.

    3. At this time, there is no consensus on the type and extent of organ system failure and/or dysfunction that is needed to make the diagnosis.

    4. This lack of uniformity in definition is demonstrated by the many different definitions and scoring systems currently used to assess organ system function.

  B. Risk factors associated with a higher incidence of MSOF

    1. Sepsis and uncontrolled infective states.

    2. Shock and prolonged hypotension.

    3. Bowel infarction.

    4. Hepatic dysfunction.

    5. Increased age.

    6. Alcohol abuse.

  C. Incidence

    1. The exact incidence of MSOF is variable, and seems to depend to some extent on the definition and scoring systems used.

    2. A limited number of studies, mostly in surgical and postoperative patients, have attempted to define the exact incidence of MSOF in given clinical settings and with different underlying risk factors.

    3. A review by Dorinsky and Gadek et al. evaluated the incidence of organ system dysfunction in patients with the adult respiratory distress syndrome (ARDS) and found the frequency of various organ system involvement to be as follows:

      a. Renal—40–55%

      b. Hepatic—12–95%

      c. Central nervous system—7–30%

      d. Hematologic—0–26%

      e. Gastrointestinal—7–30%

      f. Cardiac—10–23%

II. Etiology

  A. Result of improved ability to resuscitate critically ill patients.

  B. Found in hypermetabolic clinical states.

III. **Pathophysiology**

The pathophysiology of MSOF is uncertain. Currently, there are a number of potential hypotheses.

A. A maldistribution of blood flow which contains oxygen, as well as substrates to support organ and cellular functions, may be instrumental in the production of organ system dysfunction.

1. The maldistribution may be the result of decreased delivery, impaired metabolism, or a combination of these factors.

a. Ischemia of the organ system may be the result of decreased cardiac output, decreased systemic perfusion pressure, or selective alteration in the perfusion of an individual organ system.

b. Microthrombi composed of platelets, leukocytes, and fibrin may obstruct the small capillaries and impair the delivery of blood and substrate to the tissues.

(1) These lesions are similar to those previously described in ARDS, which may be an early manifestation of MSOF.

(2) The microthrombi may reflect limited or full-blown disseminated intravascular coagulation (DIC).

c. Adequate blood flow may reach the tissues, but the tissues and/or cells may be unable to utilize the oxygen and substrates.

B. A circulating humoral agent or another mediator in the bloodstream may directly or indirectly alter organ system function.

1. A myocardial depressant, termed *myocardial depressant substance*, has been detected in the serum of some patients with severe sepsis and septic shock, and is presumed to be at least partly responsible for reversible biventricular cardiac failure.

C. The permeability defect that is characteristic of the injury noted in both sepsis and ARDS appears to be related to endothelial cell injury, which can lead to loss of integrity of the vascular endothelium.

1. This process has been termed *malignant intravascular inflammation* and is a result of diffuse injury to the endothelial cells or a panendothelial cell injury.

2. This defect in the vascular endothelium can lead to organ edema and subsequent dysfunction.

D. Organ toxicity is related to the direct effect of the underlying process (such as infection) or the direct toxicity of released mediators (such as the endothelial cell injury produced by tumor necrosis factor).

E. Bacterial/toxin translocation

1. Loss of the intestinal mucosal barrier function may occur from ischemia or loss of cell function related to mucosal cell death or injury.

2. The terminal ileum and cecum are reservoirs for gram-negative bacteria and their toxic products, such as endotoxin.

3. The bacteria and/or their toxic products or mediators may translocate through or between the dysfunctional mucosal barrier cells and enter the mesenteric lymph system. If they are not adequately neutralized by the mesenteric lymph nodes, they may enter the systemic circulation and the liver, where they can trigger the systemic inflammatory response and produce the syndrome of MSOF.

IV. **Diagnosis**

A. Clinical manifestations

1. Patients at risk

a. Sepsis

b. Trauma

c. Postoperative states

d. Hypermetabolic states

e. Shock states

f. Elderly

g. Bowel infarction/hepatic dysfunction

B. Pattern of specific organ system involvement

1. Pulmonary system

a. Hypoxemia

b. Respiratory muscle dysfunction

(1) Respiratory fatigue

(2) Hypercapnic respiratory failure

c. ARDS

d. Nosocomial infection

2. Cardiovascular system

a. Hypotension/shock

b. Decreased contractility/myocardial depression

c. Congestive heart failure

d. Tachy-bradyarrhythmias

3. Hepatic system

a. Clinical manifestations

(1) Transaminitis

(2) Hyperbilirubinemia

(3) Prolonged prothrombin time

(4) Hepatic encephalopathy

b. Pathophysiology

(1) Possibly related to changes in hepatic blood flow

(2) Increased tissue lactate/pyruvate ratio

4. Gastrointestinal system
   a. Stress ulceration
      (1) Pathogenesis may be related to:
          (a) Alteration in mucosal blood flow
          (b) Hypoxia of the gastric mucosal cells
          (c) Disruption of the gastric mucosal barrier
   b. Bowel ischemia and translocation
      (1) Described as "fuel of MSOF."
      (2) Nutritional deficiency can promote translocation.
      (3) Concept supported by a finding endotoxemia in non-gram-negative infectious states, as reported by Danner et al.
   c. Pancreatitis
      (1) Risk related to small vascular surface area, decreased perfusion, and/or increased venous pressure.
      (2) Associated release of proteolytic enzymes and mediators.
      (3) Unsuspected pancreatitis in 16% of postmortem examinations.
   d. Ileus
5. Renal system
   a. Clinical presentation
      (1) Acute tubular necrosis
      (2) Acute renal failure
          (a) Oliguric renal failure
          (b) Nonoliguric renal failure
   b. Renal dysfunction related to:
      (1) Tubulointerstitial disease
      (2) Glomerular injury
      (3) Tubular injury
      (4) Interstitial injury
      (5) Drug effects
      (6) Infections
   c. Pathophysiology
      (1) Overall decrease in renal blood flow, despite supranormal cardiac output.
      (2) Minimal morphologic changes may produce marked functional changes.
6. Neurologic system
   a. Altered mental status (change in Glascow Coma Scale (GCS)
      (1) Alterations in mental status may take a variety of forms in the critically ill, ranging from Intensive Care Unit (I.C.U.) psychosis to coma.

(2) The Glascow Coma Scale has been used as an objective tool to evaluate the degree of neurologic dysfunction.
   b. Critical illness polyneuropathy
      (1) Clinical manifestations
          (a) Weakness
          (b) Muscle wasting
          (c) Impaired deep tendon reflexes
          (d) Polyneuropathy
          (e) May take 3–6 months to recover
          (f) May be responsible for prolonged debilitated state or for inability to wean patient from mechanical ventilatory support
      (2) Pathophysiology
          (a) Axonal degeneration of motor and sensory fibers
          (b) Results in denervation atrophy of limb and respiratory muscles
7. Metabolic
   a. Hypermetabolism
      (1) Catabolic state
      (2) Increased lactate production
   b. Alterations in glucose and oxygen use
      (1) Increased lactate production
      (2) Hyperglycemia from increased hepatic gluconeogenesis
   c. Endocrinopathies
      (1) Euthyroid "sick" syndrome
      (2) Relative insulin resistance
C. Diagnostic studies
   1. No specific test is available for MSOF.
   2. Monitor with appropriate tests of organ system function, using laboratory, radiologic, and clinical parameters.
D. Significance of organ system involvement
   1. A number of surgical studies have demonstrated that there is increased mortality when specific organ systems are involved in MSOF.
   2. A study in patients with ARDS has demonstrated that hepatic dysfunction is associated with increased mortality.
   3. A large multicenter study by Knaus and Wagner has demonstrated that there is an increased mortality rate associated with dysfunction of three or more organ systems. In addition, the longer the duration of the dysfunction, the greater the mortality.
      a. The mortality rate in this large study (2840 patients) was 100% when three or more organ systems were dysfunctional for 5 or more days (figure 2).

E. Scoring systems
1. Many different scoring systems have been proposed to try to define and quantify objectively the degree of organ system dysfunction.
2. Unfortunately, at this time, there is no uniformly acceptable scoring system that can be applied to all critically ill patients and predict the outcome.

V. **Management of Organ System Dysfunction**
A. Identify and treat the underlying predisposing condition.
1. A high incidence of infection and sepsis requires an aggressive approach to diagnosis and management.
B. Restore and maintain hemodynamic stability and adequate tissue oxygen delivery and utilization.
1. Fluid resuscitation is one of the initial measures employed to restore or maintain the intravascular volume. The means employed for fluid resuscitation are still a subject of controversy. Any of the following may be used:
a. Crystalloid solutions
b. Colloid solutions
c. Blood and blood products
d. Starch and other volume expanders
2. Vasopressor and inotropic therapy may be necessary to support and maintain the systemic arterial blood pressure once the intravascular volume has been restored.
a. The goal of therapy is to achieve an adequate blood pressure and cardiac output.
b. It is important to remember that tissue oxygen delivery is the product of the cardiac output and the arterial oxygen content.
C. Ensure adequate oxygenation and ventilation.
1. Supplemental oxygen should be administered as necessary to correct any hypoxemia.
2. Early support with mechanical ventilation may be beneficial by avoiding the need for emergent intubation and ventilatory support in patients prone to the development of acute respiratory failure. These include:
a. Patients with underlying severe lung disease or prior pulmonary compromise who may be at increased risk for the development of acute respiratory failure.

b. Patients who exhibit respiratory muscle dysfunction related to the injury state and may be at risk for developing hypercapnic respiratory failure.
c. Patients who may benefit from a reduction in the work of breathing or from a reduction in oxygen consumption.
(1) Spontaneous ventilation may require as much as 21% of the cardiac output to supply the respiratory muscles.
(2) The use of controlled or assisted ventilation may allow for redistribution of the available cardiac output to support other vital organs and possibly prevent further organ system dysfunction or even exacerbation of current organ system dysfunction.
D. Nutritional support is still controversial, but current beliefs support a possible beneficial role for early institution of enteral nutrition.
1. The enteral route is preferred to maintain the integrity of the normal intestinal mucosal barrier and possibly prevent the translocation of intestinal bacteria and bacterial products into the systemic circulation.
a. A normal diet with normal fiber content appears to maintain the intestinal barrier function best in experimental animal studies of translocation.
b. Glutamine is also an important amino acid dietary component involved in the proper maintenance of intestinal barrier function.
2. Arginine is important as a cofactor for the proper function of the macrophage system and the ability to produce cytokines.
3. Omega-3 fatty acids appear to be important in immune system function.
4. Proper nutritional therapy may also be important in counterbalancing the hypermetabolic processes associated with MSOF.
E. Prevent complications of critical illness.
1. Stress ulcers may complicate the course of these critically ill patients. The use of prophylactic regimens can decrease the incidence of stress-related gastrointestinal bleeding. A number of prophylactic regimens have been used to prevent stress ulcers. These include:
a. Enteral nutrition

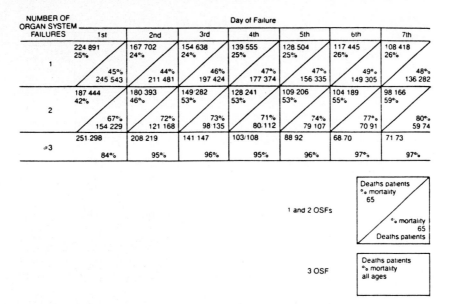

Figure 41-1. Admission of 2405 ICU patients with MSOF to 27 French hospitals. (From Knaus and Wagner, 1989)

b. H2 blockers

c. Cytoprotective agents (Sucralfate)

d. Antacid therapy to increase the gastric pH above 3.5.

2. Deep vein thrombosis and pulmonary emboli may be prevented by:

   a. Subcutaneous heparin

   b. Pneumatic compression stockings

3. Nosocomial infections

   a. May be related to loss of acidity in the stomach with the proximal migration of intestinal flora into the pharynx, where they are eventually aspirated into the lower airways.

   b. The use of cytoprotective agents for stress ulcer prophylaxis may be less likely to result in nosocomial pneumonia.

   c. Attempts to prevent the development of nosocomial pneumonia using gut decontamination have been successful in several studies, but the technique is still controversial and is viewed as experimental.

4. Pulmonary barotrauma

   a. Occurs in 5–15% of mechanically ventilated patients.

   b. Etiology related to the rupture of small alveoli and appears to be related to alveolar distention. It is not certain whether peak or mean airway pressure is more important in the production of pulmonary barotrauma.

5. Complications from invasive monitoring and invasive procedures

F. Specific therapy

1. At this time, there is no specific approved therapy for established MSOF or dysfunction other than support and therapy directed at the underlying or predisposing condition.

2. Recent trials using monoclonal antibodies to endotoxin in patients with suspected gram-negative infections have demonstrated improved resolution of established MSOF compared to placebo control.

3. Further studies are needed to confirm this observation. If proven to be beneficial, specific monoclonal antibody therapy directed at the mediator(s) thought to be responsible for the production of the organ injury may become the specific therapy of the future.

VI. **Prognosis**

A. Dependent on the organs involved.

B. Increased mortality rates with an increasing number of organ systems involved and a greater duration of involvement (Figures 41-1 and 41-2).

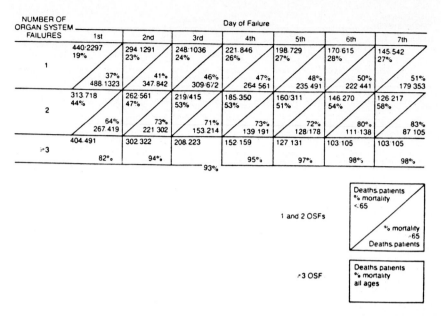

Figure 41-2. Admission of 5248 ICU patients with MSOF to 40 French and U.S. hospitals. (From Knaus and Wagner, 1989)

Bibliography

Barton R, Cerra FB. The hypermetabolism: Multiple organ failure syndrome. *Chest* 96:1153–1160, 1989.

Bersten A, Sibbald WJ. Circulatory disturbances in multiple systems organ failure. *Crit Care Clin* 5:233–254, 1989.

Danner RL, Elin RJ, Hosseini JM, Wesley RA, Reilly JM, Panillo JE. Endotoxemia in Human Septic Shock. *Chest*: 169–175, 1991.

Dorinsky PM, Gadek JE. Mechanisms of Multiple Non-Pulmonary Organ Failure in ARDS. *Chest* 96:885–892, 1989.

Fry DE. Multiple system organ failure. *Surg Clin North Am* 68:107–122, 1988.

Knaus WA, Wagner DP. Multiple systems organ failure: Epidemiology and prognosis. *Crit Care Clin* 5:221–232, 1989.

Macho JR, Luce JM. Rational approach to the management of multiple systems organ failure. *Crit Care Clin* 5:379–392, 1989.

Marshall JC, Christou NV, Horn R, et al. The microbiology of multiple organ failure: The proximal gastrointestinal tract as an occult reservoir of pathogens. *Arch Surg* 123:309–315, 1988.

Pinsky MR, Matuschak GM. Multiple systems organ failure: Failure of host defense homeostasis. *Crit Care Clin* 5:199–220, 1989.

CHAPTER 42

Trauma Management for the Internist

Eric Gluck, M.D.
James E. Calvin, M.D.

I. Types
  A. Blunt
    1. Majority of injury not caused by disruption of the skin but by sudden decelerations
    2. Automobile accidents leading cause
    3. Coup and contracoup effects
  B. Penetrating
    1. Loss of integument protection
    2. Disruption of internal viscera
    3. Bullet projectiles are the leading cause
      a. Damage proportional to the velocity of the projectile

II. Evaluation
  A. Physical exam
    1. Detailed exam deferred until the ABC's are evaluated
    2. A—Airway
      a. Control of the airway should be obtained as soon as possible.
      b. Always assume that there is a possible neck injury.
      c. Nasal intubations favored in instances of neck injuries (assuming that there are no associated facial injuries as well).
      d. Oral intubation should be performed only by experienced persons using the two-person technique, one stabilizing

the neck and the other performing the intubation.
      e. Adequate ventilation is often obtainable temporarily by mask until the appropriate personnel are available.
    3. B—Breathing
      a. Mechanical ventilation indicated once the airway is established.
      b. Tension pneumothorax is a possibility even in patients without obvious lung trauma.
        (1) Associated with decreased breath sounds, hyperresonance, deviation of the trachea, hypotension, displacement of the point of maximal impulse (PMI)
      c. Flail chest
        (1) Results from two or more fractured ribs on the same side at some distance apart.
        (2) "Pendulluft" ventilation may develop because of inability to maintain negative intrapleural pressure during spontaneous respirations.
        (3) Positive-pressure ventilation will reverse blood gas abnormalities.
      d. Patients are prone to gastric aspiration.

e. Many patients with lung contusion will develop hemoptysis. These patients are at especially high risk of air embolism.

4. C—Circulation
  a. Blood volume vs. systemic pressure
    (1) Twenty-five percent reduction in blood volume leads to significant hypotension.
    (2) Fifty percent reduction in blood volume leads to death.
  b. Fluid resuscitation
    (1) Shock persisting for >30 min leads to increased mortality.
    (2) Large volumes of normal saline (3000 ml) should be infused over the first few minutes to restore circulating volume.
    (3) Inability to control pressure with volume resuscitation should be an immediate indication for surgery.
    (4) Consider use of non-type-specific blood if blood pressure cannot be controlled with infusion of 3 liters of crystalloid. Obviously, type-specific blood is preferred if available.
    (5) Pressors are relatively contraindicated in shock from volume depletion unless accompanied by myocardial injury.
  c. Shock with elevated central venous pressure consider:
    (1) Pericardial tamponade
    (2) Pneumothorax
    (3) Myocardial contusion
    (4) Myocardial infarction
    (5) Air embolization

B. Laboratory
  1. X-rays—chest, lateral cervical spine, pelvis.
  2. Serum—electrolytes, arterial blood gases.
  3. Complete blood count, type, and cross match.
  4. Intravenous pyelogram and electrocardiogram if possible.

C. Scoring systems
  1. Used in making triage decisions, assessment of quality assurance, management of resources, systematic study of possible therapeutic interventions
    a. Revised Trauma Score (Table 42-1)

III. Specific Organ Trauma
A. Head
  1. Blunt trauma
    a. Injury caused by concussive forces (coup and contra-coup), increases in intracranial pressure, or disruption of vascular integrity.
  2. Penetrating trauma
    a. Depressed skull fractures.
    b. High-velocity objects.
  3. Epidural hematomas

Table 42-1. Trauma Score

Respiratory rate	10–24	4
	25–35	3
	>35	2
	0–9	1 ___
Respiratory effort	Normal	1
	Shallow, retractive	0 ___
Systolic blood pressure	>90	4
	70–90	3
	50–69	2
	<50	1
	No carotid pulse	0 ___
Capillary refill	Normal	2
	Delayed	1
	Absent	0 ___

Glasgow Coma Scale

Eye opening		
Spontaneous	4	
To voice	3	
To pain	2	
None	1	
Verbal response		
Oriented	5	
Confused	4	
Inappropriate words	3	
Incomprehensible words	2	
None	1	
Motor Response		
Obeys commands	6	
Localizes	5	
Withdraws	4	Total GCS
Abnormal flexion	3	Points
Abnormal extension	2	14–15 5
None	1	11–18 4
		8–10 3
		5–7 2
Total GCS Points	_____	3–4 1 ___

TOTAL TRAUMA SCORE ___

Reproduced with permission from Boyd CR, Tolson MA, Copes WS. Evaluating Trauma Care: The TRISS Method. *J Trauma* 27(4):370–378, 1987.

    a. Most commonly associated with linear fractures over the middle meningeal artery distribution, dural sinuses, and foramen magnum.

    b. Fewer than 40% patients have the classic lucid interval

    c. Most injuries commonly occur over the temporal lobe, causing contralateral hemiparesis.

    d. Epidural hematomas associated with loss of consciousness, ipsilateral pupillary dilation, contralateral hemiparesis, and third nerve palsy.

    e. Fifty percent mortality.

    f. Usually requires immediate neurosurgical attention.

4. Subdural hematoma

    a. Acute—cortical contusion results in disruption of cortical vessel and expanding mass of blood.

    b. Chronic—slowly progressive lesion associated with lethargy, confusion, and eventual hemiparesis.

    c. Requires surgical drainage.

5. Intracerebral hematoma

    a. Intracerebral collection of blood which may cause a mass effect. May require surgical drainage.

    b. Symptoms depend on location and size.

6. Basilar skull fracture

    a. Associated with cerebrospinal fluid (CSF) leakage into sinuses.

    b. Nasal tubes are contraindicated.

    c. Meningitis is a common complication and should be assumed in all patients with fever and basilar fracture.

7. Depressed skull fracture

    a. Brain tissue directly injured by the inner table of the skull.

    b. High risk of bacterial contamination.

8. Intracranial pressure monitoring

    a. Indications

      (1) Closed head injury.

      (2) Encephalopathies.

      (3) Reye's syndrome.

    b. Contraindications

      (1) Coagulopathy.

      (2) Reduced platelet count.

      (3) Immunosuppression is a relative contraindication.

    c. Techniques

      (1) Subarachnoid bolts

        (a) In subarachnoid space through a Burr hole.

        (b) Requires fair amount of maintenance.

        (c) Fairly high incidence of infection.

        (d) May underestimate real intracranial pressure (ICP).

      (2) Epidural catheters

        (a) Unable to sample fluid with this catheter.

        (b) Lowest incidence of infection.

        (c) Difficult to place.

      (3) Ventricular catheters

        (a) Can sample CSF.

        (b) Fairly easy to insert.

        (c) Significant incidence of infection.

        (d) Most reliable.

        (e) Can make only three passes to avoid injury to cerebral tissue.

    d. Treatment of elevated ICP

      (1) Hyperventilation

        (a) Most rapid means of lowering ICP.

        (b) Alkalotic pH causes cerebral vasoconstriction and decreased cerebral blood flow.

        (c) Reduced flow decreases intracerebral blood volume and pressure.

        (d) Further increases in pH result in impairment in oxygen delivery and extraction.

        (e) Optimal PCO_2 is about 25.

        (f) Effect lasts for only about 48 hr and is then compensated for.

        (g) Hyperventilation should be removed slowly to avoid rebound increases in ICP.

      (2) Diuretics

        (a) Decrease intravascular volume.

        (b) May reduce production of CSF.

      (3) Steroids

        (a) Are more effective in cases of ICP related to tumors than other causes.

        (b) Mechanism may be related to decreased production of CSF and antiedema effect.

      (4) Mannitol

        (a) Decreases intracerebral water and pressure by establishing an osmotic diuresis.

        (b) Usual dose is 50 g.

        (c) Should aim for a serum osmotic pressure of 320 mOsm.

(d) Can paradoxically increase the ICP by causing intravascular expansion if given too rapidly.

(e) Will slowly diffuse across the blood-brain barrier, decreasing its own efficacy after about 48 hr.

B. Chest
  1. Blunt
    a. Rib fractures
      (1) Upper ribs infrequently involved, since they have high tensile strength and are well protected.
        (a) Fracture of the upper ribs should result in careful evaluation of underlying major vessels.
      (2) Lower ribs are quite flexible and usually do not fracture.
        (a) If fracture occurs, evaluate intra-abdominal contents carefully.
      (3) Middle ribs most commonly affected. Nondisplaced fractures difficult to find.
      (4) Management concerns concomitant injury and relief of pain.
      (5) May result in flail chest with impaired ventilation.
    b. Lung contusion
      (1) Collection of blood within the lung parenchyma.
      (2) Appear within 6 hr of the injury.
      (3) Result in $\dot{V}/\dot{Q}$ abnormalities, causing hypoxia and hemoptysis.
      (4) Usually resolves within 5–10 days.
      (5) Can resolve with cyst formation.
    c. Pneumothorax/pneumomediastinum
      (1) Can result from puncture via fractured rib or from rupture due to excessive intra-alveolar pressure at time of impact.
      (2) Usually requires thoracotomy drainage.
    d. Bronchial tear
      (1) Trachea and right mainstem bronchus most likely sites.
      (2) Associated finding—hemoptysis, pneumothorax, subcutaneous emphysema, nonresolving air leak, atelectasis.
      (3) Frequently associated with bilateral pneumothoraces.
      (4) Bronchoscopy is highest-yielding procedure.

      (5) Complications—stenosis, infection, nonresolving air leak.
    e. Hemothorax
      (1) Thoracentesis needed to confirm diagnosis.
      (2) Drainage indicated in effusions greater than 500 ml.
      (3) Causes—rupture of intercostal or internal mammary blood vessels, rib fractures, esophageal rupture.
      (4) Continued drainage is an indication for exploration of the chest.
      (5) Complications—fibrothorax, trapped lung, infection.
    f. Diaphragmatic injuries
      (1) Result from sudden increase in intrathoracic pressure at time of impact.
      (2) More common on right than on left side.
      (3) Signs—air-fluid levels in chest on upright posteroanterior chest film, bowel sounds in the chest, atelectasis.
      (4) Diagnosis—computed tomography (CT) of the chest, contrast study.
    g. Major blood vessel trauma
      (1) Associated with sudden deceleration injuries.
      (2) Coronary arteries and aortic valve can be involved as well.
      (3) Diagnosed via CT scan or aortagram, but suspected by reduced definition of the aortic knob.
      (4) Signs—uneven blood pressures in extremities, stroke, dysphagia, hoarseness due to recurrent laryngeal nerve pressure.
      (5) Treatment—surgical.
    h. Cardiac contusion—see below
    i. Esophageal rupture
      (1) Associated with high-impact trauma.
      (2) Left-sided effusion with elevated amylase-level.
      (3) High mortality rate if left untreated.
      (4) Not easily detected by endoscopy.
      (5) Diagnosis usually made via CT scan and thoracentesis.
      (6) Complications—hypotension, shock, infection and mediastinitis.
  2. Penetrating
    a. See below

      b. Usually results in hemopneumothorax.

      c. Plain upright film shows linear air-fluid level without meniscus sign.

      d. Treatment—surgical.

C. Cardiac

  1. Penetrating lesions

      a. Cardiac tamponade

          (1) Jugular venous distention.

          (2) Pulsus paradoxus.

          (3) Hypotension.

          (4) Two-dimensional echocardiography showing pericardial effusion with ventricular collapse.

      b. Exsanguination.

      c. Coronary artery laceration.

      d. Valvular injury

          (1) New regurgitant murmur.

          (2) Large V-wave apparent on right heart catheter.

  2. Blunt trauma

      a. Injury or disruption of the valves

          (1) Supportive therapy.

          (2) Intra-aortic balloons may be of use in patients with mitral regurgitation but are contra-indicated in patients with aortic regurgitation.

          (3) Surgery indicated for significant injuries.

      b. Myocardial contusion

          (1) Fifty-five percent for right ventricle vs. 20% for left ventricle.

          (2) Echocardiography.

          (3) Majority of patients require only clinical observation and electrocardiographic monitoring. Patients with low cardiac output should be treated with inotropes and vasodilators if necessary.

      c. Rupture of intraventricular septum

          (1) Initially, may be managed medically if patient is hemodynamically stable.

          (2) Spontaneous closure has been reported.

          (3) Surgery indicated for unstable patients.

      d. Free wall rupture

          (1) Will usually require thoracotomy.

          (2) Pericardiocentesis helpful, but false-negatives are common.

      e. Late pericarditis

      f. Coronary artery laceration

D. Spinal trauma

  1. Presentation

      a. Present with hypotension with normal heart rate.

      b. Damage can occur due to vascular disruption, contusion, or compression (from bone fragments or blood).

      c. Motor vehicle accidents are the leading cause.

      d. Useful adage: C3, C4, and C5 keep the diaphragm alive.

          (1) Injuries above C4 result in paradoxical abdominal thoracic movements with respiration.

      e. In persons with suspected injuries, all potential movement of the spine should be prevented.

  2. Initial management

      a. Judicious use of fluid for volume expansion.

      b. Ensure adequate ventilation and oxygenation.

      c. Immobilize spine.

      d. Diagnostic neurologic evaluation and complete set of x-rays.

      e. Consultation with neurosurgical service.

E. Intra-abdominal trauma

  1. Diagnostic tests

      a. CT scan—useful in assessing integrity of spleen, liver, and kidneys, as well as in the evaluation of postsurgical abscesses.

      b. Lavage—useful in assessing intraperitoneal bleeding and contamination.

          (1) More than 100,000 red blood cells, more than 500 white blood cells, food particles, bacteria, elevated amylase and bile levels are indications for laparotomy

  2. Penetrating intra-abdominal injuries

      a. Strong likelihood of disrupting small or large bowel.

      b. Antibiotic therapy should include anaerobic as well as gram-negative aerobic coverage.

      c. Exploration is almost always indicated.

F. Long bones

  1. Fat emboli syndrome

      a. Can be delayed for up to 48 hr.

      b. Hypoxemia, diffuse infiltrates on chest x-ray, thrombocytopenia, coagulopathy.

      c. Occasionally, fat droplets are demonstrated in the urine.

      d. Treatment—ventilator support. Massive steroids are reported to be efficacious.

Bibliography

American College of Surgeons. Advances in trauma life support course. Chicago: American College of Surgeons, 1989.

Anderson DK, Demediuk P, Saunders RD, et al: Spinal cord injury and protection. *Ann Emerg Med* 1985; 14:816.

Halpern P, Greenstein A, Melamed Y, et al: Arterial air embolism after penetrating lung injury. *CCM* 1983; 11:392.

Gaffney FA, Thal ER: Hemodynamic effects of medical anti-shock trousers. *J Trauma* 1981; 21:931.

CHAPTER 43

Drug Overdose and Poisoning

Jerrold B. Leikin, M.D.
Paul K. Hanashiro, M.D.

I. **Importance of Toxicology in the Practice of Medicine**
  A. Eight million Americans are poisoned each year.
  B. In 1992 regional poison centers reported 1,864,188 calls, with about 60% involving children under the age of 6. There were 705 fatalities reported.
  C. Blood lead levels over 30 µg/dl are found in 4% of children between the ages of 6 months and 5 years.
  D. Cocaine is the most common cause of drug-related emergency department visits (18.2% of persons killed in motor vehicle accidents in New York City in 1988 tested positive for cocaine.)
  E. According to the National Institute on Drug Abuse, over the period 1985–1988:
    1. There were no metropolitan areas where cocaine presentations decreased.
    2. Drug abuse deaths involving cocaine almost tripled.
    3. Steady increases were noted in heroin, methamphetamine, marijuana, and phencyclidine (PCP) use in the overall DAWN (Drug Abuse Warning Network) system (Tables 43-1 to 43-3).

  F. 7,500,000 Americans use sedative/hypnotics.
  G. 500,000 Americans are opioid dependent.
  H. 560,000 Americans are arrested each year for violating drug laws.
  I. Iatrogenic disease involving medications in hospitals is frequently encountered (36% of 815 consecutive patients seen on a general medicine service in one survey).
  J. Cutaneous drug eruptions are noted in 2–3% of hospitalized patients.
  K. 41% of graduating high school seniors in 1992 stated that they had used an illicit drug at least once in their lifetime.
  L. Annual use of marijuana in 1992 was 21.9% among senior high school students and 7.2% among eighth grade students. National annual marijuana use in the general population is 9.6%.
  M. Lifetime cocaine use occurred in 6.1% of all high school seniors graduating in 1992.
  N. 10,000,000 Americans are considered "alcoholic."
  O. National prevalance of annual cocaine use was estimated to be 3.1 per cent in 1991.
  P. A 1990 Illinois Youth Survey reported an annual stimulant usage rate of 3.7% among Chicago-area students.

Table 43-1.   Drugs mentioned most frequently by emergency rooms in 1989

Drug Name	No. of Mentions	Percent of Total Episodes	Relative Increase or Decrease since 1989
Cocaine	102,727	25.7	Decreased
Alcohol in combination	123,758	30.9	Increased
Heroin/morphine	36,576	9.1	Decreased
Marijuana/hashish	16,492	4.1	Decreased
Acetaminophen	30,885	7.7	Increased
Aspirin	21,982	5.5	Increased
Diazepam	14,852	3.7	Increased
Ibuprofen	15,628	3.9	Increased
Alprazolam	16,465	4.1	Increased
Methamphetamine/speed	4,980	1.2	Decreased
Acetaminophen + codeine	7,236	1.8	Increased
OTC sleep aids	6,434	1.6	Increased
Amitriptyline	8,785	2.2	Increased
Dephenhydramine	6,836	1.7	Increased
Hydrocodone	5,089	1.3	Increased
Lorazepam	7,009	1.8	Increased
D-Propoxyphene	7,919	2.0	Increased
LSD clonazepam	6,563	1.6	Increased
Fluoxetine	6,954	1.7	Increased

Data are based on frequencies of drug mentions and a weighted raw mergency room episode estimate of 400,079. Individual drugs were frequently mentioned in combination with other drugs.
Source: NIDA, Drug Abuse Warning Network (May 1992 data file).

II. Differential Diagnosis of the Toxic Patient

A. Coma of toxic origin
1. Symmetric motor response with symmetric reflexes.
2. Symmetric pupillary response to light.
3. Venous pulsations present on fundoscopic exam.
4. Caloric testing reveals an intact reflex.
5. Neck is supple.
6. Breathing pattern may be regular, or Kussmaul respiration may be noted; usually there is no Cheynes-Stokes respiration.
7. Focal neurologic signs are absent.
8. Anisocoria is not a feature.
9. Slurred speech is usually associated with drug overdose rather than trauma related.

B. Toxin-induced seizures
1. Usually status in nature until specific antiseizure medications or antidotes are administered (Table 43-4).
2. Usually resistant to single antiseizure drug therapy.
3. Metabolic acidosis is greater than if associated with seizure alone.
4. Focal seizures less common than generalized seizures.

5. Propoxyphine and meperidine are the only opioid agonists that cause seizures.

C. Neuropsychiatric symptoms
1. Patients usually are disoriented.
2. Level of consciousness is fluctuating.
3. Hallucinations are usually visual or tactile.
4. Pseudohallucinations (patients realize that they are hallucinating) or illusionary phenomena may appear (especially with LSD).
5. Motor exam may reveal asterixis or myoclonus.

III. Evaluation of the Poisoned Patient

A. History
1. Clinical utility between history and laboratory findings ranges from 25% to 86% in concordance.
2. Type of exposure
   a. Always assume maximal number of pills ingested from bottle in quantifying exposure (worse possible scenario).
   b. Mechanism of exposure should be ascertained (i.e., inhalation, ingestion, dermal).
   c. Time since exposure.
   d. Circumstances surrounding toxin exposure.

Table 43-2. Ten Most Frequently Mentioned Drugs in the Total DAWN System by Sex, Race, Age, Drug Concomitance, and Drug Use Motive (1991)

Drug	Sex		Ethnicity				Age			Drug Concomitance			Drug Use Motive				
	Male	Female	White	Black	Hispanic	Other	6–17	18–34	Over 35	Alone	Not Alone	Most Common Drug	Dependence	Suicide	Psychic effect	Recreational Use	Other
Alcohol in combination	70,136	52,316	70,679	35,279	9,062	1,017	5,280	70,998	45,883	—	123,758	Cocaine	41,869	48,521	8,235	10,867	14,265
Cocaine	67,640	34,266	29,644	56,933	9,148	523	2,166	68,521	30,734	43,454	59,273	Alcohol	6,367	6,703	2,086	14,955	12,616
Heroin/Morphine	24,084	12,177	13,639	15,424	5,220	183	64	18,480	17,462	15,837	20,739	Cocaine	28,763	1,176	352	2,857	3,328
Acetaminophen	8,993	21,427	21,260	4,702	2,215	2,708	10,008	15,944	4,460	16,349	20,227	Alcohol	396	24,669	3,073	227	2,520
Aspirin	7,065	14,727	15,473	3,003	1,519	175	7,341	10,521	3,874	10,376	11,606	Alcohol	214	17,076	2,625	138	1,930
Marijuana/Hashish	11,489	4,794	8,149	5,706	1,410	95	2,041	11,248	2,915	3,348	13,144	Alcohol	7,185	1,280	565	4,541	2,920
Alprazolam	4,967	11,377	14,371	757	477	47	603	7,421	8,311	3,309	13,156	Alcohol	1,440	11,607	1,896	337	1,085
Ibuprofen	4,522	11,062	10,101	3,058	1,262	1,207	4,701	8,538	2,372	—	—	Alcohol	—	—	—	—	—
Diazepam	6,442	8,334	12,068	1,000	690	85	532	6,757	7,483	3,119	11,733	Alcohol	2,387	8,791	1,647	415	1,612
Amitriptyline	3,665	5,083	6,878	919	508	49	571	4,868	4,338	2,811	5,974	Alcohol	187	7,547	4,163	—	1,497

Table 43-3. Drugs mentioned most frequently by medical examiners in 1989

Drug Name	No. of Mentions	Percent of Total Episodes
Cocaine	3618	50.52
Alcohol in combination	2778	38.79
Heroin/morphine	2743	38.30
Codeine	840	11.73
Methadone	450	6.28
Diazepam	428	5.98
Amitriptyline	382	5.33
Nortriptyline	304	4.24
D-Propoxyphene	282	3.94
Marijuana/hashish	246	3.43
Diphenhydramine	238	3.32
Acetaminophen	217	3.03
Lidocaine	212	2.96
PCP/PCP combinations	211	2.95
Desipramine	192	2.68
Doxepin	191	2.67
Methamphetamine/speed	191	2.67
Unspec. benzodiazepines	177	2.47
Phenobarbital	173	2.42
Aspirin	127	1.77
Imipramine	127	1.77
Quinine	119	1.66

Data are based on raw frequencies of drug mentions and a total raw medical examiner episode count of 7162. Excluded are deaths in which AIDS was reported and deaths in which only "drug unknown" was mentioned.

Source: NIDA, Drug Abuse Warning Network (May 1990 data file).

3. Occupational history may be critical.
4. Obtain a separate history from a second observer (relative, friend, paramedic) whenever possible.

B. Physical examination
1. Primarily dependent on toxidrome recognition, which is the symptom, and on physical examination complexes associated with specific toxic agents (Table 43-5).
2. Vital signs
   a. Can differentiate between adrenergic/anticholinergic (elevated vital signs) and sedative/hypnotic ingestion (depressed vital signs).
   b. Hyperthermia can be a hallmark of major complications associated with amphetamines, cocaine, salicylates, theophyllines, monoamine oxidase inhibitors, phencyclidine, and anticholinergics.
   c. Hypothermia is most commonly associated with opiate agents, along with sedative/hypnotics, barbiturates, carbon monoxide, phenothiazines, and oral hypoglycemic agents.
3. Odors can provide identification of toxins, such as the following:

a. Bitter almonds, macaroons, or silver polish—cyanide
b. Garlic—arsenic, phosphorus, selenium, thallium, organophosphate insecticide
c. Mothballs—naphthalene
d. Peanuts—vacor (RH-787)
e. Rotten eggs—hydrogen sulfide, mercaptans, disulfiram
f. Shoe polish—nitrobenzene
g. Violets—turpentine
h. Sweet—acetone
i. Rotten Cabbage—carbon disulfide
j. Wintergreen—methylsalicylate
4. Ocular findings
   a. Nystamus
      (1) Horizontal
         (a) Alcohol
         (b) Carbamazepine
         (c) Lithium
         (d) Meprobamate
         (e) Primidone
         (f) Quinine
         (g) Solvents
      (2) Rotary, horizontal, or vertical
         (a) Phencyclidine
         (b) Phenytoin

Table 43-4. Specific Agents Useful to Treat Seizures (Addition to General Antiseizure Treatment Unless Otherwise Noted)

Toxin	Therapeutic Agent	Dose (Adult)
Anticholinergics or antihistamines	Physostigmine	1–2 mg slow IV push (may repeat in 20 min); no faster than 1 mg/min.
Camphor	In refractory seizures: lipid hemodialysis using soybean oil along with antiseizure medications	
Cyanide	Amyl nitrite	
	Sodium nitrite	10 ml of 3% solution IV over 3–5 min; 50 ml of 25% solution.
	Sodium thiosulfate (may repeat sodium nitrite and sodium thiosulfate if symptoms persist)	
Lead	British anti-lewisite (BAL) Dimeraprol	75 mg/m^2
	CaNa$_2$-EDTA	1500 mg/m^2/day
Isoniazid, Hydrazine	Pyridoxine (phenytoin is relatively contraindicated)	Gram for gram of isoniazid ingested (for unknown ingestions, patient should receive 5 grams IV)
Insulin/oral hypoglycemics	Dextrose	50 ml of 50% dextrose (25 g)
	Glucagon	5 to 10 mgm IV bolus followed with 2–10 mg/hr infusion
Propoxyphene	Naloxone	2 mg IV in an adult; repeat every 2–3 min
Salicylate or Lithium	Hemodialysis	
Carbon monoxide	Hyperbaric Oxygen	
Lindane	Hemoperfusion	

          (c) Sedative/hypnotic
     b. Mydriasis
         (1) Anticholinergics (not reactive to light)
         (2) Glutethimide
         (3) Meperidine
         (4) Sympathomimetics (reactive to light)
     c. Miosis
         (1) Cholinergic agents (including organophosphates and mushrooms)
         (2) Chloral hydrate
         (3) Clonidine
         (4) Endosulfan
         (5) Nicotine
         (6) Opiates
         (7) Phenothiazines
  C. Laboratory evaluation
    1. "Three gaps of toxicology"
      a. Anion gap: [Na$^+$ + K$^+$] − [Cl + HCO$_3$] (> 12 mEq/liter)

(1) Acetazolamide
(2) Amiloride
(3) Ammonium Chloride
(4) Ascorbic Acid
(5) Benzalkonium chloride
(6) Bialaphos
(7) Butylglycol
(8) Carbon monoxide
(9) Carbon Tetrachloride
(10) Centrimonium Bromide
(11) Chloramphenicol
(12) Colchicine
(13) Cyanide
(14) Dapsone
(15) Dimethyl sulfate
(16) Dinitrophenol
(17) Endosulfan
(18) Epinephrine (intravenous overdose)
(19) Ethanol
(20) Ethylene glycol

Table 43-5. Examples of Toxidromes

Toxidromes	Pattern	Example of Drugs
Sedative-Hypnotic	Manifested by sedation with progressive deterioration of central nervous system function. Coma, stupor, confusion, apnea, delirium or hallucinations may accompany this pattern.	Ethanol Opiates Barbiturates Methadone Benzodiazephines Glutethimide Meprobamate Methocarbamol Quinazolines Tricyclic Antidepressants Propoxyphene Fentanyl Ethchlorvynol Anti-convulsants Antipsychotics Gamma Hydroxybutyric acid
Narcotic	Altered Mental Status, unresponsiveness, shallow respirations, slow respiratory rate or periodic breathing, miosis, bradycardia, hypothermia.	Opiates Propoxyphere Dextromathorphan Pentazocine
Stimulant	Restlessness, excessive speech and motor activity, tachycardia, tremor and insomnia-may progress to seizure. Other effects noted include euphoria, mydrasis, anorexia and paranoia.	Amphetamines Ephedrin/pseudoephedrine Phencyclidine Cocaine Caffeine (Xanthines) Methylphenidate Nicotine Methcathinone
Seizuregenic	May mimic stimulant pattern with hyperreflexia and tremors being prominent signs.	Strychnine Lidocaine Cocaine Xanthines Isoniazid Chlorinated hydrocarbons Anticholinergics Camphor Phencyclidine Gamma Hydroxybutyric acid
Hallucinogenic	Perceptual distortions, synethesias, depersonalization and derealization.	Cannabinoids Cocaine Indole Alkaloids Phenothiazines Phencyclidine Amphetamines Gamma Hydroxybutyric acid Psilocybin Mescaline Ibogaine Peyote Nutmeg

Table 43-5. Continued

Toxidromes	Pattern	Example of Drugs
Anticholinergic	Fever, ileus, flushing, tachcardia urinary retention, inability to sweat, visual blurring, and mydriasis. Central manifestations include myoclonus, Choreoathetosis, toxic psychosis with Illiputian hallucinations, seizures and coma.	Tricyclic Antidepressants Benztropine Antihistamines Phenothiazines Propantheline Methylpyroline Jimson weed
Cholinergic	Characterized by Salivation, Lacrination, Urination, Defecation, Gastrointestinal cramps and emesis ("SLUDGE"). Bradycardia and bronchoconstriction may also be seen.	Organophosphates Carbanates Pilocarpine
Extrapyramidal	Choreoathetosis, hyperreflexia, trismus, opisthotonos, rigidity and tremor.	Phenothiazines Haloperidal
Solvent	Lethargy, Confusion, Dizziness, Headache, restlessness, Incoordination, derealization, depersonalization.	Hydrocarbons Acetone Toluene Naphthaline Trichloroethane Chlorinated Hydrocarbons
Serotonin	Confusion, restlessness, myoclonus diaphoresis, tremor, hyperreflexia ataxia, diarrhea.	Fluoxetine Sertraline L-Tryptophan Phenelzine Tranylcypromine Isoniazid Paroxetine

(21) Fenoprofen
(22) Flouroacetate
(23) Formaldehyde
(24) Glycol ethers
(25) Hydrogen sulfide
(26) Ibuprofen (ingestion >300 mg/kg)
(27) Iron
(28) Isoniazid
(29) Iodine
(30) Ketamine
(31) Ketoprofen
(32) Massive ingestions of acetaminophen (75–100 g)
(33) Methanol
(34) Methenamine mandelate
(35) Monochloroacetic acid
(36) Nalidixic acid
(37) Naproxen
(38) Niacin
(39) Outdated tetracycline
(40) Papaverine
(41) Paraldehyde
(42) Pennyroyal oil

(43) Pentachlorophenol
(44) Phenformin
(45) Phosphoric acid
(46) Propylene glycol
(47) Salicylates
(48) IV sorbitol
(49) Strychnine
(50) Tienilic acid
(51) Toluene
(52) Tranylcypromine
(53) Vacor
(54) Verapamil

b. Toxic causes of osmolar gap—Osmolar gap equals difference between measured osmolality (by freezing point depression) and calculated osmolality

$$\frac{(1.86 \times Na^+ [urea/2.8] + [Glucose/18])}{0.93}$$

A gap >10 mOsm/kg H_2O is considered significant.
(1) Ethanol
(2) Ethylene glycol

(3) Glycerol

(4) Hypermagnesemia (greater than > 9.5 m/Eq/liter)

(5) Isopropanol

(6) Mannitol

(7) Methanol

(8) Sorbitol

c. Toxic causes of oxygen saturation gap (difference between calculated and measured oxygen saturation is > 5%)

(1) Carbon monoxide

(2) Cyanide (possible)

(3) Hydrogen Sulfide (questionable)

(4) Methemoglobin

2. Laboratory toxicologic analysis

a. Thin-layer chromatography—least sensitive, least specific, and qualitative only.

(1) Barbiturates

(2) Opiates

b. Enzyme multiplied immunoassay technique (EMIT)—fastest test (turnaround time of about 20 min) but least specific.

(1) Urine—drugs of abuse

(2) Serum

(a) Acetaminophen

(b) Antibiotics

(c) Alcohol

(d) Antiepileptic agents

(e) Tricyclic antidepressants

c. Gas chromatography—limited to organic compound determination, but more sensitive.

(1) Barbiturates

(2) Benzodiazepine

(3) Cocaine

(4) Phencyclidine

d. High-performance liquid chromatography—not restricted to volatile compounds.

(1) Aminoglycosides

(2) Antiarrhythmic agents (type I)

(3) Antiepileptic agents

(4) Theophylline

(5) Tricyclic antidepressants

e. Gas chromatography with mass spectrometry is used primarily in confirmatory testing. Very sophisticated and sensitive (measured in nanograms).

(1) Drugs of abuse

(2) Barbiturates

f. Gas chromatography with double use of mass sepectrometry (used for increased sensitivity) can be utilized for compounds

that are very potent and thus found in only minute amounts in the body.

(1) LSD

(2) Fentanyl

g. Spectroscopy (either ultraviolet, fluorescence, or nuclear magnetic resonance)

(1) Quinine

(2) Imipramine

h. Atomic absorption spectroscopy can give either qualitative or quantitative heavy metal determinations.

(1) Aluminum

(2) Arsenic

(3) Cadmium

(4) Copper

(5) Lead

(6) Mercury

IV. **Therapeutic Approach**

A. Stabilization of the patient

1. Airway/breathing indications for endotracheal intubation in the toxic patient.

a. Protection of the airway in the obtunded patient with an absent oral gag reflex to prevent aspiration.

b. Controlled ventilation in patients who demonstrate respiratory depression.

c. Tracheal-bronchial toilet.

d. Use of positive end-expiratory pressure (PEEP) therapy for patients at risk for developing toxin-induced adult respiratory distress syndrome (ARDS).

2. Circulation—may require fluid challenge.

3. Oxygen (100%)—only relative contradiction is paraquat intoxication (can promote pulmonary fibrosis).

4. Dextrose—50 g given IV to reverse the effects of drug-induced hypoglycemia seen in:

a. Albuterol (in infants)

b. Ethanol

c. Chlorpromazine

d. Haloperidol

e. Insulin and oral hypoglycemic agents

f. Methanol

g. Propranolol

h. Salicylates

i. Tetracyclines

5. Thiamine: 50 to 100 mg IV or IM to prevent Wernicke's encephalopathy. Should be administered prior to dextrose administration.

6. Naloxone—a specific opiate antagonist (6-Allylnorovymorphone).

a. Initial adult dosage should be 2 mg intravenously, although intramuscular, subcutaneous, intratracheal, and sublingual routes may be utilized. Up to eight may be required. (Pediatric dose is 0.1 mg/kg up to 20 kg body weight).

b. Boluses may be repeated every 3 to 5 min.

c. If patient relapses into an obtunded state, a naloxone drip may be administered.

   (1) At two-thirds of the naloxone dose that has revived the patient at an hourly rate or

   (2) Mix 4 mg of naloxone in 1 liter of crystalloid solution and administer at a rate of 100 ml/hr (0.4 mg/hr).

B. Prevention of absorption

1. Decontamination

   a. Ocular—irrigate with normal saline for 30–40 min through a Morgan therapeutic lens. In alkali burns, necessary to monitor pH (<8) of runoff solution.

   b. Skin—involves removal of substance with nonabrasive soap. Separate drainage areas are desirable for contaminated runoff. Should be considered for:

      (1) Acid or alkali exposures

      (2) Aniline dyes

      (3) Dimethylsulfoxide

      (4) Dioxin

      (5) Formaldehyde

      (6) Herbicides

      (7) Hydrocarbons

      (8) Hydrofluoric acid

      (9) Mace

      (10) Methanol

      (11) Methylene chloride

      (12) Organophosphates and carbamates

      (13) Petroleum products (including Benzene)

      (14) Phenols

      (15) Radiation

      (16) Sulfides/sulfites

   c. Gastric decontamination

      (1) Emesis—only by means of syrup of ipecac

         (a) Adult Dose of 30 ml accompanied by 8–16 ounces of fluid (may be repeated in 20 min if no emesis has occurred) Pediatric dose for children over one year old is 15 ml of ipecac syrup with 4 to 6 ounces of fluid.

         (b) Most effective if utilized within 30 min of ingestion in an awake and alert patient. After this period, may decrease drug absorption by only 30–40%.

         (c) Contraindications

            (i) Children under 6 months of age

            (ii) Central nervous system (CNS) depression or convulsions

            (iii) Absence of a gag reflex

            (iv) Ingestion of corrosive agents

            (v) Ingestion of seizuregenic agents

            (vi) Ingestion of < 1 ml/kg of hydrocarbon agents.

            (vii) Hemorrhagic diathesis

         d. While home use of ipecac within twenty minutes is quite efficacious, use in the hospital setting has markedly decreased.

2. Gastric lavage—through a No. 28 to No. 40 French Ewald tube, with the patient in the left lateral decubitus position and the feet elevated 15 degrees.

   a. Normal saline or tap water may be utilized at a rate of 1.5 ml/kg/run (not to exceed 250 ml/run), with an additional 1 to 2 liters after clearing.

   b. Essentially as effective as emesis in removal of toxins.

   c. Contraindications

      (1) Acid or alkali exposure

      (2) Hydrocarbon ingestion of < 1 ml/kg

      (3) Hemorrhagic diathesis

      (4) Airway requires protection if CNS depression is present or gag reflex is absent.

3. Use of adsorbants—activated charcoal.

   a. Odorless, tasteless, and insoluble agent with a surface area of up to 3000 m^2/g in some preparations.

   b. Binding of toxins occurs within minutes of contact through intermolecular attraction (van der Waals forces). May decrease drug absorption by 80% when given within 5 min and by 33% when given at 1 hr.

   c. Elemental (heavy metal) toxins, acids/alkalis, and hydrocarbons are poorly adsorbed by activated charcoal.

   d. Dose of roughly 1 g/kg is utilized, usually with a cathartic (see Subsection 4).

e. Is being utilized more often as sole agent for gastric decontamination.

4. Cathartics—major purpose is to promote drug expulsion through gastrointestinal tract by decreasing gastrointestinal transit time. (Note that activated charcoal is a constipating agent.) Common cathartic agents are:

   a. Sorbitol 70% (50 ml adult dosage)

   b. Magnesium sulfate 10% (15–20 g)

   c. Magnesium citrate (300 ml)

   d. Sodium sulfate 10% (15–20 g)

   e. Phospho soda (30 ml diluted 1–4)—contraindicated in children.

5. Whole bowel irrigation (WBI)

   a. Can reduce drug absorption by up to 67%, with catharsis occurring within 4 hr.

   b. Can be performed with administration of GOLYTELY (polyethylene glycol electrolyte lavage solution) at an adult infusion rate of 2 liters/hr.

   c. May be useful in elemental iron, lead, zinc sulfate, enteric-coated aspirin, lithium, ampicillin or cocaine "body-packer" ingestion.

   d. Major contraindications include bowel obstruction, adynamic ileus, perforation, and hemorrhage. May decrease the efficacy of activated charcoal.

C. Antidote administration

An antidote is defined as any drug that increases the median lethal dose (LD_{50}) of a toxin. A list of some relevant antidotes is included in Table 43-6.

D. Enhancement of elimination

1. Multiple dosing of activated charcoal

   a. Mechanisms of action

     (1) Adsorption of drugs excreted through the biliary system, thus re-entering the gastrointestinal tract through enterohepatic circulation.

       (a) Carbamazepine

       (b) Digitoxin

       (c) Glutethimide

       (d) Phenobarbital

     (2) Diffusion of drugs from systemic circulation into the gastrointestinal tract, thus forming a concentration gradient (intestinal dialysis).

       (a) Methotrexate

       (b) Salicylates

       (c) Theophylline

b. Characteristics of toxins by which multiple dosing of activated charcoal appears to be most efficacious.

   (1) Low volume of distribution (<1 liter/kg)

   (2) Uncharged

   (3) Lipophilic

   (4) Low protein binding

   (5) Undergoes enterohepatic recirculation (not essential)

   (6) Adsorbs well onto activated charcoal

   (7) Prolonged half-life of the drug

c. Dosage is 1 g/kg initially, followed by 0.5 g/kg every 2 to 4 hr. Cathartics should not be administered more than once per day. Most of the complications associated with this modality can be attributed to overzealous use of cathartics.

d. Decreases of 40–60% in serum half-life have been demonstrated.

2. Forced diuresis

   a. Saline diuresis to promote renal excretion of the toxin.

     (1) Complications include:

       (a) Pulmonary edema

       (b) Increased intracranial pressure

       (c) Electrolyte abnormalities

     (2) Useful in

       (a) Bromides

       (b) Chromium

       (c) Cis-platinum

       (d) Cimetidine (questionable)

       (e) Hydrazine

       (f) Iodine and the Iodides

       (g) Isoniazid (questionable)

       (h) Lithium

       (i) Potassium chloroplatinite

       (j) Thallium

     (3) Urine flow rate of 300 ml/hr should be maintained.

   b. Alkaline diuresis

     (1) To promote the ionic form of drugs that are weak acids or bases, thus decreasing tubular reabsorption.

     (2) Useful

       (a) 2,4-D chlorophenoxyacetic acid

       (b) Fluoride

       (c) Mephobarbital

       (d) Methotrexate

       (e) Phenobarbital

       (f) Primidone

       (g) Quinolone antibiotics

Table 43-6. Poison Control Center antidote chart

Antidote	Poison/Drug	Indications	Dosage	Comments
N-Acetylcysteine (Mucomyst®)	Acetaminophen	1. Unknown quantity ingested and < 24 hr has elapsed since the time of ingestion or unable to obtain serum acetaminophen levels within 12 hours of ingestion. 2. Greater than 7.5 g of acetaminophen acutely ingested. 3. Serum acetaminophen level greater than 140 μg/ml at 4 hr postingestion. 4. Ingested dose > 140 mg/kg.	Dilute to 5% solution with carbonated beverage, fruit juice or water, administer orally *Loading:* 140 mg/kg one dose *Maintenance:* 70 mg/kg for 17 doses, starting 4 hr after the loading dose and given every 4 hr thereafter unless assay reveals a nontoxic serum level.	SGOT, SGPT, bilirubin, prothrombin time, creatinine, BUN, blood sugar, and electrolytes should be obtained daily if a toxic serum acetaminophen level has been determined *Note:* Activated charcoal has been shown to absorb acetylcysteine in vitro and may do so in patients. Serum acetaminophen levels may not peak until 4 hr postingestion, and therefore serum levels should not be drawn earlier.
Amyl nitrate, sodium nitrite, sodium thiosulfate (Cyanide Antidote Package®)	Cyanide	Begin treatment at the first sign of toxicity if exposure is known or strongly suspected.	Break ampule of amyl nitrate and allow patient to inhale for 15 sec, then take away for 15 sec; use a fresh ampule every 3 min. Continue until injection of sodium nitrate 300 mg can be injected at 2.5–5 ml/min. Then immediately inject 12.5 g of 25% sodium thiosulfate, slow IV.	If symptoms return, treatment may be repeated at half the normal dosages. For pediatric dosing see package insert. Do NOT use methylene blue to reduce elevated methemoglobin levels. Oxygen therapy may be useful when combined with sodium thiosulfate therapy.

Table 43-6. Continued

Antidote	Poison/Drug	Indications	Dosage	Comments
Atropine	Organophosphate and carbamate insecticides; Mushrooms containing Musarine (Inocybe or Clitocybe)	Myoclonic seizures, severe hallucinations, weakness, arrhythmias, excessive salivation, involuntary urination and defecation.	*Adult:* 2 mg IV *Child:* 0.05 mg/kg IV Repeat dosage every 10 min. until patients respiratory status is stabilized.	Caution should be used in patients with narrow angle glaucoma, cardiovascular disease, or pregnancy. Plasma and erythrocyte cholinesterase levels will be depressed from normal. Atropine should only be used when indicated otherwise use may result in anticholinergic poisoning.
	Digoxin	Bradyarrhythmias, heart block.	*Adult:* 0.6 mg/dose IV. *Child:* 10–30 μg/kg/dose up to 0.4 mg/dose IV.	
Calcium EDTA (calcium disodium versenate)	Lead	Symptomatic patients or asymptomatic children with blood levels > 50 μg/dl.	50–75 mg/kg/day deep IM or slow IV infusion in 3 to 6 divided doses for up to 5 days.	If urine flow is not established, hemodialysis must accompany calcium EDTA dosing. In most cases, the IM route is preferred.
Calcium gluconate	Hydrofluoric acid	Calcium gluconate gel 2.5% for dermal exposures of HF of < 20% conc. SC injections of calcium gluconate for dermal exposures of HF in > 20% conc. or failure to respond to calcium gluconate gel.	Massage 2.5% gel into exposed area for 15 min. Infiltrate each square centimeter of exposed area with 0.5 ml of 10% calcium gluconate SC using a 30-gauge needle.	Injections of calcium gluconate should not be used in digital area. With exposures to dilute concentrations of HF, symptoms may take several hours to develop. Calcium gluconate gel is not currently available. Contact your regional poison control center for compounding instructions.

Deferoxamine (Desferal®)	Iron	SI level exceeds TIBC, SI > 350 µg/dl and TIBC is unavailable. Inability to obtain SI in a reasonable time and patient is symptomatic.	*Mild Symptoms:* 90 mg/kg IM up to 1 g every 48 hr. *Symptoms:* 10–15 mg/kg/hr IV, not to exceed 6 g in 24 hr.	Passing of vin rosé-colored urine indicates free iron was present. Therapy should be discontinued when urine returns to normal color. Monitor for hypotension, especially when giving deferoxamine IV.
Digoxin immune fab (Digibind®)	Digoxin Digitoxin Oleander Foxglove Lilly of the Valley (?) Red Squill (?)	Life-threatening cardiac arrhythmias, progressive bradyarrhythmias, 2nd- or 3rd-degree heart block unresponsive to atropine, serum digitoxin level > 10 mg/ml or potassium levels > 5 mEq/L.	Multiply serum digitoxin concentration by 5.6 and multiply the result by the patient's weight in kilograms divide this by 1,000 and divide the result by 0.6. This gives the dose in number of vials to use. For other dosing methods, see package insert.	Monitor potassium levels, continuous ECG. *Note:* Digibind interferes with free serum digitoxin/digoxin levels.
Dimercaprol (BAL in oil)	Arsenic, lead, mercury	Any symptoms due to arsenic exposure.	3–5 mg/kg/dose deep IM every 4 hr until GI symptoms subside and patient switched to D-penicillamine.	Patients receiving dimercaprol should be monitored for hypertension, tachycardia, hyperpyrexia and urticaria. Used in conjunction with calcium EDTA in lead poisoning.
	All patients with symptoms or asymptomatic children with blood lead levels > 70 µg/dl.		3–5 mg/kg/dose deep IM every 4 hr for 2 days then every 4–12 hr for up to 7 additional days.	

Table 43-6. Continued

Antidote	Poison/Drug	Indications	Dosage	Comments
		Any symptoms due to mercury and patient unable to take D-penicillamine.	3–5 mg/kg/dose deep IM every 4 hr for 48 hours, then 3 mg/kg/dose every 6 hr, then 3 mg/kg/dose every 12 hr for 7 more days.	
Ethanol	Ethylene glycol or methanol	Ethylene glycol or methanol blood levels > 20 mg/dl. Blood levels not readily available and suspected ingestion of toxic amounts. Any symptomatic patient with a history of ethylene glycol or methanol ingestion.	*Loading Dose:* 7.6–10 ml/kg IV ethanol in DSW over 1 hr. *Maintenance Dose:* 1.4 ml/kg/hr IV of 10% ethanol in DSW. Maintian blood ethanol level of 100–130 mg/dL.	Monitor blood glucose, especially in children, as ethanol may cause hypoglycemia. Do not use 5% ethanol in D_5W, as excessive amounts of fluid would be required to maintain adequate ethanol blood levels. If dialysis is performed, adjustment of ethanol dosing is required.
Flumazenil (Romazicon®)	Benzodiazepine	As adjunct to conventional management of benzodiazepine overdose.	.2 mgm IV over 30 seconds; wait another 30 seconds then give an additional .3 mgm IV over 30 seconds. Additional doses of .5 mgm over 30 seconds at 1 minute intervals up to a cumulative dose of 3 mgm.	Onset of reversal usually within 1–2 minutes. Contraindicated in patients with epilepsy, increased intracranial pressure or coingestion of a seizuregenic agent (i.e., cyclic antipressant).
Methylene Blue	Methemoglobin inducers (i.e., nitrites, phenazopyridine)	1. Cyanosis 2. Methemoglobin level greater than 30% in an asymptomatic patient.	1–2 mg/kg (0.1 to 0.2 ml/kg) per dose. I.V. over 2–3 minutes. May repeat doses as needed clinically. Injection can be given as 1% solution or diluted in normal saline.	Treatment can result in falsely elevated methemoglobin levels when measured by co-oximeter. Large doses (greater than 15 mg/kg) may cause hemolysis.

Antidote	Indication	Dose	Comments
Leucovorin (Citrovorum Factor, Folinic Acid)	Methotrexate induced bone marrow depression (Methotrexate serum level greater than 1 × 10^{-8} mol/L); may also be useful in pyrimethamine-trimethoprim bone marrow depression.	Dose should be equal to or greater than the dose of methotrexate ingested. Usually 15 to 100 mg/m² is given I.V. or orally every six hours for eight doses.	Most effective if given within one hour post exposure. May not be effective to prevent liver toxicity. Monitor methotrexate levels. May enhance the toxicity of fluorouracil.
Glucagon	Propranolol; Hypoglycemic Agents. 1. Propranolol-induced cardiac dysfunction and hypotension. 2. Treatment of hypoglycemia.	.5 to 1 mgm SQ, IM or IV. May repeat after 15 minutes.	May potentiate the effects of oral anticoagulants. Require liver glycogen stores for hyperglycemia response. Intravenous glucose must also be given in treatment of hypoglycemia.
Naloxone (Narcan®)	Opiates (e.g., heroin, morphine, codeine). Coma or respiratory depression from unknown cause or from opiate overdose.	Give 0.8–2.0 mg IV bolus. Doses may be repeated if there is no response, up to 10 mg.	For prolonged intoxication, a continuous infusion may be used. See package insert for details.
D-penicillamine (Cuprimine®)	Arsenic, lead, mercury. Following BAL therapy in symptomatic acutely poisoned patients. Asymptomatic patients with excess lead burden. Patient symptomatic from mercury exposure or excessive levels.	100 mg/kg/day up to 2 g in 4 divided doses for 5 days. 1–2/day in 4 divided doses for 5 days. Adult: 250 mg PO four times daily. Child: 100 mg/kg/day up to 1 g daily in 4 divided doses. Given for 3–10 days.	Possible contraindication for patients with penicillin allergy. Monitor heavy metal levels daily in severely poisoned patients. Monitor CBC and renal function in patients receiving chronic D-penicillamine therapy. Dosages given are for short-term acute therapy only.

Table 43-6. Continued

Antidote	Poison/Drug	Indications	Dosage	Comments
Physostigmine salicylate (Antilirium®)	Atropine and anticholinergic agents, cyclic antidepressants	Myoclonic seizures, severe arrhythmias	*Adult:* 0.5–2 mg slow IV push. *Child:* 0.5 mg slow IV push. Repeat as requires for life threatening symptoms.	Dramatic reversal of anticholinergic symptoms after IV use. Should not be used just to keep patient awake. *Contraindications:* asthma, gangrene, physostigmine use in cyclic antidepressant-induced cardiac toxicity is controversial. *Extreme caution is advised—* should be considered only in the presence of life-threatening anticholinergic symptoms.
		Refractory seizures or arrhythmias unresponsive to conventional therapies.	Same as above	
Pralidoxime (2-Pam, Protopam®)	Organophosphate Insecticides	An adjunct to atropine therapy for treatment of profound muscle weakness, respiratory depression, muscle twitching.	*Adult:* 2 g IV at 0.5 g/min. or infused in 250 ml N.S. over 30 min. *Child:* 25–50 mg/kg in 250 ml saline over 30 min.	Most effective when used in initial 24–36 hr after the exposure. Dosage may be repeated in 1 hr, followed by every 8 hr if indicated.
Pyridoxine (Vitamin B₆)	Isoniazid Monomethylhydrazine containing mushrooms (Gyromitra)	Unknown overdose or ingested amount > 80 mg/kg.	Pyridoxine IV in the amount of INH ingested or 5 g if amount is unknown given over 30–60 min.	Cumulative dose of pyridoxine is arbitrarily limited to 40 g in adults and 20 g in children.
Succimer (Chemet®)	Lead Arsenic (?) Mercury (?)	Asymptomatic children with venous blood lead of 45 to 69 mcg/dl.	10 mg/kg or 350 mg/m² orally every 8 hrs for 5 days. Reduce to 10 mg/kg or 350 mg/m² every 12 hours for an additional 2 weeks.	Monitor liver function; emits "rotten egg" sulfur odor.

Vitamin K₁/Phytonadione	Large acute ingestion of warfarin rodenticides. Chronic exposure or greater than normal prothrombin time.	*Adult:* 10 mg IM *Child:* 1–5 mg IM With severe toxicity, vitamin K₁ may be given IV. (Adult up to 10 mg; child 1–5 mg). Diluted in saline or glucose at a rate not to exceed 5% of total dose per minute.	Vitamin K therapy is relatively contraindicated for patients with prosthetic heart valves unless toxicity is life-threatening.
Coumarin Derivatives Indandione Derivatives			
Antivenin (*Cortalidae*) polyvalent (equine origin)	Mild, moderate to severe symptoms and history of envenomation by a pit viper. *Mild:* Local swelling (progressive) pain, no systemic systems. *Moderate:* Ecchymosis and swelling beyond the bite site, some systemic symptoms and/or lab changes. *Severe:* Profound edema involving entire extremity, cyanosis, serious systemic involvement, significant lab changes.	*Mild:* 3–5 vials of antivenin in 250–500 ml of N.S. *Moderate:* 6–10 vials of antivenin in 500 ml of N.S. *Severe:* Minimum of 10 vials in 500 to 1,000 ml of N.S. Administer over 4–6 hr. Additional antivenin should be given on the basis of clinical response and continuing assessment of severity of the poisoning.	Draw blood for type and cross-match, hematocrit, BUN, electrolytes, CBC, platelets, coagulation profile. DO NOT administer heparin for possible allergic reaction.

Source: Rush Poison Control center, Rush-Presbyterian-St. Luke's Medial Center, Chicago, IL. 60612. Reproduced by permission.
CBC = complete blood count; D₅W = 5 percent dextrose in water; EDTA = ethylenediaminetetra-acetic acid; HF = hydrofluoric acid; INH = isoniazide; N.S. = normal saline; SI = serum iron.

       (h) Salicylates
- (3) Alkalinization of urine can be achieved through administration of 44 to 88 mEq/liter of sodium bicarbonate to tritiate to a urine pH of 7.5 to 8.0
- (4) Urine acidification should not be utilized due to production of metabolic acidosis and rhabdomyolysis-induced renal failure. Drugs in which elimination is increased in an acidic urine include:
  - (a) Amphetamine
  - (b) MAO inhibitor
  - (c) Phencyclidine
  - (d) Quinine/Quinidine

3. Hemodialysis
   a. Effective in correcting metabolic abnormalities and promoting excretion of drugs with the following characteristics:
   - (1) High water solubility
   - (2) Low lipid solubility
   - (3) Low plasma protein binding
   - (4) Low volume of distribution
   - (5) Low molecular weight

   b. Should be started very early in the course of significant methanol, ethylene glycol, or Thallium toxicity.

   c. Other Drugs or Toxins in which hemodialysis is useful:
   - (1) Acyclovir
   - (2) Aminophylline
   - (3) Ammonium chloride
   - (4) Amphetamine
   - (5) Anilines
   - (6) Atenolol
   - (7) Boric acid
   - (8) Bromides
   - (9) Bromisoval
   - (10) Calcium
   - (11) Carbromal
   - (12) Carisoprodol
   - (13) Chloral hydrate
   - (14) Chromium
   - (15) Dapsone
   - (16) Disopyramide
   - (17) Ethanol
   - (18) Fluoride
   - (19) Formaldehyde
   - (20) Glycol ethers
   - (21) Hydrochlorothiazide
   - (22) Isoniazil
   - (23) Isopropanil (acetone)
   - (24) Ketroprofen
   - (25) Lithium
   - (26) Magnesium
   - (27) Iodides
   - (28) Meprobamate
   - (29) Metal-chelate compounds
   - (30) Methaqualone
   - (31) Methotrexate
   - (32) Methyldopa
   - (33) Methyprylon
   - (34) Monochloroacetic acid
   - (35) Nadolol
   - (36) Oxalic acid
   - (37) Paraldehyde
   - (38) Phenobarbital
   - (39) Phosphoric acid
   - (40) Potassium
   - (41) Procainamide
   - (42) Quinidine
   - (43) Salicylates
   - (44) Sotalol
   - (45) Strychnine
   - (46) Thiocyanates

   d. Drugs in which hemodialysis may be useful
   - (1) Amantadine
   - (2) Amanita Phalloides
   - (3) Captopril
   - (4) Cimetidine
   - (5) Enalapril
   - (6) Famotidine
   - (7) Hydrazine
   - (8) Phenelzine
   - (9) Ranitidine
   - (10) Tranylcyproming

   e. Peritoneal dialysis has not been shown to be useful in adults for drug removal.

4. Charcoal hemoperfusion
   a. Through the pumping of blood through a charcoal cannister, thereby increasing drug clearance.

   b. Less dependent on molecular weight, water solubility, or plasma protein binding characteristics of the toxin but highly dependent on ability of charcoal to act as adsorbent.

   c. Drugs in which charcoal hemoperfusion is useful include:
   - (1) Aminophylline
   - (2) Barbiturates (especially phenobarbital and chloral hydrate)
   - (3) Bromisoval
   - (4) Bromoethylbutyramide
   - (5) Camphor
   - (6) Carbromal

(7) Chloramphenicol
(8) Dapsone
(9) Disopyramide
(10) Ethchlorvynol
(11) Glutethimide
(12) Lindane
(13) Meprobamate
(14) Methaqualone
(15) Methotrexate
(16) Paraquat/Diquat
(17) Thallium
d. Drugs in which charcoal hemoperfusion MAY be useful include:
(1) Atenolol
(2) Amanita Phalloides
(3) Colchicine
(4) Carbon tetrachloride
(5) Diltiazem

(6) Ethylene Oxide
(7) Isoniazid
(8) Metroprolol
(9) Methyprylon
(10) Nadolol
(11) Oxalic acid
(12) Phenelzine
(13) Procainamide
(14) Quinidine
(15) Sotalol
(16) Verapamil
e. Adverse reactions include:
(1) Hypotension
(2) Hypocalcemia
(3) Infection
(4) Thrombocytopenia
E. Support and monitoring for adverse effects. Table 43-7 lists criteria for admission to an intensive care unit.

Table 43-7. Criteria for admission of the poisoned patient to the ICU

Respiratory depression (P_{CO_2} > 45 mm Hg)
Emergency intubation
Seizures
Cardiac arrhythmia
Hypotension (systolic blood pressure < 80 mm Hg)
Unresponsiveness to verbal stimuli
Second- or third-degree atrioventricular block
Emergent dialysis or hemoperfusion
Increasing metabolic acidosis
Tricyclic or phenothiazine overdose manifesting with anticholinergic signs, neurologic abnormality, *or* QRS duration > 0.12 sec
Administration of pralidoxime in organophosphate toxicity
Pulmonary edema induced by drugs or toxic inhalation (ARDS)
Drug-induced hypothermia or hyperthermia, including neuroleptic malignant syndrome
Hyperkalemia secondary to digitalis overdose
Body packers and stuffers
Concretions secondary to drugs
Emergent surgical intervention
Antivenom administration in *Crotalidae*, coral snake or arthropod envenomation
Need for continuous infusion of Naloxone

Source: Kulling P, Persson H. Role of the intensive care unit in the management of the poisoned patient. Med Toxicol 1986;1:375–386; Brett AS, Rothschild N, Gray R, Perry R, Perry M. Predicting the clinical course in intentional drug overdose: Implication for use of the intensive care unit. Arch Intern Med 1987;147:133–137; Callaham M. Admission criteria for tricyclic antidepressant ingestion. West J Med 1982;137:425–429. Adapted with permission.

Bibliography

Brett AS, Rothschild N, Gray R, et al. Predicting the clinical course in intentional drug overdose: Implications for use of the intensive care unit. *Arch Intern Med* 147:133–137, 1987.

Bryson PD. *Comprehensive Review in Toxicology,* ed 2. Rockville, MD, Aspen Publications, 1989.

Callaham M. Admission criteria for tricyclic antidepressant ingestion. *West J Med* 137:425–429, 1982.

Committee on Environmental Health: Lead Poisoning: From Screening to Primary Prevention. Pediatrics. 1993:92:176–183.

Ellenhorn MJ, Barceloux DG. *Medical Toxicology: Diagnosis and Treatment of Human Poisoning.* Elsevior Press, New York, 1988.

Everson GW, Bertaccini EJ, O'Leary JO. Use of whole bowel irrigation in an infant following iron overdose. *Am J Emerg Med* 9:366–369, 1991.

Garrettson LK, Geller RJ. Acid and Alkaline Diuresis: When are they of value in the treatment of poisoning?, *Drug Safety* 5:220–232, 1990.

Goldfrank LR. *Toxicologic Emergencies,* ed 4, Norwalk, CT, Appleton-Century-Crofts, 1990.

Goldfrank LR. The expanding role of the toxicologist in modern medicine. *Hosp Physician* 27:11–12, 1991.

Jacobsen D, McMartin KE. Methanol and ethylene glycol poisoning: Mechanism of toxicity, clinical course, diagnosis and treatment. *Med Toxicol* 1:309–334, 1986.

Kirshenbaum LA, Sitan DS, Tenenbein M. Interaction between whole-bowel irrigation solution and activated charcoal: Implications for the treatment of toxic ingestions. *Ann Emerg Med* 19:1129–1132, 1990.

Kulig K, Bar-Or D, Cantrill SV, et al. Management of acutely poisoned patients without gastric emptying. *Ann Emerg Med* 14:562–567, 1985.

Kulig K. Initial Management of Ingestions of Toxic Substances N.E.J.M. 326:1677–1681, 1992.

Kulling P, Persson H. Role of the intensive care unit in the management of the poisoned patient. *Med Toxicol* 1:375–386, 1986.

Leikin JB, Hanashiro PK. Approach to toxicology, in Parrillo J (ed): *Current Therapy in Critical Care Medicine,* ed 2. Philadelphia, BC Decker, 1991. pp 320–325.

Leikin JB, Krantz AJ, Zell-Kanter M, et al. Clinical features and management of intoxication due to hallucinogenic drugs. *Med Toxicol Adverse Drug Exp* 4:324–350, 1989.

Linden C. Activated charcoal. *Clin Toxicol Rev* 9:1–6, 1987.

Litovitz TL, Holm KC, Clancy C, et al. 1992 Annual Report of the American Association of Poison Control Centers National Data Collection System. *Am J Emerg Med* 11:494–555, 1993.

McCarron MM. The role of the laboratory in treatment of the poisoned patient: A clinical perspective. *J Anal Toxicol* 4:142–145, 1983.

Merrigian KS, Woodard M, Hedges JR, et al. Prospective evaluation of gastric emptying in the self-poisoned patient. *Am J Emerg Med* 8:479–483, 1990.

National Institute on Drug Abuse. *Data From the Drug Abuse Warning Network. Annual Data—1989* Series I. Number 9. Rockville, MD, U.S. Department of Health and Human Services, 1990.

National Institute on Drug Abuse, Data from the Drug Abuse Warning Network, Annual Emergency Room Data, 1991. Series 1, Number 11-A Rockville, MD, U.S. Department of Health and Human Services, 1992.

Nice A, Leikin JB, Maturen A, et al. Toxidrome recognition to improve efficiency of emergency urine screens. *Ann Emerg Med* 17:676–680, 1988.

Noji EK, Kelen EK. *Manual of toxicologic emergencies.* Chicago, Year Book Medical Publishers, 1989.

Notarianni, L. A Reassessment of the Treatment of Salicylate Poisoning. *Drug Safety* 7:292, 1992.

Rumack BH, Spoerke DS. Poisindex information system. Denver, Micromedex, Inc., Vol. 78 edition expires November 30, 1993

Shannon M. Cathartics. *Clin Toxicol Rev* 8:1–2, 1986.

Shesser R, Jotte R, Olshaker J. The contribution of impurities to the acute morbidity of illegal drug use. *Am J Emerg Med* 9:336–342, 1991.

Spivey WH, Roberts JR, Derlet RW. A clinical trial of escalating doses of flumazenil for reversal of suspected benzodiazepine overdose in the emergency department. *Ann Emerg Med* 22:1813–1821, 1993.

Sternbach H. The serotonin syndrome. *Am J Psychiatr* 148:705–713, 1991.

Tueth, MJ. The serotonin syndrome in the emergency department. *Ann Emerg Med* 22:1369, 1993.

Hypothermia

Jerrold B. Leikin, M.D.
Paul K. Hanashiro, M.D.

I. **Definition**
Hypothermia is a core temperature of less than 35°C (95°F).

II. **Etiology**
Hypothermia occurs when there is a decrease in heat production, an increase in heat loss, or a combination of these two states.
  A. Increased heat loss to the environment
    1. Cold water immersion
    2. Wet clothing/inadequate protection in cold environment
    3. Dermal dysfunction
      a. Erythrodermas
      b. Burns
    4. Ethanol use
    5. Barbiturate use
  B. Decrease in heat production.
    1. Hypothyroidism-myxedema
    2. Malnutrition-marasmus
    3. Neuromuscular diseases
    4. Extremes of age
    5. Hypoadrenalism
    6. Hypopituitarism
    7. Hypoglycemia
    8. Immobilization
  C. Combination of above factors

  1. Impaired thermoregulation
    a. Cerebrovascular accidents
    b. Parkinson's disease
    c. Cerebellar lesions
    d. Wernicke's encephalopathy
    e. Trauma
      (1) Head trauma
        (a) Basilar skull fractures
        (b) Chronic subdural hematoma
      (2) Spinal cord transection
    f. Anorexia nervosa
  2. Drug-induced
    a. Carbon monoxide
    b. Phenothiazines
    c. Benzodiazepines
    d. Tricyclic antidepressants
    e. General anesthetics
    f. Heroin
    g. Glutethimide
    h. Organophosphates
    i. Clonidine
  3. Infections
    a. Gram-negative sepsis
    b. Pneumonia
    c. Bacterial endocarditis
    d. Brucellosis

   e. Syphilis
   f. Miliary tuberculosis
4. Other diseases
   a. Pancreatitis
   b. Uremia
   c. Diabetic ketoacidosis
   d. Congestive heart failure
   e. Portal vein thrombosis

III. **Pathophysiology**
A. Mechanisms of heat loss
   1. Conduction—heat transfer by direct contact, accounting for 2–3% normally but increasing by 5 times in wet clothes and by 32 times in cold water immersion.
   2. Convection—heat transfer through air, accounting for 10–15% of heat loss.
   3. Radiation—heat transfer by infrared radiation, accounting for 65% of body heat loss.
   4. Evaporation of water from the skin's surface and respiratory tract, accounting for 20% loss of body heat.
B. Mechanism of heat production
   1. Basal heat production is about 50 Kcal/m^2 of body surface area per hour.
   2. Shivering in response to a cold stress can increase heat production by twofold to fivefold. It can be suppressed by barbiturates, ethanol, phenothiazines, and hypoglycemia. Fatigue and glycogen depletion are causes of the limitation of shivering to a few hours as effective heat production.
C. Multisystem response to cold exposure
   1. Central nervous system
      a. Preoptic anterior hypothalamus regulates the response.
      b. Decreased cerebral function and lethargy, leading to coma.
      c. Cerebral blood flow decreases 6–7% for every 1°C drop in temperature.
      d. Unconsciousness due solely to hypothermia rarely occurs at core temperatures above 28°C, so other causes need to be investigated in the mildly hypothermic, comatose individual.
   2. Cardiovascular effects
      a. Decrease heart rate and cardiac output.
      b. Hypotension can occur at 25°C even though systemic arterial resistance may be increased.
      c. Atrial fibrillation and bradycardia may be present at temperatures below 32°C reverting back to normal upon rewarming.

   d. Osborne waves; J-point elevation and S-T-positive deflection may be present (80% occurrence when core temperature is below 34°C [93°F]).
   e. Ventricular fibrillation and asystole can occur at temperatures below 25°C.
3. Respiratory changes
   a. Hypoventilation with respiratory depression.
   b. Bronchorrhea leading to aspiration pneumonitis.
4. Circulatory changes
   a. Elevation of hematocrit due to:
      (1) Plasma loss.
      (2) Splenic contraction.
   b. Decreased peripheral leukocyte and platelet counts.
   c. Increased viscosity.
   d. Shift in oxyhemoglobin dissociation curve to the left.
5. Gastrointestinal changes
   a. Ileus and constipation.
   b. Decreased rectal tone.
   c. Abdominal distention.
6. Genitourinary changes.
   a. Increase in dilute urine flow (cold diuresis) may result in volume depletion.
   b. Anuria may develop.
7. Coagulopathies can occur at temperatures below 28°F.
8. Endocrine changes.
   a. Inhibition of insulin production may result in hyperglycemia.
   b. Hypoglycemia may develop from depleted glycogen stores caused by shivering.
   c. Stimulates release of thyroxine from thyroid.
   d. Norepinephrine is released.
   e. Suppression of antidiuretic hormone (ADH) release.
   f. Corticosteroid hormones are released.

IV. **Diagnosis**
The degree of temperature depression accounts for the clinical signs seen. A high index of suspicion must be present. Rectal thermometers (low reading) should be routinely utilized.
A. History—may not be dramatic in terms of exposure. Therefore, hypothermia must be considered in any hypotensive and/or lethargic patient. A combination of inadequate clothing, prolonged exposure to a cool environment, extremes of age, and/or alcohol

ingestion is more than sufficient to result in clinically significant hypothermia.

B. Clinical signs and physical findings—described primarily in Section III. Decreased heart sounds, dilated pupils responding sluggishly to light, and delayed or absent deep tendon reflexes are prominent clinical findings, along with a change in mentation.

C. Diagnostic tests
1. Complete blood count—may demonstrate hemoconcentration secondary to volume depletion. Platelets and white blood cell count may be decreased secondary to sequestration. All of these parameters normalize with fluid administration and rewarming, provided that no other pathology is present. The hematocrit increases 2% for every 1°C fall in temperature.
2. Arterial blood gas test—usually shows metabolic (lactate) acidosis and/or respiratory acidosis. As circulation is reestablished, metabolic acidosis may temporarily worsen as underperfused areas give up metabolic wastes to the general circulation. Blood gases may be interpreted in terms of core temperature, although the clinical utility of this redetermination is increasingly being called into question.
   a. PO_2 drops by 7.2% for every 1°C drop.
   b. PCO_2 drops by 4.4% for every 1°C drop.
   c. pH increases by 0.015 for every 1°C drop.
3. Electrolytes—hyper- or hypoglycemia may occur in prolonged hypothermia, while hyperkalemia may be related to the length of asystole.
4. Amylase—hyperamylasemia can occur and may correlate with mortality.
5. Electrocardiogram—may show characteristic Osborne wave. Prolongation of P-R, QRS, and Q-T intervals may occur with diminution of P waves. Re-entry arrhythmia are common. T waves may be inverted. All of these problems resolve with rewarming.

V. Treatment

Rewarming: Generally, hypothermia of slow onset should be treated with slow rewarming, whereas sudden-onset hypothermia calls for more rapid rewarming.

A. Passive external rewarming—attempts to minimize heat loss and maximize retention of basal heat production by removing the patient from the cold environment and wrapping him or her in insulating material (blankets or plastic wrap). This method is simple and readily available, and often the only method available at distant rescue sites. Disadvantages are slowness and reliance on the patient's already impaired physiologic reserves. In the hospital setting, room temperature should be 25°–32.9°C (77–90°F). Rewarming rates of 0.5 to 2°C/hr are optimal. This is the method of choice in the mildly hypothermic patient (32°C) with no serious metabolic or cardiac disturbances.

B. Active external rewarming—attempts heat transfer to external surfaces of the patient's body (preferably the thorax) by wrapping the patient in electric warming blankets (or in sleeping bags with normothermic rescuers) or by immersion of the patient in a warm (40°C) bath. While it is more rapidly effective in raising temperature than passive rewarming, several problems exist with this method.
1. "After drop" phenomenon—rapid peripheral warming results in vasodilation, sudden shunting of cold blood to an already cold, compromised heart, and an increased likelihood of arrhythmias (especially ventricular arrhythmias).
2. Hypovolemic shock may be precipitated by external vasodilation in an already volume-depleted patient.
3. The difficulties of resuscitating, evaluating or monitoring patient immersed in a tub of water are self-evident.
4. Thermal burns from heating blankets may occur more readily in underperfused areas.
5. Not efficacious in patients with chronic hypothermia.
6. Increased skin temperature may cause shivering to cease and thus decrease internal heat production.

C. Active core rewarming—attempts to warm the core of the body preferentially by utilizing access to large surface areas, including the gastrointestinal tract, peritoneum, alveolar surface, and general circulation.
1. Delivery of heated, humidified oxygen is a useful adjunct to core rewarming techniques that utilize the large surface area of alveoli. Oxygen should be 100% humidified and heated to 42–46°C and frequently checked by a thermometer at the

mask to avoid airway burns or irritation. A rewarming rate of 1°–2.5°C/hour can be expected. This method can be used as an adjunct to passive rewarming in the mildly hypothermic, hypovolemic patient, but it is not useful for the normovolemic (i.e., submersion), hypothermic patient because pulmonary edema may occur.

2. Intravenous fluid warming using a blood-warming coil maintained at 37°–45°C allows added heat transfer while supplying needed volume expansion, glucose, and electrolytes. Not recommended as a single method of rewarming but useful as an adjunct to other techniques.

3. Peritoneal dialysis with heated (43°C) dialysate. Correction of metabolic acidosis by alkaline dialysate with regulation of potassium level and removal of dialyzable toxins can occur. Previous abdominal surgery and trauma are contraindications. Usual flow rate of 6 liters/hr can be achieved, and an hourly rise of 1°–2°C can occur.

4. Hemodialysis offers the same advantages as peritoneal dialysis with more rapid results, but requires placement of a temporary shunt as well as specialized machinery and personnel.

5. Gastrointestinal or high colonic lavage with warm solutions is simple and readily available but may not offer any more advantages over heated, humidified inhalation.

6. Extracorporeal venovenous rewarming may be an effective and simple method in actively warming and recirculating blood and I.V. fluids.

7. Cardiopulmonary bypass is being utilized more frequently for severe hypothermia. With external warming of blood to 40°C, it is capable of raising the core temperature by 10°–12°C per hour. Anticoagulation and local vascular trauma are the major complications.

8. Open Thoracotomy (internal cardiac massage) with mediastinal irrigation (resulting in core rewarming of about 8° c/minute) has been utilized successfully in the setting of hypothermic cardiac arrest.

VI. **Patient Monitoring**

A. In the field, the patient should be ventilated and oxygenated before being transported. Intubation is a relatively safe procedure in the hypothermic patient.

B. Core temperature should be monitored with a rectal probe (inserted 15 cm) or an esophageal thermistor (inserted 43 cm). Rectal temperature changes may lag behind esophageal changes. Do not monitor with oral or tympanic probes. Urinary temperatures are unreliable.

C. Continuous cardiac monitoring is essential. Supraventricular arrhythmias that do not compromise the circulation should be observed while rewarming and metabolic correction proceed. Ventricular arrhythmias should be treated with the usual techniques, remembering that the hypothermic heart is relatively refractory to DC countershock and drugs. Asystole may be correctable after rewarming. Defibrillation should be utilized only when the core temperature is above 31°C. Bretyllium may be particularly effective for ventricular fibrillation. Cardiopulmonary resuscitation should be utilized in patients with asystole or ventricular fibrillation (not bradycardia), and chest thrusts should be performed at half the rate of normothermic patients.

D. Electrolyte abnormalities require correction and monitoring. Use potassium-free solutions; do not use Ringer's lactate solution. Attention should be directed to glucose, potassium, phosphorus, bicarbonate, and pH. The patient should be kept mildly acidotic during rewarming.

E. If the patient fails to rewarm, consider adrenocortical dysfunction; 250 mg of hydrocortisone or 30 mg/kg of methylprednisolone intravenously may be required.

F. Usually, inotropic agents are not necessary to support blood pressure. Central venous pressures should not be increased dramatically during resuscitation.

G. Monitor for complications.
   1. Pneumonia
   2. Renal failure/acute tubular necrosis
   3. Pancreatitis (pancreas is the only organ that shows lesions of hypothermia)
   4. Coagulopathies
   5. Diabetic ketoacidosis
   6. Gastrointestinal bleeding
   7. Ileus
   8. Hypotensive episodes due to vasculature regulation dysfunction
   9. Pulmonary edema
   10. Hemolysis/myoglobinuria
   11. Seizures

Table 44A-1   Differences between Hypothermia and Hyperthermia

Hypothermia	Hyperthermia
1. No good animal model for study.	Good animal model for study (canine).
2. Specific lesions seen in only one organ (pancreas).	Lesions seen in virtually every organ except one (pancreas).
3. Warming should be controlled.	Rapid cooling effective in lowering mortality.
4. Clinical signs correlate with degree of temperature depression.	Clinical signs do not correlate with degree of hyperthermia.
5. Endotracheal intubation safe to use.	Endotracheal intubation may be arrhythmogenic.
6. Most cardiac medications not useful (except possibly for brethyllium in converting ventricular fibrillation).	Cardiac medications are useful, although potent vasopressors should be avoided.
7. No physiologic adaptive changes to a cold stress.	Acclimatization is a factor in adapting to heat stress.
8. Level of rise of amylase may be useful prognostic factor.	Level of rise of SGOT may be a useful prognostic factor.
9. Hypoventilation.	Hyperventilation.
10. Avoid Ringer's lactate solution.	May use Ringer's lactate solution.
11. Tachycardia followed by sinus bradycardia.	Sinus tachycardia is universal.
12. Hypothalamic lesions can result in hypothermia.	Cerebral lesion can result in hyperthermia.
13. Pathognomonic electrocardiographic changes (Osborn wave).	No pathognomonic electrocardiographic changes.
14. Less likely to cause ischemic cardiac event.	May cause ischemic cardiac event.
15. Constipation/Ileus usually seen.	Diarrhea is frequently seen.

Table 44A-2.   Similarities Between Hypothermia and Hyperthermia

1. Extreme age groups particularly affected.
2. Disseminated intravascular coagulation can occur with either condition.
3. Phenothiazines, glutethimide, general anesthetics, and tricyclic antidepressants can cause either condition.

12. Adrenal insufficiency
13. Increased potassium excretion and alkalosis
14. Hypophosphatemia
15. Hematuria

VII. Prognosis

It should be remembered that successful recovery may follow prolonged cardiac arrest because of decreased oxygen requirements during cardiac arrest. No meaningful evaluation of neurologic damage or other derangements can be made until the patient is normothermic. Survival can be correlated with levels of hypoxia, infection, amylase, or drug overdose. It has been suggested that profound hyperkalemia (> 10 mmol/liter) may be a prognostic factor for irreversibility. The lowest accidental hypothermia survival has been recorded at 15.2°C (58.8°F); with induced hypothermia, survival has been documented at 9°C (48.2°F).

Bibliography

Auerbach PS. Some people are dead when they're cold and dead. *JAMA* 264:1856–1857, 1990.

Bangs CC. Hypothermia and frostbite. *Emerg Med Clin North Am* 2:475–487, 1984.

Brunette DD, Biros M, Mlinek EJ, et al. Internal cardiac massage and mediastinal irrigation in hypothermic cardiac arrest. *Am J Emerg Med* 10:32–34, 1992.

Danzl DF. Accidental hypothermia. In: Rosen P (ed), St Louis, CV Mosby Co, ed 3. 1992, pp 913–943.

Danzl DF, Pozos RS, Auerbach PS, et al. Multicenter hypothermia survey. *Ann Emerg Med* 16:1042–1055, 1987.

Danzl DF, Pozos RS, Hamlet MP. Accidental hypothermia. In: Auerbach PS (ed), St Louis, CV Mosby Co, 1989, pp 35–76.

Gregory J, Bergstein J, Aprahamian C, et al. Comparison of three methods of rewarming from hypothermia: Advantages of extracorporeal blood warming. *J Trauma* 31:1247–1252, 1991.

Miller JW, Danzl DF, Thomas DM. Urban accidental hypothermia: 135 cases. *Ann Emerg Med* 9:456–461, 1980.

Orts A, Alcuraz C, Delaney KA, et al. Bretylium tosylate and electrically induced cardiac arrhythmias during hypothermia in dogs. *Am J Emerg Med* 10:311–316, 1992.

Reuler JB. Hypothermia: Pathophysiology, clinical settings, and management. *Ann Intern Med* 89:519–527, 1978.

Schaller MD, Fischer AP, Perret CH. Hyperkalemia: A prognostic factor during acute severe hypothermia. *JAMA* 264:1842–1847, 1990.

Shields CP, Sirsmith DM. Treatment of moderate to severe hypothermia in an urban setting. *Ann Emerg Med* 19:1093–1097, 1990.

Sterba JA. Efficacy and safety of prehospital rewarming techniques to treat accidental hypothermia. *Ann Emerg Med* 20:896–901, 1991.

Swain JA. Hypothermia and blood pH. *Arch Intern Med* 146:1643–1646, 1988.

Chapter 44-B

Hyperthermia

Jerrold B. Leikin, M.D.
Paul K. Hanashiro, M.D.

I. **Definition**
Hyperthermia is a core temperature above 40.5°C (105°F).
II. **Etiology**
Essentially due to heat accumulation through heat production and/or an inability to dissipate heat through cooling mechanisms.
  A. Heat production
    1. Environment
    2. Metabolic factors
    3. Shivering
    4. Drugs associated with increased heat production
      a. Amphetamines
      b. Monoamine oxidase (MAO) inhibitors
      c. Phencyclidine
      d. Cocaine
      e. Antipsychotic (neuroleptic malignant syndrome)
      f. Salicylates
      g. Dinitrophenol
      h. Halothane (malignant hyperthermia)
      i. Lysergic acid diethylamide (LSD)
      j. Ethanol withdrawal (delirium tremens)
    5. Conditions associated with increased heat production
      a. Seizures
      b. Exertion
      c. Labor
      d. Thyrotoxicosis
  B. Cooling mechanisms
    1. Radiation (65% of normal heat loss)
    2. Convection (12% of normal heat loss)
    3. Insensible water loss through lungs
    4. Sweating
      a. Accounts for almost all heat loss at ambient temperatures greater than 35°C (95°F)
      b. Dependent on humidity of air
    5. Cutaneous vasodilation
    6. Drugs associated with impairment of cooling compensation mechanisms.
      a. β-blockers
      b. Anticholinergics
      c. Antihistamines
      d. Ethanol
      e. Tricyclic antidepressants
      f. Phenothiazine
      g. Glutethimide

h. Phenols
i. MAO inhibitors
7. Conditions associated with impairment of thermoregulation
  a. Cardiovascular diseases
  b. Extremes of age
  c. Obesity
  d. Burns
  e. Cystic fibrosis
  f. Systemic infections
  g. Dehydration (at least 3%)
  h. Previous history of heat stroke
  i. Scleroderma

III. Pathophysiology—Response to Heat Exposure

A. First response to elevated core temperature is peripheral vasodilatation, which necessitates an increase in cardiac output (up to 20%).
B. Vaporization (heat loss through evaporation) accounts for 30% of heat dissipation.
  1. Insensible water loss
  2. Sweating
    a. Fluid losses depend upon acclimatization (from 1.5 liters/hr in unacclimatized persons to 3 liters/hr in acclimatized persons).
    b. Dependent on humidity for effectiveness of heat loss. At humidity levels greater than 75%, evaporation decreases; heat loss does not occur at humidity levels greater than 90%.
    c. Shunting of circulation to skin and muscle.
      (1) Renal blood flow decreases 50%.
      (2) Liver function decreases 30%.
      (3) Lactic acidosis occurs.
      (4) Splanchnic vasoconstriction occurs.
      (5) Clotting abnormalities—thrombocytopenia, as well as with disseminated intravascular coagulation.
C. Acclimatization—may take up to 2 weeks to adapt to hot climates. With repeated heat exposure, four processes take place.
  1. More efficient sweating, with more fluid loss but less sodium or chloride loss.
  2. Myocardial changes—less tachycardia, along with decreased cardiac output to heat exposure.
  3. Increased muscle glycogen storage in mitochondria, resulting in decreased heat production.
  4. Activation of aldosterone secretion, which results in retention of sodium and loss of potassium. This results in increased plasma volume.

IV. Heat Illness Spectrum

Unlike hypothermia, the degree of temperature rise does not correlate with the nature of clinical signs seen.
A. Heat cramps—muscle cramps due to sodium loss. Occur in muscles used for heavy exertion (legs and abdomen). Onset is often delayed while patient is resting; muscles usually not damaged.
B. Heat edema—usually occurs only in dependent limbs of elderly persons. Pitting edema may occur.
C. Heat tetany—usually limited to carpopedal spasm but can be associated with other forms of heat illness. Serum calcium is normal but respiratory alkalosis usually occurs.
D. Heat syncope—occurs following exertion in unacclimatized individuals early in the course of heat exposure. May be caused by peripheral venous pooling due to a decrease in vasomotor tone. These patients are usually not dehydrated; in fact, their plasma volume may be increased.
E. Heat exhaustion—due to inadequate fluid intake following fluid loss from sweating. Dehydration may take the form of hypernatremia (water depletion seen with massive sweat loss) or hyponatremia (sodium depletion seen with compensation for fluid losses with hypotonic solutions). Patient may complain of fatigue, weakness, orthostasis, nausea, headache, or weakness, but cerebral function is essentially intact. Thirst is a hallmark of hypernatremic heat exhaustion, as is profuse sweating. Core temperature may be only mildly elevated. Only mild elevations of liver enzymes may occur.
F. Heat stroke—loss of thermoregulatory mechanism resulting in immediate, life-threatening emergency, with core temperatures usually greater than 41°F. Manifestations associated with heat stroke are central nervous system dysfunction (coma, seizures) due to heat exposure (either external or internal). Myocardial infarction, acute tubular necrosis, rhabdomyolysis, extremely elevated liver function tests, petechiae, cerebral edema, and disseminated intravascular coagulation (DIC) are common. These patients may not be sweating. Heat stroke may take two forms:
  1. Exertional—usually occurring in young individuals during exercise in a hot environment. Onset is rapid, so dehydration

may not occur. These patients may sweat profusely, but they cannot dissipate heat well due to the high humidity. Hypoglycemia and DIC may be pronounced, along with hypocalcemia.

2. Classic heat stroke—occurs most commonly during heat waves, affecting the elderly and infants. Most of these patients have chronic underlying disease processes (i.e., cardiovascular abnormalities, cystic fibrosis) which result in impaired thermoregulation. Significant dehydration may occur over a period of many days, and sweating may cease.

G. Neuroleptic malignant syndrome—idiosyncratic reaction in about 1% of patients taking neuroleptics (regardless of the duration of use). It is characterized by high fever (temperature over 106°F), muscle rigidity (unlike heat stroke), labile hypertension leukocytosis, profuse sweating, and marked elevation of creatine phosphokinase (CPK).

V. Differential Diagnosis

A. Heat cramps
   1. Hypocalcemic tetany
   2. Neuroleptic malignant syndrome
B. Heat edema
   1. Cardiogenic
   2. Thyroid insufficiency
C. Heat tetany
   1. Hypocalcemic tetany
   2. Hyperventilation
D. Heat syncope
   1. Cardiovascular-related syncope
   2. Hypovolemia
E. Heat exhaustion
   1. Heat stroke
   2. Hepatitis
F. Heat stroke
   1. Seizures
   2. Trauma
   3. Cerebrovascular accident
   4. Thyroid storm
   5. Other forms of heat illness
   6. Malaria
   7. Delirium tremens
   8. Systemic infections (especially meningitis)
G. Neuroleptic malignant syndrome
   1. Oculogyric crisis
   2. Rapid withdrawal of levodopa in patients with Parkinson's disease
   3. Polymyositis
   4. Anticholinergic toxicity
   5. Lethal catatonia

VI. Treatment and Monitoring

Always remove patient from hot environment.

A. Heat cramps—provide rest and salt replacement, either by oral ingestion of balanced salt solutions (1/4 teaspoon of salt per quart of water) or IV 0.9 normal saline solution. Do not massage the extremities.
B. Heat edema—self-limited; no specific treatment needed.
C. Heat tetany—resolves when hyperventilation resolves.
D. Heat syncope—usually resolves when patient is placed in a supine position in a cool environment.
E. Heat exhaustion—primary treatment is replacement of fluids with normal saline. Volume replacement should be guided by monitoring blood urea nitrogen (BUN) creatinine, serum electrolytes, and orthostatic vital signs. The serum glucose level should also be assessed.
F. Heat stroke
   1. Assessment of airway, breathing and circulation. Endotracheal intubation should be provided in comatose patients with administration of 100% oxygen. Fluids should be administered intravenously. Urinary catheters should be placed to monitor urine output.
   2. Insertion of high rectal thermometer probe to monitor temperature. Glass thermometers may be dangerous if seizures develop.
   3. Initiate cooling therapy; if temperature is above 41°C (106°F), cool patient rapidly (to below 39.8°C [102°F] within 1 hr of presentation). Methods of cooling include:
      a. Ice water soaks to areas of maximal heat transfer (axilla and groin). All restrictive clothing must be removed prior to institution of cooling techniques.
      b. Evaporative cooling by means of wetted sheets placed over patient near an air current (large fan) (0.32°C/min). Goal of cooling is to achieve core temperature of 38.5°C (101°F) may be as effective as iced peritoneal lavage. Do not administer aspirin or alcohol baths.
      c. Central cooling techniques such as cold peritoneal lavage (0.56°C/min) iced gastric lavage (0.15°C/min) is effective for rapid cooling.

4. Monitor patient for seizure activity and control shivering. Shivering can occur if skin temperature decreases below 28°C and may lead to seizure activity. Shivering may be suppressed by administering chlorpromazine, 25–50 mg IV.

5. Monitor EKG, CBC, platelet counts, prothrombin time/partial thromboplastin time, electrolytes, calcium, CPK, BUN, creatinine; arterial blood gases, phosphate, amylase, liver function tests, and glucose.

6. Urine output should be monitored, as well as urine orthotolidine test for myoglobin. Mannitol (25 mg IV) may be given if oliguria occurs. Sodium bicarbonate should also be administered if urine is acidic. Dialysis may be necessary if renal failure occurs (which may be seen in 10% of patients, especially those with exertional heat stroke).

7. For hypotension, avoid norepinephrine, since it can cause cutaneous vasoconstriction. Dopamine or dobutamine may be given, but the hypotension usually responds to cooling and fluid administration. Central venous pressure monitoring to a level of 12 cm of water is the goal.

G. Neuroleptic malignant syndrome—rapid cooling and supportive therapy, as described for heat stroke. Severe muscle rigidity may be treated with dantrolene (0.8 to 3 mg/kg IV every 6 hr up to 10 mg/kg/day). Thermoregulatory abnormalities along with extrapyramidal reactions may be responsive to bromocriptine mesylate (2.5 to 7.5 mg orally every 8 hr). Diphenhydramine (50 mg IV) and/or amantadine HCl (100 mg p.o. twice a day) can also be utilized.

VII. **Prognosis**

Heat cramps, heat edema, heat tetany, heat syncope, and heat exhaustion generally respond to symptomatic measures. Factors correlating with a poor prognosis in heat stroke include:

A. Advanced age.

B. Presence of debilitating diseases.

C. Prolonged duration of hyperthermia prior to initiation of treatment.

D. Coagulopathies (prolonged prothrombin time).

E. Patients who are comatose for longer than 10 hr.

F. Serum glutamic oxaloacetic transaminase level greater than 1000 IU/liter within 24 hr.

G. Rectal temperature greater than 42.2°C (108°F) indicates a poor prognosis, although survival has been documented at a temperature of 46.5°C (115.7°F).

Bibliography

Cantor RM. Heat illness from mild to malignant. *Emerg Med* 23:93–100, 1991.

Hubbard RW, Matthew CB, Durkot MJ. Novel approaches to the pathophysiology of heatstroke: The energy depletion model. *Ann Emerg Med* 16:1066–1075, 1987.

Leikin JB, Barron S, Engle J, et al. Treatment of neuroleptic malignant syndrome with diphenhydramine. *Vet Hum Toxicol* 30:58–59, 1988.

Olson KR, Benowitz NL. Environmental and drug-induced hyperthermia: Pathophysiology, recognition, and management. *Emerg Clin North Am* 2:459–474, 1984.

Parsons KT, Anderson RJ. Pathogenesis and management of renal failure due to physical exertion and exertional heatstroke. *IM: Internal Medicine for the Specialist* 5:55–60, 1984.

Syverud SA, Barker WJ, Amsterdam JT, et al. Iced gastric lavage for treatment of heatstroke: Efficacy in a canine model. *Ann Emerg Med* 14:424–432, 1985.

Vicario SJ, Okabajue R, Haltom T. Rapid cooling in classic heatstroke: Effect on mortality rates. *Am J Emerg Med* 4:394–398, 1986.

White JD, Kamath R, Nucci R, et al. Evaporation versus Iced Peritoneal Lavage Treatment of Heatstroke: Comparative Efficacy in a Canine Model. *Am J Emerg Med* 11:1–3, 1993.

Yarbrough B. Heat illness. In Emergency Medicine: *Concepts and Clinical Practice* ed 3. Rosen P (ed), St Louis, CV Mosby Co, 1992, pp 944–964.

CHAPTER 45

Drugs Used in Critical Care Medicine

Catherine M. MacLeod, M.D., F.R.C.P.(C), F.A.C.P., F.C.P.

I. **Drugs Used to Manage Cardiovascular Function**
   A. Drugs used in shock
      1. Sympathomimetic drugs
         a. Predominant myocardial effects
         b. Predominant vascular effects
         c. Effects on myocardium and vasculature
   B. Drugs used in hypertensive emergencies and urgencies
      1. Parenteral direct vasodilators
      2. Parenteral calcium channel blockers
      3. Parenteral drugs affecting sympathetic tone
         a. Adrenergic receptor blockers
         b. Ganglion blockers
         c. Central-acting sympatholytics
   C. Drugs used in severe congestive heart failure (See Drugs Used in Cardiac Disease)
   D. Drugs used to treat arrhythmias (See Drugs Used in Cardiac Disease)
   E. Drugs used in acute myocardial infarction (See Drugs Used in Cardiac Disease)
II. **Drugs Used to Manage Respiratory Function**
   A. Drugs used in bronchoconstrictive disorders
      1. Sympathomimetics
      2. Anticholinergic agents
      3. Methylxanthines
      4. Glucocorticoids
   B. Drugs used in ventilator support
      1. Neuromuscular blocking agents
      2. Benzodiazepines
      3. Phenothiazines and related neuroleptic agents
   C. Drugs used in pulmonary embolic disease
      1. Parenteral anticoagulants
      2. Thrombolytic agents
III. **Parenteral Drugs Used to Manage Neuropsychiatric Dysfunction**
   A. Drugs used in seizure disorders
      1. Hydantoins
      2. Benzodiazepines
      3. Barbiturates
      4. Other anticonvulsant agents
   B. Drugs used to treat increased intracranial pressure
      1. Osmotic diuretics
      2. Glucocorticoids
   C. Drugs used to treat mental status changes
      1. Benzodiazepines
      2. Phenothiazines and related neuroleptic agents
IV. **Parenteral Drugs Used to Treat Common Nosocomial Infections**

411

V. **Parenteral Drugs Used for Supportive Care**
   A. Drugs used for sedation and sleep
      1. Benzodiazepines
      2. Phenothiazines and related neuroleptic agents
   B. Anesthetic drugs for special procedures
      1. Barbiturates
      2. Opioids
      3. Parenteral anesthetic agents
   C. Analgesics
      1. Opioids
      2. Nonsteroidal anti-inflammatory drugs
   D. Drugs used to control gastrointestinal function
      1. Parenteral antiemetic and prokinetic agents
      2. Parenteral antihistamines—H_2 blockers
   E. Drugs used to treat acute hypersensitivity reactions
      1. Parenteral antihistamines—H_1 blockers
      2. Glucocorticoids
   F. Drugs used to treat malignant hyperthermia
      1. Direct skeletal muscle relaxant

VI. **Issues in Drug Therapy**
   A. Common drug adverse events in critical care units
      1. Thrombocytopenia
      2. Fever
      3. Confusion
   B. Monitoring drug therapy

Sympathomimetic Drugs
   I. **Classification**
      A. Prominent myocardial effects (β_1 stimulation)
         1. Dobutamine ($\beta_1 \gg \beta_2 > \alpha_1$ stimulation) (Dobutrex)
         2. Isoproterenol ($\beta_1 = \beta_2$ stimulation) (Isuprel)
      B. Prominent vascular effects (α_1 stimulation)
         1. Norepinephrine ($\alpha_1 > \beta_2 > \alpha_2$ stimulation) (Levophed)
         2. Mephentermine ($\alpha_1 = \beta_1 = \beta_2$ stimulation) (Wyamine)
         3. Metaraminol ($\alpha_1 > \beta_1$ stimulation) (Aramine)
         4. Phenylephrine (α_1 stimulation) (Neosynephrine)
         5. Methoxamine (α_1 stimulation) (Vasoxyl)
      C. Effects on myocardium and vasculature (α and β stimulation)
         1. Epinephrine
            a. Low dose ($\beta_1 = \beta_2$ stimulation)
            b. Intermediate dose ($\beta_1 = \beta_2 > \alpha_1$ stimulation)
            c. High dose ($\alpha_1 > \beta_1 > \beta_2$ stimulation)
         2. Dopamine (Intropin)
            a. Low dose (D_1 stimulation)
            b. Intermediate dose ($D_1 = \beta_1 > \beta_2$ stimulation)
            c. High dose ($\alpha_1 > \beta_1 > \beta_2 = D_1$ stimulation)

II. **Mechanism of Action**
   A. Drugs of this class stimulate one or more adrenergic receptors, which are glycoproteins located in cell membranes. The receptors are subdivided by tissue location, cellular effect, and ability to be blocked by specific agents. The subdivisions include alpha-(α-), beta-(β-), and dopaminergic (D) receptors.
   B. Stimulation of α_1-receptors in vascular smooth muscle causes release of free calcium ions from intracellular stores and activation of calcium channels, increasing the number of calcium ions available for myosin–actin interaction and, therefore, contraction of the peripheral vascular smooth muscle. Stimulation of β_1-receptors in myocardial cell membranes causes activation of adenylyl cyclase to increase cyclic adenosine monophosphate (cAMP), which increases myocardial contraction and conduction. β_2-receptors on smooth muscle cells of the bronchi, and of arterioles supplying skeletal muscle and parts of the mesentery, mediate relaxation when stimulated via cAMP-mediated inactivation of protein kinases required for contraction. D_1-receptors are found in the vascular smooth muscle of the renal, mesenteric, and coronary circulations; stimulation of these D_1-receptors causes active vasodilation. This effect causes increased renal, mesenteric, and coronary blood flow, an increased glomerular filtration rate, and increased sodium excretion.
   C. Drugs with prominent α_1-stimulating ability cause increased peripheral vascular resistance and reflex slowing of the heart rate via increased parasympathetic tone. Agents stimulating β_1-receptors increase myocardial contractility and heart rate. Drugs with prominent β_2-stimulating properties cause bronchial and skeletal arteriolar smooth muscle relaxation. Drugs with combined action have dose-related responses, depending on the affinity for receptors. The pattern of re-

ceptor activation for each agent is outlined in the classification above.

III. Indications

A. Alpha$_1$ stimulation (phenylephrine, metaraminol, methoxamine, mephentermine)
   1. Treatment of shock states with peripheral vasodilation.
   2. Treatment of acute supraventricular tachyarrhythmias by enhanced reflex vagal tone.

B. Beta$_1$ stimulation (dobutamine, intermediate-dose dopamine, isoproterenol)
   1. Treatment of hypotension or shock associated with failure of the myocardium, except for isoproterenol.
   2. Emergency treatment of idioventricular bradyarrhythmias with hypotension.

C. Combined α_1 and β_1 stimulation (norepinephrine, high-dose dopamine)
   1. Treatment of severe hypotension with significantly impaired myocardial function to maintain coronary and cerebral circulation.

D. Combined β_2, β_1, and α_1 stimulation (epinephrine)
   1. Treatment of anaphylaxis, cardiopulmonary arrest

E. Dopamine stimulation (dopamine)
   1. Treatment of congestive heart failure with impaired renal function secondary to decreased renal blood flow.

IV. Complications

A. Alpha$_1$ stimulation (phenylephrine, metaraminol, methoxamine, mephentermine)
   1. Central nervous system (CNS)—stimulation with mephentermine
   2. Cardiovascular (CV)—myocardial ischemia
   3. Other—tissue necrosis with extravasation

B. Beta$_1$ stimulation (dobutamine, dopamine, isoproterenol)
   1. CNS—excitation
   2. CV
      a. Tachycardia/arrhythmias (isoproterenol > dopamine > dobutamine)
      b. Myocardial ischemia mainly with isoproterenol
   3. Gastrointestinal (GI)—nausea and vomiting with dopamine
   4. Hematology—platelet function inhibition with dopamine and dobutamine

C. Combined α_1 and β_1 stimulation (norepinephrine, high-dose dopamine)
   1. CNS—stimulation
   2. CV—myocardial ischemia and arrhythmias
   3. Hematology—platelet aggregation with norepinephrine
   4. Other—tissue necrosis with extravasation

D. Combined α_1, β_1, and β_2 stimulation (epinephrine)
   1. CNS—anxiety, excitation
   2. CV—tachycardia, arrhythmias, myocardial ischemia
   3. GI—nausea and vomiting
   4. Metabolic—hypokalemia, hyperglycemia, lactic acidosis

V. Significant Drug Interactions

Drug	Interacting Drug	Effect	Mechanism
All	β-blockers	Severe ↑ BP	Unopposed α action
	General anesthetics	Arrhythmias	↑ sensitivity
	Insulin	↓ insulin effect	Antagonism
	MAO inhibitors	Severe ↑ BP	↑ norepinephrine release
	Theophylline	Arrhythmias	Additive
	Tricyclic antidepressants	Severe ↑ BP	↓ reuptake of norepinephrine

VI. Contraindications

A. Dobutamine: hypertrophic cardiomyopathy, hypovolemia (prior to correction).

B. Isoproterenol: septic shock, hypovolemia (prior to correction), ventricular ectopic activity, myocardial ischemia.

C. Dopamine: pheochromocytoma, tachyarrhythmias, ventricular ectopy.

D. Epinephrine: myocardial ischemia and cardiac arrhythmias (except in cardiac arrest).

E. Norepinephrine: peripheral vascular disease, acidosis, significant hypoxia.

F. All α_1 stimulants: peripheral vascular disease, acidosis, significant hypoxia.

Drugs Used to Treat Hypertensive Emergencies or Urgencies

I. **Classification**
   A. Parenteral direct-acting vasodilators
      1. Nitroprusside (Nipride)
      2. Nitroglycerin (high-dose) (Nitrostat)
      3. Diazoxide (Hyperstat)
      4. Hydralazine (Apresoline)
   B. Parenteral calcium channel blockers
      1. Nicardepine (Cardene)
   C. Parenteral adrenergic blocking agents
      1. Labetalol—α_1- and β blockers (Normodyne, Trandate)
      2. Phentolamine—α-blocker (Regitine)
   D. Parenteral sympatholytic agents
      1. Methyldopa (Aldomet)
   E. Parenteral ganglion blocker
      1. Trimethaphan (Arfonad)
   F. Parenteral angiotensin-converting enzyme inhibitors
      1. Enalaprilat

II. **Mechanism of Action**
   A. As noted above in the classification, these drugs have different mechanisms to decrease blood pressure, as well as different time courses of action.
   B. Nitroprusside and high-dose nitroglycerin relax the smooth muscle of arterioles and veins by releasing nitric oxide to activate guanylate cyclase and initiate a cascade of enzyme changes that results in decreased actin–myosin interaction. Their onset of action is within 1 min.
   C. Diazoxide and hydralazine cause hyperpolarization of arteriolar smooth muscle cells to decrease tone; diazoxide acts within 1–5 min and hydralazine within 10 min.
   D. Nicardepine blocks "L" calcium channels of arteriolar smooth muscle to decrease availabe intracellular free calcium and so diminish actin–myosin interaction. It acts within 2–3 min.
   E. Labetalol is a nonspecific β-blocker and a specific α_1-blocker, with the α_1-blocking action being more important for rapid control of hypertension; the onset of action is within 5–10 min.
   F. Phentolamine is a nonspecific, competitive antagonist of norepinephrine (NE) at α-receptors and so prevents the vasoconstricting action of NE; it acts within 15 sec.

G. Methyldopa is metabolized to its active derivative in the CNS and stimulates α_2-receptors to decrease sympathetic outflow; its effect is seen in 30 min to 2 hr after parenteral administration.
H. Trimethaphan blocks both sympathetic and parasympathetic systems by competitively inhibiting acetylcholine binding in the ganglia; its activity is seen within 1 min.
I. Enalaprilat is an angiotensin-converting enzyme (ACE) inhibitor which prevents the formation of the vasoconstricting angiotensin II and allows accumulation of the vasodilating bradykinin; it acts within 15 min.

III. **Indications**
For hypertensive emergencies, blood pressure (BP) must be reduced within minutes with parenteral antihypertensive agents.
   A. Hypertensive encephalopathy—nitroprusside, labetalol, diazoxide.
   B. Hypertension with dissecting aneurysm—nitroprusside, labetalol, trimethophan.
   C. Pheochromocytoma crisis—phentolamine, labetalol.
   D. Hypertensive emergency with angina—nicardepine, nitroglycerin.
   E. Hypertensive emergency with congestive heart failure (CHF)—nitroglycerin, nitroprusside, enalaprilat.
   F. Severe hypertension or hypertensive urgency requires more gradual reduction of BP, such as parenteral hydralazine, methyldopa, lower-dose labetalol, or the use of oral agents.

IV. **Complications**
   A. Nitroprusside
      1. CV—rebound hypertension on discontinuing therapy.
      2. Metabolism—thiocyanate or cyanide toxicity with prolonged use.
   B. Nitroglycerin
      1. CNS—headache
      2. CV—palpitations, tolerance, withdrawal syndrome
      3. GI—nausea, vomiting
      4. Hematology—methemoglobinemia
   C. Diazoxide
      1. CV—excessive hypotension
      2. Metabolism—hyperglycemia
   D. Hydralazine
      1. CNS—peripheral neuritis
      2. CV—angina, tachycardia, edema
      3. Immune—systemic lupus erythematosus (SLE) with high-dose, prolonged therapy
   E. Labetalol

1. CNS—confusion, altered sleep
2. CV—CHF, bradyarrhythmias
3. Pulmonary—bronchoconstriction in predisposed patients
F. Phentolamine
  1. CV—tachycardia, angina, severe hypotension
  2. Other—flushing
G. Methyldopa
  1. CNS—sedation, depression, altered sleep
  2. CV—edema, bradycardia, rebound hypertension

3. GI—liver function abnormalities
4. Immune—drug fever, SLE
H. Trimethaphan
I. Autonomic nervous system (ANS)—major effects of parasympathetic block
J. Enalaprilat
  1. CV—angina with excessive hypotension
  2. Genitourinary (GU)—proteinuria, renal failure (with renal artery stenosis)
  3. Hematology—agranulocytosis
  4. Immune—angioedema, fever
  5. Other—hyperkalemia, dry cough

V. Significant Drug Interactions

Drug	Interacting Drug	Effect	Mechanism
Nitroglycerin	Heparin	↓ anticoagulation	Unknown
	NE	↓ effect of each drug	Antagonism
Hydralazine	β-blockers	↑ β-blockade	Unknown
Labetalol	Cimetidine	↑ β-blockade	↓ metabolism
	Hypoglycemics	Severe hypoglycemia	↓ symptoms and ↓ metabolic response
Phentolamine	Sympathomimetics	↓ vasoconstriction	Antagonism
Methyldopa	CNS depressants	↑ CNS depression	Additive
	Haloperidol	Disorientation	Additive
	Levodopa	Psychosis	Additive
	Sympathomimetics	↑ pressor effect	Additive peripheral effects
Enalaprilat	K$^+$-sparing diuretic	Hyperkalemia	Additive
	Lithium	↑ lithium toxicity	↓ excretion

VI. Contraindications

A. Nitroprusside should be avoided in patients with atrioventricular (AV) shunts, coarctation of the aorta, hypothyroidism, or encephalopathy unrelated to hypertension.

B. Nitroglycerin should not be used in patients with cerebral hemorrhage or trauma, hypertrophic cardiomyopathy, hyperthyroidism, or severe anemia.

C. Hydralazine is contraindicated in patients with cerebrovascular accidents, coronary insufficiency, or aortic aneurysm.

D. Nicardepine should not be used in patients with hypersensitivity to the drug or its congeners, i.e., nifedipine and nimodepine.

E. Labetalol is precluded in patients with bronchospasm, CHF, or brittle diabetes mellitus.

F. Phentolamine is used with caution in patients with depleted intravascular volumes.

G. Methyldopa should be avoided in patients with CNS depression, altered mental state, or AV node dysfunction.

H. Enalaprilat must not be used in patients with bilateral renal artery stenosis or significant hyperkalemia.

Bronchodilating Agents
I. Classification
A. Sympathomimetics
  1. Inhalational agents
    a. Albuterol (salbutamol) (Proventil, Ventolin)
    b. Epinephrine (Adrenalin and others)
    c. Metaproterenol (Alupent)
    d. Terbutaline (Brethine)
  2. Parenteral agents
    a. Anhydrous theophylline
    b. Aminophylline (theophylline ethylenediamine)
B. Inhalational anticholinergics
  1. Ipratropium (Atrovent)

II. Mechanism of Action
A. The above agents all cause bronchial smooth muscle dilation by different mechanisms. The sympathomimetics stimulate β$_2$-receptors of

Table 45-1. Dose and Handling of Drugs Used to Manage Cardiovascular Function

Class Drug/Dose	Onset of Action	Elimination	Elimination t½	Duration of Action
Parenteral Sympathomimetics				
Dobutamine < 5 min IV: 2.5–15 µg/kg/min	1–2 min	Hepatic metabolism	2 min	

Isoproterenol
IV: 0.01–0.1 µg/kg/min
Inhaled: 1 inhalation,
  repeated in 2–5 min
  q4–6h
	< 5 min
	
	< 5 min
		Metabolism in liver,
		lungs, other tissue
			< 5 min	10 min IV up to 3 hr via
				inhalation

Dopamine
IV: 0.5–2 µg/kg/min
  (low dose)
2–19 µg/kg/min
  (intermediate dose)
20–50 µg/kg/min (high dose)
	< 5 min	Metabolism via MAO and
		catechol-*O*-methyl
		transferase in liver,
		kidneys, plasma
			2 min	< 10 min

Epinephrine
IV: 1–5mcg/kg rapid
  infusion (low dose)
5–10 µg/kg rapid
  infusion (intermediate
  dose)
> 10 µg/kg rapid
  infusion (high dose)
	Rapid	As for dopamine	1 min	1–2 min

Norepinephrine IV: 2–12 µg/min	Rapid	As for dopamine	1 min	1–2 min

Mephentermine
IV: 30–45 mg single
  dose, with 30 mg,
  repeat dose PRN
Infusion of 1 mg/ml
  solution at variable rate
	Very rapid	Hepatic metabolism	NA	15–30 min

Metaraminol
IV: 0.5–5 mg injection
  followed by infusion of
  0.2 mg/ml at variable rate
	1–2 min	Hepatic metabolism	NA	20 min

Phenylephrine IV: 0.2 mg q10–15 min Infusion of 0.05 mg/ml at 0.1–0.18 mg/min	Very rapid	Hepatic and GI metabolism	NA	15–20 min

Drug / Dosage	Onset	Metabolism / Excretion	Half-life	Duration
Methoxamine IV: 3–5 mg by slow injection for ↓ BP; 10 mg by slow injection for arrhythmias	Very rapid	Hepatic metabolism and renal excretion	NA	5–15 min

Parenteral Drugs for Hypertensive Emergencies and Urgencies

Drug / Dosage	Onset	Metabolism / Excretion	Half-life	Duration
Nitroprusside IV: initial 0.5 µg/kg/min titrate up to 10 µg/kg/min	5 sec	Red blood cell conversion to nitric oxide and cyanide, then metabolized to thiocyanate	< 3 min	5 min
Nitroglycerin IV: initial 10–20 µg/min titrate up to 200 µg/min	< 1 min	Metabolism	1–4 min	5–20 min
Diazoxide IV: 1–3 mg/kg, repeated q1–15 min up to 1.2 g/day	1 min	50% renal excretion	21–36 hr (↑ with ↓ renal function)	2–12 hrs
Hydralazine IV: 10–40 mg, repeated prn to effect	10–20 min	11–14% renal excretion Metabolism in liver and blood	2–4 hr	3–4 hr
Nicardipine IV: initial 5 mg/hr, titrate to effect	2–3 hr	Metabolism	0.75 hr	No data
Labetalol IV: 20 mg/2 min, then 40–80 mg q10 min to 300 mg	5–10 min	Metabolism	4–8 hr	4–6 hr
Phentolamine IV: initial 1–5 mg, then 0.5 mg/kg/min infusion	< 15 sec	13% renal excretion	19 min	20 min
Methyldopate IV: 0.25–1 g over 30–60 min, then q6h	0.5–2 hr	30% CNS metabolism 40% liver metabolism 30% renal excretion	2 hr (↑ with ↓ renal function)	10–16 hr
Trimethaphan IV: 1–4 mg/min with titration to effect	< 1 min	Renal excretion	No data	10–15 min
Enalaprilat IV: 1.25 mg over 5 min q6h	15 min	Renal excretion	11 hr (↑ in ↓ renal function)	6 hr

bronchial smooth muscle cells to increase intracellular adenylyl cyclase activity and inactivate protein kinases required for actin–myosin interaction. Increased cAMP inhibits the release of mediators of immediate hypersensitivity from mast cells, as well as histamine, leukotrienes, and slow-reacting substance of anaphylaxis from inflammatory cells. These agents may inhibit phospholipase A_2 in pulmonary tissue.

B. The cardiac effects of these agents are dependent on the agent selected and on the dose given. Epinephrine is a nonspecific stimulant of adrenergic receptors. Metaproterenol is more specific for β_2-receptors than for β_1-receptors. Albuterol and terbutaline are specific for stimulation of β_2-receptors at therapeutic doses, but at high doses, both β_1- and β_2-receptors are stimulated.

C. Theophylline relaxes smooth muscle of the bronchi, blood vessels, biliary ducts, GI tract, and uterus. It enhances myocardial contractility and conduction rate, improves skeletal muscle function, and decreases inflammatory responses related to mast cell and neutrophil functions. These effects are the result of competitive inhibition of adenosine receptors on cell membranes and within cells, inhibition of intracellular phosphodiesterase to increase cAMP, and possibly inhibition of prostaglandin and/or leukotriene release and effect.

D. Ipratropium is effective only when parasympathetic activity is a major factor causing or maintaining bronchoconstriction. This drug competitively inhibits the stimulatory action of acetyl choline on bronchial smooth muscle and mast cells.

III. **Indications**

A. These drugs are indicated for the treatment of bronchospasm from asthmatic attacks or reversible bronchoconstriction associated with chronic obstructive pulmonary disease.

B. Sympathomimetics may be used for short-term prophylaxis of acute episodes of bronchoconstriction. Epinephrine may be used parenterally to treat anaphylaxis with bronchospasm because of its ability to stimulate α_1- and β_1- as well as β_2-receptors.

C. Theophylline preparations are used to reverse acute bronchospasm and to maintain bronchial relaxation over time. They may prevent secondary inflammatory responses and improve diaphragmatic function.

D. Iprotropium is used in patients with elevated parasympathetic tone, primarily in chronic lung disease.

IV. **Complications**

A. Sympathomimetics
1. CNS—mental status changes, restlessness, tremors, dizziness, headache, paresthesias, insomnia, hallucinations, seizures
2. CV—angina, palpitations, hypertension, arrhythmias
3. GI—dry mouth, heartburn, anorexia, nausea, vomiting
4. GU—difficulty in urination or dysuria
5. Other—severe myalgias, paradoxical bronchospasm, fever, flushing of face or skin

B. Aminophylline: allergic reaction to ethylenediamine component, occurring up to 24 hr after administration

C. All theophylline preparations (related to blood levels)
1. CNS—headache, dizziness, confusion, irritability, seizures
2. CV—tachycardia, palpitations, arrhythmias, angina, hypotension, flushing
3. GI—nausea, vomiting, abdominal cramps

D. Ipratropium: stomatitis and skin rashes

V. **Significant Drug Interactions**

Drug	Interacting Drug	Effect	Mechanism
Sympathomimetics	β-blockers	Severe ↑ BP	Unopposed α action
	General anesthetics	Arrhythmias	↑ sensitivity
	Insulin	↓ insulin effect	Antagonism
	MAO inhibitors	Severe ↑ BP	↑ NE release
	Theophylline	Arrhythmias	Additive
	Tricyclic antidepressants	Severe ↑ BP	↓ reuptake NE
Theophylline	Allopurinol	↑ theophylline	↓ metabolism
	Barbiturates	↓ theophylline	↑ metabolism
	Carbamazepine	↓ effect both drugs	↑ metabolism
	Cimetidine	↑ theophylline	↓ metabolism

Drug	Interacting Drug	Effect	Mechanism
	Ciprofloxacin, enoxacin, ofloxacin	↑ theophylline	↓ metabolism
	Erythromycin	↑ theophylline	↓ metabolism
	Halothane	↑ arrhythmias	Synergism
	Pancuronium	Arrhythmias	Additive
	Phenytoin	↓ effect both drugs	↑ metabolism
	Verapamil	↑ theophylline	↓ metabolism
Ipratropium	Drugs with anticholinergic effects	↑ anticholinergic effect	Additive

VI. Contraindications

A. Sympathomimetic drugs should be avoided or used with caution in patients with cardiac arrhythmias, significant coronary artery disease, hypertension, hyperthyroidism, pheochromocytoma, or sensitivity to sympathomimetics.

B. Theophylline should not be used in patients with cardiac tachyarrhythmias (particularly ventricular arrhythmias), uncontrolled hypertension, severe cardiac disease, sensitivity to xanthines, or, for aminophylline, sensitivity to ethylenediamine.

C. Iprotropium should be used with caution in patients with prostatic hypertrophy (acute urinary retention) or glaucoma of the angle-closure type.

Parenteral Glucocorticosteroids

I. Classification

A. With mineralocorticoid activity
1. Hydrocortisone (Solucortef)

B. With slight mineralocorticoid activity
1. Methylprednisolone (Solumedrol)

C. With no mineralocorticoid activity
1. Dexamethasone (Decadron)

II. Mechanism of Action

A. Glucocorticoids (glucocorticosteroids or corticosteroids) bind with variable affinity to cytoplasmic steroid receptors whose number and responsiveness vary in different cell populations. After binding, the complex moves into the nucleus to alter transcription of certain gene segments.

B. In cells associated with inflammation and the immune response, glucocorticoids cause the synthesis of proteins which inhibit the action of phospholipase A_2, and so decrease the formation of prostaglandins and leukotrienes. The same proteins inhibit release of platelet-activating factor, tumor necrosis factor, and interleukin-1. Glucocorticoids may also be important in the inhibition of humoral factors involved in inflammation, such as macrophage migration-inhibition factor.

C. Catabolic changes in carbohydrate and protein metabolism correlate with anti-inflammatory action. There is catabolism of lymphoid tissue, muscle, bone marrow, and subcutaneous tissue.

D. There is a direct effect of glucocorticoids on receptors in the CNS, usually resulting in stimulation manifested by euphoria, insomnia, and restlessness.

E. Glucocorticoids increase red blood cells and neutrophils by increasing release from the bone marrow and decreasing efflux from the circulation. Lymphocytes, monocytes, eosinophils, and basophils are decreased in peripheral blood by redistribution. The T-lymphocytes decrease is greater than the B-lymphocyte decrease.

F. These effects are delayed in onset after parenteral or oral administration. Usually 4 to 6 hr are required to demonstrate a glucocorticoid effect.

III. Indications

Glucocorticoids are important as replacement therapy in adrenal insufficiency, particularly agents with mineralocorticoid (sodium-retaining) activity. They may be useful anti-inflammatory agents in severe hypersensitivity or inflammatory processes, mainly those agents with little or no mineralocorticoid activity. Immune suppression has been an indication for these drugs. They exert cytolytic action on malignant lymphocytic cells.

IV. Complications

A. CNS

1. Confusion, excitement, delirium, disorientation, euphoria (most common change), hallucinations, manic-depressive episodes, depression, paranoia
2. Seizures with rapid IV administration
B. CV—edema, cardiac arrhythmias with rapid IV administration

C. GI—mucosal irritation with ulceration
D. Metabolic (with long-term administration)—Cushing's syndrome, hypokalemia, osteoporosis, avascular necrosis of bone in predisposed patients, myopathy, tissue atrophy
E. Other—duration-dependent withdrawal

V. Significant Drug Interactions

Drug	Interacting Drug	Effect	Mechanism
All	Drugs ⬆ K$^+$ loss (amphotericin, diuretics)	Hypokalemia	Additive
	Ethacrynic acid	⬆ risk of gastric bleeding	Additive
	Phenytoin	⬇ steroid effect	⬆ metabolism
	Rifampin	⬇⬇ steroid effect	⬆ metabolism
	Theophylline	⬆ theophylline toxicity	Unknown

VI. Contraindications

Glucocorticoids should be avoided in ongoing infections except severe *Pneumocystis carinii* pneumonia in human immunodeficiency virus (HIV)–infected patients, tubercular meningitis, or pediatric meningitis. They should be used with caution in patients with myasthenia gravis. They should not be used in ocular herpes simplex virus.

Neuromuscular Blocking Agents

I. Classification

A. Depolarizing block
1. Succinyl choline (Anectine)
B. Nondepolarizing block
1. Atracurium (Tracrium)—mild histamine release
2. Doxacurium (Nuromax)
3. Pancuronium (Pavulon)—vagolytic, histamine release
4. Tubocurarine—histamine release, mild ganglion block

II. Mechanism of Action

A. Succinyl choline (suxamethonium) competes with acetyl choline for binding at nicotinic receptors on the postjunctional motor end plate. After binding, succinyl choline causes depolarization of the muscle and initial muscle cell contraction. It is not metabolized by acetylcholinesterase in the neuromuscular junction. The greater affinity of succinyl choline for the receptor, and its prolonged time of exposure to the receptor, cause prolonged partial depolarization and subsequent muscle relaxation.
B. The nondepolarizing agents also compete with acetyl choline at the motor end plate, but do not have intrinsic activity and therefore do not cause any depolarization. The block may be overcome by increased concentrations of acetyl choline.

III. Indications

These agents produce skeletal muscle relaxation or paralysis for endotracheal intubation, surgical procedure, or controlled ventilatory support in intubated patients. They are used to paralyze muscles in patients with persistent convulsions or status epilepticus who cannot tolerate other medications and in whom persistent muscle contraction is life-threatening.

Note: These agents have no sedative or analgesic properties.

IV. Complications

A. CV
1. Bradycardia (vagal stimulating activity)
2. Cardiac arrhythmias (with succinyl choline and tubocurarine)
3. Hypotension (ganglion-blocking action or histamine release)
4. Flushing of the skin (rapid administration of agents that release histamine)
5. Hypertension (atracurium and pancuronium)
6. Tachycardia (succinyl choline, atracurium, and pancuronium)
B. Other
1. Anaphylactoid reactions with agents releasing histamine
2. With succinyl choline, laryngospasm, malignant hyperthermia, myoglobinuria and myoglobinemia, and muscle pain

V. Significant Drug Interactions

Drug	Interacting Drug	Effect	Mechanism
All neuromuscular (NM) blockers	Aminoglycosides	↑ NM block	Additive
	Clindamycin	↑ NM block	Additive
	Furosemide	↑ NM block	? ↓ K$^+$
	Local anesthetics (incl. lidocaine, procainamide, quinidine)	↑ NM block	Additive
	Digoxin	↑ arrhythmias	Unknown
Succinyl choline	ACE inhibitors	hyperkalemia	Additive
	K$^+$-sparing diuretics		
	Cyclophosphamide	↑ NM block	Inhibition plasma
	MAO inhibitors		Pseudocholinesterase
Nondepolarizing blockers (e.g., diuretics)	Drugs ↓ K$^+$	↑ NM block	↓ K$^+$

VI. Contraindications

A. None of these agents should be used in patients with a history of myasthenia gravis or previous allergic reaction to the agents.

B. Patients sensitive to histamine release should not receive agents that release histamine.

C. Succinyl choline should be avoided in patients with severe trauma, burns, or digoxin toxicity because of the increased risk of cardiac arrhythmias. It should not be used in patients with a family or personal history of malignant hyperthermia. Patients with fractures or muscle spasm should not receive this drug.

Parenteral Hydantoins

I. Classification

A. Phenytoin (Dilantin)

II. Mechanism of Action

A. The major effect is on the sodium channels of excitable cell membranes, such as neurons and the His-Purkinje system. Sodium fluxes across cell membranes are decreased and sodium channels are maintained longer in an inactivated state after depolarization. This effect is much more pronounced in membranes undergoing repetitive depolarization and is voltage dependent.

B. At higher concentrations, phenytoin delays activation of potassium channels, which slows repolarization and increases the refractory period. Calcium channel responsiveness is also slowed.

C. In the nervous system, there is decreased spread of seizure activity from a focus, and maximal seizure activity is reduced. In ischemic myocardium, ventricular conduction is normalized and abnormal ventricular automaticity is decreased. Another activity is inhibition of collagenase synthesis.

III. Indications

Phenytoin can be used for seizures of any type except absence seizures. It is of value in the treatment of status epilepticus, although its onset of action is somewhat slower than that of the benzodiazepines. Other uses include trigeminal neuralgia, ventricular arrhythmias (particularly those that are digoxin induced), relaxation of skeletal muscle, and epidermolysis bullosa.

IV. Complications

Most toxicity is related to the tissue level, which correlates with the blood concentration. The unpredictable pharmacokinetics seen with increasing dose, at a point which varies among patients, is caused by saturation of metabolism, changing the kinetics from the usual first order to concentration-independent zero order; with the change, small dose increments cause large increases in blood level, increasing the risk of toxicity and prolonged duration of activity.

A. CNS—nystagmus, ataxia, confusion, muscle weakness, increased seizure frequency, slurred speech, tremors, irritability

B. CV—periarteritis nodosa, cardiac arrhythmias and hypotension with rapid IV administration, thrombophlebitis at the site of the IV injection

C. GI—vomiting, cholestatic jaundice, hepatitis

D. Immune—fever, systemic lupus erythematosus, toxic epidermal necrolysis, hypersensitivity syndrome with fever, hepatitis, rashes, lymphadenopathy, nephritis, rhabdomyolysis, pulmonary infiltrates or fibrosis

Table 45-2. Dose and Handling of Drugs Used to Manage Respiratory Function

Class Drug/Dose	Onset of Action	Elimination	Elimination t½	Duration of Action
Sympathomimetic Bronchodilators				
Albuterol	5–15 min	Metabolism	3.8 hr	3–6 hr
Inhalation via nebulizer or intermittent positive-pressure breathing (IPPB): 1.25–5 mg in 2–5 ml normal saline q4–6h				
Epinephrine	3–5 min	Metabolism	Short	1–3 hr
Inhalation via nebulizer: 1% solution q1–2min prn				
Subcut: 0.2–0.5 mg q20min to q4h; titrate up to 1 mg q20min to q4h	6–15 min	Metabolism	Short	< 1–4 hr
IV: 0.1–0.25 mg slowly q5–15 min				
Metaproterenol	5–30 min	Metabolism	NA[3]	2–6 hr
Inhalation via nebulizer or IPPB: 1.3–2.25 mg q3–4h				
Terbutaline	5–30 min	Metabolism	NA[3]	3–6 hr
Inhalation via aerosol: 0.2–0.5 mg q4–6h				
Subcut: 0.25 mg, repeat in 15–30 min if needed	< 15 min	Metabolism	NA[3]	1.4–4 hr
Anticholinergic Agents				
Ipratropium	5–15 min	Metabolism	2 hr	3–6 hr
Oral inhalation: initial 40–80 μg; maintenance 18–40 μg q4–6h				

Drug / Dose	Onset	Metabolism/Elimination	Half-life	Duration
Methylxanthines				
Theophylline IV: load: 5 mg/kg over 15–20 min (no previous theophylline) Maintenance: 0.2–0.7 mg/kg/hr (rate dependent on hepatic metabolic activity)	Rapid	Hepatic microsomal metabolism	9 hr (4–5 hr for smokers; 24 hr in CHF, ↓ hepatic function, COPD)	6–12 hr
Aminophylline IV: load: 7–7.5 mg/kg over 15–20 min (no previous theophylline) Maintenance: 0.25–0.9 mg/kg/hr IV infusion (rate dependent on hepatic metabolic activity)	As above	Hydrolyzed in blood to release active theophylline, which is then metabolized by hepatic microsomal enzymes	As above	As above
Neuromuscular Blocking Agents				
Succinyl choline IV: 0.6–1.5 mg/kg	0.5–1 min	Metabolism by blood pseudocholinesterase—first metabolite succinyl monocholine active	4–10 min (↑ with genetic deficiency psuedocholinesterase, liver disease, starvation, cytotoxic drugs)	4–10 min
Tubocurarine IV: 0.1–0.3 mg/kg; then 0.05–0.1 mg/kg in 5 min if required	< 1 min *(4–10)	Hepatic metabolism (50%) Renal excretion (50%)	1.5–2 hr	1–1.5 hr
Pancuronium IV: 0.04–0.1 mg/kg; then 0.01 mg/kg q20–60 min	< 1 min *(2–7)	Renal excretion (70%) Hepatic metabolism (30%)	2 hr	< 1 hr

(continued)

Table 45-2. Continued

Class Drug/Dose	Onset of Action	Elimination	Elimination t½	Duration of Action
Doxacurium IV: 0.05–0.08 mg/kg; then 0.005–0.025 mg/kg q30–60 min	4–5 min *(3–10)	Renal excretion Biliary excretion	1.5–2 hr	1–2 hr
Atracurium IV: 0.4–0.5 mg/kg (0.3–0.4 mg/kg by slow injection with allergy-prone patients); then 0.08–0.1 mg/kg in 20–45 min *or* 0.004–0.008 mg/kg/min infusion	< 2 min *(2–7)	Metabolized by nonspecific esterases in plasma to laudanosine (CNS stimulant), which is metabolized in the liver and/or excreted via the kidney	20 min	~1 hr
Parenteral Glucocorticosteroids				
Dexamethasone IV: load: 10–20 mg maintenance: 0.5–9 mg q4h to qd		Hepatic microsomal metabolism	3 hr	Up to 3 days
Hydrocortisone IV: 100–500 mg q2–6h until response obtained		Hepatic microsomal metabolism	1.5–2 hr	Up to 1.5 days
Methylprednisolone IV: 10–40 mg; repeat PRN		Hepatic microsomal metabolism	2.5 hr	Up to 1.5 days

*Time to peak effect

E. Hematologic—blood dyscrasias (including agranulocytosis), thrombocytopenia

F. Other—Peyronie's disease, osteomalacia with prolonged use

V. Significant Drug Interactions

Drug	Interacting Drug	Effect	Mechanism
Phenytoin	Aminodarone	↑ phenytoin toxicity	Unknown
	Antidepressants (tricyclic)	↑ phenytoin toxicity	Unknown
	Drugs ↓ cytochrome P_{450} metabolism	↑ phenytoin level	↓ metabolism
	Lithium	↑ lithium toxicity	? synergistic
	Opiates	↓ analgesia	↑ metabolism
	Phenothiazines	↓ phenytoin effect	? antagonism
	Valproic acid	↑ phenytoin toxicity	Protein binding

VI. Contraindications

Phenytoin should be avoided in patients with significant cardiac arrhythmias at or above the AV node, such as sick sinus syndrome or second- or third-degree AV block. Previous hypersensitivity reaction to hydantoins precludes the use of phenytoin.

Parenteral Benzodiazepines

I. Classification

A. Long-acting agents
   1. Diazepam (Valium)
B. Intermediate-acting agents
   1. Lorazepam (Ativan)
C. Short-acting agents
   1. Midazolam (Versed)

II. Mechanism of Action

Benzodiazepines potentiate the actions of gamma-amino butyric acid (GABA) within the CNS by binding to specific receptors at sites in close proximity to GABA-controlled chloride channels. Activation of these channels results in hyperpolarization of the neuronal membrane. The receptors vary in affinity for different benzodiazepines at different locations within the CNS, and some agonists may act as partial agonists at different sites. The highest concentration of receptors is in the cerebral cortex, and the lowest concentration is the spinal cord.

III. Indications

A. Diazepam decreases anxiety and produces short-term sedation and, at higher doses, anesthesia. It has proven benefit in controlling status epilepticus. Other uses include skeletal muscle relaxation, induction of amnesia states, and alcohol withdrawal.

B. Lorazepam is used to treat anxiety states, insomnia, restlessness, alcohol withdrawal, status epilepticus, and chemically induced nausea and vomiting.

C. Midazolam is indicated for short-term sedation and amnesia, induction of anesthesia, and muscle relaxation.

D. None of the benzodiazepines has proven analgesic properties.

IV. Complications

A. CNS—confusion, ataxia, dizziness, withdrawal syndrome

B. CV—hypotension, phlebitis at the injection site (except midazolam)

C. Other—respiratory depression, rarely apnea (may require intubation for ventilator support), paradoxical effects
   Note: Toxicity may be reversed with flumazenil, an IV benzodiazepine antagonist with a short half-life (< 1 hr).

V. Significant Drug Interactions

Drug	Interacting Drug	Effect	Mechanism
All	Aminodarone	↑ CV toxicity	Unknown
	β-blockers	↑ CNS effects	↓ metabolism
	Cimetidine	↑ CNS effects	↓ metabolism
	Digoxin	↑ digoxin effect	↓ clearance
	Theophylline	↓ CNS effect	Antagonism
	Zidovudine (AZT)	↑ AZT toxicity	↓ glucuronidation

VI. Contraindications

Benzodiazepines should be avoided in patients with hypersensitivity to benzodiazepines, as well as those in coma or shock or with myasthenia gravis.

Parenteral Barbiturates

I. Classification
   A. Long-acting
      1. Phenobarbital (Luminal)
   B. Ultra-short-acting
      1. Thiopental (Pentothal)

II. Mechanism of Action

The barbiturates produce general depression of the CNS by binding to pre- and postsynaptic GABA nerve endings to enhance the inhibitory effects of GABA. At higher concentrations, calcium-dependent action potentials in nerve fibers are suppressed. Barbiturates have no analgesic properties, and responses to pain may be elicited even with anesthetic doses of the drugs.

III. Indications
   A. Phenobarbital is used to treat both tonic-clonic and simple partial epilepsy, seizures from any cause, and status epilepticus. Its use in cases of refractory cerebral hypertension is uncertain. The onset of action is slow, but the effect is long-lasting.

   B. Thiopental, rapidly active but short-lived, is used for general anesthesia; its use in refractory cases of seizures, cerebral ischemia, and increased intracranial pressure is controversial.

IV. Complications
   A. Phenobarbital
      1. CNS—respiratory depression or apnea at high doses; confusion, particularly in the elderly; paradoxical excitement; increased pain perception; drug dependence
      2. CV—hypotension and shock at high doses
      3. Immune—hypersensitivity reactions including exfoliative dermatitis and Stevens-Johnson syndrome
      4. Hematology—thrombocytopenia
      5. Other—thrombophlebitis at the injection site
   B. Thiopental
      1. CNS—respiratory depression, excitation with involuntary muscle movement, emergence delirium
      2. CV—hypotension with rapid administration, cardiac arrhythmias
      3. Immune—allergic reactions
      4. Other—laryngospasm, thrombophlebitis at the injection site

V. Significant Drug Interactions

Drug	Interacting Drug	Effect	Mechanism
Both	All drugs metabolized by cytochrome P_{450}	↓ drug level	↑ metabolism
	Rifampin	↓ barbiturate effect	↑ metabolism
Phenobarbital	Valproic acid	↑ Phenobarbital effect	↓ metabolism
Thiopental	Sulfonamides	↑ thiopental effect	↓ binding

VI. Contraindications

The main contraindications to barbiturates are previous hypersensitivity reactions to any of these agents. Depressed respiration may be worsened; intubation with respiratory assistance is recommended in these circumstances.

Other Parenteral Agents for Seizure Control

I. Classification
   A. Acetazolamide (Diamox)—carbonic anhydrase inhibitor
   B. Magnesium sulfate—electrolyte
   C. Paraldehyde (Paral)—hypnotic-sedative

II. Mechanism of Action

Acetazolamide is a carbonic anhydrase inhibitor; magnesium tends to depress intracellular metabolic activity; paraldehyde decreases neuronal activity by unknown mechanisms. These diverse agents are capable of producing generalized CNS depression by mechanisms which are poorly understood. They may be useful in seizures unresponsive to other anticonvulsant therapy because of their different mechanisms of action.

III. Indications
   A. Acetazolamide is used in seizures of any type uncontrolled by other agents. It has been used to treat increased intracranial pressure, malignant glaucoma in conjunction with other agents, altitude sickness, hypo- and hyperkalemic familial periodic paralysis, and toxicity from weakly acidic drugs.
   B. Magnesium sulfate is frequently used to treat seizures associated with toxemia of preg-

nancy, seizures associated with acute nephritis in children, and Torsade de Pointes ventricular tachycardia.

  C. Paraldehyde is reserved for the treatment of seizures or status epilepticus uncontrolled with other medications, particularly in association with tetanus, eclampsia, and poisoning with convulsant drugs.

IV. Complications
  A. Acetazolamide
    1. CNS—sedation, confusion, convulsions
    2. GI—diarrhea, cholestatic jaundice
    3. Metabolic—metabolic acidosis, hypokalemia

    4. Hematology—blood dyscrasias
    5. Other—crystalluria
  B. Magnesium sulfate
    1. CNS—hypoventilation, decreased reflexes, hypotonia, hypothermia
    2. CV—hypotension, bradycardia, cardiac arrhythmias
  C. Paraldehyde
    1. CNS—confusion
    2. CV—bradycardia
    3. Respiratory—pulmonary edema
    4. Metabolic—metabolic acidosis
    5. Immune—skin rashes
    6. Other—thrombophlebitis

V. Significant Drug Interactions

Drug	Interacting Drug	Effect	Mechanism
Acetazolamide	Drugs causing $\downarrow K^+$	Hypokalemia	Additive $\downarrow$
	Ciprofloxacin	Crystalluria/ $\uparrow$ nephrotoxicity	$\downarrow$ urine solubility of Ciprofloxacin
	Digoxin	$\uparrow$ arrhythmias	$\downarrow K^+$
	Lithium	$\uparrow$ lithium toxicity	$\downarrow$ renal excretion
	Neuromuscular (NM) blockers	$\uparrow$ NM block	$\downarrow K^+$
	Quinidine	$\uparrow$ quinidine effects	$\downarrow$ renal excretion
Magnesium sulfate	Digoxin	$\uparrow$ risk of cardiac arrhythmias	Altered ion fluxes
Paraldehyde	Drugs $\downarrow$ CNS function	$\uparrow$ CNS depression	Additive

VI. Contraindications
  A. Acetazolamide: severe hypersensitivity to sulfonamides or sulfonamide-related diuretics such as thiazides, furosemide, and bumetanide
  B. Magnesium sulfate: heart block, myocardial dysfunction, renal failure
  C. Paraldehyde: sensitivity to paraldehyde

Osmotic Diuretics
I. Classification
  A. Mannitol (Osmitrol)
II. Mechanism of Action
  A. Mannitol is a polyglycan with high osmolality that is freely filtered by the glomerulus but is not reabsorbed or secreted by the renal tubule.
  B. In the proximal tubule it causes an osmotic-related decrease in water reabsorption, accompanied by decreased Na^+ reabsorption.
  C. It stimulates renal prostaglandin production to increase medullary blood flow, which de-

creases the ability of the loop of Henle to reabsorb Na^+.
  D. In the cerebral circulation, it may decrease the movement of vascular fluid into the brain tissue by its osmotic effect, and it may interfere with local prostaglandin production to dampen inflammatory effects in the brain.

III. Indications
Mannitol is used in the management of cerebral edema and increased intracranial pressure.

IV. Complications
Fluid and electrolyte imbalances are the major adverse effects, along with hyponatremia, hyperkalemia, fluid overload, and edema. In addition, the following effects are seen:
  A. CV—chest pain, palpitations with tachyarrhythmias, pulmonary congestion and/or edema.
  B. Immune—chills or fever, rashes, urticaria
  C. Other—irritation at the injection site, with tissue necrosis

V. Significant Drug Interactions

Drug	Interacting Drug	Effect	Mechanism
Mannitol	Digoxin	$\uparrow$ risk of digoxin toxicity	$\downarrow$ K$^+$

VI. Contraindications

Mannitol should be avoided in patients with renal failure or anuria. It should not be used in patients with severe dehydration, pulmonary edema, or intracranial bleeding.

Parenteral Phenothiazines and Related Neuroleptic Agents

I. Classification
- A. Phenothiazines
  1. Chlorpromazine (Thorazine)
  2. Fluphenazine (Prolixin)
- B. Butyrophenones
  1. Droperidol (Inapsine)
  2. Haloperidol (Haldol)

II. Mechanism of Action
- A. Neuroleptic agents antagonize dopaminergic (D$_2$) neurotransmission in the limbic, mesocortical, and hypothalamic systems. Little tolerance develops to this antagonism. The drugs have varying degrees of dopamine antagonistic action in the basal ganglia, resulting in differences in extrapyramidal side effects. The antagonism at the D$_2$ receptors in the chemoreceptor trigger zone produces an antiemetic action.
- B. Phenothiazines and, to a lesser extent butyrophenones, exhibit other blocking actions. They may produce an α-adrenergic block both centrally and peripherally, antihistaminic effects, blockage of tryptaminergic transmission, and antimuscarinic effects. The cardiovascular manifestations of these actions include peripheral vasodilation and tachycardia. The seizure threshold is lowered by phenothiazines but not by butyrophenones.

III. Indications
- A. Acute psychosis: all agents
- B. Sedation: chlorpromazine, droperidol
- C. Anesthesia adjunct: droperidol (with fentanyl)
- D. Nausea and vomiting: chlorpromazine, droperidol, haloperidol
- E. Pain: fluphenazine (adjunct)
- F. Tetanus: chlorpromazine with barbiturate
- G. Acute intermittent porphyria: chlorpromazine
- H. Intractable hiccoughs: chlorpromazine

IV. Complications
- A. CNS
  1. Sedation (most frequent with chlorpromazine and droperidol)
  2. Extrapyramidal effects (most frequent with haloperidol)
  3. Neuroleptic malignant syndrome consisting of fever, convulsions, tachypnea, dyspnea, tachycardia with or without other arrhythmias, hypertension or hypotension, severe muscle stiffness, weakness (most frequent with haloperidol)
- B. ANS—anticholinergic effects such as dry mouth, blurred vision from cycloplegia and mydriasis, tachycardia, constipation, urinary retention (most frequent with chlorpromazine)
- C. CV—hypotension (most frequent with chlorpromazine and droperidol)
- D. GI—cholestatic jaundice with fever, myalgia, arthralgia, fatigue, nausea, vomiting, or diarrhea
- E. Other—galactorrhea, photosensitivity, agranulocytosis, priapism

V. Significant Drug Interactions

Drug	Interacting Drug	Effect	Mechanism
Phenothiazines	Antidepressants, tricyclics (TCA)	$\uparrow$ toxicity from TCA	$\downarrow$ metabolism
	Clonidine	Organic brain syndrome	Unknown
	MAO inhibitors	$\uparrow$ risk of neuroleptic malignant syndrome	Additive
	Opiates	$\uparrow$ opiate toxicity	Toxic metabolites
	Valproic acid	$\uparrow$ valproic effect	$\downarrow$ metabolism
Haloperidol	β-blockers	$\downarrow\downarrow$ BP	Unknown
	Lithium	Encephalopathy, fever	Unknown
	Methyldopa	Dementia	Unknown
	Drugs $\uparrow$ cytochrome P$_{450}$ activity	$\downarrow$ haloperidol effect	$\uparrow$ metabolism

VI. Contraindications

The neuroleptics should be avoided in patients with severe cardiovascular disease, severe CNS depression, and coma. Phenothiazines should not be used in patients with a history of sensitivity to any phenothiazine or with previous neuroleptic malignant syndrome. Patients with Parkinson's disease will have a worsening of their disease when given neuroleptics.

Parenteral Anesthetic Agents

I. Classification
A. Etomidate (Amidate)
B. Ketamine (Ketalar)
C. Propofol (Dipravan)

II. Mechanism of Action

These agents cause sedation or hypnosis by unknown mechanisms. Etomidate may exert a GABA-like inhibitory effect in the brain stem reticular activating system. Ketamine produces a neuroleptic-like analgesia which is best explained by a dissociation of transmission between the thalamocortical and limbic systems, with inhibition of afferent transmission from the medial medullary reticular formation. Its analgesic effect may be caused by an opioid-like action at receptors in the spinal cord. No data explain the mechanism of action of propofol, a very lipid-soluble di-isopropylphenol.

III. Indications

All three drugs are used to induce and maintain anesthesia and/or sedation. Ketamine is used to produce a dissociative state of analgesia as well.

IV. Complications
A. Etomidate
1. CNS—myoclonus on injection; sedation/hypnosis with no analgesia, causing increased sympathetic activity
2. CV—mild hypotension, increased sympathetic activity
3. GI—nausea, vomiting
4. Respiratory—hiccoughs, brief, transient apnea
5. Endocrine—suppression of adrenal synthesis of cortisol and other steroid hormones for up to 6–8 hr after discontinuing medication
6. Other—pain at the injection site

B. Ketamine
1. CNS—tonic-clonic movements; mild respiratory depression; increased intracranial pressure; vivid dreams or nightmares; delirium; hallucinations with or without psychosis on emergence from the drug effect, with recurrences for several days to weeks
2. CV—sympathomimetic effects (increased blood pressure, heart rate, and peripheral vascular resistance)
3. Other—increased salivary secretions

C. Propofol
1. CNS—postadministration headache
2. CV—hypotension
3. Immune—allergic reactions from histamine release or allergy to solubilizing vehicle with bronchospasm, erythema, and hypotension
4. Other—apnea; mild pain at the injection site; nosocomial infection with multiple-dose vials left at room temperature

V. Significant Drug Interactions

Drug	Interacting Drug	Effect	Mechanism
All	Drugs ↓ CNS function	↑ CNS depression	Additive
Etomidate and ketamine	Drugs ↓ BP	↑ hypotension	Additive
Ketamine	Anesthetics, inhaled	↑ duration of ketamine	↓ metabolism

VI. Contraindications
A. Etomidate should be avoided in patients with sepsis (decreased adrenocorticosteroid response), transplantation, or a history of hypersensitivity to etomidate.
B. Ketamine is contraindicated in patients with severe cardiovascular disease, poorly controlled hypertension, recent myocardial infarction, stroke, cerebral trauma, intracranial mass or hemorrhage, schizophrenia or acute psychosis, thyrotoxicosis, or a history of ketamine hypersensitivity.
C. Propofol should not be used in patients with compromised cardiovascular function or with a history of hypersensitivity to propofol or its emulsion vehicle.

Parenteral Opioid Analgesics and Antagonists

I. Classification
A. Pure agonists
1. Morphine
2. Meperidine (pethidine) (Demerol)
3. Hydromorphone (Dilaudid)

Table 45-3. Dose and Handling of Drugs Used to Manage Neuropsychiatric Disorders

Class Drug/Dose	Onset of Action	Elimination	Elimination t½	Duration of Action
Parenteral Hydantoins				
Phenytoin IV: 10–15 mg/kg at ≤ 50 mg/min Then after 12–24 hr, 100 mg q6–8h	Within 5 min of end of administration	Hepatic microsomal metabolism At high concentrations, changes from first-order (concentration-dependent) to zero-order (concentration-independent) kinetics	6–24 hr (dose dependent) (prolonged with genetic enzyme deficiency or at high concentrations)	12–24 hr
Parenteral Barbiturates				
Phenobarbital IV slow injection (high dose): 10–20 mg/kg; repeat PRN for status epilepticus (moderate dose): 100–320 mg up to 600 mg qd	5 min, up to 15 min	Hepatic metabolism via microsomal enzymes; 25–50% excreted unchanged via kidney	80–120 hr	10–12 hr
Thiopental IV: 50–100 mg; repeat PRN or give 3–5 mg/kg as single dose 1.5–3.5 mg/kg for cerebral hypertension; repeat PRN	30–60 sec	Hepatic with some CNS and renal metabolism; 5% transformed to active pentobarbital	11.6 hr (8.5 min for redistribution)	10–30 min (after single dose)
Parenteral Benzodiazepines				
Diazepam IV: 5–10 mg Repeat q10–15min up to max. of 30 mg	Rapid	Metabolized to active metabolites: nordiazepam, oxazepam	30–60 hr 60–106 hr 5–8 hr	Depends on redistribution and effect required; ↑ duration with multiple doses
Lorazepam IV: 2–4 mg over 5 min; repeat 2 mg over 1–2 min q4h	Rapid	Metabolized by conjugation	9–19 hr	Variable with redistribution
Midazolam IV: 1.5–2.5 mg over 2 min, up to 5 mg over 2 min	1–5 min	Metabolized to active metabolites: 1-hydroxymidazolam, 4-hydroxymidazolam	1.3–2.5 hr 2–3 hr 2–3 hr	Variable with redistribution; ↑ with multiple doses

Other Parenteral Agents for Seizure Control

Agent and Dosage	Onset	Metabolism/Excretion	Half-life	Duration
Acetazolamide IV: 10–20 mg/kg q2–4 h	2 min	Renal excretion	NA	4–5 hr
Magnesium sulfate IV: 1–4 g 10–20% solution at 0.5–1 ml/min	Immediate	Renal excretion	Proportional to concentration and glomerular filtration rate	30 min; ↑ with ↓ renal function
Paraldehyde NG tube: Up to 12 ml (diluted to 10% solution) q4h Per rectum: 10–20 ml IM (deep): 5–10 ml IV (very slow): 0.1–0.15 ml/kg (diluted with normal saline)	< 15 min < 15 min < 15 min Very rapid	Hepatic metabolism (70–90%) Lung elimination	3.4–9.8 hr	8–12 hr

Osmotic Diuretics

Agent and Dosage	Onset	Metabolism/Excretion	Half-life	Duration
Mannitol IV: 50–100 g infusion of 5–25% solution	1–3 hr	80% renal excretion	100 min (↑ up to 36 hr with ↓ renal function)	3–8 hr

Parenteral Phenothiazines and Related Neuroleptic Agents

Agent and Dosage	Onset	Metabolism/Excretion	Half-life	Duration
Chlorpromazine IV: 5–50 mg of 1 mg/ml in normal saline at ≤ 1 mg/min IM: 25–50 mg	> 24 hr for antipsychotic effect < 1 hr for sedation < 1 hr for anti-emetic affect	Hepatic microsomal metabolism Active metabolites (7-OH metabolite)	30 hr	≥ 24 hr; depends on effect measured
Fluphenazine IM: 1.25–2.5 mg q6–8h PRN up to 10 mg/day (non-repository form)	As above	Hepatic microsomal metabolism	20 hr	12–24 hr
Droperidol 5–15 mg IV over 5 min	3–4 min as adjunct in anesthesia	Hepatic metabolism	2 hr	3–6 hr
Haloperidol IM: 2–5 mg q1h PRN, then q4–8h to total of 100 mg/day	10–20 min	Hepatic metabolism	21 hr	12–24 hr

431

      4. Fentanyl (Sublimaze, Duragesic)
      5. Sufentanil (Sufenta)
   B. Partial agonists
      1. Buprenorphine (Buprenex)
   C. Agonist-antagonists
      1. Butorphanol (Stadol)
      2. Pentazocine (Talwin)
   D. Antagonists
      1. Naloxone (Narcan)
II. **Mechanism of Action**
   A. Opioid agents binds to opioid receptors to produce their effects. Receptors are classified as μ, κ, δ, σ, or ϵ, depending on site and response. For μ, κ, and δ receptors, the binding response causes increased potassium channel conductance, with hyperpolarization and decreased release of excitatory neurotransmitters.
   B. The μ_1 high-affinity receptors are located in the limbic system, thalamus, striatum, hypothalamus, and midbrain. They mediate analgesia and, indirectly, euphoria. The μ_2 low-affinity receptors are located in the same areas as the μ_1 receptors but cause respiratory depression and sedation, and perhaps gastrointestinal effects. The κ receptors are located in the spinal cord and mediate analgesia; they may cause an alteration of calcium channels to inhibit calcium influx. The δ receptors are located in the cerebral cortex and myenteric plexus. They mediate gastrointestinal dysfunction and respiratory depression. Stimulation of σ receptors may result in an increase in D_2 receptor activation with dysphoria, hallucinations, and delirium. The sites and function of the ϵ receptors are not yet well defined.
   C. Opioids may function as full agonists, partial agonists, agonist-antagonists, or full antagonists at each of the various receptors.

III. **Indications**
   A. Agonists and partial agonists are used to produce analgesia for moderate to severe pain, as adjuncts to local or general anesthesia, for acute pulmonary edema, and rarely for cough and diarrhea. They may be given by the epidural or intrathecal route for pain relief, as an intermittent injection, or as a continuous infusion with a pump for chronic or postoperative pain. A new patient-controlled IV pump (morphine or meperidine) has improved analgesia in postoperative patients. Transdermal and transbuccal patches (fentanyl) are being developed.
   B. Antagonists are used as antidotes for undesired effects of opioid agonist administration.

IV. **Complications**
   A. CNS—respiratory depression, confusion
   B. CV—hypotension with high doses
   C. GI—biliary spasm, particularly with pure agonists; constipation
   D. GU—decreased urination from urinary retention or increased antidiuretic hormone level
   E. Immune—anaphylactoid reaction with rapid IV administration of agents, causing histamine release
   F. For pure agonists—euphoria, drug craving, drug abuse, drug dependence; muscle rigidity with high doses
   G. For agonist-antagonists—dysphoria, nightmares, hallucinations, restlessness, psychosis related to σ-receptor activity
   H. For meperidine—CNS excitation with restlessness, agitation, combativeness, seizures with accumulation of the toxic metabolite, normeperidine, particularly in renal dysfunction
   I. For fentanyl and sufentanil—muscle rigidity, hypertension and tachycardia (fentanyl)

V. **Significant Drug Interactions**

Drug	Interacting Drug	Effect	Mechanism
All	Cimetidine	↑ opioid toxicity	↓ metabolism
	MAO inhibitors	Toxic interactions	Unknown
	Rifampin	↓ opioid effect	↑ metabolism
Morphine	Zidovudine (AZT)	↑ toxicity of both drugs	↓ clearance
Meperidine	Acyclovir	↑ meperidine effect	↓ renal excretion
	Sympathomimetics	↑ risk of seizures	Additive
	MAO inhibitors	Encephalopathy + autonomic dysfunction	Interaction of MAO inhibitor and normeperidine
Partial agonist/antagonist	Pure agonist	Withdrawal syndrome	Antagonism

Table 45-4. Dose and Handling of Parenteral Direct Skeletal Muscle Relaxant

Drug/Dose	Onset of Action	Elimination	Elimination t½	Duration of Action
Dantrolene 1 mg/kg IV rapid push Repeat PRN to max of 10 mg/kg (may start with 2.5–3 mg/kg in life-threatening situations)	Rapid	Hepatic microsomal metabolism	4–8 hr	NA

VI. Contraindications

A. The opioids should be avoided in patients with pseudomembranous enterocolitis (retention of toxin) or respiratory depression (unless intubated)

B. Patients with renal dysfunction should not be given meperidine, as the toxic metabolite will accumulate.

Parenteral Nonsteroidal Anti-Inflammatory Drugs

I. Classification

A. Ketorolac (Toradol)

II. Mechanism of Action

A. The activation of phospholipase A_2 initiates a metabolic cascade which forms leukotrienes by the lipooxygenase pathway, and prostaglandins (PGs) and thromboxane by the cyclooxygenase pathway.

B. The leukotrienes, PGs, and/or thromboxane are involved in the inflammatory response, temperature regulation, platelet aggregation, peripheral pain fiber stimulation, and renal regulation of the glomerular filtration rate and intrarenal blood flow.

C. The nonsteroidal anti-inflammatory drugs (NSAIDs), including ketorolac, inhibit the cyclooxygenase enzyme, decreasing the production of all PGs and thromboxane.

III. Indications

Ketorolac may be given parenterally to patients with moderate to severe pain when oral drug administration is not feasible and when opiate drugs not tolerated or not indicated.

IV. Complications

A. CNS—drowsiness, dizziness, headache

B. GI—nonspecific upset, gastric mucosal irritation, possibly hepatic dysfunction

C. GU—edema from decreased sodium and water excretion

D. Immune—possible anaphylactoid reactions

E. Other—increased risk of bleeding, diaphoresis, possibly acute renal failure

V. Significant Drug Interactions

Drug	Interacting Drug	Effect	Mechanism
All NSAIDs	Acetaminophen	↑ renal toxicity	Additive
	Glucocorticoids	↑ risk of GI ulcer/bleed	Additive
	Drugs ↓ hemostasis	↑ risk of bleeding	Additive
	Diuretics	↓ diuretic effect	↓ renal PGs
	Antihypertensives	↓ hypotensive effect	↓ renal PGs

VI. Contraindications

Hypersensitivity to aspirin, other NSAIDs, or ketorolac precludes the use of this agent. The drug should be used with caution in patients with active bleeding sites or bleeding diatheses.

Parenteral Antiemetic and Prokinetic Agents

I. Classification

A. Antiemetics

1. Antihistamines—H_1 blockers (see Antihistamines)
2. Butyrophenones (see Neuroleptics)
3. Glucocorticoids (see Glucocorticoids)
4. Metoclopramide (Reglan)
5. Ondansetron (Zofran)
6. Phenothiazines
   a. Prochlorperazine (Compazine)
   b. Other antiemetic phenothiazines (see Neuroleptics)

Table 45-5. Dose and Handling of Parenteral Drugs Used for Supportive Care

Class Drug/Dose	Onset of Action	Elimination	Elimination t½	Duration of Action
Other Parenteral Anesthetic Agents				
Etomidate IV: bolus: 0.2–0.6 mg/kg over 30–60 sec	< 60 sec	Hepatic hydrolysis	1.5–4 hr	3–5 min
Ketamine IV: induction: 1–2 mg/kg bolus or 0.5 mg/kg/min maintenance: 0.01–0.05 mg/kg/min	15–30 sec	Hepatic metabolism to active metabolite (norketamine), then inactive metabolites	2–3 hr	5–10 min
Propofol IV: induction: 1.5–3.0 mg/kg at rate of 40 mg/10 sec Maintenance: 0.1–0.2 mg/kg/min (for sedation, 1–6 mg/kg/hr)	< 60 sec	Hepatic metabolism Lung elimination	1–3 hr but slow terminal elimination of 3–12 hr	3–10 min
Parenteral Opioid Analgesics and Antagonists				
Morphine IV: 4–10 mg by slow injection q4h IM/SC: 10–20 mg q4h Per rectum: 20–30 mg q4–6h (suppository)	< 5 min 10–30 min 20–60 min	Hepatic metabolism with renal excretion of active metabolite Morphine-6-glucuronide	2 hr 3–4 hr	4–5 hr
Meperidine IV: slow injection 50–150 mg q3–4h Infusion: 15–35 mg/hr IM/SC: 50–150 mg q3–4h	1 min 10–15 min	Hepatic metabolism with renal excretion of metabolites; normeperidine has CNS toxicity	2–4 hr 15–30 hr	2–4 hr

Drug / Dose	Onset	Half-life	Metabolism/Excretion	Duration
Hydromorphone IV: slow injection 0.5–1 mg q3h IM/SC: 1–4 mg q3–6 h Per rectum: 3 mg q4–8h (suppository)	10–15 min 15 min 30–60 min	2–3 hr	Renal excretion of inactive metabolites	4–6 hr
Fentanyl IV: 2–20 µg/kg (0.07–1.4 g/kg as adjunct for minor procedure; 20–100 µg/kg for major surgery)	1–2 min	3.6 hr (↑ up to 16 hr in elderly)	Hepatic metabolism; 10–25% excreted unchanged in urine	0.5–1 hr
cutaneous: 25–100 µg/hr by patch	?1–2 hr	15–20 hr		Up to 24–48 hr/patch
Sufentanil IV: low dose— 0.5–1 µg/kg; then 10–25 µg mod. dose: 2–8 µg/kg; then 10–50 µg PRN	< 1 min	2.7 hr	Hepatic metabolism	5 min 0.7–2.9 hr
Buprenorphine IV: 0.3 mg slow q6h, up to 0.6 mg IM: 0.3–0.6 mg q6h	< 15 min 15 min	2–3 hr	Hepatic metabolism	6 hr (up to 10 hr in some patients)
Butorphanol IV: 0.5–2 mg q3–4 h up to 0.6 mg IM: 1–4 mg q3–4 h	2–3 min 10–30 min	2–4 hr	Renal excretion of inactive metabolites	2–4 hr
Pentazocine IV: 30 mg q3–4 h IM/SC: 30 mg q3–4 h	2–3 min 15–20 min	2–3 hr	Renal excretion—up to 25% as intact drug	2–3 hr

(continued)

435

Table 45-5. Continued

Class Drug/Dose	Onset of Action	Elimination	Elimination t½	Duration of Action
Naloxone		Hepatic metabolism	1–1.7 hr	45 min
IV: 0.1–0.2 mg IV q2–3 min	< 1 min			
IM/SC: 0.4–2 mg	2–5 min			
Parenteral NSAIDS				
Ketorolac	10 min	> 50% renal excretion < 50% hepatic metabolism Renal dysfunction	4–6 hr; ↑ with ↑ age	5–6 hr
Load: IM–60 mg, then 15–30 mg q6h				
May be given IV				
Parenteral Antiemetic and Prokinetic Agents				
Metoclopramide	1–3 min	Hepatic metabolism (70%) Renal excretion (30%)	4–6 hr	1–2 hr
Antiemetic: IV—1.0–2.0 mg/kg q2–3 h				
Prokinetic: IV—10 mg				
Ondansetron	10–15 min	Hepatic microsomal metabolism	4 hr	3–4 hr
IV: 0.15 mg/kg over 15 min				
Repeat × 2 at 4-hr interval				
Trimethobenzamide	? 20–30 min	Hepatic metabolism		
IM: 200 mg tid or qid				
Parenteral H₂ Blockers				
Cimetidine	NA	75% renal excretion 25% hepatic metabolism	1.6–2.1 hr	6–8 hr (nocturnal) 4–5 hr (basal)
IV: 300 mg over ≥ 5 min q6–8 h *or* 37.5 mg/hr infusion				
Famotidine	NA	65–70% renal excretion of unchanged drug 30–35% hepatic microsomal metabolism	2.5–3.5 hr	10–12 hr (nocturnal and basal)
IV: 20 mg over ≥ 2 min q12 h				

Drug / Dose	Onset	Metabolism	Half-life	Duration
Ranitidine IV: 50 mg over ≥ 5 min q6–8h *or* 0.125–0.25 mg/kg/hr infusion	NA	70% renal excretion of unchanged drug 30% hepatic microsomal metabolism	2–2.5 hr	13 hr (nocturnal) 4 hr (basal)

Prenteral antihistamines and H$_1$ Blockers

Drug / Dose	Onset	Metabolism	Half-life	Duration
Brompheniramine IV: 10 mg q8–12h	< 5 min	Hepatic microsomal metabolism	25 hr	3–12 hr
Chlorpheniramine IV: 5–40 mg	< 5 min	Hepatic microsomal metabolism	14–25 hr	4–8 hr
Cyclizine IM: 50 mg q4–6 h	20–30 min	Hepatic microsomal metabolism	NA	4–6 hr
Hydroxyzine IM: 50–100 mg q4–6 h PRN	20–30 min	Hepatic microsomal metabolism	2.5–3.4 hr	4–6 hr
Dimenhydrinate IV: 50 mg over 2 min q4h PRN IM: 50 mg q4h PRN	< 5min	Hepatic microsomal metabolism	NA	3–6 hr
Diphenhydramine IV: 10–50 mg	< 5 min	Hepatic microsomal metabolism	1–4 hr	6–8 hr
Promethazine IV: 25–50 mg; repeat in 2–4 hr PRN	<5 min	Hepatic microsomal metabolism	10–14 hr	6–12 hr (anti-histaminic) 2–8 hr (sedative)

437

Table 45-6.   Differential Diagnosis of Confusion and Agitation in the Critical Care Unit

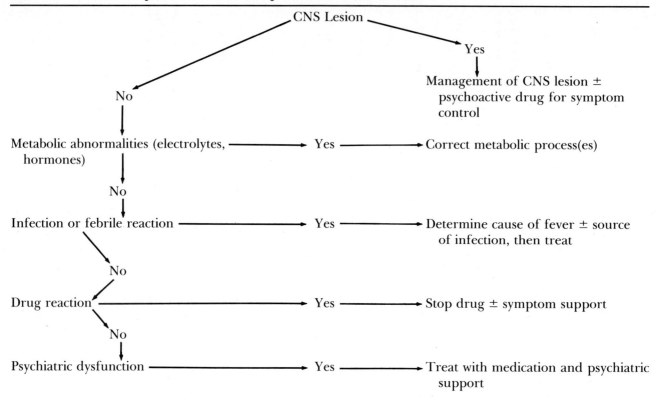

Common Drugs Causing Confusion and/or Agitation

Acetazolamide	Digoxin	Mexiletine
Acyclovir	Disopyramide	Nitroprusside (cyanide,
Antihistamines	Encainide	thiocyanate)
Aspirin	Flecainide	Opioids (N.B. meperidine)
Atropine	Fluconazole	Paraldehyde
Barbiturates (elderly)	Hydralazine	Phenoxybenzamine
Benzodiazepines	Ketamine	Phenytoin
β-blockers	Labetalol	Procainamide
β-blocker withdrawal	Lidocaine	Quinidine
Bronchodilators*	Loop diuretics	Tocainide
Clonidine	Methyldopa	Trimethobenzamide
Corticosteroids	Metoclopramide	

*Includes sympathomimetics, methylxanthines, and anticholinergics.

       7. Trimethobenzamide (Tigan)
   B. Prokinetic agents
       1. Metoclopramide (Reglan)
       2. Cisapride (investigational)
II. Mechanism of Action
   A. The butyrophenones, phenothiazines, and benzamides (metoclopramide and trimethobenzamide) inhibit D_2 receptors in the chemoreceptor trigger zone (CTZ) to decrease centrally mediated nausea and vomit-

ing. Metoclopramide has a prokinetic effect on the stomach by increasing the release of, or sensitivity to, acetylcholine at the myenteric neuroeffector junction.
   B. Ondansetron and cisapride affect serotonin (5-HT) receptors. Ondansetron inhibits $5\text{-}HT_3$ receptors in the brain and GI tract to decrease nausea and vomiting. Cisapride blocks $5\text{-}HT_2$ receptors in the GI tract, producing hypermotility.

Table 45-7. Differential Diagnosis of Fever in the Critical Care Unit

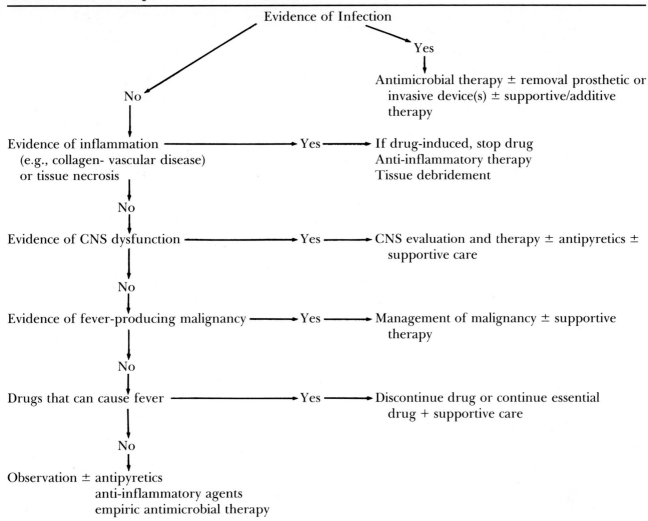

Drugs Causing Fever in the Critical Care Unit

ACE inhibitors	Nitroglycerin
Acetazolamide	Penicillins
Amphotericin B	Phenothiazines*
Aspirin	Phenytoin
Bronchodilators†	Procainamide
Cephalosporins	Quinidine
Hydralazine	Rifampin
Mannitol	Streptokinase
Methyldopa	Succinyl choline*

*Causes malignant hyperthermia.
†Sympathomimetics, methylxanthines, and anticholinergics (high doses).

III. Indications

A. Metoclopramide controls and/or treats centrally mediated nausea and vomiting, gastric hypomotility or paresis, reflux esophagitis, and persistent hiccoughs. It has been used for prophylaxis of aspiration pneumonitis prior to surgical procedures.

B. Ondansetron effectively controls drug-induced nausea and vomiting.

C. Trimethobenzamide is used to treat vomiting.

Table 45-8. Differential Diagnosis of Thrombocytopenia in the Critical Care Unit

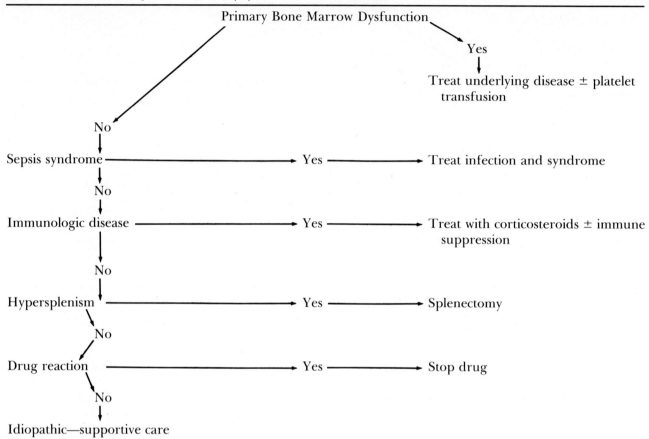

Drugs Causing Thrombocytopenia in the Critical Care Unit

Acetaminophen	Famotidine	Penicillins
Acetazolamide	Fluconazole	Pentamidine
Amrinone	Flucytosine	Phenobarbital
Antihistamines	Ganciclovir	Phenytoin
Cephalosporins	Heparin—mild, severe	Procainamide
Cimetidine	Hydralazine	Quinidine
Cotrimoxazole-	Loop diuretics	Ranitidine
(trimethoprim-sulfamethoxazole)	Mexiletine	Thiazide diuretics
		Tocainide

D. Cisapride is used to treat gastrointestinal paresis or severe constipation.

IV. **Complications**
   A. Metoclopramide
      1. CNS—extrapyramidal effects, tardive dyskinesia, agitation, sedation, akathisia
      2. Metabolic—galactorrhea, methemoglobinemia with red blood cell enzyme deficiencies
   B. Ondansetron
      1. CNS—possibly extrapyramidal effects
      2. GI—constipation, mild liver enzyme abnormalities
      3. Immune—bronchospasm, rashes
   C. Trimethobenzamide
      1. CNS—mental depression, convulsions, opisthotonos
      2. GI—hepatic dysfunction, Reye's syndrome
      3. Immune—allergic reactions, mainly rashes
      4. Hematology—blood dyscrasias

Table 45-9. Therapeutic Drug Monitoring

Although therapeutic drug monitoring generally refers to assessment of blood concentrations of specific drugs at designated times after drug administration, the main focus should be the clinical status of the patient. Blood sampling for determination of drug concentration is of value only when clinical conditions or potential clinical problems warrant this testing, and when plasma concentrations have been shown to correlate with the clinical effect. Such clinical situations include:

1. Use of relatively toxic drugs whose handling differs significantly among patients, so that dose does not correlate with therapeutic effect or toxicity *and* accumulation could lead to serious toxicity.
2. Effectiveness of drug therapy is not easy to measure clinically, and blood level data assist in providing the most likely therapeutic benefit with the least toxicity.
3. Addition of drugs to previous therapy could alter drug handling or clinical effects of the previous therapy, i.e., preventable toxic drug interactions.
4. Emergence of clinical symptoms and/or signs which are consistent with either drug toxicity or a worsening disease state.
5. Lack of clinical response to the drug therapy to document patient compliance.
6. Determination of a dosing schedule of a relatively toxic drug which is optimal for a patient with potentially altered durg handling.

To provide maximal information, blood concentration data for a drug should be correlated with the clinical condition of the patient and should be sampled at specific times in relation to drug administration. However, if drug toxicity is suspected, blood sampling should be done as soon as possible. Data about specific drugs used frequently in the critical care unit are outlined in Table 45-10.

V. Significant Drug Interactions

Drug	Interacting Drug	Effect	Mechanism
Metoclopramide	Carbamazepine	Neurotoxicity	Unknown
	Hydroxyzine	Neurotoxicity	? additive
	Hepatotoxic drugs	↑ hepatotoxicity	? additive
Ondansetron	Drugs ↑ cytochrome P_{450} metabolism	↓ ondansetron effect	↑ metabolism
	Drugs ↓ cytochrome P_{450} metabolism	↑ ondansetron toxicity	↓ metabolism
Trimethobenzamide	Ototoxic drugs	↓ ototoxic symptoms	CNS effect

VI. Contraindications
A. A history of hypersensitivity to particular agent precludes further use.
B. With metoclopramide, a history or the presence of epilepsy, GI hemorrhage, or pheochromocytoma obviates its use.

Parenteral Antihistaminic H₂ Blockers
I. Classification
A. Cimetidine (Tagamet)
B. Famotidine (Pepcid)
C. Ranitidine (Zantac)
II. Mechanism of Action
These agents competitively inhibit the histamine-induced response of H_2 receptors, found in the stomach, vascular smooth muscle, bronchial smooth muscle, and heart. This action blocks the histamine-induced secretion of gastric acid and decreases the volume of gastric secretions. It also blunts histamine-induced vasodilation and cardiac stimulation.

III. Indications
The following are clinical situations in which these drugs are used: prophylaxis and treatment of duodenal ulcers; treatment of gastric ulcers; treatment of reflux esophagitis; treatment of upper GI bleeding; prophylaxis or treatment of stress-induced gastric mucosal damage; treatment of Zollinger-Ellison syndrome; prophylaxis of aspiration pneumonia; treatment adjunct of systemic mastocytosis; treatment adjunct of multiple endocrine adenomata; adjunct to NSAID drug therapy in rheumatoid arthritis to decrease GI symptoms; adjunct to H_1 blockers in urticaria or cutaneous allergic disorders.

Table 45-10. Therapeutic Drug Monitoring in Critical Care

Drug/Administration	Timing of Blood Sampling*	Therapeutic Blood Concentration†	Clinical Monitoring
Digoxin			
IV load		0.5–2.0 ng/ml (10% of patients require and tolerate levels of up to 2–4 ng/ml; 10% of patients toxic at levels < 2 ng/ml)	Cardiac monitoring Blood monitor for K^+, Mg^{+2}, Ca^{+2}, PO_2
IV maintenance	6–8 hr after last administration		
Lidocaine			
IV load (lack of response)	20–30 min postload	2–5 µg/ml	Cardiac monitoring CNS symptoms and signs
IV maintenance (if > 12–24 hr)	12–24 hr after onset	2–5 µg/ml	
Procainamide			
IV load	0.5–1 hr postload	4–12 µg/ml	Cardiac monitoring Immune markers if therapy chronic
IV maintenance	0.5–1 hr after infusion	4–12 µg/ml (up to 16 µg/ml in some patients) NAPA:‡ 10–30 µg/ml or PA + NAPA ≤ 35 µg/ml	
Phenytoin			
IV load	2–4 hr postload	Total: 10–20 µg/ml Free: 1–2 µg/ml§	Cardiac monitoring Seizure frequency CNS signs/symptoms
IV maintenance	Prior to dose 24 hr after start of therapy		

Drug / Dosing	Sampling time	Desired concentration	Monitoring
Quinidine			
IV load ± maintenance	0.5–1 hr postdose	2–5 µg/ml	Cardiac monitoring BP monitoring CNS and GI symptoms
Theophylline			
IV load	Preload	< 10 µg/ml to give load	Cardiac monitoring Respiratory status CNS status
IV load	15 min after end of IV load	10–16 µg/ml (up to 20 µg/m in some patients)	
IV maintenance	6–12 hr after start; q24h thereafter	10–16 µg/ml (up to 20 µg/ml in some patients)	GI symptoms
Amikacin			
IV peak	1 hr after 30-min infusion	20–30 µg/ml	Renal function
IV trough	0.5 hr prior to infusion	< 10 µg/ml	Vestibular/auditory status
Gentamicin/Tobramycin			
IV peak	1 hr after 30-min infusion	4–8 µg/ml (up to 10–12 µg/ml in some patients)	Renal status
IV trough	0.5 hr prior to infusion	0.5–1 µg/ml	Vestibular/auditory status
Vancomycin			
IV peak	1–2 hr after 60-min infusion	25–40 µg/ml	BP and symptoms during infusion
IV trough	0.5 hr prior to infusion	5–10 µg/ml	Renal function Vestibular/otic status

* Blood sampling should be done at any time when drug toxicity is suspected.
† Adverse effects may be seen at levels below the stated minimal desired concentration, and efficacy may require levels above the stated maximal desired concentrations.
‡ N-Acetylprocainamide.
§ Free levels should be measured when abnormal protein binding occurs (e.g., hypoalbuminemia, renal dysfunction).

IV. **Complications**
   A. CV—hypotension with rapid IV injection, cardiac arrhythmias
   B. GI—rarely hepatitis
   C. Other

1. Cimetidine—antiandrogenic activity, increased serum prolactin
2. Famotidine—anorexia, tinnitus
3. Ranitidine—slightly increased serum prolactin, blurred vision

V. **Significant Drug Interactions**

Drug	Interacting Drug	Effect	Mechanism
All	Drugs bone marrow function	↑ risk of neutropenia	Additive
Cimetidine	Drugs metabolized by cytochrome P_{450} system	↑ effect of drug	↓ metabolism
	Captorpril	Neuropathy (in renal failure)	Additive
	Digoxin	↑ digoxin effect	Unknown

VI. **Contraindications**
Patients with sensitivity to any H_2 blocker or hepatic cirrhosis with portal systemic encephalopathy should not receive H_2 blockers.

Parenteral Antihistamines: H₁ Blockers

I. **Classification**
   A. Alkylamines
      1. Brompheniramine (Dehist)
      2. Chlorpheniramine
   B. Piperazines
      1. Cyclizine (Marezine)
      2. Hydroxyzine (Vistaril)
   C. Ethanolamines
      1. Dimenhydrinate (Dramamine)
      2. Diphenhydramine (Benadryl)
   D. Phenothiazines
      1. Promethazine (Phenergan)

II. **Mechanism of Action**
Histamine is released from storage sites, primarily in tissue mast cells, in response to various triggers. It acts on H_1 histamine receptors located in arterioles and capillaries; on smooth muscle cells of the bronchi and intestinal tract; and in dermal tissue and in the CNS to cause rapid-onset, short-duration vasodilation, increased capillary permeability, bronchoconstriction, increased intestinal muscle tone, cutaneous itchiness or burning pain, and stimulation of CNS vestibular connections and the chemoreceptor trigger zone (CTZ). The H_1 blockers diminish these histamine-induced responses.

III. **Indications**
   A. The H_1 blockers are used in the symptomatic therapy of allergic reactions associated with excess histamine release, as well as for mild anxiety or insomnia.
   B. In addition, specific agents have been used to treat other conditions:
      1. Diphenhydramine—dyskinesia from Parkinson's disease or from drugs (central anticholinergic effect), cough, emesis, vertigo
      2. Hydroxyzine—anxiety, nausea or emesis, vertigo
      3. Promethazine—analgesia adjunct, motion sickness (therapy or prophylaxis), vertigo, nausea or emesis

IV. **Complications**
   A. CNS—sedation, confusion (rarely, stimulation with insomnia, hallucinations, seizures), anticholinergic effects (dry mouth and throat, facial flushing, dyspnea, tachycardia, blurred vision)
   B. CV—hypotension, tachycardia
   C. Hematology—blood dyscrasias
   D. Other
      1. Dimenhydrinate and diphenhydramine—increased sedation and anticholinergic activity
      2. Promethazine—extrapyramidal effects

V. **Significant Drug Interactions**

Drug	Interacting Drug	Effect	Mechanism
All	CNS depressants	↑ CNS depression	Additive
	Anticholinergic drugs	↑ anticholinergic effects	Additive

VI. Contraindications
These drugs should not be used in patients with intolerance to H_1 blockers or to anticholinergic effects.

Direct Skeletal Muscle Relaxants
I. Classification
A. Dantrolene (Dantrium)
II. Mechanism of Action
Dantrolene acts directly on skeletal muscle cells to uncouple excitation from contraction by decreasing Ca^{+2} release from sarcoplasmic reticulum in response to excitation. This process decreases the metabolic requirements of the cells and so de- creases heat production. Reflex activity is reduced more than voluntary muscle action because "fast" twitch muscle fibers are more affected.

III. Indications
Dantrolene given intravenously is used to treat malignant hyperthermia syndrome resulting from the administration of neuroleptic, anesthetic, or neuromuscular blocking drugs.

IV. Complications
A. CNS—euphoria, dizziness, lightheadedness, drowsiness, fatigue
B. GI—hepatotoxicity including fatal hepatitis, severe diarrhea
C. Other—muscle weakness

V. Significant Drug Interactions

Drug	Interacting Drug	Effect	Mechanism
Dantrolene	CNS depressants	↑ CNS depression	Additive
	Verapamil (? other Ca^{+2} channel blockers)	Ventricular fibrillation or cardiovascular collapse	? severe ↓ K^+

VI. Contraindications
Caution should be used in administering dantrolene to patients with active hepatitis, hepatic cirrhosis, or sensitivity to the drug.

Bibliography

Benumuf JL (ed). *New Anesthetic Drugs*. Anesthesia Clinics of North America: Vol 6 (2). Philadelphia, WB Saunders, 1988.

Blumer JL, Bond GR (eds). *Toxic Effects of Drugs Used in the ICU*. Critical Care Clinics: Vol 7 (3). Philadelphia, WB Saunders, 1991.

Chernow B (ed). *The Pharmacological Approach to the Critically Ill Patients*. Baltimore, Williams and Wilkins, 1988.

Drug Information for the Health Care Professional USP D1 1993 United States Pharmacopeial Convention, Rockville, MD.

Dukes MNG (ed). *Meyer's Side Effects of Drugs*. Amsterdam, Elsevier, 1988.

Parrillo JE (ed). *Critical Care Medicine*, ed 2. Baltimore, Williams and Wilkins, 1990.

Rizack MA. *Handbook of Adverse Drug Interactions*. New Rochelle, NY, Medical Letter, 1987.

SECTION 6

Infectious Disease

CHAPTER 46-A

Arthropod-Borne Disease

Jeffrey A. Nelson, M.D.

Bibliography

Spach DH, Liles WC, Campbell GL, et al. Tick-borne diseases in the United States. *N Engl J Med* 329:936–947, 1993.

Oldfield EC III, Rodiev GR, Gray GC. The endemic infectious diseases of Somalia. *CID* 16:S132–S157, 1993.

Oldfield EC III, Wallace MR, Hyams KC, et al. Endemic infectious diseases of the Middle East. *Rev Infect Dis* 13: S199–S217, 1991.

Table 46A-1. Arthropod-borne diseases (United States)

Disease	Vector	Organism	Geography	Clinical Clue	Laboratory	Treatment
Babesiosis	Tick	*Babesia microti*	New England Upper Midwest	Asplenic	Anemia, parasitized RBCs	Clindaymcin and quinine
Colorado tick fever	Tick	*Orbivirus*	Rocky Mountains	Biphasic illness	Leukopenia	Supportive
Ehrlichiosis	Tick	*Ehrlichia canis*	Southeast, South central		Leukopenia Transaminase elevation	Tetracycline
Encephalitis						
Eastern	Mosquito	alphavirus	Atlantic/Gulf states	Encephalopathy	CSF lymphocytosis	Supportive
LaCrosse	Mosquito	Bunyavirus	North central	Encephalopathy	CSF lymphocytosis	Supportive
St. Louis	Mosquito	Flavivirus	Throughout	Encephalopathy	CSF lymphocytosis	Supportive
Venezuelan	Mosquito	Alphavirus	Texas/Florida	Encephalopathy	CSF lymphocytosis	Supportive
Western	Mosquito	Alphavirus	West of Mississippi	Encephalopathy	CSF lymphocytosis	Supportive
Endemic typhus (murine)	Flea	*Rickettsia typhi*	Urban South-east	Central rash	Serology	Tetracycline
Epidemic typhus	Worldwide louse, United States?	*Rickettsia prowazeki*	East	Axillary rash in winter	Serology	Tetracycline
Lyme disease	Tick	*Borrelia burgdorferi*	New England, Upper Midwest California	Bull's-eye rash, facial palsy, large joint arthritis	Serology	Doxycycline (early), ceftriaxone (late)
Plague	Flea	*Yersinia pestis*	Southwest	Focal lymph-adenopathy	Serology	Streptomycin or chloramphenicol
Relapsing fever	Tick	*Borrelia* sp.	Rocky Mountains	Relapsing fever course	Peripheral smear spirochetes	Doxycycline
Rickettsial pox	Mouse Mite	*Rickettsia akari*	Urban	Papule/eschar, papulovesicular rash	Serology	Tetracycline
Rocky Mountain spotted fever	Tick	*Rickettsia rickettsii*	Southeast Throughout	Peripheral rash	Serology	Tetracycline or chloramphenicol
Tularemia	Tick	*Francisella tularensis*	South central Throughout	Ulcer, lymphadenopathy	Serology	Streptomycin or tetracycline

Table 46A-2. Arthropod-borne diseases (Foreign Traveler)

Disease	Vector	Organism	Geography	Clinical Clue	Laboratory	Treatment
Bartonellosis	Sand fly	*Bartonella bacilliformis*	Andes Mountains	Pallor, icterus; skin nodules (late disease)	Anemia, peripheral smear reveals organisms on RBCs	Chloramphenicol
Boutonneuse fever	Tick	*Rickettsia conorii*	Africa, Southern Europe	Eschar at bite site	Serology	Doxycycline or ciprofloxacin
Chagas disease	Reduviid bug	*Trypanosoma cruzi*	Mexico, Central and South America	Periorbital edema (acute); cardiomyopathy megaesophagus (chronic)	Blood smear (early); serology (late)	
Dengue fever	Mosquito	Flavivirus	Tropical America, Asia, Africa	Petechiae, hemorrhage	Disseminated intravascular coagulation, thrombocytopenia	Supportive
Filariasis	Mosquito	*Wuchereria bancrofti, Brugia malayi, B. timori*	Tropics, Southeast Asia, Indonesia	Lymphatic obstruction	Blood smear (see Microfilaria)	Diethylcarbamazine
Leishmaniasis	Sand fly	*Leishmania* spp. (visceral)	Worldwide	Fever, weight loss, hepatosplenomegaly	Anemia, leukopenia, + bone marrow aspirate	Antimonial compounds
		Leishmania sp. (cutaneous), *Leishmania* (*braziliensis, mexicana*)	Asia, Africa (Old World), Central America, South America (New World)	Chronic ulcer	Amastigote in tissue	Antimonial compounds

(continued)

Table 46A-2. Continued

Disease	Vector	Organism	Geography	Clinical Clue	Laboratory	Treatment
Loiasis	Fly	Loa loa	Central and West Africa	Subcutaneous swellings (Calabar), conjunctivitis, worm in eye	Microfilariae in daytime blood, eosinophilia	Diethylcarbamazine
Malaria	Mosquito	*Plasmodium* spp.	Worldwide	Fever, rigors	parasites in RBCs	See Chapter 48M
Onchocerciasis	Black fly	*Onchocerca volvulus*	Africa, Central and South America	Pruritic rash, skin nodules, keratitis	Eosinophilia, skin snip, microfilariae	Ivermectin
Scrub typhus	Mite	*Rickettsia tsutsugamushi*	East Asia	Ulcer, lymphadenopathy	Serology	Tetracycline or chloramphenicol
Sleeping sickness	Fly	*Trypanosoma brucei gambiense*	West Africa	Chancre (early), lymphadenopathy, encephalopathy (late)	Nodal aspirate	Suramin (early)
		Trypanosoma brucei rhodesiense	East Africa	Fever, rash, tachycardia, encephalopathy	Peripheral smear	Arsenicals (late)
Yellow fever	Mosquito	Flavivirus	South America, Africa	Black vomit, jaundice, oliguria	Serology	Suppportive

452

Zoonoses

James Levin, M.D.
Stuart Levin, M.D.

Bibliography

Del Brutto OH, Sotelo J. Neurocysticercosis: An update. *Rev Infect Dis* 10:1075–87, 1988.

Elliot DL, Tolle SW, Goldberg L, Miller J. Pet associated illness. *N Engl J Med* 313:985–95, 1985.

Hirsch MS, Moellering RC, Pope HG, Poskanzen DC. Lymphocytic-choriomeningitis-virus infection traced to a pet hamster. *N Engl J Med* 291:610–12, 1974.

Lamb R. Anthrax. *Br Med J* 1:157–60, 1973.

Pinner RW, Schuchat A, Swaminathan B, et al. Role of foods in sporadic listeriosis: II. Microbiologic and epidemiologic investigation. *JAMA* 267:2046–50, 1992.

Sawyer LA, Fishbein DB, McDade JE. Q fever: Current concepts. *Rev Infect Dis* 9:935, 1987.

Schuchat A, Denver KA, Wenger JD, et al. Role of foods in sporadic listeriosis: I. Case-control study of dietary risk factors. *JAMA* 267:2041–45, 1992.

Table 46B-1. Reservoir, Modes of Transmission, and Clinical Syndromes for Selected Zoonoses

Disease (Organism)	Animal Reservoir	Mode of Transmission	Clinical Syndrome
Anthrax (*Bacillus anthracis*)	Goats, sheep, cattle, horses, and other herbivores	1. Direct contact with animals or their raw products (e.g., hides, hair/wool, bones). 2. Inhalation of spores, especially during processing of goats hair (e.g., wool-sorter's disease). 3. Ingestion (rare).	1. Cutaneous (95% of cases): papule (pruritic) evolving to eschar with surrounding edema. 2. Inhalation (very high mortality): hemorrhagic mediastinal adenitis; bloody meningitis. 3. Ingestion: bloody diarrhea, adenitis, sepsis.
Brucellosis (*Brucella abortus, B. suis, B. melitensis, B. ovis, B. canis*)	Cattle, swine, goats, dogs, sheep, and other animals	1. Direct contact with infected tissue. 2. Ingestion of contaminated meat or unpasteurized dairy products. 3. Inhalation of infectious aerosols.	1. Fever of unknown origin: lymphadenopathy and splenomegaly in 10–30% of cases. 2. Relapsing and chronic diseases. 3. Focal infection: osteomyelitis, splenic abscess, endocarditis.
Pasteurellosis (*Pasteurella multocida*)	Cats, dogs, and other domesticated animals and birds	1. Majority of cases occur after animal bites.	1. Focal soft tissue infections (e.g., cellulitis) after animal bite or scratch. 2. Respiratory infections in patients with underlying pulmonary disease (e.g., pneumonia, sinusitis, empyema, bronchitis).
Leptospirosis (*Leptospira canicola, L. icterohaemorrhagiae, L. pomona*, etc.)	Dogs, cattle, swine, rodents, wild mammals, cats	1. Contact with infected animals' urine via water and soil. 2. Direct animal contact.	1. Biphasic illness: Anicteric disease (90% of cases) a. "Septicemic" phase characterized flu-like symptoms. b. "Immune" phase characterized by recurrent fever, severe headache, nausea, vomiting, and splenomegaly. Meningitis common in this phase. 2. Icteric disease (Weils' syndrome): fever, jaundice, hepatorenal failure, hemorrhage, vascular collapse, high mortality.

Rabies	In United States, bats, racoons, skunks most common sources. Outside United States, dogs account for 90% or more of rabies exposures to humans.	1. Bite from infected animals or mucous membrane exposure.
		2. "Nonbite" rabies (inhalation)
		  a. Environment contains high concentration of virus (e.g., caves, laboratories)
		  b. Rare cases after corneal transplants
			1. Four distinct periods (nearly 100% fatal)
			  a. Incubation period 20–90 days.
			  b. Prodrome:
			    a. Nonspecific complaints with fever.
			    b. Pain or paresthesia at site of exposure suggestive.
			  c. Acute neurologic period: Agitation, hydrophobia, aerophobia, seizures, meningeal signs, hallucination.
			  d. Coma

Lymphocytic choriomeningitis	Rodents	1. Aerosols. 2. Direct contact with rodents. 3. Rodent bites.	1. Nonspecific febrile illness, Grippe syndrome. 2. Aseptic meningitis. 3. Focal disease: orchitis, myopericarditis, arthritis.

Listeriosis (*Listeria monocytogenes*)	Almost any animal, including humans, can carry the organism	1. Direct animal contact.
		2. Food-borne transmission.
		3. Transplacental
			1. Nonspecific febrile illness in pregnancy.
			2. Granulomatosis infantiseptica:
			  a. Transplacentally acquired infection.
			  b. Characterized by disseminated abscesses or granulomas in multiple organ systems.
			3. Sepsis of unknown origin: Adults and neonates.
			4. Meningoencephalitis
			5. Focal infection:
			  a. Osteomyelitis/septic arthritis.
			  b. Endocarditis.
			  c. Conjunctivitis.
			  d. Ulcerating skin lesions.
			  e. Cervical adenitis.
			  f. Peritonitis.
			  g. Abscess.

(continued)

Disease (Organism)	Animal Reservoir	Mode of Transmission	Clincal Syndrome
Q-fever (*Coxiella burnetti*)	Most common are cattle, sheep, goats	1. Inhalation of infected aerosols. 2. Ingestion of contaminated dairy products. 3. Direct contact with infected animals or their tissues (especially placentas).	1. Self-limited febrile illness. 2. Atypical pneumonia syndrome. 3. Hepatitis a. May mimic viral hepatitis. b. Granulomatous hepatitis. c. Incidental finding in patients with pneumonia. 4. Endocarditis—chronic Q-fever. a. One of many causes of culture-negative endocarditis. b. Usually involves diseased or prosthetic valves.
Psittacosis (*Chlamydia psittaci*)	Psittacine birds are the major reservoir, but virtually any species of bird may serve as the host	1. Inhalation of infective aerosols of dried excretion. 2. Direct contact with infected tissues, plummage.	1. Atypical pneumonia syndrome: Macular rash, occasional lobar consolidation, splenomegaly (10–70%).
Cysticercosis (*Taenia solium*)	Swine	1. Ingestion of food or water contaminated with human feces containing eggs. 2. Autoinfection from anus to mouth. 3. Reverse peristalsis and internal infection (less likely).	1. Most common clinical manifestation is CNS dysfunction, usually manifested by seizures, headache, hemiparesis, papilledema, or other focal findings. 2. Other manifestations include subcutaneous nodules, ocular cysticercosis, heart block, etc.
Trichinosis (*Trichinella spiralis*)	Swine	1. Ingestion of inadequately processed pork which is infested with cysts.	1. Enteric phase: Diarrhea, nausea, vomiting, abdominal pain resembling acute food poisoning; occasional maculo-papular rash and pneumonitis. 2. Migratory (invasive) phase: a. Severe myalgia. b. Periorbital edema. c. Remittant fever. d. Splinter hemorrhages. e. Conjunctival hemorrhages. 3. Encystment stage: Only in striated muscle 4. Complications: Congestive heart failure and meningoencephalitis.

Disease	Reservoir/Hosts	Transmission	Clinical Features
Echinococcosis (*Echinococcus granulosus, E. multilocularis*)	Dogs definite host; sheep, buffalo, pigs, camels, moose, and deer are intermediate hosts	1. Ingestion of contaminated food/water. 2. Direct contact with contaminated dog feces.	1. After ingestion of the egg, an oncosphere is released, which penetrates the intestinal wall and invades various organs throughout the body, forming hydatid cysts. 2. The organs most commonly involved are the liver (50%) and lungs (40%), but any organ system can be affected. 3. Symptoms can be due to pressure of enlarging cyst (especially in brain, eyes, spinal cord) or to rupture of cyst, causing anaphylactic shock, peritonitis, urticaria, fever. 4. Cysts can be mistaken for tumors or abscesses in the involved organ system. 5. Aspiration of cysts or mechanical/traumatic rupture should be avoided to prevent dissemination of daughter cysts and anaphylaxis.

Toxocariasis (*Toxocara canis*)	Dogs, especially puppies infected in utero	1. Ingestion of soil contaminated with eggs.
		2. Direct contact with puppies.
			1. Visceral larva migrans:
			  a. Due to heavy infection.
			  b. Mainly seen in young children (< 6 years of age).
			  c. Presents with fever, asthma, hepatomegaly most commonly, although other organ systems can also become involved (e.g., CNS, heart, kidney).
			  d. Pathologically, multiple granulomas are sometimes seen surrounding live larvae.
			2. Ocular toxocariasis:
			  a. Seen in older children.
			  b. Presents as a solid mass near the macula. Strabismus is most common presenting symptom.
			  c. Retinal detachment and endophthalmitis also seen.

Occupational Infections

Joseph Bick, M.D.
Stuart Levin, M.D.

Bibliography

Ariza J, Pujol J, Valverde J, et al. Brucellar sacroiliitis: Findings in 63 episodes and current relevance. *CID* 16:761–765, 1993.

Centers for Disease Control. Rabies prevention—United States, 1991. *MMWR* 40:1–19, 1991.

Gold WL, Salit IE. *Aeromonas hydrophila* infections of skin and soft tissue: Report of 11 cases and review. *CID* 16:69–74, 1993.

Jackson LA, Kaufman AF, Adams WG, et al. Outbreak of leptospirosis associated with swimming. *Pediatr Infect Dis J* 12:48–54, 1993.

Staskiewicz J, Lewis CM, Colville J, et al. Outbreak of *Brucella melitensis* among microbiology laboratory workers in a community hospital. *J Clin Microbiol* 29:287–290, 1991.

Winn RE, Anderson J, Piper J, et al. Systemic sporotrichosis treated with itraconazole. *CID* 17:210–217, 1993.

Table 46C-1. Occupational Infections.

Occupation	Organism/Disease	Mechanism of Acquisition
Agricultural Workers		
Dairy farmers	Bovine pustular stomatitis (ORF)	Contact with lesions on cornea/mucous membranes of sheep, goats
	Brucella spp.	Contact with tissue, blood, urine, aborted fetuses, or placentas of sheep, pigs, cattle, goats, dogs; ingestion of milk/dairy products
	Coxiella burnettii (Q fever)	Inhalation of aerosolized placental tissues, birth fluids, or excreta of cattle, sheep, goats, cats
	Milker's nodule virus	Contact with lesions on teets/udders Fecal-oral contact in fields
Field workers	*Ascaris lumbricoides*	Fecal-oral contact in fields fertilized with human feces
	Bacillus anthracis (Anthrax)	Inhalation or cutaneous exposure to fertilizer made from bone meal
	Chromoblastomycoses	Skin inoculation from soil/decaying wood
	Clostridium tetani	Inoculation of spores into skin by puncture would contaminated with soil or feces
	Leptospira spp.	Skin/mucous membrane contact with water, moist soil, or vegetation contaminated with animal urine, direct contact with animals or their urine
	Necator americanus, Ancylostoma duodenale (hookworm)	Skin inoculation with soil or water from fields fertilized with human feces
	Schistosoma spp.	Skin penetration by larval forms in contaminated water
	Sporothrix schenkii	Inoculation into skin by thorn, barb, splinter, handling peat moss
	Yersinia pestis (plague)	Flea bite from rodent or due to handling infected tissues from rodents
	Yersinia tularensis (tularemia)	Inhalation of organisms in dust or drinking water contaminated by rodent blood, urine, or tissue or fly or tick bite from rodents (e.g., skinning rabbits)
Archeologists	*Coccidioides immitis*	Inhalation of spores from soil
	Histoplasma capsulatum	Inhalation of spores from soil
	Cryptococcus neoformans	Inhalation of dust from soil contaminated with bird feces
Athletes	*Microsporum* spp., *Trichophyton* spp. (dermatophytoses)	Contact with contaminated floors, shower stalls, etc.
Butchers	*Bacillus anthracis* (anthrax)	Skin contact with tissue, hair, hide
	Erysipelothrix rhusiopathiae (erysipeloid)	Contact with raw meat/fish

Occupation	Organism/Disease	Mechanism of Acquisition
	Yersinia tularensis (tularemia)	Inoculation of skin, eye, or oropharynx with tissue or blood from wild or domestic animals
Construction/demolition/ excavation Workers	*Clostridium tetani*	Inoculation of spores into skin by puncture wound contaminated with soil or feces
	Coccidioides immitis	Inhalation of spores from soil
	Histoplasma capsulatum	Inhalation of spores from soil
	Cryptococcus neoformans	Inhalation of dust from contaminated soil
Cooks	*Diphyllobothrium latum* (fish tapeworm)	Tasting raw/inadequately cooked fish
	Hepatitis A	Fecal-oral contact, contaminated food
	Salmonella species	Hand-mouth contact with fecally contaminated meat, poultry, eggs, egg products
	Trichinella spiralis	Hand-mouth contact with raw/undercooked meat (especially pork)
Dishwashers/bartenders	*Candida albicans*	Excessive water exposure; predisposition: intertrigo or paronychia
Divers	*Aeromonas*	Skin/wound exposure to contaminated water
	Hepatitis A	Fecal-oral contact in contaminated water
	Mycobacterium marinum (swimming pool granuloma)	Skin wound exposure to contaminated water
	Trichobilharzia spp., *Schistosoma* spp. (swimmer's itch)	Skin contact with fluke in water
	Vibrio spp.	Wound exposure to contaminated seawater
Fishermen, fish handlers	*Erysipelothrix rhusiopathiae* (erysipeloid)	Skin contact with raw seafood
	Mycobacterium marinum (swimming pool granuloma)	Skin contact with contaminated water
Gardener/florists	*Bacillus anthracis* (anthrax)	Inhalation or cutaneous exposure to fertilizer made from bone meal
	Clostridium tetani	Skin inoculation with spores by puncture wound contaminated with soil or feces
	Sporothrix schenkii	Skin inoculation by barb, thorn, splinter, sphagnum moss
Grainery workers	*Aspergillus* spp.	Inhalation of airborne conidia from stored grains, hay
	Rickettsia typhi (murine typhus)	Rat flea bite
Health care workers	See Chapter 53B	
Hunters/trappers/foresters	*Bacillus anthracis* (anthrax)	Skin contact with tissue, hair, hide, inhalation of spores
	Borrelia burgdorferi (Lyme disease)	Tick bite

(continued)

Occupation	Organism/Disease	Mechanism of Acquisition
	Leptospira spp.	Skin/mucous membrane contact with water, moist soil, or vegetation contaminated with urine, direct contact with animals or their urine
	Rabies	Exposure to saliva by bite, scratch, or licking of open skin
	Rickettsia rickettsii (RMSF)	Tick bite
	Trichinella spiralis	Eating raw/undercooked meat (fox, wolf, bear, walrus)
	Yersinia pestis (plague)	Flea bite, handling infected tissues (rodents)
	Yersinia tularensis (tularemia)	Inoculation of skin, eyes, or oropharynx with tissue or blood; inhalation of dust; fly or tick bite
Laboratory workers	See Chapter 53B	
Pet shop workers/ veterinarians/animal handlers	*Bacillus anthracis* (anthrax)	Contact with animal skins, inhalation of spores
	Brucella species	Contact with tissues, blood, urine, aborted fetuses, or placentas; inhalation in stables (cattle, sheep, pigs, goats, dogs)
	Afipia felis (cat scratch bacillus)	Lick, bite, or scratch (usually cat)
	Coxiella burnetii (Q-fever)	Aerosolization of placental tissues, birth fluids, excreta of infected animals, direct contact with animals (cattle, sheep, goats, cats)
	Cryptosporidium species	Hand-mouth contamination with feces
	Dirofilaria immitis (dog heart worm)	Mosquito bite
	Echinococcus spp.	Hand-mouth contact with dog feces
	Erysipethrix rhusiopathiae (erysipeloid)	Skin contact
	Leptospira spp.	Skin or mucous membrane contact with animals or urine
	Pasteurella multocida (cellulitis)	Cat bite
	Campylobacter spp. (DFF-2) (bacteremia)	Dog bite
	Rabies virus	Exposure to saliva by bite, scratch, or licking of open skin
	Salmonella spp.,	Hand-mouth contact with feces from dogs, cats, birds, turtles; animal feeds
	Toxoplasma gondii	Fecal-oral (cat)
Prison workers	*Mycobacterium tuberculosis*	Inhalation of aerosolized droplets
Poultry handlers	*Chlamydia psittaci* (psittacosis)	Inhalation of desiccated bird droppings, direct contact with turkeys, ducks, geese, squab
	Erysipelothrix rhusiopathiae	Skin contact with meat
	New Castle disease	Inoculation of conjunctiva
	Salmonella spp.	Hand-mouth contact with fecally contaminated poultry, eggs, egg products, animal feeds

Occupation	Organism/Disease	Mechanism of Acquisition
Ranchers/shepherds	Bovine pustular stomatitis (ORF)	Contact with mucous membranes, lesions on udders (sheep, goats, reindeer)
	Coxiella burnetii (Q-fever)	Aerosolization of placental tissues, birth fluids, and excreta, contact with animals
	Cryptosporidium spp.	Hand-mouth contamination with animal feces
	Echinococcus spp.	Hand-mouth contact with dog feces, ingestion in fecally contaminated food or water
	Rabies virus	Exposure to saliva by bite, scratch, or licking of open skin
	Rickettsia rickettsii (RMSF)	Tick bite
	Yersinia tularensis (tularemia)	Inoculation of skin, eyes, or oropharynx with tissue or blood, inhalation of dust, tick bite
Sewer workers	*Leptospira* spp.	Skin or mucous membrane contact with water, moist soil, or vegetation contaminated with urine, contact with animals or urine
	Necator americanus, Ancylostoma duodenale (hookworm)	Skin penetration during exposure to soil/water
Spelunkers	*Histoplasma capsulatum*	Inhalation of spores
	Rabies	Exposure to saliva of bats by bite, scratch, or licking of open skin
Slaughterhouse workers, meat packers	*Brucella* spp.	Contact with tissues, blood, urine, aborted fetuses, placentas (sheep, pigs, cattle, goats)
	Coxiella burnetii (Q-fever)	Aerosolization of placental tissues, excreta, contact with animals (cattle, sheep, goats, cats)
	Erysipelothrix rhusiopathiae (erysipeloid)	Skin contact with infected meat
Weavers, wool and hide handlers	*Bacillus anthracis* (anthrax)	Skin contact with tissues, hair, wool, hides, or their products, inhalation of spores
	Brucella spp.	Contact with tissues, blood, urine, aborted fetuses, or placentas, inhalation in stables
	Coxiella burnetii (Q-fever)	Aerosolization of placental tissues, birth fluids, or excreta, contact with animals (cattle, sheep, goats)

Food Poisonings

Larry J. Goodman, M.D.

Bibliography

Centers for Disease Control. Viral agents of gastroenteritis: Public health importance and outbreak management. *MMWR* 39 April (No. RR-5), 1990.

Centers for Disease Control. CDC surveillance summaries. *MMWR* 39 (No. SS-1), March 1990.

Table 46D-1. Vehicle, Clinical Symptoms/Findings, and Diagnosis of Selected* Foodborne Poisons

Syndrome	Vehicle	Incubation Period	Symptoms	Duration	Diagnosis
Scombroid (histamine fish poisoning)	Tuna, mackeral yellowjack, bluefish, mahi mahi	<1 hr	Flushing, headache, dizziness, cramps, and occasional diarrhea	Hours	Histamine level of 100 mg in 100 g of fish flesh
Ciguatera	Sea bass, grouper, snapper, amberjack	1–6 hr	Paresthesias, temperature dysesthesias, abdominal pain, weakness, headache	Days–months	Clinical syndrome, ciguatoxin isolation from fish
Paralytic shellfish poisoning	Mussel, clam, scallop	<1 hr	Paresthesias, ataxia, vertigo, paralysis, cranial nerve palsy	Hours–days	Clinical syndrome, identification of the toxin (saxitoxin) in molluscs
Neurotoxic shellfish poisoning	Mussels and clams	<3 hr	Paresthesias, ataxia, vertigo	Hours–days	Clinical syndrome, identification of the toxin in molluscs
Amnesiac shellfish poisoning	Mussels	<48 hr	Diarrhea, abdominal pain, headache, loss of short-term memory, seizures	Hours–years	Domoic acid isolated from mussels
Puffer fish poisoning	Puffer fish	Hours	Lethargy, nausea and vomiting, paresthesias, hypotension, bradycardia, paralysis	Hours–days	Tetrodotoxin isolation
Botulism	Home-canned foods, occasional commercial food outbreaks	12–48 hr	Nausea, vomiting, diarrhea, urinary retention, dilated pupils, ptosis, cranial nerve palsies	Weeks–months	Identification of *Clostridium botulinum* from stool, food, or one of the toxins (usually A, D, or E) from serum, stool, or food

*A foodborne illness is defined as the development of gastrointestinal or neurological symptoms in 2 or more people after a common meal. (See Ch 48G for a discussion of diarrheal pathogens).

Waterborne Skin, Soft Tissue, and Systemic Infections

Jeffery Semel, M.D.

Bibliography

Blacklow NR, Greenberg HB. Viral gastroenteritis. *N Engl J Med* 325:252–362, 1991.

Craun GF. Waterborne giardiasis in the United States: A review. *Am J Public Health* 69:817–819, 1979.

Fang GD, Uy VL, Vickers RM. Disease due to Legionellaceae (other than *L. pneumophila*). Historical, microbiological, clinical, and epidemiological review. *Medicine* 68:116–131, 1989.

Guerrant RL, Bobak DA. Bacterial and protozoal gastroenteritis. *N Engl J Med* 325:327–340, 1991.

Ma P, Visvesvara GS, Martinez AJ, et al. *Naegleria* and *Acanthamoeba* infections: Review. *Rev Infect Dis* 12:490–512, 1990.

Maki DG. Infections due to infusion therapy, in Bennett JV (ed): *Hospital Infections*, ed. 2. Boston, Little, Brown, 1986, pp 561–580.

Pitlik S, Berger SA, Huminer D. Non-enteric infections acquired through contact with water. *Rev Infect Dis* 9:54–63, 1987.

Ramia S. Transmission of viral infections by the water route: Implications for developing countries. *Rev Infect Dis* 7:180–188, 1985.

Rhame FS. The inanimate environment, in Bennett JV (ed): *Hospital Infections*, ed. 2. Boston, Little, Brown, 1986, pp 223–250.

Snyder MB, Siwicki M, Wireman J, et al. Reduction in *L. pneumophila* through heat flushing followed by continuous supplemental chlorination of hospital hot water. *J Infect Dis* 162:127–132, 1990.

Table 46E-1. Waterborne Nosocomial Infections

Organism(s)	Type of Infection	Mode of Transmission	Author/(Year)
Pseudomonas cepacia	Bloodstream	Water bath/thaw cryoprecipitate	Rhame (1979)
Enterobacter sp.	Bloodstream	Contaminated dextrose-containing infusate	Maki (1976)
P. cepacia	Bloodstream	Distilled water used to flush blood gas analyzer	Henderson (1988)
Flavobacterium meningosepticum	Meningitis	Environmental colonization of nursery	Thong (1981)
Legionella micdadei	Pneumonia	Nebulizer used in respiratory therapy	Gorman (1980)
Acinetobacter sp.	Pneumonia, bloodstream	Aerosol from room humidifier	Smith (1977)
Legionella sp.	Postoperative sternal wound	Exposure to tap water	Lowry (1991)
Mycobacterium fortuitum	Sternal wound, endocarditis	Cold water bath for cardioplegia	Kuritsky (1983)

468

Table 46-2. Diagnostic/Therapeutic Considerations—Waterborne Infections

Primary Organ System	Agent	Incubation Period	Salient Clinical Features	Diagnosis	Therapy
Enteric	Norwalk and related viruses	1–2 days	Nausea, vomiting, myalgia, diarrhea of 24- to 48-hr duration	Electron microscopy	Supportive
	Hepatitis A	15–45 days	Hepatitis	Serology	Supportive
	Vibrio cholera	1–3 days	Diarrhea, dehydration	Culture	Rehydration, tetracycline
	Salmonella typhi	10–14 days	Enteric fever, abdominal pain, gastrointestinal (GI) bleeding, perforation	Culture of blood, stool, bone marrow	Ampicillin, chloramphenicol, quinolones
	Giardia lamblia	7–14 days	Bloating, diarrhea, weight loss	Light microscopic examination of stool	Metronidazole, quinacrine
	Cryptosporidium sp.	2–14 days	Similar to those of Giardia	Light microscopic examination of stool	Supportive
Cutaneous	Aeromonas hydrophila, Plesiomonas shigelloides, Edwardsiella tarda	1–3 days	Wound infection after freshwater trauma, often involves the tendon, muscle, ligament. Also occult GI pathogen.	Culture	Imipenem, ampicillin/sulbactam
	Vibrio vulnificus, aglynolyticus	1–3 days	Wound infection after saltwater trauma. Secondary bullous and hemorrhagic cutaneous lesions. Liver disease predisposes patient to infection. May also be acquired by ingestion.	Culture of wound and blood	Tetracycline, chloramphenicol
	Pseudomonas aeruginosa	1–3 days	"Hot tub folliculitis" of aprocrine sweat glands: axillary, inguinal, breast	Culture	Quinolone
	Mycobacterium marinum	2–8 weeks	Enlarging papule (usually on the hand); spread via lymph glands or along tendon sheaths	Culture	Ethambutol, rifampin

(continued)

Table 46-2. Continued

Primary Organ System	Agent	Incubation Period	Salient Clinical Features	Diagnosis	Therapy
	Schistosoma sp.	4–8 weeks	Swimmer's itch; Katayama fever; chronic intestinal, liver, bladder infection	Histology, light microscopic examination of stool (searching for eggs)	Praziquantel
Central nervous system	*Leptospira* sp.	7–12 days	First phase is influenza-like, conjunctivitis; second phase, "immune": meningitis, rash, hepatitis, renal	Culture, serology	Penicillin, tetracycline
	Enterovirus (echo, coxsackie, polio), ameba	Variable	Aseptic meningitis, cardiac, pleural	Culture	Supportive
	Naegleria fowleri	2–5 days	Acute meningitis	Wet mount examination of cerebrospinal fluid	Amphotericin B
	Acanthamoeba sp.	?	Granulomatous amebic encephalitis (GAE), with or without skin or pulmonary lesions; patient usually immunocompromised; amebic keratitis	Histology	?
				Histology, culture	Topical miconazole, propamidine, debridement
Respiratory	*Legionella* sp.	2–10 days	Early toxicity with minimal cough, diarrhea, mental status change; increased risk in immunocompromised patients; progressive multilobar infiltrate	Culture, serology, direct fluorescent antibody	Erythromycin, tetracycline
	Atypical mycobacteria	Variable	Pulmonary, skin, nosocomial	Culture	Variable

Fulminant Skin/Soft Tissue Infection

Jeffery Semel, M.D.

Community Acquired Skin and Soft Tissue Infections

I. Problems

Infections of the skin and skin structures vary from localized processes such as impetigo or furunculosis to rapidly progressive soft tissue infections such as cellulitis or fasciitis. Localized soft tissue infections may be associated with systemic manifestations via toxin production (e.g., toxic shock syndrome).

II. Differential Diagnosis

A. *Impetigo* is a superficial bacterial infection (group A β-hemolytic streptococcus, *Staphylococcus aureus*), usually vesicular or pustular, often with a thin amber crust. Impetigo is seen most often in children, frequently in the summer.

B. *Cellulitis* (sometimes referred to as *erysipelas*) is an infection of the skin and/or subcutaneous structures (group A β-hemolytic streptococcus, *S. aureus* enterobacteriaceae, *Pseudomonas ceruginosa*, anaerobes, often polymicrobial, aeromonas sp., vibrio sp., *Pasteurella multocida*). Cellulitis may occur anywhere on the body but is most often seen on the extremities (lower > upper) or face. Typically, examination reveals a homogeneous area of erythema varying in color from pink to deep purple. Purulence is generally minimal but may occur at the portal of entry. Later, blister formation may occur. Streaks of lymphangitis may be present proximal to the involved area.

C. *Necrotizing fasciitis* is a severe infection of the subcutaneous superficial and/or deep fascia (anaerobes with or without streptococci and Enterobactericaea or group A β-hemolytic streptococcus, with or without *S. aureus*). Any body part may be involved, although the leg, groin, and abdominal wall are most frequently affected. Pain is usually prominent initially. Examination shows erythema, induration, a lack of sharply demarcated borders, and tenderness. Over time, the involved area may turn brown or gray and become anesthetic. Blisters or cutaneous gangrene may occur in some areas. Crepitance may be present when anaerobic or facultative bacteria are involved. Necrotizing fasciitis occurring around the male genital organs is termed *Fournier's gangrene*. This latter disease usually begins in the scrotum and may progress to the perineum and the abdominal wall.

D. *Clostridial myonecrosis* is caused by gram-positive, anaerobic bacteria (*Clostridium perfringes, septicum, hemolytium, novi*), which are found naturally in soil as well as in the normal intestinal and genitourinary flora of animals. Over 60 species of clostridia exist. *C. perfringens* is the best-known and most frequently isolated strain of *Clostridium*. Clostridial soft tissue infections vary in severity. Clostridia are often found as part of the polymicrobial flora of decubitus ulcers or lower extremity infections in patients with diabetes or peripheral vascular insufficiency. *Clostridium* species have also been associated with crepitant cellulitis. In this condition there is abundant gas formation in the soft tissues, but minimal pain and toxicity, and progression is not rapid. In clostridial myonecrosis (gas gangrene), progression may be fulminant. The incubation period is usually 1 to 4 days but may be as short as a few hours. Pain is the first symptom. Initially, examination shows pallor, edema, and tenderness. Crepitation is present. Later, the wound assumes a bronze or magenta color. A thin, brown discharge witha "sweet odor" may weep from bullae andblisters. Progressive gangrene occurs, and systemic toxicity is common (septic shock,intravascular hemolysis due to clostridial α-hemolysin).

E. *Toxic shock syndrome* (TSS) is a rapidly progressive, multisystem disorder caused by toxin(s) elaborated by *S aureus* (SA). Toxic shock toxin 1 (TSST-1), an exoprotein, and enterotoxins A, B, C, D, and E have been found to be elaborated by strains of SA isolated from patients with TSS. In 1980, large numbers of female patients with TSS were described. This condition was later found to be associated with the use of hyperabsorbable tampons during menstruation. The subsequent removal of these tampons from the market led to a decrease in the number of menstruation-associated cases and to the awareness that TSS may occur in a wide variety of SA infections (the local site of SA infection is often inconspicuous). The onset of TSS is generally abrupt. Initial symptoms include high fever, myalgias, vomiting, and diarrhea. The hallmarks of TSS are hypotension and a desquamating skin rash. A diffuse, erythematous rash develops which is often described as a "sunburn." Seven to 10 days later, the involved areas desquamate, especially the palms and soles. In addition, there may be oral, conjunctival, and vaginal hyperemia. Laboratory abnormalities include leukocytosis (with immature white blood cells), thrombocytopenia, abnormal urinary sediment and azotemia, abnormal liver function tests, elevated creatinine phosphokinase (CPK), and hypocalcemia. There are five major criteria for the diagnosis of TSS:

1. Temperature > 38.9°C.
2. Systolic blood pressure < 90 mmHg.
3. Rash with subsequent desquamation.
4. Involvement of three or more organ systems (gastrointestinal, muscular, mucous membranes, renal, liver, blood central nervous system).
5. Other diseases are excluded.

When desquamation occurs, three criteria are necessary for diagnosis. Serum antibody production against the offending TSS toxin has been shown to be deficient in many cases and may help to explain the development of recurrent TSS in some patients. The differential diagnosis includes scarlet fever or streptococcal toxic shock, Kawasaki syndrome (especially if the patient is < 2 years old), rickettsial infection, measles, and leptospirosis.

III. **Diagnostic/Therapeutic Approach**

A. An initial diagnostic impression is formed after evaluation of the history and physical examination. Predisposing conditions; the appearance and location of the infection; presence or absence of purulence, crepitation, or lymphangitis; and exposure to water or soil are examples of factors that are helpful in determining the etiology.

B. Initial broad-spectrum therapy may be necessary until the exact microbial etiology can be determined.

C. In cellulitis, isolation of an organism may be difficult. Aspiration of the area of cellulitis itself has a very low microbiologic yield. Crusted lesions, furuncles, blisters, and subcutaneous abscesses, however, should be looked for and, if found, drained and sent for Gram's stain and culture.

D. For cellulitis, surgical intervention is ordinarily not required unless complications such as myonecrosis or fasciitis occur.

E. In clostridial myonecrosis, the presence of gas can be confirmed by soft tissue radiography and further defined, if necessary, by computed tomography. Gram's stain of purulent material reveals "boxcar"-shaped, gram-positive rods, absence of spores (in *C. perfringens* infections), and few white blood cells. Prompt surgical intervention is essential to halt the progress of the infection. At surgery, myonecrosis may be confirmed by the finding of pale tissue which fails to bleed. Wide excision of all necrotic tissue must be performed, with healthy tissue margins achieved. The use of hyperbaric oxygen as an adjunctive form of therapy has been advocated by some, though its efficacy is still unproven. The use of this modality should not delay surgical therapy.

F. Hemodynamic monitoring is essential in the management of TSS. A decrease in systemic vascular resistance and leakage of fluid out the intravascular space will occur in severe cases. Adequate intravenous fluids must be provided. Cultures should be obtained from blood, mucous membranes, and any clinically relevant area or wound. Any vaginal tampon, contraceptive device, or wound packing should be removed and cultured. Sutures should be removed or loosened from any suspected surgical site.

Bibliography

Broome CV. Epidemiology of toxic shock syndrome in the United States. *Rev Infect Dis* 11:S14–S21, 1989.

Chesney JP. Clinical aspects and spectrum of illness of toxic shock syndrome. *Rev Infect Dis* 11:S1–S7, 1989.

Klontz KC, Lieb S, Schreiber M, et al. Syndromes of *Vibrio vulnificus* infections. Clinical and epidemiological features in Florida cases, 1981–1987. *Ann Intern Med* 109:318–323, 1988.

Peter G, Smith AL. Group A streptococcal infections of the skin and pharynx. *N Engl J Med* 297:311–317, 365–370, 1977.

Schlivert PM. Role of TSST-1 in TSS: Overview. *Rev Infect Dis* 11:S107–109, 1989.

Semel JD, Trenholme GM. *Aeromonas hydrophila* water-associated traumatic wound infections: A review. *J Trauma* 30:324–327, 1990.

Stevens DL, Tanner MH, Winship J, et al. Severe group A streptococcal infections associated with a toxic shock-like syndrome and scarlet fever toxin A. *N Engl J Med* 321:1–7, 1989.

Styrt B, Gorbach SL. Recent developments in the understanding of the pathogenesis and treatment of anaerobic infections. *N Engl J Med* 321:240–246, 298–302, 1989.

Weinstein L, Barza M. Gas gangrene. *N Engl J Med* 289:1129–1134, 1973.

Approach to the Patient with Fever, Pain in the Mouth or Throat, and Stridor

Larry J. Goodman, M.D.

I. **Problems**

Infections involving the mouth or throat are extremely common and typically benign. Rarely, complications of these common processes can lead to rapidly progressive, life-threatening syndromes. These conditions are characterized by local pain and combinations of dysphonia, dysphagia, dysphagia, trismus, and inspiratory stridor.

II. **Differential Points of Selected Syndromes** (Table 47B-1)

A. Peritonsillar abscess may mimic accute mononucleosis.

B. Diphtheria is included in the differential diagnosis of a pustular pharyngitis (e.g., group A *Streptococcus*, acute mononucleosis, gonorrhea, adenovirus).

C. Tetanus, strychnine poisoning, and phenothiazine reactions each may present with similar findings.

III. **Diagnostic/Therapeutic Approach**

A. In each of these syndromes, airway assessment and management is the primary concern. Antibiotics are an important adjunct to treatment of these syndromes. Antimicrobial therapy should be directed against the most common etiologic organisms (Table 47B-1). In the neutropenic host, fungi may also be among the etiological agents for each of these processes except the toxin-mediated ones.

B. Surgical drainage is usually not necessary in Ludwig's angina or peritonsillar abscess.

C. Retropharyngeal abscess often requires careful suction drainage.

D. Antitoxins should be administered for the toxin-mediated processes.

1. Diphtheria antitoxin (DAT) and botulinium antitoxin are made of equine hyperimmune serum. From 10% to 20% of persons may be allergic to horse protein. All individuals should be questioned concerning known allergies and tested with a diluted test dose (e.g., 1:10 dilution DAT on the conjunctiva). For botulism, polyvalent antitoxin (A, B, E) should be used unless the toxin type is known.

2. Tetanus immune globulin is produced from human serum.

E. Patients with tetanus and diphtheria should also receive a primary vaccination series since these infections are not immunogenic.

Table 47B-1. Emergency Syndromes Presenting with Head and Neck Symptoms

Syndrome	Etiology/Organisms	History/Symptoms	Physical Examination	Complications
Ludwig's angina	Mixed infection, mouth flora	Poor dentition or recent tooth extraction	Fever, involvement of sublingual and submandibular spaces, trismus, drooling, and strider (late)	Swelling of involved space(s) leading to airway obstruction
Peritonisllar abscess	Group A streptoccus, anaerobes, *Eikenella corrodens*, diptheria	Throat pain and dysphagia	Tonsillar swelling with one tonsil near the midline	May track to the mediastinum and/or pericardium; less commonly to the lateral neck
Retropharyngeal abscess	Mixed infection, *Staphylococcus* spp.	Fever and neck pain	Tonsils usually normal; trismus; abscess bulges toward mouth and may be difficult to detect on examination	Rupture of abscess into airway or penetration inferiorly (mediastinum) or posteriorly (base of brain)
Epiglottitis	*Haemophilus influenzae* (rarely, *Streptococcus pneumoniae* or fungi in compromised host)	More common and more serious in children; fever and dysphagia	Fever and epiglottal swelling	Airway obstruction
Diphtheria	*Corynebacterium diphtheria* (toxin)	Unvaccinated patient	Pharyngitis with rapid accumulation of pus (over hours) and development of gray pseudomembrane	Airway obstruction, distant effect(s) of the toxin (palsies and cardiac abnormalities)
Tetanus	*Clostridium tetanui* (toxin)	Unvaccinated (or no recent booster) and tetanus-prone injury	Trismus, dysphagia, and posterior neck pain are early findings	Generalized tetanus
Botulism	*Cl. botulinum* (toxin)	Ingestion of home-canned food or other contaminated foodstuff	Dry throat, dysphonia, dysphagia, diplopia, and dilated pupils	Other cranial nerve palsies and/or ascending paralysis

Bibliography

deMarie S, Tjon A, Tham RTO, et al. Clinical infection and non-surgical treatment of parapharyngeal space infections complicating throat infections. *Rev Infect Dis* 6:975–982, 1989.

Levin S, Goodman LG, Fuhrer J. Fulminant community-acquired infectious diseases: Diagnostic problems. *Med Clin North Am* 70(5):967–986, 1986.

Wolf M, Strauss B, Kronenberg J, et al. Conservative management of adult epiglottitis. *Laryngoscope* 100:183–185, 1990.

Overwhelming Pneumonia

John Segreti, M.D.

I. **Definition**
Community-acquired pneumonia resulting in acute respiratory failure.

II. **Pathophysiology**
   A. Diffuse pulmonary infection resulting in increased permeability of alveolocapillary membranes and noncardiogenic pulmonary edema.
   B. Localized pneumonia with sepsis related to bacteremia or indirect activation of mediators of inflammation (e.g., tumor necrosis factor [TNF], interleukin-2 [IL-2], etc.) leading to acute respiratory distress syndrome (ARDS) (Figure 47C-1).

III. **Clinical Presentation**
   A. Tachypnea and dyspnea association with hypoxemia, hypocapnia, and a widened alveolar-arterial oxygen gradient seen in patients with respiratory failure.
   B. Fever, chills, tachycardia, and mental status changes may also be seen.
   C. Leukocytosis with immature forms is most common, but leukopenia and normal counts are also possible.

D. Disseminated intravascular coagulation (DIC), metabolic acidosis, and renal failure may be seen.
E. Chest radiograph shows diffuse interstitial and/or alveolar infiltrate.

IV. **Infectious Etiologies**
   A. Viruses
      1. Primary influenzae A and B
      2. Adenoviruses.
      3. Respiratory syncytial virus.
      4. Measles virus (rubella).
      5. Varicella.
      6. Herpes simplex virus (HSV).
   B. Bacteria
      1. *Streptococcus pneumoniae.*
      2. Mycoplasma pneumonia.
      3. Anaerobic necrotizing pneumonia.
      4. Group A streptococci (*Streptococcus pyogenes*).
      5. Legionellosis.
      6. Melioidosis (*Pseudomonas pseudomallei*).
      7. Plague (*Yersinia pestis*).
      8. Tularemia.
      9. Miliary tuberculosis.

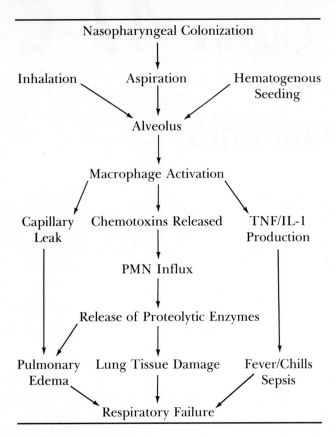

Figure 47C-1 Pathophysiology of overwhelming community-acquired pneumonias.

C. Fungi
   1. *Histoplasmosis capsulatum.*
   2. *Coccidioides immitis.*
   3. *Blastomyces dermatitidis*
D. Parasites
   1. *Pneumocystis carinii.*
   2. *Strongyloides stercoralis.*
V. Differential Diagnoses
   A. ARDS related to noninfectious etiology (drowning, cardiovascular accident, hemorrhagic pancreatitis, etc.).
   B. Massive pulmonary emboli.
   C. Hypersensitivity pneumonitis.
   D. Lymphatic spread of tumor.
   E. Vasculitis/autoimmune disease.
   F. Intrapulmonary hemorrhage.

Bibliography

Segreti J, Bone RC. Overwhelming pneumonia. *Disease-a-Month* 33:1–59, 1987.

CHAPTER 48-A

Fever of Undetermined Origin

Mary K. Hayden, M.D.
Stuart Levin, M.D.

I. **Definition**

In their classic article on the subject, Petersdorf and Beeson defined fever of unknown origin (FUO) as an illness of greater than 3 weeks' duration with a temperature higher than 101°F (38.3°C) on several occasions and an uncertain diagnosis after 1 week of study in the hospital. Today it is reasonable to consider a patient to have FUO after some period of intensive outpatient evaluation. This definition is useful in helping to eliminate acute self-limited infections and febrile illnesses of obvious cause, which have a different differential diagnosis and approach.

II. **Differential Diagnosis**

A. Most FUOs are uncommon presentations of common diseases.

B. Infection (22–40%)

1. Abscess is one of the most frequently identified infectious processes producing FUO. Sites include intra-abdominal, hepatic, subphrenic, paraovarian, and prostatic locations. Dental and brain abscesses are less frequent causes.

2. Biliary tract infection has been implicated, including ascending cholangitis, frank empyema of the gallbladder, and infection of the pancreatic duct. Localized pain and tenderness can be absent, and liver function tests may be normal.

3. Subacute bacterial endocarditis (SBE) can produce FUO, although the proportion of cases of SBE in more recent reviews has diminished. A heart murmur may not be heard. Blood cultures can be negative if the causative organism is fastidious or slow-growing or if the patient received prior antibiotic therapy. Other intravascular sources of infection include bacterial mycotic aneurysm and septic thrombophlebitis.

4. Osteomyelitis, in particular vertebral, maxillary, or mandibular bone infection, can present with few symptoms other than fever.

5. Bacterial infection of the renal parenchyma rarely causes FUO, as it is usually detected easily in the urine. However, perinephric abscess may cause bacteriuria intermittently or not at all. Anatomic abnormalities of the kidney may lead to obstruction and prolonged fevers.

6. Extrapulmonary and miliary tuberculosis are common causes of FUO; some studies

have found *Mycobacterium tuberculosis* to be the microorganism most often isolated from patients with FUO. The chest x-ray can be normal and the purified protein derivative (PPD) test nonreactive.

7. Miscellaneous infectious causes include bacterial sinusitis and virus-related subacute thyroiditis. Numerous infections with intracellular pathogens such as brucellosis, toxoplasmosis, malaria, disseminated histoplasmosis, candidiasis, and psittacosis can cause FUO. Typhoid fever occasionally presents with fever alone. Elderly patients with cytomegalovirus (CMV) or Epstein-Barr virus (EBV) infection may not manifest pharyngitis or lymphadenopathy. Other infections considered in the differential diagnosis but rarely seen include bartonellosis, listeriosis, "relapsing fever" due to *Borrelia* species, visceral leishmaniasis, and Whipple's disease.

C. Neoplasm (15–31%)

1. Hodgkin's disease and non-Hodgkin's lymphoma are the most frequent malignancies identified in association with FUO. Peripheral lymphadenopathy can be absent. Pel Ebstein fever is seen in fewer than half of the patients with Hodgkin's disease and can be seen in other febrile disorders. Aleukemic and preleukemic leukemia, especially monocytic, can occasionally present as FUO, as can sarcoma, malignant histiocytosis, and angioimmunoblastic lymphadenopathy.

2. The solid tumors most commonly associated with FUO are renal cell and hepatocellular carcinoma, with adenocarcinoma of the breast, colon, stomach, and disseminated carcinomatosis occasionally being found.

D. Collagen vascular disease (9–18%)

1. In older studies, systemic lupus erythematosus (SLE), acute rheumatic fever, and rheumatoid arthritis (RA) were common, but more recently, Still's disease and polyarteritis nodosum have been more frequently reported. Temporal arteritis, with or without polymyalgia rheumatica, should be considered in patients older than 60 years of age with FUO. Wegener's granulomatosis, systemic vasculitis, and hypersensitivity angiitis have also been identified as causes.

E. Drug fever

1. Most drugs, including many antibiotics and some nonsteroidal anti-inflammatory agents, have been implicated as causes of fever and can sometimes cause FUO. Rash and eosinophilia are each seen in only about 20% of cases. The time to resolution of the fever after discontinuation of the drug is dependent upon the drug's half-life.

F. Occupational causes

1. "Monday morning fever" is an idiosyncratic reaction to metal fumes resulting in fever, chills, pulmonary symptoms, and leukocytosis. It usually occurs after a worker is reexposed to the causative environment after an absence of ≥24 hr. "Polymer fume fever" is a similar syndrome.

G. Factitious fever

1. This occurs when a patient fabricates fever by manipulating a thermometer. The person usually appears well. A variant of this condition is seen in a patient who injects or consumes foreign material which produces fever. This diagnosis is classically made in a young female health care worker with FUO and is almost never seen in the elderly.

H. Miscellaneous causes

1. Granulomatous causes of FUO include sarcoidosis, granulomatous hepatitis, and idiopathic granulomatosis. Inflammatory bowel disease, tropical sprue, dissecting aneurysm, thrombophlebitis, retroperitoneal hematoma, and pulmonary embolism all occasionally cause FUO. Familial etiologies include familial Mediterranean fever, periodic fever, and Fabry's disease. Thyrotoxicosis, Addison's disease, and abnormally elevated progesterone levels are endocrine etiologies of FUO.

I. Prolonged FUO

1. One study of 347 patients who had FUO for more than 6 months reported that 27% had no fever documented during a 2-week hospital stay. Granulomatous hepatitis, malignancy, Still's disease, and infection were the most frequently identified causes.

III. **History and Physical Examination**

A. Document that fever exists.

B. The pattern of fever is usually not helpful, with a few exceptions including tertian and quartan fever seen in malaria, the fever seen every 21 days in cyclic neutropenia, and fever occurring on alternate days in a patient receiving alternate-day steroid therapy.

C. Any clinical, laboratory, or radiologic abnormality noted during the evaluation should be aggressively pursued and the standard systematic investigation abandoned. ("Go where the money is.")

D. A careful, complete history is important to obtain clues to the diagnosis and to direct the evaluation. Symptoms which may be transient, such as rashes and hematuria, should be sought. Occupational exposure, travel, pets, medications, and infectious contacts are all important. If the initial history is unrevealing, serial interviews should be obtained.

E. A thorough physical exam is mandatory and should be repeated at regular intervals during the evaluation. Areas of special concern include the following:

1. Skin. Particular attention should be paid to nail beds, skin folds, scrotum, scalp, and the area under the breasts. Look for peripheral stigmata of SBE, rashes which may be evanescent, and lesions which can be biopsied.

2. Lymph nodes. Biopsy of enlarged or otherwise abnormal nodes may provide a diagnosis.

3. Teeth. Examine for the presence of an abscess or for periodontal disease, which is a risk factor for endocarditis.

4. Cardiac exam. Murmurs associated with SBE can be intermittent or inaudible, especially in right-sided infection.

5. Abdomen. Tenderness, masses, and organomegaly should be sought.

6. Rectal and prostate or pelvic exams should be performed to evaluate for a tumor or an occult abscess.

7. Ophthalmologic exam. All patients should receive a complete evaluation, including fundoscopic and slit lamp exams, to look for corneal, conjunctival, uveal tract, and retinal lesions which might provide a clue to a systemic illness.

IV. **Diagnostic Tests**

A. Abnormalities discovered in routine hematologic and biochemical studies can be useful guides for further evaluation but are not usually diagnostic.

B. Serologic studies can be suggestive or even diagnostic of some infectious diseases, including CMV, EBV, toxoplasmosis, psittacosis, leptospirosis, brucellosis, and Lyme disease.

Because of the low specificity of some of these tests, they should be sent when there is clinical or laboratory evidence of a particular illness, rather than as screening studies. Serum should be obtained at the time of the patient's first evaluation and saved as an early or acute-phase sample. This can be studied later if information emerges which implicates a disease not initially considered. Titers should be repeated at intervals to look for a rise.

C. Culture of blood, urine, other relevant and available body fluids, and biopsy material should be sent for aerobic, anaerobic, fungal, mycobacterial, or viral culture as indicated by the clinical picture. Up to six specimens of blood should be collected over several days to look for low-grade bacteremia or fungemia. The microbiology laboratory should be informed if a slow-growing or fastidious organism is suspected so that appropriate modifications of the usual isolation protocol can be made if necessary.

D. Except for a PPD, skin tests for microorganisms are generally not helpful. The patient's ability to form delayed-type hypersensitivity reactions should be evaluated concomitantly so that a negative PPD can be properly interpreted.

E. Most collagen vascular diseases which may involve fever and for which accurate serologic tests exist, such as SLE and RA, no longer commonly cause FUO. Therefore, screening batteries of tests for autoantibodies are frequently low in yield. However, as with serology for infections, they can be diagnostic in the appropriate clinical setting. A nonspecific abnormality of complement or rheumatoid factor may provide a clue to a disease such as SBE or vasculitis.

F. Acute-phase reactants such as the sedimentation rate, C-reactive protein, fibrinogen, haptoglobin, and other β_2-globulins are often nonspecifically elevated in patients with FUO and so are of limited utility. In addition, they may be low or normal in a patient with a serious cause of FUO.

G. Radiologic exams

1. The tests to be performed and the order in which to perform them should be dictated by the clinical scenario. All can give false-positive or false-negative results.

2. Plain x-rays. Repeating a chest x-ray which was found to be normal early in the evaluation of FUO may be helpful in detecting a

slowly evolving pulmonary process. Dental and sinus x-rays can diagnose infection in these areas.

3. Computed tomography (CT) scanning can reveal an intra-abdominal, subphrenic, hepatic, pancreatic, or prostatic abscess or retroperitoneal pathology. Enlarged lymph nodes in the chest or abdomen can sometimes be seen. Hepatosplenomegaly which is not clinically evident can be detected, although this finding is often nonspecific.

4. Ultrasonography is particularly useful in identifying biliary or urinary tract disease. Echocardiography can visualize valvular vegetations and atrial tumors. Transesophageal echocardiography may be particularly useful to evaluate structures not easily seen by standard two-dimensional echocardiography.

5. Radionuclide scanning. ^{99m}Tc sulfur colloid scanning of the liver and spleen has been useful in diagnosing liver and splenic abnormalities. Whole-body gallium citrate (^{67}Ga) and ^{111}In granulocyte scans can localize abscesses, some lymphomas, and other neoplasms. Bone scans are sensitive means of identifying osteomyelitis and osteoblastic bone tumors.

H. Invasive procedures

1. If noninvasive evaluation has not led to a diagnosis, percutaneous liver or bone marrow biopsy may be diagnostic, even without evidence of disease in these organs. However, hepatic or bone marrow granulomas can be formed in a multitude of disorders, including hypersensitivity reactions, collagen vascular diseases, and infections, so this finding is nonspecific.

2. Skin, muscle, and nerve biopsies can lead to a diagnosis of vasculitis. Temporal artery biopsy is the gold standard for the diagnosis of temporal arteritis.

3. Exploratory laparotomy is less often necessary now due to the advent of more sensitive radiologic techniques. It should be performed only if there is firm evidence of abdominal pathology. Good communication with the surgical team is essential to ensure that tissue specimens are processed for maximal information.

I. Trials of empiric therapy in patients with FUO without a diagnosis are generally discouraged, but they may be considered in circumstances where a strong suggestion of a particular disease exists but definitive proof is lacking.

1. Such trials are of most benefit when the drugs used for empiric therapy have a limited spectrum of activity against specific pathogens (e.g., isoniazid and ethambutol as a trial of therapy for tuberculosis).

2. One should avoid using broadly active anti-inflammatory agents when attempting a trial of therapy for presumed infection, as fever may be the only sign or symptom to monitor for response.

3. Corticosteroids and other immunosuppressive anti-inflammatory drugs should be used with caution in trials of therapy, generally after infectious causes of FUO have been largely eliminated from consideration.

Bibliography

Aduan RP, Fanci AS, Dale DC, et al. Fevere of unknown origin (FUO): A prospective study of 347 patients. *Clin Research* 26:558A, 1978.

Deal WB: Fever of unknown origin: Analysis of 34 patients. *Postgrad Med J* 50:182, 1971.

Gleckman R, Crowley M, Esposito A: Fever of unknown origin: a view from the community hospital. *Am J Med Sci* 274:21, 1977.

Howard P, Hahn HH, Palmer RL, et al. Fever of unknown origin: a prospective study of 100 patients. *Tex Med* 73:56, 1977.

Jacoby GA, Swartz MN. Fever of undetermined origin. *N Engl J Med* 289:1407, 1973.

Knockaert DC, Vanneste LJ, Vanneste SB, et al. Fever of unknown origin in the 1980's: An update of the diagnostic spectrum. *Arch Int Med* 152:51, 1992.

Larson EB, Featherstone HJ, Petersdorf RG. Fever of undetermined origin: Diagnosis and follow-up of 105 cases, 1970–1980. 61:269, 1982.

Mackowiak PA, LeMaistre CF. Drug fever: A critical appraisal of conventional cases. *Ann Intern Med* 106:728, 1987.

Mandell GL, Douglas RG, Bennett JE (eds). Fever of unknown origin. Dinavello CA, Wolff SM, *in Principles and Practice of Infectious Diseases*, ed 3. New York, Churchill Livingstone, 1990.

Sheon RP, Van Ommen RA. Fever of obscure origin: Diagnosis and treatment based on a series of sixty cases. *Am J Med* 34:486, 1963.

CHAPTER 48-B

Mononucleosis Syndromes

Constance A. Benson, M.D.

I. Definition

Mononucleosis is a systemic illness characterized by fatigue, fever, pharyngitis, cervical or generalized lymphadenopathy with or without hepatosplenomegaly, and a variety of rashes accompanied by a constellation of laboratory abnormalities, which may include one or more of the following: anemia, mononuclear leukocytosis, atypical lymphocytosis, thrombocytopenia, abnormal liver function studies, an elevated erythrocyte sedimentation rate, and circulating autoantibodies.

A. A host of systemic symptoms or signs of organ involvement may also be recognized, including myalgia, arthralgia, headache, lethargy, nausea, vomiting, anorexia, abdominal pain, jaundice, or aseptic meningitis, depending on the specific etiology.

II. Differential Diagnosis

A. Most common etiologies: Epstein-Barr virus (EBV), cytomegalovirus (CMV), and *Toxoplasma gondii* are the most common causes of the mononucleosis syndrome in adolescents and adults.

B. Other infectious etiologies: acute human immunodeficiency virus (HIV) infection, secondary syphilis, tuberculosis, other granulomatous infections such as histoplasmosis, cryptococcosis, blastomycosis, coccidioidomycosis, or other fungal infections, cat-scratch disease, tularemia, acute viral hepatitis, human parvovirus B19, and occasionally acute rubella in the adult.

C. Noninfectious etiologies: lymphoma, sarcoidosis, metastatic carcinoma, leukemia, adult Still's disease, systemic lupus erythematosus, and some other collagen vascular diseases.

III. Specific Organisms

A. EBV

1. EBV is a member of the Herpesviridae.

2. Epidemiology

a. EBV is a widespread, prevalent virus. By adulthood, 90 to 95% of individuals are seropositive for EBV.

b. Most EBV-associated mononucleosis infections develop in persons exposed to the virus in adolescence, with symptomatic disease occurring most frequently in persons between the ages of 15 and 25.

c. EBV is transmitted by direct contact with infectious secretions, most often saliva. EBV may persist in the oro- and nasopharyngeal epithelial cells of persons with mononucleosis for prolonged periods (up to 18 months or more) following resolution of symptoms. EBV is also transmitted by blood product transfusion.

3. Diagnosis
   a. History and clinical presentation
      (1) The most common symptoms of mononucleosis are sore throat, fever, and lymphadenopathy. Systemic symptoms including myalgia, headache, fatigue, anorexia, nausea, abdominal pain, and jaundice may occur.
      (2) Fever is present in more than 90% of symptomatic persons. A variety of skin rashes have been associated with EBV mononucleosis; a diffuse maculopapular rash is the most common. In up to 90% of patients with EBV mononucleosis who receive concomitant ampicillin during acute infection, a morbilliform rash occurs which mimics (but should not be construed as) an allergic reaction to ampicillin.
      (3) Symptoms resolve without consequences over a 2- to 4-week period. The pharyngitis remits earlier, followed by a more gradual decline in fever. Fatigue, often described as a *neurasthenia*, may be prolonged for weeks to months, with intermittent waxing and waning. However, there is no correlation between EBV antibody titers and the *chronic fatigue syndrome*, formerly suggested to be the result of chronic active EBV infection.
   b. Clinical signs and physical findings
      (1) An exudative pharyngitis, often with palatal petechiae, is present in about one-third of patients.
      (2) Posterior cervical lymphadenopathy is the most common physical finding. However, other cervical, axillary, or inguinal nodal groups may also be enlarged.
      (3) Splenomegaly is seen in up to one-half of symptomatic persons; hepatomegaly and jaundice are much less common but can also be seen.
   c. Laboratory data
      (1) Peripheral blood lymphocytosis is present in most patients at the time clinical symptoms occur. The number and proportion of lymphocytes are maximal between the second and third weeks of symptoms. Atypical lymphocytes, which may comprise as many as 30% of the total, are commonly seen.
      (2) Neutropenia, usually mild, is seen in the majority of patients; up to 50% may also have mild thrombocytopenia.
      (3) Mild elevations of liver transaminases, alkaline phosphatase, and bilirubin (up to 1.5- to 2-fold) are common.
      (4) Circulating autoantibodies, such as mixed cryoglobulins with anti-i or anti-I specificity, may be present in the majority of patients but are rarely of clinical or prognostic significance. They may occasionally be associated with hemolysis.
   d. Diagnostic tests
      (1) Heterophile antibodies (sheep red blood cell agglutinins) are the basis of the commercially available *monospot* test and are present in about 90% of patients at the time of onset of symptoms. This is usually the diagnostic test of choice.
      (2) EBV-specific antibodies: While rarely necessary to establish the diagnosis, antibodies to the viral capsid antigen (VCA) and EBV nuclear antigen (EBNA) are the most clinically useful specific antibody tests. IgM antibody to VCA generally signals acute or recent infection; a fourfold rise in IgG antibody or new seroconversion measured in the sera of acute and convalescent patients may also be helpful in the diagnosis of recent infection.
      (3) EBV may be isolated from peripheral blood mononuclear cells or oro- or nasopharyngeal secretions from nearly all patients with acute mononucleosis. However, viral shedding is quite common among healthy persons without active mononucleo-

sis, making this of little diagnostic benefit.

4. Treatment
   a. Treatment requires only supportive measures in the immunologically normal individual. Recovery without sequelae is the rule. Strenuous physical activity should be limited during the first few weeks of illness, especially when splenomegaly is present, Antipyretics, hydration, and rest may also be beneficial.
   b. Adjunctive corticosteroids have been recommended by some for patients with imminent airway obstruction related to tonsillar engorgement and pharyngeal edema or for those with severe hematologic manifestations. If these are used, recommended doses are 60 to 80 mg of prednisone or its equivalent daily, to be rapidly tapered over 1 to 2 weeks.
   c. Although acyclovir and intravenous immunoglobulins have been advocated by some as therapy for EBV mononucleosis, there is no convincing evidence to support the use of these or any other antiviral drugs.
5. Prognosis and complications
   a. Most cases of EBV mononucleosis are benign and self-limited in the normal host. While complications are rare and also usually self-limited, deaths have been reported.
   b. The risk of splenic rupture, particularly following trauma, is increased when lymphocytic infiltration results in rapid capsular expansion and splenic enlargement.
   c. Neurologic complications may include aseptic meningitis, encephalitis, transverse myelitis, Guillain-Barré syndrome, optic or retrobulbar neuritis, cranial nerve palsies, mononeuritis multiplex, seizures, and psychosis.
   d. Cardiac complications are unusual, but ST- and T-wave electrocardiographic abnormalities, pericarditis, and myocarditis have been reported in a small number of patients.
   e. A potentially fatal, overwhelming EBV infection has been reported in patients with the familial X-linked recessive immunodeficiency syndrome (Duncan syndrome). EBV-associated lympho-

proliferative disorder, due to unrestricted viral replication, is seen in transplant recipients and others treated with immunosuppressive agents, particularly cyclosporine, OKT3 monoclonal antibody, and antilymphocyte globulins. This may progress to EBV-associated lymphoma.
   f. Malignant transformation of EBV-infected epithelial cells or B lymphocytes is associated with nasopharyngeal carcinoma, Burkitt's lymphoma, and some types of primary B-cell lymphoma.

B. CMV
1. CMV is a member of the Herpesviridae.
2. Epidemiology
   a. The seroprevalence of CMV in adults ranges from 40% to 100%. In the United States, the infection rate reaches a maximum both in early infancy and in late adolescence or young adulthood.
   b. CMV mononucleosis occurs in adults usually between the ages of 18 and 65; the median age is 29 years.
   c. CMV transmission to immunologically normal adults is thought to occur through contact with infected saliva, possibly via respiratory secretions, and through sexual contact. Virus can also be transmitted via blood product transfusion and in utero.
3. Diagnosis
   a. History and clinical presentation: CMV-induced mononucleosis is similar in presentation to EBV-induced mononucleosis. Fever is the dominant symptom and may be prolonged for up to 6 weeks. Exudative pharyngitis with sore throat is less prominent and less severe than with EBV-associated mononucleosis.
   b. Clinical signs and physical findings: Also in contrast to EBV-induced mononucleosis, posterior cervical lymphadenopathy is less common and generalized lymphadenopathy more common. Splenomegaly is seen but is usually mild; hepatomegaly and jaundice are rare.
   c. Laboratory data
      (1) Peripheral blood lymphocytosis is less prominent than with EBV mononucleosis but may be present in one-half of patients. Atypical

lymphocytes may comprise up to 50% of the total.

  (2) Mild elevations of liver transaminases or transient autoantibodies, such as mixed cryoglobulins, rheumatoid factor, cold agglutinins, or antinuclear antibodies, may also be detected.

d. Diagnostic tests

  (1) Heterophile antibody studies are negative.

  (2) Commercially available and commonly used serologic tests include indirect fluorescent antibody (IFA), anticomplement immunofluorescent antibody (ACIF), and enzyme-linked immunosorbent (ELISA, EIA) assays. To be diagnostically useful, serologic tests must demonstrate a fourfold rise in antibody level or convert from negative to positive. IgM antibody may be an indicator of recent infection, although it may not be present during the acute infection or may persist for a prolonged period, making it a less reliable diagnostic test.

  (3) Culture of blood, urine, respiratory tract secretions, or other normally sterile body fluids may be useful. However, some persons may shed virus in such body fluids for prolonged periods after resolution of symptoms and in the absence of clinically apparent end-organ disease.

  (4) Histologic demonstration of CMV viral inclusions or CMV antigens in tissue may provide supportive evidence of acute infection.

  (5) Ultimately, the diagnosis requires the presence of a compatible clinical syndrome coupled with serologic, culture, and/or histologic demonstration of virus in involved tissue.

4. Treatment

a. As with EBV-associated mononucleosis, therapy for CMV mononucleosis is largely supportive. Most infections are subclinical or benign and self-limited, although fever, lymphadenopathy, and fatigue may be prolonged for several weeks.

b. Ganciclovir, a nucleoside analog similar in structure and mechanism of action to acyclovir, is active against CMV. It has been successfully used and is approved for treatment of CMV disease in immunosuppressed hosts but is not recommended for the treatment of CMV mononucleosis in the otherwise normal host. Foscarnet, a pyrophosphate analog, approved for the treatment of CMV retinitis, has not been evaluated for and is not recommended for the treatment of CMV mononucleosis.

5. Prognosis and complications: Most immunologically intact adults have benign disease from which they recover without consequences. Rarely, interstitial pneumonia, hepatitis, pancreatitis, epididymitis, oophoritis, and neurologic sequelae, such as those described in association with EBV, may occur in otherwise healthy adults with CMV mononucleosis.

C. *Toxoplasma gondii*

1. *T. gondii* is an obligate intracellular protozoan.

2. The cat is the definitive host; humans are incidental hosts. The life cycle of the organism is maintained in the cat following ingestion of either trophozoites or oocysts. Humans can be infected through ingestion of oocysts, usually via food or soil contaminated by infected cat feces. Transmission can also occur through blood product transfusion, transplantation of infected organs or tissues, or in utero.

3. Epidemiology

a. *T. gondii* is worldwide in environmental distribution. The seroprevalence in adults ranges from 3% to 70% in the United States. Probably fewer than 1% of cases of mononucleosis are due to *T. gondii*.

4. Diagnosis

a. History and clinical presentation

  (1) Fewer than 20% of acutely infected adults develop symptoms. The most common syndrome is one of asymptomatic cervical lymphadenopathy.

  (2) Symptoms, when present, include fever, fatigue, myalgia, sore throat, and, rarely, a maculopapular rash. Abdominal pain may accompany abdominal lymphadenopathy.

b. Clinical signs and physical findings

(1) Cervical lymphadenopathy is the most common finding, although generalized lymphadenopathy may occasionally be noted. Nodes are usually well delineated and non-tender.

(2) Hepatosplenomegaly, atypical rash, exudative pharyngitis, or unilateral chorioretinitis may be present but are rare.

c. Laboratory data: Atypical lymphocytosis, involving fewer than 10% of circulating lymphocytes, may be present during the symptomatic phase of acute infection. Other laboratory abnormalities are uncommon; mild elevations in liver transaminases have been reported.

d. Diagnostic tests: Acute infection can be diagnosed by culturing *T. gondii* from blood or other body fluids; histologic demonstration of trophozoites in tissue; detection of antigen in body fluids or tissue; or serologic tests indicating antibody seroconversion, a fourfold rise in IgG antibody titer, or the presence of IgM antibody. Lymph nodes, if biopsied, may yield a characteristic architecture which can be readily recognized by an experienced histopathologist.

5. Treatment: Similar to mononucleosis due to other pathogens, toxoplasmic mononucleosis is a benign, self-limited syndrome which does not require treatment in the nonimmunosuppressed adult.

Bibliography

Adler SP. Transfusion-associated cytomegalovirus infections. *Rev Infect Dis* 5:977, 1983.

Andersson J, Britton S, Ernberg I, et al. Effect of acyclovir on infectious mononucleosis: A double-blind, placebo-controlled study. *J Infect Dis* 153:283, 1986.

Aronson MD, Komaroff AL, Pass TM, et al. Heterophil antibody in adults with sore throat. Frequency and clinical presentation. *Ann Intern Med* 96:505, 1982.

Baron DN, Bell JL, Demmett WN. Biochemical studies on hepatic involvement in infectious mononucleosis. *J Clin Pathol* 18:209, 1965.

Betts RF, George SD, Rundell BR, et al. Comparative activity of immunofluorescent antibody and complement-fixing antibody in cytomegalovirus infection. *J Clin Microbiol* 4:151, 1976.

Brooks RG, McCabe RE, Remington JS. Role of serology in the diagnosis of toxoplasmic lymphadenopathy. *Rev Infect Dis* 9:1055, 1987.

Cameron D, MacBear LM. *A Clinical Study of Infectious Mononucleosis and Toxoplasmosis.* Baltimore, Williams & Wilkins, 1973, p 8.

Carter RL. Granulocyte changes in infectious mononucleosis. *J Clin Pathol* 19:279, 1966.

Carter RL. Platelet levels in infectious mononucleosis. *Blood* 25:817, 1965.

Chandler SH, Handsfield HH, McDougall JK. Isolation of multiple strains of cytomegalovirus from women attending a clinic for sexually transmitted diseases. *J Infect Dis* 155:655, 1987.

Chou S. Newer methods for diagnosis of cytomegalovirus infection. *Rev Infect Dis* 12(Suppl 7):S727, 1990.

Cohen JI, Corey GR. Cytomegalovirus infection in the normal host. *Medicine* 64:100, 1985.

Cotton PB, Webb-Peploe MM. Acute transverse myelitis as a complication of glandular fever. *Br Med J* 1:654, 1966.

Dorfman RF, Remington JS. Value of lymph node biopsy in the diagnosis of acute acquired toxoplasmosis. *N Engl J Med* 289:878, 1973.

Frishman W, Kraus ME, Zabkar J, et al. Infectious mononucleosis and fatal myocarditis. *Chest* 72:535, 1977.

Gautier-Smith PC. Neurological complications of glandular fever (infectious mononucleosis). *Brain* 88:323, 1965.

Gilbert JW, Culebras A. Cerebellitis in infectious mononucleosis. *JAMA* 220:727, 1972.

Grierson H, Purtilo DT. Epstein-Barr virus infections in males with the X-linked lymphoproliferative syndrome. *Ann Intern Med* 106:538, 1987.

Grose C, Henle W, Henle G, et al. Primary Epstein-Barr virus infections in acute neurologic diseases. *N Engl J Med* 292:392, 1975.

Henle G, Henle W, Clifford P, et al. Antibodies to Epstein-Barr virus in Burkitt's lymphoma and control groups. *JNCI* 43:1147, 1969.

Hoagland RJ. Infectious mononucleosis. *Am J Med* 13:158, 1952.

Hoagland RJ. Mononucleosis and heart disease. *Am J Med Sci* 248:1, 1964.

Ho M. Cytomegalovirus, in Mandell GL, Douglas RG Jr, Bennett JE (eds), *Principles and Practice of Infectious Diseases,* ed 3. New York, Churchill Livingstone, 1990, p 1159.

Ho M. Epidemiology of cytomegalovirus infections. *Rev Infect Dis* 12(Suppl 7):S701, 1990.

Horwitz CA, Henle W, Henle G, et al. Heterophil-negative infectious mononucleosis and mononucleosis-like illness. Laboratory confirmation of 43 cases. *Am J Med* 63:947, 1977.

Horwitz CA, Moulds J, Henle W, et al. Cold agglutinins in infectious mononucleosis and heterophil-antibody-negative mononucleosis-like syndromes. *Blood* 50:195, 1977.

Johnson JD, Holliman RE. Incidence of toxoplasmosis in patients with glandular fever and in healthy blood donors. *Br J Gen Pract* 41:375, 1991.

Kaplan ME. Cryoglobulinemia in infectious mononucleosis: Quantitation and characterization of the cryoproteins. *J Lab Clin Med* 71:754, 1968.

Katz BZ, Raab-Traub N, Miller G. Latent and replicating forms of Epstein-Barr virus DNA in lymphomas and lymphoproliferative diseases. *J Infect Dis* 160:589, 1989.

Klemola E, Kaariainen L, von Essen R, et al. Further studies on cytomegalovirus mononucleosis in previously healthy individuals. *Acta Med Scand* 182:311, 1967.

Klemola E, von Essen R, Henle G, et al. Infectious-mononucleosis-like disease with negative heterophil agglutination test. Clinical features in relation to Epstein-Barr virus and cytomegalovirus and antibodies. *J Infect Dis* 121:608, 1970.

Luft BJ, Remington JS. Acute *Toxoplasma* infection among family members of patients with acute lymphadenopathic toxoplasmosis. *Arch Intern Med* 144:53, 1984.

Mason WR Jr, Adams EK. Infectious mononucleosis. An analysis of 100 cases with particular attention to diagnosis, liver function tests, and treatment of selected cases with prednisone. *Am J Med Sci* 236:447, 1958.

McCabe RE, Brooks RG, Dorfman RF, et al. Clinical spectrum in 107 cases of toxoplasmic lymphadenopathy. *Rev Infect Dis* 9:754, 1987.

McCabe RE, Remington JS. *Toxoplasma gondii*, in Mandell GL, Douglas RG Jr, Bennett JE (eds), *Principles and Practice of Infectious Diseases*, ed 3. New York, Churchill Livingstone, 1990, p 2090.

Miller G, Niederman JC, Andrews LL. Prolonged oropharyngeal excretion of Epstein-Barr virus after infectious mononucleosis. *N Engl J Med* 288:229, 1973.

Patel BM. Skin rash with infectious mononucleosis and ampicillin. *Pediatrics* 40:910, 1967.

Pereira MS, Blake JM, Macrae AD. EB virus antibody at different ages. *Br Med J* 4:526, 1969.

Preiksaitis JK, Brown L, McKenzie M. The risk of cytomegalovirus infection in seronegative transfusion recipients not receiving exogenous immunosuppression. *J Infect Dis* 157:523, 1988.

Pullen H, Wright N, Murdock J McC. Hypersensitivity reactions to antibacterial drugs in infectious mononucleosis. *Lancet* 2:1176, 1967.

Rao N, Waruszewski DT, Ho M, et al. Evaluation of the anticomplement immunofluorescence test in cytomegalovirus infection. *J Clin Microbiol* 6:633, 1976.

Remington JS, Barnett CG, Meikel M, et al. Toxoplasmosis and infectious mononucleosis. *Arch Intern Med* 110:744, 1962.

Schooley RT, Dolin R. Epstein-Barr virus (infectious mononucleosis), in Mandell GL, Douglas RG Jr, Bennett JE (eds), *Principles and Practice of Infectious Diseases*, ed 3. New York, Churchill Livingstone, 1990, p 1172.

Shapiro SC, Dimich I, Steier M. Pericarditis as the only manifestation of infectious mononucleosis. *Am J Dis Child* 126:662, 1973.

Shepp DH, Hackman RC, Conley FK, et al. *Toxoplasma gondii* reactivation identified by detection of parasitemia in tissue culture. *Ann Intern Med* 103:218, 1985.

Shuster EA, Beneke JS, Tegtmeier GE, et al. Monoclonal antibody for rapid laboratory detection of cytomegalovirus infections: Characterization and diagnostic application. *Mayo Clin Proc* 60:577, 1985.

Silverstein A, Steinberg S, Nathanson M. Nervous system involvement in infectious mononucleosis. The heralding and/or major manifestation. *Arch Neurol* 26:353, 1972.

Straus SE. The chronic mononucleosis syndrome. *J Infect Dis* 157:405, 1988.

Straus SE, Cohen JI, Tosato G, et al. NIH conference. Epstein-Barr virus infections: Biology, pathogenesis, and management. *Ann Intern Med* 118:45, 1993.

Sumaya CV, Ench Y. Epstein-Barr virus infectious mononucleosis in children. I. Clinical and general laboratory findings. *Pediatrics* 75:1003, 1985.

Sumaya CV, Ench Y. Epstein-Barr virus infectious mononucleosis in children. II. Heterophil antibody and viral-specific responses. *Pediatrics* 75:1011, 1985.

Sullivan JL, Medveczky P, Forman SJ, et al. Epstein-Barr-virus induced lymphoproliferation. Implications for antiviral chemotherapy. *N Engl J Med* 311:1163, 1984.

Swinnen LJ, Costanzo-Nordin MR, Fisher SG, et al. Increased incidence of lymphoproliferative disorder after immunosuppression with the monoclonal antibody OKT3 in cardiac transplant recipients. *N Engl J Med* 323:1723, 1990.

Zaia JA. Epidemiology and pathogenesis of cytomegalovirus disease. *Semin Hematol* 27(2, Suppl 1):5, 1990.

Ulcer/Node Syndromes

Jeffrey M. Lisowski, M.D.
Stuart Levin, M.D.

I. Definition

The ulcer-node syndromes consist of a heterologous collection of infectious diseases clinically related by presentations involving ulcerative cutaneous lesions at the site of inoculation and concomitant regional lymphadenitis. Ulcer and lymphadenopathy may be equally prominent manifestations of the specific illness (e.g., tularemia) or either cutaneous or nodal involvement may predominate (e.g., cutaneous involvement with sporotrichosis and nodal involvement with plague).

II. Ulcer and Node Involvement

A. Tularemia

1. The organism

Tularemia is a clinically variable, febrile illness caused by the small, gram-negative coccobacillus *Francisella tularensis*.

2. Epidemiology

a. *F. tularensis* has been isolated throughout the northern hemisphere. In the United States, most case reporting comes from Arkansas, Tennessee, Texas, Oklahoma, and Mississippi.

b. U.S. exposure typically involves rabbits, hares, muskrats and ticks.

c. Acquisition requires contact with infected animal tissue or body fluid, bites from infected animals or arthropods, inhalation of contaminated aerosols, or ingestion of contaminated foods or liquids.

d. Tick-borne cases, which are increasing in incidence, predominate in the summer months, while rabbit-associated disease peaks in the winter.

3. Pathogenesis

a. Cutaneous inoculation results in entry-site papule formation within 2 weeks, quickly followed by same-site ulcer formation, with fever and regional necrotizing granulomatous adenopathy.

b. Bacteremia and intracellular organism survival within the reticuloendothelial system lead to disseminated organ involvement with necrotizing granuloma formation.

c. Inhalation results in nonspecific systemic symptoms (fever, malaise, headache), as well as respiratory complaints of nonproductive cough with substernal chest pain; radiographic evidence of pneumonia or adenopathy may or may not be present.

d. Ingestion is associated with fever, pharyngeal mucosal inflammation, and cervical adenopathy.

4. Diagnosis
   a. History and clinical presentation
      (1) History of wild animal or tick exposure.
      (2) Disease presentation falls into six categories: ulceroglandular, glandular, typhoidal, pleuropulmonary, oculoglandular, or oropharyngeal.
   b. Laboratory data and diagnostic tests
      (1) Gram stain identification of the organism in sputum, ulcer exudate, or nodal tissue is rare.
      (2) Culture requires enriched media and presents aerosolization risks to laboratory personnel.
      (3) Serology is most helpful in diagnosis. A fourfold rise between acute and convalescent tularemia agglutination titers or a single titer greater than 1:160 is diagnostic of prior or current infection. Titers begin to rise after 2 weeks and may remain elevated for years.

5. Treatment
   Streptomycin is the drug of choice, with gentamicin, tetracycline, and chloramphenicol suggested alternatives.

B. Cat-scratch disease (CSD)
   1. The organism: Several agents have been proposed as the cause of CSD, but current studies implicate a small, gram-negative bacillus seen best after Warthin-Starry stain of early cutaneous and nodal lesions.
   2. Epidemiology
      a. CSD occurs worldwide, with temperate climate seasonal predominance between September and March.
      b. Eighty percent of cases involve youths less than 21 years of age; there is a male predominance.
      c. A history of a recent cat scratch or bite (typically involving a kitten) is seen in 75%. Other animal associations occur rarely and include dogs and monkeys. Implicated animals show no evidence of disease.
   3. Pathophysiology
      a. Cutaneous inoculation is followed in 2 weeks by regional lymphadenitis exhib-

iting granulomatous lymphoid hyperplasia, with or without suppuration.
      b. Similar granulomatous involvement has been seen in liver and osteolytic bone lesions.

4. Diagnosis
   a. History and clinical presentation
      (1) Often, an exposure to cats within the last 3 to 10 days.
      (2) Subsequent development of a papule or pustule at the inoculation site lasting for 1 to 3 weeks, with accompanying low-grade fever, malaise, headache, and sore throat in less than 30%.
      (3) Slow development of painful regional adenopathy 2 weeks after exposure. Head, neck, and axillary nodes are most frequently involved. Single-node involvement in one area is seen in 50%, multiple area involvement occurs in one-third, and suppurative complications occur in 20%. Lymphadenopathy usually lasts for 2 to 4 months.
      (4) Rashes, including erythema multiforme and erythema nodosum, occur occasionally.
      (5) Less common presentations include an oculoglandular syndrome with conjunctivitis and periauricular lymphadenitis, encephalitis with unusual cerebrospinal fluid changes and clinical resolution by 6 months, hepatic granulomas without hepatomegaly or dysfunction, and osteitis.
   b. Laboratory data and diagnostic tests
      (1) Mild leukocytosis is seen, with 10–20% developing eosinophilia.
      (2) Although Warthin-Starry staining of involved tissue may reveal small bacilli, routine culture conditions may produce negative results. To date, isolation outside of experimental laboratories has not occurred.

5. Treatment
   CSD is historically not responsive to antimicrobial therapy, but the disease remains self-limited.

6. Prognosis and complications
   CSD resolves spontaneously, with apparent lifelong immunity. Complications in-

clude sinus tract formations after suppurative or chronic lymphadenopathy lasting for several years.

III. Primarily Ulcer Involvement

A. Sporotrichosis

1. The organism: Sporotrichosis is the cutaneous and/or extracutaneous fungal disease caused by the dimorphic saprophyte *Sporothrix schenckii*. Yeast forms are seen both on enriched culture media and in vitro, while growth as a mold occurs on simple culture media.

2. Epidemiology

a. *S. schenckii* has been isolated from soil, healthy plants, organic debris, and domestic animals.

b. Sporotrichosis often occurs in the setting of exposure to thorny plants such as rose or barberry bushes or sphagnum moss, whereby cutaneous injury sustained from such a plant allows for a portal of spore entry.

c. Occupational exposure risk groups include gardeners, farmers, and miners.

d. Cutaneous sporotrichosis, a disease without gender predilection, is seen primarily in individuals less than 30 years of age. In contrast, extracutaneous sporotrichosis is predominantly a disease of older men with outdoor occupations. A specific immunodeficiency is not associated with this disease, although one-third of patients have a history of alcohol abuse.

3. Pathophysiology

a. After gaining access through a cutaneous wound, spores elicit a subcutaneous granulomatous reaction, with nodulation and ulceration at the site of entry and secondary nodular lesion formation along proximal lymphatic channels.

b. Regional lymphatic involvement manifests as lymphangitis; however, lymphadenitis is rare.

c. Dissemination is rare, but when seen, it is often associated with an immunocompromised state.

d. Histopathologically, involvement is confined to the dermis, with stellate microabscess formation. The histopathologic "asteroid" seen in some series consists of fungal forms surrounded by a periodic acid–Schiff-staining body.

4. Diagnostic tests

Diagnosis depends on organism isolation from skin, joint fluid, or sputum. Blood cultures are rarely positive. Histopathologic diagnosis lacks specificity secondary to the variability of tissue yeast forms.

5. Treatment

Cutaneous sporotrichosis is successfully treated with iodides. Extracutaneous disease currently requires systemic amphotericin B, but except for osteoarticular disease, it is difficult to cure.

IV. Primarily Node Involvement

A. Plague

1. The organism

a. *Yersinia pestis* (formerly *Pasteurella pestis*) is a gram-negative bacillus of the family Enterobacteriaceae with bipolar staining characteristics.

b. The organism grows aerobically on most culture media but, as with all *Yersinia* species, calcium is required for growth at 37°C.

2. Epidemiology

a. The organism can be found worldwide, with most reported cases of plague occurring in endemic regions of Africa, Asia, and South America. Plague is endemic to the semirural southwestern United States (primarily New Mexico but also Arizona, Colorado, Utah, and California).

b. Plague is primarily a disease of rodents, with transmission through rodent flea bites. Human infection is incidental after being bitten by an infected flea. Human acquisition is also possible after the handling of contaminated tissue or, rarely, via person-to-person spread through an aerosolized inoculum in situations of plague pneumonia.

c. In the United States, most cases occur between May and October and involve individuals less than 20 years of age. Attack rates are significantly greater among Native Americans living in endemic areas.

3. Pathophysiology

a. Infected fleas will regurgitate organisms during attempts to ingest blood meals.

b. After inoculation, organisms travel via lymphatics to regional lymph nodes. Femoral node involvement is more common than axillary or cervical node involvement and reflects the propensity of fleas to target specific areas.

c. *Yersinia* species evade host defenses by surviving and multiplying intracellularly after monocyte phagocytosis.

d. Transient recurrent bacteremia is common acutely and allows for dissemination with multisystem involvement; subsequent high-grade bacteremia with endotoxin release is responsible for the syndrome of septicemic plague.

4. Diagnosis

a. History and clinical presentation

(1) Residence in or travel to endemic areas, as well as rodent and/or flea exposure, may be elicited.

(2) A number of distinct plague syndromes have been described, although the presentations may be variable and may include overlap. The most common presentations involve bubonic and septicemic plagues. Pneumonic plague may be seen as a complication of bubonic or septicemic syndromes, with pulmonary seeding after hematogenous spread, or, more rarely, through inhalation. Meningitis, pharyngitis, and gastroenteritis syndromes occur less commonly.

(3) Malaise, fever with chills, and headache develop after a 2-day to 1-week incubation period. These systemic symptoms typically herald the onset of bubo formation.

(4) When the patient presents with a bubo, associated pain may lend to posturing and immobilization of the involved area.

(5) Cutaneous involvement at the site of flea inoculation is the exception rather than the rule and may include papules, vesicles, pustules, and eschars.

b. Clinical signs and physical findings

(1) Bubonic plague: The most common and identifiable presentation of *Y. pestis* infection. Noteworthy is the development of the painful bubo, which consists of inflamed, edematous regional lymph nodes producing a very tender, nonfluctuant mass with overlying skin distention, mild erythema, and warmth. The acutely developing, painful bubo, its lack of an associated lymphangitis, the typical absence of an associated cutaneous lesion, and the commonly fulminant course in complicated disease help to distinguish plague from other nodal syndromes. Tender and mild hepatosplenomegaly can be present. Diffuse purpuric lesions with associated distal extremity gangrene ("black death") can be the result of systemic disease with vasculitis.

(2) Septicemic plague: A rapidly overwhelming sepsis with a high bacteremic load can complicate bubonic plague or progress without bubo formation, as seen in 25% of cases.

(3) Pneumonic plague: Can be primary after organism inhalation (now rare) or secondary after hematogenous dissemination. Symptoms include fever, lymphadenopathy, cough with purulent bacilli-containing sputum, chest pain, and possible hemoptysis. Chest x-ray findings include consolidation and possible cavitation. Inhalation disease is rapidly fatal in the absence of therapy.

(4) Meningitis syndrome: Can be a late sequela (after 1 week) of initially uncomplicated or inadequately treated bubonic plague. Seen more often in association with axillary bubo involvement. Occasionally develops without node involvement.

c. Laboratory data
Peripheral white blood cell count elevation can progress to a myelocytic leukemoid reaction in children. Thrombocytopenia can accompany disseminated intravascular coagulation, but bleeding complications are rare. Elevations in serum bilirubin and liver transaminase levels can occur.

d. Diagnostic tests

(1) Diagnostic tests include blood and possible sputum culture, bubo aspiration for Gram and Wayson stains, culture, and acute and convalescent titer evaluation.

(2) Nonsuppuration of the bubo may require repetitive injection and as-

piration of sterile saline for specimen harvest.

    (3) On Wayson stain, *Y. pestis* appear as light blue bacilli with dark polar bodies.

    (4) Laboratory personnel must strictly adhere to policies preventing skin contamination or culture aerosolization.

5. Treatment

Streptomycin remains the drug of choice. Tetracycline and chloramphenicol are considered alternative therapies.

6. Patient monitoring

Plague is an internationally quarantinable disease. Strict respiratory isolation is required for at least 48 hr after institution of therapy in patients with an associated cough or evidence of pneumonia.

7. Prognosis and complications

Untreated, plague mortality is greater than 50%. Complications such as nonbubonic septicemic plague and pneumonia are associated with more fulminant disease and higher mortality possibly secondary to delays in diagnosis and treatment. High-density bacteremia with septicemic plague is a poor prognostic indicator. Meningitis also carries a higher fatality to case ratio. Relapses are rare.

Bibliography

Barnes AM, Quan TJ. *Yersinia pestis.* In Gorbach SL, et al (eds): *Infectious Diseases.* Philadelphia, W.B. Saunders, 1992, p 1285–1291.

Bennett JE. Sporotrichosis. In Mandell GL, Douglass RG Jr, Bennett JE (eds): *Principles and Practices of Infectious Diseases,* ed 3. New York, Churchill Livingstone, 1990, p 1972–1974.

Boyce JM. Recent trends in the epidemiology of tularemia in the U.S. *J Infect Dis* 131:197–199, 1975.

Boyce JM. Tularemia. In Mandell GL, Douglass RG Jr, Bennett JE (eds): *Principles and Practices of Infectious Diseases,* ed 3. New York, Churchill Livingstone, 1990, p 1742–1745.

Butler T. *Yersinia pestis.* In Mandell GL, et al (eds): *Principles and Practices of Infectious Diseases,* ed 3. New York, Churchill Livingstone, 1990, p 1748–1754.

Crook LD, Tempest B. Plague: A clinical review of 27 cases. *Arch Intern Med* 152:1253–1256, 1992.

Evans ME, Gregory DW, Schaffner W, et al. Tularemia: A 30 year experience with 88 cases. *Medicine* 64:251–269, 1985.

Fischer GW. Cat scratch disease. In Mandell GL, et al (eds): *Principles and Practices of Infectious Diseases,* ed 3. New York, Churchill Livingstone, 1990, p 1874–1877.

Hadfield TL. Cat scratch disease. In Gorbach SL, et al (eds): *Infectious Diseases.* Philadelphia, W.B. Saunders, 1992, p 1318–1322.

Muchmore HG, Scott EN. Sporotrichosis. In Gorbach SL, et al (eds): *Infectious Diseases.* Philadelphia, W.B. Saunders, 1992, p 1923–1926.

Sanford JP. Tularemia. In Gorbach SL, et al (eds): *Infectious Diseases.* Philadelphia, W.B. Saunders, 1992, p 1281–1285.

CHAPTER 48-D

Bacterial Meningitis

Alan A. Harris, M.D.

I. Definition

Meningitis is an inflammatory process of the pia-arachnoid

A. Clinical presentation

1. Meningitis classically presents with altered sensorium, headache, fever, and stiff neck. Do not wait for signs of nuchal rigidity to suspect meningitis. The presentation does not distinguish bacterial from viral pathogens.

2. Infants and children are more likely to present with focal findings, i.e., deafness or seizures. In adults, onset with seizures is a clue that *Listeria monocytogenes* is the etiology.

B. Etiology/epidemiology/pathophysiology

1. Pathogens are predictable by age group. Group B streptococci and enteric gram-negative rods are frequent during the neonatal period. *Haemophilus influenzae*, followed by *Neisseria meningitides* and *Streptococcus pneumoniae*, occur in childhood. During adolescence, *N. meningitides* is most common, followed by *S. pneumoniae*. During adulthood, *S. pneumoniae* and *N. meningitides* remain most common but switch places. In patients above 50 years of age, there appears to be an increase in *H. influenzae* and gram-negative rods.

a. Other pathogens may have associated clues—e.g., T-cell immunosuppression and *L. monocytogenes*, and *Staphylococcus aureus* and gram-negative rods with bacteremia from another focus and/or trauma.

2. Colonization of the nasopharynx antedates invasive disease with *H. influenzae*, *N. meningitides*, and *S. pneumoniae*. Asymptomatic chronic carriers are less likely to develop disease than are those who acquired the organism more recently. In the absence of nasal trauma involving the cribriform plate, meningitis occurs secondary to bacteremia rather than by direct extension.

a. Pili permit attachment, and capsules resist complement and phagocytic destruction. Lack of sufficient normal cerebrospinal fluid (CSF) antibody or phagocytic activity facilitates early replication of organisms.

3. Membrane components of bacteria in CSF cause central nervous system (CNS) glia cells and astrocytes to release cytokines such as interleukin-1 (IL-1) and tumor necrosis fac-

tor (TNF). There is damage to the blood vessels, white blood cell–endothelial interaction, and disruption of the blood-brain barrier. The end result is increased intracranial pressure coupled with cerebral edema and decreased cerebral blood flow.

C. Diagnosis is dependent on lumbar puncture.

1. Changing focal neurologic signs or edema and shift of the midline on CNS scan are contraindications to lumbar puncture.

 a. Not every lumbar puncture requires an antecedent scan.

2. Coagulation defects or thrombocytopenia dictate caution but do not absolutely preclude lumbar puncture.

3. Cisternal or ventricular taps by appropriate personnel can be done when a local problem, such as cellulitis or anatomic deformity, precludes lumbar puncture.

4. CSF analysis is the goal of lumbar puncture. This analysis is the only definitive way in which to diagnose meningitis and establish an etiology.

 a. CSF cell counts ≥ 1000/cc, the majority of which are polymorphonuclear neutrophils (PMNs), should be considered bacterial meningitis until proven otherwise.

  (1) When the tap is traumatic, allow 1 white blood cell for each 500 red blood cells, i.e., about two times the ratio in blood. The patient's own ratio should be calculated to adjust for severe anemia and/or leukocytosis. Each 700 red blood cells will increase CSF protein by 1 μg%.

  (2) Enteroviruses, herpes simplex, and *Mycobacterium tuberculosis* have been associated anecdotally with cell counts ≥ 1000/ml.

  (3) When cell counts are under 1000/ml, and especially when they are under 500/ml, and a majority are PMNs, the etiology may be bacterial, viral, fungal, mycobacterial, or noninfectious. In a *clinically stable* patient in whom therapy has not been started, a repeat lumbar puncture after 8–12 hr should show an increase in lymphocytes or PMN, pointing to a viral or bacterial process, respectively. Remember that *L. monocytogenes* got its name because of the mononuclear cellular response it may generate.

 b. CSF sugar is usually less than both 40 μg% and 40% of simultaneous blood sugar.

 c. CSF protein is usually greater than 150 μg%, is higher than in viral meningitis, and is not a distinguishing etiologic parameter.

 d. Gram stain and culture are positive 80–90% of the time. Except in centers studying meningitis, the overall sensitivity and specificity of a Gram stain are approximately 40–50%.

  (1) Blood cultures are positive 20–50% of the time in patients who have not received oral antibiotics prior to consideration and diagnosis of meningitis.

 e. Counterimmunoelectrophoresis, latex agglutination, or coagglutination tests to detect bacterial antigens in CSF are available for *S. pneumoniae*, *H. influenzae* B, *N. meningitides*, group B β-hemolytic streptococci, and *Escherichia coli* K1 antigen. These rapid methodologies add approximately 7% to the overall microbiologic diagnosis and, unlike Gram stain and culture, do not require viable organisms.

 f. A positive limulus test for endotoxin indicates a gram-negative agent but is not organism specific. The test requires a pyogen-free system. Anaerobic gram-negatives and some fungi also produce endotoxin.

 g. CSF pH, lactate, C-reactive protein, and inflammatory intermediaries, such as IL-1 and TNF, have been used to distinguish bacterial from nonbacterial etiologies. These tests are not currently in general use.

D. Therapy should be initiated promptly when the diagnosis is definite or highly suspect.

1. Initial therapy based on CSF formula and clinical status will be empiric by age group (Table 48D-1) and/or the presence of underlying disease or traumatic injury. When the organism is known, a specific regimen should be implemented.

2. Duration of therapy is best decided by the clinical course, but anticipated minimums are: *H. influenzae*, 7–10 days; *N. meningitides*, 7 days; *S. pneumoniae*, 10–14 days; gram-negative rods, 21 days; and *L. monocytogenes*, 14 days in a normal host and 21 days in an immunosuppressed patient.

3. Dexamethasone seems destined to have a role in the therapy of bacterial meningitis. The exact niche of steroids, based on age, organism, and associated antimicrobial ther-

Table 48D-1. Empiric Therapy by Age Group

Age	Therapy Options*
Neonate (< 2 months)	Ampicillin + gentamicin Ampicillin + third-generation cephalosporin
6 months to 3 years	Third-generation cephalosporin Ampicillin + chloramphenicol
Child–young adult	Third-generation cephalosporin
> 30 years old	Penicillin Chloramphenicol
Elderly or immuno-compromised	Ampicillin or penicillin + third-generation cephalosporin Intrathecal aminoglycoside + IV piperacillin or ticarcillin Bactrim

*This table is not intended to be comprehensive or exhaustive.

apy, is still being evaluated. The therapeutic toxic ratio is not determined. Duration will likely vary from 3 to 4 days.

  a. When administered, steroids should be given prior to or at the same time as the first dose of the antimicrobial agent.

  b. Adults and children with pneumococcal meningitis have diminished mortality and hearing loss.

  c. Steroid use in childhood meningitis has been associated with diminished sensorineural hearing loss.

  d. A poll of program directors in pediatric infectious disease programs revealed that in children with bacterial meningitis 17% always used dexamethasone, while 60% used it sometimes.

E. Prophylaxis, when indicated, is directed at either the patient, household members or other close contacts, or the general population.

  1. Household contacts of patients with *N. meningitides* should receive rifampin, 10 mg/kg up to 600 mg orally q12h for 2 days. Start as soon as possible. Do not culture the nasopharynx routinely prior to starting prophylaxis.

    a. Health care workers giving cardiopulmonary resuscitation should also receive prophylaxis.

    b. Give rifampin to the index case.

    c. I recommend immunizing the case and household contacts with quadrivalent A, C, Y, and W135 meningococcal vaccines.

    (1) There is no current vaccine for group B meningococcus.

  d. Sulfa is acceptable in the unusual circumstance when the infecting strain is already known to be susceptible.

  e. Minocycline prophylaxis has a high rate of vestibular toxicity.

  2. Household contacts of patients with *H. influenzae* meningitis or invasive disease, such as epiglottitis, should be given rifampin prophylaxis if there is another child less than 4 years of age in the home. The daily dose is 20 μg/kg up to a maximum of 600 μg, once a day for 4 days.

    a. *H. influenzae* immunization status should be checked and vaccine administered according to current guidelines.

    b. Adults working in day care centers should receive prophylaxis as household contacts when an outbreak occurs in the center.

  3. Twenty-three valent pneumococcal vaccine should be given according to current public health guidelines. Whether this will decrease the incidence of meningitis due to *S. pneumoniae* in those over 65 years of age or with sickle cell anemia is not yet known.

  4. I recommend immunization for *S. pneumoniae*, *N. meningitides*, and *H. influenzae* in a patient with recurrent bacterial meningitis.

    a. Patients with this syndrome should be evaluated for a CSF leak and for deficiencies of globulin and complement

  5. Oral penicillin should be considered in patients with traumatic CSF rhinorrhea. Efficacy is greatest during the first 2 weeks postinjury. Leaks which do not close spontaneously in 6 months should be surgically corrected. Large leaks may require early surgery.

F. Follow-up/prognosis

  1. Repeat lumbar puncture at 24–48 hr is usually performed in pediatric meningitis, as the Gram stain and culture have been shown to be of prognostic value. This is not standard practice in adult patients.

  2. Repeat lumbar puncture should be performed if the etiologic agent or clinical course is unusual or if there is little efficacy or pharmacokinetic information pertaining to the therapeutic agent(s) selected.

  3. Complications of the acute process which require management are seizures, inappropriate antidiuretic hormone secretion, and increased intracranial pressure.

   a. Brain abscess is a rare sequela.

   b. Subdural effusions and empyemas rarely occur as a complication of nontraumatic meningitis in adults. Empyemas require drainage. Effusions need intervention only if there is a mass effect.

4. Outcome is dependent on the etiologic agent, the patient's age, and the state of consciousness at the time of diagnosis.

   a. Neonates and adults ≥50 years of age have the highest mortality.

   b. Pneumococcal and gram-negative rod meningitis are worse than *H. influenzae*, which is worse than meningococcal meningitis.

   c. Sequelae include deafness, seizures, learning deficits, hydrocephalus, and mental retardation.

Bibliography

Benson CA, Harris AA, Levin S. Acute bacterial meningitis: General aspects, in Harris AA (vol ed), Vinken PJ, Bruyn GW, Klawans HL (eds): *Handbook of Clinical Neurology: Infections of the Central Nervous System*. New York, Elsevier Science Publishers, Inc., 1988, pp 1–19.

Carpenter RR, Petersdorf RG. The clinical spectrum of bacterial meningitis. *Am J Med* 33:262–275, 1962.

Harris AA, Levin S. Brain abscess, In *Infectious Diseases in Medicine and Surgery*. Gorbach SL, Bartlett JG, Blacklow NR (eds), W.B. Saunders Company, Harcourt Brace Jovanovich, Inc., Philadelphia, 1992, pages 1197–1206.

Tunkel AR, Wispelwey B, Scheld WM. Bacterial meningitis: Recent advances in pathophysiology and treatment. *Ann Intern Med* 112:610–623, 1990.

Whitley RJ. Viral encephalitis. *N Engl J Med* 323:242–249, 1990.

Whitley RJ, Cobbs CG, Alford CA, et al. Diseases that mimic herpes simplex encephalitis. *JAMA* 262:234–239, 1989.

Sinusitis, Pharyngitis, and Otitis

Jeffrey A. Nelson, M.D.

I. **Definition**

Inflammation of the membranes lining the sinus cavities.

II. **Etiology**

A. Acute

The two most important pathogens continue to be *Streptococcus pneumoniae* and *Haemophilus influenzae*. *Moraxella catarrhalis* has had an increased role in recent years.

B. Chronic

1. Anaerobic bacteria play an important role in chronic sinusitis. *Streptococcus* and *Bacteroides* species are the most frequent isolates.

2. Gram-negative aerobic organisms also must be considered, particularly in a compromised host or a hospitalized patient.

3. *Aspergillus fumigatus* can cause invasive disease in the compromised host, and *Mucor* must be considered in the diabetic patient. These two infections can often be acute in an abnormal host.

III. **Pathophysiology**

A. The filtering role and the general milieu of the sinuses are maintained by regulated production of mucus and active ciliary transport of trapped foreign materials toward draining ostia.

B. Overproduction of secretions, impaired ciliary transport, or reduced ostia diameter can facilitate the accumulation of mucus and debris in the sinus and create an optimal environment for secondary infection.

C. The list of potential predisposing conditions is long and includes allergic responses, viral infections, septal abnormalities, nasal polyps, smoking, foreign bodies, and tumors.

IV. **Diagnosis**

A. History

1. Acute sinusitis may manifest with significant pain over the involved sinus. This pain may be exacerbated by a supine position.

2. Chronic sinusitis may lack this pain but may present with symptoms of excessive tearing, pain with chewing, throat discomfort, chronic cough, and halitosis.

3. Historical clues which can raise one's suspicion for sinusitis include a history of allergies, long-standing use of decongestants, smoking, recent dental problems,

nasogastric tube placement, and nasotracheal intubation.

B. Physical exam
   1. Fever and chills are common with acute disease but are seen less frequently with chronic illness. Purulent drainage can be observed in both settings.
   2. Black or necrotic material may be seen with mucormycosis.
   3. Septal abnormalities, nasal polyps, foreign bodies, and dental disease should all be considered.
   4. Physical findings may include signs related to complications of sinusitis. These may involve a cellulitis, ocular complaints suggestive of an orbital extension, seizures or mental status changes supportive of an intracranial process, or focal swellings suggestive of a Pott's putty tumor with underlying osteomyelitis.

C. Diagnostic tests
   1. Sinus roentgenograms are usually an adequate means of establishing a diagnosis in uncomplicated presentations.
   2. Culturing of nasal secretions has little utility and aspiration methods are typically reserved for refractory disease, since the pathogens of acute disease have remained the same for several years.
   3. Chronic disease, presentations with signs of orbital or intracranial extension, or disease in a compromised host should be evaluated further. This may involve the combined use of nasal endoscopy and computed tomography to further define the process. These presentations may also require varying degrees of surgical intervention for culture, biopsy, and sometimes debridement.

V. **Differential Diagnosis**
   A. Acute sinusitis
      1. Acute sinusitis involving the maxillary and frontal sinuses does not usually cause a serious diagnostic dilemma.
      2. Sinusitis involving the ethmoid and sphenoid areas can be more difficult. If headache is the predominant symptom, one may confuse this with more common etiologies for headaches.
      3. Computed tomography has done much to aid us in evaluating these more difficult cases.
   B. Chronic sinusitis
      Chronic sinus difficulties should make one

consider potential predisposing factors including anatomic abnormalities, local obstructive lesions such as polyps and tumors, cystic fibrosis, hypogammaglobulinemia, ciliary dysfunctional syndromes such as Kartagener's, and vasculitic processes such as Wegener's granulomatosis.

VI. **Treatment**
   A. Acute sinusitis
      1. Common antibiotic choices include amoxicillin, 500 mg p.o. q8h; cefaclor, 500 mg p.o. q6h; and cefuroxime axetil, 250 mg p.o. q12h. Penicillin-allergic patients may receive trimethoprim-sulfamethoxazole, one double-strength tablet p.o. bid. Tetracyclines will not cover *S. pneumoniae*, and erythromycin, penicillin, and first-generation cephalosporins will not cover *H. influenzae*. Because of the increasing incidence of β-lactamase-producing organisms, there is increasing support for the use of agents with β-lactamase inhibitors as initial empiric therapy. Amoxicillin-clavulanate, 250–500 mg p.o. q8h, will cover these resistant therapeutic failures seen with the other agents. Treatment courses with any of the regimens is typically for 2 weeks.
      2. In addition to antimicrobial therapy, therapeutic intervention may involve the use of vasoconstrictive agents such as phenylephrine.
      3. Antihistamines and steroids do not play a significant role in resolution of the acute process, but they may reduce further episodes if an allergic component is suspected.
      4. Acute disease in the compromised host warrants broader coverage for *Staphylococcus aureus* and gram-negative organisms, imaging with computed tomography, and consultation with an otolaryngologist to obtain culture and biopsy specimens.
      5. Empiric antifungal therapy may be considered in compromised hosts. An infectious disease consultation should be sought in these patients.
   B. Chronic sinusitis
      1. Chronic disease often involves anaerobic bacteria such as *Streptococcus* and *Bacteroides* species. Gram-negative organisms also have a role, particularly in a compromised host or nosocomial acquisition.

2. Empiric therapy should include coverage for these pathogens, but treatment may be tailored with culture information. These patients should have aspirates obtained or material from endoscopic evaluation sent for culture.

3. Surgical intervention to improve drainage may have a role in some patients.

4. In a compromised host, debridement may be necessary for therapeutic success (e.g., *Mucor* in a diabetic patient, invasive *Aspergillus* in a neutropenic host).

VII. Follow-Up
A. Acute sinusitis

1. Therapeutic responses usually occur within 5 to 7 days. If the response is inadequate, compliance, absorption, or suspected resistance may make one reconsider antimicrobial therapy. This is particularly true if an agent without a β-lactamase inhibitor was chosen as the initial therapy.

2. The patient should be followed closely for any signs or symptoms suggestive of more extensive disease. Acute disease in the compromised host should be monitored on a daily basis in the hospital setting.

3. Refractory disease deserves further evaluation for anatomic abnormalities, the possible presence of resistant organisms, possible allergic contributions to disease, and possible immunologic abnormalities.

B. Chronic sinusitis

1. Chronic sinusitis is still often related to drainage problems and ostia patency. An otolaryngologist should evaluate the patient, and a combination of endoscopy and computed tomography may identify a surgically corrective abnormality.

2. Culture information must also be obtained in these patients.

VIII. Prognosis
A. Acute sinusitis

1. In the absence of contiguous extension of disease to the orbit or intracranial areas, immunocompetent patients generally will do well with appropriate early antimicrobial therapy.

2. Compromised hosts require urgent evaluation, imaging, culture, and histolytic evaluation if their course is to be altered.

B. Chronic sinusitis

Attention to correctable anatomic defects, allergy problems, and other predisposing factors, as well as careful monitoring for drainage difficulties, should improve the course of these patients. Consultation with an otolaryngologist is recommended.

Pharyngitis

I. Definition
Inflammatory process involving the throat.

II. Etiology
A. Infectious causes include a number of viral and bacterial agents: rhinovirus, coronavirus, adenovirus, respiratory syncytial virus, parainfluenza virus, influenza, coxsackie, cytomegalovirus, Epstein-Barr virus, herpes, *Corynebacterium diphtheriae*, *C. hemolyticum*, *Neisseria gonorrhea*, *Chlamydia pneumoniae*, *Mycoplasma pneumoniae*, *Yersinia enterocolitica*, *Francisella tularensis*, *H. influenzae*, and *Treponema pallidum*. Fungi such as *Candida albicans* can also be considered.

B. Noninfectious etiologies include collagen vascular diseases, Behcet's disease, pemphigoid, Kawasaki's syndrome, and drug-induced damage.

III. Diagnosis
A. History

1. A few historical questions may narrow the scope of consideration. An immunization history may be helpful if diphtheria is suspected.

2. A sexual history may lead one to consider herpes, syphilis, and *N. gonorrhoeae*.

3. Wild animal exposure would raise the suspicion of tularemia.

4. A history of dysphagia should make one suspect *H. influenzae*. Hoarseness can be a clue to *C. pneumoniae*.

5. Recognition of an outbreak of pharyngitis in a group with common meal exposure should make one suspect streptococci.

B. Physical exam

a. A few physical signs may be helpful. The presence of a membrane makes diphtheria a strong etiologic candidate.

b. A maculopapular rash on the extremities should make one consider *C. hemolyticum*, human immunodeficiency virus, enteroviruses, and syphilis in a young adult patient.

c. Conjunctivitis with pharyngitis in a young adult may suggest adenovirus.

    c. Soft palate ulceration is seen with coxsackie viruses.

    d. Significant cervical lymphadenopathy in an adult with pharyngitis makes Epstein-Barr virus a possible candidate.

    e. One should always consider some of the head and neck processes which may compromise the airway when seeing a patient with pharyngitis.

    f. Any significant tongue elevation should make one think of Ludwig's angina, usually due to mixed mouth organisms.

    g. Significant unilateral tonsillar swelling may signify the presence of a peritonsillar abscess.

    h. The posterior pharyngeal wall should also be seen and, if necessary, appropriate radiologic evaluation considered for a retropharyngeal process.

    i. All of these syndromes can move rapidly through facial planes and occlude the airway.

    j. Inability to handle secretions should raise the suspicion of epiglottitis and potential airway compromise.

C. Diagnostic

    1. Though many of the etiologic viruses can be isolated if appropriate cultures are obtained, the processes are primarily self-limited and a culture would offer little additional information. Herpes isolation may be an exception to this general rule.

    2. Serologic evaluation for Epstein-Barr virus, cytomegalovirus, or human immunodeficiency virus may be useful in the appropriate clinical setting.

    3. Convalescent titers may be required.

    4. Bacterial pathogens such as streptococci and *H. influenzae* may be cultured easily. *N. gonorrhoeae* can be cultured on special media, as can *C. diphtheriae*. *C. pneumoniae* is usually evaluated serologically. Rapid screens for group A streptococci are specific but lack the desired sensitivity. If the result is positive, culture can be avoided, but if it is negative, a culture should be obtained.

IV. Treatment

A. After historical and clinical clues point to uncomplicated pharyngitis, the primary consideration is whether to institute therapy for group A streptococci immediately or await culture information.

B. Since the major reason to treat streptococcal pharyngitis is to prevent the cardiac sequelae of rheumatic fever, either course is reasonable.

C. Appropriate treatments include penicillin or erythromycin. Tetracycline and trimethoprim-sulfamethoxazole should not be used. Therapy must be given for 10 days.

V. Patient Monitoring

A. With streptococcal pharyngitis, follow-up cultures in asymptomatic patients who have complied with a 10-day course are not routinely recommended.

B. Clinical resolution of the primary process is perhaps the best measure of the efficacy of therapy.

Otitis

I. Definition

Inflammatory processes that involve the ear can be divided into those which occur behind the tympanic membrane (otitis media) and those which involve the auditory canal and contiguous structures (external otitis). These syndromes can be further characterized as acute or chronic.

II. Etiology

A. Acute otitis media

    1. This process is most often seen in children under the age of 3. Primary bacterial pathogens include *S. pneumoniae*, *H. influenzae*, and *Branhamella catarrhalis*.

B. Chronic otitis media

    1. The spectrum of pathogens in chronic middle ear disease expands to include *P. aeruginosa* and *Staph. aureus*. Other considerations include tuberculous otitis, sarcoidosis, syphilis, and the presence of a cholesteatoma.

C. External otitis

    1. *Staph. aureus* and *P. aeruginosa* are primary considerations. Staphylococcal involvement may be more focal and may evolve from an infected hair follicle. Occasionally, *Strep. pyogenes* may enter the outer ear structures and present as erysipelas. *P. aeruginosa* is often the pathogen when a diffuse external canal process is present. Frequently, this will occur in warm weather in conjunction with a history of swimming.

2. Fungi occasionally will contribute to inflammatory processes of the external canal. *Aspergillus* can be seen as a focal process, but it may be invasive in the setting of diabetes, steroid use, or immunodeficiency states. *Candida albicans* in a child may be seen in patients with mucocutaneous candidiasis syndrome.

3. Malignant invasive disease is most often attributed to *P. aeruginosa*. This process most often occurs in diabetics, and most patients are over 50.

III. Pathophysiology

A. Otitis media

1. The middle ear milieu is dependent on eustachian tube function. Processes which alter this canal's ability to keep nasopharyngeal pathogens from the middle ear may also impede drainage of materials once focal inflammation begins. Perhaps the most frequently implicated inciting event is a viral upper respiratory condition. In adults, nasopharyngeal tumors need to be considered.

2. External canal infections are often preceded by local skin maceration. This may be due to local trauma, cotton swabs, hearing aids, or repeated wetting from frequent water exposure ("swimmer's ear"). Invasive processes are most often seen in the setting of diabetes or some degree of immune suppression.

IV. Diagnosis

A. Otitis media in a child with fever, otalgia, and fluid behind the tympanic membrane should create little diagnostic dilemma.

1. In the absence of fluid, pneumatic otoscopy can reveal evidence of altered tympanic membrane mobility.

2. Cultures are rarely necessary in acute disease, but with refractory or recurrent processes, an aspirate may occasionally be useful. If obtained, cultured for fungi and mycobacterial pathogens should be sent.

3. In the adult with recurrent or refractory disease, an ear, nose, and throat exam should be performed by a specialist.

B. External otitis may offer purulent material for culture.

1. *P. aeruginosa* is often found: In a normal host, it may be managed with local therapy such as cortisporin otic suspension and maintenance of a dry canal.

2. Focal *Staph. aureus* infections will usually resolve with oral antimicrobial therapy.

3. Compromised hosts, including those with diabetes, with external canal infections should undergo further evaluations. Though a number of these patients may have resolution of their problem with local therapy or oral antimicrobials, one should pursue further diagnostic studies.

4. Imaging procedures such as magnetic resonance imaging and gallium scanning may be useful to evaluate bony involvement. If present, intravenous therapy for at least 4 to 6 weeks and careful monitoring are needed. Surgical debridement may be necessary.

V. Differential Diagnosis

While infectious etiologies represent the majority of otitis media and external otitis, noninfectious etiologies such as sarcoidosis, tumor, and primary skin or cartilage disorders such as psoriasis, discoid lupus, or polychondritis must be considered.

VI. Treatment

A. Otitis media

1. Acute disease can be treated with empiric antimicrobial therapy directed at the major pathogens. Because of the increasing number of β-lactamase-producing *Haemophilus* and *Branhamella* organisms, agents more resistant to these effects may need to be considered. Amoxicillin-clavulanate (Augmentin) may be the preferred agent to cover the common pathogens, including resistant strains. A dose of 250 mg tid is standard.

2. Chronic disease may involve organisms from the external canal, and coverage for *Staph. aureus* and *P. aeruginosa* must be considered. Noninfectious etiologies must also be considered. Therapy should be dictated by aspirate results and by consultation with an ear, nose, and throat specialist.

B. Otitis externa

1. Mild disease may resolve by maintaining dry conditions within the canal to promote healing. Topical treatment may be considered with antibiotic/steroid combinations such as cortisporin otic suspension, but these agents can be sensitizing and may create their own inflammatory response.

2. More severe cases should be cultured and treated with an agent to cover *Staphylococcus* and *Pseudomonas*.
3. Refractory patients and those with diabetes, on steroid therapy, or with an immunocompromised status need intravenous therapy, consultation with an otolaryngologist, and imaging studies such as magnetic resonance to determine the extent of the disease process.

VII. **Patient Monitoring**

A. Otitis media
1. Acute disease should be resolve in 72 hr after initiation of therapy. Residual fluid may present for weeks. Patients who do not respond should have therapy reconsidered. If the initial regimen did not include a β-lactamase-resistant agent, this should be initiated.
2. Chronic disease should be managed by an otolaryngologist.

B. Otitis externa
1. Abnormal hosts need careful follow-up exams, and initial therapy should take place in the hospital.
2. Occasionally, normal hosts will also have invasive disease. If prompt resolution does not occur, further examination with a consultant and imaging procedures should be considered.

Bibliography (Sinusitis)

Brook I. Bacteriology of chronic maxillary sinusitis in adults. *Ann Otol Rhinol Laryngol* 98:426–428, 1989.

Slavin RG. Management of sinusitis. *J Am Geriatr Soc* 39:212–217, 1991.

Stafford CT. The clinician's view of sinusitis. *Otolaryngol Head Neck Surg* 103:870–874, 1990.

Bibliography (Pharyngitis)

Huovinen P, Lahtonen R, Ziegler T, et al. Pharyngitis in adults: The presence and co-existence of viruses and bacterial organisms. *Ann Intern Med* 110:612–616, 1989.

Mayosmith MF, Hirsch PJ, Wodzinski SF, et al. Acute epiglottitis in adults. *N Engl J Med* 314:1133–1139, 1986.

Rubin J, Yu VL. Malignant external otitis: Insights into pathogenesis, clinical manifestations, diagnosis, and therapy. *Am J Med* 85:391–398, 1988.

Van Hane GF, Shurin PA, Marchant CD, et al. Acute otitis media caused by *Branhamella catarrhalis:* Biology and therapy. *Rev Infect Dis* 9:16–27, 1987.

Bibliography (Otitis)

Johnson MP, Ramphal R. Malignant external otitis: Report on therapy with ceftazidine and review of therapy and prognosis. *Rev Infect Dis* 12:173–180, 1990.

Celin SE, Bluestone CD, Stephenson J, Yilmuz HM, Collins JJ. Bacteriology of acute otitis media in adults. *JAMA* 266:2249–2252, 1991.

Schwartz LE, Brown RB. Purulent otitis media in adults. *Arch Intern Med* 152:2301–2304, 1992.

Chapter 48-F

Infective Endocarditis

Mitchell Goldman, M.D.
Denise C. Weaver, M.D.
Stuart Levin, M.D.

I. Definition

A. Infective endocarditis (IE) is the infection of the endocardial surface of the heart by microorganisms.
1. Although bacteria remain the most common microorganisms causing IE, other infecting agents include fungi, rickettsiae, chlamydiae, and possibly viruses.
2. Disease characteristically affects the valvular structures; however, the mural endocardium or septum may also be involved. In addition, infection of the vascular endothelial lining of arteriovenous shunts, patent ductus arteriosus, and coarctation of the aorta are included in the definition of IE.

II. Epidemiology

A. Incidence: The incidence of IE is 2–4/ 100,000 person-years. IE accounts for 1–5 cases per 1,000 hospital admissions.
B. Patient characteristics
1. Age: Currently, the majority of patients with IE are more than 50 years of age. Patients with a history of parenteral drug use have a mean age of 29 years.
2. Sex: Male patients presently outnumber female patients by nearly 2:1. Even larger male:female ratios are seen in patients over age 60 and among intravenous drug users (IDUs).
3. Predisposing cardiac lesions: Recent series demonstrate a decline in the incidence of rheumatic and congenital heart disease, and the emergence of mitral valve prolapse and degenerative calcified lesions of the mitral and aortic valves as the major predisposing cardiac lesions. A substantial number of patients have no underlying cardiac disease. Prosthetic valve endocarditis (PVE) accounts for 10–30% of cases in some institutions. In addition, patients with a prior history of endocarditis are also at risk for recurrent infection.
   a. Among those with native valve endocarditis (NVE), 30% have prolapsed mitral valve (particularly redundant valves), 25% have no valvular disease (especially among IDUs), 20% have degenerative mitral and aortic valves (the most commonly identified abnormality in those above age 60), 13% have congenital valvular disease, 6% have rheu-

matic valvular disease, and 5% have hypertrophic cardiomyopathy.

    4. Nosocomial endocarditis: In addition to infection in individuals with intracardiac prostheses, hemodialysis shunts, or intracardiac pacemaker wires, IE occurs more frequently in seriously ill hospitalized patients, many of whom are immunocompromised. These hosts include the elderly, cancer patients, and transplant recipients who are subjected to intravascular access procedures including central venous catheters and monitoring devices.

III. Etiologic Agents

A. General: The following table lists the most frequent organisms causing endocarditis in various populations. It must be noted that wide local variations exist.

B. Culture-negative endocarditis is inflammation of the endocardium associated with negative blood cultures. Infectious and noninfectious etiologies are listed below. Approximately 5% of endocarditis cases are culture-negative.

    1. Prior antimicrobial therapy is the most common factor associated with culture-negative IE.

    2. Nutritionally deficient and fastidious bacteria may be associated with initial culture negativity. These organisms are slow-growing and/or require special media for growth. Included in this group are the following:

      a. HACEK organisms.

      b. Nutritionally deficient streptococci

      c. *Brucella* spp.

      d. *Neisseria* spp.

      e. *Corynebacterium* spp.

      f. Acid-fast organisms such as *Mycobacterium* and *Nocardia* spp.

    3. Fungal endocarditis.

    4. *Coxiella burnetii* (Q fever).

    5. *Chlamydia* spp.

    6. Right-sided endocarditis.

    7. Uremia.

    8. Noninfectious endocardial diseases.

      a. Myxoma.

      b. Rheumatic fever.

      c. Lupus (Libman-Sacks) nonbacterial verrucous endocarditis.

      d. Marantic endocarditis.

      e. Carcinoid syndrome.

      f. Endocardial fibroblastosis.

      g. Loeffler's endocarditis.

IV. Pathogenesis

A. Endothelial disruption abnormality

    1. The valve surface must be altered to allow for bacterial attachment, as well as for release of a cascade of mediators.

    2. Preexisting causes of endothelial disruption include mitral valve prolapse, degenerative valvular disease, rheumatic valvular disease, and congenital valvular lesions.

    3. Acquired causes of endothelial disruption include instrumentation (Swan-Ganz catheters, pacemakers, etc.) and turbulent flow from a high-pressure to a low-pressure zone. This "jet effect" ultimately erodes and exposes the endothelial surface along the low-pressure side of the valves, such as the atrial surface of the mitral valve and the ventricular surface of the aortic valve. These are the most frequent sites of localization for vegetations. Lesions with small pressure gradients, such as large ventricular septal defects, are less likely to disrupt endothelium.

B. Formation of platelet/fibrin mesh or nonbacterial thrombotic endocarditis occurs at the site of endothelial disruption.

C. Bacteria in the bloodstream become trapped and then colonize the endothelial thrombus.

    1. Although spontaneous bacteremia has been well documented, dental, gastrointestinal, or genitourinary manipulations promote bacteremia. Bacteremia itself is usually insufficient to cause IE in the absence of an existing endothelial thrombus. The likelihood of developing IE depends on the virulence characteristics of the organisms, such as the ability to avoid immune defenses or to produce a dextran coating that allows bacteria to adhere to innate surfaces.

D. Propagation of infection: The endothelial thrombus provides a protective sheath allowing microorganisms to evade host defenses and to continue to grow and multiply. Microorganisms that have a tendency to aggregate platelets and become deeply sequestered, and to which the host does not have preexisting antibodies, are more likely to survive.

V. Diagnosis

A. Clinical presentation/history

    1. General: The signs and symptoms of IE are quite variable, and any organ system may be involved. The clinical manifesta-

tions are the result of a varying mix of four major processes: cardiac involvement (valvular dysfunction and local complications), system infection (constant bacteremia and metastatic foci of infection), embolization (bland, thrombotic, or septic), and circulating immune complexes.

2. Subacute IE presents with the classic triad of heart failure, heart murmur, and fever in only 40% of patients. Often there is an insidious onset of symptoms that may include fatigue, anorexia, weakness, fever, night sweats, arthralgias, myalgias, and neurologic changes. Central nervous system findings predominate in 20% and may include stroke, delirium, or coma, especially in the elderly. Musculoskeletal complaints, including asymmetric polyarthritis or monoarticular arthritis, can be seen in 45% of patients and may be the dominant symptom in 15%, mimicking systemic lupus erythematosus, polyarteritis, or rheumatoid arthritis.
   a. Although the onset of subacute IE may be related to an antecedent event such as dental work, in the majority of cases no such event can be identified. Symptoms are often present for weeks to months before diagnosis.

3. Patients with acute IE present within several days to a week after the onset of illness. Fever, chills, arthralgias, myalgias, and back pain are common, and patients appear toxic. A history of a noncardiac focus of infection that predates the endocarditis may be present.

4. The following clinical syndromes or presentations should raise a high index of suspicion for left-sided IE:
   a. Fever of unknown origin.
   b. A heart murmur with fever and/or heart failure.
   c. High-grade or persistent bacteremia.
   d. Vegetations seen on echocardiogram.
   e. Cardiovascular accident, with or without fever.
   f. Any streptococcal meningitis.
   g. Splenic infarction of unknown etiology.
   h. Febrile glomerulonephritis.
   i. Febrile vascular aneurysm.
   j. Skin-mucosal signs (Osler nodes, Janeway lesions, proximal nail bed splinter

hemorrhages, fundoscopic Roth spots, clubbing).
   k. New or changing heart murmurs.

5. Right-sided endocarditis may present with a predominance of pulmonary findings. Clinical clues suggesting the presence of right-sided disease include:
   a. Multiple pulmonary infiltrates, with or without cavities or pleural effusions.
   b. Recurrent pneumonia.
   c. Any pulmonary infiltrate with positive blood cultures for staphylococci or *Pseudomonas* spp.

B. Clinical signs/physical findings
   1. Fever is present in 90% of patients. While the temperature rarely exceeds 103°F, it may do so in acute IE.
   2. Heart murmurs are present in more than 85% of patients, although the development of new or changing murmurs is uncommon.
   3. Other cardiac findings may include congestive heart failure (usually from valvular insufficiency), heart block/arrhythmias due to intracardiac extension of infection involving the conduction system, and pericarditis.
   4. Peripheral signs are found in less than 50% of patients with IE with the exception of splenomegaly, which may be seen in 50–60% of cases. These include the following:
      a. Osler nodes are small, painful, nodular lesions in the pads of fingers or toes and are believed to be due to deposition of immune complexes. They are seen in 10–25% of patients with IE.
      b. Janeway lesions are painless, hemorrhagic, macular lesions that are due to septic emboli.
      c. Eye findings including conjunctival petechiae and retinal hemorrhages (Roth spots).
      d. Splenomegaly.

C. Diagnostic tests
   1. Blood cultures: Blood cultures remain the single most important diagnostic test. In patients who have not received prior antibiotic therapy, the initial specimens obtained will yield the etiology 90% of the time. If antibiotics have been given within the preceding 2 weeks, the yield is halved. To enhance the microbiologic yield, multiple blood cultures should be obtained

from different sites over time. Maximum blood volume should be utilized to detect low-grade bacteremia. Cultures should be held for a minimum of 7 days, although a longer incubation period or the use of nutritionally supplemented media should be requested if the presence of fastidious organisms is suspected.

2. Hematologic: Anemia is found in 75–90% of patients with subacute IE. The hemoglobin in patients with acute IE is most often normal. Leukocytosis is seen in less than one-third of cases.

3. Erythrocyte sedimentation rate (ESR): An elevated sedimentation rate is almost invariably seen (mean, 57 mm/hr Westergren). A normal ESR in the absence of chronic renal failure, congestive heart failure, or disseminated intravascular congestion argues against IE.

4. Circulating immune complexes: As constant antigenemia is associated with IE, tests such as the Raji cell assay are often strikingly abnormal. Similarly, elevated rheumatologic factor and depressed complement levels are often found in patients with IE.

5. Urinalysis: Urine sediment is usually active in patients with IE. More than 50% of patients have proteinuria because of glomerular involvement, but only 15% have red blood cell casts. Microscopic hematuria is seen in 30–50% of cases.

6. Imaging studies
   a. Chest radiography: Cardiomegaly and interstitial edema may be present if valvular dysfunction impairs left ventricular function; the presenting feature of right-sided endocarditis is often septic pulmonary emboli.
   b. Liver-spleen scan: The presence of splenic infarcts supports the diagnosis of IE.
   c. Echocardiography: Sonographic examination of valvular structures to detect vegetations is an extremely useful study. However, a negative echocardiogram does not exclude IE. Nonvalvular endocarditis, right-sided vegetations, and prosthetic valve IE are more difficult to diagnose using this technology.
   d. Transesophageal echocardiography (TEE): A transducer introduced into the esophagus is in closer proximity to the heart, enhancing images and increasing both the sensitivity and specificity of the sonographic examination. As the test is invasive, it should not be used for screening. It is particularly useful in diagnosing perivalvular disease, prosthetic valve dysfunction, right-sided disease, cardiac clots or tumors, and aortic dissection. TEE images are attenuated as they pass through tissue, so the distal left ventricle is poorly visualized. Complications such as aspiration, esophageal injury, bleeding, and arrhythmias may occur. Positioning the scope requires experience.

VI. Treatment
   A. Medical therapy
      1. General concepts
         a. Antibiotics should be given intravenously at doses which will maintain high therapeutic levels.
         b. Antibiotics should be bactericidal for the etiologic organism(s).
         c. Prolonged therapy is indicated, as bacteria are sequestered in platelet/fibrin networks, valves are avascular, and vegetations often have high inocula of organisms in quiescent or low replicative phases.
         d. The decision to initiate antibiotic therapy depends on the clinical scenario. If the disease is rapidly progressive or acute in onset, therapy should be initiated on a presumptive basis after appropriate cultures are obtained. However, if the presentation is subacute, it may be prudent to withhold therapy until the results of the culture are known.
      2. Antibiotic therapy depends on the etiologic agent. Empiric treatment should be guided by the likeliest implicated organisms, as outlined in Table 48F-1.

VII. Monitoring
   A. Tests for effectiveness of therapy
      1. Minimum inhibitory concentration is useful for initial selection and dosing of antibiotics and is influential in selecting combination therapy.
      2. Minimum bactericidal concentration is the concentration of drug necessary to kill an inoculum of the offending organism. Ad-

Table 48F-1. Prevalence of Organisms in Infective Endocarditis

	NVE (%)	IDU%	Early (<2 mos) PVE (%)	Late (>2 mos) PVE (%)
Streptococci	55	5–10	5	35
Viridans	35	5	<5	25
Strep. bovis	15	<5	<5	<5
Other sp.	<5	<5	<5	<5
Staphylococci	25	50	50	30
Coagulase +	23	50	20	10
Coagulase −	<5	<5	30	20
Enterococci	10	8	<5	<5
Gram-negative aerobic bacilli	<5	5	20	10
Fungi	<5	5	10	5
Polymicrobial	<1	5	5	5
Culture-negative	5–10	5	<5	<5

equate therapy of IE requires the use of an agent which is bactericidal for the implicated organism.

3. Serum kill or serum bactericidal level is the maximum dilution of the patient's serum containing antibiotics that kill 99.9% of a standard inoculum of the causative organism. This takes into account the patient's ability to distribute, metabolize, and eliminate the chosen antibiotic. Peak serum bactericidal activity at a dilution of >1:8 has been correlated with a favorable clinical outcome. Controversy continues about the clinical relevance of these levels.

4. Checkerboard or time kill curves are useful to evaluate antibiotic synergy.

B. Surveillance blood cultures are essential throughout the early course of therapy to ensure eradication of the organism.

C. Continuing clinical evaluation is necessary to monitor for signs of ongoing infection, that is, annular disease (may be suggested by the presence of conduction disturbances), cardiac decompensation, or systemic emboli.

D. Posttreatment monitoring

1. Recurrent disease is a particular problem among parental drug users. Patients with persistent or chronic dental pathology are also at risk of recurrent bacteremia and endocarditis. It is important to identify and eradicate extracardiac infection.

2. Relapsing disease may be a consequence of residual perivalvular disease, failure to eradicate infection or a foreign body, use of nonbactericidal antimicrobial treatment, or short-course therapy.

Bibliography

McKinsey DS, Ratts TE, Bisno AL. Underlying cardiac lesions in adults with infective endocarditis: The changing spectrum. *Am J Med* 82:681–688, 1987.

Hermans PE. The clinical manifestations of infective endocarditis. *Mayo Clin Proc* 57:15–21, 1982.

Scheld WM, Sande MA. Endocarditis and intravascular infection. In Mandell GL, Douglass RG Jr, Bennett JE (eds): *Principles and Practices of Infectious Diseases*, ed 3. New York, Churchill Livingstone, 1990, p 670–706.

Durack DT. Infective and noninfective endocarditis. In Hurst JW, Schlant RC, Rackley CE, et al (eds): *The Heart Arteries and Veins*, ed 7. New York, McGraw-Hill, 1990, p 1230–1255.

Van Scoy RE. Culture-negative endocarditis. *Mayo Clin Proc* 57:149–154, 1982.

Mügge A, Daniel WG, Frank G, et al. Echocardiography in infective endocarditis: Reassessment of prognostic implications of vegetation size determined by the transthoracic and transesophageal approach. *J Am Coll Cardiol* 14:631–638, 1989.

Weinstein L. Life-threatening complications of infective endocarditis and their management. *Arch Intern Med* 146: 953–957, 1986.

Bisno AL, Dismukes WE, Durack DT, et al. Antimicrobial treatment of infective endocarditis due to viridans streptococci, enterococci, and staphylococci. *JAMA* 261:1471–1477, 1989.

CHAPTER 48-G

Gastrointestinal Infections

Larry J. Goodman, M.D.

I. Definition
Diarrhea is usually defined as a change in stool consistency from formed to watery or soft. The specimen typically conforms to the shape of the container in which it is placed. In published studies, three to four loose stools per day are usually required to meet entrance criteria. Such a strict definition is not necessary in the typical clinical setting.

II. Overview
A. Worldwide, infectious diarrheal diseases account for more morbidity and mortality than any other disease process.
B. In the United States, practice audits suggest that infectious diarrhea is second only to respiratory illnesses as a reason to seek medical evaluation.
C. Historically, outbreaks of diarrheal diseases have played important and occasionally pivotal roles in military conflicts.

III. Epidemiology
A. Increased incidence in children. Approximately 5 million deaths per year (worldwide) in children under 5 years of age are attributed to diarrheal disease. Breast feeding appears to be protective, with an increased incidence of diarrhea observed at the time of weaning.
B. A second (but less marked) increase is seen in young adults. This is primarily true for bacterial pathogens, especially *Campylobacter jejuni*.
C. Nearly all pathogens are acquired by the oral route and may be transmitted from person to person primarily via fecal-oral spread. Factors contributing to acquisition and/or transmission include:
   1. Poor sanitation.
   2. Lack of water treatment facilities or limited water supply.
   3. Crowding.
   4. Poor personal hygiene.
D. Animals are important reservoirs for many enteric pathogens.
E. Temperate climates have a marked seasonality in the frequency of diarrheal disease. Bacterial pathogens are more common in the summer/fall, and viral etiologies predominate in the winter.

IV. Etiology
A. A large number of organisms have been implicated as etiologic agents of diarrhea. Fig. 48G-1 lists the most common ones.

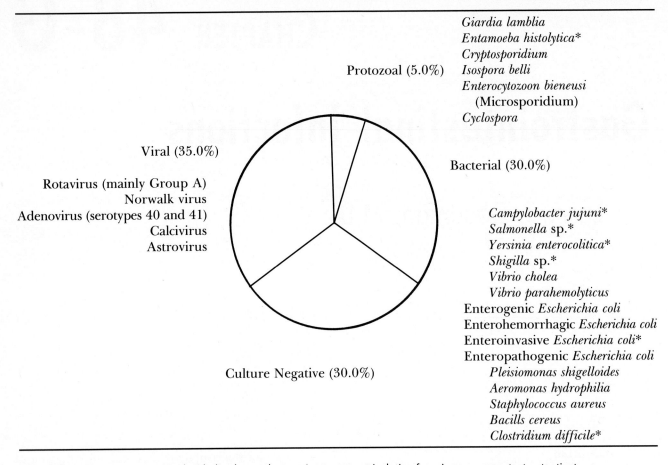

Protozoal (5.0%)   *Giardia lamblia*
                   *Entamoeba histolytica**
                   Cryptosporidium
                   Isospora belli
                   Enterocytozoon bieneusi
                      (Microsporidium)
                   Cyclospora

Viral (35.0%)

Rotavirus (mainly Group A)
Norwalk virus
Adenovirus (serotypes 40 and 41)
Calcivirus
Astrovirus

Bacterial (30.0%)

                   *Campylobacter jujuni**
                   Salmonella sp.*
                   *Yersinia enterocolitica**
                   Shigilla sp.*
                   Vibrio cholea
                   Vibrio parahemolyticus
Enterogenic *Escherichia coli*
Enterohemorrhagic *Escherichia coli*
Enteroinvasive *Escherichia coli**
Enteropathogenic *Escherichia coli*
                   Pleisiomonas shigelloides
                   Aeromonas hydrophilia
                   Staphylococcus aureus
                   Bacills cereus
                   *Clostridium difficile**

Culture Negative (30.0%)

Figure 48G-1 Organisms associated with diarrhea and approximate percent isolation from immunocompetent outpatients
*Organisms most commonly producing afebrile syndrome with white blood cells & red blood cells in the stool.

B. Typically, a pathogen is identified in only about one-third to one-half of cases. Reasons for this low diagnostic yield include the following:
  1. It is difficult to identify the pathogen from among the millions of nonpathogens present in stool.
  2. Pathogen viability is lost during transportation and storage.
  3. Identification of some pathogens requires specialized procedures (e.g. plasmid analysis, electron microscopy) that are not available in many laboratories.
  4. To increase cost efficiency, specimens are typically screened for only the most common potential pathogens.

V. **Pathophysiology**
  A. Overview
     Essentially all enteric pathogens are acquired by oral ingestion. The development of diarrhea and related symptoms depends on an interaction between the virulence fac-

tors of the organism, the quantity of organism ingested, and host defenses.
  B. Organism virulence factors
     1. *Enterotoxins.* An enterotoxin is a product excreted by the organism (exotoxin) that has a direct effect on the bowel mucosa (usually via stimulation of cyclic adenine monophosphate or cyclic guanosine monophosphate) leading to a net movement of fluid into the gut lumen. This action does not cause mucosal bleeding, nor does it stimulate a local or systemic inflammatory response. The small bowel is the usual site of action. The choleratoxin of *Vibrio cholera* and the heat-labile and heat-stable toxins of enterotoxigenic *Escherichia coli* are examples of enterotoxins. *Clostridium perfringens* and *Bacillus cereus* also may cause disease via enterotoxin release.
     2. *Cytotoxins.* These products destroy mucosal cells and trigger an inflammatory response. The usual sites of action are the

colon and the distal small bowel. Red and white blood cells are usually seen in the stool, and the patient may be febrile. *Shigella* (shigatoxin), *C. difficile*, and some strains of *E. coli* (shiga-like toxin, verotoxin) are believed to cause diarrhea via this mechanism.

3. *Neurotoxins.* Neurotoxins cause gastrointestinal symptoms by a direct effect on the neuromuscular juncture (e.g., *Botulinum* toxin), the autonomic nervous system (e.g., *Staphylococcus aureus*, β-toxins), or the emetic center of the brain (e.g., the emetic toxin of *B. cereus*).

4. *Attachment/adhesion factors.* These are structures (e.g., fimbria) or antigens that prolong contact of the organism with the mucosal cell.

C. Quantity of organism ingested. The infections dose of various enteric pathogens varies widely, from fewer than 100 organisms (*Shigella*, *Giardia lamblia*, and *Entamoeba histolytica*) to 10^5 organisms for *Salmonella* and as high as 10^8 organisms for *V. cholera*. If very large quantities of organisms are ingested, the incubation period may be shortened.

D. Host factors. Host factors that are important for the prevention of enteric infection include:

1. Gastric acidity. Normal stomach acidity kills most ingested pathogens. This is probably the most important host defense.

2. Small bowel motility. Constant small bowel movement decreases contact time between the organism and the mucosal surface.

3. Endogenous microflora. Other organisms take up attachment sites, compete for nutrients, and may produce chemicals toxic to some pathogens.

4. Local antibody production (coproantibody).

VI. Diagnosis

A. A history is useful in directing the workup toward the most likely pathogens and providing an initial assessment of the severity of disease. The following should be assessed:

1. Frequency and consistency of stools.

2. Presence of gross blood or pus, suggestive of an invasive pathogen.

3. Associated symptoms
   a. Fever—suggests an invasive pathogen
   b. Nausea and/or vomiting—more commonly associated with a small bowel, enterotoxigenic, or viral process.
   c. Characteristics of pain—focal or very severe pain is unusual in most uncomplicated infectious diarrheal illnesses. When it occurs, consider gut ischemia, toxic megacolon, mesenteric adenitis, typhlitis (in the neutropenic patient), appendicitis, or other processes.

4. Fluid intake, weight changes, dizziness— clinical assessment of the state of hydration.

5. Travel history—may suggest the possibility of organism(s) infrequently found at the location of the examination.

6. Food ingestion history/incubation period—most useful during the evaluation of an outbreak when more than one person is ill and a meal has already been implicated; of limited use in the evaluation of sporadic cases of diarrhea.

B. Clinical signs and physical findings

1. State of hydration—blood pressure and pulse (orthostatic changes), mentation, skin turgor, and mucous membrane examination assist in this evaluation.

2. Temperature.

3. Abdominal examination—in most infectious diarrheal illnesses, this examination is essentially normal. Occasionally patients have diffuse abdominal tenderness or hyperactive bowel sounds. Hypoactive or absent bowel sounds, focal tenderness, rebound tenderness, or a mass are all unusual and should suggest complications or other processes.

C. Diagnostic tests

1. Stool examination for cells (See Fig. 48G-1).

2. Other microscopic tests
   a. Wet mount and trichrome stain—generally for ova and parasites.
   b. Acid-fast stain—for *Cryptosporidium*, *Isospora belli*, *Cyclospora* spp, and *Mycobacterium* spp.
   c. Dark-field examination—may detect the "darting motility" of *Campylobacter* or *Vibrio* spp.
   d. Gram stain—may detect curved, gram-negative rods suggestive of *Campylobacter* or *Vibrio* spp.
   e. Stool cultures.
   f. Toxin assays
      (1) Cytotoxic effect on cell culture.
      (2) Enzyme-linked immunosorbent assay.
      (3) Enzyme immunoassay.

(4) Nucleic acid probes.
  g. Electron microscopy—primarily for viral diagnosis.
  h. Proctoscopy/colonoscopy—particularly useful in the diagnosis of *C. difficile* (pseudomembranes), amebiasis (biopsy may reveal organisms), inflammatory bowel disease (biopsy), and sexually transmitted diseases involving the gastrointestinal tract (usually confined to the distal 15 cm, including gonorrhea, lymphogranuloma venereum, herpes simplex, and syphilis).

VII. Differential Diagnosis
  A. Fig. 48G-1 presents the differential diagnosis of common diarrhea syndromes (see also Ch 46D & 49D).
  B. The differential diagnosis of diarrhea lasting for over 3 weeks includes the following:
    1. Usually afebrile diseases
      a. *G. lamblia*
      b. *Cryptosporidium*
      c. Tropical sprue
      d. Postinfective malabsorption syndrome
      e. Hyperthyroidism, diabetic diarrhea, glucagonoma, serotonin- or histamine-secreting tumors, medullary carcinoma of the thyroid.
    2. Febrile diseases
      a. Amebiasis
      b. *I. belli*
      c. *C. difficile*
      d. Pericolonic abscess
      e. Inflammatory bowel disease

VIII. Treatment
  A. Rehydration
    1. Oral.
    2. Intravenous.
  B. Antimicrobial therapy of acute syndromes
    1. May shorten the acute illness by 1 to 2 days if instituted early.
    2. Appropriate therapy shortens the duration of excretion of many pathogens, thereby decreasing the risk of secondary transmission.
    3. Antimicrobial sensitivity patterns vary widely, and no single agent is effective against all pathogens.
  C. Antimotility agents
    1. Most are effective in decreasing the symptoms and the frequency of diarrhea in afebrile, watery diarrhea syndromes.
    2. In invasive processes, there is some concern that these agents may increase the contact time between the pathogen and the mucosa and worsen the illness.
  D. Bismuth compounds
    1. Useful in watery diarrhea syndromes. They shorten the illness, possibly by binding the toxin in the gut or via the action of salicylate.
    2. Bismuth subsalicylate may be associated with symptoms of salicylism, particularly in patients concomitantly taking aspirin.

IX. Patient Monitoring
  A. State of hydration.
  B. Risk of systemic infection.
    1. Primarily seen in invasive syndromes. Organisms in blood may be part of normal bowel flora (e.g., *E. coli*) entering via a mucosal lesion caused by an enteric pathogen (e.g., *C. jejuni*).
  C. Stool cultures
    1. Follow-up cultures are particularly important in persons who remain symptomatic (a second pathogen may be present) and in patients with job restrictions or immunocompromising illnesses.

X. Prognosis
  A. Most enteric infections produce a self-limited syndrome lasting for 1 to 5 days. If patients maintain an adequate state of hydration, complications are rare.
  B. Risk factors for complications include:
    1. Underlying malnourished/immunocompromised state
    2. Extremes of age.

Bibliography

Asirkoff B, Bennett JV. Effect of antibiotic therapy in acute salmonellosis on the fecal excretion of *Salmonellae*. *N Engl J Med* 281:636–640, 1969.

DiJohn D, Levine MM. Treatment of diarrhea. *Infect Dis Clin North Am* 2:719–745, 1988.

DuPont HL. Diarrheal diseases: an overview. *Am J Med* 78(Suppl 6B):64–64, 1985.

Goodman LJ, Trenholme GM, Kaplan RL, et al. Empiric antimicrobial therapy of domestically acquired acute diarrhea in urban adults. *Arch Intern Med* 150:541–546, 1990.

Guerrant RL, Bobak DA. Bacterial and protozoal gastroenteritis. *N Engl J Med* 325:327–338, 1991.

Blacklow N, Greenberg H. Viral gastroenteritis *N Engl J Med* 325:252–264, 1991.

Taylor DN, Sanchez JL, Candler W, et al. Treatment of travelers' diarrhea: Ciprofloxacin plus loperamide compared with ciprofloxacin alone: A placebo-controlled, randomized trial. *Ann Intern Med* 114:731–734, 1991.

CHAPTER 48-H

Urinary Tract Infections

John Segreti, M.D.

Acute Urinary Tract Infections (UTIs) in Adult Women

I. **Definitions**
- A. Lower UTI—cystitis/urethritis/dysuria frequency syndrome
- B. Upper UTI—pyelonephritis, renal abscess, perinephric abscess
- C. Bacteriuria—bacteriuria in the urine
- D. Significant bacteriuria—$\geq 10^5$ bacteria/per milliliter
- E. Asymptomatic bacteriuria—significant bacteriuria without symptoms

II. **Epidemiology**
- A. Affects 10–20% of adult women at some point during their lives.
- B. Accounts for about 5 million physician visits per year.
- C. Accounts for about $1 billion per year in national health care costs.
- D. *Escherichia coli* is the most common pathogen, followed by other Enterobacteriaceae, *Staphylococcus saprophyticus*, and *Enterococcus*.

III. **Pathophysiology**
- A. Bacterial virulence factors
  1. Bacterial adherence to uroepithelial cells via bacterial adhesins (fimbriae/pili)
  2. Lipopolysaccharide, which is probably responsible for the inflammatory response in the bladder and kidney. Endotoxin may also decrease ureteral peristalsis, resulting in vesicoureteral reflux.
  3. Capsular polysaccharide (K antigen), which inhibits complement attachment, and therefore phagocytosis, by polymorphonuclear leukocytes (PMNs).
  4. Serum resistance appears to be related to the presence of lipopolysaccharide.
  5. Hemolysins—proteins toxic to erythrocytes, PMNs, monocytes, and possibly renal tubular cells.
- B. Host defenses
  1. Antibacterial properties of urine include high oxygen tension (toxic to obligate anaerobes), low and high osmolality, high urea concentration, and low pH.
  2. Antiadherence mechanisms—bacterial interference, Tamm-Horsfall protein, urinary immunoglobulins, and glycoaminoglycan.
  3. Micturition—interferes with bacterial attachment by providing mechanical flushing of the mucosal surfaces.

4. Phagocytic cells such as macrophages and PMNs.

C. Risk factors for UTI
1. Obstruction appears to be the most important factor predisposing to infections due to:
   a. Incomplete flushing.
   b. Increased residual volume, which promotes bacterial growth.
2. Calculi
   a. May produce partial or complete obstruction.
   b. May damage the mucosal surface, facilitating bacterial adherence.
   c. Protected environment for bacteria.
3. Vesicoureteral reflux
   a. Usually observed in patients with congenital anomalies and bladder neck obstruction, as well as in pregnant women.
   b. Results in UTI infection and causes renal damage even in the absence of infection.
4. Diabetes mellitus
   a. UTI more frequent in patients with neuropathy and delayed bladder emptying.
   b. More severe renal disease, especially in diabetics with nephrosclerosis.
5. The elderly
   a. Obstruction is more common with age, especially in men.
   b. Reduced antiadherence defenses with age.
   c. Higher incidence of instrumentation in the elderly.

D. Risk factors in young women with normal urinary tracts.
1. Contraceptive method—*E. coli* bacteriuria is more common in women using a diaphragm with spermicidal jelly or a spermicidal foam with a condom.
2. Women with recurrent UTI are more likely to be Lewis blood group nonsecretors.

IV. **Pathogenesis**
A. Hematogenous spread to the kidney is uncommon but may be seen with *Salmonella*, *Mycobacterium tuberculosis*, *Staph. aureus*, and *Candida*.
B. Ascending route is the most common pathway.
1. Periurethral area and urethra are colonized with gram-negative bacilli.

2. Massage of the urethra forces bacteria into the bladder.
3. Bacteria multiply in the bladder and then may pass up the ureters to the kidneys, especially in the presence of vesicoureteral reflux.

V. **Diagnosis of Lower UTI**
A. Dysuria is the cardinal symptom.
B. Frequency, nocturia, urgency, and suprapubic pain may be present.
C. Ten percent of patients have suprapubic tenderness.
D. Differential diagnosis includes vaginitis in women, as well as gonococcal, *Chlamydia*, and/or herpes simplex virus genital infections.
E. Urine culture
1. Most patients with UTI have more than 100,000 bacteria per milliliter of urine.
2. Some women with dysuria/pyuria syndrome have 10^2–10^4 bacteria per milliliter.
F. Urinalysis
1. Pyuria (>10 white blood cells per milliliter) is usually present.
2. Hematuria occurs in 40–60%.
3. Presence of nitrite is very specific but is not a sensitive test for bacteriuria.
4. Esterase detection is very sensitive but not specific.
5. High pH may be a clue to infection with a urea-splitting organism (e.g., *Proteus*, *Klebsiella*).
G. Gram stain of unspun urine may be very helpful. The presence of one bacterium per oil immersion field correlates with $\geqslant 10^5$ bacteria/per milliliter of urine.

VI. **Diagnosis of Upper UTI**
A. Flank, low back, or abdominal pain may be present.
B. Fever and chills are often present and usually indicate upper rather than lower UTI.
C. Up to one-third of patients only have symptoms of uncomplicated acute cystitis.
D. White blood cell casts are seen on urinalysis.
E. Bladder washout—the bladder is drained, and antibiotic solution is instilled and drained 30 min later. Six subsequent quantitative cultures are obtained at 15-min intervals. If the colony count increases from culture 2 to culture 6, UTI may be present. This is a very good and reproducible test; however, it is too time-consuming, costly, and invasive for routine use.

F. Selective ureteral catheterization is the most reliable method of localization. However, it is not without risk and is not recommended for routine use.

G. Ultrasound examination may be able to replace intravenous pyelography (IVP) in the search for anatomic abnormalities.

H. Computed tomography scan may be helpful if renal or perinephric abscess is suspected.

I. IVP should be normal in lower UTI. Pyelonephritis may show changes, including caliceal blunting; however, the test is nonspecific, and it is difficult to differentiate acute from chronic disease.

J. Biopsy of the kidney is unreliable, as pyelonephritis is a focal disease and is often missed by blind biopsy.

K. Detection of antibody-coated bacteria may be useful in localizing the infection, but it is not widely available. Fluorescent antibody test—UTI infection stimulates local antibody formation. In general, lower UTI does not. Using fluorescein-tagged antihuman globulin and finding bacteria coated with antibody is suggestive of upper UTI. Generally, there is an 85% correlation. Most notable false-positive results occur in men with prostate infections and in young girls. Other problems include the fact that the patient must be untreated at the time of the test, and technician time and training are involved.

L. Urine culture. In general, the presence of $>10^5$ bacteria in a clean catheter specimen is associated with infection. If there is significant delay between the times of collection and plating, 10^2–10^3 bacteria may become 10^5, giving a false-positive result. Three cultures, each with 10^5 or more of the same bacteria, are associated with a 95–97% chance of being significant. Finding an average of one bacterium per high-power field on a fresh, unspun Gram stain correlates very well with the presence of 10^5 bacteria in culture.

VII. **Therapy**

A. Lower UTI—A 3-day course of therapy is associated with an incidence of adverse reactions similar to that seen with single-dose therapy and with efficacy comparable to that of a 7- to 10-day course of therapy.

B. Upper UTI—A 14-day course is as effective as a 6-week course but appears to be more effective than shorter courses of therapy.

C. Initial antibiotic choice should be based on local susceptibility data and then adjusted when in vitro susceptibility data are available.

VIII. **Posttherapy Procedures**
Posttherapy cultures not necessary except in those patients with persisting symptoms, pregnancy, a recent indwelling catheter, diabetes, or other immunosuppressing conditions.

IX. **Recurrent UTI**

A. Persistence of bacteria (relapse)—The same organism is reisolated after apparently successful therapy. Causes include infected calculi, chronic bacterial prostatitis, infected cyst, medullary sponge kidneys, and other anatomic abnormalities. It usually requires a surgical procedure for correction or chronic suppressive antibiotic therapy.

B. Reinfection accounts for the vast majority of recurrent infections. It is usually caused by different organisms.
   1. In women, reinfection is related to periurethral colonization.
   2. In men, reinfection is usually associated with an anatomic or functional urinary tract abnormality.

C. Treatment of recurrent reinfections in women
   1. Low-dose, continuous antimicrobial prophylaxis for about 6 months. Many remissions are followed by reinfection after discontinuation of therapy.
   2. Self-initiated intermittent therapy—A 3-day course of empiric antibiotics is taken as soon as symptoms begin.
   3. Postintercourse antibiotics should be taken if sexual intercourse appears to be a risk factor for reinfection.

Prostatitis

I. **Definitions**

A. Bacterial prostatitis—associated with UTI symptoms, positive cultures of prostatic fluid, and the presence of white blood cells in prostatic secretions.
   1. Acute prostatitis—abrupt febrile illness associated with constitutional symptoms.
   2. Chronic bacterial prostatitis—subtle condition with relapsing UTI.

B. Nonbacterial prostatitis—white blood cells in prostatic secretions but prostate fluid cultures negative.

C. Prostatodynia—no UTI, prostate fluid cultures negative, and no white blood cells in prostatic secretions.

II. Etiology

A. Community-acquired bacterial prostatitis—*E. coli* is most common, followed by *Klebsiella* and *Proteus*.

B. Hospital-acquired prostatitis—*Staph. aureus*, multiresistant gram-negative bacilli, and enterococci.

C. Nonbacterial prostatitis—*Chlamydia* and genital mycoplasmas may play a role, though this has not been documented.

D. Rarely, prostatitis is due to *Mycobacteria*, *Blastomyces*, or gonococci.

III. Pathogenesis

A. Intraprostatic reflux of urine may be the most important factor leading to bacterial prostatitis.

B. Ascending urethral infection—facilitated by both indwelling urethral catheters and condom catheters. May follow transurethral resection of the prostate.

C. Pathogenesis of nonbacterial prostatitis and prostatodynia is unknown.

IV. Diagnosis

A. Examination of prostatic fluid and semen shows >15 white blood cells per high-power field and macrophages containing fat droplets (oval fat bodies) indicating prostatic inflammation.

B. Bacterial culture and localization:

Tube 1	2	3	4
1st voided urine	mid stream culture	expressed prostatic secretion	1st void after massage

1. Bacterial prostatitis indicated if culture of tube 3 or 4 has more bacteria than culture of tube 1 or 2.
2. If tubes 1 or 2 have high bacterial counts, then a short course (2–3 days) of antibiotics should be given before cultures are repeated.
3. Chronic bacterial prostatitis is associated with relapsing or recurrent UTI.

V. Treatment

A. Acute bacterial prostatitis—pathogen specific antibiotics for at least 30 days.

B. Chronic bacterial prostatitis—pathogen-specific antibiotics for 4–16 weeks; results in 30–40% cure rates.

C. Suppressive therapy may be necessary for patients who are not medically cured.

D. Nonbacterial prostatitis may respond to tetracycline or erythromycin given for 14 days.

E. Most antibiotics penetrate poorly into prostatic fluid. Trimethoprim and quinolones achieve the highest levels of penetration.

Asymptomatic Bacteriuria

I. Definition

Two separate clean-voided urine specimens with $\geq 10^5$ bacteria per milliliter of the same organism in the absence of symptoms.

II. Asymptomatic Bacteriuria in Young, Nonpregnant Women

A. Prevalence is about 5%.

B. Up to 30% of patients may become symptomatic within one year, but pyelonephritis is rare.

C. Usually not associated with renal damage.

D. Short-course antibiotic therapy does not seem to alter the natural history; therefore, this treatment is not recommended.

III. Asymptomatic Bacteriuria in Pregnancy

A. Prevalence ranges from 2.5 to 15%.

B. From 20% to 40% of untreated women with bacteriuria develop pyelonephritis. This disease is probably related to dilation of the ureters and renal pelvis starting in the first trimester, which facilitates reflux of infected urine.

C. Associated with a higher incidence of prematurity, low-birth-weight infants, and perinatal death.

D. Appropriate treatment lowers the incidence of pyelonephritis to about 3%.

IV. Asymptomatic Bacteriuria in Men

A. Incidence increases after age 50, most likely as a result of prostatic hypertrophy and urinary tract instrumentation.

B. Unclear if the source of bacteriuria is localized to the bladder, kidneys, or prostate.

C. In the absence of obstruction, men with asymptomatic bacteriuria do not develop renal damage.

D. If infection is localized to the prostate, then antimicrobial therapy is indicated (see above).

E. If infection not localized to the prostate, then antibiotic use is controversial.

V. Asymptomatic Bacteriuria in the Elderly

A. Asymptomatic bacteriuria present in 20–50% of women and in 5–35% of men over 65 years of age.

B. The highest frequency occurs in institutionalized elderly patients who require nursing care, especially for fecal or urinary incontinence.

C. The clinical significance of this condition is unclear.

D. In the absence of obstruction, no treatment is required.

Bibliography

Johnson JR, Stamm WE. Urinary tract infections in women: Diagnosis and treatment. *Ann Intern Med* 111:906–917, 1989.

Komaroff AL. Urinalysis and urine culture in women with dysuria. *Ann Intern Med* 104:212–218, 1986.

Krogfelt KA. Bacterial adhesion: Genetics, biogenesis, and role in pathogenesis of fibrial adhesins of *Escherichia coli*. *Rev Infect Dis* 13:721–735, 1991.

Kunin CM. Duration of treatment of urinary tract infections. *Am J Med* 71:849–854, 1981.

Lipsky BA. Urinary tract infections in men: Epidemiology, pathophysiology, diagnosis, and treatment. *Ann Intern Med* 110:138–150, 1989.

Nicolle LE, Bjornson J, Harding GKM, MacDonell JA. Bacteriuria in elderly institutionalized men. *New Engl J Med* 309:1420–1425, 1983.

Nicolle LE, Mayhew WJ, Bryan L. Prospective randomized comparison of therapy and no therapy for asymptomatic bacteriuria in institutionalized elderly women. *Am J Med* 83:27–33, 1987.

Safrin S, Siegel D, Black D. Pyelonephritis in adult women: Inpatient versus outpatient therapy. *Am J Med* 85:793–798, 1988.

Stamm WE, Counts GW, Wagner KF, et al. Antimicrobial prophylaxis of recurrent urinary tract infections: A double-blind, placebo-controlled trial. *Ann Intern Med* 92:770–775, 1980.

Stamm WE, McKevitt M, Counts GW. Acute renal infection in women: Treatment with trimethoprimsulfamethoxazole or ampicillin for two or six weeks—a randomized trial. *Ann Intern Med* 106:341–345, 1987.

Stamm WE, Hooton TH. Management of Urinary Tract Infections in Adults. *New Engl J Med* 329:1328–1334, 1993.

Strom BL, Collins M, West SL, et al. Sexual activity, contraceptive use, and other risk factors for symptomatic and asymptomatic bacteriuria—a case-control study. *Ann Intern Med* 107:816–823, 1987.

Wong ES, McKevitt M, Running K, et al. Management of recurrent urinary tract infections with patient-administered single-dose therapy. *Ann Intern Med* 102:302–307, 1985.

Zhanel GG, Harding GKM, Guay DRP. Asymptomatic bacteriuria—which patients should be treated? *Arch Intern Med* 150:1389–1395, 1990.

Chapter 48-I

Sexually Transmitted Diseases

Constance A. Benson, M.D.

Gonorrhea

I. Etiology

The etiology is *Neisseria gonorrhoeae*.

A. Gonococci are small, nonmotile, gram-negative diplococci.

B. The organism grows optimally when immediately inoculated on modified Thayer-Martin or chocolate agar medium and incubated at 37°C in 5% CO_2. Colonies grow within 24–48 hr but lose viability after 48 hr.

C. Virulence factors involved in the pathogenesis of gonococcal disease include:

1. Pili—piliated gonococci attach to mucosal surfaces more readily than non-piliated organisms.

2. Outer membranes, which contain lipopolysaccharides, protein, and phospholipids, may be associated with serum resistance and allow dissemination (outer membrane proteins I, II and III).

3. "Auxotype"—characteristic that determines strain variation by the ability to grow on media lacking certain nutrients (e.g., AHU⁻ auxotype requires arginine, hypoxanthine, and uracil for growth).

The AHU auxotype may be associated with asymptomatic infection in men and disseminated infection in women.

4. Extracellular products—production of proteases that cleave and inactivate IgA on mucosal surfaces.

II. Epidemiology

A. More than 500,000 cases per year in the United States are reported to the Centers for Disease Control. The attack rate is highest in the 15- to 24-year age group, with a male:female ratio of 1.5:1.

B. Transmission occurs through sexual contact with an infected partner; the risk increases with increasing numbers of exposures. After a single exposure, the transmission rate from an infected male to a female through genital intercourse is about 50%, and the transmission rate from an infected female to a male through genital intercourse is about 20%. The risk triples after more than four exposures.

1. Organisms may also be transmitted by oral-genital contact, rectal intercourse, and nonsexual contact (perinatal transmission).

C. Penicillinase-producing strains of *N. gonor-rhoeae* (PPNG) have substantially increased in incidence in urban areas since 1980; the incidence is currently ~10% in major urban centers.
  1. Penicillinase production may be either plasmid or chromosomally mediated.
  2. Plasmid or chromosomally mediated tetracycline resistance has also been reported in association with scattered outbreaks of gonococcal disease.

III. **Pathogenesis**
  A. Following contact, organisms attach or adhere to noncornified epithelial surfaces through the interaction of pili or outer membrane proteins.
  B. Following penetration to submucosal tissue, a brisk polymorphonuclear leukocyte (PMN) response is triggered, with engulfing and intracellular killing of organisms, sloughing of epithelium, and development of submucosal microabscesses.
  C. If untreated, PMNs are replaced with a mononuclear and lymphocytic infiltrate.
  D. Organisms able to evade host defenses may invade the bloodstream or spread to contiguous structures.

IV. **Clinical Presentation: History and Physical Findings**
  A. Male genital infection: Within 2–7 days after exposure to an infected partner, men may experience a purulent urethral discharge, usually copious, milky, and heaviest in the morning, accompanied by urethral irritation, erythema, and dysuria. Infection may be asymptomatic in 5–60% (depending on gender, virulence factors, etc.) and may persist if untreated. Additional local manifestations include epididymitis, prostatitis, periurethral abscess, and penile lymphangitis.
  B. Female genital infection: The most frequent initial site of infection is the endocervix. Asymptomatic infection may be more common in women. Symptoms, when they are present, include endocervical discharge, dysuria, urinary frequency, and menstrual irregularities. Cervical erythema, friability, and mucopurulent discharge may be present on exam. Additional local manifestations include urethritis, vaginitis, and periurethral gland abscesses.
  C. Extragenital manifestations
    1. Pharyngitis: Usually acquired through orogenital contact; most infections are asymptomatic, but some may be associated with odynophagia, tonsillar exudate, and cervical lymphadenitis.
    2. Proctitis: Approximately 30–50% of infected women have positive rectal cultures, usually as a result of contamination from cervical secretions. This is usually not symptomatic. Symptomatic proctitis occurs most commonly in those who engage in anal intercourse. Signs and symptoms include pruritus, tenesmus, purulent discharge, and rectal friability and bleeding.
    3. Conjunctivitis: This is seen most often in neonates born through an infected birth canal or in adults through inadvertent autoinoculation of the eye.
    4. Pelvic inflammatory disease: This occurs in 10–20% of women with endocervical infection. Contiguous spread results in salpingitis, tuboovarian abscesses, pelvic peritonitis, and perihepatitis. The most consistent symptom is lower abdominal or pelvic pain. Exam will generally reveal adnexal tenderness, pain on manipulation of the cervix, and a mucopurulent cervical discharge. A palpable adnexal mass may be present.
    5. Disseminated gonococcal infection: This syndrome occurs in 1–3% of patients and is the leading cause of acute septic arthritis in young adults. The initiating infection may be asymptomatic in 80%. Local infection appears to occur up to 7–30 days prior to dissemination. Dissemination may be triggered by menstruation in women. The onset is subacute; migrating polyarthralgia, pustular skin lesions, and tenosynovitis are the most common symptoms and signs, later followed by septic complications which may include septic arthritis, endocarditis, meningitis, pneumonitis, and osteomyelitis. Patients with terminal complement deficiencies have an increased incidence of bacteremic neisserial infection.
    6. Neonatal infection: Transmitted in utero following rupture of membranes, during passage through an infected birth canal, or in the postpartum period from mother to infant. Neonatal ophthalmia or purulent conjunctivitis has been associated with blindness when untreated; systemic dissemination of infection can occur.

V. Diagnostic Tests

A. Gram's stain of urethral/cervical smears revealing typical intracellular gram-negative diplococci is 90% sensitive and 98% specific in symptomatic men, 60% sensitive in asymptomatic men, and 50–70% sensitive and 90% specific in symptomatic women under optimal circumstances of specimen collection and laboratory technique.

B. Specimens for culture should be obtained from infected sites with calcium alginate swabs and inoculated immediately on appropriate media.

C. Rapid enzyme immunoassays are associated with a yield, sensitivity, and specificity approximately those of the Gram's stain.

VI. Differential Diagnosis

A. Purulent *Chlamydia trachomatis* genital infections most closely mimic the presentation of gonococcal disease.

B. Herpes simplex virus (HSV) may cause sexually transmitted mucopurulent cervicitis, urethritis, proctitis, exudative pharyngitis, and ocular infections; HSV is usually distinguished by its characteristic ulcerative mucosal lesions.

C. Vaginitis or other genital syndromes due to *Trichomonas* spp., *Candida* spp., or bacterial vaginosis may mimic gonococcal vaginitis or local mucosal infection.

VII. Treatment

Recommended first-line therapy is ceftriaxone in a single 250-mg intramuscular dose combined with a 7-day course of tetracycline for treatment of potential *Chlamydia* coinfection.

VIII. Monitoring

Tests of cure cultures are recommended 7 days after therapy. Sexual partners should be *treated*.

Syphilis

I. Etiology

The etiology is *Treponema pallidum.*

A. *T. pallidum* is a member of the family Spirochaetaceae.

B. The organism cannot be routinely cultivated in vitro; it has been cultivated under research conditions.

II. Epidemiology

A. The organism is acquired by direct inoculation through contact with infected lesions, by transfusion, and in utero. Infection is most contagious in the early stages of disease.

B. Disease is most frequent among the 15- to 30-year age group. The incidence in the United States fluctuated between 21,000 and 30,000 cases per year until the advent of the acquired immunodeficiency syndrome epidemic, which has been accompanied by a rise in the annual number of new cases and an attendant rise in congenital syphilis.

III. Pathogenesis

A. The organism penetrates skin or mucous membranes, spreads to local lymphatics and then to the bloodstream, and finally disseminates widely.

B. The incubation period for primary disease varies according to the size of the inoculum, with a median of 3 weeks and a range of 3–90 days.

C. The most prominent pathologic finding at all stages of the disease is an obliterative endarteritis with endothelial and fibroblast proliferation, which can occur in any tissue or organ system. The pathology closely follows the clinical course.

IV. Clinical Presentation: History and Physical Findings

A. *Primary syphilis:* At the site of inoculation, a chancre begins as a single painless papule that erodes and indurates, with a smooth base and raised, firm borders. Persons with a previous history of syphilis often fail to develop noticeable primary lesions.

  1. Regional lymphadenopathy will generally accompany the primary lesion. In the absence of therapy, the chancre heals within 3–6 weeks; however, regional lymphadenopathy may persist for a longer period.

B. *Secondary syphilis:* This stage results from local replication and subsequent dissemination of spirochetes and lasts until the host immune response intervenes. It begins 2–8 weeks after the appearance of the primary chancre.

  1. Clinical manifestations span a wide spectrum.

    a. Skin rash (90%): Macular, maculopapular, papular, or pustular lesions involving the palms and soles; condylomata lata and atypical chancres are also seen.

    b. Mucous membranes (70%): Lesions include mucous patches, erosions, and aphthous ulcers.

    c. Constitutional symptoms (70%): Fever, malaise, pharyngitis, anorexia, weight loss, arthralgias, and headache.

d. Central nervous system (CNS): Asymptomatic (8–33%); symptomatic (1–2%). Manifestations may include headache, meningismus, aseptic meningitis, diplopia, tinnitus, vertigo, and cranial nerve II–VIII deficits.

e. Renal (rare): Glomerulonephritis, nephrotic syndrome.

f. Granulomatous hepatitis (rare).

g. Musculoskeltal syndromes (rare): Arthritis, osteitis, and periostitis.

C. *Latent syphilis:* This stage is arbitrarily divided into "early latent," which usually applies to the first 1–4 years after infection when infectious relapse can occur, and "late latent," which is associated with relative resistance to infectious relapse or reinfection. It is a period when there are no clinical manifestations of disease but when specific treponemal antibody tests are positive.

D. *Late syphilis:* A multisystem indolent granulomatous inflammatory disease causing clinical symptoms years after initial infection.

1. Asymptomatic neurosyphilis is a condition in which no CNS symptoms are present but one or more abnormalities of the cerebrospinal fluid (CSF), including cell count, protein, glucose, or a positive CSF Venereal Disease Research Laboratory (VDRL) or fluorescent treponemal antibody absorbed assay are found.

2. Symptomatic neurosyphilis is divided into meningovascular and parenchymatous disease.

a. Meningovascular disease is an inflammatory endarteritis obliterans affecting the blood vessels of the brain, meninges, and spinal cord. Manifestations range from hemiplegia or progressive neurologic deficits to focal or generalized seizures. Symptoms occur 5–10 years after the onset of untreated syphilis.

b. Parenchymatous disease results from destruction of nerve cells primarily in the cerebral cortex. *General paresis* refers to personality changes, affectational changes, hyperactive reflexes, Argyl Robertson pupil (which reacts on accommodation but not in response to light), changes of sensorium, decreases in recent memory

or judgment, and speech abnormalities; this syndrome occurs 15–20 years after onset of syphilis. *Tabes dorsalis* involves demyelinization of the posterior column, dorsal roots, and dorsal root ganglia, resulting in an ataxic gait, foot slap, paresthesias, bladder dysfunction, impotence, and loss of position, vibratory, deep pain, and temperature sensation; this syndrome occurs 25–30 years after the onset of untreated syphilis.

c. Special localized forms of neurosyphilis include:

(1) Syphilitic otitis, which may include sensorineural hearing loss and/or cochleovestibular dysfunction.

(2) Syphilitic eye disease, which may manifest as uveitis, diffuse chorioretinitis, or vasculitis involving the eye.

E. Other manifestations of late syphilis

1. Cardiovascular syphilis: aortitis with a predilection for the ascending aorta; the incidence is thought to approach 10% in untreated patients.

2. Gummatous syphilis is a granulomatous inflammatory disease resulting in slowly progressive tissue destruction within any organ system; however, gummas are most commonly found in skeletal, skin, and mucocutaneous tissues.

F. Anecdotal data suggest that there may be an accelerated course of progression of syphilis and a higher rate of CNS involvement in patients coinfected with human immunodeficiency virus (HIV). This has implications for diagnosis and therapy.

G. Congenital syphilis

1. Transmission of syphilis in utero can occur in infected pregnant women during any stage of syphilis but is most likely during early infection.

2. Infection of the fetus before the fourth month of gestation is rare.

3. Treatment of the mother during the first 4 months of pregnancy usually ensures that the fetus will not be infected. Fetal infection may result in intrauterine fetal demise, neonatal disease, or latent infection.

4. Clinical manifestations of congenital syphilis include a constellation of signs and symptoms, depending on the timing of in utero infection.

a. Early: Osteochondritis, snuffles, rash, anemia, hepatosplenomegaly, jaundice, neurologic abnormalities, lymphadenopathy, and mucous patches.

b. Late: Frontal bossing, short maxilla, saddle nose deformity, protruding mandible, interstitial keratitis, eighth nerve deafness, high palatal arch, Hutchinson's incisors, Mulberry molars, sternoclavicular thickening, bilateral painless swelling of knees, saber shins, and flaring scapulas.

5. If the untreated child survives the first 6–12 months, late or latent disease may occur, manifestations of which may be progression of neonatal lesions or development of cardiovascular disease or neurosyphilis.

V. **Diagnostic Tests**

A. Dark-field microscopic exam of serous transudate from moist lesions (with the exception of mouth lesions, which may contain oral spirochetes).

B. Silver stains of tissue biopsy specimens for detection of spirochetes.

C. Serologic tests

1. Nontreponemal tests: IgG and IgM antibody directed against a cardiolipin-cholesterol-lecithin antigen produced by host tissue interaction with *T. pallidum*. These tests include VDRL, rapid plasma reagin (RPR), and automated reagin tests. They are used as screening tests, are most useful during secondary and primary syphilis, and can be used to follow therapy.

2. The FTA-abs assay is an indirect immunofluorescent assay which detects specific antibody to *T. pallidum* antigens.

Once positive, it remains positive for life and is primarily used to verify the diagnosis. The treponemal hemagglutination-*T. pallidum* and micro-hemagglutination-T. pallidum tests are easier, less expensive, and less time-consuming than the FTA but less sensitive in the diagnosis of primary syphilis.

3. Serologic tests may be falsely negative or difficult to interpret for those with HIV coinfection; repeat testing or the use of more direct tissue staining of biopsy specimens may be necessary in suspicious cases.

4. False-positive serologic tests, both nonspecific and specific treponemal assays, can occur in a number of other conditions, including other spirochetal infections, viral infections, autoimmune diseases, pregnancy or chronic liver disease.

VI. **Differential Diagnosis**

A. Primary syphilis must be differentiated from HSV, chancroid, early granuloma inguinale, lymphogranuloma venereum, venereal warts, and, rarely, other infections causing genital ulcers.

B. Secondary syphilis is associated with protean and extensive manifestations mimicking those of numerous other diseases.

C. The differential diagnosis of late syphilis depends on the site of localization, with other granulomatous inflammatory diseases or vasculitides being those principally considered.

VII. **Treatment** (See Table 48I-1)

A. CSF exam is advisable for patients with secondary or later stages of disease, for those with a positive specific treponemal antibody test and no previous therapy, and for those with HIV coinfection.

Table 48I-1. Treatment of Syphilis*

Stage	Patients Not Allergic to Penicillin	Patients Allergic to Penicillin**
Early syphilis (primary, secondary)	Procaine PCN plus probenecid or doxycycline or amoxicillin plus probenecid or ceftriaxone or benzathine penicillin G	Doxycycline or tetracycline hydrochloride or erythromycin (stearate, ethylsuccinate, or base)
Late syphilis (tertiary), neurosyphilis, or HIV infection, especially late-stage disease	Aqueous crystalline penicillin (by IV injection) or procaine penicillin plus probenecid or amoxicillin plus probenecid, doxycycline, or ceftriaxone.	Chloramphenicol

*Adapted from Tramont EC. pg. 1806 (ref.).

**Syphilis during pregnancy should be treated with a penicillin regimen; desensitization may be necessary for those who are penicillin-allergic.

VIII. Monitoring

A. Follow-up nontreponemal tests should be repeated at 3, 6, and 12 months after therapy of early or congenital syphilis; those with later-stage disease should be retested at the end of 24 months as well. Retreatment should be considered when the clinical signs and symptoms persist despite therapy or when nontreponemal antibody titers rise after an initial decline or remain positive 1–3 years after therapy, depending on the stage.

B. After therapy of neurosyphilis, follow-up CSF exams should be repeated every 3 to 6 months for at least 3 years.

Bibliography

Brunham RC, Paavonen J, Stevens CE, et al. Mucopurulent cervicitis—the ignored counterpart in women of urethritis in men. *N Engl J Med* 311:1–6, 1984.

Centers for Disease Control and Prevention. Pelvic inflammatory disease: Guidelines for prevention and management. *MMWR* 40(RR-5):1–25, 1991.

Centers for Disease Control and Prevention. 1989 Sexually transmitted diseases treatment guidelines. Recommendations and reports. *MMWR* 38(S-8):1–43, 1989.

Clark EG, Danbolt N. The Olso study of the natural course of untreated syphilis. *Med Clin North Am* 48:613, 1964.

Corey L, Adams HG, Brown ZA, et al. Genital herpes simplex virus infections: Clinical manifestations, course, and complications. *Ann Intern Med* 98:958–972, 1983.

Corey L, Holmes KK. Genital herpes simplex virus infections: Current concepts in diagnosis, therapy, and prevention. *Ann Intern Med* 98:973–983, 1983.

Dallabetta G, Hook EW III. Gonococcal infections. *Infect Dis Clin North Am* 1:25–54, 1987.

Eron LJ, Judson F, Tucker S, et al. Interferon therapy for condylomata acuminata. *N Engl J Med* 315:1059–1064, 1986.

Fife KH, Rogers RE, Zwickl BW. Symptomatic and asymptomatic cervical infections with human papillomavirus during pregnancy. *J Infect Dis* 156:904–911, 1987.

Gourevitch MN, Selwyn PA, Davenny K, et al. effects of HIV infection on the serologic manifestations and response to treatment of syphilis in intravenous drug users. *Ann Intern Med* 118:350–355, 1993.

Hansfield HH. *Neisserina gonorrhoeae*, in Mandell GL, Douglas RG Jr, Bennett JE (eds): *Principles and Practice of Infectious Diseases*, ed 3. New York, Churchill Livingstone, 1990, pp 1613–1631.

Holtom PD, Larsen RA, Leal ME, et al. Prevalence of neurosyphilis in human immunodeficiency virus-infected patients with latent syphilis. *Am J Med* 93:9–12, 1992.

Hook EW III. Syphilis and HIV infection. *J Infect Dis* 160:530–534, 1989.

Hook EW III, Handsfield HH. Gonococcal infections in the adult, in Holmes KK, Mardh P-A, Sparling PF, et al (eds):

Sexually Transmitted Diseases, ed 2. New York, McGraw-Hill, 1990, pp 149–160.

Hook EW III, Holmes KK. Gonnococcal infections. *Ann Intern Med* 102:229–243, 1985.

Hook EW III, Jones RB, Martin DH, et al. Comparison of ciprofloxacin and ceftriaxone as single-dose therapy for uncomplicated gonorrhea in women. *Antimicrob Agents Chemother* 37:1670–1673, 1993.

Hook EW III, Marra CM. Acquired syphilis in adults. *N Engl J Med* 326:1060–1069, 1992.

Hooper RR, Reynolds GH, Jones OG, et al. Cohort study of venereal disease: I. The risk of gonorrhea transmission from infected women to men. *Am J Epidemiol* 108:136–144, 1978.

Hooton TM, Rogers E, Medina TG, et al. Ciprofloxacin compared with doxycycline for nongonococcal urethritis. Ineffectiveness against *Chlamydia trachomatis* due to relapsing infection. *JAMA* 264:1418–1421, 1990.

Hooton TM, Wong ES, Barnes RC, et al. Erythromycin for persistent or recurrent nongonococcal urethritis. A randomized, placebo-controlled trial. *Ann Intern Med* 113:21–26, 1990.

Kahn JC, Walker CK, Washington AE, et al. Diagnosing pelvic inflammatory disease. *JAMA* 266:2594–2604, 1991.

Kaplowitz LG, Baker D, Gelf L, et al. Prolonged continuous acyclovir treatment of normal adults with frequently recurring genital herpes simplex virus infection. *JAMA* 265:747–751, 1991.

Kiviat NB, Koutsky LA, Paavonen JA, et al. Prevalence of genital papillomavirus infection among women attending a college student health clinic or a sexually transmitted disease clinic. *J Infect Dis* 159:293–302, 1989.

Koutsky LA, Holmes KK, Critchlow CW, et al. A cohort study of the risk of cervical intraepithelial neoplasia grade 2 or 3 in relation to papillomavirus infection. *N Engl J Med* 327:1272–1278, 1992.

Koutsky LA, Stevens CE, Holmes KK, et al. Underdiagnosis of genital herpes by current clinical and viral-isolation procedures. *N Engl J Med* 326:1533–1539, 1992.

Kulhanjian JA, Soroush V, Au DS, et al. Identification of women at unsuspected risk of primary infection with herpes simplex virus type 2 during pregnancy. *N Engl J Med* 326:916–920, 1992.

Lukehart S, Hook EW III, Baker-Zander SH, et al. Invasion of the central nervous system by *Treponema pallidum*. Implications for diagnosis and therapy. *Ann Intern Med* 109:855–862, 1988.

Macnab JCM, Walkinshow SA, Cordiner JW, et al. Human papillomavirus in clinically and histologically normal tissue of patients with genital cancer. *N Engl J Med* 315:1052–1058, 1986.

Martin DH, Mroczkowski TF, Dalu ZA, et al. A controlled trial of a single dose of azithromycin for the treatment of chlamydial urethritis and cervicitis. *N Engl J Med* 327:921–925, 1992.

Masi AT, Eisenstein BI. Disseminated gonococcal infection (DGI) and gonococcal arthritis (GCA): II. Clinical manifestations, diagnosis, complications, treatment and prevention. *Semin Arthritis Rheum* 10:173–197, 1981.

Mertz GJ, Benedetti J, Ashley R, et al. Risk factors for the sexual transmission of genital herpes. *Ann Intern Med* 116:197–202, 1992.

Mertz GJ, Jones CC, Mills J, et al. Long-term acyclovir suppression of frequently recurring genital herpes simplex virus infection. A multicenter double-blind trial. *JAMA* 260:201–206, 1988.

O'Brien JA, Goldenberg DL, Rice PA. Disseminated gonococcal infection: A prospective analysis of 49 patients and a review of the pathophysiology and immune mechanisms. *Medicine* 62:395–406, 1983.

Peterson HB, Walker CK, Kahn JG, et al. Pelvic inflammatory disease: Key treatment issues and options. *JAMA* 266:2605–2611, 1991.

Rockwell DH, Yobs AR, Moore MB. The Tuskeegee study of untreated syphilis; the 30th year of observation. *Arch Intern Med* 114:792, 1964.

Ronald AR, Albritton W. Chancroid and *Haemophilus ducreyi*, in Holmes KK, Mardh P-A, Sparling PF, et al. (eds): *Sexually Transmitted Diseases*, ed 2. New York, McGraw-Hill, 1990, pp 263–272.

Schwarcz SK, Zenilman JM, Schnell D, et al. National surveillance of antimicrobial resistance in *Neisseria gonorrhoeae*. JAMA 264:1413–1417, 1990.

Scieux C, Barnes R, Bianchi A, et al. Lymphogranuloma venereum: 27 cases in Paris. *J Infect Dis* 160:662–668, 1989.

Sparling PF. Biology of *Neisseria gonorrhoeae*, in Holmes KK, Mardh P-A, Sparling PF, et al. (eds): *Sexually Transmitted Diseases*, New York, McGraw-Hill, 1990, pp 131–148.

Stamm WE, Holmes KK. *Chlamydia trachomatis* infections of the adult, in Homes KK, Mardh P-A, Sparling PF, et al. (eds): *Sexually Transmitted Diseases*, New York, McGraw-Hill, 1990, pp 181–194.

Stamm WE, Koutsky LA, Benedetti JK, et al. *Chlamydia trachomatis* urethral infections in men. Prevalence, risk factors, and clinical manifestations. *Ann Intern Med* 100:47–51, 1984.

Straus SE, Rooney JF, Sever JL, et al. Herpes simplex virus infection: Biology, treatment, and prevention. *Ann Intern Med* 103:404–419, 1985.

Tramont EC. *Treponema pallidum* (Syphilis), in Mandell GL, Douglas RG Jr, Bennett JE (eds): *Principles and Practice of Infectious Diseases*, ed 3. New York, Churchill Livingstone, 1990, pp 1794–1808.

Wasserheit JN, Bell TA, Kiviat NB, et al. Microbial causes of proven pelvic inflammatory disease and efficacy of clindamycin and tobramycin. *Ann Intern Med* 104:187–193, 1986.

Wong ES, Hooton TM, Hill CC, et al. Clinical and microbiological features of persistent or recurrent nongonococcal urethritis in men. *J Infect Dis* 158:1098–1101, 1988.

Table 481-2. Other Common Sexually Transmitted Diseases

Syndrome	Etiology	Transmission	Clinical Symptoms	Sequelae	Diagnosis	Treatment
Genital herpes	Herpes simplex virus type 1 or 2	Direct contact with infected lesions or secretions	Painful vesiculo-pustular rash with subsequent ulceration, shallow-based painful ulcers. Primary lesions heal in a mean of 14–21 days; recurrent lesions heal in a mean of 3–10 days; first clinical episode in patients with prior HSV antibody is less severe than true primary episodes.	Primary: Fever, sacral radiculo-myelitis, cervicitis, urethritis, aseptic meningitis, regional lymphadenitis, involvement of other con-tiguous sites. Recurrent HSV: Recurrences seen in 50–80%, more common with HSV-2; frequency of recurrences is variable; less likely to be associated with extragenital manifestations.	Viral culture, characteristic cytopathic changes in tissue or cells (as seen in Tzanck's smear); serology generally not helpful	Acute: Acyclovir, foscarnet (for resistant virus; Chronic suppression: Acyclovir
Genital chlamydia infection	*Chlamydia trachomatis* (D-K strains)	Direct contact with infected secretions	Women: Mucopurulent cervicitis, acute urethral syndrome, proctitis, pelvic inflammatory disease (PID). Men: Non- or post-gonococcal urethritis, epididymitis, proctitis.	Women: PID (infertility, chronic pelvic pain, ectopic pregnancy)	Culture, direct antigen detection	Tetracycline, doxycycline, erythromycin, azithromycin, clarithromycin

Lympho-granuloma venereum	*Chlamydia trachomatis* (L1-L3 strains)	Direct contact with infected secretions	Stage 1: Painless vesiculopapular skin lesions at the site of contact. Stage 2: Regional painful periadenitis with suppuration. Stage 3: Chronic fistulae, fibrosis, interruption of local lymphatic drainage.	Systemic dissemination, metastatic foci of infection, aseptic meningitis, septic arthritis, hepatitis, conjunctivitis, erythema nodosum	Culture	Same as for genital chlamydia infection but may require longer duration
Genital warts	Human papillomavirus	Direct contact with infected epithelial surface	Painless, exophytic or flat papulonodular skin lesions (condylomata); penis, vulva, perianal, vagina, cervix, urethra	Cervical, vulvar, vaginal, or penile intraepithelial neoplasia or frank carcinoma (DNA types 16, 18, 31, 35, and others)	PAP smear, colposcopy, tissue biopsy, HPV-DNA probe for antigen detection, or visual appearance	Chemical or physical ablation (topical podophyllin, 5-fluorouracil or trichloro-acetic acid; cryotherapy; surgical removal; laser ablation) Interferon
Trichomoniasis	*Trichomonas vaginalis*	Direct contact with infected secretions	Women: Vaginitis with frothy, malodorous, pruritic vaginal discharge; can be asympto-matic. Men: Usually asymptomatic; occasional balanitis, urethritis		PAP smear, saline wet prep of vaginal secretions, culture	Metronidazole

(continued)

531

Table 481-2. Continued

Syndrome	Etiology	Transmission	Clinical Symptoms	Sequelae	Diagnosis	Treatment
Chancroid	*Haemophilus ducreyi*	Direct contact with infected secretions	Tender papulo-pustular lesion at site of contact, followed by ulceration and regional lymphadenopathy	Bacterial superinfection (phagodenic chancroid), suppuration with chronic draining sinus formation	Gram's stain ("school of fish"), culture	Erythromycin, ceftriaxone, trimethoprim-sulfamethoxazole, ciprofloxacin
Pelvic inflammatory disease	Polymicrobial (*Neisseria gonorrhoeae*, *Chlamydia trachomatis*, genital tract anaerobes [*Peptostreptococcus*, *Peptococcus*, *Bacteroides* spp.])	Genital sexual contact	Lower abdominal pain, purulent cervical discharge, cervical motion tenderness, adnexal tenderness or mass, fever, leukocytosis	Infertility, chronic pelvic pain, ectopic pregnancy, recurrent PID	History, physical exam, pelvic sonography, culdocentesis, laparoscopy	Cefoxitin plus doxycycline or clindamycin plus gentamicin or metronidazole plus doxycycline or therapy guided by laparoscopic culture results

Bone and Joint Infections

John Segreti, M.D.

Infectious Arthritis

I. **Definition**
Infectious arthritis is inflammation of the joint space following infection with a microorganism.

II. **Pathogenesis**
Most cases of bacterial arthritis are secondary to hematogenous spread from a distant focus. Direct inoculation secondary to trauma is unusual. Spread of infection into the joint space from a contiguous osteomyelitis is unusual in adults except in cases where the epiphyseal plate is abnormal or fractured. In the case of an infected prosthesis, infections within a year of surgery are usually acquired at the time of surgery, and infections after 1 year from surgery are often acquired via hematogenous spread.

A. Hematogenous spread of infection results from direct spread through the articular cartilage from the vascular channels at the articular margin. Infection leads to an inflammatory response with polymorphonuclear leukocytes, which migrate to the joint fluid and release enzymes destructive to the articular surface.

B. If the infection is left untreated, the joint space narrows due to destruction of the cartilage. This leads to rapid loss of the joint space and erosive damage to the cartilage and bone.

C. Untreated infection can spread to neighboring soft tissue, with abscess and sinus tract formation. Ligaments or tendons may be destroyed.

D. Infection of the hip joint in both children and adults may result in vascular compromise of the femoral head, with resultant avascular necrosis.

III. **Risk Factors**
A. Many patients with infectious arthritis have an underlying preexisting joint disease such as arthritis or trauma.

B. Intravenous drug users, as well as patients with chronic renal failure, sickle cell disease, and diabetes mellitus, are also more likely to acquire bacterial arthritis than the general population.

IV. **Clinical Features**
A. Patients with bacterial arthritis often present with pain and loss of function in the joint.

B. Many patients are febrile at the time of presentation.

C. The joint is usually tender, warm, and red.

D. A joint effusion is almost always present with bacterial infection.

E. The most common sites of involvement in adults with nongonococcal infection are the knee (50%), hip (15%), shoulder (10%), wrist, ankle, hand, foot, and elbow (<10%).

F. Intravenous drug users are also more likely to present with sternoclavicular, acromioclavicular, or sacroiliac joint involvement.

G. Tenosynovitis is a manifestation of gonococcal infection, as well as chronic arthritis due to mycobacteria and fungi.

V. Microbiology of Infected Joints

A. Almost any organism can cause infectious arthritis.

1. In patients 15 to 40 years of age, *Neisseria gonorrhoeae* accounts for the vast majority of cases.

2. In the pediatric population, *Haemophilus influenzae* is a very common cause of septic arthritis, followed by *Staphylococcus* and streptococci.

3. In adults with nongonococcal arthritis, *Staphylococcus aureus* is isolated in the majority of cases.

4. *Streptococcus*, especially groups A, B, and G, is seen in all age groups. Arthritis due to these organisms may respond slowly to therapy, with persistent synovitis and joint destruction.

5. Gram-negative bacilli are relatively uncommon except in patients with underlying malignancy, immunosuppression, intravenous drug use, and chronic debilitating diseases.

6. Anaerobes are exceedingly uncommon in nondiabetic patients with septic arthritis.

7. Polyarticular septic arthritis may occur in up to 20% of adult patients with nongonococcal septic arthritis and is usually caused by *Staph. aureus*.

8. *Pasteurella multocida* should be suspected after a cat or dog bite. *Eikenella corrodens* is often seen after human bites, including closed-fist injuries.

VI. Laboratory Features

A. The peripheral white blood cell count may be mildly elevated.

B. The erythrocyte sedimentation rate is elevated in most patients.

C. Blood cultures should be obtained, as up to one-third of patients may be bacteremic.

D. It is imperative that synovial fluid be examined.

1. An elevated synovial fluid leukocyte count is common.

2. When the synovial fluid leukocyte count exceeds 100,000 white blood cells per milliliter, infection is almost always present. However, bacterial infection can also exist with synovial fluid leukocyte counts as low as 10,000 white blood cells per milliliter.

3. The differential of the synovial fluid leukocytes is usually 95% polymorphonuclear leukocytes.

4. Synovial fluid glucose levels below 40 mg/dl are strongly suggestive of bacterial arthritis.

5. The presence of urate or calcium pyrophosphate crystals does not rule out infection, as simultaneous septic and crystal arthritis is seen.

6. Positive Gram stain may immediately suggest the etiology of the organism. However, Gram stain may not differentiate staphylococci from streptococci.

7. Joint fluid should be cultured both aerobically and anaerobically.

8. Sexually active individuals should have synovial fluid cultured for *N. gonorrhoeae*. These patients should also have pharyngeal, rectal, urethral, and/or cervical cultures for *N. gonorrhoeae*.

9. X-rays of the involved joint usually reveal only periarticular soft tissue swelling.

10. Technetium bone scans demonstrate increased asymmetric uptake due to increased blood flow to the septic joint.

11. Gallium or indium scans may be more specific for infection, especially in the presence of an underlying inflammatory arthritis or recent trauma.

12. Ultrasonography and computed tomography (CT) may be useful in identifying hip joint effusions and in distinguishing them from psoas abscesses.

VII. Differential Diagnosis of Acute Monoarticular Arthritis

The differential diagnosis is trauma, crystal disease, and, much less commonly, tumor.

VIII. Chronic Monoarticular Arthritis

These patients often present with a several-week history of joint swelling. The joint is often not very warm or tender, and range of motion may not be significantly affected.

A. Mycobacterial infections often have a granulomatous reaction on pathologic examination.

   1. *Mycobacterium tuberculosis* is often the cause of this disease. However, nontuberculous mycobacteria can occasionally cause chronic monoarticular arthritis, including *M. kansasii, marinum, gordonii, avium-intracellulare, chelonei,* and *fortuitum.*

   2. A synovial biopsy is often required for diagnosis, as synovial fluid cultures may be negative.

   3. Pathology reveals chronic inflammation with granuloma formation and giant cells.

B. Fungal arthritis is most commonly caused by *Sporothrix schenckii.*

   1. The majority of patients with this infection have a history of contact with soil or plant material, or they perform labor-intensive work.

   2. Joint infection probably follows hematogenous spread from another site of inoculation rather than by direct inoculation into the joint.

   3. Joint infections are less commonly seen with other fungi, such as *Coccidioides, Blastomyces,* and *Candida* spp.

IX. Diagnostic Approach to Patients with Possible Infectious Arthritis

A. Infectious arthritis should be suspected in anyone with joint swelling.

B. Arthrocentesis should be performed and fluid sent for cell counts, glucose level, and cultures. Fluid should also be examined for crystals, but the presence of crystals does not rule out infectious arthritis.

C. In patients with suspected gonococcal infection, pharyngeal, rectal, and urethral cultures should be obtained.

D. Blood cultures should be obtained in every patient.

E. Patients with chronic monoarticular arthritis should have a similar evaluation.

   1. Fluid should be sent for fungal and mycobacterial cultures.

   2. Often a synovial biopsy is required to visualize or grow the organisms.

   3. *Sporothrix* typically is not visualized on biopsy but will eventually grow on culture.

F. If the patient lives in an area endemic for Lyme disease or has had exposure to ticks, then Lyme disease should be considered.

X. Therapeutic Approach to Infectious Arthritis

Antibiotic therapy should be initiated immediately in patients with suspected bacterial arthritis.

A. One should not wait for return of cultures before initiating therapy.

B. Sexually active persons with suspected gonococcal arthritis should be assumed to have a penicillin-producing or other resistant *N. gonorrhoeae.* Initial therapy with a third-generation cephalosporin or possibly a quinolone is indicated.

C. In addition, therapy should be given for *Staph. aureus* and streptococci. Vancomycin is the treatment of choice for patients with suspected methicillin-resistant *Staph. aureus.*

D. If the patient is an intravenous drug user, gram-negative organisms should be suspected. Treatment with a third-generation cephalosporin effective against *Pseudomonas* may be indicated.

E. Since most antimicrobial agents achieve adequate concentrations in synovial fluid, intra-articular antibiotic administration is almost never indicated. The optimal duration of antibiotic therapy is unclear, but most patients require a 3- to 4-week course.

F. In patients with animal bites or closed-fist injuries with related septic arthritis, therapy should include coverage of *P. multocida* and *E. corrodens* with penicillin, ampicillin, ticarillin/clavulanate or ampicillin/sulbactam. Doxycycline may be an alternative in penicillin-allergic patients.

G. If a particular joint is easily accessible to repeated needle aspiration, then arthroscopic or open surgical debridement is not necessary. However, in cases of hip and possibly shoulder infection, open surgical debridement may be indicated earlier because of the difficulty of repeated aspirations of the joint.

H. Patients with chronic monoarticular arthritis due to *M. tuberculosis* usually require at least a 9-month course of isoniazid and rifampin therapy.

I. *M. kansasii* and *M. marinum* infections can also be treated with oral therapy. However, longer durations of therapy may be required as with *M. avium-intracellulare.*

J. Amphotericin B is the treatment of choice for arthritis due to most fungi.

1. The dose of amphotericin B varies, but most patients require a total dose of 1 to 2.5 g.
2. For *Candida* infections, chronic suppressive therapy with oral imidazole or triazole may be used for chronically infected patients.

Osteomyelitis

I. Definition

Osteomyelitis is an inflammatory process in bone and bone marrow.

A. It is caused primarily by pyogenic bacteria, but it may also be caused by other microorganisms including mycobacteria and fungi.
B. Classification may be either clinical, as in acute versus chronic osteomyelitis, or pathogenic, based on whether the infection is hematogenous, from a contiguous focus, or related to peripheral vascular disease.

II. Epidemiology

A. *Staph. aureus* remains the most common cause of osteomyelitis due to hematogenous spread.
B. *H. influenzae* is a significant pathogen in children.
C. The annual incidence of osteomyelitis is highest in patients under the age of 20 and rises again over the age of 60.
D. Males tend to have a slightly higher incidence of osteomyelitis than females. The reasons remain unclear.
E. Sickle cell disease predisposes patients to osteomyelitis, particularly due to *Salmonella*.
F. Bone and joint infection is also increased in patients undergoing hemodialysis and in intravenous drug users.
G. Diabetics are at much higher risk of developing osteomyelitis of the feet than the general population.

III. Pathogenesis

A. The most important feature in the pathogenesis of osteomyelitis is the ability of the microbe to adhere to bone.
B. Once established, infection is extremely difficult to cure, even with long-term antibiotic treatment.
C. In general, undamaged cells are resistant to bacterial adhesion.
D. Fibronectin and laminin may be the initial targets of bacterial adhesins. These proteins are probably not exposed unless the tissue is damaged.

E. *Staph. aureus* also appears to have receptors for collagen and sialoprotein.
F. The adherent bacteria are covered by a biofilm consisting of polysaccharide and debris, which inhibits the ability of antibiotics to kill the bacteria.
1. Diffusion of antibiotics through the biofilm is also inhibited.
2. The bacteria within the slime layer may be physiologically different from the adherent bacteria; therefore, their response to antibiotics may be altered.
G. Acute hematogenous osteomyelitis usually involves rapidly growing bone and characteristically affects the metaphysis of long bones.
H. Once infection starts, it provokes an acute inflammatory response that leads to necrosis of tissue, breakdown of bone, and removal of calcium.
I. Infection may extend to neighboring bony structures, thereby shutting off the vascular supply and causing further necrosis of bone.
J. At this point, the chronic phase of osteomyelitis is established as large segments of avascular bone separate and form sequestra.

IV. Hematogenous Osteomyelitis

A. Hematogenous osteomyelitis is usually seen in children.
B. Hematogenous osteomyelitis of the vertebrae is a disease of individuals over 50.
C. The most frequently involved bones are the long bones of the lower extremities and the humerus.
D. The most common cause of acute hematogenous osteomyelitis is *Staph. aureus*, although gram-negative bacilli are being found with increasing frequency.
E. The classic presentation of acute osteomyelitis includes abrupt onset of high fever, systemic toxicity, and local inflammation around the infected bone.
F. In adults, the symptoms may be less abrupt.
G. Once chronic osteomyelitis supervenes, systemic signs are relatively uncommon. Drainage from a sinus tract is a hallmark of chronic osteomyelitis. Sedimentation rates and white blood cell counts are frequently elevated.

V. Osteomyelitis Secondary to a Contiguous Focus of Infection

A. This form of osteomyelitis is due either to direct infection of bone from an exogenous source or to the spread of infection from a nearby infected focus.

B. The most common precipitating factor is postoperative infection.

C. Nonsurgically induced infections develop from soft tissue infections, infected teeth, or infected sinuses.

D. After animal or human bites, spread of locally inoculated organisms may occur, with development of osteomyelitis (due to *P. multocida* or *E. corrodens*).

E. Most cases of this type of osteomyelitis are seen in patients over the age of 50.

F. Any bone may be involved; however, the long bones of the lower extremities are most frequently affected.

G. Pressure sores may overlie a focus of osteomyelitis, especially in the sacral area.

H. The skull and mandible may be sites of osteomyelitis after neurosurgery, oral surgery, or dental infections.

I. Sternal osteomyelitis may be seen following median sternotomy incisions for cardiac surgery.

J. Osteomyelitis due to a contiguous focus is often associated with a polymicrobial infection.
   1. *Staph. aureus* is still the most common organism, but it is frequently part of a mixed infection.
   2. Gram-negative bacilli and anaerobes are much more common, especially when seen with a contiguous pressure sore or diabetic foot ulcer.

K. The major clinical signs are fever, swelling, and erythema in initial episodes. However, with recurrent sinus formation, drainage is most commonly seen. Patients then generally show very few systemic signs of infection.

VI. **Osteomyelitis Associated with Vascular Insufficiency**
A. These patients nearly always have diabetes or severe atherosclerosis.

B. Most patients are over 50 and have had diabetes for more than 2 years.

C. The toes or small bones of the feet are most usually affected.

D. Most infections are polymicrobial. Although staphylococci are common, gram-negative aerobic bacilli and anaerobes are also frequently recovered.

VII. **Diagnosis**
A. Plain radiography
   1. Plain x-rays are often accurate; however, their findings may lag considerably behind the activity of the disease.

2. The radiographic appearance of osteomyelitis depends on the vascular anatomy of the bone involved, the chronicity of the process, and the patient's age.

3. A periosteal reaction is less prominent in adults than in children. The earliest radiographic changes consist of metaphyseal destruction.

4. If acute osteomyelitis progresses to chronic disease, a sequestrum or involucrum may be seen. A sequestrum is a piece of necrotic bone surrounded by an area of granulation tissue. An involucrum is a periosteal envelope surrounding a focus of necrotic bone.

5. Other radiographic changes may include bone destruction, soft tissue swelling, and periosteal reaction.

B. CT has been used to evaluate osteomyelitis because of its excellent definition of cortical bone and special resolution.

C. Magnetic resonance imaging (MRI) provides more accurate and detailed information than CT or plain radiographs.
   1. On T2 weighted images, a bright MRI signal within the marrow is a sensitive indicator of active disease.
   2. MRI also offers multiplanar reconstruction to create images.
   3. Although there are few studies, MRI appears to be a very sensitive and specific imaging modality.
   4. Healing fractures and tumors may sometimes resemble osteomyelitis on MRI.
   5. Artifacts caused by joint implants may affect the quality of the image. Therefore, MRI does not appear to be very helpful in diagnosing infected joint arthroplasty.

D. Radionuclide bone scanning
   1. Bone scans give less anatomic detail than routine radiographs but more functional information.
   2. The uptake of technetium 99M is related to both osteoblastic activity and skeletal vascularity.
   3. The bone scan is generally abnormal within a few days of infection.
   4. The three-phase bone scan is the routine nuclear medicine procedure currently available. The first phase is the flow phase, consisting of 2- to 5-sec images over the area of suspected osteomyelitis while the technetium is injected. The

second phase is the blood pool image, which is obtained within 5 min after injection. In areas of inflammation, capillaries dilate, causing increased blood flow and blood pooling. The third phase, or bone image, is obtained about 3 hr later. Classically, cellulitis has increased activity in the first two phases but no focal increase in the third phase. Osteomyelitis has increased activity in the first two phases and focal increased activity in the third phase.

5. In adult patients with a normal radiograph, the three-phase bone scan is highly sensitive and specific for bone infection.

6. Infants with osteomyelitis have falsely normal bone scans 20–70% of the time.

7. The bone scan is also much less specific in cases of increased bone turnover, such as in surgery, fracture, and neuropathic osteopathy.

E. Gallium-67 citrate localizes in areas of osteomyelitis by granulocyte or bacterial uptake and by binding to lactoferrin at the site of infection.

1. Gallium-67 lacks high sensitivity and specificity when diagnosing osteomyelitis superimposed on diseases that cause increased bone turnover. Indium-111 label leukocyte scans have been used to overcome some of the limitations of gallium scanning.

F. Indium-111 leukocyte scans appear to have a sensitivity of 80–100% and a specificity of 50–100%.

1. The highest false-positive results occur in patients with underlying conditions affecting bones.

2. When using combined bone and indium-111 leukocyte studies, a sensitivity of over 80% and a specificity over 95% should be expected.

VIII. **Diagnosis of Etiologic Agents**

Since patients with osteomyelitis are committed to a prolonged course of therapy, it is important to make a precise diagnosis of the etiologic agents.

A. Blood cultures should be obtained, as up to 50% of patients with hematogenous osteomyelitis will be bacteremic.

B. In patients with chronic osteomyelitis, however, it may be difficult to isolate the responsible organism.

1. In general, culture of the sinus tract does

not appear to be very accurate in predicting the bacteriologic cause of the osteomyelitis.

2. Aspiration or biopsy of bone is the only reliable method for establishing a precise microbiologic diagnosis of osteomyelitis.

IX. **Anti-infective Agents**

Anti-infective agents for the treatment of osteomyelitis must have in vitro activity against the potential pathogens.

A. They must also be able to penetrate bone and to be given in sufficient concentration.

B. Most cases of osteomyelitis require at least 4 weeks of antibiotics. Even then, relapses years later have been reported.

C. The β-lactamase-stable cephalosporins, especially third-generation cephalosporins, offer excellent activity against gram-negative bacilli.

D. Because of the prolonged nature of intravenous therapy for osteomyelitis, there is a growing trend to complete and at times even initiate antimicrobial therapy on an outpatient basis.

E. Oral therapy offers even greater economic benefits.

1. Children with acute osteomyelitis are commonly treated with short-term parenteral therapy followed by prolonged oral therapy.

2. The development of oral quinolones with good activity against gram-negative bacilli now allows oral therapy to be used even in adults.

3. One potential problem with oral quinolones in their fairly poor activity against *Staph. aureus* and the decreasing susceptibility of *Pseudomonas aeruginosa*.

4. In vitro susceptibility testing is very important prior to initiation of oral quinolone therapy.

F. The vast majority of methicillin-resistant *Staph. aureus* and methicillin-resistant, coagulase-negative staphylococci are now resistant to quinolones, and vancomycin is the only reasonable therapy for these infections. Unfortunately, vancomycin does not penetrate well into bone. Newer therapies such as teicoplanin and daptomycin are under evaluation, but they are not yet clinically available.

X. **Other Therapies**

A. Surgical intervention is often required in chronic osteomyelitis to remove sequestra, debride necrotic and devitalized material, and obtain culture material. Improvements in surgical technique have allowed surgeons to debride infected areas extensively and then to fill in the dead space with autologous bone grafts and muscle flaps.

B. Hyperbaric oxygen may be helpful in some cases of chronic osteomyelitis. However, its routine use has not been supported by currently available studies.

XI. Complications

Complications of long-standing chronic osteomyelitis include secondary amyloidosis and epidermoid carcinoma. Carcinoma occurs in less than 1% of patients with chronic osteomyelitis, but when it does develop, amputation is often required.

Vertebral Osteomyelitis

I. Introduction

The vertebrae are the third most common bones involved in hematogenous osteomyelitis and account for a significant number of cases of osteomyelitis secondary to contiguous foci of infection.

II. Pathophysiology

The reason vertebral osteomyelitis due to hematogenous spread appears to predominate in adults is likely related to the persistence of a rich cellular bone marrow, lack of true epiphyseal growth, and the presence of a sluggish blood supply in the adult vertebrae. These factors appear to favor deposition of bacteria in the vertebrae during bacteremia. It is believed that the arterial route of spread is more likely than the venous route.

III. Microbial Etiology

A. *Staph. aureus* accounts for the majority of isolates from patients with hematogenous vertebral osteomyelitis.

B. Gram-negative aerobic bacilli may be identified in up to one-third of the cases, with *Escherichia coli* being the most common. These gram-negative bacilli usually originate in the genitourinary tract.

C. Intravenous drug users are more likely to be infected with *P. aeruginosa* in addition to *Staph. aureus* and other gram-negative organisms.

D. In certain regions of the world, *Brucella* vertebral osteomyelitis should be strongly considered.

E. Mycobacteria and fungi have also been implicated in vertebral osteomyelitis. These include *M. tuberculosis, Blastomyces dermatitidis, Coccidioides immitis,* and *Candida* spp.

F. Hematogenous vertebral osteomyelitis is usually a monomicrobial disease.

G. Contiguous osteomyelitis may have a polymicrobial infection. This is most commonly seen with infected pressure sores in postoperative patients.

H. Anaerobes are exceedingly uncommon except in contiguous osteomyelitis secondary to infected pressure sores.

I. Intervertebral disc space infections are usually acquired postoperatively and are usually due to coagulase-negative or positive staphylococci. Aerobic gram-negative bacilli, including *P. aeruginosa,* may also be seen.

IV. Clinical Manifestations

A. Neck or back pain with stiffness is present in the vast majority of patients.

B. Only half of these patients have a fever, and only slightly more have a peripheral leukocytosis.

C. The erythrocyte sedimentation rate is usually elevated, although this is not a very specific test.

D. About half of the patients with hematogenous vertebral osteomyelitis have symptoms for at least 3 months before seeking medical attention.

E. On physical examination, almost all patients have tenderness to palpation over the involved area.

F. Few patients have limitation of back motion or a positive straight-leg raising sign.

G. About 15–20% present with a neurologic deficit such as sensory, motor, or combined defects.

H. When a patient presents with back pain progressing to weakness and paralysis, a spinal epidural abscess should be suspected.

V. Risk Factor

Risk factors for vertebral osteomyelitis include male sex, a history of blunt trauma to the spine, diabetes mellitus, and intravenous drug use.

VI. Source of Infection

A. The genitourinary tract accounts for approximately 30% of the cases of vertebral osteomyelitis. Males represent the great majority of these cases.

B. Other sources of infection include soft tissue infections, respiratory tract infections, infected vascular sites, dental infections, surgical manipulations of the spine or disc, and infective endocarditis.

C. About one-third of patients with vertebral osteomyelitis have no obvious or likely source of infection.

VII. Site of Vertebral Involvement

A. The lumbar vertebrae are involved in at least half of the cases of hematogenous vertebral osteomyelitis.

B. The lower lumbar vertebrae are more commonly involved than the upper lumber vertebrae.

C. The thoracic vertebrae are involved approximately one-third of the time; the cervical vertebrae are least commonly involved.

D. In cases of osteomyelitis secondary to a contiguous focus, the sacrum is the most commonly affected area.

E. In tuberculous spondylitis, the thoracic vertebrae are most frequently involved (over 50% of the cases).

VIII. Diagnosis

A. Anterior-posterior and lateral spine films reveal irregularities of the contiguous vertebral end plates, with or without disc space narrowing, in the vast majority of cases of pyogenic vertebral osteomyelitis.

B. In intravenous drug users, there is a greater chance of films being read initially as normal.

C. If plain x-rays are normal, tomograms and bone scan are often abnormal.

D. The gallium scan is generally said to be less sensitive than the technetium scan but more specific for inflammatory processes.

E. CT may show early bony changes before these are detected on routine x-rays. In addition, the presence of paravertebral and psoas abscesses may be detected.

F. MRI appears to be even more sensitive than CT. Some investigators now consider MRI the test of choice for vertebral osteomyelitis.

IX. Identification of the Organism

Because of the number of organisms that can potentially cause vertebral osteomyelitis, identification of the microorganism is mandatory for appropriate antimicrobial therapy.

A. Up to one-quarter of patients have positive blood cultures; therefore, obtaining a blood culture is crucial.

B. For patients who are not bacteremic, it is imperative that a bone or disc biopsy, or both, be performed. This may be done with a cutting needle such as a Craig needle. Biopsy is often guided by fluoroscopy or CT scanning for accurate localization.

C. Specimens should be sent for histologic study, as well as special stains for fungi and acid-fast bacilli.

D. Cultures should be sent for aerobic and anaerobic cultures, in addition to fungal and mycobacterial cultures.

E. If *Brucella* is suspected, then the cultures should be maintained for at least 3 weeks.

F. If the biopsy culture is negative (which occurs in up to 30% of cases), a second biopsy or an open biopsy should be considered.

X. Differential Diagnosis

A. Malignancy—It is extremely rare to see disc space involvement with malignancy. Posterior elements of the spine are also commonly involved.

B. Benign discitis, which is almost exclusively seen in children (Scheuermann's disease) is a disease of adolescents, usually males, of unknown etiology.

C. Musculoskeletal strain or trauma.

XI. Management

A. In the vast majority of patients, appropriate antimicrobial therapy in addition to bed rest is sufficient.

B. If there is significant instability of the spine, immobilizing devices such as braces may be used.

C. Surgical therapy is generally not necessary unless it is necessary to evacuate a paravertebral or epidural abscess.

D. Surgical fusion is generally not necessary unless bony fusion does not occur spontaneously. The most common reason for surgical intervention is decompression of an epidural abscess to relieve neurologic symptoms.

E. Antimicrobial therapy is generally continued for at least 4 weeks and sometimes up to 8 weeks.

F. The erythrocyte sedimentation rate should be followed and should fall to pretherapy levels by the end of therapy. The treatment of tuberculosis and fungal vertebral osteomyelitis is covered in subsequent chapters.

Bibliography

Bircher MD, Tasker T, Crawshaw C, et al. Discitis following lumbar surgery. *Spine* 13:98–102, 1988.

Danner RL, Hartman BJ. Update of spinal epidural abscess: 35 cases and review of literature. *Rev Infect Dis* 9:265–274, 1987.

Deyo RA, Bigos SJ, Maravilla KR. Diagnostic imaging procedures for the lumbar spine. *Ann Intern Med* 111:865–867, 1989.

Gardner GC, Weisman MH. Pyarthrosis in patients with rheumatoid arthritis: A report of 13 cases and a review of the literature from the past 40 years. *Am J Med* 88:503–511, 1990.

Gentry LO. Osteomyelitis: Options for diagnosis and management. *J Antimicrob Chemother* 21:115–128, 1988.

Goldenberg DL, Reed JI. Bacterial arthritis. *New Engl J Med* 312:764–771, 1985.

Keenan AM, Tindel NL, Alavi A. Diagnosis of pedal osteomyelitis in diabetic patients using current scintigraphic techniques. *Arch Intern Med* 149:2262–2266, 1989.

Mackowiak PA, Jones SR, Smith JW. Diagnostic value of sinus-tract cultures in chronic osteomyelitis. *JAMA* 239: 2771–2775, 1978.

Meyers SP, Wiener SN. Diagnosis of hematogenous pyogenic vertebral osteomyelitis by magnetic resonance imaging. *Arch Intern Med* 151:683–687, 1991.

Lyme Disease

Jeffrey A. Nelson, M.D.

I. Definition
Clinical illness due to the spirochete *Borrelia burgdorferi*.

II. Etiology
B. burgdorferi is a loosely coiled spirochete that measures approximately 0.2 by 30 μm. This narrow, motile bacterium can be visualized with dark-field microscopy and cultured in an artificial medium.

III. Pathophysiology
A. Vector
   1. Transmission to humans is usually by the bite of an infected *Ixodes* tick. In the eastern and midwestern United States, the primary vector is *Ixodes scapularis*. *I. pacificus* harbors the spirochete in the western United States. Other ticks such as *Amblyomma americanum*, and additional arthropods such as flies and mosquitoes, may serve as rare vectors. *Ixodes* ticks have a 2-year life cycle including egg, larva, nymph, and adult stages. Nymphs are small (approximately 1 mm) and are most active in the spring. Adults are three times this size and are more troublesome in the fall.

B. Once introduced into the skin, spirochetes may remain localized or disseminate hematogenously to any organ. The humoral immune response to this organism may be delayed for several weeks; therefore, early serologic evaluations must be interpreted with caution. Sera surveillance efforts have suggested that asymptomatic or subclinical infection may occur.

IV. Diagnosis
A. Historical information should be obtained regarding travel to highly endemic areas (New England, western Wisconsin, Minnesota, and many areas in Europe). Because of the focal nature of infected tick habitats, any history of exposure to a wooded area may be pursued with local health authorities who have up-to-date tick distribution information. Other historical clues may be obtained by eliciting information regarding several common clinical presentations (erythema migrans rash, Bell's palsy, lymphocytic meningitis, large joint arthritis).

B. Clinical disease has been historically divided into three stages.
   1. Stage I occurs within days to weeks of the

tick bite and may consist only of constitutional symptoms. In about 50% of patients, a characteristic rash may appear at the bite site. Erythema chronicum migrans (more recently referred to as *erythema migrans*) is classically a bull's-eye, erythematous rash which expands its borders over several days to weeks. As spirochetes disseminate, similar lesions may appear elsewhere on the skin.

2. Stage II manifestations occur a few weeks to months after the bite and may involve a variety of organ systems, with musculoskeletal, neurologic, and myocardial involvement perhaps being the most well characterized. Classic neurologic manifestations involve lymphocytic meningitis, cranial neuritis, or radicular complaints similar to those seen with herpes zoster. Cardiac involvement occurs in about 10% of patients and may cause varying degrees of heart block. Cardiac involvement is usually transient, resolving over a number of weeks.

3. Stage III disease in the United States most commonly involves arthritic complaints. Large joint, asymmetric arthritis can occur abruptly and can recur over several months to years. European late Lyme disease more often involves the central nervous system. This late neurologic disease can cause subtle memory and concentration difficulties. Neurologic disease is also seen with late Lyme disease in the United States, but it appears to be less frequent. The subtle clinical nature of this disease makes the historical clues of endemic exposure, previous erythema migrans rash, lymphocytic meningitis, and large joint arthritis extremely valuable in considering further evaluation. Most patients with late Lyme disease have serologic evidence of disease.

C. Laboratory information
   1. Organisms can be grown in a complex medium developed by Barbour-Stoenner and Kelly (BSK medium). Human isolates can occasionally be obtained from blood, skin, synovial, and spinal fluids.
   2. Histologic evidence of spirochetes can be obtained by using silver staining methods. The number of spirochetes present

is small and the search is time-consuming, limiting the use of these tests.

3. Antibody detection is currently the most widely available laboratory method to identify patients with possible *Borrelia* exposure. Indirect immunofluorescence (IFA) and enzyme-linked immunosorbent assay (ELISA) methods are the most widely used techniques. Western blot procedures are less readily available, but they offer additional information regarding the patient's immune response. Cross-reactive problems in any of these serologic tests can generate false-positive results in patients with syphilis, mononucleosis, and autoimmune disease. In the appropriate setting, serology for these other illnesses may be considered. False-negative results can be seen in early disease, and perhaps in a few patients who have received early antibiotic therapy, with subsequent blunting of the normal immune response.

V. **Differential Diagnosis**
   A. A tick exposure history should make one consider:
      1. Rocky mountain spotted fever.
      2. Tularemia.
      3. Babesia.
      4. Ehrlichia.
      5. Colorado tick fever.
      6. Relapsing fever.

VI. **Treatment**
   A. Early disease in a patient over the age of 8 may be treated with doxycycline, 100 mg twice a day. Children can be given amoxicillin, 500 mg three times a day, and, if allergic to penicillin, erythromycin, 250 mg four times a day. The optimal length of therapy has not been determined, but a 2-week course is commonly given.
   B. Late manifestations including cardiac, neurologic, and arthritic difficulties can sometimes be treated orally, but intravenous therapy is preferable. Ceftriaxone, 2 g/day given intravenously, has been used. Penicillin appears to be less efficacious. Doxycycline offers an alternative to the β-lactam agents. Many clinicians extend the course of therapy from 2 to 4 weeks. It is currently unclear whether longer courses offer any advantage.

VII. **Patient Monitoring**

A. Initiation of antimicrobial therapy may elicit a Jarish-Herxheimer reaction similar to that seen in some syphilis patients. Thus, blood pressure monitoring and close observation seem warranted with initial dosing, and especially in those with early disease when the spirochete burden may be greatest.

B. Refractory symptoms can be seen in some patients. Immune-mediated factors may contribute to this condition, but long-standing disease may also cause irreversible organ damage. Any patient who does not respond to therapy should prompt the clinician to reconsider the initial diagnosis and pursue further diagnostic evaluations when clinically warranted.

C. Repeat serologic evaluations can be useful in patients with suspected early disease. Many of these patients, even if treated, will seroconvert in the weeks following their initial illness. Unlike syphilis, repeat serology should not be used to prove the efficacy of therapy. The clinical response should be followed to determine the need for any further therapeutic interventions.

VIII. Prognosis

Early initiation of appropriate antimicrobial therapy typically results in clinical resolution of Lyme disease. Long-standing disease may contribute to irreversible organ damage that will not resolve with treatment. Immune stimulation may resolve slowly and contribute to persistent symptoms. As with any treatment, a small subset of patients may fail to respond. A second agent or a slightly longer course might be efficacious in this group. In any patient without a clinical response, the initial diagnosis should also be reconsidered.

IX. Prevention

Reasonable precautions include the use of light-colored clothing, judicious use of insect repellents, and tick checks as one returns from suspect wooded areas. Tick removal can be accomplished with tweezers. Animal data suggest that tick removal within 24 hr markedly reduces the chances of spirochete acquisition. Prophylaxis for tick bites has not been routinely recommended but must be considered on an individual basis. A vaccine is presently being tested.

Bibliography

Barbour AG. Laboratory aspects of Lyme borreliosis. *Clin Microbiol Rev* 1:399–414, 1988.

Halperin JJ, Luft BJ, Anand AK, et al. Lyme neuroborreliosis: Central nervous system manifestations. *Neurology* 39:753–759, 1989.

Rahn DW, Malawista SE. Lyme disease: Recommendations for diagnosis and treatment. *Ann Intern Med* 114:472–481, 1991.

Steere AC. Lyme disease. *N Engl J Med* 321:586–596, 1989.

Tuberculosis

Alan A. Harris, M.D.

I. Definition
Clinical illness due to *Mycobacterium tuberculosis*. Refer to chapter 52C on antituberculous agents.
A. Epidemiology

Tuberculosis is a worldwide illness. Approximately 3 million people die each year. After decades of steady decline in the United States, there has been a 6–7% increase in cases during each of the last 2 years. Association with human immunodeficiency virus (HIV) infection likely accounts for one-third to one-half of this increase.

B. Pulmonary acquisition is most common. Extrapulmonary spread also occurs. The *M. tuberculosis* group includes *M. tuberculosis*, *M. bovis*, and *M. africanum*.

C. There are several schema for atypical mycobacteria. The one most commonly used is the Runyon grouping based on pigment production, rate of growth, and varying growth requirements. Disease due to these organisms may mimic that due to tuberculosis. The clinical manifestations, diagnosis, and management of disease due to the atypical strains is beyond the scope of this chapter.

II. Etiology
M. tuberculosis is an acid-fast bacillus. Standard stains include Ziehl-Neelsen, rhodamine auramine, and Kinyoun. On Gram stain, it may appear as a gram-positive bacillus.

III. Pathophysiology
A. Droplets measuring 1 to 10 μm are acquired through the respiratory route following contact with an infectious person. Rarely, the organism may be inoculated (e.g., a pathologist with prosector's wart).

B. Droplets measuring 1 to 10 μm bypass mucociliary defenses, deposit in alveoli, and stimulate an inflammatory response consisting primarily of lymphocytes and macrophages. This is followed in 4–12 weeks by conversion of the tuberculin skin test (5-tuberculin units purified protein derivative, 5-TU PPD) from negative to positive.

C. Lymphohematogenous dissemination usually occurs at the time of primary infection. There is a predilection for areas of high oxygen content—the lower upper or upper lower lobes of the lung, renal cortex, bone, and central nervous system.

D. Active disease is usually associated with reactivation of old infection. Primary progression likely accounts for no more than 15% of cases. From 10% to 20% of reactivation occurs within 3 years of infection, and the rate is then approximately 1% per year.

E. Lymphohematogenous spread may occur at the time of pulmonary reactivation, and, therefore, miliary/disseminated disease either concurrent with or years following the initial infection.

IV. **Diagnosis**

Pulmonary manifestations predominate, but signs and symptoms are protean and infection has been reported in essentially every organ in the body.

A. History

1. The clinician should seek a history of exposure to a patient with known tuberculous infection and/or active disease.

2. Fever, malaise, weight loss, and anorexia may be present for weeks to months.

3. Thoracic—cough, with or without sputum production or hemoptysis. A dull pleuritic chest pain may occur. Shortness of breath is rare unless there is miliary disease or underlying chronic pulmonary disease. Fever of undetermined origin occurs as a presentation of isolated pleural effusion.

4. Extrapulmonary lymph node—discrete, tender, or nontender, firm lymphadenopathy. A draining sinus may occur (e.g., cervical nodes with scrofula).

5. Central nervous system—headache, stiff neck, and altered sensorium. Symptoms referable to the posterior fossa, such as diplopia and ataxia, may reflect tuberculoma and/or basilar meningitis.

6. Bone—cardinal signs of inflammation with rubor, calor, dolor, and tumor. Only a mass may be present (i.e., cold abscess).

7. Genitourinary—usually no symptoms occur, but hematuria, dysuria, or symptoms of prostatic obstruction with hesitance, postvoid dribbling, and decreased strength of the stream may all be present.

B. Clinical signs and physical findings

1. Thoracic—rales and rhonchi with tuberculous pneumonia or bronchiectasis. Egophony and whispered pectoriloquy if there is a cavity communicating with the bronchial tree. Dullness to percussion may be present with either parenchymal or pleural disease. Tactile fremitus may

be increased, decreased, or normal, depending on the degree of cavitation, consolidation, and/or pleural fluid.

2. Extrapulmonary

a. Lymphatic—frequently detected by palpation during physical examination. Lymph nodes may be firm, or fluctuant.

b. Usually nontender adenopathy. A sinus tract is possible.

c. Bone—may be due to local deformity or pain. Lower thoracic and upper lumbar spines are the most common sites of involvement, along with the long bones of the lower extremities. Gibbus of the spine reflects collapse of vertebrae with anterior wedging. Cold abscess is typically found with paravertebral psoas involvement. Its initial presentation may be in the anterior thigh inferior to the inguinal ligament. Signs of spinal cord compression may be associated with vertebral or paravertebral disease.

d. Central nervous system—stiff neck, nystagmus, ataxia, alterations in sensorium, cranial nerve palsies, and papilledema. Long tract sign and crossed sensory abnormalities may be due to spinal cord compression. Signs and symptoms referable to the posterior fossa may be related to meningitis, a vasculitis associated with basilar meningitis, a space-occupying tuberculoma, or hydrocephalus.

e. Genitourinary—hematuria, renal mass, hydronephrosis, prostatic nodule, or fibrosis or nodule formation in the epididymis have all been reported.

C. Diagnostic tests

1. Skin tests—multiple puncture techniques are used for screening. Intradermal 5-TU PPD is the standard test for infection.

a. A positive skin test does not indicate active disease. Active disease may be associated with false-negative skin tests in up to 20% of patients.

b. When active tuberculosis is suspected, do not start with skin testing unless microbiologic results (smears and/or culture) are unavailable and/or already known to be negative. If tuberculin skin testing is to be used in an evaluation for active disease, one should start with a first strength (i.e., 1-TU PPD).

c. Interpretation of the 5-TU PPD test as indicative of infection is based on the number of millimeters of induration.

(1) Induration ≥5 mm—contact of active case, recent converter, abnormal chest x-ray compatible with tuberculosis in the presence of no symptoms and negative sputum, prior history of untreated tuberculosis, and at high risk for or known to be infected with HIV.

(2) Induration ≥10 mm

(a) High-risk disease—silicosis, postgastrectomy, diabetes mellitus, chronic obstructive pulmonary disease, renal failure, immunosuppressive therapy, primary immunosuppressive disease, malignancies of the lymphatic system.

(b) High-risk populations—nursing homes, shelters for the homeless, drug abuse programs, immigrants/refugees from areas with a high incidence of tuberculosis.

(3) Induration ≥15 mm—all other individuals.

d. Booster test—Many years after the primary infection, the degree of induration may decrease. Subsequent tests may "boost" the induration. If testing is done at 1-year intervals, the individual may be mistakenly identified as a recent converter. Therefore, testing for the booster phenomenon in selected populations (e.g., the elderly or individuals with any amount of induration from areas with a high incidence of tuberculosis) should be done within 2 weeks of the initial tests.

e. Bacille Calmette-Guèrin—immunization with attenuated *M. bovis* used selectively in the United States with certain high-risk populations or individuals uninfected but exposed to drug-resistant cases. Immunization results in a positive tuberculin skin test. Positivity more than 10 years following immunization should be construed as having *nothing* to do with the immunization. When active tuberculosis is suspected, the time interval for interpretation should be reduced to 5 years.

2. Radiologic studies

a. Chest—primary disease associated with parenchymal infiltration with consolidation. Calcified granulomas in lungs or intrathoracic nodes. Cavitary disease, usually in the absence of fluid levels, with a predilection for the posterior segment of the upper lobes or the superior segment of the lower lobes. An isolated cavity in the anterior segment as the sole x-ray finding should be considered malignancy until proven otherwise.

b. Central nervous system—computed tomography (CT) may show a mass lesion in the posterior fossa (i.e., tuberculoma). Tuberculoma usually is unassociated with meningitis and vice versa. Meningitis may result in hydrocephalus or cerebral edema. Atrophy occurs as a sequela.

c. Bone—cortical and medullary destruction. Erosions occur. Involvement of three contiguous vertebrae is a soft clue to tuberculosis or fungus and against pyogenic infection or malignancy.

d. Genitourinary—intravenous pyelography is usually negative in the presence of active disease. Caliectasis, calcified mass, hydroureter, focal ureteral abnormality, or adrenal calcification may be detected during the course of intravenous pyelography, ultrasonography, or CT scanning.

V. Differential Diagnosis

A. Infections

1. Fungi—histoplasmosis, coccidiomycosis, paracoccidiomycosis, blastomycosis. The likelihood depends on geographic exposure. Disease due to cryptococcosis usually enters the differential diagnosis with an isolated nodule when malignancy is the major diagnostic concern.

2. Bacterial infections—chronic pneumonias due to *Klebsiella* or *Nocardia*. *Pseudomonas pseudomallei*, the etiologic agent of melioidosis, causes disease which may exactly mimic tuberculosis in Southeast Asia.

3. Bacterial abscess associated with aspiration or endobronchial spread of pulmonary tuberculosis is rare. Tuberculous adenopathy may result in bronchial obstruction and postobstructive pneumonia or abscess.

B. Noninfectious agents
   1. Diseases of unknown etiology—sarcoid, Wegener's disease, Goodpasture's syndrome.
   2. Neoplasia—carcinoma of the breast, lung, thyroid, ovaries, testicles, and colon may all cause nodular lesions. Cavitation occurs rarely and may mimic infection.

VI. **Therapy** (see also chapter 52C on antituberculous drugs)
A. Chemoprophylaxis of individuals infected but without active disease (i.e., with positive tuberculin skin tests).
   1. Individuals ≤35 years of age—essentially all individuals with a positive PPD test should receive prophylaxis unless this is contraindicated.
   2. Individuals ≥35 years of age—those in high-risk populations or with high-risk associated diseases should receive prophylaxis unless this is contraindicated.
   3. Isoniazid (INH) is the only proven prophylactic and is 90% effective if taken as recommended.
      a. While 12 months of therapy has been the studied standard, the current goal is to administer at least 6 months of continuous therapy.
      b. HIV-infected individuals should receive therapy for 12 months.
      c. It is easier to give all individuals supplemental pyridoxine (vitamin B_6) to prevent sideroblastic anemias and peripheral neuropathy than to monitor and treat persons at risk of such complications (i.e., those with malnutrition, uremia, diabetes mellitus, or HIV infection).
   4. Infection with an INH-resistant strain of *M. tuberculosis*
      a. Concern is based on the level of INH resistance in the country where infection was acquired.
      b. Concern over contact with a known INH-resistant individual.
      c. There is currently no definitive answer; reasonable approaches have been developed.

(1) INH—acceptable for VI.A.4.a disease.
(2) Rifampin—acceptable for VI.A.4.a and VI.A.4.b disease.
(3) Rifampin and ethambutol—acceptable for VI.A.4.a and VI.A.4.b disease. I suggest not using this option, which is also an effective therapy for active disease.
(4) Doing nothing is the least preferable choice.

B. Therapy of active disease (see also chapter 52C on antituberculous agents)
   1. Caveats
      a. Never treat with one drug.
      b. Two drugs have never been shown to have greater efficacy than regimens with more than two drugs if the organism is susceptible to the drugs being used, if INH is part of the therapy, and if therapy is continued long enough.
      c. Never add one drug to a failing regimen.
      d. Pyridoxine (vitamin B_6) should be given to anyone receiving INH.
      e. New short-course regimens are for convenience, not for improved efficacy. They are good for extrapulmonary as well as pulmonary disease. Although there are reports of efficacy, I caution against short-course regimens in treating central nervous system disease until more information is available.
      f. The traditional rationale for using more than two drugs focused on the severity of the underlying illness (i.e., central nervous system, renal, bone, multiple pulmonary cavities, cavities ≥2 cm, miliary or disseminated disease). Current practice is to shorten the therapeutic course and reduce the number of clinic visits, diagnostic tests, and need for follow-up while improving our ability to deliver medication in a labor-intense, controlled fashion.
      g. A new diagnosis of tuberculosis should result in HIV antibody testing. With improved survival in this population, relapse rates and the required duration of therapy of active tuberculosis may be greater in this group, and

there may be a need for continued suppressive therapy. The HIV-infected patient should be treated for at least 9 months.

h. Trials of antituberculous therapy for a compatible clinical syndrome in the absence of positive microbiology should avoid rifampin when possible. While the reality of clinical medicine makes trials of therapy necessary, they are a suboptimal way to arrive at a clinical conclusion. The antimicrobial spectrum and the immunosuppressive activity of rifampin may make a response difficult to interpret. Due to the morbidity and mortality of miliary and central nervous system disease, rifampin will likely be used empirically. This decision is based on the presence of greater and earlier microbicidal activity when INH and rifampin are used in combination.

i. These caveats apply only to *M. tuberculosis* sensitive to therapeutic agents. The therapy of resistant *M. tuberculosis* and atypical mycobacteria is driven by susceptibilities, requires multidrug regimens with otherwise infrequently used agents, and contains no short-course therapy recommendations. Many atypical strains, especially group IV, are resistant to all antituberculous drugs but susceptible to some common antimicrobial agents.

2. Nine-month regimen—involving INH and rifampin. Following 2 months of daily therapy, the regimen may be either continued on a daily basis or altered to twice per week. The twice weekly regimen allows directly observed therapy either in the clinic or in the home. With this therapy, INH is increased to 15 mg/kg/day, with a maximum daily dose of 900 mg. The dose of rifampin remains the same.

3. Six-month therapy—initial 2 months of daily INH, rifampin, and pyrazinamide, followed by daily or twice weekly INH and rifampin for the next 4 months. With twice weekly administration, the INH dose is modified as noted immediately above.

4. Modifications of the short-course regimen

a. Ethambutol or streptomycin should be added if INH resistance is suspected or if disease appears to be life-threatening. I prefer to use ethambutol rather than streptomycin.

(1) In my opinion, ethambutol should always be administered with the other medications being given for either the 6- or 9-month regimen. In the 9-month regimen, this provides effective therapy from the onset if INH resistance is present. In either regimen, it provides effective therapy from the onset for the treatment of *M. kansasii*. While the number of cases of tuberculosis has diminished, atypical mycobacteria have accounted for an increased percentage of patients presenting with clinically suspect tuberculosis and positive acid-fast smears.

5. Ancillary therapies

a. Surgery for the mechanical complications of infection such as obstructive hydrocephalus, vertebral collapse, ureteral or urethral obstruction, and tuberculous empyema.

b. Steroids—not recommended as a standard component of therapy. They have been used for years in other countries. If an effective antituberculous regimen is used, a short course of steroids accelerates the clinical response without causing obvious detrimental effects. High doses and long courses are associated with all the complications of steroids. Recent evidence suggests that steroids have a beneficial effect when used as part of the therapy of tuberculous meningitis. This has been a matter of debate for several decades, and the issue is currently still unresolved.

c. Nutrition—rest and nutrition are important and were effective in most patients with uncomplicated pulmonary disease prior to the availability of medications. Prolonged isolation was required.

VII. Monitoring

Tuberculosis is best cared for on an outpatient basis. Hospitalization should be reserved for patients who require invasive diagnostic techniques or who have severe illness. Positive sputum microbiology alone is not an indication for hospitalization.

A. Therapeutic efficacy
   1. Clinical improvement is associated with decreased temperature, cough, and sputum production. Patients should be followed monthly.
   2. X-rays should demonstrate stabilization and subsequent improvement, although persistent abnormalities are common. If patients are doing well, monthly x-rays for the first 2 or 3 months should be obtained, followed by an x-ray at the completion of therapy.
   3. Sputum—a specimen should be checked on a monthly basis. Acid-fast bacilli seen on smears should decrease and eventually vanish. If culture negativity is not obtained by 3 months, the therapeutic regimen should be reevaluated and the duration of therapy prolonged.
   4. The patient with clinical improvement and decreased sputum production may return to work. A minimum of 2 weeks and preferably 3 weeks of therapy should have occurred. The approach to workplace contacts is not dictated by the presence or absence of a treated index case in the workplace.

B. Therapeutic toxicity
   1. Hepatitis—Hepatic function should be assessed prior to initiating therapy, and the patient should be given instruction about the signs and symptoms of hepatitis. Symptoms should be monitored monthly. Enzyme levels should be checked once or twice during therapy in patients over 35 years of age. Medications should be discontinued when symptoms are present or when normal hepatocellular enzyme levels increase more than five-fold. While INH hepatotoxicity is best known, rifampin, ethambutol, pyrazinamide, and ethionamide are all hepatotoxic. Rifampin hepatotoxicity tends to occur earlier in therapy than that due to INH. Hepatotoxicity may be increased in individuals with preexisting liver disease.
   2. Red blood cell secretions—Rifampin has been associated with red urine, tears, saliva, and stool. This may be quite disconcerting and frightening to patients. The staining of contact lenses may be permanent and may require lens replacement.
   3. Ophthalmologic changes—The patient should be counseled about blurring of vision and changes in color. There should be a baseline and monthly check of visual acuity and color vision. A decrease in the total daily dose of ethambutol from 25 to 15 mg/kg results in equivalent efficacy and reduced optic toxicity (i.e., a higher therapeutic-toxic ratio). INH can also cause optic neuritis.
   4. Hyperuricemia—This is common in patients receiving pyrazinamide and is a way to check if the medication is being taken. Ethambutol also may elevate the serum uric acid level. Clinical gout is rare.
   5. Nephrotoxicity/ototoxicity—This is a major concern in patients receiving aminoglycosides. Baseline renal function and audiometry tests should be performed. Aminoglycoside serum levels should be monitored once or twice per week after a stable regimen has been established. An audiogram should be repeated monthly. Patients should be counseled about nausea, vomiting, tinnitus, vertigo, or decreased hearing and the need to contact their physicians immediately. Dose adjustment of other antituberculous medications may be necessary in the presence of diminishing renal function.

VIII. **Prognosis**
   A. Morbidity associated with tuberculosis is rare if the diagnosis and therapy have been prompt. There may be morbidity associated with the underlying diseases predisposing to tuberculosis (i.e., silicosis, diabetes, or uremia). Surgery required for the mechanical aspects of infection has its own inherent morbidity. Central nervous system infection has the greatest associated morbidity. Motor and intellectual impairments commonly persist if they are present at the time of diagnosis. Obstructive hydrocephalus appearing during the course of successful therapy may be relieved by the addition of steroids.
   B. Mortality—Overall mortality is <10% for pulmonary disease, but increased mortality is associated with underlying illnesses. Even with excellent therapeutic agents, tuberculous meningitis and miliary tuberculosis carry mortality rates of 30% or more.

Bibliography

Bass JB, Farer LS, Hopewell, et al. Diagnostic standards and classification of tuberculosis. *Am Rev Respir Dir* 142:725–735, 1990.

Centers for Disease Control. Screening for tuberculosis and tuberculous infection in high risk populations and the use of preventive therapy for tuberculous infection in the United States: Recommendations of the Advisory Committee for Elimination of Tuberculosis. *MMWR* 39: (1990).

Division of Tuberculosis Control, Center for Prevention Services, Centers for Disease Control, et al. National tuberculosis training initiative. Core Curriculum on Tuberculosis, New York, 1990.

Green GM, Daniel TM, Ball WC (eds). Koch Centennial Supplement: 100th Anniversary of the Announcement of the Discovery of the Tubercle Bacillus by Robert Koch, March 24, 1881. *Am Rev Respir Dis* Vol. 125, March 1982.

Modilevsky T, Sattler FR, Barnes PF. Mycobacterial disease in patients with human immunodeficiency virus infection. *Arch Intern Med* 149:2201–2205, 1989.

Rieder HL, Cauthen GM, Kelly GD, et al. Tuberculosis in the United States. *JAMA* 262:385–389, 1989.

Chapter 48-M

Systemic Fungal Infections

John C. Pottage, Jr., M.D.

I. **Definition**

   A. Systemic fungal infections are characterized by blood-borne spread of the pathogen following its introduction into the body. For most systemic fungal infections, the portal of entry is the pulmonary system: fungal spores are inhaled. From the lungs there is spread via the bloodstream and lymphatics to the skin and visceral organs. Other fungi can gain access to the bloodstream via inoculation, usually infected intravenous catheters, or breaks in the gastrointestinal mucosa.

II. **Etiology**

   A. *Candida* species

     1. Specific organisms

       The majority of *Candida* infections are caused by *Candida albicans*. Other important species include *C. tropicalis, C. parapsilosis, C. krusei, C. lusitaniae,* and *Torulopsis glabrata*.

     2. Epidemiology

       Candida species are normal inhabitants of the gastrointestinal tract, vagina, and skin. Systemic infections caused by *Candida* are associated with (1) broad-spectrum antibiotics, (2) intravenous catheters, (3) colonization of the skin or mucosal surfaces with *Candida*, (4) bladder catheters, and (5) hemodialysis.

     3. Pathogenesis

       Systemic infections are usually due to *Candida* from the patient's own flora. Breaks in the skin (e.g., from intravenous catheters) or the gastrointestinal tract allow the organism access to the bloodstream. Abscesses can then be formed in the various organs. Polymorphonuclear leukocytes are involved in the early response. Both humoral and cell-mediated immunity have important roles in the body's defenses.

     4. Clinical presentation

       a. Candidemia—This is defined as a positive culture of the blood for *Candida* species without evidence of visceral organ involvement. It can be divided into transient candidemia (blood cultures positive over a period of time less than 24 hr) and persistent candidemia with blood cultures positive over a period of time greater than 24 hr. These are almost always associated with an intravenous catheter. Patients may be asymptomatic or have continuing fevers despite broad-spectrum antibacterial agents. Nonspecific complaints of fatigue, myalgias, or headaches may also be present. Signs and symptoms related to infection around the catheter site may or may not be present. A careful exam searching for signs of dissemination is mandatory.

b. Disseminated candidiasis—Disseminated candidiasis is defined as a blood-borne *Candida* infection with evidence of visceral infection. Signs and symptoms are the same as that for candidemia with the exception that evidence for visceral invasion is present. Skin lesions can be erythematous macules, papules, or pustules. A thorough eye exam to search for endophthalmitis is necessary in all patients suspected of having disseminated candidiasis. A careful cardiac exam should also be performed to look for evidence of endocarditis.

c. Hepatosplenic candidiasis—Hepatosplenic candidiasis is a form of disseminated candidiasis usually seen in patients who are severely neutropenic. Symptoms usually include persistent fever, chills, and night sweats. Tenderness over the liver and/or spleen may be present. Elevated liver function tests, including transaminases and alkaline phosphatase, are present.

5. Diagnosis

The diagnosis of *Candida* infections involves pathologic demonstration of organisms in clinical specimens and/or growth of the organism from cultures. Direct-mount or potassium hydroxide (KOH) preparations will show the presence of budding yeast forms together with pseudohyphal and hyphal forms. *Candida* is gram-positive when stained with Gram's stain. Biopsies of abscesses will show fungal forms with periodic acid-Schiff (PAS) and methenamine silver stains. Cultures for *Candida* should be obtained from the blood as well as all sites that have been biopsied, such as the skin or liver. Serologic testing has not been shown to be useful in the diagnosis of *Candida* infections. Additional radiologic testing with a chest x-ray, bone x-rays, intravenous pyelogram (IVP), computed tomography (CT) scans of the abdomen, bone scan, and/or gallium scan is obtained as needed.

6. Treatment

The intravenous catheter in all patients with candidemia or disseminated candidiasis needs to be removed. For patients with candidemia, a course of amphotericin B (500–1,000 mg) should be given. Alternatively, 200 mg fluconazole once daily for four weeks can be used. For patients with disseminated candidiasis, amphotericin B (1,000 mg) or fluconazole can be used. In patients with infection due to *Candida krusei* or *Torulopsis glabrata*, amphotericin B is the only available therapy, as these pathogens are resistant to fluconazole. In patients with hepatosplenic candidiasis, the combination of amphotericin B and 5-flucytosine is used.

B. *Cryptococcus species*

1. Etiology

The only important human pathogen is *Cryptococcus neoformans* which is divided into four serotypes, A–D. Cryptococci are characterized by round yeast forms surrounded by a polysaccharide capsule. The isthmus between mother and daughter cell is very narrow.

2. Epidemiology

Cryptococcus is a worldwide pathogen found in the soil. It has been associated with birds, particularly pigeons.

3. Pathogenesis

Cryptococcal infections are acquired through inhalation. Most initial infections are asymptomatic, though a severe pneumonia can sometimes be noted. The organism has a strong predilection for infection of the central nervous system. Other areas of the body that are frequently involved with cryptococcal infections include the bone, skin, and prostate. Cryptococcal infections are seen in patients with HIV infection, transplant patients, or those with altered cell-mediated immunity. The polysaccharide capsule is an important virulence factor for cryptococci. Infection with cryptococci frequently results in a minimal host response.

4. Clinical presentations

A history of immune compromise is present in 50% of patients with cryptococcal disease. For patients with pulmonary cryptococcosis, the findings are that of a chronic pneumonia: fevers, chills, cough, and chest pain. Cryptococcal meningitis presents with a fever, headache, stiff neck, and/or altered mental status. Often the symptoms are slight and are present for weeks.

5. Diagnosis

Yeast forms with a large capsule are strongly suggestive of cryptococci. An India ink stain will demonstrate this in spinal fluid in approximately 50% of patients. PAS stains will highlight the capsule in pathologic specimens. Antigen testing of the cerebrospinal fluid (CSF) and blood is more sensitive than India ink smears. It is positive in > 90% of the cases. Antibody testing is not useful. Culture of appropriate specimens should be performed. In all patients in whom cryptococci is isolated, a spinal tap should be performed even if there are no central nervous system (CNS) symptoms. A determination of CSF pressure should be attempted as this is an important prognostic indicator.

6. Treatment

For non-HIV-infected patients with cryptococcal infection, a 6-week course of the combination of amphotericin B and 5-flucytosine is used. In HIV-infected patients, the initial therapy is usually amphotericin B alone or in combination with 5-flucytosine followed by lifelong suppressive therapy with fluconazole. Fluconazole can be used for initial therapy in patients who have a normal mental status.

C. Histoplasmosis

1. Etiology

Histoplasma capsulatum is a dimorphic fungus that exists as a yeast form in humans.

2. Epidemiology

Histoplasma capsulatum exists as a mycelial form in the soil in endemic areas of North and South America. In North America, the endemic area is the Ohio-Mississippi River basin, areas near the Rio Grande in Texas, and a portion of central California. Areas of Central and South America also contain areas of endemicity for histoplasmosis. Certain birds such as starlings and chickens have been associated with histoplasmosis.

3. Pathogenesis

The initial site of infection for histoplas-mosis is the lower lobes of the lungs after inhalation of fungal spores. The majority of patients are asymptomatic or report a "flu-like" syndrome. From the lungs there is dissemination via the bloodstream and lymphatics to the visceral organs. The pathogenesis of histoplasmosis is very similar to that of tuberculosis. In response to a histoplasma infection, the yeast organisms are ingested by macrophages and granulomas are formed. As the organisms are destroyed, caseous necrosis develops with eventual calcification. Like tuberculosis, reactivation of infection can occur years later.

4. Clinical presentation

a. Acute pulmonary histoplasmosis—Most patients are asymptomatic or have very mild symptoms. In patients who have been exposed to a heavy inoculum of fungal spores, fevers, chills, night sweats, and cough are the predominant symptoms. Erythema nodosum and erythema multiforme are sometimes present. On physical exam, the lungs may sound clear or demonstrate rales and rhonchi. Signs of pulmonary consolidation may be present. Hepatosplenomegaly and lymphadenopathy may sometimes be seen.

b. Chronic pulmonary histoplasmosis—This usually occurs in patients with chronic obstructive lung disease in whom the upper lobes of the lungs are infected with *H. capsulatum*. Symptoms are similar to those of tuberculosis or lung cancer: fever, chills, night sweats, cough, pleuritic chest pain, fatigue, and weight loss. Exam of chest shows evidence of consolidation and/or cavitation, usually in the upper lobes. Evidence for chronic disease may be present.

c. Disseminated histoplasmosis—This usually occurs in patients with preexisting immune compromise such as HIV infection. The disease is characterized by fatigue, fevers, night sweats, and weight loss. Symptoms specific for the various organ systems involved are also seen, including gastrointestinal symptoms relating primarily to intestinal ulcerations, anemia, meningitis, endocarditis, or adrenal insufficiency.

The physical exam is generally nonspecific, though hepatosplenomegaly is common. Ulceration of the oropharyngeal region may be seen.

   d. Focal infections—Focal areas of infection such as lymph nodes and the mediastinum are sometimes seen with infection with histoplasmosis.

5. Diagnosis

The diagnosis for histoplasmosis rests upon pathologic demonstration of organism in pathologic specimens and/or culture positivity. Histoplasmosis is seen as a small yeast (2–3 μm in diameter) intracellularly in macrophages. The methenamine silver stain highlights the organism best. *Histoplasma capsulatum* is dimorphic and is readily grown in the laboratory. Cultures can take up to 4 to 6 weeks to grow. Culture of the bone marrow is particularly useful in the diagnosis of disseminated histoplasmosis. Serology is sometimes useful. The immunodiffusion test is specific but not sensitive. *Histoplasma* antigen detection appears useful but is investigational at this time. Skin testing should not be performed as it may give a false-positive serologic response. Chest x-rays, CT scans, and gallium scans are useful in estimating the extent of the infection and identifying areas for biopsy.

6. Treatment

For life-threatening histoplasmosis, the treatment of choice is amphotericin B. The usual treatment course is 1.5 to 2.0 grams. For non-life-threatening histoplasmosis, itraconazole is used. The usual treatment course if 400 mg/day for a 3 to 6-month course. HIV-infected patients need to receive lifelong maintenance therapy with itraconazole in order to prevent relapses.

D. Blastomycosis

1. Etiology

Blastomyces dermatiditis is a dimorphic fungus that exists as a yeast form in humans.

2. Epidemiology

Blastomyces dermatiditis is endemic to North America in the Mississippi-Ohio River valley.

3. Pathogenesis

Like the other endemic fungus from this region, histoplasmosis, the initial site of infection for blastomycosis is in the lungs following inhalation of fungal spores. Most primary infections are asymptomatic. The organism can become blood-borne and has a predilection for causing lesions in the skin, bone, prostate, and central nervous system. Reactivation of disease has been described.

4. Clinical presentation

The initial site of infection in blastomycosis is the lung. A dense consolidating pneumonia can be seen and is often thought to be lung cancer. Nonspecific symptoms including fever, night sweats, fatigue, and weight loss are commonly seen. Dissemination of disease can lead to involvement in the skin, bone, prostate, and central nervous system. Skin lesions appear as either crusted, heaped-up lesions or as ulcerative lesions. Skin lesions are often seen on or near mucosal surfaces such as the mouth or nose. In patients with immune compromise, an overwhelming disseminated disease can occur.

5. Diagnosis

Upon direct examination of clinical specimens, *Blastomyces dermatiditis* appears as yeast cells with broad-based budding. PAS stains of pathologic specimens highlight the cell wall. Culture of specimens should be performed in all cases. Growth sometimes takes up to 4 to 6 weeks. Serology is generally not sensitive enough to be useful in the diagnosis.

6. Treatment

For life-threatening blastomycosis, amphotericin B is the treatment of choice. The usual course of therapy is 1.5 to 20 grams. Intraconazole is used in patients who do not have life-threatening disease. The usual dose is 200–400 mg/day for a 3- to 6-month period.

E. Coccidioidomycosis

1. Etiology

Coccidioides immitis is a dimorphic fungus that exists in the mycelial phase in soil and the yeast phase in humans.

2. Epidemiology

Coccidioides immitis is endemic to the desert Southwest in the United States, and Central and South America. The fungus resides in the soil.

3. Pathogenesis

Spores of *C. immitis* are inhaled and cause initial infection in the lungs. As with the other endemic fungi, most infections are asymptomatic. Dissemination to the visceral organs occurs through the bloodstream and lymphatics. The host response is similar to that seen for histoplasmosis and tuberculosis with the development of granulomas. Reactivation of disease can occur with coccidioidomycosis.

4. Clinical presentation

Most patients infected with *C. immitis* are asymptomatic. In those who develop symptoms, signs of pneumonia are seen. Nonspecific symptoms including fevers, chills, night sweats, and myalgias are common. Erythema nodosum and erythema multiforme may occur. For the most part, these symptoms will resolve. A small percentage of patients will develop chronic pulmonary coccidioidomycosis. This can be characterized as a chronic pneumonia, cavitary lung lesion, or simply a small mass-like lesion. Like the other endemic fungi, coccidioidomycosis can disseminate to other visceral organs. The central nervous system, bone and joints, and the skin are the most common sites for dissemination.

5. Diagnosis

The organism can be seen on examination of clinical specimens. The fungal form present in these specimens is a spherule which is filled with several hundred endospores. Methenamine silver stains demonstrate the spherule wall in pathologic specimens. Culture of the organism is simple and growth occurs usually within 1 week. The arthroconidia are virulent and if there is the suspicion of coccidioidomycosis, the microbiology laboratory should be notified. Serology in coccidioidomycosis is helpful and should be obtained. IgM antibodies are detected by tube precipitation or immunodiffusion. IgG antibodies are detected by complement fixation. Skin testing with coccidioidal antigen is also helpful.

6. Treatment

For life-threatening disease, the treatment is amphotericin B for a treatment course of 1.5–2.0 grams. For less severe disease, the triazoles, fluconazole and itraconazole, show activity against the fungus. The exact role of these agents is currently under investigation.

F. Invasive aspergillosis

1. Etiology

Aspergillosis is usually caused by *Aspergillus fumigatus* or *Aspergillus flavus*. The organisms grow in humans as mycelia. Aspergillosis is characterized by septated hyphae that branch at 45° angles. *Aspergillus* species are worldwide in distribution and grow in the soil and in various forms of vegetation.

2. Pathogenesis

Invasive aspergillosis is acquired via inhalation of fungal spores. For the most part, invasive aspergillosis occurs in immune-compromised hosts. The most important risk factor is neutropenia. *Aspergillus* species invade blood vessels and cause infarction and necrosis. Though most disease occurs in the lungs, spread to the visceral organs occurs, particularly the central nervous system.

3. Clinical presentation

Invasive aspergillosis is characterized as a consolidating pneumonia in a neutropenic patient. Symptoms include fevers, chills, night sweats, cough, and hemoptysis unresponsive to antibacterial antibiotics. Pleuritic chest pain is often a clue for aspergillosis. The development of cavitary disease is also seen with aspergillosis. In patients in whom spread to other organ systems such as the central nervous system, skin, or bone has occurred, focal signs and symptoms will also be present.

4. Diagnosis

The organism is readily demonstrated upon examination of pathologic specimens. Methenamine silver stains show the septated hyphae invading blood vessels. Growth from cultures of lung tissue is also important in confirming the diagnosis. Positive growth from sputum samples without demonstration of tissue invasion is difficult to interpret. Serologic methods of diagnosis are being investigated.

5. Treatment

The treatment of choice for invasive aspergillosis is amphotericin B for a treatment course of 2–3 grams. Itraconazole has *in vitro* activity against aspergillosis; however, its use in the treatment of invasive aspergillosis is investigational.

G. Mucormycosis

1. Etiology

Mucormycosis is caused by fungal species of the genera *Rhizopus, Absidia,* and *Mucor.* These organisms appear as mycelia in humans and are characterized by non-septated hyphae that branch at 90° angles.

2. Epidemiology

The fungi that cause mucormycosis are worldwide in distribution and live in the soil and vegetation.

3. Pathogenesis

The pathogenesis of mucormycosis is similar to that of aspergillosis with inhalation of fungal spores and resultant local invasion of blood vessels with subsequent infarction and necrosis. Patients with uncontrolled acidosis such as diabetics or those with renal failure are predisposed to rhinocerebral mucormycosis.

4. Clinical presentation

a. Rhinocerebral mucormycosis—This occurs in patients with uncontrolled acidosis. It is characterized as an invasive sinusitis with local extension into the bone, palate, and central nervous system. The most common symptoms include altered mental status and cranial nerve abnormalities. Evidence of invasion with proptosis or draining ulcers are also seen.

b. Pulmonary mucormycosis—This is characterized by the same symptomatol-ogy as invasive pulmonary aspergillosis. It occurs primarily in patients who are neutropenic.

5. Diagnosis

Demonstration of nonseptated large hyphae with 90° angles branching is characteristic in biopsy specimens. Growth from cultures of biopsy specimens is also important.

6. Treatment

Treatment of mucormycosis requires surgical debridement of necrotic tissue, correction of underlying disease states, and amphotericin B (2- to 3-gram course).

Bibliography

Bradsher RW. Blastomycosis: *Clinical Infectious Diseases* 14(Suppl 1):582–90, 1992.

Komshian SV, Uwaydah AK, Sobel JD, et al: Fungemia caused by Candida species and Torulopsis glabrata in the hospitalized patient: Frequency, characteristics and evaluation of factors influencing outcome. *Reviews of Infectious Disease* 11:379–90, 1989.

Perfect JR. Cryptococcosis. *Infectious Disease Clinics of North America* 3:77–102, 1989.

Wey SB, Mori M, Pfaller MA, et al: Risk factors for hospital-acquired candidemia: A matched case control study. *Archives of Internal Medicine* 149:2349–53, 1989.

Wheat LJ. Histoplasmosis. *Infectious Disease Clinics of North America* 2:841–859, 1988.

Malaria

Gordon M. Trenholme, M.D.

I. **Definition**

Parasitic infection caused by protozoa of the genus *Plasmodium* associated with fever, chills, and hemolytic anemia.

II. **Etiology**

P. falciparum, P. vivax, P. ovale, P. malariae

III. **Incidence**

A. Two-fifths of the world's population live in malarious areas (Figure 48N-1, Table 48N-1).

B. In the United States, approximately 1,000 cases, almost all imported, are reported yearly to the Centers for Disease Control.

IV. **Pathophysiology**

A. Life cycle

1. Transmission to humans usually occurs by the bite of an infected *Anopheles* mosquito, or, rarely, by transfusion of infected red blood cells or transplacentally from mother to fetus.

2. Hepatic stage—Within 1 hr after the bite of an infected mosquito, the parasite infects hepatocytes. Parasites replicate asexually in the hepatocytes for periods ranging from days to weeks. They then emerge to infect the red blood cells. The patient is entirely asymptomatic during the hepatic stage. Liver function studies and physical examination are normal. A persistent hepatic stage is responsible for relapse due to *P. vivax* and *P. ovale*.

3. Red blood cell stage—After emerging from hepatocytes, parasites attach to receptors on the red blood cell membrane, invade red blood cells, and utilize hemoglobin and nutrients to replicate asexually. The reproductive cycle in the red blood cell lasts for 48 hr for all species except *P. malariae*, for which it is 72 hr. All symptoms are related to this stage.

a. Hemolytic anemia is due to destruction of red blood cells by parasites.

b. Splenomegaly is due to stimulation of the reticuloendothelial system by release of fragmented red blood cells and parasites.

c. Thrombocytopenia is usually immune mediated but may be secondary to disseminated intravascular coagulation.

d. Fever and chills are related to release of cytokines in response to the red blood cell stage.

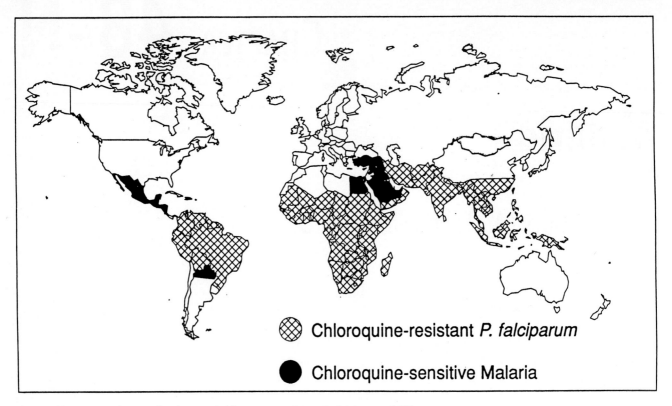

Figure 48N-1. Distribution of malaria and chloroquine-resistant *P. falciparum,* 1991.

B. Multiorgan dysfunction is seen only with *P. falciparum* and is primarily related to intravascular sequestration of parasitized red blood cells, with subsequent deficient oxygen delivery to peripheral tissues.

V. Diagnosis

A. History

1. Travel to rural areas of tropical or semitropical areas except in Africa, where malaria can be acquired in both rural and urban locales.

2. Periodic symptoms are strongly suggestive of malaria. However, symptoms may occur daily during the initial period of infection with all species. The occurrence of symptoms every other day suggests infection with *P. vivax* and *P. ovale.* Symptom occurrence every third day suggests infection with *P. malariae.*

B. Clinical signs and physical findings

1. A classical malaria paroxysm consists of severe chills followed by headache, nau-

Table 48N-1. Malaria Cases Yearly in the United States by Distribution of Species and Area of Acquisition

Area of Acquisition	Species of *Plasmodium*				
	Vivax	*Falciparum*	*Malariae*	*Ovale*	**Total**
Africa	5*	38	2	1	46
Asia	20	4	1	<1	25
Central America and Caribbean	11	1	1	0	13
Mexico	13	<1	<1	<1	13
South America	1	<1	0	0	2
Total	52	43	4	1	100

*Percentage of total cases.

sea, vomiting, and a high fever spike. It is periodic for all species except *P. falciparum*, in which a paroxysm usually occurs daily.

2. Pallor related to anemia may be present.
3. Although splenomegaly occurs in 50% of patients, peripheral lymphadenopathy is never due to malaria.
4. Cerebral malaria is indicated by coma and/or encephalopathic features. It occurs only with infection with *P. falciparum*.
5. Hypoglycemia due to decreased hepatic gluconeogenesis may be a complication of severe falciparum malaria.

C. Diagnostic tests
1. A thin smear of the peripheral blood will show intraerythrocytic parasites in almost all patients.
2. Only intraerythrocytic ring forms are seen on the peripheral smear of *P. falciparum*.
3. If >3% of red blood cells are parasitized, one should strongly consider *P. falciparum*.
4. A thick smear should be ordered only if thin smears are negative. Erythrocytes are not evident on a thick smear.
5. No serologic tests are useful.
6. Eosinophilia is not seen unless there is concomitant helminth infection.
7. In cerebral malaria, the cerebrospinal fluid and a computed tomography scan of the brain are usually normal.

VI. Differential Diagnosis
A. Daily fever acquired in the tropics may be due to
1. Typhoid fever.
2. Dengue.
3. Amebic liver abscess.
4. Trypanosomiasis.
5. Acute schistosomiasis.
6. Typhus.
7. Miliary tuberculosis.

B. Fever occurring every other day has a very limited differential diagnosis and usually is related to alternate dosing of a medication (e.g., corticosteroids).

VII. Treatment
A. *P. falciparum*
1. IV quinidine gluconate is the preferred treatment for patients:
   a. With parasite counts >5%.
   b. Unable to tolerate oral medications.
   c. With signs or symptoms of cerebral dysfunction.

2. IV quinidine is given until the patient is markedly improved, which generally requires at least 72 hr. The patient should then be treated with tetracycline for 7 days.
3. For patients with mild disease acquired in Central America or Haiti, oral chloroquine may be used.
4. Mild disease acquired anywhere except Central America or Haiti can be treated with either mefloquine or pyrimethamine/sulfadoxine.
5. Empiric antibiotic therapy for gram-negative bacteremia is indicated for patients with severe falciparum malaria until bacterial blood cultures are known to be negative.

B. *P. vivax* and *P. ovale* are treated with chloroquine followed by primaquine.
C. *P. malariae* is treated only with chloroquine.
D. Potential indications for exchange transfusion include:
1. >10% parasitemia.
2. Cerebral malaria with >5% parasitemia.

VIII. Patient Monitoring
A. A red blood cell thin smear with determination of parasite counts should be repeated at least daily or more frequently if there is concern about the patient's course during the acute phase of malaria.
B. Quinidine levels should be maintained at 2–6 μg/ml.
C. As with any other severe infection, a patient with *P. falciparum* may need maximum supportive therapy and careful monitoring of hemodynamic and renal function.
D. All patients who receive primaquine should have glucose-6-phosphate deficiency excluded before administration of this drug.

IX. Prognosis
A. Excellent with early, appropriate therapy.
B. Directly related to parasitemia.
1. <2–3%—minimal morbidity and mortality.
2. >5%—increased morbidity.
3. >10%—increased mortality.

C. Cerebral malaria is usually associated with no residual neurologic damage if the patient survives.

X. Prevention
A. Prophylaxis is recommended for travelers who will stay overnight in rural areas of countries with malaria except for travelers to Africa, who should receive prophylaxis regardless of their itinerary.

Table 48N-2. Treatment of Malaria

Agent	Route	Dose
Quinidine gluconate	IV	10 mg/kg load given over 1–2 hr, then 0.02 mg/kg/min × ~3 days
Quinine sulfate	Oral	650 mg q8h × ~3 days
Chloroquine phosphate	Oral	1,000 mg initially, then 1,000 mg in 8 hr and 500 mg in 24 and 48 hr
Mefloquine hydrochloride*	Oral	1 g, single dose
Pyrimethamine/sulfadoxine*	Oral	3 tabs, single dose
Tetracycline†	Oral	250 mg q6h × 7 days
Primaquine phosphate	Oral	27 mg each for 14 days

* Not to be used for severe malaria.
† Only after administration of quinidine or quinine.

Table 48N-3. Prevention of Malaria

Agent	Dose	Sequence
Mefloquine hydrochloride	250 mg	250 mg weekly. Begin 1 week before and continue until 4 weeks after leaving endemic area.
Chloroquine phosphate	500 mg	500 mg weekly as above.
Doxycycline	100 mg	100 mg b.i.d. daily. Begin day before and continue until 4 weeks after leaving endemic area.

B. Mefloquine is the agent of choice for prophylaxis of travelers to all malarious areas except those countries north of the Panama Canal. If mefloquine cannot be used, doxycycline is an alternative.

C. Chloroquine can be used for prophylaxis of travelers to malarious areas north of the Panama Canal.

D. In addition to prophylactic drugs, travelers should use topical insecticides and appropriate protective clothing.

E. Although the preceding measures are very useful, individuals should still be aware that they may develop malaria.

F. Patients with prolonged exposure to areas endemic for *P. vivax* may take a course of primaquine after completing chloroquine prophylaxis.

Bibliography

Grau GE, Taylor TE, Molyneux ME, et al. Tumor necrosis factor and disease severity in children with falciparum malaria. *N Engl J Med* 320:1586–1591, 1989.

Hoffman SL. Prevention of malaria. *JAMA* 265:398–399, 1991.

Lobel HO, Bernard KW, Williams SL, et al. Effectiveness and tolerance of long-term malaria prophylaxis with mefloquine. *JAMA* 265:361–364, 1991.

Miller KD, Greenberg AE, Campbell CC. Treatment of severe malaria in the United States with a continuous infusion of quinidine gluconate and exchange transfusion. *N Engl J Med* 321:65–70, 1989.

Neva FA, Sheagren JN, Shulman R, et al. Malaria: Host-defense mechanisms and complications. *Ann Intern Med* 73:295–306, 1970.

Trenholme GM. Malaria. Harris AA (Vol. ed.), Vinken PJ, Bruyn GW, Klawans HL (eds), Elsevier Science Publishing Co., Inc. *Handbook of Clinical Neurology* 8:365–375, 1988.

CHAPTER 48-O

Sepsis

David Simon, M.D.
Gordon M. Trenholme, M.D.

I. **Definition**
Sepsis is a systemic inflammatory response to infectious agents and/or their products, with evidence of dysfunction in one or more organ systems. Progression to shock and death occurs in a significant number of affected patients (Table 48O-1).

II. **Etiology**
A. Gram-negative bacteria: All gram-negative organisms may produce sepsis in the proper clinical setting. The incidence of gram-negative organisms producing sepsis or septic shock varied from 30% to 80% in recent studies.
   1. *Escherichia coli, Klebsiella* species, and *Pseudomonas aeruginosa* account for nearly 80% of gram-negative blood isolates.
   2. *Proteus, Enterobacter, Serratia,* and *Bacteroides* species represent other major blood isolates.
B. Gram-positive bacteria: These organisms accounted for 5–24% of isolated organisms in recent studies. *Staphylococcus aureus,* coagulase-negative staphylococci, and streptococci species may produce sepsis. The incidence of sepsis secondary to these

pathogens is increasing, primarily in the granulocytopenic patient.
   1. Toxic shock syndrome is a toxin-mediated syndrome produced by specific strains of *Staph. aureus* associated with fever, desquamative rash, hypotension, multiorgan dysfunction, and death in 5–10% of those affected.
   2. Toxic "strep" syndrome may occur in the setting of soft tissue infection caused by *Strep. pyogenes.* Bacteremia is common, and strains that produce the toxin exotoxin A, are frequently isolated. Mortality approaches 30%.
C. Other organisms
   1. Fungi such as *Candida* species, *Aspergillus,* and *Cryptococcus* may cause multiorgan failure and shock.
   2. Rickettsial infection such as Rocky Mountain spotted fever may be fulminant, with a clinical picture of sepsis.

III. **Incidence**
Precise figures are not available. Recent estimates suggest that approximately 400,000 cases of sepsis occur yearly in the United States. One-half of these patients develop shock.

Table 480-1.   Definitions of Sepsis Syndrome and Septic Shock

Sepsis	Severe Sepsis	Septic Shock

Clinical evidence of infection
  Tachypnea (>20 breaths/min; >10 liters/min with mechanical ventilation)
  Tachycardia (>90 beats/min)
  Hyperthermia (>38.3°C) or hypothermia (<35.6°C)
	Sepsis plus evidence of inadequate organ perfusion, including one or more of the following:
	  Hypoxemia (P_aO_2/FIO$_2$ ≤280 with no other pulmonary or cardiovascular disease as the cause)
	  Elevated plasma lactate level (above upper limit of normal for the testing laboratory)
	  Oliguria (<0.5 ml/kg body weight for at least 1 hr in patients with catheters)
	  Acute alteration in mental status
		Sepsis with hypotension (sustained decrease in systolic blood pressure <90 mmHg or a drop >40 mmHg for at least 1 hr, when volume replacement is adequate and the patient is taking no antihypertensive medication, in the absence of other causes of shock such as hypovolemia, myocardial infarction, and pulmonary embolism)

IV. **Pathophysiology**

Sepsis is a complex host response to infection. The interaction of the microorganism or its products with the host may produce an overwhelming inflammatory response and may lead to myocardial depression, endothelial dysfunction, multiorgan failure, and death.

A. Endotoxin is a complex lipopolysaccharide (LPS) found in the outer cell membrane of gram-negative bacteria. Endotoxin initiates the inflammatory response in the development of sepsis secondary to gram-negative bacteria. The interaction of LPS with humoral pathways and the stimulatory effect of LPS on monocytes/macrophages is responsible for the generation of an array of bioactive substances. The complex interplay of these molecules with poorly defined host factors is responsible for the development of sepsis.

1. Humoral pathway activation by LPS

   a. Endotoxin can activate the alternative complement pathway, producing the anaphylatoxins C3a and C5a.

      (1) C3a and C5a activate neutrophils which secrete arachidonic acid metabolites (leukotrienes, thromboxane), oxygen radicals, and lysosomal enzymes that may contribute to endothelial cell damage and capillary leakage.

      (2) C3a and C5a stimulate mast cell release of vasodilatory mediators which may contribute to hypotension.

   b. Endotoxin activates Factor XII of the coagulation cascade, which may lead to consumption of coagulation factors and development of disseminated intravascular coagulation. Factor XII also stimulates the production of bradykinin, a potent hypotensive agent.

2. Cellular activation by LPS

   a. Monocytes/macrophages contain several binding sites for LPS on their cell surface. One binding site is the CD14 antigen. The ability of LPS to bind to CD14 first requires LPS to bind with an acute phase serum protein, lipopolysaccharide-binding protein (LBP). The LPS-LBP complex then binds to CD14 receptors on monocytes/macrophages. This binding triggers the synthesis of cytokines such as tumor necrosis factor (TNF α) and interleukins (IL-1, IL-6). These substances appear to play a central role in the pathophysiology of sepsis.

   b. Polymorphonuclear cells, endothelial cells, and platelets contribute a host of vasoactive and cytotoxic substances during sepsis (i.e., platelet-activating factor and leukotrienes). The release of these agents may be directly due to endotoxin challenge or may occur in response to molecules generated by the action of LPS on humoral pathways or mononuclear cells.

B. Other bacterial products are capable of initiating inflammatory reactions independent of the effects of endotoxin.
   1. Toxic shock syndrome toxin-1.
   2. Exotoxin A.
   3. Hemolysins.
   4. Bacterial proteases.

V. Diagnosis

A. The diagnosis of sepsis syndrome and/or septic shock is made as defined by the clinical criteria presented in Table 48O-1.

B. Laboratory data: Any or all of the following may be present at the onset or during the course of sepsis:
   1. Leukopenia/leukocytosis.
   2. Thrombocytopenia.
   3. Prolonged prothrombin time or partial thromboplastin time; presence of fibrin split products (disseminated intravascular coagulation).
   4. Elevated serum lactate level.
   5. Elevated serum transaminase levels secondary to shock liver.
   6. Rising blood urea nitrogen/serum creatinine levels.
   7. Abnormal chest x-ray demonstrating a possible nidus of infection and/or a pattern consistent with adult respiratory distress syndrome.
   8. Blood cultures are positive in only 30–40% of patients with sepsis.
   9. The characteristic hemodynamic profile in sepsis reveals an elevated cardiac index with decreased systemic vascular resistance.

VI. Differential Diagnosis

Noninfectious causes of syndromes that may mimic sepsis include multiple trauma, acute pancreatitis, recurrent pulmonary emboli, transfusion or other anaphylactic reactions, and aortic dissection.

VII. Treatment

Therapy is directed to optimize cardiac output and systemic oxygen delivery. The administration of broad-spectrum antibiotics and possible surgical intervention are used to treat the underlying infection.

A. Rapid volume repletion with crystalloids/colloids is initiated.

B. Sympathomimetic amines may be required to improve cardiovascular function.
   1. Dopamine (5–15 µg/kg/min).
   2. Norepinephrine (0.05–20 µg/kg/min) is an alternative agent for patients who remain hypotensive on maximum dopamine dose.
   3. Dobutamine (2–25 µg/kg/min) may be useful in patients who are not hypotensive to increase cardiac output.

C. Ventilator-assisted respiration may be required for adequate oxygenation.

D. Hemodialysis may be needed for patients with deterioration in renal function.

E. Empiric broad-spectrum antibiotics are administered quickly after the collection of appropriate specimens for culture. Antibiotic selection is based on the suspected site of infection, suspected organism, acquisition of the suspected organism, and host factors (e.g., degree of immunodeficiency, as in neutropenia, asplenia, or AIDS (Table 48O-2). Maximum use of available culture data and Gram stains may provide useful information for decisions concerning antibiotic selection.

F. Corticosteroid therapy has been shown to have no clinical utility in the treatment of sepsis or septic shock. Higher secondary infection rates have been observed in patients treated with corticosteroids in placebo-controlled trials.

G. Immunotherapy
   1. Antiserum to endotoxin: The endotoxin molecule consists of three regions based on structural and immunogenic properties. The O-side chains are a series of complex oligosaccharides. The core oligosaccharide and Lipid A regions have structural similarity in many strains of gram-negative organisms. Lipid A is responsible for many of the toxic effects of endotoxin. Antiserum-antibody directed against these structural determinants appear protective against bacteremias caused by a wide range of organisms.
      a. Human antiserum directed against Lipid A of J5 *E. coli* improved survival in patients with gram-negative bacteremia. Mortality decreased from 39% to 22% in recipients of J5 antiserum.
      b. Antiserum to J5 was administered

Table 480-2. Empiric Antibiotic Selection

	Suspected Source of Sepsis				
	Lung	**Abdomen**	**Skin/Soft Tissue**	**Urinary Tract**	**Central Nervous System**
Major community-acuired pathogens	*Pneumococcus, Haemophilus, Klebsiella*	Enteric gram-negative rods, *Bacteroides* spp.	Gram-positive bacteria, *Staph. aureus*, streptococci, gram-negative rods	*E. coli, Klebsiella, Proteus*	*Neisseria meningitidis, H. influenzae Pneumococcus*
Empiric antibiotic therapy	Third-generation cephalosporin + erythromycin	Aminoglycoside + cleocin or ampicillin/sulbactam	Vancomycin ± third-generation cephalosporin	Aminoglycoside + ampicillin	Ceftriaxone or cefotaxime
Major nosocomial pathogens*	Enteric gram-negative rods, *Staph. aureus*	Enteric gram-negative rods, *Bacteroides* spp. + *Candida* spp.	Gram-positive bacteria, *Staph. aureus*, streptococci, gram-negative rods	*E. coli + Klebsiella, Proteus + P. aeruginosa, Enterobacter*	Enteric gram-negative rods (GNR), *P. aeruginosa, Staphylococcus aureus.*
Empiric antibiotic therapy	Antipseudomonal + β-lactam + aminoglycoside ± vancomycin	Aminoglycoside + imipenem ± amphotericin B	Vancomycin ± third-generation cephalosporin	Aminoglycoside + third-generation cephalosporin	Third-generation cephalosporin ± vancomycin

*Empiric antibiotic selection for hospital-acquired sepsis should be based on antibiotic resistance patterns for bacteria at the specific institution. Antibiotic regimen can be modified 48–72 hours later based on culture and antibiotic susceptibility results.

prophylactically to surgical patients who were at high risk for development of sepsis. The development of shock was decreased in this group despite similar rates of infection to gram-negative organisms.

2. Monoclonal antibody (MAb) to LPS endotoxin: MAbs (IgM) directed against the Lipid A portion of J5 *E. coli* have been developed and evaluated in placebo-controlled clinical trials. The studies reveal that MAb therapy is effective in subsets of patients with severe gram-negative infection. The mechanism of action of these agents is unknown.

   a. HA-1A (centoxin) treatment improved survival in patients with gram-negative bacteremia and sepsis. Mortality decreased from 49% to 30% in this patient population. If shock was present, mortality declined from 57% to 33% in the HA-1A-treated group. No benefit was seen with HA-1A treatment in patients without gram-negative bacteremia or in patients with sepsis due to gram-positive bacteria or fungi.

   b. E5 is a murine MAb similar to HA-1A in antigenic specificity. E5 treatment reduced mortality in patients with gram-negative infection who were not in shock when the study began. Resolution of organ dysfunction occurred more quickly in this subgroup of patients.

3. MAb to tumor necrosis factor (TNF): TNF synthesis and release by mononuclear cells appears to be a pivotal mediator in the development of sepsis. Agents which antagonize the biological effects of TNF may be effective in the treatment of sepsis.

VIII. Prognosis

Estimates indicate that 50–80% of patients who develop shock will die. The underlying disease of the host, source and type of infection, and choice of antimicrobial chemotherapy appear to be important determinants of the clinical outcome.

Bibliography

Bone RC. The pathogenesis of sepsis. *Ann Intern Med* 115:457–469, 1991.

Greenman RL, Schein RMH, Martin MA, et al. A controlled clinical trial of E5 murine monoclonal IgM antibody to endotoxin in the treatment of gram-negative sepsis. *JAMA* 266:1097–1102, 1991.

Parillo JE. Septic shock in humans. *Ann Intern Med* 113:227–420, 1990.

Stevens DL, Tanner MH, Winship J, et al. Severe group A streptococcal infections associated with a toxic shock-like syndrome and scarlet fever toxin A. *N Engl J Med* 321:1–7, 1989.

Wright SD, Ramos RA, Tobias PS, et al. CD14, a receptor for complexes of lipopolysaccharide (LPS) and LPS binding protein. *Science* 249:1431–1433, 1990.

Young LS. Gram-negative sepsis. In Mandell GL, Douglas RG Jr, Bennett JE (eds): *Principles and Practices of Infectious Diseases.* New York, NY, Churchill Livingstone Inc., 1990, pp 611–636.

Ziegler EJ, Fisher CJ, Sprung CL, et al. Treatment of gram-negative bacteremia and septic shock with HA-1A human monoclonal antibody against endotoxin. *N Engl J Med* 324:429–436, 1991.

CHAPTER 48-P

Respiratory Viral Infections

John C. Pottage, Jr., M.D.

I. **Definition**

Respiratory infections caused by viruses can be divided into two groups: upper respiratory infections and lower respiratory infections. Included in upper respiratory infections are the cold, pharyngitis, laryngotracheobronchitis (croup), sinusitis, and laryngitis. Included in the lower respiratory tract infections are bronchitis, bronchiolitis, and pneumonia.

II. **Etiology**

The specific etiology of viral respiratory infections is presented in Tables 48P-1 and 48P-2

III. **Diagnosis**

The major concern in patients with viral respiratory disease is to distinguish between viral and bacterial pathogens. The diagnosis of viral disease is centered around culture of respiratory secretions, detection of viral antigen in respiratory secretions, and/or serology. Cultures for bacterial pathogens should also be performed. See Tables 48P-1 and 48P-2.

IV. **Therapy**

The treatment of most viral respiratory infections is supportive. Amantadine is used for early treatment of influenza A infections. Ribavirin is useful in the treatment of bronchiolitis. Because it is difficult to clinically distinguish viral from bacterial infections, antibacterial agents are often started empirically. See Tables 48P-1 and 48P-2.

Table 48P-1. Upper Respiratory Viral Infections

Clinical Syndrome	Symptoms	Viral Etiology	Other Pathogens	Diagnosis	Treatment
Cold	Rhinorrhea, sneezing, sore throat, low-grade fever	Rhinovirus Coronavirus Adenovirus Parainfluenza virus Influenza virus Respiratory syncytial virus (RSV)	*Mycoplasma pneumoniae*	Usually based on clinical characteristics. Sinus x-ray to rule out sinusitis	Supportive care with decongestants, aspirin, acetaminophen
Pharyngitis	Cold symptoms, sore throat, fevers, chills, cervical lymphadenopathy	Adenovirus Rhinovirus Coronavirus Influenza virus Epstein-Barr virus Herpes simplex virus Coxsackie virus	Group A β-hemolytic streptococci *Mycoplasma pneumoniae*	Throat culture to rule our group A β-hemolytic streptococci; Monospot; serology	Penicillin if positive for group A streptococci, otherwise supportive care with antipyretics, throat gargles
Laryngotracheo-bronchitis (Croup)	Cold symptoms, rhinorrhea, sore throat, hoarseness, distinctive barking cough	Parainfluenza Influenza virus RSV	*Mycoplasma pneumoniae*	X-ray of neck; antigen detection of respiratory secretions, viral culture of respiratory secretions	Supportive care with close observation for signs of respiratory failure; corticosteroids are controversial
Sinusitis	Cold symptoms, headache, fever, erythema, and tenderness over involved sinuses	Rhinovirus Adenovirus Influenza virus	Bacteria: *Streptococcus pneumoniae Haemophilus influenzae Branhamella catarrhalis* Anaerobes *Staphylococcus aureus*	Transillumination of sinuses. X-ray of sinuses	Supportive measures with decongestants, antipyretics for viral causes. Antibiotics for bacterial causes
Laryngitis	Cold symptoms, hoarseness	Rhinovirus Influenza virus Parainfluenza virus Adenovirus RSV Coxsackie virus	*Chlamydia pneumoniae* Group A streptococcus	Made on clinical basis	Supportive measures

Table 48P-2. Lower Respiratory Viral Infections

Clinical Syndrome	Symptoms	Viral Etiology	Other Pathogens	Diagnosis	Treatment
Bronchitis	Cough, cold symptoms, fever	Influenza virus Adenovirus Rhinovirus Parainfluenza virus	Bacteria: *Streptococcus pneumoniae, Haemophilus influenzae, Branhamella catarrhalis, Bordetella pertussis*	Gram's stain and culture of respiratory secretions, serology; CXR to rule out pneumonia	Symptomatic treatment; antibiotics to cover bacterial pathogens
Bronchiolitis	Cough, cold symptoms, wheezing, tachypnea on physical exam	Respiratory syncytial virus Parainfluenza virus	*Mycoplasma pneumoniae*	CXR, rapid methods of detection of viral antigen in respiratory secretions	Ribavirin; close observation for respiratory failure
Pneumonia	Cough, cold symptoms, fever, sore throat, myalgias, pleuritic chest pain, shortness of breath	Influenza virus Adenovirus Respiratory syncytial virus	Bacteria: *Streptococcus pneumoniae, Haemophilus influenzae, Mycoplasma pneumoniae, Chlamydia pneumoniae*	CXR, Gram's stain, and bacterial culture of respiratory secretions	Amantadine or rimantadine for influenza A, appropriate antibacterial agents; close observation for respiratory failure

573

Outbreaks of Nosocomial Infection

Alan A. Harris, M.D.

I. Definition

Nosocomial infections are those acquired during hospitalization and are neither present nor incubating at the time of admission.

A. Some institutions may use onset of infection more than 48–72 hr following admission as part of their definition. This has flaws in that community-acquired diseases with long incubation periods (e.g. varicella) may begin late in a hospitalization. Alternatively, diseases acquired in the hospital and involving long incubation periods (e.g. posttransfusion hepatitis) may have onset several months following hospital discharge.

B. Endemic events are those which occur with an expected background frequency. Of the common nosocomial infections, urinary tract (40–50%), surgical wound (20–30%), respiratory tract (15–20%), and primary bacteremias (2–5%) all occur endemically.

C. Epidemics represent an increased incidence over the expected background. Endemic diseases may become epidemics. Epidemics may occur at the common sites of infection with unusual organisms or devices. Epidem-

ics of unusual diseases have also occurred in hospitals.

1. A single case of botulism is an epidemic.

2. For epidemiologic investigatory purposes, a single wound infection with group A *Streptococcus* may be considered an epidemic.

D. Gram-positive cocci and gram-negative aerobic rods have been etiologic in 80–90% of nosocomial infections over the past four decades.

1. The future portends infection with non-aeruginosa pseudomonads, multiantibiotic-resistant *Klebsiella* and *Enterobacter* species, *Candida* species and other fungi, *Staphylococcus epidermidis*, and enterococci—both vancomycin susceptible and resistant.

E. Host parameters are important risk factors for acquisition of nosocomial infection, such as diabetes mellitus, invasive procedures, inserted devices, antimicrobial therapy, steroids/immunosuppressive therapy, the extremes of age, and male gender.

F. Transmission of nosocomial pathogens may

occur through any of the traditional routes—contact, water or food vehicles, airborne, or human disseminators.

1. The major route of patient-to-patient spread is through contact with the hands of hospital personnel.
2. Disseminators of *Staph. aureus* and group A β-hemolytic streptococci may cause point or longitudinal outbreaks. Dissemination is usually associated with nasal or pharyngeal carriage but may also occur from vaginal and/or anal colonization.
3. Airborne spread is most commonly associated with usual community pathogens (e.g. influenza, varicella, measles, and tuberculosis). Potable water supplies frequently may contain *Legionella*. Do not survey for the organism unless this is part of quality control or there is evidence of nosocomial occurrence.

II. **Outbreaks of Nosocomial Infection**
   A. Outbreak connotes a higher than expected frequency of occurrence. A single case of postoperative group A streptococcal wound infection warrants investigation; a single case of postoperative *Escherichia coli* urinary tract infection does not. Thresholds for individual organisms or sites of infection will determine the level of epidemiologic investigatory activity.
   B. The investigative approach to outbreaks is similar for community and hospital occurrences.
      1. Establishing the presence of an outbreak is of prime importance. A cluster of an organism rarely causing nosocomial infection, or a usual pathogen with an unusual antimicrobial susceptibility pattern, are frequently the first indicators.
         a. The corollary is that outbreaks with common nosocomial pathogens with usual antimicrobial susceptibility patterns may not be detected early.
      2. The diagnosis must be verified.
      3. A case count should be obtained. Recognize that this preliminary information will be inexact. The case count will depend on the case definition.
         a. The case definition should be developed early and will evolve over time. Initially, it may be purely clinical and/or microbiologic. Over time, antimicrobial susceptibility patterns or testing, phage typing, biotyping, se-

rology, or plasmid analysis may all become part of the definition.
         b. A case definition must be both sensitive and specific. During the early investigation, specificity is extremely important. Too broad a case definition will result in an expanded case count and obscure analysis of the outbreak due to inclusion of noncases.
      4. Data should be organized in terms of time, place, and person. Graphic display may facilitate interpretation. Expected incubation periods, when known, should define the window of transmission. The graphic display may, therefore, assist in determining whether transmission is ongoing.
      5. An estimate should be made of the population at risk.
      6. A hypothesis concerning the source of the problem and the method of spread should be offered. Statistical analysis will require control groups.
      7. The hypothesis should be tested and control measures implemented. Like the case count, these measures will likely change over time as the database is expanded and the analyses are refined.
      8. The goal is to stop the transmission of disease and the occurrence of new cases. It should be readily apparent that diseases with a short incubation period will require action prior to knowledge of all the scientific data or a true case count.

III. **Association of Nosocomial Infections**
   Nosocomial infections have been associated with all of the following pathogens. The known usual routes of acquisition of each organism may suggest the source of the outbreak. This list is not intended to be inclusive. The information does not pertain to the usual sites of nosocomial infection with the usual hospital-acquired pathogens.
   A. Airborne infections spread by the airborne route—measles, varicella, tuberculosis, *Bordetella pertussis*, *Pasteurella pestis*, *Legionella pneumophila*, *L. micdadei*, *Neisseria meningitidis*, *Aspergillus fumigatus*, *Pseudomonas aeruginosa*, and *Pneumocystis carinii*.
   B. Recently identified gastrointestinal pathogens—*Clostridium difficile*, adenovirus 34, rotavirus, Norwalk agent, *Campylobacter jejuni*, and *E. coli* 0157:H7.
   C. Unusual pathogens in renal transplant pa-

tients—*Ureaplasma urealyticum*, JC or BK papovavirus, and *Gardnerella vaginalis*.

D. Unusual pathogens in bone marrow transplant recipients—rotavirus, coxsackie A virus, adenovirus 34, and cytomegalovirus.

E. Old community pathogens which are new hospital pathogens—*Nocardia asteroides* (pneumonia), *A. fumigatus* (pneumonia, skin or sinus), *Rhizopus* or *Mucor* (pneumonia, skin or sinus), *N. meningitidis* (bacteremia, meningitis, pneumonia), *Streptococcus agalactiae* (meningitis), and *Chlamydia psittaci* (pneumonia).

F. New community pathogens which are new nosocomial pathogens—*L. pneumophila* (pneumonia, soft tissue infections), *L. micdadei* (pneumonia), *Staph. aureus* (toxic shock syndrome), *Cl. difficile* (pseudomembranous colitis), *C. jejuni* (diarrhea), and *Mycobacterium chelonei* (sternal osteomyelitis, infected breast implants, and bacteremia).

G. Viral hospital outbreaks caused by common viruses—influenza A, influenza B, respiratory syncytial virus, parainfluenza 3, rhinovirus, hepatitis A, Norwalk agent, rotavirus, rubella, herpes simplex virus, and varicella zoster.

H. Rare viral hospital-acquired infections—rabies (corneal transplantation), Jakob-Creutzfeld (corneal transplantation), ebola virus, lassa fever virus, and marburg virus.

I. Nosocomial parasitic infections—*Strongyloides stercoralis* (transplanted kidney), *Toxacara canis*, *Entamoeba histolytica* (colonoscopy), *Toxoplasma*, *Trichosporon* species, and Norwegian scabies.

J. Outbreaks associated with contaminated fluids or instruments—*Enterobacter agglomerans* (IV fluids), *Candida albicans* (hyperalimentation fluid), *Pseudomonas cepacia* (chlorohexidine, dialysis fluid, and arterial pressure transducers), *P. maltophila* (evacutubes), *Rhizopus* and *Aspergillus* (contaminated plaster dressings and tape), *Achromobacter xylosoxidans* (diagnostic tracer equipment), and group B *Streptococcus* (radioactive tracer).

K. Infection following blood transfusions.
1. Viral infections have included cytomegalovirus, Epstein-Barr virus, hepatitis B, hepatitis C, non-A non-B hepatitis, and Colorado tick fever.
2. Parasitic infections include babesiosis, malaria, toxoplasmosis, trypanosomiasis, and filariasis.
3. Bacterial infections include brucellosis, bartonellosis, gram-negative endotoxemia, and salmonellosis (following platelet transfusions).

Bibliography

Bennett JV, Brachman PS. Hospital Infections. Boston, Little, Brown, 1986.

Haley RW, Culver DH, White JW, et al. The nationwide infection rate: A new need for vital statistics. *Am J Epidemiol* 121:159, 1985.

Harris AA, Levin S, Trenholme GM: Selected aspects of hospital acquired infections in the 1980's. *Amer J Med* 77:3–10, 1984.

Mandell GL, Douglass RG Jr, Bennett JE (eds): Principles and Practices of Infectious Diseases, ed 3. New York, Churchill Livingstone, 1990, p 2176–2257.

Wenzel RP. Handbook of Hospital Acquired Infections. Boca Raton, Florida, CRC Press, 1981.

Chapter 49-B

Nosocomial Urinary Tract Infection

John Segreti, M.D.

I. **Pattern of Infection**

The most common nosocomial infections are urinary tract infections (UTIs), accounting for 40% of all such infections.

A. Most nosocomial UTIs are related to the use of urinary catheters and subsequent bacteriuria.

B. The catheter represents an entryway for microorganisms to the bladder; it also offers bacteria and fungi a sanctuary. The presence of a catheter appears to increase the ability of bacteria to adhere to uroepithelial cells and also adversely affects polymorphonuclear neutrophil function.

C. In the presence of a catheter, the incidence of bacteriuria is 5–10% per day.

II. **Short-Term Catheterization (<30 Days)**

A. Bacteriuria occurs in 10–30% of short-term catheterized patients.

B. Risk factors include duration of catheterization, female gender, diabetes mellitus, and periurethral colonization.

C. Organisms enter the bladder either through the lumen of the catheter or along its external surface.

D. *Escherichia coli* is the most common species

isolated, followed by other Enterobacteriaceae, *Pseudomonas*, *Staphylococcus*, and *Enterococcus*. Yeast may be seen especially during or after antibiotic use.

E. Complications include fever, pyelonephritis, and bacteremia. It is estimated that 2–4% of patients with catheter-associated bacteriuria develop bacteremia.

F. Prevention

1. Avoid urethral catheterization by utilizing suprapubic catheterization, external condom devices, or intermittent clean catheterization whenever possible.

2. Prevention of bacteriuria

a. Remove the catheter as soon as possible.

b. Maintain a closed system to postpone bacteriuria.

c. Prevent bacterial entry by limiting the separation of the catheter-collection tube junction, by avoiding contamination of the collection bag, and possibly by periurethral or urethral cleansing (the last option has not been shown to be effective).

3. Bacterial inhibition or killing after entry

a. Use of an antiseptic in the collection bag

does not seem to affect the incidence of bacteriuria.

    b. Continuous or intermittent irrigation of the catheter with an antibacterial substance is cumbersome and has not been shown to be effective.

    c. Systemic antibiotics postpone but do not prevent bacteriuria. When bacteriuria occurs, it usually involves an organism resistant to the antibiotic used.

G. Treatment

    1. Asymptomatic catheterized patients with bacteriuria usually do not require antibiotics.

    2. Patients with fever and/or signs of bacteremia require systemic antimicrobial therapy effective against aerobic gram-negative bacilli until culture results are available.

III. Long-Term Catheterization (>30 Days)

A. Epidemiology—patients with spinal cord lesions and nursing home residents.

B. Microbiology—*Providentia, Pseudomonas, Proteus* and *Morganella,* in addition to *E. coli, Klebsiella, Enterococcus,* and *Candida.* Up to 90% of patients have more than one bacterial strain.

C. Complications include inadvertent catheter removal, leaking, and obstruction. The material causing obstruction is composed of bacteria, Tamm-Horsfall protein, glycocalyx, and crystals.

D. Prevention of bacteriuria

    1. Condom catheterization for men with urinary incontinence may avoid infection. However, some studies do not confirm this finding.

    2. Intermittent catheterization for patients with spinal cord lesions appears to be safe and effective.

E. Candiduria can usually be ignored and usually clears with removal of the catheter. Specific treatment may be necessary in the presence of symptoms, with persistence after removal of the catheter, and in the presence of upper UTI.

F. Treatment—In general, only symptomatic (febrile) patients require antibiotics.

    1. Upper tract symptoms—Organism-directed antibiotics for 2 weeks. If reinfection occurs, treat each episode separately. Consider ultrasound scan or intravenous pyelogram examination to look for stones or anatomic abnormalities which may require surgical intervention.

    2. Lower tract symptoms—Consider removing the catheter. If infection persists after removal of the catheter, give a short course of organism-specific antibiotics.

    3. Candiduria—Most patients do not need treatment.

        a. If upper tract symptoms or fever are present, consider systemic antifungal therapy and ultrasound or computed tomography scan to look for fungal balls, renal abscess, or perinephric abscess.

        b. If no symptoms are evident but pyuria is present and repeat cultures grow *Candida,* then bladder irrigation with amphotericin may be indicated. Systemic fluconazole may be effective. However, relapse with either treatment is common unless the catheter is removed.

Bibliography

Burke JP, Garibaldi RA, Britt MR, et al. Prevention of catheter-associated urinary tract infections: Efficacy of daily meatal care regimens. *Am J Med* 70:655–658, 1981.

Daifuku R, Stamm WE. Bacterial adherence to bladder uroepithelial cells in catheter-associated urinary tract infection. *New Engl J Med* 314:1208–1213, 1986.

Garibaldi RA, Burke JP, Britt MR, et al. Meatal colonization and catheter-associated bacteriuria. *New Engl J Med* 303:316–318, 1980.

Garibaldi RA, Burke JP, Dickman ML, et al. Factors predisposing to bacteriuria during indwelling urethral catheterization. *New Engl J Med* 291:215–219, 1974.

Harding GKM, Nicolle LE, Ronald AR, et al. How long should catheter-acquired urinary tract infection in women be treated? A randomized controlled study. *Ann Intern Med* 114:713–719, 1991.

Platt R, Polk BF, Murdock B, et al. Mortality associated with nosocomial urinary-tract infection. *New Engl J Med* 307:637–642, 1982.

Platt R, Polk BF, Murdock B, et al. Prevention of catheter-associated urinary tract infection: A cost-benefit analysis. *Infect Control Hosp Epidemiol* 10:60–64, 1989.

Platt R, Polk BF, Murdock B, et al. Risk factors for nosocomial urinary tract infection. *Am J Epidemiol* 124:977–985, 1986.

Stark RP, Maki DG. Bacteriuria in the catheterized patient. What quantitative level of bacteriuria is relevant? *New Engl J Med* 311:560–564, 1984.

Turck M, Stamm W. Nosocomial infection of the urinary tract. *Am J Med* 70:651–654, 1981.

Warren JW, Platt R, Thomas RJ, et al. Antibiotic irrigation and catheter-associated urinary-tract infections. *New Engl J Med* 299:570–573, 1978.

Chapter 49-C

Nosocomial Pneumonia

Gordon M. Trenholme, M.D.

I. Definition
A. *Nosocomial* indicates that the infection is acquired during hospitalization.
 1. It is not incubating or present on admission to the hospital.
 2. An infection which develops after 72 hr of hospitalization.
B. Pneumonia is a lower respiratory tract infection which involves the lung parenchyma.
 1. Bronchitis is a lower respiratory tract infection that involves the bronchi but not the lung parenchyma.
 2. Anatomically, the lower respiratory tract is the portion distal to the larynx.
 3. In normal individuals, the lower respiratory tract has no residual flora.

II. Etiology
A. Common etiologies
 1. Enteric gram-negative rods
  a. *Klebsiella pneumoniae*
  b. *Pseudomonas aeruginosa*
  c. *Escherichia coli*
  d. *Enterobacter* spp.
 2. *Staphylococcus aureus*
B. Uncommon etiologies
 1. Coagulase-negative staphylococci

2. Anaerobes
3. Enterococci
4. *Streptococcus pneumoniae*
5. *Legionella* species are unusual except in the following situations:
 a. Renal or cardiac transplants.
 b. An endemic focus of *Legionella* in the hospital.
6. *Candida albicans*
 a. Disseminated *C. albicans* frequently invades the lung and other major organs.
7. *Aspergillus*
 a. In patients with prolonged neutropenia.
8. Viruses
 a. During an influenza outbreak in the community, transmission between personnel and patients may occur.

III. Pathophysiology
A. Colonization
 1. During hospitalization following any severe illness, receptors for aerobic gram-negative bacilli are unmasked on upper respiratory epithelial cells.
 2. Aerobic gram-negative bacilli attach to these receptors and replicate without an inflammatory response.

B. Aspiration
   1. Organisms from the upper respiratory tract are aspirated into the lower respiratory tract.
   2. Conditions which favor aspiration and interfere with the normal ciliary clearing mechanism of the lower respiratory tract
      a. Intubation
      b. Nasogastric suction
      c. Sedation
   3. In unusual circumstances, microorganisms may be introduced directly into the lung by contaminated ventilatory apparatus.
C. Bronchitis
   1. Organisms in the lower respiratory tract replicate and induce an inflammatory response.
   2. The inflammatory response is associated with mobilization of polymorphonuclear leucocytes in an attempt to limit the infection. If this fails, parenchymal invasion occurs.
D. Pneumonia
   1. Parenchymal invasion of the lung by microorganisms occurs because of a failure of defense mechanisms. These mechanisms may be mechanical, such as endobronchial obstruction, or intrinsic, such as neutropenia.
   2. The inflammatory response results in an area of poor ventilation with continued perfusion and may result in hypoxemia and tachypnea.
   3. The inflammatory response caused by microorganisms results in the release of cytokines and a systemic response with fever and tachycardia.
   4. If the pneumonia is due to a particularly virulent organism or if the host is unable to localize the infection to the lung, bacteremia may occur.
E. Hematogenous pneumonia
   1. Rarely during a bacteremia associated with an infection at a nonpulmonary site, the lung may be seeded and pneumonia may develop. More frequently, bacteremia is associated with adult respiratory distress syndrome (ARDS) and pulmonary infiltrates with hypoxemia.

IV. **Diagnosis**
A. Predisposing historical factors for a nosocomial pneumonia include:
   1. Thoracic or abdominal surgery.
   2. Surgery over 4 hr duration.
   3. Intubation.
   4. Obesity.
   5. Neutropenia.
   6. Hospitalization in an intensive care unit.
B. Clinical signs may include fever, chills, purulent sputum, tachypnea, cyanosis, nasal flaring, mental confusion, pleuritic chest pain, cough, and shallow respirations.
C. Physical findings include tachypnea, tachycardia, and cyanosis.
   1. Pulmonary auscultation generally reveals rales but may also show consolidation.
   2. Pleural effusion may be present.
   3. A pleural friction rub is uncommon and should suggest a pulmonary infarct.
D. Diagnostic tests
   1. Sputum Gram stain
      a. Must consist of material from the lower respiratory tract.
      b. Should show a large number of white blood cells, a small number of epithelial cells, and microorganisms.
      c. Purulent sputum without microorganisms suggests *Legionella*.
   2. Sputum culture
      a. Very difficult to avoid contamination with upper respiratory flora.
      b. Isolation of *C. albicans* from sputum usually reflects colonization, not infection.
   3. Bronchoscopy with bronchoalveolar lavage involving quantitative cultures may help distinguish pathogens from contaminants.
   4. Chest x-ray should show new or increasing pulmonary infiltrates.
      a. Infiltrates are dependent upon obstruction and/or an inflammatory response and thus may be minimal in a neutropenic patient.
   5. Blood cultures should be obtained, as 10% of patients are bacteremic.
   6. If a pleural effusion is present, thoracentesis should be done, as 5–10% of patients may have an empyema.
   7. Needle aspiration of the lung may be done to establish a definite diagnosis, but this procedure is associated with a high incidence of pneumothorax and bleeding.
   8. Open lung biopsy will determine the etiology in 80% of patients, but it is reserved for patients in whom other procedures

have not established a diagnosis and who are not responding to empiric therapy.

9. Serologic tests are useful for *Legionella* and influenza.

V. Differential Diagnosis

A. Septic pulmonary emboli may be seen with septic thrombophlebitis or nosocomial right-sided endocarditis.

B. Pulmonary infarction.

C. ARDS is difficult to distinguish from pneumonia, particularly since pneumonia may cause ARDS and ARDS may be complicated by pneumonia.

1. ARDS is accompanied by fever and pulmonary infiltrates but usually does not include purulent sputum.

D. Cytotoxic lung reaction to medications such as bleomycin.

VI. Treatment

A. Broad-spectrum antibiotics are usually required because of the difficulty in identifying a pathogen from sputum cultures.

1. Third-generation cephalosporins, quinolones, and aminoglycosides have been used successfully, either alone or in combination.

2. If a pathogen is identified, directed therapy may be given.

3. If methicillin-resistant S. aureus (MRSA) are isolated, then vancomycin is the agent of choice.

4. *Legionella* should be treated with erythromycin. Quinolones may be an alternative.

B. Supportive measures such as oxygen and mechanical ventilation may be necessary.

C. Therapy is usually continued for at least 2 weeks.

1. Recent studies indicate that after a favorable clinical response, a therapeutic course may be completed with an oral quinolone if the pathogen is susceptible.

VII. Patient Monitoring

A. A favorable therapeutic response is indicated by a decrease in fever, improved oxygenation, and clearing white blood cells from the sputum.

B. If the patient is intubated, it may be difficult to clear the pathogen from the sputum.

C. Repeat sputum cultures during therapy will usually indicate the appearance of resistant organisms. If the patient is improving, these organisms should not prompt a change in therapy.

D. If aminoglycosides are used, careful attention to their levels is necessary. One study indicated that a gentamicin level of at least 8 μg/ml was necessary for a favorable response.

VIII. Prevention

A. Prophylactic parenteral antibiotics do not prevent nosocomial pneumonia.

B. In intubated patients, attempts to decrease pharyngeal colonization by oral administration of nonabsorbable antibiotics have met with moderate success in preventing pneumonia.

IX. Prognosis

A. Nosocomial pneumonia is a serious illness. It is the leading infectious cause of death in hospitalized patients.

B. Parenchymal destruction of lung tissue with residual damage after recovery is common.

Bibliography

Garibaldi RA, Britt MR, Coleman ML, et al. Risk factors for post-operative pneumonia. *Am J Med* 70:677–680, 1981.

Gross PA, Neu HC, Aswapokee P, et al. Deaths from nosocomial infections: Experience in a university hospital and a community hospital. *Am J Med* 68:219–223, 1980.

Johanson WG Jr, Pierce AK, Sanford JP, et al. Nosocomial respiratory infections with gram-negative bacilli. *Ann Intern Med* 77:701–706, 1972.

Pennington JE. nosocomial respiratory infection, in Mandell GL, Douglas RG Jr, Bennett JE (eds): *Principles and Practices of Infectious Diseases*, ed 3. Churchill Livingston, Inc., 1990, New York, pp 2199–2204.

Pugin J, Auckenthaler R, Lew DP, et al. Oropharyngeal decontamination decreases incidence of ventilator-associated pneumonia: A randomized, placebo-controlled, double-blind clinical trial. *JAMA* 265:2704–2710, 1991.

Approach to the Patient with Nosocomial Diarrhea

Larry J. Goodman, M.D.

I. **Problem**

The development of watery or purulent stools or the isolation of an enteric pathogen during hospitalization.

II. **Differential Diagnosis**

The differential diagnosis of nosocomial diarrhea includes both infectious and noninfectious processes. *Clostridium difficile* is the most common identified infectious pathogen in this setting, although almost any of the organisms described previously (see Chapter 48) may be the causative agent. Diarrhea is also a common side effect of many medications.

A. Outbreak versus Pseudo-outbreak: A pseudo-outbreak is suggested by the identification of an uncommonly large number of isolates of a single pathogen, usually from geographically separate patients without symptoms. These pseudo-outbreaks are due to contamination at some point in the acquisition and processing of a specimen and account for 10–15% of all nosocomial outbreaks.

B. Sources of nosocomial enteric pathogens
1. Spread from an inadequately isolated, infected patient.
2. An infected health care worker.

3. Food may be the source of a nosocomial outbreak involving geographically separate patients.
4. Other vehicles—human milk, carmine used as a stool marker, pancreatin, platelets and suction apparatus have all been vehicles for nosocomial *Salmonella* infections.
5. Patient's flora—*C. difficile* may be present on admission or acquired in the hospital. Medications may modify the stool milieu, increasing *C. difficile* growth and toxin production.

III. **Focus of History and Physical**

A. New medications (i.e., stool softeners).
B. Risk factors for *C. difficile* diarrhea include:
1. Increased age.
2. More severe underlying disease.
3. Antibiotics (particularly penicillins and cephalosporins).
4. Enemas.
5. Gastrointestinal stimulants.
6. Stool softeners.
C. Abdominal examination—signs of abdominal perforation or toxic megacolon.

IV. **Diagnostic Approach**

The diagnostic approach for nosocomial diarrhea

is similar to that for community-acquired diarrheal disease, with the following exceptions:

A. The patient should be placed on enteric isolation while the workup is in progress.

B. Review new medications and preparations given for procedures.

C. For an immunocompetent host developing diarrhea in the hospital, C. *difficile* should be the primary diagnostic consideration. Initial studies should, therefore, be aimed at identifying this pathogen. If possible, discontinue antimicrobial therapy, hydrate, and observe. If antibiotics are necessary, and C. *difficile* infection is proven or highly likely initiate the specific treatment (metronidazole 500 mg orally three times a day or vancomycin 125 mg orally four times daily).

Bibliography

Bartlett JG. Antibiotic-associated pseudomembranous colitis. *Rev Infect Dis* 1:530–539, 1979.

Goodman LJ, Harris AA. Nosocomial gastrointestinal infections. *J Nosocom Infect* 2:2–6, 1985.

Johnson S, Hoomman SR, Bettin KM, et al: Treatment of asymptomatic *Clostridium difficile* (fetal excretus) with vancomycin or metronidazole. *Ann Intern Med* 117:297–302, 1992.

Kunz LJ, Ouchterlony OTG. Salmonellosis originating in a hospital. *N Engl J Med* 253:761–763, 1955.

McFarland LV, Surawicz CM, Stamm WE. Risk factors for *Clostridium difficile* carriage and C. *difficile*—associated diarrhea in a cohort of hospitalized patients. *J Infect Dis* 162:678–784, 1990.

Weinstein RA, Stamm WE. Pseudoepidemics in hospitals. *Lancet* 2:862–864, 1977.

CHAPTER 49-E

Postprocedural Wound Infections

Alan A. Harris, M.D.

I. **Background**

Infections at injection sites, as well as at IV catheter sites, while puncture rather than incisional, generate many of the same concerns as do surgical incisions. This discussion pertains to superficial infections related to the wound and surrounding soft tissues, not those occurring deep in the operative site.

A. These infections comprise 20–30% of all nosocomial infections.

1. In addition to potential mortality, diagnostic/therapeutic intervention, with incision and drainage and/or antimicrobial therapy, result on average in a 5- to 7-day prolongation of the hospital stay. These infections are, therefore, the most costly of all nosocomial infections.

2. The wound classification system used for several decades is currently undergoing revision.

   a. The old system classified the likelihood of wound infection based on whether the wound was clean, clean contaminated, contaminated, or dirty.

   b. The newer system assigns points based on an anesthesiology risk score above 3, duration of the procedure above the 75th percentile, and whether the wound is contaminated or dirty. The maximum wound risk score is, therefore, 3.

   c. Preliminary validation of the new categorization indicates that it is more predictive of the likelihood of wound infection, as well as of nosocomial infection at other sites.

II. **Differential Diagnosis**

The diagnosis of wound infection seems straightforward. Pus at the incision site is the single most reliable criterion. Cardinal signs of inflammation are suggestive but not pathognomonic. The differential diagnosis includes:

A. Allergy to soap, antiseptic, or dressing.

B. Soft tissue bleeding.

C. Allergic or toxic reaction to suture material.

D. Superficial dermatophytic infection.

III. **History and Physical Examination**

The focus of the history and physical examination should be on the patient, the operative personnel, and, in the presence of trauma or outbreaks, the environment.

A. Wound infections usually occur at the time of surgery.

B. In the presence of trauma or a perforated viscus, infection is likely already incubating or evident.

C. Infections following clean procedures are usually associated with β-hemolytic streptococci or *Staphylococcus aureus*. *Staph. epidermidis* has evolved from a usual contaminant to a major cause of prosthetic device infections. Recently this organism has increased in virulence and can be an etiology of postoperative wound infections.

D. Infections following procedures adjacent to or compromising mucosal surfaces mandate consideration of the normal flora at these sites as potential etiologic agents. As with trauma or contaminated procedures, these infections are frequently polymicrobial.

E. Rarely, infection at another site (e.g., the vascular line or urinary tract) may result in bacteremic seeding of a fresh wound.

F. Relative to environmental exposures:
   1. *Staph. aureus* and/or β-hemolytic steptococci (i.e. groups A, B, and C) are usually spread from person to person.
      a. Infection in a single patient is usually due to the patient's organism other than one acquired in hospital.
      b. Clusters should be considered and sought.
      c. Personnel with staphylococcal or streptococcal infections and/or weeping dermatitis should not be involved in hands-on patient care or the handling of devices inserted in patients.
   2. Trauma and soil exposures should suggest non–group A β-hemolytic streptococci, gram-negative aerobes, anaerobes with special concern for *Clostridium* and *Bacteroides*, and atypical mycobacteria.
   3. Trauma associated with water exposure should heighten one's concern for *Aeromonas hydrophila*, noncholera vibrios, and atypical mycobacteria.

G. Time of onset of infection following surgery is suggestive of the etiologic agent.
   1. When onset occurs within 48 hr of a clean procedure, group A β-hemolytic streptococci or clostridia should be considered etiologic until proven otherwise. The secretions in either of these infections are usually serous rather than purulent. Clostridia are rare if the surgery is not related to the abdomen or a juxtaposed mucous membrane.

2. Onset of *Staph. aureus* postoperative wound infections usually occurs at 3 to 7 days and gram-negative rods or fungi at 5 to 10 days. However, there is overlap between the time of onset of staphylococcal and gram-negative aerobic infections.
   3. In the presence of trauma/contamination, the inoculum size of any organism present may be quite large. The time of onset of infection is not predictive of the pathogen.

H. In outbreaks, the suspected source may also suggest a likely pathogen.
   1. When personnel are colonized and shedding, the usual organisms have been *Staph. aureus* and either group A or group B β-hemolytic streptococci. There has been a recent outbreak due to *Rhodococcus*.
      a. A single case of group A streptococcal infection warrants investigation to ensure that no hospital personnel are transmitting the organism asymptomatically or that a cluster was not previously undetected.
   2. The hands of all personnel should be considered weapons. While possibly due to any organism, outbreaks are usually associated with *Staph. aureus* or gram-negative aerobic bacilli.
   3. *Staph. aureus*, β-hemolytic streptococci, and gram-negative rods have colonized solutions applied topically or used for injection. Outbreaks associated with atypical mycobacteria and *Legionella* species should also be considered in these settings.
      a. Injections from multidose vials should be avoided.
      b. The *Legionella* outbreak was unique in that infection at the operative site was associated with postoperative use of potable water containing the organism and was used to clean the skin in a routine fashion.
   4. Occlusive pressure dressings have caused infection due to *Rhizopus* or *Mucor*. In the orthopedic setting, these dressings should not be considered sterile.

IV. **Diagnostic Approach**
A. An initial guess at the etiologic agent should be based on the prehospitalization epidemiologic circumstances, the operative procedure, and the time of onset of the infection.
B. A Gram stain and culture should be obtained.
   1. A negative Gram stain does not exclude infection.

   a. Remember to culture for anaerobes when the circumstances are correct.

2. Initial antibiotic selection should be based on the Gram stain, the likely pathogens, known hospital flora and susceptibility patterns, and in-hospital antibiotics (if any) administered previously to the patient.

3. Eradication of infections around foreign materials will likely require their removal (e.g., sutures or vascular lines).

4. Prevention is better than diagnosis and cure. When possible, it is preferable to eradicate infections at other sites prior to surgery and perform skin preparations at an appropriate time prior to the procedure. Prophylactic antibiotics, when indicated, should be given 30–60 min prior to surgery.

Bibliography

Altemeier WA, Burke JF, Pluitt BA Jr, et al. *Manual on Control of Infection in Surgical Patients.* Philadelphia, JB Lippincott, 1976, pp 29–30.

Condon RE, Haley RW, Lee JT Jr, et al. Does infection control control infections? *Arch Surg* 123:250–256, 1988.

Culbertson WR, Altemeier WA, Gonzalez LL, et al. Studies on the epidemiology of postoperative infection of clean operative wounds. *Ann Surg* 154:599–610, 1961.

Kaiser AB. Postoperative infections and antimicrobial prophylaxis, in Mandell GL, Douglas RG Jr, Bennett JE (eds): *Principles and Practice of Infectious Diseases*, ed 3. Churchill Livingstone, New York, 1990, pp 2245–2257.

Olson M, O'Connor M, Schwartz ML. Surgical wound infections: A 5-year prospective study of 20,193 wounds at the Minneapolis VA Medical Center. *Ann Surg* 199:253–259, 1984.

Schaffner W, Lefkowitz LB, Goodman JS. Hospital outbreak of infections with group A streptococci traced to an asymptomatic anal carrier. *N Engl J Med* 280:1224–1225, 1969.

CHAPTER 49-F

Device-Related Bacteremia

Jeffrey A. Nelson, M.D.

I. Problem

Recent advances in the therapy of many chronic illnesses have created a population of patients who frequently benefit from the use of long-term vascular access. Additionally, technologic strides in the management and monitoring of many acute disease states have created a second group of patients who require transient vascular access. These two patient populations contribute to more than 25,000 vascular access–related bacteremias per year. This translates into prolonged hospital stays, a huge economic burden, and significant morbidity and mortality.

II. Differential Diagnosis

Numerous portals of entry are possible when these access devices are used.

A. Monitoring lines such as arterial and Swan-Ganz catheters have numerous side ports, require frequent flushing, and may (in the case of Swan-Ganz catheters) be used for a variety of infusions. All of these manipulations are potential sources of contamination.

B. Peripheral and central access lines may also be the recipients of pathogens introduced by contaminated fluid, nonsterile spiking of containers, and junctional contamination.

C. Monitoring and access lines also present a risk, as they breach skin integrity and afford access to the bloodstream. Therefore, the skin preparation, the size of the catheter, the material it is made of, the method of insertion (percutaneous or cutdown), the location (groin versus other site), the length of use, and the dressing materials all have variable degrees of impact on the predisposition to catheter infection, both local and systemic.

III. Historical and Physical Clues

A. Several historical hints may be helpful.

1. *Serratia*, *Pseudomonas cepacia*, and *Citrobacter* species have been associated with infusate contamination.

2. Lipid supplementation has been associated with *Malassezia furfur* infections.

3. Parenteral nutrition is a risk factor for *Candida* bacteremia.

4. A clustering of patients with an unusual organism may suggest infusate contamination.

5. Sepsis refractory to broad-spectrum ther-

apy should make one consider the possibility of a catheter-related infection.

B. Certain physical exam findings may suggest a line source.
   1. Local phlebitis at a current or a recent line site.
   2. Unilateral edema in an extremity with a concurrent line or previous access site.
   3. The presence of pulmonary emboli.
   4. Fungal endophthalmitis.

IV. Diagnostic Approach

When evaluating a patient for possible line-related infection, one should consider the following:

A. If no other obvious focus of infection can be found, a line-related infection must be considered. Staphylococcal organisms are the most frequent pathogens, but gram-negative organisms including *Pseudomonas aeruginosa* may also be seen. Initial therapy usually includes vancomycin and an antipseudomonal agent.

B. Tunnel infection in long-term indwelling catheters (e.g., Hickman) reduces the likelihood of cure without catheter removal.

C. The presence of a documented thrombus at the end of the catheter reduces the likelihood of a medical cure.

D. Certain bloodstream isolates are more refractory to cure without removal (*Bacillus* and *Candida* species). Most fungal line infections dictate removal of the catheter.

E. If the isolate can be cleared from the bloodstream with antimicrobials, it may be reasonable to treat with an appropriate antibiotic for 2 weeks and attempt a medical cure. Careful follow-up and repeat blood cultures are needed.

F. In essential long-term lines where the source of bacteremia is questionable, an indium or gallium scan may be helpful to document the catheter as a source. Sensitivity of these scans for catheter infection is often low, but positive findings or the identification of another occult process can occasionally be useful.

G. Studies such as computed tomography and ultrasound can aid in documenting a thrombus.

H. Obtaining simultaneous quantitative cultures from the central line and the periphery has been useful at some institutions.

I. If the catheter is removed, some microbiology laboratories offer quantitative tip cultures. Problems with appropriate collection, transport, and evaluation have limited this approach to documenting the catheter as a source of bacteremia.

Bibliography

Maki DG. Pathogenesis, prevention, and management of infections due to intravascular devices used for infusion therapy. In: Bisno AL, Waldvogel FA, eds. *Infectious Associated With Indwelling Medical Devices.* Washington, DC, American Society of Microbiology, 1984, pp 161–177.

Maki DG, Ringer M. Risk factors for infusion-related phlebitis with small peripheral venous catheters. A randomized controlled trial. *Ann Intern Med* 114:845–854, 1991.

Maki DG, Ringer M, Alvarado CJ. Prospective randomized trial at povidone-iodine, alcohol, and chlorhexidine for prevention of infection associated with central venous and arterial catheters. *Lancet* 338:339–343, 1991.

Infection Associated with Diabetes, the Elderly, Malnutrition and Alcohol Use

John Segreti, M.D.

Diabetes

I. The Problem

A. It is widely believed that patients with diabetes mellitus have an increased susceptibility to bacterial and fungal infections, and that infections in diabetics tend to be more severe and more difficult to control.

1. Foot infections are a common and serious problem in patients with diabetes.
2. Bacteriuria appears to be more common in diabetic women, and complications such as pyelonephritis, renal papillary necrosis, and perinephric abscess seem to occur more often.
3. Rare infections such as rhinocerebral mucormycosis, emphysematous cholecystitis, and invasive otitis externa occur almost exclusively in diabetics.

B. Patients with poorly controlled diabetes mellitus have a number of abnormalities of polymorphonuclear leukocyte (PMN) function which are reversible with insulin treatment.

1. In general, these defects alone do not appear to predispose diabetics to infection.

2. When coupled with neuropathy and arterial vascular disease, in which the delivery of blood flow and oxygen to the tissue is reduced and the arrival of PMNs is delayed, the growth of organisms may be promoted and the oxygen-dependent bactericidal function of PMNs reduced.

3. Alterations in the composition of resident flora are seen in diabetics, but the reasons for these changes are unknown. Diabetics have a higher prevalence of oropharyngeal colonization by gram-negative bacilli and an increased rate of carriage of *Candida*.

C. The neurologic, vascular, and metabolic complications of diabetes predispose patients to infection.

1. Neurogenic bladder causes stasis and urinary retention that often requires catheterization.
2. Sensory neuropathies lead to wounds which may be ignored.
3. Ischemia and gangrene predispose patients to extensive infections of the extremities.
4. Altered states of consciousness associated

with diabetic ketoacidosis or hypoglycemia may predispose to aspiration pneumonia and/or lung abscess.

II. **Urinary Tract Infections**

A. Adult diabetic women are two to four times
more likely to have bacteriuria than matched
nondiabetic controls.

B. There appears to be no difference between
diabetic and nondiabetic patients in the
pathogenesis of urinary tract infection.

C. Complications of urinary tract infections appear to be more common in diabetics, including renal papillary necrosis, perinephric abscess, and emphysematous pyelonephritis.

D. Emphysematous pyelonephritis is a necrotizing infection often caused by a facultative
gram-negative bacillus such as *Escherichia coli*
or other Enterobacteriaceae.

E. Factors believed to contribute to the increased prevalence of urinary tract infection
and its complications include diabetic neuropathy leading to neurogenic bladder, increased frequency of catheterization and instrumentation, diabetic microangiopathy,
poor glucose control, recurrent bouts of
vaginitis, and empiric PMN function in the
presence of high concentrations of urinary
glucose.

III. **Pneumonia**

A. Patients with altered consciousness due to
either ketoacidosis or hypoglycemia are more
prone to aspiration.

B. Diabetics are more likely to have oropharyngeal colonization with gram-negative bacilli;
therefore, gram-negative bacillary pneumonias appear more commonly.

C. Pneumococcal and *Haemophilus influenzae*
pneumonias do not occur more frequently in
diabetic patients.

IV. **Skin and Soft Tissue Infections**

Diabetics appear to be predisposed to necrotizing infections, particularly of the lower extremities.

A. Necrotizing fasciitis is a rare, rapidly progressive infection involving primarily subcutaneous tissue, particularly the superficial and
deep fascia.

1. This infection is caused by either *Streptococcus pyogenes* or a mixture of facultative
and anaerobic bacteria.

2. The portal of microbial entry in the diabetic is usually at the site of minor trauma
or an ischemic or neuropathic foot ulcer.

3. The inflammatory process progresses

rapidly, with sequential skin color changes
from red to purple to patches of blue/gray.

4. Subcutaneous gas is often present and the
patient appears toxic, with temperature
elevation frm 102°F to 105°F.

5. Prompt diagnosis is essential, as is empiric
antibiotic therapy and surgery.

B. Synergistic necrotizing cellulitis is a more
severe and life-threatening disease than fasciitis alone.

1. This infection occurs mainly in the lower
extremities and perineum at sites of subcutaneous infection.

2. There is often involvement of the skin and
muscle, as well as subcutaneous tissue and
fascia.

3. Cultures usually show evidence of polymicrobial infection with anaerobic streptococci, *Bacteroides* species, and facultative
gram-negative bacilli.

C. Gas gangrene or myonecrosis is a rapidly
progressive, life-threatening toxemic infection of skeletal muscle due primarily to
Clostridium perfringens.

1. Gas is produced when a muscle injury is
contaminated with spores of this bacterium.

2. The usual incubation period is 2–3 days
but may be as short as 6 hr.

3. Typically, the onset is very acute, with pain
as the earliest symptom. Patients are often
febrile, although hyperthermia may occur. Shock and jaundice may be present,
and *C. perfringens* bacteremia occurs in
about 15% of patients.

4. Treatment consists of emergency surgical
debridement and antibiotic therapy.

D. Invasive external otitis is seen almost exclusively in elderly diabetic patients.

1. Microangiopathy and vascular insufficiency are believed to predispose patients
to this infection.

2. Typically there is severe, persistent pain
and tenderness around the ear and mas-
toid, pus draining from the external auditory canal, and no fever or leukocytosis.

3. Life-threatening disease may result from
spread of infection to the sigmoid sinus,
jugular bulb, base of the skull, meninges,
and brain.

4. *Pseudomonas aeruginosa* is the most common bacterium; however, *Aspergillus, Staphylococcus,* and *Candida* have occasionally
been isolated.

E. Rhinocerebral mucormycosis is an infection

seen almost exclusively in diabetics with ketoacidosis.

1. Infection may involve many different molds
commonly found in the environment.
2. Spores are inhaled via the respiratory tract
and are deposited as hyphae in the nasal
turbinates.
3. In the presence of acidosis, fungal growth
is promoted.
4. Patients with invasive mucormycosis typically present with sudden onset of perior-
bital or perinasal pain, often with conjunctival swelling, fever, and cellulitis.
5. Occasionally there is loss of extraocular
muscle function and proptosis.
6. Complications include cerebral abscess,
cavernous sinus thrombosis, internal carotid artery thrombosis, and death.
7. Aggressive therapy with correction of
metabolic abnormalities, amphotericin B,
and surgical debridement are necessary.
Despite this therapy, mortality remains
high.

V. Tuberculosis

A. Currently there is no evidence that tuberculosis occurs more frequently in diabetics.
B. However, it is suggested that tuberculosis in
diabetics is more likely to be atypical.

VI. Emphysematous Cholecystitis

Emphysematous chyolecystitis is a rare infection
characterized by gas in or around the gallbladder.

A. Diabetes is present in over one-third of reported cases.
B. Infection is usually polymicrobial, with
Clostridium species, Enterobacteriaceae, and
microaerophilic and aerophilic streptococci
frequently isolated from cultures.
C. Treatment consists of cholecystectomy and
broad-spectrum antibiotics.

VII. Diabetic Foot Infections

A. Foot infections are extremely common and
are a serious problem in diabetics.
B. The major factors predisposing to infection
are ischemia and neuropathy.
C. Foot infections usually begin in the toenail
bed, beneath the plantar callouses, or in ulcers.
D. Once established, these infections may
spread to contiguous areas of bone and joint.
E. Neuropathy due to diabetes probably predisposes to many of these infections.
1. Damage to sensory nerves decreases the
ability to recognize trauma.

2. Autonomic neuropathy results in decreased sweating and dry skin, which is
more easily traumatized, colonized, and
invaded by skin flora.
3. The most common complication of diabetic neuropathy is the formation of ulcers. These occur most often over weight-
bearing areas of the foot. These lesions
may go unnoticed for an extended period
of time because of the lack of symptoms.
F. Ischemia is second to neuropathy in predisposing to infection.
1. The ischemic foot is usually dry, scaly, and
cool.
2. It may show small, dry, atrophic ulcers
with skin necrosis.
G. These infections are often polymicrobial, involving staphylococci, streptococci, facultative gram-negative bacilli, and anaerobes.
1. Unfortunately, superficial swabs of these
ulcers often fail to give accurate information about the causative agents.
2. Deep cultures obtained at the time of
debridement are more likely to result in
an accurate diagnosis.
H. Osteomyelitis is often present beneath these
ulcers, and most patients with diabetic foot
ulcers should be treated empirically as having osteomyelitis.
I. Unfortunately, radiographic and nuclide
studies are often not very helpful in distinguishing soft tissue infection from bone infection. White cell–labeled indium scans may
be more effective in distinguishing osteomyelitis from soft tissue infection.
J. Bone biopsy for microscopic and microbiologic diagnosis should be considered.
K. Therapy usually requires antibiotics given in
combination with surgical incision and drainage.
1. Debridement should be extensive enough
to excise all gangrenous and infected tissue.
2. It is important that the vascular compromise be corrected, if possible, to improve
the chances of healing.

The Elderly

I. The Problem

A. It appears that the elderly have an increased
susceptibility to infections.

1. It has been shown that T-cell function is impaired in some older individuals.
   a. With age, the capacity to induce lymphocyte deterioration declines.
   b. In addition, anergy, or the inability to respond to delayed skin reactions, is more prevalent in the aged than in younger individuals. This situation appears to be associated with changes in T-cell function.
   c. The number of circulating T cells is normal, but the number of T suppressor cells is reduced. There is also evidence that interleukin-2 is decreased.
   d. In addition, the elderly are less likely to respond to new antigens when immunized. B cells from older patients fail to respond with specific antibody production in vitro when exposed to foreign antigen. This may be due to T-cell changes, as well as to B-cell defects.
   e. Neither complement function nor polymorphonuclear neutrophil function appears to be altered with age.
2. Therefore, it is unlikely that alteration of immune mechanisms plays a critical role in increasing the susceptibility of the elderly to infection.
3. The elderly tend to have other underlying diseases which may affect the ability to resist infections, such as diabetes mellitus and atherosclerosis, as well as malignant diseases.
4. Elderly patients are more likely to be placed in high-risk environments such as hospitals and nursing homes where invasive procedures may need to be done, such as endotracheal intubation, urinary catheterization, and IV lines, which also predispose to infection.
   a. When cerebrovascular accidents occur, patients may become bedridden, leading to the development of pressure sores.
   b. These patients are also more likely to aspirate, resulting in pneumonia.
B. The elderly respond differently to infection.
   1. Elderly patients are less likely to present with fever or leukocytosis. This may instead present with hypothermia, confusion, altered consciousness, or inability to maintain adequate oral intake.
   2. Therefore, it is imperative that infection be considered in elderly patients who present with these symptoms.

II. **Common Infections**
Infections which are seen more frequently in the elderly include:
A. Infective endocarditis: This is probably related to the increased incidence of calcification of heart valves, especially the aortic valve, as well as a higher incidence of bacteremia.
B. Pulmonary tuberculosis: This is more likely to reactivate in the elderly. The elderly are also at a higher risk of developing a primary infection. This is likely related to the alteration of T-cell function in the elderly.
C. The elderly are more likely to be colonized in the oropharynx with gram-negative bacilli. Therefore, when pneumonia does occur, gram-negative bacilli need to be considered even in community-acquired pneumonias.
D. In the elderly, bacteriuria occurs more often in both men and women.
   1. In men, this is most likely related to the incidence of prostatic hypertrophy and urinary obstruction.
   2. Host defense mechanisms, including antiadherent mechanisms, decline with age.
E. Herpes zoster infection is much more common in the elderly, with a peak incidence between 50 and 70 years of age. Infection is caused by spontaneous reactivation of latent virus in the dorsal root ganglion.

Malnutrition and Alcohol Use

I. **The Problem**
A. Malnutrition results primarily in defects in T-cell function, leading to increased susceptibility to intracellular pathogens such as *Mycobacterium tuberculosis*.
B. Alcohol use appears to be associated with an increased risk of infection.
   1. Granulocytopenia due to direct bone marrow suppression can result from overwhelming alcohol use.
   2. Prolonged excessive alcohol ingestion may also cause nutritional deficiencies of folic acid and vitamin B_{12}, resulting in the arrest of megaloblastic granulocyte maturation.
   3. There is also evidence that PMN function is impaired in the presence of ethanol.
   4. If cirrhosis complicates alcohol use, hypersplenism and portal hypertension may result.

II. Common Infections

A. Common bacteria associated with excessive alcohol use include *Streptococcus pneumoniae* and aerobic gram-negative bacilli.

B. Lower respiratory infections appear to be more common in alcohol abusers.

1. This pattern is most likely related to the change in mental status associated with alcohol use and possibly also to the occurrence of seizures seen with alcohol withdrawal.

2. Patients who abuse alcohol are more likely to be colonized in the oropharynx with aerobic gram-negative bacilli.

C. *Strep. pneumoniae* is unique in its ability to cause fulminant disease in the alcoholic patient.

1. It is unclear which aspects of the host response are altered in the alcoholic patient to explain the increased incidence of pneumococcal illness.

2. Given the importance of splenic function in preventing pneumococcal infection, it appears reasonable to conclude that altered splenic function plays a role.

3. Patients with cirrhosis are more prone to spontaneous bacterial peritonitis as well as bacteremia, probably due to shunting of blood away from the liver through portal systemic collaterals or to impaired intracellular killing of bacteria by hepatic Kupffer cells.

D. Patients with cirrhosis, regardless of the etiology, are also more likely to be infected with unusual organisms such as *Aeromonas hydrophila, Pasteurella multocida, Yersinia enterocolitica,* and *Vibrio vulnificus.*

1. This may be due to the relative iron overload seen in cirrhotic patients, which may be a virulence factor for these organisms.

2. *V. vulnificus* and *V. alginolyticus* infections are usually associated with salt water. These organisms may cause skin and soft tissue infections in cirrhotic patients receiving trauma in saltwater environments, and may also cause gastroenteritis and bacteremia after ingestion of raw oysters. Therefore, patients with cirrhosis should be advised to avoid trauma in saltwater areas and to avoid ingestion of raw seafood.

Bibliography

Bagdade JD, Segreti J. The infectious emergencies of diabetes. *Endocrinologist* 1:155–162, 1991.

Creditor MC. Hazards of hospitalization of the elderly. *Ann Intern Med* 118:219–223, 1993.

Newman LG, Waller J, Palestro CJ, et al. Unsuspected osteomyelitis in diabetic foot ulcers—diagnosis and monitoring with indium III oxyquinolone leukocyte scanning. *JAMA* 266:1246–1251, 1991.

Saltzman RL, Peterson PK. Immunodeficiency of the elderly. *Rev Infect Dis* 9:1127–1139, 1987.

Saviteer SM, Samsa GP, Rutala WA. Nosocomial infections in the elderly: Increased risk per hospital day. *Am J Med* 84:661–666, 1988.

Young CL, MacGregor RR. Alcohol and host defenses: Infectious consequences. *Infections in Medicine,* p 163–175, September 1989.

Infections in Patients Immunosuppressed Due to Neutropenia or Cytotoxic Chemotherapy

Constance A. Benson, M.D.

Infections in Neutropenic Patients

I. Risk of Infection

A. The incidence of infection appears to be directly related to the absolute neutrophil count (ANC) and the duration of neutropenia.

B. The risk of any infection increases when the ANC declines below 1,000 cells/mm^3; there is an increased risk of life-threatening infection when the ANC is <500 cells/mm^3; the risk of rapidly fatal bacteremia due to gram-negative bacilli markedly increases when the ANC is <100 cells/mm^3.

II. Differential Diagnosis

A. Frequency*

Documented Infection	Percent
Single—gram-negative bacteremia	13–15
Single—gram-positive bacteremia	10–15
Viral/fungal infection	5–10
Polymicrobial bacteremia	3

*Adapted from Meunier, F. (ref.)

B. Common sites of infection*

Site	Percent
Oropharynx	25
Respiratory tract	25
Skin, soft tisue, indwelling catheters	15
Perineal/Perirectal	10
Urinary tract	~–10
Gastrointestinal tract	5

*Adapted from Meunier, F. (ref.)

C. Source and specific pathogens

Infection	Common Pathogens
Pneumonia	*Pseudomonas aeruginosa, Klebsiella* spp., *Escherichia coli, Enterobacter* spp., *Staphylococcus aureus, Aspergillus* spp., *Mucor* spp.
Anorectal lesions	*P. aeruginosa, E. coli,* enteric anaerobes
Pharyngitis	Mixed oral flora, gram-negative bacilli, *Candida* spp., *S. aureus*

Continued

Infection	Common Pathogens
Oral ulcers	*Candida*, herpes simplex virus (HSV), cytomegalovirus (CMV), mixed anaerobes, gram-negative bacilli
Esophagitis	*Candida*, HSV, CMV, gram-negative bacilli
Skin/soft tissue (including catheter related)	Gram-negative bacilli (icthyma gangrenosum), streptococci, *S. aureus*, skin flora (*Corynebacterium* spp., coagulase-negative staphylococci), enterococci, HSV
Urinary tract infection	*E. coli*, Enterobacteriaceae, enterococci
Hepatitis	NANB (hepatitis C), CMV, Epstein-Barr virus, hepatitis B

*Adapted from Meunier, F. (ref.)

D. Special cases
  1. Hickman or tunneled catheter infections may present with fever, often in the absence of localized erythema, tenderness, or purulent drainage around the catheter exit site or tunnel.
    a. Etiology: Coagulase-negative staphylococci, *Corynebacterium* JK, *S. aureus*, gram-negative bacilli, *Candida* spp., other fungi, and enterococci are frequently recovered in blood cultures.
    b. Relative indications for catheter removal
      (1) Refractory bacteremia.
      (2) Tunnel infection (difficult to treat) unresponsive to therapy after 72 hr.
      (3) Fungemia.
      (4) Septic complications (e.g., emboli).
      (5) Gram-negative bacilli are harder to eradicate than gram-positive, antibiotic-susceptible organisms and may require removal of the catheter.
    c. Localized exit-site infections, even with bacteremia, are sometimes curable with antibiotic therapy alone.

III. **Focus of the History and Physical Examination**
  A. A thorough exam conducted daily, with particular attention to skin, catheter sites, the perianal area, oral cavity, lungs, and abdomen, is necessary.

IV. **Diagnostic Tests**
  A. Chest radiography, culture of any suspicious lesions, and panculture of blood and other body fluids for bacteria, viruses, and fungi should be done.
  B. Other diagnostic studies are dependent on clinical and laboratory findings.

V. **Approach to Therapy**
  A. Rapid initiation of empiric antibiotic therapy is essential. Appropriate and early antibiotic administration has been convincingly shown to decrease mortality due to gram-negative bacteremia.
  B. The first febrile episode is usually due to endogenous bacterial flora. Early empiric therapy with agents active against gram-negative bacilli and *P. aeruginosa* is recommended.
  C. Empiric antimicrobial therapy: Regimens should be guided by epidemiologic and clinical data, and should be amended to provide appropriate therapy when an organism(s) is (are) isolated and antibiotic susceptibilities are determined.
    1. Standard initial therapy: Aminoglycoside plus an antipseudomonal β-lactam (e.g., amikacin plus ceftazidime).
      a. Some have advocated initial monotherapy with an antipseudomonal β-lactam; however, this approach remains controversial. Antipseudomonal quinolones, administered alone or in combination with other agents, are under investigation and may be useful especially in β-lactam-allergic patients.
    2. If the fever and clinical symptoms fail to respond after 48–72 hr, the addition of antistaphylococcal agents such as vancomycin is recommended, particularly for those with indwelling catheters or other disruption of mucosal or skin integrity.
      a. Some recommend the addition of vancomycin to the initial regimen; there appears to be no substantial difference in survival when vancomycin is added initially or after 48–72 hr.
  D. During prolonged and profound neutropenia, fungal infection and bacterial superinfection with antibiotic-resistant organisms become more common; *Candida* fungemia or deep tissue infection and invasive aspergillosis are the most commonly seen fungal infections.
    1. A fourth empiric therapeutic agent, often added for patients who remain febrile for 5–7 days after initiation of broad-spectrum antimicrobial regimens, is amphotericin B

or IV fluconazole. Fluconazole, however, is inactive against *Aspergillus* species.

E. Depending on the clinical findings and the suspected source of infection, the usual suggested duration of therapy is 10–14 days if the patient responds to therapy and is afebrile. Some advocate continuation of broad-spectrum therapy until the neutropenia resolves, particularly if the fever and clinical symptoms do not respond.

F. A general pattern, which has emerged based on collective experience from clinical trials of febrile, neutropenic patients, suggests that about 20% will have microbiologically documented bacteremia; 20% will have a microbiologically documented site of infection without bacteremia; 20% will have a clinically documented site of infection without microbiologic confirmation (e.g., pneumonia on chest x-ray); 20% will have suspected infection without a documented source or site; and in 20% fevers will be unrelated to infection (e.g., drug induced).

VI. **Preventive Measures**

A. Hand washing, use of gloves or other barriers in appropriate settings, and immaculate housekeeping appear to be useful.

B. The use of a low-bacterial cooked diet, control of the water supply, limitation of plants, and the installation of laminar air flow, when available, may be beneficial.

C. Gut decontamination

1. The use of various agents to decontaminate the gut is based currently on the premise that anaerobic flora should be left intact to allow resistance to colonization of the gastrointestinal tract with other exogenous gram-negative bacilli.

2. Examples: Trimethoprim-sulfamethaxazole has been used; however, its use has been associated with the emergence of resistant gram-negative bacilli and delayed engraftment due to marrow suppression by trimethoprim. Quinolones suppress aerobic gram-negative bacilli but may create selection pressure, with emergence of gram-positive organisms such as *S. aureus*, viridans streptococci, and pneumococci.

D. Viral suppression: Daily use of acyclovir prevents HSV infections and decreases CMV reactivation in patients known to be seropositive or previously infected.

E. Fungal suppression: Some studies suggest a benefit of prophylactic fluconazole; data are as yet inconclusive.

F. Immunomodulation: IV immunoglobulin used in conjunction with acyclovir appears to decrease CMV reactivation, particularly when CMV-hyperimmune globulin is used. Recombinant granulocyte-colony stimulating factor (G-CSF) and granulocyte-macrophage-colony stimulating-factor (GM-CSF) have been used with some success in decreasing infection rates and reducing the number of febrile days by accelerating marrow recovery and ameliorating neutropenia associated with chemotherapy. Varicella-zoster immune globulin or vaccine has been useful in preventing varicella-zoster among susceptible persons exposed to the virus.

Infections in Patients Receiving Cytotoxic Chemotherapy

I. **Risk of Infection**

A. Cyclosporine: This drug has a highly selective ability to inhibit activation of T cells, primarily T-helper lymphocytes.

1. Cyclosporine causes a rapid and profound inhibition of interleukin-2 (IL-2) production by T-helper lymphocytes. It also appears to reduce the production and release of other lymphokines in response to antigenic stimuli. Higher concentrations inhibit expression of receptors for IL-2 and induction of cytotoxic T cells while sparing expression of suppressor T-cell function.

2. These effects are associated with an increased risk of infection due to organisms which require intact T-helper cell function for their containment.

B. Cytotoxic agents: Included in this category is a broad range of agents customarily used for cancer chemotherapy and/or for their effect in suppressing certain immunologic responses. In general, they have in common the ability to cause myelosuppression resulting in neutropenia. For most patients, the risk of infection is related to the degree of neutropenia induced. However, some agents also are able to induce changes in cell-mediated immune function. For example, methotrexate may inhibit replication and function of T lymphocytes; cyclophosphamide is cytotoxic for lymphoid cells and their precursors, hence its usefulness in combinations active against lymphomas and lymphoblastic leukemia.

C. Antilymphocyte globulins and monoclonal antibodies used for immunosuppression:

These agents chiefly act to block lymphocytic function (OKT3 blocks the function of all lymphocytes bearing the CD3 surface receptor) or to destroy lymphoid cells (antithymocyte globulin).

D. The effect of these agents on immune function is most profound when they are used in combination regimens. In such instances, their immunosuppressive effect is broad and the associated risk of infection due to specific pathogens or types of pathogens is difficult to predict.

II. Differential Diagnosis

A. The relatively specific effect of cyclosporine on T-helper lymphocyte function, and that of OKT3 on CD3 lymphocyte function, may result in an enhanced risk of infection due to intracellular pathogens. DNA viruses such as herpesviruses, adenovirus, and papovaviruses, mycobacteria, fungi, *Listeria*, *Nocardia*, and other intracellular pathogens are seen with increased frequency in patients receiving prolonged therapy with these agents. However, these drugs are rarely used alone; consequently, the infections seen span a wider spectrum than might be expected purely on the basis of interference with the function of a specific portion of the immune system.

B. Acute infection in patients treated with cytotoxic chemotherapy is more often caused by bacterial pathogens related to myelosuppression-induced neutropenia. Later infections may be due to viral, fungal, and intracellular pathogens normally influenced by cell-mediated immune function.

III. Approach to Therapy

In addition to providing initial broad-spectrum antimicrobial treatment, as discussed in previous sections, or specific therapy for subsequently identified infectious agents, attention must often be given to modifying the doses of cytotoxic drugs. The aim here is to decrease, if possible, the degree of immunosuppression to allow the host immune responses to recover sufficiently to aid in the attack on infection.

Bibliography

Balfour HH, Chace BA, Stapleton JT, et al. A randomized, placebo-controlled trial of oral acyclovir for the prevention of cytomegalovirus disease in recipients of renal allografts. *N Engl J Med* 320:1381–1388, 1989.

Bowden RA, Fisher LD, Rogers K, et al. Cytomegalovirus (CMV)-specific intravenous immunoglobulin for the prevention of primary CMV infection and disease after marrow transplant. *J Infect Dis* 164:483–487, 1991.

Calabresi P, Chabner BA. Antineoplastic agents, in Gilman AG, Rall TW, Nies AS, Taylor P (eds): *The Pharmacological Basis of Therapeutics*, ed 8. New York, Pergamon Press, 1990, pp 1209–1263.

Donowitz GR. Infections in bone marrow transplant recipients (update 12), in Mandell GL, Douglas RG Jr, Bennett JE (eds): *Principles and Practice of Infectious Diseases*, ed 3, update 12. New York, Churchill Livingstone, 1992, pp 3–12.

Emanuel D, Cunningham I, Jules-Elysee K, et al. Cytomegalovirus pneumonia after bone marrow transplantation successfully treated with the combination of ganciclovir and high-dose intravenous immune globulin. *Ann Intern Med* 109:777–782, 1988.

EORTC International Antimicrobial Therapy Cooperative Group. Empiric antifungal therapy in febrile granulocytopenic patients. *Am J Med* 86:668–672, 1989.

Fox BC, Sollinger HW, Belzer FO, et al. A prospective, randomized, double-blind study of trimethoprim-sulfamethoxazole for prophylaxis of infection in renal transplantation: Clinical efficacy, absorption of trimethoprim-sulfamethoxazole, effects on the microflora, and the cost-benefit of prophylaxis. *Am J Med* 89:255–274, 1990.

Ganser A, Ottmann OG, Erdmann H, et al. The effect of recombinant human granulocyte-macrophage colony-stimulating factor on neutropenia and related morbidity in chronic severe neutropenia. *Ann Intern Med* 111:887–892, 1989.

GIMEMA Infection Program. Prevention of bacterial infection in neutropenic patients with hematologic malignancies. A randomized, multicenter trial comparing norfloxacin with ciprofloxacin. *Ann Intern Med*, 115:7–12, 1991.

Goodman JL, Winston DJ, Greenfield RA, et al. A controlled trial of fluconazole to prevent fungal infections in patients undergoing bone marrow transplantation. *N Engl J Med* 326:845–851, 1992.

Handschumacher RE. Immunosuppresive agents, in Gilman AG, Rall TW, Nies AS, et al (eds): *The Pharmacological Basis of Therapeutics*, ed 8. New York, Pergamon Press, 1990, pp 1264–1276.

Haynes RC Jr. Adrenocorticotropic hormone: Adrenocorticosteroids and their synthetic analogues, inhibitors of the synthesis and actions of adrenocortical hormones, in Gilman AG, Rall TW, Nies AS, et al (eds): *The Pharmacological Basis of Therapeutics* ed 8. New York, Pergamon Press, 1990, pp 1442–1444.

Ho M, Dummer JS. Risk factors and approaches to infections in transplant recipients, in Mandell GL, Douglas RG Jr, Bennet JE (eds): *Principles and Pratice of Infectious Disease*, ed 3. New York, Churchill Livingstone, 1990, pp 2284–2291.

Ho M, Dummer JS, Peterson PK, et al. Infections in solid organ transplant recipients, in Mandell GL, Douglas RG Jr, Bennett JE (eds): *Principles and Practice of Infectious Disease*, ed 3. New York, Churchill Livingstone, 1990, pp. 2294–2303.

Hughes WT, Armstrong D, Bodey GP, et al. Guidelines for the use of antimicrobial agents in neutropenia patients with unexplained fever. *J Infect Dis* 161:381–396, 1990.

Karp JE, Merz WG, Hendricksen C, et al. Oral norfloxacin for prevention of gram-negative bacterial infections in patients with acute leukemia and granulocytopenia. A randomized, double-blind, placebo-controlled trial. *Ann Intern Med* 106:1–7, 1987.

Meunier F. Infections in patients with acute leukemia and lymphoma, in Mandell GL, Douglas RG Jr, Bennett JE (eds): *Principles and Practice of Infectious Diseases*, ed 3. New York, Churchill Livingstone, 1990, pp 2265–2276.

Meyers JD. Infections in marrow transplant recipients, in Mandell GL, Douglas RG Jr, Bennett JE (eds): *Principles and Practice of Infectious Diseases*, ed 3. New York, Churchill Livingstone, 1990, pp 2291–2294.

Meyers JD, Reed EC, Shepp DH, et al. Acyclovir for prevention of cytomegalovirus infection and disease after allogeneic marrow transplantation. *N Engl J Med* 318:70–75, 1988.

Pizzo PA. Empirical therapy and prevention of infection in the immunocompromised host, in Mandell GL, Douglas RG Jr, Bennett JE (eds): *Principles and Practice of Infectious Diseases*, ed 3. New York, Churchill Livingstone, 1990, pp 2303–2312.

Pizzo PA, Hathorn JW, Hiemenz J, et al. A randomized trial comparing ceftazidime along with combination antibiotic therapy in cancer patients with fever and neutropenia. *N Engl J Med* 315:552–558, 1986.

Reed EC, Bowden RA, Dandliker PS, et al. Treatment of cytomegalovirus pneumonia with ganciclovir and intravenous cytomegalovirus immunoglobulin in patients with bone marrow transplants. *Ann Intern Med* 109:783–788, 1988.

Reed EC, Wolford JL, Kopecky KJ, et al. Ganciclovir for the treatment of cytomegalovirus gastroenteritis in bone marrow transplant patients. A randomized, placebo-controlled trial. *An Intern Med* 112:505–510, 1990.

Rubin RH, Tolkoff-Rubin NE. Antimicrobial strategies in the care of organ transplant recipients. Antimicrob Agents Chemother 37:619–624, 1993.

Sanders JW, Powe NR, Moore RD. Ceftazidime monotherapy for empiric treatment of febrile neutropenic patients: A metaanalysis. *J Infect Dis* 164:907–916, 1991.

Singh N, Dummer JS, Kusne S, et al. Infections with cytomegalovirus and other herpesviruses in 121 liver transplant recipients: Transmission by donated organ and the effect of OKT3 antibodies. *J Infect Dis* 158:124–131, 1988.

Smyth RL, Scott JP, Borysiewicz LK, et al: Cytomegalovirus infection in heart-lung transplant recipients: Risk factors, clinical associations, and response to treatment. *J Infect Dis* 164:1045–1050, 1991.

Sullivan KM, Kopecky KJ, Jocom J, et al. Immunomodulatory and antimicrobial efficacy of intravenous immunoglobulin in bone marrow transplantation. *N Engl J Med* 323:705–712, 1990.

Winston DJ, Ho WG, Bruckner DA, et al. Beta-lactam antibiotic therapy in febrile granulocytopenic patients. A randomized trial comparing cefoperazone plus piperacillin, ceftazidime plus piperacillin, and imipenem alone. *Ann Intern Med* 115:849–859, 1991.

Wolff SN, Fay JW, Herzig RH, et al. High-dose weekly intravenous immunoglobulin to prevent infections in patients undergoing autologous bone marrow transplantation or severe myelosuppressive therapy. A study of the American Bone Marrow Transplant Group. *Ann Intern Med* 118:937–942, 1993.

CHAPTER 50-C

Approach to Infections in the Injectable Drug User

Larry J. Goodman, M.D.

I. **Problem**

Patients who abuse injectable drugs frequently become infected. While opiates and other agents may affect immune function in animals or in vitro systems, the significance of the drug's direct effect in clinically altering the host's immune status remains questionable. Rather, most of the infections seen appear to result from injecting a pathogen from the skin, drug, diluent used (e.g., tap water), mouth (licking the needle or sucking the injection site), or previous user of the needle and/or syringe (blood). Malnutrition, alcoholism, and other adverse conditions affecting many injectable drug users (IDUs) may modify the patient's response to the infection. Today, the IDU is also at high risk for infection with human immunodeficiency virus (HIV), with over 50% of IDUs in some cities being infected with this virus.

II. **Differential Diagnosis**

Mouth and skin organisms account for the majority of infections in the IDU. Blood-borne pathogens and pathogens acquired from the drug/diluent are also important. Table 50C-1 reviews the most likely etiologic agents for typical presen-

tations. This differential diagnosis must be further broadened to include opportunistic pathogens in the patient infected with HIV.

III. **Focus of the History and Physical Examination**
   A. History
      1. Symptoms
      2. Specific drug use history
      3. Routes and sites of injection
      4. Mechanism of mixing/preparing the injection
      5. Shared materials
      6. HIV status, (PPD) status, tuberculosis exposure
      7. Ill contacts
   B. Physical examination
      1. Symptomatic area(s)
      2. Skin lesions/adenopathy
      3. Peripheral manifestation of endocarditis
      4. Heart murmur
      5. Neurologic examination
   C. Relatively occult processes
      1. Necrotizing fasciitis
      2. Compartmental syndrome
      3. Osteomyelitis (e.g., symphysis pubis)
IV. **Diagnostic Approach** (See Table 50C-1)

Table 50C-1. Selected Differential Diagnoses of Infection Syndromes in the IDU

Site/Syndrome	Common Etiologic Agent(s)/Processes	Other Diagnostic Considerations	Diagnostic Tests
Skin abscess	*Staphylococcus* spp, *Streptococcus* spp., mixed anaerobic, HACEK* organisms, *Pseudomonas aeruginosa, Candida* spp. (particularly *C. parasilosis*)	Necrotizing fascitis, compartment syndrome, endocarditis, wound diphtheria, tetanus	1. Gram stain and culture 2. Blood culture 3. Plain x-rays; assess for gas in soft tissues, bony changes, foreign body 4. Incision and drainage exploration
Cough/pulmonary symptoms	1. Community-onset pneumonia (e.g., *Streptococcus pneumoniae*) 2. Aspiration pneumonia; rule out lung abscess 3. Tuberculosis	1. Emboli (right-sided endocarditis, phlebitis secondary to injections) 2. Opportunistic infections related to HIV (e.g., pneumocystis carinii pneumonia) 3. Heart failure due to endocarditis	1. Sputum Gram stain, acid-fast stain, culture 2. Blood culture 3. Chest x-ray 4. Bronchoscopy, echocardiogram, venous studies for clot
Hepatitis	Hepatitis A, B, or C	1. Delta hepatitis 2. Granulomatous hepatitis 3. Cytomegalovirus, herpes simplex virus, or Epstein-Barr virus if infected with HIV	1. Serology 2. Consider liver biopsy

Focal neurologic disease	1. Embolus from the heart (endocarditis) 2. Encephalitis (e.g., herpes simplex virus) 3. Brain abscess 4. Basilar meningitis (e.g., tuberculosis)	1. Meningovascular syphilis 2. Diphtheria 3. Tetanus 4. Spinal and/or perispinal infection 5. Toxoplasmosis, lymphoma, cryptococcal disease in HIV-infected patients	1. Computed tomography or magnetic resonance imaging scan of the brain 2. If no contraindication, perform spinal tap 3. Consider biopsy if focal area is identified
Endocarditis	1. *Staphylococcus* spp. 2. *Streptococcus* spp. 3. *Enterococcus* 4. *Pseudomonas aeruginosa*	1. Fungi—*Candida* spp., *Aspergillus* 2. HACEK organisms 3. Other gram-negative rods	1. Blood culture 2. Echocardiogram 3. Ophthalmologic exam, liver/spleen scan.
Wasting syndrome	1. Endocarditis 2. Lung abscess 3. Tuberculosis	1. Acquired immunodeficiency syndrome 2. HIV-associated lymphoma, disseminated *Mycobacterium avium* complex, cryptococcal disease, adrenal insufficiency	1. HIV 2. PPD/anergy 3. Chest x-ray 4. Echocardiogram 5. Cryptococcal antigen 6. Consider bone marrow and/or liver biopsy to assist in diagnosis of miliary tuberculosis if other tests are negative

*HACEK organisms include *Haemophilus* spp., *Actinobacillus actinomycetemcomitans*, *Cardiobacterium hominis*, *Eikenella*, and *Kingella*.

Bibliography

MMWR. Hepatitis A among drug abusers. *MMWR* 37:297–305, 1988.

Ponzetta A, Suf LB, Buskell-Bales Z, et al. Hepatitis B markers in United States drug addicts with special emphasis on the delta hepatitis virus. *Hepatology* 4:1111–1115, 1984.

Tuazon CU, Sheagren JN. Increased rate of carriage of *Staphylococcus aureus* among narcotic addicts. *J Infect Dis* 129:725–727, 1974.

Weisse AB, Heller DR, Cchimenti RJ, et al. The febrile parenteral drug user: A prospective study in 121 patients. *Am J Med* 94:274–280, 1993.

CHAPTER 51

Human Immunodeficiency Virus: Epidemiology, Pathophysiology, Immunology, Diagnostic Tests, Infectious and Malignant Complications

Joseph Bick, M.D.
Harold A. Kessler, M.D.
Constance A. Benson, M.D.

I. Background

Acquired immunodeficiency syndrome (AIDS) has been generally defined as a reliably diagnosed disease indicative of underlying cellular immune deficiency in an individual with no known predisposing cause, that is, underlying disease affecting the immune system or drugs known to affect cellular immunity.

A. Prior to 1984, any life-threatening opportunistic infection or unusual malignancy (Table 51-1) presenting in a person meeting the above criteria was usually classified as AIDS, according to the Centers for Disease Control (CDC) epidemiologic definition derived in 1981.

B. Human immunodeficiency virus (HIV) was established as the etiologic agent of AIDS in 1984.

1. The definition of AIDS has been modified to include evidence of infection with HIV.

2. Future modification of case definition may include the degree of immune suppression based on the absolute number of CD4 lymphocytes.

II. Etiology

The etiology is HIV-1 or HIV-2. HIV-2 is found predominantly is West Africa. HIV-2 has been imported into Europe through West African contact but is rare (only 12 cases under investigation) in the United States.

A. HIV is a member of the Lentivirinae subfamily of the Retroviridae.

1. Reverse transcriptase (RT) is a unique polymerase enzyme found in all retroviruses.

a. RT activity results in translation of the single-stranded RNA genome into sin-

Table 51-1. Infections, Malignancies, and Neurologic
Syndromes Most Commonly Associated with
Advanced HIV Infection and AIDS

Viruses
   Chronic mucocutaneous herpes simplex virus
   Disseminated varicella-zoster virus (shingles)
   Cytomegalovirus (retinitis, colitis, or other
      documented organ involvement)
   Epstein-Barr virus (oral hairy leukoplakia, B-cell
      lymphoma)
   Papillomavirus (cervical or rectal neoplasia)
   Papovavirus (JC virus–induced progressive
      multifocal leukoencephalopathy)
Bacteria
   Pneumococcus pneumoniae (bacteremia)
   Haemophilus influenzae (bacteremia)
   Salmonella (recurrent bacteremia)
   Mycobacterium tuberculosis (extrapulmonary)
   Mycobacterium avium-intracellulare (disseminated)
   Other atypical mycobacteria (extrapulmonary)
   Cat scratch bacillus (epithelioid angiomatosis)
Fungi
   Candida (esophagitis)
   Histoplasmosis (disseminated)
   Coccidioidomycosis (disseminated)
   Cryptococcus neoformans (meningitis, pneumonia,
      disseminated)
   Other disseminated fungal infections
      (blastomycosis, aspergillosis)
Protozoa
   Pneumocystis carinii pneumonia (recently classified
      as a fungus)
   Toxoplasmosis (predominantly encephalitis)
   Cryptosporidiosis
   Isospora belli
   Leishmaniasis
Malignancies
   Kaposi's sarcoma
   B-cell lymphomas (groin and extranodal
      common)
Neurologic Syndromes
   AIDS dementia complex
   Peripheral sensory neuropathy
   Chronic meningitis
   Inflammatory polyradiculoneuropathy
   Myopathy (inflammatory and noninflammatory)

---

gle-stranded DNA, which is critical to
the replication strategy of all retroviruses.
   2. HIV-1 and HIV-2 are closely related but
      immunologically distinct.
      a. Differences are found predominantly in
         the envelope glycoproteins.

B. HIV-1 structure (see Figure 51-1)
   1. Lipid-enveloped, single-stranded RNA vi-
      rus.
   2. A 120,000-MW envelope glycoprotein
      (gp120) binds predominantly to the cluster
      domain 4 (CD4) antigen complex, which
      acts as a receptor for the virus.
      a. CD4 is a membrane protein found pre-
         dominantly in T-helper/inducer lym-
         phocytes and cells of monocyte/
         macrophage lineage.
      b. Alternative receptors for HIV-1 include
         Fc receptors and CR2 (complement 3d)
         receptors.
   3. The RNA genome consists of three main
      structural genes; gag (nucleocapsid), pol
      (polymerase), and env (envelope).
      a. Major gag region protein is a
         24,000-MW (p24) protein which arises
         following cleavage of a p55 precursor
         protein by a protease enzyme coded for
         in the pol region.
      b. Pol gene codes for three enzymes: re-
         verse transcriptase, protease, and endo-
         nuclease (integrase).
      c. Env gene codes for a precursor
         160,000-MW glycoprotein (gp160)
         which is cleaved into a gp41 transmem-
         brane glycoprotein, which anchors the
         gp120 to the lipd envelope of the virus.
C. Replication strategy (see Figure 51-2)
   1. Attachment: receptor-specific gp120–CD4
      interaction.
      a. Fusion of virus and cell plasma mem-
         branes, with nucleocapsid insertion.
   2. Uncoating of nucleocapsid.
   3. Reverse transcription of virus RNA
      complementary DNA (cDNA).
   4. Circulization and migration of double-
      stranded cDNA into the nucleus.
   5. Integration of cDNA into the host cellular
      genome.
   6. Transcription of cDNA into the virion
      RNA and virion mRNA.
   7. Translation of mRNA into virion struc-
      tural proteins.
      a. Posttranslational cleavage of structural
         precursor proteins by the protease en-
         zyme.
      b. Glycosylation of envelope proteins and
         insertion into the host cell plasma mem-
         brane.
   8. Assembly of virion RNA and nucleocapsid
      proteins into the core (nucleocapsid) parti-
      cle.

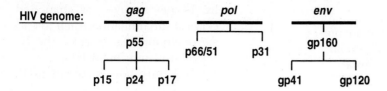

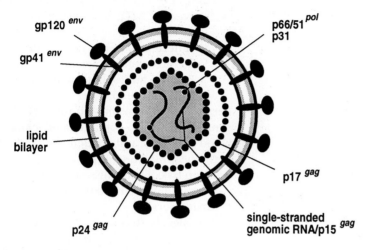

Major HIV-1 Proteins in Western Blot Analysis

gp160 - env precursor glycoprotein

gp120 - Envelope glycoprotein

p66 - Reverse transcriptase

p55 - Core precursor protein

p51 - Reverse transcriptase

gp41 - Transmembrane glycoprotein

p31 - Endonuclease

p24 - Major core protein

p17 - Core protein

Figure 51-1. HIV-1 Structure

9. Final maturation, with envelopment of the core particle by the plasma membrane containing virion glycoproteins.

D. Inactivation of HIV
   1. The HIV virus is relatively labile and loses infectivity on exposure to extremes of heat, drying, soap/detergents, bleach, and common household antiseptics.

III. Epidemiology
   A. Modes of transmission are via sexual or paren-

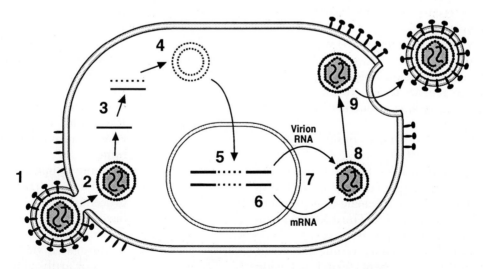

1	Attachment	4	Circularization	7	Translation
2	Uncoating	5	Integration	8	Core Particle Assembly
3	Reverse Transcription	6	Transcription	9	Final Assembly / Budding

Figure 51-2. Replication Strategy

Table 51-2. HIV Transmission: Global Summary

Type of Exposure	Efficiency per Single Exposure	Percentage of Global Total
Blood transfusion	>90%	3–5
Perinatal	30%	5–10
Sexual intercourse	0.1–1.0%	70–80
Vaginal		60–70
Anal		5–10
Intravenous drug use	0.5–1.0%	5–10
Health care setting	<0.5%	<0.01

Source: Adapted from Chin J. Plenary Address, VIIth International AIDS Conference, World Health Organization, June 19, 1991, Florence, Italy

teral mucous membrane or percutaneous inoculation of infected blood, blood products, semen, or vaginal secretions (Table 51-2).

1. HIV has also been isolated from cerebrospinal fluid, saliva, tears, breast milk, and urine.
   a. Viral titers in saliva, tears, breast milk, and urine are very low.
   b. Transmission by saliva, tears, or urine are not well documented and, if they occur, must be rare events.
      (1) Orogenital transmission is rarely reported.
   c. Transmission from mother to infant and from infant to mother through breast feeding has been documented.
2. Vertical transmission from mother to offspring occurs in approximately 30% of pregnancies.
   a. Predisposing factors are still unidentified.
3. Sexual transmission is bidirectional, that is, male to female, female to male, male to male, and, in at least one instance, female to female.
   a. Rectal intercourse is considered to pose a greater risk of transmission.
   b. Although male-to-female transmission has been suggested to be a more efficient route than female-to-male transmission, data from Third World countries suggest otherwise.
   c. Illicit drugs such as cocaine and crack, which induce hypersexual behavior, have been associated with an increased prevalence of infection.
   d. Sexually transmitted diseases which cause genital ulcerations, such as syphi-

lis, herpes simplex, or chancroid, or cervical inflammation, such as *Chlamydia* or gonorrhea, increase the risk of sexual transmission of HIV.
   (1) HIV infection is spread predominantly through heterosexual transmission in Third World countries.
   (2) There is a 1:1 ratio of male:female cases of AIDS in Third World countries.
   (3) There has been a rapid increase in heterosexual transmission in the United States, both male to female and female to male.
4. Percutaneous transmission through intravenous drug use, contaminated blood or blood products, and accidental inoculation in the health care setting.
   a. High risk of transmission due to sharing of contaminated needles by intravenous drug users.
      (1) Bleach decontamination may decrease the risk of transmission.
      (2) Needle exchange programs in Europe have had some success in decreasing transmission.
   b. Introduction of screening tests for HIV antibody in April 1985 dramatically reduced the risk of transmission via blood transfusion. Self-deferral of potential blood donors with known high-risk behaviors for HIV infection are also critical to decreased transmission by blood transfusion.
      (1) The CDC currently estimates that the risk of infection following blood transfusion is approximately 1 in 100,000.
      (2) Heat pasteurization of blood clotting factors, starting in January 1987, has essentially eliminated HIV transmission through this route.
      (3) Immune globulin preparations produced using current recommended procedures in the United States have not been implicated in HIV transmission.
      (4) Transmission via organ transplantation or artificial insemination has occurred, but the risk currently is believed to be similar to that for blood transfusion.
   c. The risk of transmission to health care

professionals through high-risk exposure has been approximately 0.3% in the United States.

(1) Transmission has occurred primarily through hollow-core needlestick exposures.

(2) Sharp injuries also carry a high risk of transmission.

(3) Solid-core needlestick exposures in the surgical setting appear to carry a much lower risk.

(4) Mucous membrane (of the eyes or mouth) contamination or prolonged blood exposure to abnormal or abraded skin may also pose a risk of accidental transmission.

(5) Transmission from an infected health care worker to a patient is a rare event and has been documented from a dentist with AIDS to six patients.

(a) Circumstances of transmission are currently under investigation.

5. Arthropod-borne transmission has not been established.

B. Prevalence and incidence of HIV infection and AIDS

1. As of July 1, 1991, AIDS has been reported from 163 countries.

a. The greatest number of cases were reported from the United States, South America, Western Europe, Africa, and the Caribbean.

b. Recent reports of cases from India and Southeast Asia and high rates of other sexually transmitted diseases in these geographic regions suggest the potential for an explosive increase in AIDS over the next 5 to 10 years.

c. Worldwide, as of July 1, 1991, 372,802 cases of AIDS have been reported.

2. From 8 to 10 million people with HIV infection are currently estimated worldwide.

a. By the year 2000, approximately 40 million people will be infected, according to World Health Organization projections.

b. Infection will spread to a significantly greater degree in Third World countries, with a slowly declining incidence in the United States and Western Europe.

c. Approximately 1 million people in the United States are infected with HIV-1.

(1) Estimates based upon data from serosurveys of military applicants, blood donors, college students, hospital admissions, and newborn infants.

(2) Seroprevalence of HIV antibodies varies greatly, depending on the geographic location and demographics of the population being studied.

(3) Major epicenters of HIV-infected individuals in the United States continue to be large urban areas in the coastal regions, although decentralization of new HIV infections into the interior states is occurring rapidly.

3. As of May 31, 1991, 179,136 cases of AIDS were diagnosed in the United States.

a. CDC projects 390,000 to 480,000 cases by 1993.

b. The yearly increase in the number of new cases has recently begun to plateau. This is due in part the introduction of zidovudine (AZT) in 1987 and the resultant delay in the progression rate of HIV infection to AIDS secondary to the antiviral properties of the drug.

(1) The projected decrease in AIDS cases does not indicate a decline in the number of HIV-infected individuals.

C. Changing epidemiology of AIDS

1. Original high-risk groups included homosexual and bisexual males, intravenous drug users, individuals with blood clotting disorders and those transfused with blood or blood products prior to April 1985, sexual partners of persons in the above groups, and infants born to HIV-infected mothers.

2. Introduction of HIV infection into the heterosexual population predominantly through bisexual males and intravenous drug users has resulted in a shift of new HIV infections to childbearing females and the pediatric population (Table 51-3).

3. High-risk behavior modification of homosexual males has resulted in a <2% incidence of new HIV infections in this population.

4. The 15- to 24-year age groups of both

Table 51-3. Changing Epidemiology of Reported Adult AIDS Cases in the United States in 1990

Risk Group	Percent of Total Cases	
	1985	**1990**
Homosexual and bisexual males	65	55
Homosexual and intravenous drug users	8	5
Intravenous drug users	17	23
Blood transfusion recipients	2	2
Hemophiliacs	1	4
Heterosexuals	1	6
Perinatal population	1	2
Unknown	6	6
Demographics		
White	60	52
Black	25	30
Hispanic	14	17
Male	93	88
Female	7	12

homosexual males and heterosexual individuals are less likely to practice safe sex and are at great risk of an increasing incidence of HIV infection.

    5. In 1990, the incidence of AIDS increased most rapidly in the heterosexual transmission risk group.

IV. Immunopathogenesis and Natural History (see Table 51-4 and Figure 51-3)

    A. Acute (primary) HIV infection has an incubation period which ranges from 2 to 12 weeks.

Table 51-4. Clinical Stages of HIV Infection, CD4 Lymphocyte Counts, and Time of Progression

Clinical Stage	Time/Duration	CD4 Lymphocyte Count (/mm^3)
Acute HIV infection	1 to 2 weeks	≥750
Asymptomatic	2 to >10 years	~750 to 200
Symptomatic	0 to 5+ years	~500 to 100
Advanced HIV disease	0 to 3+ years	<200
End-stage HIV disease	0 to 2+ years	<50

1. From 30% to 70% of patients develop a nonspecific febrile viral syndrome which may be mistaken for influenza, acute mononucleosis, or rubella.

    a. Illness lasts for 4 to 14 days and spontaneously resolves.

    b. Signs and symptoms include fever, myalgias, arthralgias, pharyngitis, cervical lymphadenopathy, and truncal macular rash. Aseptic meningitis or meningoencephalitis may also be seen.

    c. Resolution of symptoms is complete, after which patients move into the asymptomatic stage of the illness.

    d. Rarely, a chronic meningitis or meningoencephalitis may develop.

2. Primary infection of CD4-bearing circulating T-helper lymphocytes probably occurs first, followed by a viremic stage and subsequent infection of tissue macrophages.

    a. As the immune response to HIV infection evolves, the viremia is cleared and viral replication declines to a low persistent level, predominantly in CD4-bearing T-helper lymphocytes and macrophages.

      (1) Dissemination of virus occurs throughout all tissues of the body, and the macrophage probably acts as a reservoir of infection.

    b. Initially, the immune response probably involves natrual killer (NK) cells, followed by HIV antigen processing in monocyte/macrophages which present HIV antigens to T-helper lymphocytes in association with HLA-DR receptors. This ultimately results in subsequent immune responses, which can be measured via cytotoxic T lymphocytes and antibody-dependent cellular cytotoxic and humoral (antibody) immune responses.

    c. HIV-specific antibodies can be detected by 6 to 12 weeks following infection in 90% of individuals.

    d. Delayed antibody responses of up to 44 months have been documented rarely by some investigators, but >95% of infected people will develop antibodies by 6 months.

3. Biologic effects of HIV infection on T-helper lymphocytes and monocytes/macrophages are different.

    a. Infection of T-helper lymphocytes is

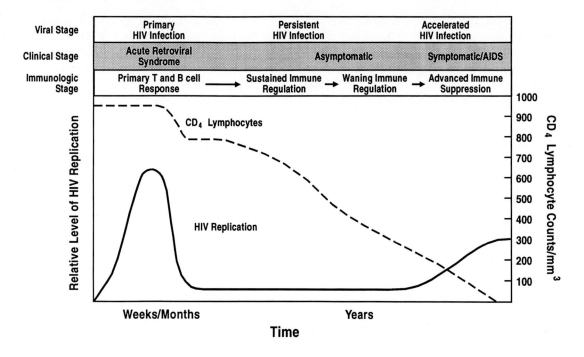

Figure 51-3. Natural History of HIV Infection

cytopathic and results in slow, progressive destruction of the T-helper lymphocyte population over many years.

  b. Infection of cells of the monocyte/macrophage lineage results in chronic productive infection without cell death. Biologic effects on the macrophage include decreased intracellular killing, defects in antigen presentation, decreased expression of HLA-DR antigens, prostaglandin-mediated suppression of lymphocyte blastogenesis and NK cell function, and a decreased migratory response.

  (1) Chronic infection of brain macrophages is a critical event in the long-term effects of HIV on the central nervous system.

B. The asymptomatic stage of HIV infection follows the primary infection stage and can last for periods ranging from 2 to more than 10 years.

  1. CD4 lymphocyte counts decline by 50 to 100 cells/mm^3 per year of infection during this stage.

  2. The risk of developing symptomatic disease increases as CD4 cell counts approach 200–250 cells/mm^3.

  3. Viral replication, as measured by the number of surrogate markers or direct virologic markers, remains at a low level until CD4 cell counts decline below 200–300 cells/mm^3 or <20–25% T-helper lymphocytes.

C. Symptomatic HIV infection generally manifests itself as the CD4 lymphocyte count declines to <200–250 cells/mm^3. Patients may progress from asymptomatic infection to an AIDS-defining illness without prior development of HIV-related systemic signs and symptoms.

  1. The systemic effects can include:

    a. Unexplained fever, weight loss, night sweats, and diarrhea.

    b. Chronic dermatitides such as seborrhea and eosinophilic folliculitis.

    c. Recurrent severe aphthous ulcers involving the mouth, esophagus, or stomach.

    d. Cervical atypia and a high incidence of cervical interepithelial neoplasia.

    e. Anal intraepithelial neoplasia, more commonly in males.

    f. Neurologic complications including distal, symmetrical sensory neuropathy, neurocognitive deficits, inflammatory polyradiculoneuropathy, and chronic meningitis or meningoencephalitis.

2. Non-AIDS deficiency infections can include:
   a. Dermatomal herpes zoster.
   b. Oral hairy leukoplakia secondary to reactivated Epstein-Barr viral infection of lingual buccal mucosal cells.
   c. Frequently recurrent oral or genital herpes simplex.
   d. Pulmonary tuberculosis.
   e. Neurosyphilis.
   f. Superficial dermatophyte infections of the skin and skin appendages.
   g. Oral candidiasis or recurrent recalcitrant vaginal candidiasis.
   h. Severe recurrent purulent sinusitis.
3. Viral replication and the presumed total body viral burden are increased in this stage of HIV infection, as measured by quantitative viral cultures of peripheral blood mononuclear cells and by plasma and surrogate markers such as plasma HIV antigen levels, β_2-microglobulin, and neopterin levels.
   a. Increased viral replication leads to accelerated destruction of CD4 lymphocytes, which in turn accelerates progressive immune deficiency.
4. Progressive immune deficiency can be measured by functional impairments, in addition to declining numbers of CD4 lymphocytes.
   a. T-cell blastogenesis to common recall antigens, cytotoxic T-lymphocyte activity, antibody-dependent cell-mediated cytotoxicity, and CD8 cytotoxic/suppressor cell down-regulation of HIV replication are all impaired as the disease progresses.

D. AIDS
1. The risk of developing an AIDS-defining illness increases significantly when the CD4 lymphocyte count declines to <20% or 200–250 cells/mm^3.
2. The mean survival for patients with AIDS has increased from 12 months in 1985 to greater than 24 months currently.
   a. The increase in survival is felt to be due primarily to the introduction of antiretroviral therapy with AZT in 1987 and, to a lesser extent, to the routine use of prophylaxis against *Pneumocystis carinii* pneumonia (PCP).
3. Mortality increases significantly when the CD4 lymphocyte count declines to <50 cells/mm^3.

a. The mean survival in a small cohort of patients with <50 cells/mm^3 CD4 lymphocytes is 12 months, as recently reported by Yarchoan et al.

V. **Diagnosis** (see Table 51-5)
A. The diagnosis of HIV infection is dependent upon the identification of individuals with high-risk behaviors or exposure to HIV infection.
   1. Identification of risk requires appropriate history-taking skills on the part of the physician.
   2. Sexual and drug use histories should be obtained in all routine encounters.
   3. The sexual history should include the number of casual sexual contacts over the last 5 to 10 years and whether the individual has sex with men, women, or both.
      a. Success in obtaining reliable information is increased if the history is elicited in a dispassionate, nonjudgmental way.
      b. A history of any sexually transmitted disease is an important risk factor for HIV infection.
   4. A history of blood or blood products exposure prior to April 1985 should also alert the physician to the risk of HIV infection.
B. Virologic diagnosis of HIV infection is made by isolation of HIV from cocultures of either the patient's peripheral blood mononuclear cells or plasma with healthy donor peripheral blood mononuclear cells.

Table 51-5. Methods for Detecting HIV Infection

Anti-HIV Antibody
   Enzyme immunoassays
   Western blot
   Immunofluorescence assays
   Radioimmunoprecipitation
   Latex agglutination
   Whole blood immunoassay
HIV Antigen
   Enzyme immunoassays
HIV Nucleic Acids
   Polymerase chain reaction
   In situ hybridization
HIV Culture
   Coculture of peripheral blood mononuclear cells
   Plasma culture
Detection of Immunodeficiency
   Flow cytometry for lymphocyte subset analysis
   In vitro lymphocyte functional assays

1. Isolation rates vary with the stage of disease, culture technique, and immunologic status of the patient.

    a. Isolation of HIV is greatest during the primary infection stage, prior to the development of an immunologic response to the infection, and in later stages of the infection as the T-helper cell count declines below 20% or 200/mm^3

    b. Culture is expensive, of limited availability, and can take up to 4 weeks to obtain a result.

    c. The demonstration of plasma viremia is a good indicator of the level of viral replication or viral load.

2. HIV proviral DNA or mRNA in the patient's peripheral blood mononuclear cells can be demonstrated using the polymerase chain reaction (PCR) method.

    a. This method is highly sensitive but is not yet automated, and therefore is very expensive and not widely available.

    b. The high sensitivity of this test can also lead to false-positive results due to cross-contamination within the laboratory.

    c. This method may be most useful in the diagnosis of HIV infection in newborns in whom passive antibody transfer from an infected mother makes serological diagnosis impossible.

    d. PCR can also be useful in diagnosis prior to the development of antibodies to HIV.

    e. Quantitation of the PCR technique may be useful in assessment of the level of viral replication and the efficacy of antiretroviral therapy.

3. Demonstration of HIV in tissues through in situ hybridization molecular techniques is also available but is generally limited to research laboratories.

C. Serologic diagnosis of HIV is accomplished through the demonstration of either antibodies to HIV or HIV antigen in the plasma or serum.

    1. HIV antibodies are most commonly demonstrated by enzyme immunoassay (EIA) and confirmed by immunoblot (Western blot) or immunofluorescent (IFA) methods.

        a. Commercially available EIAs are highly sensitive (99.6%) and specific (99.6%), but when used as screening tests in a low-incidence population, they have a false-positive rate of 50–75%.

        b. Confirmation by immunoblot assay, with demonstration of HIV-specific antibodies to at least one HIV protein from each of two different major HIV genes (env, pol, or gag), is necssary to establish the diagnosis of HIV infection (see Figure 51-1).

        c. Most common false-positive EIAs are due to the presence of isolated cross-reacting antibodies to the gag region proteins (i.e., p55, p24, or p17).

        d. Isolated antibody bands to the gag region protein(s) usually remain stable or disappear on subsequent testing 1 to 3 months later and are not indicative of HIV infection.

    2. HIV p24 antigen (the major nucleocapsid protein) can be detected in the plasma or serum by EIA in some patients with HIV infection.

        a. Antigen detection is probably indicative of the presence of infectious viral particles.

        b. Antigen detection is very sensitive in vitro, but antibodies to the p24 protein (anti-p24) in an infected patient can form immune complexes with the p24 and result in a negative test.

        c. HIV p24 antigen detection is most common in the acute retroviral syndrome and in advanced HIV infection.

        d. HIV p24 antigen in the plasma or serum is a surrogate marker for increased viral replication and is associated with an increased risk of disease progression.

        e. Quantitative HIV p24 antigen levels has also been used to evaluate the efficacy of antiretroviral drugs.

VI. **Infectious and Malignant Complications of HIV Disease**

A. *Pneumocystis carinii* pneumonia

    1. Etiology-*Pneumocystis carinii*

    2. Epidemiology

        a. *P. carinii* pneumonia (PCP) occurs in 60–85% of all patients with AIDS; the risk increases as the CD4 cell count declines below 200/mm^3 >200–250/mm^3.

        b. The organism is ubiquitous, usually acquired in childhood; two-thirds of normal children have antibody to *P. carinii* by 2–4 years of age.

3. Pathogenesis
   a. HIV-infected patients may either acquire new primary infection or reactivate latent infection as immunosuppression progresses. Pulmonary alveolar macrophages harbor *P. carinii*; when organisms are triggered to replicate, an intense lymphocytic inflammatory response with release of chemical mediators promotes diffuse lung damage.
4. Clinical presentation: History and physical findings
   a. The most common presentation is the acute or subacute onset of progressive dyspnea, fever and nonproductive cough.
   b. Pulmonary exam may be normal at rest; with exertion or in those with moderate to severe disease, tachypnea, tachycardia, and diffuse rales may be present.
5. Diagnostic tests
   a. Hypoxemia, the most characteristic laboratory abnormality, may range from mild or moderate (room air arterial oxygen [pO2] of >70–80 and alveolar-arterial oxygen gradient <35 mm Hg) to severe ([pO_2] < 70 mm Hg and alveolar-arterial oxygen gradient >35 mm Hg).
   b. Chest radiographs show diffuse, bilateral interstitial infiltrates; up to 5% of patients with early disease may have a normal chest x-ray; atypical presentations with nodular, cavitary, or upper lobe localization may occur, particularly in those receiving systemic prophylaxis or aerosolized pentamidine. Disseminated or extrapulmonary disease occurs but is uncommon; this complication is most frequent among those receiving no or only aerosol pentamidine prophylaxis.
   c. Histopathologic demonstration of organisms in tissue or bronchoalveolar samples remains the gold standard diagnostic test.
   d. Other diagnostic tests and their relative yields include:
      (1) Induced sputum: 55–80%
      (2) Bronchoscopy with bronchoalveolar lavage: 90–98%
      (3) Transbronchial biopsy: 95–100%
      (4) Open lung biopsy: 95–100%
   e. The yield may be substantially reduced in patients receiving prophylaxis.

   f. Gallium scanning may be a useful adjunct study in patients with mild to moderate symptoms and a normal chest x-ray.
6. Treatment
   a. Standard therapy:
      (1) Trimethoprim-sulfamethoxazole (TMP-SMX: 15–20 mg/kg/d IV (of TMP component) every 6 hours in divided doses for those with normal renal function.
      (2) Pentamidine: 4 mg/kg/d single IV dose infused over at least 60 minutes.
      (3) TMP-SMX at 15 mg/kg/d and pentamidine 3 mg/kg/d have been found to be nearly equal in efficacy and associated with reduced toxicity.
   b. Adjunctive corticosteroids: Currently recommended for those with moderate to severe disease as defined by room air pO_2 of <70 mm Hg or arterial-alveolar O_2 gradient of >35 mm Hg.
      (1) Dose: Prednisone or prednisolone 40 mg every 12 hours orally or IV for days 1–5, 40 mg every 24 hours for days 6–10, and 20 mg every 24 hours for days 11–21.
   c. Alternative therapeutic regimens:
      (1) TMP 15 mg/kg/d + dapsone 100 mg/d.
      (2) Aerosolized pentamidine 600 mg over 30 min daily.
      (3) Primaquine 30 mg/d + clindamycin 1,800–2,400 mg/d in divided doses.
      (4) Atovaquone 750 mg TID
   d. Investigational salvage therapy
      (1) Trimetrexate: 45 mg/M^2/d (with leucovorin)
   e. Adverse reaction rates overall for standard therapy range from 20% to 50%; these include rash, fever, neutropenia, thrombocytopenia, renal unsufficiency, hepatitis, pancreatitis, (pentamidine), dysglycemia (pentamidine)
   f. At least 14–21 days of therapy should be given; relapse rates may be higher in those who receive shorter courses of therapy.
7. Prophylaxis
   a. Overall relapse rates following first episode PCP are 26–55% within 1 year in the absence of any prophylaxis.
   b. Prophylaxis is recommended for all HIV-infected patients with CD4 cell counts <200/mm^3, for any HIV-in-

fected person with one or more HIV-related symptoms regardless of CD4 cell count, and for those who have had a prior episode of PCP.

    c. Recommended prophylactic regimens:

       (1) TMP-SMX: One DS (double strength) tab once daily, recent studies suggest less frequent dosing schedules, 2–3×/week, may be effective.

       (2) Aerosol pentamidine 300 mg/month.

       (3) Dapsone: 50 mg/d; less frequent dosing may also be effective.

    d. Aerosolized pentamidine is associated with a higher breakthrough rate than TMP-SMX in patients who have had a prior episode of PCP.

B. Cytomegalovirus disease

  1. Etiology: Cytomegalovirus (CMV)

  2. Epidemiology

    a. Ubiquitous; seroprevalence among HIV-infected adults ranges from 60% to 100%; transmitted by contact with infected body fluids, sexual contact, transfusion, donor organ, and transplacental and perinatal modes.

    b. CMV disease occurs in patients with advanced immunosuppression, usually with CD4 counts <100 cells/mm^3; it is the first opportunistic infection for 6–10%, CMV retinitis accounts for 70% of all ocular disease among HIV-infected patients.

  3. Pathogenesis

    a. As most HIV-infected patients have previously acquired but latent CMV infection, disease results from reactivation with subsequent viral replication and spread. The site of viral latency is thought to be circulating and tissue mononuclear cells. Secondary viremia then results in disseminated infection to other organ systems.

    b. Disease manifestations depend on the sites of localization following viremia.

  4. Clinical presentation: History and physical findings

    a. Chorioretinitis is the most common manifestation occurring in 15% to 20% of patients with AIDS; seen most frequently in those with CD4 lymphocytes <100 cells/mm^3. Retinitis may be unilateral or bilateral and is commonly sight-threatening. Presenting symptoms include floaters, decreased visual acuity, and visual field defects; may be asymptomatic.

    b. GI tract disease occurs in 5–10% of patients with AIDS; common presentations include hepatitis, ulcerative disease involving the esophagus or colon (associated with odynophagia or diarrhea with or without blood, respectively) and papillary stenosis with sclerosing cholangitis (associated with abdominal pain, fever, markedly elevated alkaline phosphatase with or without hyperbilirubinemia and characteristic abnormalities by endoscopic retrograde cholangiopancreatography [ERCP] or cholangiography).

    c. Encephalitis or encephalopathy; CMV has a predilection for infecting ependymal cells of brain and spinal cord resulting in fever, mental status change, seizures, progressive dementia or myelopathy with paraparesis or other focal deficits. This may be clinically indistinguishable from, but less common than other causes of encephalopathy, myelopathy, or dementia in patients with AIDS.

    d. Pneumonitis: a substantial proportion of patients with AIDS shed CMV in respiratory secretions, urine, and blood in the absence of end organ disease; a diagnosis of CMV pneumonitis, therefore, requires histologic demonstration of characteristic viral inclusions in tissue specimens, in addition to a clinically compatible syndrome of diffuse interstitial pneumonitis on chest x-ray, fever, dyspnea, and absence of other pathogens.

  5. Diagnostic tests

    a. Seroconversion or a fourfold rise in IgG antibody titer is rare in HIV-infected patients; serodiagnosis is usually not helpful.

    b. Virus isolation is presumptive evidence of active infection but should be supported by histopathologic demonstration of characteristic viral inclusions or immunologic staining of viral antigens in tissue specimens obtained from clinically involved organ systems.

    c. Diagnosis of retinitis is based on the characteristic ophthalmologic lesions of the retina—creamy white or yellow exudates obscuring vascular structures and accompanied by retinal hemorrhages.

6. Treatment

a. Phosphonoformate (foscarnet): Recommended induction doses are 60 mg/kg IV every 8 hours or 90 mg/kg IV Q 12h for 14 days for those with normal renal function. Doses must be adjusted for rises in serum creatinine or changes in creatinine clearance or weight. Maintenance therapy is required to prevent relapse. Recommended maintenance doses are 90 mg/kg/d to 120 mg/kg/d 7 days/week.

(1) Toxicities include anemia; renal insufficiency; metabolic disturbances of calcium, magnesium, phosphorus, and potassium; neurotoxicity; and rarely neutropenia.

b. Ganciclovir: The induction dose is 5 mg/kg IV every 12 hours for 14 days; doses must be adjusted for renal failure. The recommended doses for maintenance therapy are 5 mg/kg/d 7 days per week or 6 mg/kg/d 5 days per week.

(1) The major toxicity of ganciclovir is bone marrow suppression (neutropenia 45–55%, thrombocytopenia 25%); mutagenesis or teratogenesis has been reported in animal studies.

c. For retinitis the response rate is 75%–90% with stabilization and/or healing of existing lesions and delay in the development of new lesions. The mean time to progression on maintenance therapy ranges from 45 to 60 days.

(1) While foscarnet and ganciclovir have equal efficacy in the treatment of CMV retinitis, foscarnet is associated with a possible survival advantage (a median of 12 months for foscarnet versus 8 months for ganciclovir from the time of retinitis diagnosis in one study).

(2) Similar response rates have been reported with ganciclovir treatment of CMV colitis and esophagitis, although diarrhea may persist. Prospective trials evaluating response of CMV pneumonitis in persons with AIDS to ganciclovir or foscar-

net have not been reported. Response of neurologic disease to ganciclovir has been disappointing.

(3) Intravitreal and oral forms of ganciclovir are under investigation for therapy of CMV retinitis.

(4) As yet, no effective prophylactic regimen has been developed to prevent CMV disease in patients with AIDS; high-dose, formulations of acyclovir, valacyclovir, and oral ganciclovir are under investigation.

C. Other herpesvirus infections (key points pertaining to HIV-infected patients)

1. Herpes simplex virus (HSV)

a. Clinical presentation: Similar to non-HIV-infected individuals but may be associated with prolonged or persistent mucocutaneous outbreaks characterized by atypical enlarging painful perirectal or perineal ulcers.

(1) HSV may also cause organ-invasive disease such as pneumonitis, esophagitis, or other GI tract disease.

b. Diagnostic tests: Culture of appropriate specimens or biopsy of involved organs.

c. Treatment

(1) Acyclovir: Standard dose for acute treatment is 200–400 mg orally every 4 hours 5×/d for 7 days or 5 mg/kg IV every 8 hours for 7 days (for those with normal renal function).

(2) Acyclovir resistance has become increasingly common among HIV-infected patients; this should be suspected in the setting of enlarging or persisting lesions unresponsive to standard or high-dose oral or IV acyclovir.

(3) Alternative therapies for acyclovir-resistant HSV include high-dose or continuous infusion IV acyclovir 10 mg/kg every 8 hours (doses must be adjusted for renal insufficiency) or IV phosphonoformate (foscarnet) 40 mg/kg every 8 hours for 10–21 days.

2. Varicella-zoster virus (VZV)

a. Clinical presentation: Zoster in a single or multidermatomal distribution is the most common HIV-related presentation; rarely, disseminated cutaneous disease may be seen associated with prolonged or recurrent skin lesions. Organ involvement is unusual but VZV esophagitis and acute retinal necrosis have been rarely reported in patients with AIDS.

   (1) Primary varicella can be seen in HIV-infected adults; it may be severe and disseminate to multiple organ systems in those with advanced immunodeficiency.

  b. Diagnostic tests: The clinical appearance, virus culture, and biopsy of involved sites.

  c. Treatment: Acyclovir 800 mg orally every 4 hours 5×/d or 10 mg/kg IV every 8 hours for 7–10 days (for those with normal renal function).

3. Epstein-Barr virus (EBV)

  a. Clinical presentation: EBV has been linked with oral hairy leukoplakia (OHL) and primary B-cell lymphoma.

   (1) OHL is an oral lesion characterized by adherent, white, frondlike projections along the lateral surface of the tongue, occasionally extending to the dorsal or ventral surface or on to the buccal mucosa; lesions are painless and may remit spontaneously. This lesion has also been linked to human papillomavirus.

  b. Diagnostic tests: Biopsy of tissue with immunohistochemical staining, electronmicroscopy, DNA hybridization studies.

  c. Treatment: OHL may respond to acyclovir or zidovudine; antiviral treatment does not appear to alter the course of EBV-associated B-cell lymphoma.

D. *Mycobacterium avium* complex disease

1. Etiology

  a. Microorganisms of the *M. avium–M. intracellulare* complex (MAC).

2. Epidemiology

  a. MAC organisms are ubiquitous, found in soil, water, domestic and wild animals, milk, and other foodstuffs. Most organisms are probably acquired by inhalation or ingestion; there is no evidence to suggest person-to-person transmission.

  b. *M. avium* accounts for >90% of atypical mycobacterial infections in patients with AIDS. The incidence of clinical disease; ranges from 18% to 43%; au-

topsy studies suggest that up to 60% of AIDS patients will have MAC disease present at the time of death.

  c. Disease occurs chiefly among those with advanced immunosuppression with CD4 lymphocyte counts <75 cells/mm^3.

3. Pathogenesis

  a. The pathogenesis of MAC disease is poorly defined; a proportion of patients may be colonized in the absence of invasive disease while others appear to develop disseminated disease shortly after the acquisition of infection with no prior evidence of colonization.

  b. Whether MAC disease results from reactivation or recent acquisition of new infection has not been established.

  c. Intracellular infection within macrophages successfully evades immune response. Histopathologically, large numbers of organisms are seen with little local reaction; rarely a granulomatous inflammatory response is present.

4. Clinical presentation

  a. Disease most often presents with disseminated disease involving multiple organs; nonspecific symptoms and signs include fever, diarrhea, sweats, hepatosplenomegaly, lymphadenopathy, weight loss, and wasting.

   (1) Lymph nodes, spleen, liver, and GI tract are the most commonly involved organs; high-grade mycobacteremia is present in 80–90%; chronic diarrhea with malabsorption may be a manifestation of GI tract invasion. Splenomegaly and intra-abdominal lymphadenopathy may be associated with chronic abdominal pain.

5. Diagnostic tests

  a. Blood culture (radiometric detection system) or isolation of the organism from appropriate normally sterile clinical specimens.

  b. Acid-fast bacteria (AFB) smears and stains of involved tissue are nonspecific as *Mycobacterium tuberculosis*, *Mycobacterium kansasii*, and other atypical mycobacterial infections may also be seen with increased frequency among HIV-infected patients.

6. Treatment

  a. As yet, no specific regimen has been

proved uniformly successful in eradicating MAC disease with a sustained clinical and microbiologic response.

b. In vitro susceptibility data indicate that amikacin, clofazimine, the rifamycin derivatives rifampin and rifabutin, ethambutol, ciprofloxacin, sparfloxacin, some newer quinolones and the macrolides, clarithromycin and azithromycin have substantial activity against MAC; MAC organisms are not uniformly susceptible to all of these agents.

c. Several regimens have had clinical and microbiologic efficacy in limited studies. Recommended regimens include: Clarithromycin 500 mg BID or azithromycin 500 mg once per day. Combined with one or more of the following:

(1) Oral ethambutol 15 mg/kg/d

(2) Oral clofazimine 100–200 mg/d

(3) Oral rifampin or rifabutin 600 mg/d

(4) Oral ciprofloxacin 500–750 mg twice per day.

(5) IV amikacin 10–15 mg/kg/d in single or divided doses

d. Oral clarithromycin twice per day or azithromycin once per day have clinical and microbiologic efficacy as single agents in short-term clinical trials; resistance does occur with single drug use, however, the most appropriate other drugs to use in combination with the macrolides has not been established.

e. In general, when AFB are recovered from a patient with HIV infection who has a clinical disease compatible with mycobacterial infection, empiric therapy is recommended with four or more drugs including isoniazid, rifampin, ethambutol, and pyrazinamide, until final identification of the pathogen is available.

(1) This regimen will generally suffice for initial treatment of *M. tuberculosis* or *M. kansasii* infections; once culture confirmation is available treatment regimens can be appropriately altered. The decision whether or not to add empiric therapy for MAC disease prior to identification of MAC is one of judgment based on the clinical presentation and severity of illness.

E. Other mycobacterial infections—Selected aspects in HIV-infected patients

1. Etiology *Mycobacterium tuberculosis*

a. Epidemiology: Tuberculosis is the most common HIV-related infection worldwide; the incidence of tuberculosis has increasd in the U.S. by more than 15% since 1985. HIV-related tuberculosis is thought to contribute at least one-third of all new tuberculosis cases in the U.S. The incidence of multidrug resistant tuberculosis has also increased, particularly in urban areas such as New York City and Miami.

(1) Due to its greater virulence, tuberculosis is generally diagnosed among HIV-infected patients with >100 cells/mm^3; more often patients have CD4 counts in the range of 300–500 cells/mm^3. Patients who are HIV-infected and tuberculin skin test positive are more likely to reactivate and develop clinically active tuberculosis than are persons who are not HIV-infected. HIV-infected persons exposed to tuberculosis are more likely to become infected and to develop active tuberculosis more quickly than those not HIV-infected.

b. Pathogenesis (see Chapter 48L Mycobacterial Infections).

c. Clinical presentation

(1) The clinical presentation is dependent on the degree of immunosuppression. For patients coinfected with HIV who do not have AIDS or advanced immunosuppression, signs and symptoms resemble those in non-HIV-infected populations; chronic cavitary, upper lobe pneumonia is the most common presentation.

(2) Tuberculosis in patients with AIDS or with profound immunosuppression is characterized by atypical presentations with cutaneous anergy to purified protein derivative of tuberculin (PPD), diffuse atypical or interstitial pulmonary infiltrates, and disseminated or extrapulmonary disease.

(3) Multidrug-resistant tuberculosis, especially in those with profound

immunosuppression, is likely to have a more aggressive course with atypical and often disseminated disease, rapid progression, and mortality rates in excess of 70 to 80% over a median of 4 to 16 weeks if inadequately treated.

(4) The most common extrapulmonary site of involvement with tuberculosis is the lymphoreticular system with diffuse or localized lymphadenopathy, hepatosplenomegaly and/or bone marrow invasion; blood cultures may be positive in 20–40% of patients.

(5) Most patients with extrapulmonary disease will also have pulmonary involvement.

d. Diagnostic tests: Chest radiographs generally reflect the localized or disseminated nature of the disease; those with higher CD4 cell counts will likely have upper lobe infiltration with cavitary disease while those with advanced immunosuppression will more likely have atypical patterns, lower lobe infiltrates, or miliary disease.

(1) Sputum smears for AFB are positive in one-third to one-half of HIV-infected patients with culture-proven pulmonary tuberculosis, however, sputum cultures will be positive in 90–95%. The use of radiometric detection systems may decrease the time to positive culture.

(2) Among persons with CD4 counts below $500/mm^3$, the presence of cutaneous anergy varies inversely with the CD4 cell count. For those with counts <50 cells, 80% may be anergic. For HIV-infected persons, a PPD skin test (5 tuberculin units [TU] strength by the Mantoux method) of ≥ 5 mm of induration should be regarded as a positive PPD skin test.

(3) Blood or bone marrow cultures or culture of tissue biopsies or specimens from involved sites may assist in the diagnosis.

e. Treatment: In general, HIV-infected patients with a positive AFB sputum smear should be treated for tuberculosis pending culture results.

(1) Treatment of tuberculosis in patients with HIV infection is effective; conversion of sputum cultures to negative within 3 months of initiation of appropriate therapy occurs for >90%; lifelong therapy is probably not required.

(2) The excess mortality often reported among HIV-infected patients with tuberculosis may be a consequence of underlying immunosuppression and other HIV-related illnesses.

(3) Initial therapy should include INH 300 mg/d with pyridoxine, rifampin 600 mg/d (450 mg for those weighing <50 kg), and pyrazinamide 20–30 mg/kg/d; and either ethambutol (15–25 mg/kg/d) or streptomycin (1 gm IM/d); for patients from endemic areas at high risk for multidrug resistance, addition of a fifth and/or sixth drug has been advocated, pending susceptibility testing results.

(4) After the first 2 months of therapy, for patients who appear to be clinically responding, INH and rifampin alone may be continued for a total of 9 months or at least 6 months following conversion of cultures to negative.

(5) For INH-resistant or multidrug resistant disease treatment should continue for 18 to 24 months or for 12 months following conversion of cultures to negative.

(6) Adverse reactions to antimycobacterial agents appear to be more common among HIV-infected patients than non-HIV-infected patients; reported rates range from 5% to 24%. The types of reactions are similar to those seen with these drugs in other populations.

(7) Compliance should be assured with directly observed therapy when possible, especially for those with INH-resistant or multidrug resistant tuberculosis.

(8) All initial isolates should be tested for antimycobacterial drug susceptibility; treatment regimens should be modified according to susceptibility results to assure that the pa-

tient receives at least two to three drugs to which their isolate is susceptible.

f. Prophylaxis: All persons known to be HIV-infected should have a PPD tuberculin skin test (5 TU PPD by the Mantoux method). Persons with HIV infection should also be evaluated for delayed type hypersensitivity (DTH) anergy at the time of PPD testing; this should be carried out using at least two additional DTH antigens (*Candida*, mumps, or tetanus toxoid) administered preferably by the Mantoux method. Any induration to a DTH antigen measured at 48–72 hours is regarded as a positive response.

(1) Those with a positive ($\geq$5 mm induration) PPD reaction are considered to be infected with *M. tuberculosis* and should be considered for INH prophylaxis after active tuberculosis has been excluded.

(2) Anergic, tuberculin-negative persons whose risk of active tuberculosis is $\geq$10% (e.g., known contacts of infectious tuberculosis patients, IDUs, prisoners, homeless persons, migrant laborers, and persons born or residing in areas with high endemic rates of tuberculosis) should also be considered for INH prophylaxis after active tuberculosis is excluded.

(3) INH 300 mg/d with pyridoxine for a duration of 12 months is currently recommended. Studies of shorter duration of INH and shorter courses with two or more drugs are underway.

g. Infection control measures are important and should be followed regardless of HIV status. Respiratory isolation procedures should be instituted for suspected cases of active pulmonary tuberculosis. A chest x-ray and PPD/anergy skin testing should be done prior to initiation of aerosolized pentamidine treatment.

2. *Mycobacterium kansasii*—Selected aspects in HIV-infected patients

a. Epidemiology: In the U.S. the highest incidence appears to occur in the South and Midwest with outbreaks of disease among HIV-infected patients in Chicago and other urban areas.

(1) *M. kansasii* appears to be somewhat more common among urban IDU patients with HIV infection and among those with underlying chronic pulmonary disease.

b. Clinical presentation: The most common presentation is an insidious progressive pulmonary disease that closely resembles pulmonary tuberculosis. Extrapulmonary disease or disseminated disease has also been reported, usually among those with more advanced immunosuppression.

c. Diagnostic tests: Culture of appropriate clinical specimens.

d. Treatment: *M. kansasii* is predictably susceptible to rifampin and ethambutol and relatively resistant to INH; combination drug regimens containing rifampin have been the most effective. Emergence of resistance to rifampin has developed during therapy with two-drug rifampin-containing regimens, therefore, INH is usually included.

(1) The usually recommended duration of therapy is 18–24 months.

3. Other atypical mycobacterial infections

a. Among HIV-infected individuals, sporadic cases of localized or disseminated disease due to *M. xenopi, M. chelonei, M. fortuitum, M. marinum,* and other atypical mycobacteria have been reported. M *genovense*, a newly described species, may also cause disseminated disease in those with advanced immunosuppression.

b. Therapy for disease due to these organisms must be individualized and will generally depend on the clinical manifestations, availability of culture or nucleic acid probe identification, and on antimycobacterial susceptibility testing.

F. Candidiasis

1. Etiology—*Candida albicans*

2. Epidemiology

a. *Candida* spp. are normal commensals of humans commonly found on skin, in the GI tract, respiratory tract, and female genital tract.

b. Some form of mucocutaneous candidiasis occurs in virtually 100% of HIV-infected patients at some point during their disease course. The risk of mucocutaneous disease rises as the CD4 lymphocyte count declines below 350 cells/mm^3 although some may experience mild or intermittent disease at CD4 counts above this level; once the CD4 count declines below 200 cells/mm^3, the risk of invasive disease rises.

3. Pathogenesis
   a. Most infections are endogenous in origin resulting from reactivation in the face of progressive immunosuppression.
4. Clinical presentation
   a. White mucocutaneous patches or plaques are the most common lesions seen; may precede and are a prognostic indicator of progression to AIDS.
      (1) Lesions are most often seen in the oral cavity, although refractory or recurrent *Candida* vaginitis is common among women with HIV infection.
   b. *Candida* esophagitis is the first AIDS-defining infection for ~12–15% of individuals; it may be more common in women with AIDS.
      (1) Clinical symptoms and signs include fever, odynophagia, nausea, ulcerative plaques demonstrated by upper gastrointestinal (UGI) radiograph or endoscopy; disease is usually but not always accompanied by oral thrush.
5. Diagnostic tests
   a. Wet mount/KOH prep with microscopic examination or culture of samples obtained from mucocutaneous plaques will yield yeast forms; histopathologic demonstration of organisms in tissue biopsy specimens will confirm the etiology of esophageal lesions.
6. Treatment
   a. Chronic mucocutaneous disease: Clotrimazole oral troches, one taken orally 5×/d; nystatin swish and swallow 5×/d; ketoconazole 200–400 mg/d; fluconazole 100–200 mg/d, itraconazole 200 mg/d.
   b. Vaginal candidiasis: Clotrimazole or other triazole/imidazole vaginal troches or cream, one application each bedtime for 7–10 days.
   c. *Candida* esophagitis: Ketoconazole 200 mg orally twice per day; fluconazole 100–200 mg orally every day; amphotericin B 20 mg IV every day for 10 days.
   d. Repeated intermittent or chronic maintenance therapy may be required.
   e. When using ketoconazole or itraconazole, gastric acidity is required for adequate absorption.
      (1) Concurrent use of antacids, H$_2$ blockers or the presence of achlorhydria will impair absorption; fluconazole does not require the presence of gastric acid for absorption.

G. Cryptococcosis (See chapter on Systemic Fungal Infections)
H. Histoplasmosis. (See chapter on Systemic Fungal Infections)
I. Toxoplasmosis
   1. Etiology—*Toxoplasma gondii*
   2. Epidemiology
      a. Worldwide distribution; 30–40% of HIV-infected adults are seropositive for *T. gondii*. Of those who are seropositive, it is estimated that 30–40% will develop acute toxoplasmic encephalitis. Toxoplasmic encephalitis is estimated to occur in 6–10% of patients with AIDS.
   3. Pathogenesis
      a. Disease is thought to be due to reactivation of latent infection; fewer than 10% of all cases represent new infection in patients seronegative for *T. gondii*.
      b. The trigger for reactivation is thought to be progressive immunosuppression with impairment of immune surveillance.
      c. Tissue cysts, persisting in latent viable form, are the likely source for recrudescence; once triggered, trophozoites within cysts proliferate with cyst rupture, trophozoite tissue invasion, production of severe necrotizing lesions, and eventual local tissue destruction.
   4. Clinical presentation
      a. Toxoplasmic encephalitis is the most common disease manifestation in patients with AIDS. Fever, headache, mental status changes, focal neurologic deficits, and seizures are common symptoms.
      b. Extraneurological disease may be seen in patients with AIDS; manifestations include miliary or nodular lung disease, chorioretinitis, and lymphoreticular, testicular, or GI tract lesions.

5. Diagnostic tests
   a. CSF parameters are usually normal although elevated protein and a mild lymphocytic pleocytosis may be seen. Computerized Tomographic or Magnetic Resonance (MRI) imaging characteristically reveals multiple white matter parenchymal enhancing lesions; single mass lesions can be seen, but are less common. MRI appears to be more sensitive.
   b. The definitive diagnosis is based on histologic demonstration of tachyzoites in tissue biopsy specimens and/or growth of organisms in tissue culture.
   c. While a small percentage of patients will be seronegative in the presence of clinical disease, the absence of antibody should raise doubt regarding the diagnosis.
   d. The presumptive diagnosis of toxoplasmic encephalitis is based on the clinical presentation, positive serology, the characteristic appearance of lesions on CT or MR imaging, and the clinical and CT or MR response to specific therapy.
6. Treatment
   a. The current treatment of choice is pyrimethamine combined with sulfadiazine or triple sulfa. Leucovorin is also administered to ameliorate pyrimethamine-associated bone marrow suppression.
      (1) Pyrimethamine: Loading dose 50 mg twice a day for 2 days; 50–100 mg/d, thereafter.
      (2) Sulfadiazine or triple sulfa: Loading dose 75 mg/kg (4 gm); 100 mg/kg/d (8 gm).
      (3) Leucovorin: 10 mg/d; adjust upward for leukopenia.
   b. Duration of therapy is generally prolonged, from 2 to 6 months. Most respond to initial treatment within 2–6 weeks, however, relapse is common following discontinuation of therapy, suggesting the need for longer-term maintenance therapy.
      (1) In the absence of brain biopsy confirmation, empiric therapy can be initiated. An objective response noted on repeat CT or MR imaging and a clinical response should be apparent within 2–6 weeks; if no response is seen or lesions increase with appropriate therapy, biopsy should be considered to look for alternative pathogens. Concurrent use of steroids may make interpretation of repeat scans difficult.
      c. The high rate of hypersensitivity reactions to sulfa agents may prompt alternative therapies.
      d. Alternative regimens include pyrimethamine combined with clindamycin (2,400 mg/d) or other macrolides; these regimens are under investigation.
      e. The most appropriate maintenance and prophylactic regimens have yet to be established; some have advocated continuation of primary therapy indefinitely, the use of pyrimethamine alone, and the use of less potent inhibitors alone or in combination.
         (1) Prophylaxis with pyrimethamine alone has not been successful but pyrimethamine plus dapsone and Trimethoprim-sulfamethoxazole have been shown to reduce the incidence of both toxoplasmosis and *P. carinii* pneumonia.
J. Cryptosporidiosis
   1. Etiology—*Cryptosporidium parvum*
      a. This organism is a coccidian protozoan. When the oocyte matures, it releases four motile sporozoites, which are thought to be the infectious form of the organism.
   2. Epidemiology
      a. Probably a ubiquitous animal pathogen with humans as incidental hosts; common cause of diarrhea worldwide in normal hosts. The exact incidence or prevalence in patients with AIDS is unknown. Geographic location may influence the incidence; disease is more common in New York, Miami, the Caribbean, and the southeastern United States, but occurs sporadically elsewhere.
      b. Organisms can be transmitted from person to person.
   3. Pathogenesis
      a. Oocysts sporulate in the host and release sporozoites which implant in host epithelial cells of the intestinal tract.
      b. Histologic changes induced include blunting or denuding of villi, deepen-

ing of crypts, and a mixed cellular infiltration of the lamina propria.

   c. Inflammatory infiltration of the biliary tract with necrosis can be seen with cryptosporidial cholecystitis.

   d. The profuse secretory diarrhea and malabsorption are thought to be due to the combined effect of a possible enterotoxin or to destruction of the brush border.

4. Clinical presentation

   a. Most patients have a severe diarrheal illness with frequent, voluminous (1–20 liters/d), watery bowel movements, crampy abdominal pain, malabsorption, and profound weight loss.

   b. Cryptosporidial cholecystitis results in right upper quadrant abdominal pain, nausea, and vomiting. Laboratory studies demonstrate cholestasis with marked elevation of alkaline phosphatase; gall bladder wall thickening and irregularities of bile ducts may be seen on ultrasound or radiographic imaging.

5. Diagnostic tests

   a. A modified acid-fast stain of stool demonstrating oocysts confirms the diagnosis.

   b. Histopathologic demonstration of organisms in intestinal or biliary tract biopsies.

6. Treatment

   a. There currently is no known uniformly effective therapy for cryptosporidial infection.

   b. Experimental oral therapy with the macrolide spiramycin has been disappointing.

     (1) Anecdotal reports and small retrospective studies suggest that paromomycin, a nonabsorbable oral aminoglycoside, may be beneficial in doses ranging from 500 mg three times a day to 500 mg four times a day.

     (2) Somatostatin and octreotide have been useful adjuncts in slowing GI tract motility and decreasing diarrhea. Letrazuril, azithromycin and hyperimmune bovine colostrum are under investigation for therapy.

K. Isosporiasis

1. Etiology—*Isospora belli*

   a. A coccidian protozoan similar to *Cryptosporidium*; large (20–30 microns), oval, acid-fast oocysts.

2. Epidemiology

   a. More common in Caribbean patients with AIDS and in the southeastern United States; occurs in fewer than 0.2% of AIDS patients reported to the CDC in the U.S.

3. Pathogenesis

   a. Infection of the intestinal tract results in atrophic mucosa with villous changes and an eosinophilic infiltration of the lamina propria.

   b. The mechanism by which *Isospora* causes diarrhea is probably similar to that associated with cryptosporidiosis.

4. Clinical presentation

   a. Similar to cryptosporidiosis; chronic, profuse, watery diarrhea associated with malabsorption and continuous passage of oocysts.

5. Diagnostic tests

   a. Saline wet mount microscopic exam or a thin stool smear stained with modified Kinyoun stain may be used to demonstrate oocysts.

6. Treatment

   a. Trimethoprim-sulfamethoxazole (160 mg TMP–800 mg SMX) 4 times daily for 10 days then twice daily for 3 weeks.

   b. The relapse rate may be as high as 50%; some may need chronic suppressive therapy.

   c. Alternatives: Metronidazole, pyrimethamine-sulfadiazine.

L. Other selected infections occurring among HIV-infected individuals

1. Recurrent bacterial infection

   a. A number of bacterial pathogens are or have been associated with more frequent and often recurrent infections among those with HIV disease than may be noted among the general population.

   b. *Salmonella* spp. have been associated with relapsing bacteremia and GI tract disease; now seen with reduced frequency possibly related to antibacterial activity of zidovudine and other prophylactic antibiotics.

   c. *Streptococcus pneumoniae* may cause bacteremic pneumonia, meningitis, endocarditis and multiorgan system disease; morbidity and mortality appear to be higher in HIV-infected persons than in non-HIV-infected patients.

d. *Haemophilus influenzae* has been associated with pneumonia, endocarditis, and bacteremia with metastatic foci of infection.

e. *Staphylococcus aureus* bacteremia, seen particularly in those with indwelling vascular catheters, and recurrent or severe staphylococcal skin and soft tissue infections appear to occur more frequently in HIV-infected patients.

f. Bacillary Angiomatosis due to *Rochalimea* spp. (Cat scratch bacillus) infection can cause skin and mucosal lesions that may mimic Kaposi's sarcoma and may be associated with disseminated disease; or bacillary peliosis hepatis is included in the spectrum of infections caused by these organisms.

g. Other sporadic or recurrent bacterial infections due to *Nocardia*, *Legionella*, *Listeria*, *Campylobacter*, *Clostridium difficile*, and *Shigella* species have been reported.

h. Anecdotal reports suggest that pelvic inflammatory disease may be more severe and associated with more frequent complications among HIV-infected women.

2. Syphilis (See chapter on Sexually Transmitted Diseases)

3. Other viral infections

   a. Human papillomavirus (HPV): Lesions in HIV-infected patients may be large, recurrent, or refractory to therapy; HPV may be associated with anogenital intraepithelial dysplasia or carcinoma among men and with cervical intraepithelial neoplasia (CIN) or carcinoma among women with HIV infection. Intralesional or systemic alpha-interferon may be a useful alternative treatment for patients with condylomata refractory to conventional therapy. Cervical or intravaginal lesions in women may require laser or surgical ablation.

      (1) Preliminary studies suggest there may be an accelerated progression of HPV to CIN in HIV-infected women. Pap smear and exam should be done every 6 to 12 months; colposcopy may be a useful component of the exam particularly if Pap smears are abnormal.

b. The JC papovavirus is the etiologic agent of progressive multifocal leukoencephalopathy (PML). In patients with AIDS, this is usually a disease of brain parenchyma; multiple or single white matter or mass lesions are demonstrated on CT or MRI of brain and spinal cord. Clinically, patients present with mental status changes, focal neurologic deficits, seizures and/or a progressive dementia complex often indistinguishable from that caused by HIV. There is currently no effective therapy.

c. Poxviruses cause molluscum contagiosum; multiple umbilicated wartlike skin lesions, often refractory to therapy, are seen in patients with HIV infection.

d. Human T-cell lymphotropic virus types I and II (HTLV-I/II) may occur as a coinfection among HIV-infected injection drug users (IDUs); the clinical significance is as yet unknown; transmission routes are similar to those of HIV.

e. Vaccinia virus has been associated with disseminated infection after smallpox vaccine administration to HIV-infected military personnel and following the administration of an HIV vaccine prepared in incompletely neutralized vaccinia vector.

f. Adenovirus has been recovered from the stool and GI tract of patients with AIDS and diarrhea. It has also been detected in tissue samples from HIV-infected patients with interstitial pneumonitis. Its contribution as a causative agent is unclear.

4. Other Protozoan Infections

   a. *Giardia lamblia* infection may cause diarrhea, malabsorption, and weight loss; clinical responses to metronidazole therapy are generally good.

   b. Leishmaniasis has been associated with visceral disease and localized rectal disease; acquired in geographic regions where *Leishmania* are endemic.

   c. Disseminated strongyloidiasis

   d. Microsporidiosis

      (1) *Microsporidia* are coccidian protozoa reported with increasing frequency in patients with HIV infection. These protozoa have been implicated in sporadic cases of keratoconjunctivitis, hepatitis, invasive

small bowel disease with diarrhea, and myositis. Treatment trials in this population are in progress; some investigators have reported success with albendazole.

M. Neoplastic complications of AIDS

1. Kaposi's sarcoma (KS)

    a. Kaposi's sarcoma (KS) is the most common of the neoplastic complications of AIDS. Currently, it is estimated that from 15% to 20% of gay men with HIV infection have or will develop KS; KS is distinctly uncommon but occasionally occurs in HIV-infected women and children.

    b. The clinical manifestations of KS span the spectrum from localized cutaneous lesions to widespread visceral disease. Cutaneous KS is the most frequent and visible presentation, causing characteristic purple, raised or palpable, nodular skin lesions. They can occur anywhere, although most appear on the lower and upper extremities, face, and anterior and posterior trunk.

        (1) Lesions are generally painless, may begin singly but with progression multiply, coalesce into larger lesions, and occasionally will have central pallor.

        (2) Their onset may be insidious and undetected until they become larger, or more numerous, or appear in a cosmetically noticeable location. For some, cutaneous lesions rapidly progress. Mucocutaneous surfaces, such as the oral cavity and anal canal, are also common sites of involvement.

        (3) The most common sites of visceral or organ system involvement are the lung, gastrointestinal tract, lymph nodes, and liver. Symptoms of pulmonary involvement include persistent nonproductive cough and progressive dyspnea. Chest radiographs may show subtle increases in interstitial markings, nodular densities, frank interstitial infiltration, and/or pleural effusions.

        (4) Gastrointestinal tract involvement may occur at any level and may remain asymptomatic unless lesions erode mucosal surfaces and bleed or their enlarging bulk creates obstructive changes. Infiltrative KS within the gastrointestinal mucosa may cause diarrhea, malabsorption, and wasting.

    c. The diagnosis of KS is based on the appearance of the lesions and the characteristic histopathologic changes in biopsied tissue. Visceral disease generally requires biopsy confirmation; pulmonary disease may be particularly difficult to diagnose in that samples obtained by bronchoalveolar lavage may not contain abnormal cells. Transbronchial, open lung, or pleural biopsy may be necessary.

    d. Treatment of KS depends on the location and extent of disease. Isolated cutaneous disease may require no therapy if lesions are few, not rapidly progressive, and not cosmetically obvious. For large lesions or those strategically located in an area of discomfort or cosmetic concern, local irradiation may diminish the size and appearance. For more extensive or rapidly progressive cutaneous disease, systemic interferon-alpha or single agent cytotoxic chemotherapy may be beneficial. Interferon-alpha doses shown to be effective alone range from 10 million to 20 million units/d. The overall tumor response rate ranges from 40% to 60% depending on the underlying immune status of the patient; those with CD4$^+$ lymphocyte counts of greater than 400 cells/mm^3 at the initiation of therapy are likely to have more substantial and durable responses.

        (1) Zidovudine or antiretroviral therapy alone does not appear to influence the progression of KS. Interferon-alpha doses of 5 million to 10 million units/d combined with a total daily dose of 600 mg of zidovudine appeared to be relatively well tolerated and associated with substantial antitumor effect in one study.

        (2) Cytotoxic agents used as single drug therapy include adriamycin, bleomycin, VP-16, and the *Vinca rosea* alkaloids, vincristine and vinblas-

tine. Doses must be individualized; response rates vary with doses, extent of disease, and underlying host status.

(3) For those with visceral or extensive or rapidly progressive cutaneous involvement, combination chemotherapy is generally recommended. However, the myelosuppressive effect of multiple cytotoxic agents often precludes continuation of zidovudine and chemotherapeutic doses are often limited by the poor bone marrow reserve of patients with advanced HIV-related immunosuppression.

2. Non-Hodgkin's lymphoma (NHL)
   a. NHL is a neoplastic complication of HIV infection which appears to occur with increasing frequency as survival of patients with HIV disease is prolonged. While NHL is more likely to occur in patients with advanced HIV disease, it may be the initial AIDS-defining illness or HIV-related event in those with higher CD4$^+$ lymphocyte counts. The incidence is not well delineated; estimates range from 2% to 3%. Some investigators have suggested that NHL, particularly primary central nervous system lymphoma, may be a consequence of malignant transformation of EBV-infected lymphocytes.
      (1) Prolonged zidovudine use does not appear to be associated with the occurrence of NHL; the apparent increase in incidence is likely related to prolonged survival following zidovudine or antiretroviral therapy and other cofactors.
   b. The clinical presentation of NHL is dependent on the site of involvement. Central nervous system localization is a common primary site. Symptoms of headache, focal neurologic deficits, and seizures predominate. A single space occupying mass is most often seen on brain imaging studies. Without histologic confirmation, such lesions are difficult to distinguish from other mass lesions due to opportunistic infections such as toxoplasmosis, PML, or CNS tuberculosis.
      (1) Involvement of lymphoid tissue outside the central nervous system

has become increasingly more common. Gastrointestinal mass lesions, splenic disease, bone marrow infiltration, and peripheral nodal disease may produce diarrhea, abdominal pain, weight loss, splenomegaly, pancytopenia, and enlarging nodal masses, respectively.

(2) Rarely, intraoral or other mucocutaneous enlarging ulcers have been an initial manifestation of NHL in this population.

(3) Laboratory abnormalities reflect the site or sites of involvement; anemia or pancytopenia and elevated serum lactate dehydrogenase levels may be clues to the presence of bone marrow infiltration or high tumor burden.

c. The definitive diagnosis of NHL requires biopsy and histologic examination of involved tissue. Histologically, these are often high-grade, immunoblastic, or large B-cell tumors.

d. Appropriate therapy for NHL requires radiation, cytotoxic chemotherapy, or the combination of both. Consultation with an oncologist is recommended. Combinations of methotrexate, adriamycin, cyclophosphamide, vincristine, prednisone, and bleomycin (MACOP-B), and of cyclophosphamide, vincristine, methotrexate, etoposide, and cytarabine (COMET-A) have been associated with favorable initial response rates; the durability of the tumor response appears short-lived and poor marrow reserve often limits the tolerability of therapy.

3. Other neoplastic diseases
   a. Other malignancies reported among patients with HIV infection include EBV-associated Burkitt's lymphoma; malignant melanoma; peripheral T-cell lymphoma; carcinoma of the anus, rectum, cervix, or genital tract, presumably related in part to concomitant HPV or other sexually transmitted cofactors; and Hodgkin's disease.

Bibliography

Araujo FG, Huskinson J, Remington JS: Remarkable in vitro and in vivo activities of the hydroxynaphthoquinone

566C80 against tachyzoites and tissue cysts of *Toxoplasma gondii Antimicrob Agents Chemother* 35:293–299, 1991.

Bartlett JG, Feinberg J: Update on management of opportunistic infections in patients with HIV infection. *Infect Dis Clin Prac* 2:233–246, 1993.

Benson CA, Ellner JJ: *Mycobacterium avium* complex infection and AIDS: Advances in theory and practice. *Clin Infect Dis* 17:7–20, 1993.

Bermudez MA, Grant KM, Rodvien R, et al: Non-Hodgkin's lymphoma in a population with or at risk for acquired immunodeficiency syndrome: Indications for intensive chemotherapy. *Am J Med* 86:71–76, 1989.

Bozzette SA, Sattler FR, Chiu J, et al: A controlled trial of early adjunctive treatment with corticosteroids for *Pneumocystis carinii* pneumonia in the acquired immunodeficiency syndrome. *N Engl J Med* 323:1451–1457, 1990.

Centers for Disease Control and Prevention: Risk for cervical disease in HIV-infected women—New York City. *MMWR* 39:846–849, 1990.

Centers for Disease Control and Prevention: Purified protein derivative (PPD)-tuberculin anergy and HIV infection: Guidelines for anergy testing and management of anergic persons at risk of tuberculosis. *MMWR* 40:27–33, 1991.

Centers for Disease Control and Prevention: Recommendations for prophylaxis against *Pneumocystis carinii* pneumonia for adults and adolescents infected with human immunodeficiency virus. *MMWR* 41(RR-4): 1–11, 1992.

Chaisson RE, Griffin DE: Progressive multifocal leukoencephalopathy in AIDS. *JAMA* 264:79–82, 1990.

Cohn JA, McMeeking A, Cohen W, et al: Evaluation of the policy of empiric treatment of suspected *Toxoplasma* encephalitis in patients with the acquired immunodeficiency syndrome. *Am J Med* 86:521–527, 1989.

Dieterich D, Chachoua A, Lafleur F, et al: Ganciclovir treatment of gastrointestinal infections caused by cytomegalovirus in patients with AIDS. *Rev Infect Dis* 10(Suppl 3):S532–S537, 1988.

Eversole LR, Stone CE, Beckman AM: Detection of EBV and HPV DNA sequences in oral "hairy" leukoplakia by in situ hybridization. *J Med Virol* 26:271–277, 1988.

Gill PS, Rarick M, McCutchan JA, et al: Systemic treatment of AIDS-related Kaposi's sarcoma: Results of a randomized trial. *Am J Med* 90:427–433, 1991.

Goldstein JD, Dickson DW, Moser FG, et al: Primary central nervous system lymphoma in acquired immune deficiency syndrome. A clinical and pathologic study with results of treatment with radiation. *Cancer* 67:2756–2765, 1991.

Horsburgh CR Jr: *Mycobacterium avium* complex infection in the acquired immunodeficiency syndrome. *N Engl J Med* 324:1332–1338, 1991.

Jacobson MA, Cello JP, Sande MA: Cholestasis and disseminated cytomegalovirus disease in patients with the acquired immunodeficiency syndrome. *Am J Med* 84:218–224, 1988.

Jacobson MA, Mills J: Serious cytomegalovirus disease in the acquired immunodeficiency syndrome (AIDS). Clinical findings, diagnosis and treatment. *Ann Intern Med* 108:585–594, 1988.

Kaplan LD, Abrams DI, Feigel E, et al: AIDS-associated non-Hodgkin's lymphoma in San Francisco. *JAMA* 261:719–724, 1989.

Katlama C: Evaluation of the efficacy and safety of clindamycin plus pyrimethamine for induction and maintenance therapy of toxoplasmic encephalitis in AIDS. *Eur J Clin Microbiol Infect Dis* et al: 10:189–191, 1991.

Kessler HA, Bick JA, Pottage JC Jr, AIDS: Part II. Disease-a-Month 38:693–764, 1992.

Kreinik G, Burstein O, Landor M, et al: Successful management of intractable cryptosporidial diarrhea with intravenous octreotide, a somatostatin analogue. *AIDS* 5:765–767, 1991.

Krown SE: Interferon and other biologic agents for the treatment of Kaposi's sarcoma. *Hematol Oncol Clin North Am* 5:311–322, 1991.

Krumholz HM, Sande MA, Lo B: Community-acquired bacteremia in patients with acquired immunodeficiency syndrome: Clinical presentation, bacteriology, and outcome. *Am J Med* 86(6 Pt 2):776–779, 1989.

Levine B, Chaisson RE: *Mycobacterium kansasii:* A cause of treatable pulmonary disease associated with advanced human immunodeficiency virus (HIV) infection. *Ann Intern Med* 114:861–868, 1991.

Luft BJ, Remington JS: Toxoplasmic encephalitis. *J Infect Dis* 157:1–6, 1988.

Masur H and the Public Health Service Task Force on Prophylaxis and Therapy for *Mycobacterium avium* complex: Recommendations on prophylaxis and therapy for disseminated *Mycobacterium avium* complex disease in patients infected with the human immunodeficiency virus. *N Engl J Med* 329:898–904, 1993.

Medina I, Mills J, Leoung G, et al: Oral therapy for *Pneumocystis carinii* pneumonia in the acquired immunodeficiency syndrome. A controlled trial of trimethoprim-sulfamethoxazole versus trimethoprim-dapsone. *N Engl J Med* 323:776–782, 1990.

Montgomery AB: *Pneumocystis carinii* pneumonia in patients with the acquired immunodeficiency syndrome. Pathophysiology and therapy. *AIDS Clin Rev* 127–143, 1991.

National Institutes of Health—University of California Expert Panel for Corticosteroids as Adjunctive Therapy for Pneumocystis Pneumonia: Consensus statement on the use of corticosteroids as adjunctive therapy for pneumocystis pneumonia in the acquired immunodeficiency syndrome. *N Engl J Med* 323:1500–1504, 1990.

Northfelt DW, Kahn JO, Volberding PA: Treatment of AIDS-related Kaposi's sarcoma. *Hematol Oncol Clin North Am* 5:297–310, 1991.

Palefsky JM, Gonzales J, Greenblatt RM, et al: Anal intraepithelial neoplasia and anal papillomavirus infection among homosexual males with group IV HIV disease. *JAMA* 263:2911–2916, 1990.

Phair J, Munoz A, Detels R, et al: The risk of *Pneumocystis carinii* pneumonia among men infected with human immunodeficiency virus type 1. *N Engl J Med* 322:161–165, 1990.

Post MJ, Hensley GT, Moskowitz LB, et al: Cytomegalic inclusion virus encephalitis in patients with AIDS: CT, clinical and pathologic correlation. *Am J Radiol* 146:1229–1234, 1986.

Relman DA, Loutit JS, Schmidt TM, et al: The agent of

bacillary angiomatosis. An approach to the identification of uncultured pathogens. *N Engl J Med* 323:1573–1580, 1990.

Rutherford GW, Schwarcz SK, Lemp GF, et al: The epidemiology of AIDS-related Kaposi's sarcoma in San Francisco. *J Infect Dis* 159:569–572, 1989.

Safrin S, Assaykeen T, Follansbee S, et al: Foscarnet therapy for acyclovir-resistant mucocutaneous herpes simplex virus infection in 26 AIDS patients: Preliminary data. *J Infect Dis* 161:1078–1084, 1990.

Safrin S, Crumpacker C, Chatis P, et al: A controlled trial comparing foscarnet with vidarabine for acyclovir-resistant mucocutaneous herpes simplex in the acquired immunode-ficiency syndrome. The AIDS Clinical Trials Group. *N Engl J Med* 325:551–555, 1991.

Soave R, Johnson WE: *Cryptosporidium* and *Isospora belli* infections. *J Infect Dis* 157:225–229, 1988.

Studies of Ocular Complications of AIDS Research Group, in Collaboration with the AIDS Clinical Trials Group: Mortality in patients with the acquired immunodeficiency syndrome treated with either foscarnet or ganciclovir for cytomegalovirus retinitis. *N Engl J Med* 326:213–220, 1992.

Tappero JW, Mohle-Boetani J, Koehler JE, et al: The epidemiology of bacillary angiomatosis and bacillary peliosis. *JAMA* 269:770–775, 1993.

Antibacterial Agents

Catherine M. MacLeod, M.D., F.R.C.P.(C), F.A.C.P., F.C.P.

β-Lactam Antibiotics

I. Classification

All members of this group of antibiotics possess a β-lactam ring. They include oral and parenteral penicillin and cephalosporin derivatives, carbapenems, and monobactams.

A. Penicillins
1. Narrow spectrum
   a. Penicillin G—oral and parenteral
   b. Penicillin V (Pen-Vee)—oral
   c. Procaine Penicillin (Wycillin)—parenteral
   d. Benzathine Penicillin (Bicillin)—parenteral
2. Aminopenicillins
   a. Ampicillin (Omnipen)—oral and parenteral
   b. Amoxicillin (Amoxil)—oral
   c. Ampicillin-sulbactam (Unasyn)—parenteral
   d. Amoxicillin-clavulanate (Augmentin)—oral
3. Carboxypenicillins
   a. Carbenicillin indanyl (Geocillin)—oral
   b. Ticarcillin-clavulanate (Timentin)—parenteral

4. Penicillinase-resistant
   a. Cloxacillin (Tegopen)—oral
   b. Dicloxacillin (Dynapen)—oral
   c. Methicillin (Staphcillin)—parenteral
   d. Nafcillin (Unipen)—oral and parenteral
   e. Oxacillin (Prostaphlin)—oral and parenteral
5. Extended-spectrum
   a. Azlocillin (Azlin)—parenteral
   b. Mezlocillin (Mezlin)—parenteral
   c. Piperacillin (Pipracil)—parenteral
B. Cephalosporins
1. First generation
   a. Cefadroxil (Duracef)—oral
   b. Cefazolin (Ancef)—parenteral
   c. Cephalexin (Keflex)—oral
   d. Cephradine (Velocef)—oral and parenteral
2. Second generation
   a. Cefaclor (Ceclor)—oral
   b. Cefotetan (Cefotan)—parenteral
   c. Cefoxitin (Mefoxin)—parenteral
   d. Cefuroxime (Zinacef)—parenteral
   e. Cefuroxime axetil (Ceftin)—oral
3. Third generation
   a. Cefixime (Suprax)—oral

b. Cefoperazone (Cefobid)—parenteral
c. Cefotaxime (Claforan)—parenteral
d. Ceftazidime (Fortaz)—parenteral
e. Ceftriaxone (Rocephin)—parenteral

C. Monobactams
  1. Aztreonam (Azactam)—parenteral
D. Carbapenems
  1. Imipenem-cilastatin (Primaxin)—parenteral

II. Mechanism of Action and Resistance

A. β-Lactam antibiotics are usually bactericidal. Peptidoglycan, which is essential for maintaining bacterial cell shape and integrity, requires at least 30 enzymatic processes for completion. β-Lactams, as well as glycopeptides, inhibit enzymes involved in this cell wall synthesis. β-Lactams inhibit mainly the transpeptidases, but also interfere with earlier steps in the synthetic process, which causes accumulation of precursor substances having an antibacterial effect. They bind to a variety of proteins, the penicillin-binding proteins (PBP), which act as enzymes for peptidoglycan synthesis. The binding inactivates the enzyme function.

B. Resistance to β-lactams is mediated by:
  1. Inactivation of the drug prior to binding to its target PBPs by β-lactamases (e.g., ampicillin-resistant *Hemophilus influenzae*). This resistance may be overcome by the addition of β-lactamase inhibitors such as sulbactam, clavulanate, or tazobactam.
  2. Alteration of the PBPs to decrease affinity for the β-lactam (e.g., methicillin-resistant staphylococci).
  3. Alteration of the composition of the outer bacterial layer to prevent access of the drug to its binding sites (e.g., ceftazidine-resistant *Pseudomonas aeruginosa*).

III. Spectrum of Activity

A. Narrow-spectrum penicillins: Non-β-lactamase-producing gram-positive and gram-negative cocci, both aerobic and anaerobic (except enterococci); *Treponema pallidum*

B. Aminopenicillins: As for (A), plus enterococci, non-β-lactamase-producing *H. influenzae*, *Listeria monocytogenes*, some *Eschericia coli*, and *Proteus mirabilis*. Addition of β-lactamase inhibitor expands the spectrum of activity.

C. Carboxypenicillins: As for (B), plus additional Enterobacteriacreae, some non-lactose-fermenting gram-negative bacilli (at high doses); also many anaerobes.

D. Penicillinase-resistant penicillins: β-lactamase-producing gram-positive cocci, mainly aerobic.

E. Extended-spectrum penicillins: As for (C), plus additional activity against gram-negative bacilli, including *P. aeruginosa*.

F. First-generation cephalosporins: Gram-positive aerobic cocci including penicillinase-producing staphylococci, *E. coli*, *Klebsiella pneumoniae*, and other common Enterobacteriaceae.

G. Second-generation cephalosporins: As for (F), plus some extension of gram-negative aerobic spectrum and some anaerobes, including some *Bacteroides fragilis* species.

H. Third-generation cephalosporins: Greatly enhanced aerobic gram-negative bacilli spectrum, including some nonlactose fermenters; ceftazidime and cefoperazone have activity against *P. aeruginosa*, while cefoperazone and probably cefotaxime (with its active metabolite) have some anaerobic activity. There is some reduction in gram-positive activity compared to (F) or (G).

I. Monobactams (aztreonam): Aerobic gram-negative bacilli, including *P. aeruginosa*.

J. Carbapenems (imipenem-cilastatin): Greatest spectrum of activity, including gram-positive and gram-negative cocci and bacilli, as well as anaerobes; some enterococcal activity.

IV. Indications

Infections caused by organisms with known or presumed sensitivity to the chosen β-lactam. With central nervous system (CNS) infections, cephalosporins must be chosen carefully, as not all of them penetrate the brain in adequate concentrations to treat CNS infections.

V. Complications

A. CNS
  1. Excitation with a potential for seizures may occur at high doses of any β-lactam, or with therapeutic doses of imipenem, in the presence of renal failure.

B. Gastrointestinal
  1. *Clostridium difficile*-associated diarrhea is linked to the use of broad-spectrum cephalosporins.
  2. High doses of ceftriaxone may cause biliary sludge, with a syndrome resembling cholecystitis.
  3. Mild abnormalities of liver transaminases are seen with the use of β-lactams.

C. Hematologic
  1. β-Lactams infrequently cause leukopenia

from direct suppression of bone marrow white cell maturation.

2. High doses of all penicillins are associated with some degree of platelet dysfunction.

3. Cephalosporins with the methylthiotetrazole (MTT) side chain (i.e., cefoperazone, cefotetan) may be associated with hypoprothrombinemia.

D. Immunologic

1. Methicillin is associated with allergic nephritis.

2. Approximately 5% of patients who receive β-lactams develop a morbilliform skin eruption. This is not IgE mediated and may subside with continued administration. In some patients, this morbilliform eruption may progress to toxic epidermal necrolysis.

3. Fever may be associated with administration of any β-lactam and is particularly frequent during the third or fourth week of prolonged therapy.

4. IgE-mediated reactions, including urticaria, wheezing, and hypotension, occur within minutes of β-lactam administration. These reactions generally preclude administration of any β-lactam.

5. Almost all patients with infectious mononucleosis who receive ampicillin develop a morbilliform skin rash.

E. Sodium and potassium imbalance

1. Many β-lactams are administered parenterally as sodium salts. The administration of ticarcillin (~5 mg Na$^+$/per gram of ticarcillin) may be associated with a significant sodium load and may exacerbate congestive heart failure or hypokalemia.

VI. **Interactions**

A. Penicillins should not be mixed with aminoglycosides.

B. Allopurinol and ampicillin.

C. Cephalosporins which possess the MTT side chain are associated with an Antabuse-like reaction with concomitant use of alcohol.

VII. **Contraindications**

A. All β-lactams except aztreonam are contraindicated in any patient with an IgE-mediated reaction to any penicillin, cephalosporin, or carbapenem.

B. Procaine penicillin is contraindicated in patients with an allergic reaction to local anesthetics.

C. Imipenem is contraindicated in patients with seizure disorders.

Aminocyclitols

I. **Classification**

A. Aminoglycosides

1. Streptomycin

2. Gentamicin (Garamycin)

3. Tobramycin (Nebcin)

4. Amikacin (Amikin)

5. Netilmicin (Netromycin)

6. Neomycin

B. Spectinomycin (Trobicin)

II. **Mechanism of Action and Resistance**

A. The aminocyclitols all bind to ribosomes to inhibit protein synthesis and are bactericidal.

B. 1. Resistance to streptomycin is primarily mediated by changes in the 12S segment of the 30S subunit to prevent binding of streptomycin.

2. Conjugation of aminoglycosides to inactive substances by enzymes produced by plasmid-encoded genes is the most common mechanism of resistance. Acetylation, adenylation, and phosphorylation enzymes have been identified in resistant bacteria.

III. **Spectrum of Activity**

A. Gentamicin, tobramycin, amikacin, and netilmicin are active against most aerobic, gram-negative bacilli.

B. Streptococci and anaerobic organisms are resistant to aminoglycosides.

C. Spectinomycin is active against *Neisseria gonorrhoeae*.

IV. **Indications**

A. Streptomycin

1. Therapy for *Mycobacterium tuberculosis*.

2. In combination with penicillin for therapy and prophylaxis of endocarditis caused by *Enterococcus faecalis* and *Streptococcus viridans*.

3. Alternate therapy for infections caused by *Brucella* species.

4. Therapy for infections with *Francisella tularensis* and *Yersinia pestis*.

B. Neomycin

1. Preoperative oral administration to decrease bowel flora in gastrointestinal surgery.

C. Gentamicin, tobramycin, netilmicin, and amikacin are used as therapy for susceptible gram-negative infections. Gentamicin may be used as adjunctive therapy in the treatment of staphylococcal endocarditis.

D. Spectinomycin

1. Treatment of *N. gonorrhoeae* infections in

patients allergic to β-lactams or with resistant organisms.

  a. Single-dose therapy for uncomplicated infections or 3-day therapy with twice-a-day injections for disseminated infections is effective.

  b. Not effective against pharyngeal gonococcal infections, syphilis, or *Chlamydia trachomatis*.

V. Complications
A. Aminoglycosides
1. Central nervous system
  a. Ototoxicity, both auditory and vestibular neuritis.
  b. Neuromuscular blockage by interference with blockade of release of acetylcholine and postsynaptic blockade of acetylcholine receptors.
2. Nephrotoxicity is similar to that of acute tubular necrosis and is reversible.
3. Allergic reactions are very unusual and are almost always due to another medication.
B. Spectinomycin
1. Central nervous system: Dizziness.
2. Other: Pain at the infection site.

VI. Contraindications
Although extremely unusual, previous significant allergic reactions to any aminoglycoside preclude subsequent use.

Fluoroquinolones

I. Classification
A. All antibiotics have a fluorine atom on position 6 of the quinolone ring.
1. Ciprofloxacin (Cipro)—oral and parenteral
2. Norfloxacin (Noroxin)—oral
3. Ofloxacin (Floxin)—oral and parenteral

II. Mechanism of Action and Resistance
A. The bactericidal activity of the fluoroquinolones is from the inhibition of DNA gyrase in bacterial cells. DNA synthesis and cell division are decreased, and certain proteins associated with the "SOS" response are generated; these proteins may have lethal effects on the bacterial cell. The SOS response is a complex cascade of gene activations resulting from damage to or inhibition of DNA.
B. Resistance to fluoroquinolones can occur during therapy, particularly with infections

due to *P. aeruginosa* and *Staphylococcus aureus*. Resistance occurs through mutation of the gene coding for DNA gyrase, causing decreased binding affinity for the quinolone–DNA complex binding. Decreased bacterial cell penetrability has also been seen.

III. Spectrum of Activity
These antibiotics have broad-spectrum capabilities against most gram-negative aerobic organisms, including nonlactose fermenters like *P. aeruginosa*, staphylococci, some streptococci, and some unusual organisms such as mycobacteria, *Chlamydia, Mycoplasma, Legionella, Rickettsia,* and *Coxiella.* Enterococci are not affected, and *Streptococcus pneumoniae* is variably affected.

IV. Indications
Because of good penetration into tissues including the prostate, biliary system, bone, joint spaces, upper and lower respiratory tracts, and soft tissues, infections at these sites caused by susceptible organisms may be treated with this group of drugs.

V. Complications
A. CNS: Increase in excitatory impulses, causing agitation, restlessness, bad dreams, hallucinations, psychosis, and seizures.
B. Gastrointestinal: Nausea, vomiting, diarrhea.
C. Other: Arthralgias.

VI. Contraindications
A. Caution should be used in treating infections with fluoroquinolones in patients with CNS disorders such as seizures.
B. Children under 12 years of age should avoid taking these drugs because of the possible damage to cartilage.

Macrolide Antibiotics

I. Classification
A. Azithromycin (Zithromax)—oral
B. Clarithromycin (Biaxin)—oral
C. Erythromycin (E.E.S., E-Mycin, Ilosone)—oral and parenteral

II. Mechanism of Action and Resistance
A. The macrolides bind tightly to the 50S ribosomal subunit of susceptible bacteria to inhibit ribosome-dependent protein synthesis. The action may be bacteriostatic or bactericidal, depending on the organism.
B. Resistance to macrolides results from:
1. Decreased permeability through the bacterial cell envelope.
2. Altered target site on the ribosome.

3. Inactivation by esterases produced mainly by the Enterobacteriaceae.

III. Spectrum of Activity

Most common gram-positive cocci including β-lactamase-producing staphylococci, some gram-negative rods such as *Hemophilus* and *Legionella* species, gram-negative cocci such as *Neisseria* and *Moraxella*, many anaerobes including *Bacteroides* species, *Mycoplasma pneumoniae*, and for the newer agents, *Chlamydia* species, some atypical mycobacteria, and *Toxoplasma*.

IV. Indications

A. Newer macrolides (clarithromycin and azithromycin) have been shown to be more acid stable, resulting in better and more predictable absorption and possibly decreased gastrointestinal effects, longer duration of action, higher tissue concentrations (except in cerebrospinal fluid), and an improved safety profile.

B. Clinical indications
1. Upper and lower respiratory tract infections caused by susceptible organisms.
2. Sexually transmitted infections.
3. Community-acquired skin and soft tissue infections.

V. Complications

A. Central nervous system
1. Ototoxicity, mainly auditory, with large IV doses of erythromycin lactobionate or with very large and prolonged oral dosing in patients with renal failure.

B. Gastrointestinal
1. Abdominal cramping and discomfort, diarrhea, nausea, and vomiting, mainly with erythromycin from its motilin action.
2. Cholestatic jaundice with erythromycin estolate.

C. Other
1. Phlebitis at the site of IV infection.

VI. Contraindications

A. Previous significant hypersensitivity reactions to macrolides.

B. Caution needed in treating patients with renal impairment when large doses are required.

Glycopeptides

I. Classification

Vancomycin is a glycopeptide that is unique among the currently available antimicrobials.

A. Vancomycin (Vancocin)—(oral) parenteral

II. Mechanism of Action and Resistance

A. Vancomycin is bactericidal against most susceptible organisms except *Enterococcus faecium* and *E. faecalis*. It inhibits synthesis of the bacterial cell wall by binding with important precursors.

B. Resistance to vancomycin among gram-positive cocci is extremely rare. Recently, vancomycin-resistant enterococci have been described.

III. Spectrum of Activity

A. Gram-positive aerobic and anaerobic bacteria.

IV. Indications

A variety of gram-positive organisms are susceptible to vancomycin but are often amenable to less costly antimicrobial therapy. Some indications for the use of this agent include:

A. Therapy for methicillin-resistant staphylococci
1. Vancomycin is the agent of choice for these infections.
2. Treatment for enterococcal endocarditis
3. This drug offers a therapeutic option for patients who are penicillin allergic.
4. In addition to vancomycin, an aminoglycoside must be administered for predictable cidal activity in this setting.

B. Treatment for *C. difficile* colitis
1. Metronidazole therapy is less expensive, but oral vancomycin is preferred in more severely compromised patients.

C. Therapy for *Corynebacterium* JK bacillus bacteremia
1. This organism has been reported to cause sepsis in patients with underlying neoplastic disease, neutropenia, and prolonged antimicrobial therapy. It is often susceptible only to vancomycin.

V. Complications

Reactions to vancomycin may be local or systemic and include the following:

A. Histamine related
1. If the drug is given rapidly, a rash and hypotension may ensue. This "red neck" syndrome can usually be overcome by slowing the infusion rate or by administering an antihistamine.

B. Ototoxicity
1. This is an unusual problem if serum levels of vancomycin are monitored. The defect can be permanent and may be potentiated by other ototoxic agents (aminoglycosides, erythromycin, furosemide).

C. Hematologic

1. Leukopenia occurs in approximately 2% of patients.

VI. Interactions

When vancomycin is used with other nephrotoxic agents, such as aminoglycosides, the potential for renal toxicity is increased.

VII. Contraindications

There is a significant, verified allergic reaction to vancomycin.

Tetracyclines

I. Classification
   A. Short-acting
      1. Oxytetracycline (Terramycin)—oral and parenteral
      2. Tetracycline (Achromycin)—oral and parenteral
   B. Long-acting
      1. Doxycycline (Vibramycin)—oral and parenteral
      2. Minocycline (Minocin)—oral and parenteral

II. Mechanism of Action and Resistance
   A. At clinically useful blood concentrations, the tetracyclines are bacteriostatic. These antibiotics bind in a reversible manner to the 30S ribosomal subunit of susceptible organisms to block binding of aminoacyl-tRNA to the acceptor site on the mRNA–ribosome complex. Bacterial protein synthesis is thus inhibited.
   B. Resistance, both plasmid mediated and inducible, causes decreased transport of tetracyclines across bacterial cell membranes.

III. Spectrum of Activity

These antibiotics inhibit a wide variety of grampositive and gram-negative aerobes and anaerobes, both cocci and bacilli. *Chlamydia, Rickettsia, Coxiella burnetii, Mycoplasma* species, *Ureaplasma* species, and *atypical* Mycobacteria are also inhibited.

IV. Indications

Tetracyclines penetrate and accumulate in tissues and cells and have broad activity. They are used to treat a wide variety of sites, including eye, sinuses, bronchial mucosa, gingiva, cervix, prostate, and cerebrospinal fluid. However, their bacteriostatic activity and ease of development of resistance lessen their usefulness in most severe infections.

V. Complications
   A. Central nervous system: Dizziness, lightheadedness, unsteadiness, and vertigo are most

frequently seen with minocycline but occur with all agents.
   B. Gastrointestinal
      1. Nausea, vomiting, and epigastric distress are frequent.
      2. Esophageal ulcerations may occur if insufficient fluid is ingested to allow passage through the esophagus.
      3. Diarrhea.
      4. Hepatotoxicity, particularly in pregnancy or in renal dysfunction.
      5. Rarely, pancreatitis.
   C. Genitourinary
      1. Diuresis, particularly with demeclocycline.
      2. Nephrogenic diabetes insipidus.
      3. Increased azotemia or renal dysfunction from a catabolic state.
   D. Photosensitivity occurs in approximately 1% of patients who take doxycycline.
   E. Allergic reactions are rare but include morbilliform rashes to anaphylaxis.
   F. Superinfections, particularly with *Candida* species, such as vaginal and oral candidiasis, can occur.
   G. Staining of teeth can occur in children when used during the mother's pregnancy or in children under the age of 8 years.

VI. Contraindications
   A. Doxycycline and minocycline should be used cautiously in patients with hepatic function impairment.
   B. Tetracyclines other than doxycycline and minocycline should not be used in renal function impairment.
   C. Because intramuscular preparations of tetracyclines contain local anesthetics, this route should not be used in patients who are allergic to local anesthetics.

Folic Acid Metabolism Antagonists

I. Classification
   A. Sulfonamides
      1. Sulfadiazine—oral
      2. Sulfamethoxazole (Gantanol)—oral
      3. Sulfisoxazole (Gantrisin)—oral
   B. Others
      1. Trimethoprim (Proloprim)—oral
      2. Pyrimethamine (Daraprim)—oral
   C. Combinations
      1. Trimethoprim-sulfamethoxazole (Bactrim)—oral and parenteral

2. Pyrimethamine-sulfadoxine (Fansidar)—oral

II. Mechanism of Action and Resistance

A. Mechanism of Action

1. The sulfonamides are structurally similar to para-aminobenzoic acid (PABA), which is an essential precursor for bacterial synthesis of folic acid. Bacteria cannot utilize environmental folic acid. Sulfonamides competitively inhibit the enzyme dihydropteroate synthetase, which incorporates PABA into dihydropteroic acid. This latter compound is normally converted to folic acid in the bacterial cell. With decreased folic acid synthesis, nucleotide formation is decreased and bacterial growth is inhibited. These actions are bacteriostatic.

2. Trimethoprim and pyrimethamine also act on the folic acid metabolic pathway of bacteria, but at a different enzymatic step. They reversibly inhibit the enzyme dihydrofolate reductase. This action is bacteriostatic.

3. The combination of trimethoprim or pyrimethamine with a sulfonamide is bactericidal against a wide variety of organisms, both bacterial and protozoan. The combinations are synergistic in inhibiting different enzymes of the folic acid metabolic pathway.

B. Resistance: Plasmid-mediated resistance results in altered enzyme affinity and decreased bacterial cell permeability to sulfonamides. Resistance to trimethoprim is caused by changes in dihydrofolate reductase.

III. Spectrum of Activity

The combination of trimethoprim with sulfamethoxazole provides activity against most common aerobic, gram-positive and gram-negative organisms, as well as *Listeria monocytogenes*, *Nocardia*, *Moraxella catarrhalis*, *Hemophilus* species, and *Pneumocystis carinii*. Pyrimethamine with sulfadoxine is active against *Toxoplasma gondii* and *Plasmodium falciparum*.

IV. Indications

Because of the very wide distribution of these antibiotics into tissues and cells, including brain, cerebrospinal fluid, prostate, joint fluid, pleural fluid, and bronchial secretions, they are used to treat many infections, particularly when bactericidal combinations are used. The combinations also decrease the development of resistance to sulfonamides.

V. Complications

A. Sulfonamides

1. Gastrointestinal
   a. Nausea, vomiting.
   b. Hepatotoxicity.

2. Genitourinary: Crystalluria.

3. Hematologic
   a. Acute hemolysis occurs in patients with glucose-6-phosphate dehydrogenase (G6PD) deficiency when they receive certain sulfonamide preparations but not sulfamethoxazole.
   b. Leukopenia, thrombocytopenia, and anemia, which are reversible, may occur in patients with acquired immunodeficiency syndrome and in patients with limited bone marrow reserves.

4. Immunologic
   a. Erythema nodosum.
   b. Erythema multiforme, including Stevens-Johnson syndrome and toxic epidermal necrolysis. This is particularly associated with the use of a combination of pyrimethamine and sulfadoxine.
   c. Serum sickness.
   d. Vasculitis of the periarteritis type.

B. Trimethoprim

1. Central nervous system: Headache, depression, hallucinations, aseptic meningitis.

2. Gastrointestinal
   a. Anorexia, nausea, vomiting.
   b. Unusual taste.
   c. Cholestatic jaundice.

3. Hematologic: Blood dyscrasias.

4. Immunologic: Skin rashes.

C. Trimethoprim-sulfamethoxazole (cotrimoxazole): All the complications of the separate components alone are seen, but the incidence of skin reactions is greater than with either agent alone.

D. Pyrimethamine: Generally well tolerated except for occasional skin rashes and depression of hematopoiesis. May produce a megaloblastic anemia which responds to folinic acid.

VI. Contraindications

A. Sulfonamides: A history of hypersensitivity reactions to previous sulfonamide or sulfa-like drugs (such as furosemide, thiazide-type diuretics, oral hypoglycemic agents, carbonic anhydrase inhibitors, and sulfa-containing topical preparations) is a contraindication to sulfonamide use.

B. Trimethoprim: Patients with a history of hypersensitivity to trimethoprim or who are folate deficient should not receive this medication.

C. Trimethoprim-sulfamethoxazole: Patients should not receive this combination if there are any contraindications to either trimethoprim or sulfamethoxazole.

Other Antibiotics

I. Classification
A. Chloramphenicol (Chloromycetin)—oral and parenteral
B. Clindamycin (Cleocin)—oral and parenteral
C. Metronidazole (Flagyl)—oral and parenteral

II. Mechanism of Action and Resistance
A. Chloramphenicol
   1. Chloramphenicol is bacteriostatic; it inhibits protein synthesis in susceptible organisms by binding to the 50S subunit of the 70S ribosome.
   2. The most common mechanism for resistance is plasmid-mediated or inducible production of specific acetyltransferase enzymes which acetylate chloramphenicol.
B. Clindamycin
   1. Clindamycin binds to the 50S ribosomal subunit of susceptible bacteria at a site overlapping the binding sites of chloramphenicol and erythromycin, and is usually bacteriostatic.
   2. Resistance to clindamycin is most often the result of an altered 50S ribosomal subunit structure, which diminishes binding.
C. Metronidazole
   1. Under anaerobic conditions, metronidazole is reduced to the active metabolite, which forms cytotoxic products; these products inhibit nucleic acid synthesis. Metronidazole is bactericidal.
   2. Resistance is intrinsic to aerobic organisms in which metronidazole does not undergo reduction. Development of resistance in anaerobic organisms is uncommon but results from decreased uptake of the drug.

III. Indications
All three of these drugs are active against anaerobic pathogens, with metronidazole being the most active. Both chloramphenicol and metronidazole penetrate well into all tissues, including the central nervous system and cerebrospinal fluid; clindamycin does not achieve adequate concentrations in the cerebrospinal fluid.

Because of its potential to cause severe adverse effects, chloramphenicol is used only as an alternative agent in a variety of infections caused by susceptible organisms. Clindamycin has been useful in infections caused by mixed aerobic, gram-positive coccal and anaerobic bacterial infections. It may be of value against a variety of aerobic protozoan infections. Metronidazole is active only against anaerobic organisms, both bacterial and protozoan.

A. Chloramphenicol is indicated in the treatment of meningitis and anaerobic infections.
   1. Gram-positive: *Streptococcus pneumoniae*, *Listeria*.
   2. Gram-negative: Enterobacteriaceae, *N. meningitidis*, *H. influenzae*.
   3. Others: Anaerobes, spirochetes, *Rickettsiae*, *Chlamydiae*, *Mycoplasma*.
B. Clindamycin is indicated in the treatment of susceptible gram-positive infections and in combination with a broad-spectrum, gram-negative antibiotic in the treatment of mixed anaerobic and aerobic infections.
   1. Gram-positive: Staphylococci and streptococci.
   2. Anaerobe: *Bacteroides*.
   3. Others: *Toxoplasma*, *Pneumocystis*.
C. Metronidazole is indicated for anaerobic infections below the diaphragm.
   1. Bacterial: Anaerobic gram-negative rods.
   2. Protozoan: *Giardia*, *Entamoeba histolytica*.

IV. Complications
A. Chloramphenicol
   1. Central nervous system: Confusion, delirium, headache.
   2. Cardiovascular: Cardiomyopathy.
   3. Gastrointestinal: Nausea, vomiting, diarrhea, glossitis, stomatitis (generally mild).
   4. Hematologic
      a. Decreased bone marrow function from its effect on mitochondrial ribosomes, which is reversible.
      b. Aplastic anemia, possibly from initial gastrointestinal flora metabolism of drug to a precursor substance, which is further metabolized in the liver and/or bone marrow to a metabolite lethal to stem cells.
   5. Immune reactions
      a. Fever, skin rashes, anaphylaxis.
      b. Herxheimer reaction when used in the treatment of syphilis, brucellosis, and typhoid fever.

B. Clindamycin
1. Gastrointestinal
a. Pseudomembranous enterocolitis.
b. Nonspecific diarrhea, nausea, vomiting, abdominal discomfort.
2. Immune: Skin rashes, urticaria.
C. Metronidazole
1. Central nervous system
a. Seizures.
b. Dizziness, lightheadedness, vertigo.
c. Peripheral neuropathy.
2. Gastrointestinal
a. Anorexia, nausea, vomiting, abdominal discomfort.
b. Glossitis, stomatitis, dry mouth, metallic taste.
3. Hematologic: Leukopenia.

V. **Contraindications**
A. Chloramphenicol: Patients with a prior significant toxic or allergic reaction to chloramphenicol or with concurrent bone marrow depression should not receive chloramphenicol.

B. Clindamycin: Patients with significant intestinal dysfunction, particularly associated with diarrhea, should be given clindamycin with caution.
C. Metronidazole: Patients with a prior adverse reaction to metronidazole should not be given this drug.

Bibliography

Evans WE, Schentaq JJ & Jusko WJ. (editors) Applied Pharmacokinetics—Principles of Therapeutic Drug Monitoring—2nd edition. Applied Therapeutics, Inc., Spokane, WA 1986.

Gilman AG, Rall TW, Nies AS, Taylor P, eds. *Goodman and Gilman's The Pharmacological Basis of Therapeutics*, ed 8. New York, McGraw-Hill, Inc., 1990.

The Medical Letter 32:41–48, 1990.

Mandell GL, Douglas RG, Bennett JE, eds. *Principles and Practice of Infectious Diseases*, ed 3. New York, Churchill Livingstone, 1990.

USP Drug Information, ed 13. Rockville, Md., United States Pharmacopeial Convention, 1993.

Table 52A-1. Drug Interactions of Antibacterial Agents

Drug	Interacting Drug	Effect	Mechanism
β-Lactams			
Penicillins (high IV doses)	Aminoglycosides	↓ effect of aminoglycoside	Inactivation of aminoglycoside when admixed in same bag
Penicillins (all)	? Chloramphenicol, tetracyclines	? ↓ effect of penicillins	Possible antagonism of bacteriostatic and bactericidal agents
	Drugs causing ↓ K⁺	↓ K⁺	Na⁺ load of salts of penicillins ↑ renal K⁺ loss ↓ renal excretion
	Methotrexate	↑ methotrexate toxicity	
	Anticoagulants (oral) (IV) Aspirin Nonsteroidal anti-inflammatory drugs (NSAIDs) Thrombolytic agents	↑ bleeding tendency	Antiplatelet effect of high penicillin doses additive to bleeding effects of other agents
Ampicillin	Hepatotoxic medications	↑ risk of hepatotoxicity	Additive
Nafcillin	Allopurinol	↑ risk skin rash	Unknown
	Anticoagulants, oral	↓ anticoagulant effect	↑ metabolism
Cefoperazone and cefotetan	Alcohol-containing preparations	Disulfiram reaction	N-methyl thiotrazole (MTT) side chain inhibits acetaldehyde dehydrogenase
	Anticoagulants (all), thrombolytic agents, aspirin and NSAIDs	↑ risk of bleeding	MTT side chain interferes with vitamin K–dependent cofactors
Imipenemcilastatin	CNS stimulants	↑ risk of seizures	Risk of additive neurotoxicity
Aminocyclitols			
Gentamicin (and other aminoglycosides)	Amphotericin B	↑ blood gentamicin	↓ renal excretion
	Cisplatin	↑ nephrotoxicity	Additive
	Cyclosporine	↑ nephrotoxicity	Additive
	Loop diuretics	↑ nephrotoxicity	Additive
	? Ketorolac/other NSAIDs	↑ nephro/ototoxicity	Additive
		↑ aminoglycoside levels	↓ renal excretion
	Magnesium sulfate	↑ neuromuscular block	Additive
	Neuromuscular blockers	↑ neuromuscular block	Additive
	Ticarcillin/carbenicillin	↓ aminoglycoside effect	Inactivation of aminoglycosides by penicillins
Spectinomycin	Vancomycin	↑ nephro/ototoxicity	Additive
	Lithium	↑ lithium toxicity	↓ renal clearance

642

	Interacting drug	Effect	Mechanism
Fluoroquinolones			
Ciprofloxacin	Carbamazepine	↑ carbamazepine levels	↑ metabolism
	Theophylline	↑ theophylline levels	↑ metabolism
	Drugs metabolized by microsomal P$_{450}$ system of liver	Possible ↑ effect and/or toxicity of interacting drug	↑ metabolism
	Anticoagulants, oral	↑ anticoagulation	↑ metabolism
	Caffeine	↑ caffeine toxicity	↑ metabolism
	Cyclosporine	↑ risk of neurotoxicity	↑ metabolism
	Probenecid	↑ ciprofloxacin blood levels	↑ excretion
	? CNS stimulants	↑ CNS toxicity	Additive
Macrolides			
Erythromycin	Alfentanil	↑ duration of action of alfentanil	↑ metabolism
	Anticoagulants, oral	↑ anticoagulant effect	↑ metabolism
	Carbamazepine	↑ carbamazepine effect	↑ metabolism
	Chloramphenicol/clindamycin	↑ effect of chloramphenicol/clindamycin	Competition for binding sites on bacterial ribosome
	Cyclosporine	↑ cyclosporine levels	↑ metabolism
	Digoxin	↑ dogoxin effect	↑ gut metabolism of digoxin
	Ergotamine	↑ vasospasm	↑ metabolism
	Phenytoin	possible ↑ phenytoin effect	↑ metabolism
	Theophylline	↑ risk of theophylline toxicity	↑ metabolism
Glycopeptides			
Vancomycin	Aminoglycosides	↑ levels of vancomycin and aminoglycosides	Interference with renal excretion
		↑ oto/nephrotoxicity	Additive
	Amphotericin B	↑ levels of vancomycin	↓ renal excretion
		↑ risk of nephrotoxicity	Additive
	Cisplatin	↑ oto-/nephrotoxicity	Additive
	Corticosteroids	Inactivation of vancomycin	Physical incompatibility if admixed
	Cyclosporine	↑ risk of nephrotoxicity	Additive
	H$_1$-blocking agents	↓ symptoms of ototoxicity	Masking of tinnitus/vertigo
	Heparin, if admixed with vancomycin	Inactivation	Physical incompatibility

(continued)

Table 52A-1. Continued

Drug	Interacting Drug	Effect	Mechanism
Tetracyclines			
Tetracyclines (All)	Loop diuretics	↑ oto/nephrotoxicity	Additive
	Methicillin, if admixed	Inactivation of vancomycin	Physical incompatibility
	Antacids	↓ tetracycline effect	↓ oral absorption
	Anticoagulants, oral	↑ anticoagulation	Unknown
	Bismuth subsalicylate	↓ tetracycline effect	↓ oral absorption
	Cholestyramine and colestipol	↓ tetracycline effect	↓ absorption
	Contraceptives, oral	↓ contraception	↓ enterohepatic circulation
	Digoxin	↑ digoxin effect	↓ gut metabolism and absorption
	Heparin	↓ anticoagulation	Unknown
	Iron preparations	↓ tetracycline effect	↓ absorption
	Lithium	↑ lithium toxicity	↓ renal excretion
	Methotrexate	↑ methotrexate effect	Binding displacement
	Methoxyflurane	↑ risk of nephrotoxicity	Additive
	Zinc	↓ tetracycline effect	↓ absorption
Doxycycline	Alcohol	↓ doxycycline effect	↑ metabolism
	Barbituates	↓ doxycycline effect	↑ metabolism
	Carbamazepine	↓ doxycycline effect	↑ metabolism
	Phenytoin	↓ doxycycline effect	↑ metabolism
Minocycline	Tricyclic antidepressants	Local hemosiderosis	Synergism
Folic Acid Metabolism Antagonists			
Sulfonamides	Anticoagulants, oral	↑ anticoagulation	↓ metabolism
	Hypoglycemics, oral	↑ hypoglycemia	↓ metabolism
	Methotrexate	↑ methotrexate toxicity	↓ metabolism
	Monoamine oxidase inhibitors (MAOI)	↑ MAOI effect	↓ metabolism
	Phenytoin	↑ phenytoin levels	↓ metabolism
	Barbiturates	↑ sedation	↑ protein binding
	Cyclosporine	↓ effect of cyclosporine	↑ metabolism
	Local anesthetics (ester type)	↓ antibacterial effect	↑ PABA
Trimethoprim	Dapsone	↑ dapsone and trimethoprim levels	↓ metabolism and renal excretion
	Digoxin	↑ digoxin effect	↓ renal excretion
	Bone marrow–suppressing drugs	↑ leukopenia/thrombocytopenia	Additive
Pyrimethamine	Other folate antagonists	Megaloblastic anemia	Additive

Other Antibiotics	Interacting Drug	Effect	Mechanism
Chloramphenicol	Acetaminophen	↓ chloramphenicol toxicity	↓ metabolism
	Anticoagulants, oral Hypoglycemics, oral Anticonvulsants Anesthetics, IV	↑ effect of each interacting drug	↓ metabolism
Clindamycin	Antidiarrheal agents	↓ absorption	↓ absorption
	Chloramphenicol/erythromycin	↓ antimicrobial effect and ↑ GI toxicity from pseudomembraneous enterocolitis	Competition for binding sites
	Neuromuscular blockers	↑ neuromuscular blocks	Additive
	Opioid analgesics	↓ respiration	Additive and peripheral effects
Metronidazole	Alcohol	Disulfiram reaction ↑ acetaldehyde	↑ acetaldehyde
	Anticoagulants, oral Hypoglycemics Anticonvulsants	↑ effect of each interacting drug	↓ metabolism

CHAPTER 52-B

Antiviral Agents

Harold A. Kessler, M.D.

Amantadine/Rimantadine

I. **Classification**
Symmetric primary amine molecule.
II. **Mechanism of Action**
Interferes with penetration and/or uncoating of the influenza A virus nucleocapsid intracellularly.
III. **Indications**
   A. Active only against influenza A virus. Has no activity against influenza B.
   B. Prophylaxis against influenza A virus is approximately 70–90% effective.
      1. Should be used in conjunction with immunization in influenza A outbreaks among patients at high risk of adverse outcomes associated with influenza A infection.
      2. Amantadine should be utilized for 2 weeks following immunization, the time necessary for the maturation of the immune response to the vaccine.
      3. Treatment of acute influenza A infection if used in the early stages of infection (within 24–48 hr of onset of symptoms).
         a. Therapy of influenza A pneumonia is unproven.
IV. **Interactions**

Concomitant administration of antihistamines may increase central nervous system (CNS) side effects.
V. **Complications**
   A. Blood levels >1 μg/ml associated with CNS side effects including insomnia, confusion, poor concentration, nervousness, hallucinations, and depression.
   B. Additional side effects include anorexia, nausea, vomiting, blurred vision, and orthostatic hypotension.
   C. Rare side effects include seizures, leukopenia, and neutropenia.
VI. **Contraindications**
   A. Relative contraindications include a history of seizures or psychosis.
   B. Individuals such as airline pilots, bus drivers, and train engineers due to possible impairment of sustained concentration.

Ribavirin

I. **Classification**
Synthetic triazole nucleoside analog structurally related to guanosine and inosine.

II. Mechanism of Action
A. Not clearly established but appears to inhibit inosine monophosphate dehydrogenase, a critical enzyme in DNA synthesis.
B. May also cause depletion of intracellular purines such as guanosine triphosphate, which results in inhibition of RNA synthesis.

III. Indications
A. Severe respiratory syncytial virus infections in children and adults.
B. Some studies have suggested activity in influenza A and B.
C. Lassa fever virus infection.
D. Some reports of efficacy in treating severe measles infections.

IV. Interactions
May inhibit phosphorylation of zidovudine.

V. Complications
A. Hemolytic anemia with systemic administration.
B. Nausea, lethargy, headache, and increased serum bilirubin and uric acid levels have been reported after oral administration.

VI. Contraindications
A. Drug is teratogenic, mutagenic, embryotoxic, and gonadotoxic in small nonprimate animals.
B. Use in pregnancy contraindicated.
C. Health care workers exposed to the aerosol have had the drug detected in their erythrocytes.
D. Environmental exposure of health care workers should be limited.

Acyclovir (ACV)

I. Classification
Acyclic nucleoside analog of guanine.

II. Mechanism of Action
A. ACV is triphosphorylated intracellularly to its active triphosphate compound, ACV-TP.
  1. The initial phosphorylation step is dependent upon a virus-specific thymidine kinase enzyme.
  2. Di- and triphosphorylation are catalyzed by cellular kinase enzymes.
  3. The virus-dependent monophosphorylation requirement of ACV results in a high degree of selectivity for virus-infected cells.
B. ACV-TP is a potent inhibitor of viral DNA polymerase.

C. ACV-TP also is incorporated into viral DNA and results in DNA chain termination.

III. Indications
A. ACV is effective in the treatment of herpes simplex virus (HSV) and varicella-zoster virus (VZV) infections.
B. ACV is active in vitro against Epstein-Barr virus but has not shown efficacy in the treatment of acute infectious mononucleosis.
C. ACV is effective in suppression of frequently recurrent orolabial and genital herpes simplex virus infections.
D. ACV in high doses has been shown to protect against cytomegalovirus (CMV) disease in bone marrow and solid organ transplant patients in the immediate posttransplant period.

IV. Complications
A. Phlebitis when administered intravenously.
B. Reversible nephrotoxicity when given intravenously in high doses or to a dehydrated patient due to crystallization of drug in renal tubules.
C. Neurotoxicity manifesting as confusion, delirium, lethargy, tremors, seizures, and/or coma has been reported in ~1% of patients and correlates with serum concentrations >25 μg/ml.
D. Nausea, vomiting, lightheadedness, diaphoresis, and rash have also been reported.
E. ACV-resistant mutants (both HSV and VZV) causing clinical disease have been described in immunocompromised hosts.

V. Contraindications
A. No absolute contraindications unless hypersensitivity has been previously documented.
B. The drug has not been shown to be teratogenic or carcinogenic and was not mutagenic in several test systems.
C. Use during pregnancy is not approved, but pregnant women treated unknowingly during the early stages of pregnancy have not given birth to children with any specific abnormalities.

Ganciclovir (GCV)

I. Classification
Acyclic nucleoside analog of guanine.

II. Mechanism of Action
A. GCV is triphosphorylated intracellularly to its active compound, GCV-TP.

1. Host cellular kinases, as well as herpes-specific viral thymidine kinase, will initially phosphorylate the molecule to GCV-MP.

B. GCV-TP is a potent inhibitor of viral DNA polymerase.

C. GCV-TP is also incorporated into viral DNA and results in DNA chain termination.

III. Indications

A. GCV is 10 times more active in vitro against CMV and Epstein-Barr virus than ACV.

B. GCV has the same in vitro potency as ACV against HSV and VZV and is also active against human herpesvirus type 6.

C. The only approved clinical indication currently is for the treatment and suppression of CMV retinitis in patients with acquired immunodeficiency syndrome (AIDS).

D. GCV has been shown to be effective in the treatment of other types of CMV disease in highly immunocompromised patients.

E. GCV has also recently been shown to have efficacy in the prophylaxis of CMV disease in immunocompromised patients, such as transplant recipients, at high risk of CMV disease.

IV. Interactions

A. Concomitant administration of other bone marrow suppressive drugs is relatively contraindicated and should be used with extreme caution.

V. Complications

A. Bone marrow suppression, in particular neutropenia and thrombocytopenia.

B. Uncommon side effects include fever, rash, anemia, mild increases in liver function tests, nausea, vomiting, eosinophilia, increased blood urea nitrogen and creatinine, and CNS toxicity.

C. GCV-resistant CMV has been documented in highly immunocompromised patients with CMV disease.

D. HSV isolates resistant to ACV are generally also resistant to GCV.

VI. Contraindications

A. Demonstrated hypersensitivity to GCV.

B. Severe neutropenia with granulocytopenia (G-CSF or GM-CSF have been used successfully in conjunction with GCV).

C. Concomitant utilization of other marrow suppressive agents, such as AZT or oncologic/hematologic chemotherapeutic agents, is relative contraindicated and, if necessary, must be done with extreme caution.

Foscarnet

I. Classification
Inorganic pyrophosphate analog.

II. Mechanism of Action

A. Selective inhibition of viral DNA polymerase and reverse transcriptases.

B. Not dependent upon phosphorylation to be active.

III. Indications

A. Drug is active in vitro against all herpesviruses, human immunodeficiency virus (HIV), and hepatitis B viruses.

B. Currently approved for the treatment of CMV retinitis in patients with AIDS.

C. The drug is active in vivo against CMV resistant to GCV and HSV and VZV isolates resistant to ACV.

D. Foscarnet is active in vivo against HIV, which may account for the observed survival benefit (~4 months) of AIDS patients with CMV retinitis treated with foscarnet compared to those treated with GCV.

IV. Interactions
Other nephrotoxic drugs may enhance the nephrotoxicity of foscarnet.

V. Complications

A. Nephrotoxicity is the major complication.

B. Other toxicities include hypocalcemia, hypercalcemia, hypophosphatemia, hyperphosphatemia, nausea, vomiting, seizures, and anemia.

VI. Contraindications

A. Significant renal insufficiency (one case report available on dosing in a patient on hemodialysis).

B. Concomitant use of nephrotoxic drugs.

C. Foscarnet-resistant CMV and HSV isolates from patients with AIDS and clinically unresponsive disease have been documented.

Zidovudine (AZT)

I. Classification
2′,3′-dideoxynucleoside analog of thymidine.

II. Mechanism of Action

A. AZT is sequentially phosphorylated to its triphosphate, AZT-TP, by intracellular enzymes.

B. AZT-TP is the active form of the drug, which acts as a competitive inhibitor of viral reverse transcriptase and, in addition, incorporates into growing viral nucleic acid and results in chain termination.

III. Indications

A. AZT is active principally against HIV-1 but also has in vitro activity against HIV-2, human T-cell lymphotropic virus (HTLV)-1/2, and Epstein-Barr virus.

B. The drug is principally indicated for the treatment of individuals with HIV infections, irrespective of clinical disease, who have fewer than 500/mm^3 CD4 T-helper lymphocytes.

C. Therapy with AZT has been shown to delay progression to AIDS in patients with HIV infection and to prolong survival of those with AIDS.

IV. Interactions

A. Probenecid decreases renal excretion and hepatic glucuronidation.

B. Concomitant medications which suppress bone marrow, particularly those causing anemia and granulocytopenia.

V. Complications

A. Most significant toxicities are anemia and granulocytopenia. Platelet levels generally are not affected and, in fact, frequently increase.

B. Minor complications include nausea, vomiting, and headache, which tend to be self-limited.

C. Patients with more advanced stages of disease, as judged principally by CD4 lymphocyte counts <200/mm^3, are at increased risk of anemia and granulocytopenia.

D. Severe anemia (<7.0 to 8.0 hemoglobin) or granulocytopenia (<500/mm^3) can be treated by dose cessation; dose reduction to ≥300 mg/day; or transfusion of or treatment with bone marrow growth factors such as erythropoietin, G-CSF, or GM-CSF.

E. Other toxicities include a myopathy manifested principally as muscle wasting of the buttocks and proximal thighs, nail pigmentation, darkening of the skin in dark-skinned individuals, lengthening of the eyelashes, macular edema, and esophageal ulceration.

F. HIV isolates resistant to AZT have been identified in patients with advanced HIV disease who have been treated with AZT for >6 months.

VI. Contraindications

A. Demonstrated hypersensitivity (rarely observed).

B. Concomitant use of bone marrow suppressive drugs, particularly the chronic administration of GCV, interferon, or oncologic/hematologic chemotherapeutic agents.

Didanosine (ddI)

I. Classification

Purine nucleoside analog of adenosine.

II. Mechanism of Action

A. ddI is a prodrug of dideoxyadenosine.

1. Following intracellular uptake, ddI is monophosphorylated to ddI-MP and then converted to ddA-MP, which is then converted to the triphosphate (ddA-TP).

B. ddA-TP has a mechanism of action similar to that of AZT-TP. It competitively inhibits retroviral reverse transcriptase and acts as a chain terminator of viral nucleic acid synthesis.

III. Indications

A. ddI is active in vitro against HIV-1 and HIV-2, HTLV-1/2, and simian immunodeficiency virus.

B. The drug is currently indicated for the treatment of patients with advanced HIV infection or AIDS who are intolerant of AZT or are clinically failing AZT therapy.

IV. Interactions

A. The incorporated acid buffer has been shown to interfere with the absorption of drugs which require an acid environment, such as dapsone and ketoconazole.

B. Administration of concomitant medications such as those listed above should be done at least 2 hr prior to the ingestion of ddI.

V. Complications

A. ddI is less toxic to bone marrow progenitor cells than AZT, and hemologic toxicity associated with AZT generally decreases when patients are switched to ddI.

B. Pancreatitis, ranging in severity from asymptomatic increases in pancreatic serum enzyme levels to life-threatening disease, has been associated with ddI.

C. Peripheral sensory neuropathy is seen infrequently with the current doses of drug utilized.

D. Preexisting peripheral neuropathy secondary to HIV infection or a prior history of pancreatitis increases the risk of these two major toxicities.

E. Other toxicities include diarrhea (most common side effect but generally not dose limiting), xerostomia, and seizures, which are difficult to link directly to ddI.

F. HIV isolates with decreased susceptibility to ddI have been found in patients with advanced AIDS treated with ddI for several months or longer.

VI. Contraindications

A. Demonstrated hypersensitivity which is rare.

B. A history of prior or chronic pancreatitis which is clinically significant.

C. Severe preexisting peripheral neuropathy is a relative contraindication.

D. A prior history of seizures is a relative contraindication, and the drug should be used with caution.

E. Concomitant use of other drugs which can cause either a peripheral neuropathy or pancreatitis.

Dideoxycytidine (ddC)

I. Classification

Dideoxynucleoside analog of cytidine.

II. Mechanism of Action

A. Intacellular triphosphorylation to ddC-TP, which is the active form of the drug.

B. ddC-TP is a competitive inhibitor of retroviral reverse transcriptase and acts as a chain terminator when incorporated into viral nucleic acid.

III. Indications

A. ddC is approximately 10 times more potent in vitro against HIV than AZT.

B. The drug is currently approved for the treatment of patients with advanced HIV disease or AIDS who are intolerant of AZT and/or ddI or who are failing AZT therapy.

C. The drug is also approved for use in combination with AZT for patients with advanced disease.

D. The drug is not indicated as initial monotherapy for patients with advanced HIV disease or AIDS. A randomized comparative study with AZT in this patient population showed AZT to be superior in terms of overall survival.

IV. Interactions

Concomitant use of drugs which can cause a peripheral neuropathy.

V. Complications

A. The major dose-limiting toxicity is a painful peripheral neuropathy which appears to be cumulative dose related.

B. Other frequent non-dose-limiting side effects are rashes, oral aphthous ulcers, fever, and malaise, which generally resolve without stopping therapy.

C. Uncommon but possibly related additional side effects include pancreatitis, esophageal ulceration, and cardiomyopathy.

D. The development of resistance of HIV patients to ddC has rarely been reported. Preliminary in vitro data suggest cross-resistance with ddI.

VI. Contraindications

A. Demonstrated hypersensitivity which is rare.

B. Severe preexisting peripheral neuropathy.

C. Concomitant use of other drugs which can cause a peripheral neuropathy.

Interferon

I. Classification

A. Low molecular weight glycoproteins produced by all cells in response to various inducers, including viral infections.

B. Three types of interferon have been identified: α, β, and γ.

1. α- and β-interferon are produced by virtually any cell in the body.

2. γ-Interferon is produced exclusively by T lymphocytes.

II. Mechanism of Action

A. The α- and β-interferons are the predominant types with antiviral properties.

B. These interferons have no direct effect on viruses, but they induce an antiviral state in susceptible cells.

C. Interferons have broad-spectrum antiviral activity in vitro against RNA and DNA viruses.

D. The antiviral effects are variable; they depend upon the virus studied and include inhibition of:

1. Viral penetration and uncoating.

2. mRNA synthesis.

3. Translation of viral proteins.

4. Final assembly and release.

III. Indications

A. Recombinant human α-2b-interferon is the only interferon approved for the treatment of viral infections in the United States.

B. Interferon has been approved for the treatment of condyloma acuminatum (genital warts), chronic hepatitis C virus infection and chronic hepatitis B virus infection.

C. Other viral infections in which interferon has shown clinical activity include VZV infections in immunocompromised hosts, HIV, prevention of reactivated HSV following trigeminal surgery, suppression of CMV infection in renal transplant patients, and juvenile laryngeal papillomatosis.

IV. Interactions

Increases plasma half-lives of drugs metabolized by the hepatic cytochrome p450-dependent system.

V. Complications

A. Interferons are associated with a number of significant clinical toxicities, which limits their use.

B. Doses above 3 to 5 million units/day are commonly associated with a flu-like illness manifested by fevers, myalgias, chills, headache, and occasionally nausea and vomiting.

C. Bone marrow suppression manifests primarily as granulocytopenia and thrombocytopenia and can be dose limiting.

D. Neurotoxicity with somnolence, confusion, seizures, electroencephalographic abnormalities, behavior changes, and, in some cases, depression have been reported.

E. Patients with advanced liver disease due to chronic hepatitis B or C have had rapid decompensation in hepatic function following initiation of interferon therapy.

F. Local reactions at injection sites, particularly with subcutaneous injections, can be severe.

G. Patients with underlying coronary artery disease have had anginal episodes in association with the flu-like systemic reactions.

VI. Contraindications

A. Advanced liver disease with cirrhosis is a relative contraindication.

B. Severe underlying coronary artery disease.

C. Concomitant use of drugs which suppress platelets or granulocytes should be done with close monitoring.

D. A history of seizures is a relative contraindication.

Bibliography

Aronoff GR, Szwed JJ, Nelson RL, et al. Hypoxanthine-arabinoside pharmacokinetics after adenine arabinoside administration to a patient with renal failure. *Antimicrob Agents Chemother* 18:212–214, 1980.

Bradley JS, Connor JD, Compogiannis LS, et al. Exposure of health care workers to ribavirin during therapy for respiratory syncytial virus infections. *Antimicrob Agents Chemother* 34:668–670, 1990.

Connolly KJ, Hammer SM. Antiretroviral therapy: Reverse transcriptase inhibition. *Antimicrob Agents Chemother* 36:245–254, 1992.

Connolly KJ, Hammer SM. Antiretroviral therapy: Strategies beyond single-agent reverse transcriptase inhibition. *Antimicrob Agents Chemother* 36:509–520, 1992.

Hochster H, Dieterich D, Bozzette S, et al. Toxicity of combined ganciclovir and zidovudine for cytomegalovirus disease associated with AIDS: An AIDS clinical trials group study. *Ann Intern Med* 113:111–117, 1990.

Jacobson MA, van der Horst C, Causey DM, et al. In vivo additive antiretroviral effect of combined zidovudine and foscarnet therapy for human immunodeficiency virus infection (ACTG protocol 053). *J Infect Dis* 163:1219–1222, 1991.

Keating MR. Antiviral agents. *Mayo Clin Proc* 67:160–178, 1992.

McLeod GX, Hammer SM. Zidovudine: Five years later. *Ann Intern Med* 117:487–501, 1992.

Mitsuya H, Yarchoan R, Broder S. Molecular targets for AIDS therapy. *Science* 249:1533–1543, 1990.

Sachs MK. Antiretroviral chemotherapy of human immunodeficiency virus infections other than with azidothymidine. *Arch Intern Med* 152:485–501, 1992.

Sha BE, Benson CA, Pottage JC, et al. The art of antiviral treatment. Part I: AZT, ddI, and ddC. *The AIDS Reader*, p 153–160, September/October 1992.

Whitley RJ, Gnann JW. Acyclovir: A decade later. *New Engl J Med* 327:782–789, 1992.

Chapter 52-C

Antituberculous Agents

Alan A. Harris, M.D.

I. Definition
Refer also to Chapter 48L. Medications used in the therapy of infection/disease due to *Mycobacterium tuberculosis* can be broken down into first-line, second-line, and third-line categories.

A. First-line drugs are those considered the drugs of choice.

B. Second-line drugs are used in the presence of organism resistance, with toxicity precluding the use of other drugs, or after therapeutic failure.

C. Third-line drugs are those which are being used for other purposes but which may inadvertently mask or partially treat unsuspected tuberculosis. They include chloramphenicol, tetracycline, ciprofloxacin, erythromycin, and aminoglycosides used in the therapy of serious gram-negative infections (i.e., gentamicin, tobramycin, amikacin, and kanamycin).

II. First-Line Drugs
A. Isonicotinic hydrazide (INH)

1. Classification—A derivative of isonicotinic acid.

2. Mechanism of action—Interferes with the cell wall metabolism of mycolic acid. Bacteriostatic in low doses, and bactericidal in high doses and in the presence of actively replicating organisms.

3. Indications—Spectrum of activity limited to mycobacteria. Also used in the therapy of group I atypical disease and with other atypical mycobacteria based on susceptibilities.

4. Dosage—Available in oral and intramuscular formulations in both 100- and 300-mg tablets. Syrup is also available. Children should receive a single daily dose of 10–20 mg/kg/day and adults a single daily dose of 5 mg/kg/day. The maximum daily dose is 300 mg. When used twice weekly, the pediatric dose is 20–40 mg/kg/day. The adult equivalent dose is 15 mg/kg/day. The maximum daily dose on the twice-weekly schedule is 900 mg. A combination tablet of INH and rifampin is available. There will soon be a single tablet incorporating INH, rifampin, and pyrazinamide.

5. Interactions

a. Inhibits para-hydroxylation of phenytoin. Dilantin intoxication may result.

b. Phenobarbital induces metabolic degradation and may augment hepatotoxicity.

c. Noncompetitively inhibits degradation of para-aminosalicylic acid and ethionamide.

6. Complications—Hepatic enzyme elevation, hepatitis, peripheral neuropathy, and sideroblastic anemia. Rarely causes optic neuritis.
   a. Supplemental vitamin B_6 at a dose of 50–100 mg/day will prevent neuropathy and sideroblastic anemia.
   b. Less common complications include seizures, headache, and insomnia.

7. Contraindications—Known hypersensitivity or significant hepatitis.

B. Rifampin
1. Classification—A semisynthetic derivative of rifamycin B. Derived from *Streptomyces mediterranii*.
2. Mechanism of action
   a. Inhibits DNA-dependent RNA polymerase.
   b. Broadest-spectrum antibiotic known to humans. In vitro activity against mycobacteria, spirochetes, bacteria, viruses, *Rickettsia*, protozoa, and *Chlamydia*.
   c. Bactericidal in low concentrations.
3. Indications
   a. Used in the therapy of tuberculosis, as well as group I and group III atypical mycobacterial disease.
   b. May have activity against some group II organisms.
   c. Used as part of combination therapy to obtain synergy in some patients with serious infection due to *Staphylococcus aureus*.
   d. Used in eradicating nasal carriage of *Neisseria meningitidis* and *Haemophilus influenzae* B.
   e. Can be used in combination to eliminate nasal carriage of *Staph. aureus* (methicillin resistant and susceptible).
4. Dosage—Available in oral form as a 300-mg capsule. Maximum daily dose is 600 mg/day. Children receive a 10–20 mg/kg/day single daily dose and adults a 10 mg/kg/day single daily dose. Dosages do not change with a twice weekly schedule.
5. Interactions
   a. Stimulates hepatic ribosomal enzymes and enhances the metabolic degradation of many medications, including coumadin, steroids, dilantin, and oral contraceptives. Dose adjustments are necessary when rifampin is being added to or subtracted from a patient receiving these medications to avoid complications related to overdosing or underdosing.
   b. Inhibits the hepatic uptake of cholecystographic dye and may result in nonvisualization of the gallbladder.
   c. Probenecid inhibits rifampin uptake by the liver, retarding its degradation.
6. Complications
   a. Hepatotoxicity, nausea, vomiting, urticaria, and morbilliform erythematous eruptions.
   b. Red-orange discoloration of multiple body fluids, including urine and stool. Tears may permanently stain contact lenses.
   c. Associated immunologic events include light chain proteinuria and in vitro suppression of T-cell function. A flu-like syndrome, thrombocytopenia, hemolytic anemia, and immune nephritis have been reported in the presence of intermittent therapy and may be immunologically mediated.
7. Contraindications—Significant hepatitis, hypersensitivity, and immunologic events.

C. Ethambutol
1. Classification—A derivative of butanol.
2. Mechanism of Action—Unknown. Bacteriostatic at low doses against replicating organisms.
3. Indications—The spectrum of activity is limited to *Mycobacterium*. Is important in the therapy of *M. tuberculosis*, *M. kansasii*, and *M. avium* complex.
4. Dosage—Oral formulation as 100-mg and 400-mg tablets. Pediatric and adult doses are 15–25 mg/kg/day as a single dose, with a maximum of 2.5 g. When twice weekly schedules are used, the dose is 50 mg/kg on each therapeutic day.
   a. The higher daily dose is necessary when treating atypical mycobacteria or partially resistant organisms.
   b. The lower dose maintains efficacy against *M. tuberculosis* and widens the therapeutic toxic ratio by reducing optic neuritis.
5. Interactions—Interferes with renal tubular secretion of urate, with resultant hyperuricemia.
6. Complications

a. The principal adverse reaction is retrobulbar neuritis. Decreased visual acuity and red-green color blindness may occur centrally or peripherally. Fundoscopic examination is usually normal. Complications are dose related over time, with a frequency of ≤1% at a dose of 15 mg/kg/day.

b. Hepatitis.

c. Idiosyncratic reactions and skin rash are rare. Gastrointestinal intolerance is usually mild.

7. Contraindications—Known hypersensitivity. Progressive or significant optic neuritis occurs despite use of the lowest effective daily doses.

D. Pyrazinamide

1. Classification—A derivative of nicotinamide.

2. Mechanism of action—Bactericidal at slight acidic pH and effective intracellularly.

3. Indications—An important component of 6-month therapy. Not effective in the therapy of *Mycobacterium avium* complex, as the organism lacks an amidase which is necessary for activity of pyrazinamide.

4. Dosage—Total daily dose is 15–30 mg/kg given either three or four times per day. Maximum daily dose is 2–3 g. Twice weekly dosing regimens are at 50–70 mg/kg/day. Available in 500-mg tablets.

5. Complications—The best-known complication is hyperuricemia. Clinical gout is rare. The most dreaded complication is hepatitis, which may mimic that due to INH or rifampin. Hepatic dysfunction/hepatitis occurs in up to 15% of patients when doses of 3 g/day are given. Death has been reported.

6. Contraindications—Known hypersensitivity or clinically significant hepatitis.

E. Aminoglycosides

1. Classification—Only streptomycin is a first-line antituberculous aminoglycoside. Other aminoglycosides will not be discussed in depth here. All have similar end-organ toxicity and require monitoring of the kidneys, as well as the auditory and vestibular systems. Amikacin and kanamycin are also used in the therapy of gram-negative bacterial infection. Capreomycin and viomycin are available on a limited basis for the therapy of tuberculosis when resistance to streptomycin is documented.

a. Streptomycin is a derivative of *Streptomyces griseus*.

2. Mechanism of action—Inhibitor of protein synthesis through its effect on the ribosomes.

3. Indications—Last choice among the first-line antituberculous drugs. Its position is dictated by required parenteral administration and toxicities which require close monitoring. Efficacy is likely as good as or better than that of ethambutol or pyrazinamide.

4. Dosage—Must be administered intramuscularly. Pediatric dose is 20–40 mg/kg/day. Adults <60 years of age receive 15 mg/kg/day, while those >60 should receive 10 mg/kg/day. Maximum daily doses are 1 g in those <60 years of age and 750 mg in those ≥60 years of age. When twice weekly regimens are used, the dose is 25–30 mg/kg/day.

5. Complications

a. Auditory deficit or vestibular dysfunction. Decreased hearing is cumulative, regardless of which aminoglycoside is used. Patients should be monitored for vertigo, tinnitus, or decreased hearing. Baseline audiometry is recommended and should be repeated at least bimonthly.

b. Nephrotoxicity—Assess baseline renal function. Assess once or twice per week when the regimen is stabilized.

6. Contraindications—Known hypersensitivity or significant ototoxicity or nephrotoxicity.

III. **Second-Line Drugs**

A. Para-aminosalicylic acid

1. Classification—A derivative of para-aminogalicylic acid.

2. Mechanism of action—Unclear.

3. Indications—Used to treat *M. tuberculosis* in conjunction with streptomycin and INH prior to the availability of rifampin, ethambutol, and pyrazinamide.

4. Dosage—150 mg/kg/day, with a maximum daily dose of 12 g. Available in 500-mg and 1-g tablets.

5. Complications

a. Gastrointestinal disturbance with nausea, vomiting, and dyspepsia has resulted in frequent discontinuation of medications.

b. The tablets are quite large.

c. Hepatotoxicity may also occur.

d. Goiter has occurred as a result of decreased thyroidal iodine uptake.

e. Sodium loading and fluid retention are problems in patients with cardiac, hepatic, and renal disorders.

f. Rashes have been frequent and have also resulted in discontinuation of therapy.

6. Contraindications—Hypersensitivity.

B. Ethionamide

1. Classification—A derivative of thioisonicotinamide.

2. Mechanism of action—Uncertain.

3. Indications—Effective in combination with other drugs in the therapy of *M. tuberculosis*. Its use in the therapy of disease due to atypical mycobacteria should be based on susceptibilities.

4. Dosage—15–20 mg/kg/day with a maximum of 1 g. Available in 250-mg tablets.

5. Complications—Hepatotoxicity and gastrointestinal disturbance may occur.

6. Contraindications—Hypersensitivity.

C. Cycloserine

1. Classification—A derivative of *Streptomyces orchidaceous*.

2. Mechanism of action—Inhibits incorporation of *d*-alanine in cell wall synthesis. When *d*-alanine is absent from media, cycloserine also has in vitro activity against *Escherichia coli*, *Staph. aureus*, *Enterococcus*, *Nocardia*, and *Chlamydia*.

3. Indications—Effective in combination with other drugs in the therapy of *M. tuberculosis*. Its use in the therapy of disease due to atypical mycobacteria should be based on susceptibilities.

4. Dosage—15–20 mg/kg/day, with a maximum of 1 g. Available in 250-mg tablets.

5. Complications—Headaches, confusion, psychoses, somnolence, tremor, dysarthria, irritability, and seizures may occur. Central nervous system complications are frequently dose limiting, especially in the elderly. These effects are enhanced by alcohol.

6. Contraindications—hypersensitivity.

Bibliography

Bailey WC, Albert RK, Davidson PT, et al. Treatment of tuberculosis and other mycobacterial diseases. American Thoracic Society, Medical Section of the American Lung Association, 1983, pp 790–796.

Cohn DL, Catlin BJ, Peterson KL, et al. A 62-dose, 6-month therapy for pulmonary and extrapulmonary tuberculosis. *Ann Intern Med* 112:407–414, 1990.

Combs DL, O'Brien RJ, Geiter LJ. USPHS tuberculosis short-course chemotherapy trial 21: Effectiveness, toxicity, and acceptability. *Ann Intern Med* 112:397–406, 1990.

Dash LA, Comstock GW, Flynn JPG. Isoniazid preventive therapy: Retrospect and prospect. *Am Rev Respir Dis* 121:1039–1044, 1980.

Davidson PT. Treating tuberculosis: What drugs, for how long? *Ann Intern Med* 112:393–395, 1990.

Dutt AK, Moers D, Stead WW. Short-course chemotherapy for extrapulmonary tuberculosis. *Ann Intern Med* 104:7–12, 1986.

Antifungal Agents

John C. Pottage, Jr., M.D.

Amphotericin B (Amb)

I. **Definition**
Polyene antibiotic derived from *Streptomyces nodosus*.

II. **Mechanism of Action**
A. Binds to ergosterol in the fungal cytoplasmic membrane, altering the osmotic integrity of the cell.
B. Induces oxidative changes leading to cell damage.

III. **Indications**
A. Treatment of infections due to *Candida* species, *Blastomyces dermatitidis*, *Histoplasma capsulatum*, *Coccidioides immitis*, *Paracoccidioides brasiliensis*, *Aspergillus* species, and *Zygomycetes*.
B. Disseminated sporotrichosis.

IV. **Dosages**
A. Typical dose range is 0.3–1.2 mg/kg/day given IV over 4 hr in dextrose (5%) in water (D5W).
B. Usually started with a 1-mg test dose to assess the patient's febrile response.
C. Given for 6–12 weeks depending upon the fungal pathogen.

V. **Adverse Effects**
A. The most common adverse effect is fever. This is caused by a direct effect of amb on monocytes, causing a release of interleukin-1 and tumor necrosis factor. Pretreatment with antipyretics (acetaminophen) and/or corticosteroids (50–75 mg of hydrocortisone in the amb bag) can block these effects.
B. Hypokalemia and hypomagnesemia result from amb use and need to be monitored closely.
C. Renal failure due to intrarenal arterial vasospasm leading to a decreased glomerular filtration rate (GFR) occurs in virtually all patients. Attention to fluid status is important in all patients receiving amb. Concomitant use of diuretics can worsen the renal failure. Discontinuation of amb leads to a return of normal renal function is most patients. Long-term amb (>5 grams) use can lead to permanent renal tubular damage.
D. Anemia due to amb inhibition of erythropoietin is readily reversible following amb discontinuation.

Nystatin

I. Definition
Polyene antibiotic derived from *Streptomyces noursei.*

II. Mechanism of Action
A. Acts in the same fashion as amphotericin B.

III. Indications
A. Treatment of oral candidiasis (thrush)
B. Vaginal candidiasis
C. Topical *Candida* infections

IV. Dosages
A. Used as an oral suspension, cream, ointment, topical powder, and vaginal tablet.
B. For treatment of thrush, 5 ml (100,000 units/ml) is given; swich and swallow four times per day.
C. For vaginal candidiasis, one tablet per day is applied via an applicator in the vagina for 3–7 days.

Flucytosine

I. Definition
Fluorinated pyrimidine.

II. Mechanism of Action
A. Flucytosine enters the fungal cell with the aid of cytosine permease.
B. It is then deaminated to form 5-fluorouracil which then interferes with fungal DNA and RNA biosynthesis.

III. Indications
A. Primarily indicated for treatment of infections due to *Cryptococcus* and chromomycosis. Because of rapid development of resistance of fungi to flucytosine, flucytosine is usually used in combination with amphotericin B.
B. Used for treatment of serious *Candida* infections (e.g., hepatosplenic candidiasis, endocarditis) in combination with amphotericin B.

IV. Dosage
A. Usual dose is 150 mg/kg/day in four divided doses by mouth.
B. The drug is excreted renally and needs to be adjusted in patients with renal insufficiency. In these patients, blood levels should be monitored. Peak levels of between 50–100 $\mu g/ml$ should be obtained.

V. Adverse Effects
A. The most common adverse effect is gastrointestinal intolerance characterized by nausea, vomiting, and diarrhea.

B. The most serious adverse effect is leukopenia and thrombocytopenia.
C. Patients with elevated plasma levels (> 100 $\mu g/ml$) are more prone to toxicity. Levels should be closely monitored in patients with underlying renal insufficiency.

Clotrimazole

I. Definition
Imidazole antifungal agent.

II. Mechanism of Action
A. Inhibits ergosterol production by inhibiting lanosterol demethylase.
B. This interferes with normal cytoplasmic membrane function which leads to abnormal permeability properties, ultimately leading to cell death.

III. Indications
A. Dermatophytic infections
B. Cutaneous candidiasis
C. Oral candidiasis
D. Vaginal candidiasis

IV. Dosages
A. Used topically as a 1% cream, lotion, or solution.
B. For dermatophytic infections and cutaneous candidiasis: Appy locally twice per day for a 4- to 6-week course.
C. For oropharyngeal candidiasis. Give as a 10-mg troche, taken five times per day for 7–14 days.
D. For vaginitis, clotrimazole is formulated as a vaginal tablet or a 1% cream, usually given 3–7 days, once daily.

V. Adverse Effects
A. These are minimal and consist of erythema and/or pruritis at the site of application.
B. Some patients report a bad taste associated with the troches.

Miconazole

I. Definition
Imidazole antifungal agent.

II. Mechanism of Action
A. Same as that of clotrimazole.

III. Indications
A. Used primarily as a topical agent in the treatment of vaginal candidiasis.
B. IV treatment of infection due to *Pseudallescheria boydii.* These are usually mycetoma or sinusitis infections.

IV. Dosages

A. Miconazole is formulated as a 0.4–2.0% cream or a 100–200 mg suppository for treatment of *Candida vaginitis*, and applied once-daily for 3–7 days.

B. Give IV miconazole in a dosage of 600–3,000 mg/day divided into three doses. Because of possible anaphylaxis to IV miconazole, give a test dose of 200 mg at the start of therapy. Therapy is usually necessary for 2–6 months.

V. Adverse Effects

A. Topical miconazole is usually well-tolerated. Local reactions with mild erythema or pruritis clear with discontinuation of the drug.

B. The most serious reaction to IV miconazole is anaphylaxis and cardiopulmonary arrest, usually due to a hypersensitivity to the drug. For this reason, the drug is usually given at a test dose of 200 mg in appropriate clinical surroundings.

C. More common adverse effects are nausea, vomiting, fever, and phlebitis at the IV site.

Ketoconazole

I. Definition
Imidazole antifungal agent.

II. Mechanism of Action

A. Same as that for clotrimazole.

III. Indications

A. Dermatophytic infections

B. Topical and mucosal *Candida* infections, including skin infections, vaginitis, thrush, and esophagitis.

C. Non–life-threatening histoplasmosis and blastomycosis.

IV. Dosage

A. The usual dosage is 200–400 mg orally once per day. Ketoconazole requires normal gastric acidity for absorption. Antacids and H_2 blockers should not be used concurrently with ketoconazole.

B. Duration of ketoconazole therapy for treatment of *Candida* infections is 7–21 days.

C. For infections due to dermatophytes, histoplasmosis, and blastomycosis, therapy may be needed for up to 6–12 months.

V. Adverse Effects

A. The most common adverse effects are nausea, vomiting, and abdominal pain. This occurs in approximately 15% of patients and is reversible upon discontinuation of the drug.

B. An idiosyncratic hepatitis which can be fatal occurs in approximately 1/10,000 patients. Patients should be warned of this complication and liver enzymes should be monitored.

C. In addition to blocking ergosterol biosynthesis in fungi, ketoconazole in high doses blocks cholesterol biosynthesis in mammalian cells. This can lead to decreased steroid hormone production. In men, gynecomastia and loss of libido are seen; in women, menstrual abnormalities have been reported.

D. Significant drug interactions include concurrent use of rifampin (decreased ketoconazole levels), cyclosporin A (increased cyclosporin A levels), phenytoin (increased phenytoin levels), oral hypoglycemic agents (increased oral hypoglycemic agent levels), and terfenadine (increased terfenadine levels).

Fluconazole

I. Definition
Triazole antifungal agent.

II. Mechanism of Action

A. Like the imidazoles, triazole antifungal agents block ergosterol production in the fungal cytoplasmic membrane.

B. The triazoles are far more specific for the fungal enzymes and have less activity against mammalian enzymes than imidazoles.

III. Indications

A. Treatment of all forms of infections caused by *Candida* species, including candidemia and disseminated candidiasis.

1. Has little activity against *Candida krusei* and *Torulopsis glabrata* and should not be used in these infections.

B. Treatment of cryptococcal infections.

1. Particularly useful in the long-term maintenance therapy required to suppress the infection in HIV-infected patients.

IV. Dosages

A. Doses range from 100–400 mg orally taken once per day.

B. Does not require gastric acidity for absorption.

C. An IV formulation is also available, the same dosing regimens are used.

V. Adverse Effects

A. Fluconazole is well-tolerated. The most common adverse effect if gastrointestinal disturbance occurring in approximately 3–5% of patients.

B. Hepatitis has been reported, but is less common than that reported for ketoconazole.

C. Endocrinologic adverse effects are not seen.
D. Like ketoconazole, fluconazole has interactions with several other medications including phenytoin (leads to increased levels of phenytoin), rifampin (leads to decreased fluconazole levels), cyclosporin A (leads to increased cyclosporin A levels), and the oral hypoglycemic agents (leads to increased concentrations of oral hypoglycemic agents).

Itraconazole

I. **Definition**
   Triazole antifungal agent.
II. **Mechanism of Action**
   A. Same as that for fluconazole.
III. **Indications**
   A. Treatment of non–life–threatening histoplasmosis and blastomycosis
IV. **Dosages**
   A. Give 100–400 mg orally once daily. Gastric acidity is needed for full absorption. There is no intravenous formulation.

B. Treatment for histoplasmosis and blastomycosis requires therapy for at least 3 months and up to 6–12 months. A clinical response is usually seen within 1 month.
V. **Adverse Effects**
   A. Gastrointestinal disturbances.
   B. Hepatitis; liver function tests should be monitored.
   C. Hypokalemia.
   D. Drug interactions are the same as reported for ketoconazole and fluconazole.

Bibliography

Gallis HA, Drew RH, Pickard WW. Amphotericin B: 30 years of clinical experience. *Reviews of Infectious Disease.* 12:308–329, 1990.

Graybill JR. Azole therapy of systemic fungal infections. In: Holmberg K, Meyer R (eds). Diagnosis and therapy of systemic fungal infections, New York, Raven Press 1989 133–143.

CHAPTER 52-E

Antiretroviral Treatment

John C. Pottage, Jr., M.D.

I. Definition

Antiretroviral therapy is based primarily upon the patient's symptoms and the absolute CD4 lymphocyte count. At present the only available antiretroviral agents for general use are zidovudine (AZT), didanosine (ddI), and zalcitabine (ddC). The specific pharmacologic properties of these agents are listed in the chapter on antiviral therapy. Tables 52E-1, 52E-2 and 52E-3 list recommendations for various clinical situations in the HIV-infected patient. They are based partially upon recommendations made by a panel of experts convened by the National Institute of Allergy and Infectious Disease in June 1993.

Table 52E-1.   Initiation of Therapy in HIV-infected Patients

Patient Characteristics	Recommendations/Therapy
Asymptomatic CD 4 cell count >500 cells/mm^3	Observation, repeat CD4 cell count every 6 months. No antiretroviral therapy
Asymptomatic CD4 cell count 200–500 cells/mm^3	Either: 1) Observe closely, monitor CD 4 cell count every 6 months. No antiretroviral therapy 2) Start AZT monotherapy (600 mg/day)
Symptomatic CD4 cell count 200–500 cells/mm^3	Start AZT monotherapy (600 mg/day)
Symptomatic or asymptomatic CD4 cell count <200 cells/mm^3	Start AZT monotherapy or combination therapy of AZT and ddC

Table 52E-2. Therapy in Patients Who Experience
Disease Progression

Patient Characteristics	Recommendation/Therapy
Disease progression; CD4 cell count 50–500 cells/mm^3, patient on AZT	Change to ddI monotherapy or combination therapy with AZT and ddC or AZT and ddI
Disease progression; CD4 cell count <50 cells/mm^3, patient on AZT	Switch to ddI or ddC monotherapy or combination therapy with AZT and ddC or AZT and ddI

Table 52E-3. Therapy in Patients Who are Intolerant* to AZT

Patient Characteristics	Recommendation/Therapy
CD4 cell count >500 cells/mm^3	Stop therapy and observe
CD4 cell count 50–500 cells/mm^3	Switch to ddI
CD4 cell count <50 cells/mm^3	Switch to ddI, ddC or discontinue therapy

*AZT intolerance defined as inability to tolerate 300 μg of AZT per day. The usual reasons for intolerance are hematologic abnormalities, anemia, and leukopenia. Gastrointestinal intolerance occurs rarely.

Bibliography

Hirsch MS and D'Aquila RT, Therapy for human immunodeficiency virus infection. *New Engl J Med* 328:1686–1695, 1993.

Dosing of Antimicrobial Agents

Kenneth Kortas, Pharm.D.
Gordon M. Trenholme, M.D.
Catherine M. MacLeod, M.D., F.R.C.P.(C),
F.A.C.P., F.C.P.

I. Aminoglycoside Dosing

A. Approximate dosage adjustments for aminoglycosides using serum levels of aminoglycosides as guidelines.

If Peak (mcg/ml)		If Trough (mcg/ml)		Corrective Action
Gentamicin/ Tobramycin	Amikacin	Gentamicin/ Tobramycin	Amikacin	
>10	>30	<2	<10	Decrease dose
>10	>30	>2	>10	Decrease dose and/or increase dosing interval
4–10	20–30	>2	>10	Increase dosing interval
<4	<20	<2	<10	Increase dose
<4	<20	<1	<5	Increase dose and/or decrease dosing interval

B. Pharmacokinetics
1. Aminoglycosides are poorly absorbed from the GI tract and are administered by either intramuscular injection or intravenous infusion.
2. Following administration, aminoglycosides are widely distributed into most body fluids including synovial, peritoneal, ascetic, pericardial, pleural, and abscess fluids.
   a. These agents distribute slowly into the bile, feces, prostate, and amniotic fluid.
   b. Aminoglycosides distribute poorly into the central nervous system and the vitreous humor of the eye.
3. With the exception of streptomycin (35%), binding to serum proteins is less than 10% and is not considered to be clinically important.

 4. Aminoglycosides are primarily eliminated unchanged by the kidney via glomerular filtration.
   a. Renal elimination accounts for approximately 85–95% of administered dose with small amounts being found in the bile.
   b. Adjustment in interval and/or dosage is required in decreased renal function to avoid potential toxicity.
C. Specific points about aminoglycoside dosing
 1. The initial loading dose is independent of renal function.
 2. The initial dose should be designed to obtain a peak serum level above the minimum of the therapeutic range.
 3. Subsequent adjustments based on serum levels will minimize toxicity and maintain therapeutic efficacy.

II. Dosing of Antiinfective Agents in Renal and Hepatic Failure and no Dialysis (Table 52F-1)

Bibliography

Evans WE, Schentaq JJ & Jusko WJ. (editors) Applied Pharmacokinetics—Principles of Therapeutic Drug Monitoring—2nd edition. Applied Therapeutics, Inc., Spokane, WA 1986.

Gilman AG, Rall TW, Nies AS, Taylor P, eds. *Goodman and Gilman's The Pharmacological Basis of Therapeutics*, ed 8. New York, McGraw-Hill, Inc., 1990.

The Medical Letter 32:41–48, 1990.

Mandell GL, Douglas RG, Bennett JE, eds. *Principles and Practice of Infectious Diseases*, ed 3. New York, Churchill Livingstone, 1990.

USP Drug Information, ed 13. Rockville, Md., United States Pharmacopeial Convention, 1993.

Table 52F-1. Dosing of Anti-Infective Agents in Renal and Hepatic Failure and in Dialysis

| Anti-Infective Agent | Usual Adult Dose | Peak Serum Level (μg/ml) | Dose-Interval Adjustment | | | | Dialysis | |
| | | | Renal Failure-Cr. Cl. (ml/min) | | | Hepatic Failure* | H.D.† | P.D. |
			>50	50-10	<10 (Anuric)			
Acyclovir	5 mg/kg q8h	9	N.C.	5 mg/kg q12-24h	2.5 mg/kg q24h	N.C.	5 mg/kg post dialysis	2.5 mg/kg q24h
Amantadine	200 mg q24h (100 mg q24h >65 yrs.)	1.0	200 mg q24-48h	200 mg q48-72h‡	200 mg q 7 days	N.C.	N.C.	N.C.
Amikacin	7.5 mg/kg q8h	30	q12h	q24-36h	q48h	N.C.	3.75 mg/kg post H.D.	15-20 mg/liter/day in P.D. fluid
Amphotericin B	0.5 mg/kg q24h	2	N.C.	N.C.	N.C.	N.C.	N.C.	Removal by P.D. is slow; no additional dose needed
Amoxicillin	500 mg PO q8h	8	N.C.	N.C.	250 mg q12h	N.C.	250 mg postdialysis	
Amox.-clavulanate acid	500 mg PO q8h	9.7/3.9	N.C.	q12h	q24h	N.C.	250 mg postdialysis	Usual dose q24h
Ampicillin	500 mg PO q6h/2 g IV q6h	4/40	N.C.	q8h	q12h	N.C.	500 mg post-H.D.	N.C.
Ampicillin-sulbactam	3 g IV q6h	150	q6-8h	q8-12h	q24h	N.C.	1.5 g postdialysis	Usual dose q24h
Axetil	500 mg PO q12h	7.0	N.C.					
Azithromycin	500 mg x1, then 250 mg PO q24h	0.4	N.C.		N.C.	N.C. (N.K.)	N.K.	N.K.
Azlocillin	4 g IV q6h	300	N.C.	q6-8h	q8h	Daily dose 3-6 g	3 g postdialysis	q8h
Aztreonam	2 g IV q8h	250	N.C.	q8-12h	q24h	N.C.δ	0.5 g postdialysis	2 g q24h
Carbenicillin indanyl sodium 382 mg	2 tablets PO q6h	6.5	N.C.	N.C.	N.C.	N.C.	N.C.	N.C.
Cefaclor	500 mg PO q8h	12	N.C.	250-600 q8h	250 mg q8h	N.C.	250 mg postdialysis	250 mg q8-12h
Cefadroxil	1 g PO q12h	16	N.C.	500 mg q12-24h	250-500 mg q24-48h	N.C.	0.5-1 g postdialysis	0.5 g q24h
Cefamandole	1 g IV q6h	80	N.C.	1 g q6-8h	1 g q12-24h	N.C.	0.5-1 g postdialysis	0.5-1 g q12h
Cefazolin	1 g IV q8h	120	NC.	q12h	500 mg-1 g q24h	N.C.	0.5-1 g postdialysis	0.5 g IV q12h
Cefixime	200 mg PO q12h	4	N.C.	N.C.	200 mg q24h	N.C.	300 mg postdialysis	200 mg q24h
Cefonicid	1 g q24h	220	N.C.	.5 g q24h	.5 g q24h	N.C.	N.C.	N.C.
Cefoperazone	2 g q12h	250	N.C.	N.C.	1.5 g q12h	1 g q21h	1 g postdialysis	N.C.
Cefotaxime	1 g IV q8h	200	N.C.	N.C.	1-2 g q12-24h	N.C.	1-2 g postdialysis	1 g q24h
Cefotetan	2 g IV q12h	200	N.C.	1 g q12h	500 mg q12h	N.C.	1 g postdialysis	1 g q24h
Cefoxitin	2 g IV q6h	150	1-2 g q8h	2 g q8-12h	1 g q24h	N.C.	1-2 g postdialysis	1 g q24h
Ceftazidime	2 g IV q8h	160	N.C.	q12-24h	q24h	N.C.	1 g postdialysis	2 g, then 0.5 g q24h
Ceftizoxime	2 g IV q8h	120	q8-12h	q24h	500 mg q24h	N.C.	1 g postdialysis	0.5-1 g q24h

(continued)

665

Table 52F-1. Continued

| Anti-Infective Agent | Usual Adult Dose | Peak Serum Level (μg/ml) | Dose-Interval Adjustment | | | | Dialysis | |
| | | | Renal Failure-Cr. Cl. (ml/min) | | | Hepatic Failure* | H.D.† | P.D. |
			>50	50–10	<10 (Anuric)			
Ceftriaxone	2 g IV q24h	270	N.C.	N.C.	N.C.	N.C.	Usual dose postdialysis	N.C.
Cefuroxime	1.5 g IV q8h	98	N.C.	q8–12h	q24h	N.C.	Usual dose postdialysis	Usual dose q24h
Cephalexin	500 mg PO q6h	25	N.C.	N.C.	q8–12h	N.C.	250 mg postdialysis	250 mg TID
Cephalothin	2 g IV q6h	70	N.C.	q6–8h	q12h	N.C.	Usual dose postdialysis	1 g q12h
Cephapirin	2 g q6h	37	N.C.	q6–8h	q12h	N.C.	Usual dose postdialysis	1 g q12h
Cephradine	2 g IV q6h/500 mg PO q12h	26/16	N.C.	q8h	250 mg q12–24h	N.C.	Usual dose postdialysis	500 mg q6h
Chloramphenicol	12.5 mg/kg q6h	14	N.C.	N.C.	N.C.	Daily dose of 0.5–1 g	N.C.	N.C.
Chloroquine	600 mg	0.125	N.C.	N.C.	150–300 mg PO q24h	N.C.	N.C.	N.C.
Cinoxacin	500 mg PO q12h	8	N.C.	250 mg PO q12h	250 mg q24h	N.C.	N.K.	N.K.
Ciprofloxacin	400 mg IV q12h/500 mg PO q12h	3.8/2.9	N.C.	<30 ml/min q18h	q24h	N.C.	200 mg q12h postdialysis	200 mg q12h/250 mg q12h
Clarithromycin, 14-OH metabolite	500 mg PO q12h	2.4/1.0	N.C.	<30 q24h	q24h	N.C.	N.K.	N.K.
Clindamycin	900 mg IV q8h/300mg PO q6h	12/2.5	N.C.	N.C.	N.C.	Reduce daily dose by 1/3	N.C.	N.C.
Clofazimine	100 mg PO q24h	0.7	N.C.	N.C.	N.C.	N.K.	N.K.	N.K.
Cycloserine	500 mg PO BID	25	N.C.	250–500 q24h	250 mg q24h	N.C.	N.C.	N.C.
Dapsone	100 mg PO q24h	2.3 (steady state)	N.C.	N.C.	No data	N.K.	N.C.	N.K.
Dicloxacillin	500 gm PO q6h	4	N.C.	N.C.	N.C.	N.C.	N.C.	N.C.
Dideoxyinosine (ddI)	375 mg PO BID (>75 kg)	6.2	N.C.	C.I. for CR >2.5 mg/dl	C.I. for CR >2.5 mg/dl	N.K.	N.K.	N.K.
Doxycycline	100 mg q12h PO/IV	3	N.C.	N.C.	N.C.	N.C.	N.C.	N.C.
Erythromycin	500 mg IV q6h/500 mg PO q6h	8/1.7	N.C.	N.C.	50–70% of daily dose	50% of daily dose	N.C.	N.C.
Ethambutol	15/25 mg/kg q24h	2–5	N.C.	q24–36h or 7.5 mg/kg/day	q48h or 5 mg/kg/day	N.C.	Usual dose postdialysis	q48h

(continued)

Drug	Dose		GFR >50	GFR 10–50	GFR <10	Comments	Hemodialysis	CAPD/Anuric
Fluconazole	200 mg q24h IV/PO	10	N.C.	50% normal dose q24h	25% of normal dose q24h	N.C.	Usual dose postdialysis	Anuric dose
Flucytosine	150 mg/kg q24h, 0.5–1 g PO q6h	80	q6–8h	q12–24h	q24–48h	N.C.	Usual dose postdialysis	0.5–1 g q24h
Foscarnet	60 mg/kg q8h#, 90 mg/kg q24h##	500–800 uM	40–50 mg/kg q8h#, 70–80 mg/kg q24h##	10–30 mg/kg q8h#, 30–60 mg/kg q24h##	C.I.	N.C.	Redose 1/2 of dose postdialysis	N.K.
Ganciclovir	5 mg/kg q12h	8.3	80–50 ml/min, 2.5 mg/kg q12h	50–25 ml/min 2.5 mg/kg q12h	<25–1.25 mg/kg q24h	N.C.	Usual dose postdialysis	Dose q48–76h
Gentamicin	1.5 mg/kg q8h	10	q12h	q12–24h	q24–48h	N.C.	2/3 of normal dose postdialysis	3–4 liter q24h
Imipenem-cilastin	500 mg IV q6h	43	500 mg q8h	500 mg q12h	250 mg q12h	N.C.	Usual dose postdialysis	Anuric
Isoniazid	300 mg q24h	7	N.C.	N.C.	50% of dose	May require dose reduction	Usual dose postdialysis	Anuric
Itraconazole	200 mg q12h	0.6	N.C.	N.C.	50–100 q12h	N.K.	100 mg q12–24h	100 mg q12–24h
Kanamycin	7.5 mg/kg q12h	20	q24h	q24–72h	q72–96h	N.C.	2/3 of normal dose postdialysis	15–20 mg liter q24h
Ketoconazole	400 mg PO q24h	7	N.C.	N.C.	N.C.	N.K.	N.C.	N.C.
Methicillin	2 g IV q4h	80	q6h	q8h	q12h	N.C.	2 g postdialysis	N.C.
Metronidazole	500 mg IV q8h	21	N.C.	N.C.	500 mg IV q12h	250–500 mg q24h	Usual dose postdialysis	50% of daily dose
Mezlocillin	4 g IV q4–6h	255	q4–6h	q6–8h	q8h	Reduce dose by 75%	Usual dose postdialysis q8h	Anuric dose
Miconazole	1200 mg q8h	4	N.C.	N.C.	N.C.	?	N.C.	N.C.
Minocycline	100 mg q12h	3	N.C.	N.C. (N.K.)	N.C. (N.K.)	N.K. (N.C.)		
Moxalactam	2 g q8–12h	76	N.C.	q12–24h	q12–24h	?	Usual dose postdialysis	q24–48h
Nafcillin	2 g IV q4h	10	N.C.	N.C.	N.C.	Reduce dose by −50% when accompanied by renal failure		N.C.
Nalidixic acid	1 g PO q6h	30	N.C.	N.C.	Avoid	N.K.	Avoid	Avoid
Netilmicin	2 mg/kg q8h	8	q8–12h	q12–24h	q24–48h	N.C.	2/3 usual dose postdialysis	3–4 mg/liter q24h
Nitrofurantoin	100 mg PO q6h	<1.0	N.C.	Avoid	Avoid	N.K.	Avoid	Avoid
Norfloxacin	400 mg PO BID	1.6	N.C.	q12–24h	q24h or avoid	N.C.	Avoid	Avoid
Ofloxacin	400 mg PO BID	8.6	N.C.	q24h	q48h or decrease 25–50%	N.C.	100 mg BID	Anuric dose
Oxacillin	2 g IV q6h	63	N.C.	N.C.	N.C.	N.K.	N.C.	N.C.
Penicillin G	4 Mμ q6h	400	N.C.	75% of dose	1/3–1/2 of daily max. dose	N.C.	Usual dose postdialysis	Anuric dose
Penicillin V	500 mg PO q6h	4	q8h	q8h	q12h	N.C.	250 mg postdialysis	Anuric dose
Pentamidine	300 mg q24h (4 mg/kg/day)	0.5	q24–36h	q24–36h	q48h	N.C.	N.C.	N.C.

Table 52F-1. Continued

Anti-Infective Agent	Usual Adult Dose	Peak Serum Level (μg/ml)	Dose-Interval Adjustment					
			Renal Failure-Cr. Cl. (ml/min)			Hepatic Failure*	Dialysis	
			>50	50–10	<10 (Anuric)		H.D.†	P.D.
Piperacillin	4 g IV q6h	412	N.C.	q6–8h	q8h	Decrease dose by 75%	Usual dose postdialysis	q8h
Ribavarin (unapproved use)	600 mg PO q8h	1.3	N.C.	N.C.	100 mg q8h	N.C.	Usual dose postdialysis	Anuric dose
Rifampin	600 mg PO q24h	10	N.C.	N.C.	N.C.	N.K.	N.C.	N.C.
Spectinomycin	2 g IM × 1	74	N.C.	N.C.	N.C.	N.C.	N.C.	N.C.
Streptomycin	1 g q24h	50	N.C.	q24–72h	q72–96h	N.C.	0.5 g postdialysis	20–40 mg/liter q24h
Sulfamethoxazole	1 g q8h	92	q12h	q18h	q24h	N.C.	1 g postdialysis	1 g q24h
Sulfasoxazole	2 g q6h	110	q6h	q8h–12h	q12h–24h	N.C.	2 g postdialysis	3 g q24h
Temafloxacin	600 mg PO BID	7.2	N.C.	q24h	300 mg PO q24h	400 mg PO BID (based on serum levels)	N.C.	N.C.
Tetracycline	500 mg PO q6h	4.3	q8–12h	q12–24h	Not recommended	N.C.	500 mg postdialysis	N.C.
Ticarcillin	3 g IV q4h	250	1–2 g q4h	1–2 g q8h	1 g q12h	N.C.	3 g postdialysis	1 g q12h
Ticarcillin/clavulanate	3.1 g IV q6h	324/8	N.C.	q8h	q12h	N.C.	3.1 g postdialysis	3.1 g q 12h
Tobramycin	1.5 mg/kg IV q8h	10	q8–12h	q12–24h	q24–48h	N.C.	2/3 normal dose postdialysis	3–4 mg/liter q24h
Trimethoprim	100 mg PO q12h	1	q12h	q24h	q24–48h	N.C.	N.C.	N.C.
Trimethoprim/sulfamethoxazole	160/800 mg IV/PO	3.4/46, 2/40	q12h	q18h	q24–48h	N.C.	4–5 mg/kg TMP postdialysis	160/800 mg q48h
Vancomycin	1 g IV q12h	40	q24h	q48–60h	q96h	N.C.	1 g q/week	0.5–1 g q/week
Vidarabine	15 mg/kg q24h	0.2	N.C.	N.C.	10 mg/kg q24h	N.C.	Infuse postdialysis	10 mg/kg q24h
Zidovudine (AZT)	100 mg PO q4h	0.5	N.C.	q6h	q6h	N.K.	100 mg postdialysis	100 mg q6h

Abbreviations: N.C. = no change/ N.K. = not known; C.I. = contraindicated; H.D. = hemodialysis; P.D. = peritoneal dialysis.
* Some recommend dose reduction of 20–25%.
† Dose supplement to anuric dosing after H.D.
‡ With an internal range (i.e., Cr. Cl. 50–10, drug dosed at q48–72h), the q48h interval should be used with Cr. Cl. at the higher range (i.e., 50 ml/min) and the q72h interval with Cr. Cl. approaching the lower range (i.e., 10 ml/min).
δ Liver disease being acute or associated with severe hepatic failure as indicated by ascites, jaundice, and/or coagulopathies.
Induction therapy, with iv infusion over 1 hour.
Maintenance therapy, with iv infusion over 2 hours, and dose escalation with failure to suppress retinitis to: 120 mg/kg (normal renal function) OR 90–100 mg/kg (creatinine clearance > 50 ml/min) OR 50–80 mg/kg (creatinine clearance 10–50 ml/min) infused over 2 hours q24h.

CHAPTER 53-A

Antimicrobial Prophylaxis

John Segreti, M.D.

I. Definition

Antibiotics given prior to exposure to bacterial pathogens in order to prevent infection. The actual benefit of many such practices remains the subject of ongoing investigation. Therefore, the recommendations presented in Tables 53A-1 to 53A-6 are subject to change as new experimental data become available.

II. Surgical Antimicrobial Prophylaxis

A. The goal is to prevent postoperative infections, including those of wounds, the urinary tract, and the respiratory tract.

B. Antibiotics are effective only when given immediately before or during the surgical procedure. Antibiotics given hours after surgery are not effective.

Bibliography

Bergamini TM, Polk HC. The importance of tissue antibiotic activity in the prevention of operative wound infection. *J Antimicrob Chemo* 23:301–313, 1989.

Dajani AS, Bisno AL, Chung KJ, et al. Prevention of Bacterial Endocarditis. Recommendation by the American Heart Association. *JAMA* 264:2919–2922, 1990.

Geroulanos S, Oxelbark S, Turina M. Perioperative antimicrobial prophylaxis in cardiovascular surgery. A prospective randomized trial comparing two day cefuroxime prophylaxis with four day cefazolin prophylaxis. *J Cardiovasc Surg* 27:300–306, 1986.

Nichols RL. Current approaches to antibiotic prophylaxis in surgery. *Infect Dis Clin Practice* 2:149–157, 1992.

Segreti J, Levin S. The role of prophylactic antibiotics in the prevention of prosthetic device infections. *Infect Dis Clinics of North America* 3:357–370, 1989.

Table 53A-1.   Examples of Recommended Surgical Antibiotic Prophylaxis

Procedure	Antimocrobial Regimen
Elective colon procedures	Erythromycin (1 g) and neomycin (1 g) three times/day for 1 day before surgery.
Nonelective colon procedures or when patient is unable to take oral medications	Cefoxitin or cefotetan, (1 or 2 g) at the onset of surgery *or* clindamycin (600–900 mg) and either gentamicin or tobramycin (1.7 mg/kg) *or* metronidazole (1 g) and either gentamicin or tobramycin (1.7 mg/kg) at onset of surgery.
Cholecystctomy (high-risk patients—jaundice, age >60, acute symptoms, previous biliary surgery)	Prophylaxis as above.
Gastroduodenal surgery (gastric cancer, bleeding ulcer)	Prophylaxis as above.
Penetrating abdominal trauma, ruptured viscus	Require treatment, not just prophylaxis.
Vaginal or abdominal hysterectomy, cesarean section (only for nonelective, complicated surgeries)	Cefazolin (1–2 g) at onset of surgery or cefoxitin or cefotetan as above.
Head and neck surgeries	Clindamycin (900 mg IV) at onset of surgery.
Orthopedic surgery involving a prosthesis	Cefazolin (1–2 g IV) at onset of surgery. Intraoperative dose if surgery prolonged.
Cardiovascular surgery	Cefazolin (1–2 g IV) at onset of surgery or cerfuroxime (1.5 g IV) every 8 hr for up to 48 hr.

Table 53A-2.   Cardiac Conditions for Which Infective Endocarditis Prophylaxis Is Recommended

Prosthetic cardiac valves
Previous endocarditis
Congenital cardiac malformations (except isolated secundum atrial septal defect)
Rheumatic valvular disease
Hypertrophic cardiomyopathy
Mitral valve prolapse with valvular regurgitation

Table 53A-3.   Procedures for Which Infective Endocarditis Prophylaxis is Recommended

Dental procedures with bleeding
Tonsillectomy and/or adenoidectomy
Surgery involving respiratory or bowel mucosa
Rigid bronchoscopy
Gallbladder surgery
Esophageal dilatation
Sclerotherapy for esophageal varices
Cystoscopy
Urethral dilatation
Urinary catheterization with urinary tract infection present
Prostatic surgery
Incision and drainage of abscess
Vaginal hysterectomy
Vaginal delivery in presence of local infection

Table 53A-4. Prophylactic Regimens for Dental or Oral Procedures in Patients at Risk

Antimicrobial	Dosage
Amoxicillin	3 g p.o. 1 hr before the procedure, then 1.5 g p.o. 6 hr later.
Erythromycin	1 g p.o. 2 hr before the procedure, then 6 hr later.
Clindamycin	300 mg IV or p.o. 1 hr before the procedure, then 150 mg IV or p.o. six hours later.
Ampicillin	2 g IV or IM 30 min prior to the procedure, then 2 g IV or IM 6 hr later.
Vancomycin	1 g IV over 1 hr, starting 1 hr prior to the procedure.

Table 53A-5. Prophylactic Regimens for Patients at Risk Undergoing Gastrointestinal or Genitourinary Procedures

Antimicrobial	Dosage
Ampicillin	2 g IV or IM 30 min prior to the procedure, then repeat 8 hr later.
and	
gentamicin	1.5 mg/kg (not to exceed 80 mg) 30 min prior to the procedure, then repeat 8 hr later.
Vancomycin	1 g IV over 60 min 1 hr prior to the procedure.
and	
gentamicin (for penicillin-allergic patients)	1.5 mg/kg (not to exceed 80 mg) 30–60 min prior to the procedure, then repeat 8 hr later.

Table 53A-6. Other Conditions for Which Prophylactic Antibiotic Use Is Generally Accepted

Condition	Antibiotic Regimen
Prevention of recurrent rheumatic fever	Benzathine penicillin G, 1.2 million units IM every 4 weeks; or oral sulfadiazine, 1 g/day; or penicillin V, 250 mg twice/day for at least 5 years or until patient is over 25 years of age.
Recurrent cellulitis with lymphedema	Benzathine penicillin, 600,000 to 1.2 million units IM every 4 weeks; or penicillin V, 250 mg orally four times/day.
Bite wounds (especially cat and human bites)	Amoxicillin/clavulanate, 500 mg orally three times/day; or penicillin V, 500 mg orally four times/day for 5 days.

CHAPTER 53-B

Health Care Workers and Other Hospital Personnel: Infection Prevention

Alan A. Harris, M.D.

I. Employee Health Service Program

The scope of an employee health service (EHS) program encompasses preemployment and postemployment assessment of physical restrictions, allergies, and underlying diseases which affect job categorization and activities in the workplace. Acute infections are a major cause of days lost. Workplace exposures impact on lost work days, the individual's family, and potential transmission of disease to patients. Exclusion from the workplace due to concerns over communicable infections requires EHS clearance prior to returning.

II. Programs with Direct Benefit for Personnel and Secondary Benefits for Patients

A. Preemployment assessment of physical disabilities relating primarily to the spine or other parts of the musculoskeletal system which preclude certain jobs.

B. Preemployment updates of standard immunizations

1. Diphtheria-tetanus (dT) and measles-mumps-rubella (MMR).

2. Hepatitis B immunization should be strongly recommended for all those with predictable exposures to blood and body fluids. Serologic screening is not mandated, and its benefit and efficiency will depend on the cost of the individual screening test.

C. Annual programs should include:

1. Tuberculin skin testing. Baseline purified protein derivative (PPD) should be obtained at the time of employment.

a. If the test is positive, isonicotinic hydrazide (INH) prophylaxis recommended according to age, history of liver disease, or presence of other underlying illness. Supplemental vitamin B_6 is recommended for individuals at high risk for peripheral neuropathy. I suggest that it should also be given to any individual receiving INH, whether prophylactically or therapeutically.

b. Depending on the patient population or the underlying disease, current reading of an intermediate PPD test as positive will be either 5, 10, or 15 mm of induration. For baseline assessment, in the absence of a history of recent exposure, 10 mm of induration should be considered positive in hospital personnel.

    c. Annual skin testing should be performed to assess for recent conversion. Annual testing will also indicate unsuspected transmission in the hospital/clinic environment.

      (1) In the presence of contact or recent conversion, 5 mm of induration is considered positive.

      (2) Prophylactic INH recommendations in recent converters are independent of age, that is, 35 years of age is not a cutoff.

  2. Influenza immunization

    a. Health care professionals are recognized as vital community resources by the Centers for Disease Control and are recommended to receive annual influenza immunization. At present, programs are voluntary and overall participation rates are low, probably less than 20%.

      (1) During influenza epidemics, as much as 25% of the workforce will be home with illness. This occurs at a time when the most seriously ill, labor-intense patients, frequently requiring respirator care and bronchopulmonary toilet, are being admitted to the hospital.

      (2) Immunization programs should be implemented in the early fall or as soon as the current vaccine becomes available.

      (3) If immunization is delayed until influenza is already occurring in the community, amantadine prophylaxis can be used for 2 weeks while immunization takes effect. Amantadine can be used throughout the influenza season in individuals for whom vaccine is contraindicated. Amantadine prophylaxis is more cumbersome and costly, and less durable and preferable, than immunization.

III. Policies with Direct Benefits for Patient and Hospital Personnel

A. Preemployment education concerning the institution of infection control policies and procedures, availability of elective immunization such as influenza and hepatitis B, mandatory immunization such as measles, and the importance of self-reporting, with its potential for requisite work restrictions.

  1. Policy pertaining to compensation for exclusion from work precipitated by exposures or illness acquired in the workplace should be on-line and non-punitive.

    a. Hospital personnel should be found alternative work, if possible, when the disease of concern is not transmissible through the respiratory route but requires stoppage of direct patient care.

  2. Hospital discharge is a good time to immunize high-risk patients for influenza. Over the ensuing influenza season, admissions for both respiratory and myocardial illness will decline.

B. The importance of hand transmission or acquisition of infectious agents should be stressed. *Staphylococcus aureus* and herpes simplex virus are the classic examples.

  1. Patient care in the absence of barriers should be prohibited while lesions are active.

  2. Handling of insertable devices or vascular lines should be avoided.

C. Febrile diarrhea requires cultures for *Salmonella*, *Shigella*, and *Campylobacter*. In neonatal and pediatric settings, rotavirus is an important pathogen and requires use of the Rotazyme test. Individuals with positive stool cultures in the absence of diarrhea have low communicability. Local laws will apply and will vary according to the jurisdiction and the pathogen.

  1. A positive culture for *Salmonella* usually precludes work in intensive care units, in neonatal units, with high-risk geriatric or immunosuppressed patients. Depending on local law, two to three stool cultures 24 to 72 hr apart, initiated at least 48 to 72 hr following discontinuation of all antimicrobial therapy, will be required.

  2. Typhoid is distinct from other Salmonellae, and usually requires four negative stool cultures, as well as four negative urine cultures, for work clearance.

  3. Routine annual stool culture of food handlers is no longer recommended.

D. Diagnoses of specific communicable infections

  1. Group A β-hemolytic streptococci (*Streptococcus pyogenes*). Nosocomial acquisition of the organism is of greatest concern in the postoperative setting.

    a. Pharyngitis requires work restriction until completion of the first 48 hr of therapy.

b. Impetigo or cellulitis must be resolved.

c. If an individual is linked to an outbreak, all positive culture sites should be negative. One outbreak spanning more than 2 years was traced to scalp and cutaneous lesions in an operating room nurse.

2. Varicella is an ongoing annual concern. A live attenuated vaccine should be available in the future. Community and hospital exposures will occur.

   a. Lesions progress from macules to papules to vesicles to pustules that crust over for approximately 48 hr, appearing during the first 5 days of illness.

   b. Individuals will need to be restricted until no new lesions occur and all existing lesions have crusted. This usually requires 1 week from the time of onset.

3. Rubella—Fever, rash, and adenopathy are characteristic. Unfortunately, infection is asymptomatic in many individuals.

   a. It is of greatest concern when the illness occurs in the first trimester of pregnancy.

   b. Serologic screening is the best way to test for immunity but is not mandatory.

   c. Proof of immunity or immunization can be mandated as a hospitalwide policy or targeted for high-risk areas (i.e., obstetrics, gynecology, pediatrics, outpatient clinics, and/or emergency rooms).

4. Measles—resurgence has occurred during the past few years. A two-dose immunization series is now recommended by the American Academy of Pediatrics and the Advisory Committee on Immunization Practices of the Centers for Disease Control.

   a. Vaccine is recommended for those individuals born after 1956 who do not have a documented history of measles and/or positive serology.

   b. Measles immunity should be assessed at the time of employment. At present, a plan to assess existing hospital personnel is also required. Optimally, an assessment program should include all hospital personnel, students, and volunteers.

   c. Serologic screening by the institution is not obligatory.

   d. Immunization with MMR is recommended and will have spill-over benefit for rubella and mumps protection.

5. Undiagnosed rash—should be evaluated either by the individual's physician or by the EHS. Evaluation should consider the likely etiology in terms of infection, allergy, contact, or toxic eruption. This will enable an assessment of potential communicability. In the absence of a diagnosis, communicability should be assumed and exclusion from the workplace instituted.

IV. **Special Situations**

A. Hospital personnel have recognized home and/or community exposures to varicella, measles, *Salmonella*, *Shigella*, *Campylobacter*, and other known infectious agents to which the employee may be susceptible and capable of subsequent transmission in the workplace. It would be ideal for such employees to bring these exposures to the attention of the EHS, so that an assessment of susceptibility and risk can be made. Unfortunately, this is not practical at the present time, and these problems will usually come to light when hospital personnel are diagnosed as having a problem or are linked to illness in patients.

B. Potential cause of outbreaks—Whenever a cluster of cases occurs in a given patient care area/service, an assessment based on the illness, agent, and potential routes of transmission should be undertaken.

   1. In the case of *Staph. aureus*, group A β-hemolytic streptococci, or diarrheal pathogens, investigation of those individuals common to all cases will be necessary.

   2. Investigations are facilitated when the illness is an easily diagnosed febrile exanthem.

   3. Investigation of bacterial pathogens may require culturing of appropriate sites and work restrictions during and/or following the investigation.

C. Human immunodeficiency virus (HIV)—Employees infected with HIV should be encouraged to call these infections to the attention of appropriate hospital personnel.

   1. Policy and procedure should allow infected individuals to work as long as their activities do not put patients, coworkers, or themselves at risk.

   2. Infected individuals should be evaluated on a regular basis by their personal physician, and this information should be provided to an EHS physician. Alternatively, this physician can assess the individual directly.

a. The mental and physical ability of the individual with HIV infection to perform work duties should be specifically addressed.

b. An assessment should be made of communicable diseases for which these individuals are at risk and for which specific policies, irrespective of the presence or absence of HIV infection, exist (i.e., tuberculosis, *Salmonella*, *Shigella*, dermatitis, herpes simplex virus).

c. HIV-infected persons may also be precluded from caring for patients who put them at greater than usual risk for acquisition of infection (i.e., infections such as tuberculosis).

D. Cytomegalovirus—Most transmission in the community is related to sexual activity and exposure to children. Many hospital personnel will be immune based on prior asymptomatic or, rarely, symptomatic infection.

1. Concern over transmission in the workplace is greatest in neonatal units. Infants congenitally infected are known to shed the virus for several years. These infants are frequently well at birth, and infection is not suspected. Documented transmission is anecdotal.

2. When a patient is known to be actively infected or shedding the virus and an individual involved with direct care of the patient is known to be pregnant, it is preferable to separate the pregnant worker from the patient. Without any work restriction, barrier precautions should be effective and the risk is likely less than from exposures to unsuspected sources.

V. Employees Presenting with a Workplace Exposure to a Specific Infection

A. Varicella zoster—Whether preemployment serologic screening is preferable to postexposure evaluation will depend on the incidence of varicella, logistics, size of the hospital, personnel turnover, and cost. When exposure occurs and an employee's immunity is uncertain:

1. Exposed employees should be screened for a history of chickenpox. While serology or physician documentation is preferable, the characteristic rash makes the history more reliable than with other exanthematous diseases.

2. Individuals with a negative history should be screened serologically. Current methods include enzyme-linked immunosorbent assay (ELISA), the indirect fluo-

rescent antibody test, and fluorescent antibody to membrane antigen (FAMA). Approximately 20% of exposed individuals will need screening, and 80% of this group will be found to be immune. False-positive serology tests are rare.

3. Susceptible individuals will need to be excluded from the workplace from the 9th through 21st day following exposure.

a. Communicability of infection may occur 1 to 4 days prior to the onset of rash. We use 48 hr in calculating the earliest possible exposure for determining the date of work exclusion.

4. The use of varicella zoster immune globulin in otherwise healthy individuals is not a standard recommendation. It may either prevent or modify illness. The cost of a single adult dose is more than $500.

a. If 100% effective, it would obviate the need for workplace exclusion; however, its efficacy is probably no greater than 80%. Therefore, caution is needed if an individual is allowed to work.

b. As with the use of other immune serum globulins (ISGs), there is the potential of prolonging the incubation.

B. Tuberculosis—If a documented exposure occurs, all individuals with negative skin tests not tested within the previous month should be tested with 5 TU intradermal PPD. Those who are negative should be retested 8 to 12 weeks later.

1. A decision to institute INH prophylaxis should be based on tuberculin skin test positivity, not on contact, as might be done in the household setting.

C. Measles (rubeola)

1. The incubation period is 7 to 18 days and may be delayed to 21 days if ISG has been given.

2. Communicability starts in the prodromal phase of cough, coryza, and conjunctivitis and usually antedates the rash by 4 days.

a. Work restrictions of susceptible individuals should be determined by the earliest exposure.

3. Documentation of immunity requires physician diagnosis, two doses of vaccine, or a positive serology test.

4. ISG may either prevent or modify the disease if given within 6 days following exposure.

a. The dose is 0.25 ml/kg in otherwise

healthy individuals and 0.5 ml/kg for those with immunosuppressed illness. The maximum dose is 15 ml.

   b. If there is no contraindication for immunization, it should be given 3 months following the use of ISG.

5. Measles vaccine can be given within the first 72 hr after an exposure. Its efficacy is approximately 75%. This is less than the historical preventive efficacy of ISG. However, the vaccine provides durable immunity rather than the temporary protection provided by ISG.

   a. Postexposure immunization appears less likely than ISG to allow an exposed individual to be both protected and noncommunicable.

D. Blood and body fluid exposures—hepatitis B, hepatitis C, HIV, and syphilis.

1. Local wound care will usually have been accomplished before the individual reports to the EHS. If not, the area should be cleansed with soap and water, followed by either isopropyl alcohol or a 1:10 dilution of household bleach.

2. Baseline assessment of antibodies to hepatitis B virus (HBV), hepatitis C virus (HCV), and HIV should be obtained.

   a. If there is a history of immunization, then hepatitis B surface antibody is the test of choice. In the absence of a history of immunization, the screen can be for either hepatitis B surface antibody or core antibody.

     (1) Do not screen for hepatitis B surface antigen (HBsAg) unless the tested individual is being evaluated for potential linkage to nosocomial transmission to patients.

   b. The only available test for HCV is an antibody test whose sensitivity is not established. Seroconversion may take up to a year. Newer tests to evaluate for communicability of infected individuals, such as occurred with HBV testing, are anticipated.

3. Hepatocellular enzymes and hepatitis B core antibody are used as surrogate markers for non-A, non-B hepatitis.

4. Serology and enzyme determinations should be obtained on source patients when identifiable.

   a. The source patient should also be tested for HBsAg.

5. When an individual is exposed to HBsAg and/or material from a patient who is at known risk for HBV infection and who cannot be tested, the exposed individual should receive hepatitis B immune globulin (HBIG) and the first dose of the three-dose HBV immunization series. The second and third doses of vaccine should follow at 1 and 6 months.

   a. This approach is >90% protective and obviates the need for a second dose of HBIG.

   b. Two doses of HBIG 1 month apart, in the absence of immunization, are only 75% protective. Each dose of HBIG costs as much as the entire HBV primary immunization series.

   c. The need for booster doses is currently unresolved, and evaluation is ongoing. There is no current recommendation for an HBV immunization booster.

     (1) Antibody titers wane over time. Although acute HBV infection has occurred in successfully immunized individuals, such individuals with low antibody titers usually demonstrate an anamnestic response following documented HBsAg exposure.

   d. One currently available HBV vaccine has an approved postexposure four-dose regimen. Vaccine is administered at 0, 1, 2, and 12 months following exposure. While seroconversion occurs sooner, this regimen has not been shown to provide greater protection than the 0-, 1-, and 6-month regimen.

     (1) HBIG must still be administered after exposure.

6. HIV serologies should be obtained at baseline and at least at 3 and 6 months postexposure. Some programs may involve testing at 6 weeks.

   a. The need to inform source patients that they are being tested will vary according to local laws.

   b. Whether or not the source patient is prospectively notified, if this patient is found to be positive, his or her physician should be notified. A physician from the EHS, infection control department, or hospital epidemiology department should notify the personal physician. He or she should decide on who will notify the patient.

c. The use of zidovudine (AZT) prophylaxis after documented HIV exposure remains controversial. Failures have clearly been documented. Efficacy will be difficult to assess with a baseline risk of ≤0.04%.
  (1) Long-term toxicity is unknown. Vaginal and cervical cancers have been reported in animals.
  (2) If AZT is utilized, the recommended dose is 1,000–1,500 mg/day for 6 weeks—which is in excess of current recommendations for individuals known to be infected and/or diseased.
    (a) Gastrointestinal intolerance and/or marrow suppression may preclude completion of therapy in 25–33% of individuals.
7. ISG for the prevention of non-A, non-B hepatitis is unproven. The availability of hepatitis C serologies will enable us to determine whether protective antibody is present in commercial lots of ISG. This will require identification of neutralizing antibodies to HCV. Hepatitis C will not account for all cases of non-A, non-B hepatitis. We currently recommend ISG if exposure to non-A, non-B hepatitis was likely. Employees are counseled and are free to refuse treatment. Other institutions may choose not to make the offer.
8. Serologies should be repeated long enough after exposure of concern for seroconversion to have occurred.
9. Treat for syphilis if the employee is susceptible and seroconverts or if the source patient is documented to be infected.
E. Noninfectious exposures which may mimic communicable disease

1. Respiratory illness due to allergens or noxious substances. The classic noxious substance is carbon monoxide. Early symptoms include headache, nausea, and vomiting. Foodborne illness is frequently suspected.
  a. Do not forget that *Legionella* may cause outbreaks of pneumonia or fever related to cooling towers and evaporative condensers. Some cases are also associated with potable water.
2. Contact dermatitis associated with the use of commercial soaps. This usually results in clustering on single or multiple patient care units. Nurses are most frequently affected. Attack rates are highest in those who are the best hand washers.
  a. Scabies is an erythematous, pruritic eruption. A hyperinfested patient (with Norwegian scabies) is usually the source. Outbreaks may last for more than a year. Personnel may infect family members at home.

Bibliography

Balcarek KB, Bagley R, Cloud GA, et al. Cytomegalovirus infection among employees of a children's hospital. *JAMA* 263:840–844, 1990.

Benenson AS. *Control of Communicable Diseases in Man*, ed 15. Washington DC, American Public Health Association, 1990.

Bennett JV, Brachman PS. *Hospital Infections*. Boston, Little, Brown, 1979.

Fedson DS. Influenza and pneumococcal immunization strategies for physicians. *Chest* 91:436–443, 1987.

Polk BF, White JA, DeGirolami PC, et al. An outbreak of rubella among hospital personnel. *N Engl J Med* 303:542–545, 1980.

Wenzel RP. *Handbook of Hospital Acquired Infections*. Boca Raton, FL, CRC Press, 1981.

SECTION 7

Digestive Diseases

CHAPTER 54-A

Heartburn and Dysphagia

Sheldon Sloan, M.D.

I. **Definition**

Heartburn is a common symptom experienced by at least 44% of the adult population at least once a month. Although the classic symptom is described as substernal burning, sour belching, water brash, or epigastric discomfort, the underlying pathophysiology stems from reflux of gastric acid into the esophagus. The symptoms do not necessarily correlate with the severity of the disease (i.e., esophagitis).

II. **History**

The history of the patient's symptoms help guide the workup and treatment.

A. Are symptoms worse when the patient is supine, upright, or bending over?

B. Is the onset associated with meals?

C. What foods precipitate the attach (e.g., chocolate, alcohol (EtOH), spearmint, peppermint, high-fat foods, spicy foods?)

D. Has there been recent weight gain?

E. Does the patient have recalcitrant asthma or recurrent laryngitis?

F. Is there difficulty swallowing?

III. **Physical Examination**

Physical exam may be negative although some patients have tenderness in the epigastric area.

IV. **Workup**

Workup for heartburn is individualized. Patients who have mild symptoms and who respond to antacids may not need further workup. Patients with associated symptoms (e.g., asthma, laryngitis, dysphagia) should have a workup.

A. Barium esophagogram is helpful in delineating anatomy (e.g., stricture, hiatal hernia, diverticula), gross mucosal detail (e.g., moderate and severe esophagitis, neoplasm), and function (e.g., peristaltic stripping wave).

B. Endoscopy is better for delineating finer mucosal detail (e.g., mild esophagitis, Barrett's esophagus), allows the option of tissue sampling, and has therapeutic capability (e.g., dilatation, hemostasis).

C. Ambulatory 24-hr pH monitoring helps determine whether the symptoms correlate with reflux.

D. Esophageal manometry (see the discussion of esophageal motility testing in Chapter 56) measures lower esophageal sphincter tone and peristaltic function. In addition, a Bernstein test can be easily performed to determine if the patient has an acid-sensitive esophagus.

V. Treatment

See the section on gastroesophageal reflux disease in Chapter 56.

Dysphagia

I. Definition

The sensation of difficulty with swallowing is a problem usually localized to the upper alimentary tract, either in the oropharynx or the esophagus. The presence of a constant sensation unrelated to swallowing (i.e., globus histericus) is not dysphagia. The history is important to assess the nature as well as the level of involvement. If dysphagia occurs during the initiation of swallowing and is associated with aspiration (e.g., coughing, stridor, wheezing), nasal regurgitation, or impaction of food in the posterior oral pharynx, then the problem may be localized to the oral pharynx and may be classified as oropharyngeal dysphagia, also referred to as *transfer dysphagia* (see below). If the patient can swallow and clear the oropharynx, but complains of food "sticking" or has immediate regurgitation, this is most likely due to esophageal dysphagia (see below). As with oropharyngeal and esophageal dysphagia, the mechanism of poor bolus transit must be delineated as due to either a structural or a functional (motor) cause. Keeping this in mind, the history and resultant workup lead to the diagnosis.

II. Physiology of Normal Swallowing

The act of initiating swallowing (deglutition) requires sensory input at the level of the anterior tonsillar pillars. Sensory information incorporates temperature, bolus size, and bolus consistency, and this information flows through cranial nerves (V, VII, IX, X, and XII) into the solitary tract nucleus (a component of the swallowing center) located in the medulla and the pons. The efferent output of the swallowing sequence is carried through cranial nerves similar to those of afferent loop, with the addition to the dorsal motor nucleus and the nucleus ambiguus of the vagus nerve. The efferent sympathetic innervation comes from the paravertebral and cervical ganglia.

III. Pathophysiology

A. Oropharyngeal dysphagia: structural causes
 1. Carcinoma of the oropharynx or proximal esophagus.
 2. Benign esophageal tumors.
 3. Proximal esophageal webs, Zencker's diverticulum, proximal esophageal strictures.
 4. Postsurgical changes.
 5. Vertebral spur.
 6. Thyromegaly.
B. Oropharyngeal dysphagia: neurologic causes
 1. Cerebrovascular accident.
 2. Parkinson's disease.
 3. Amyotropic lateral sclerosis.
 4. Multiple sclerosis.
 5. Diabetes mellitus.
 6. Recurrent laryngeal nerve palsy.
 7. Guillain-Barré syndrome.
C. Oropharyngeal dysphagia: skeletal muscle diseases
 1. Inflammatory myopathies (e.g., mixed connective tissue disease, polymyositis, scleroderma).
 2. Muscular dystrophies.
 3. Hyper- and hypothyroidism.
 4. Myasthenia gravis.
 5. Cricopharyngeus achalasia.
D. Esophageal dysphagia
 The normal response to an initiated swallow is a sequential caudad contraction of the esophagus called *primary peristalsis*. Once a swallow is initiated in the orol pharynx, the motor activity in the esophagus, much like that in the orol pharynx, is a programmed, involuntary response. Secondary peristalsis is a nonswallow-induced sequential peristaltic sequence that is usually induced by any remaining bolus not cleared by primary peristalsis that distends the esophagus. When there is a disruption in primary peristalsis, either by a motor abnormality or by a structural abnormality, symptomatic dysphagia may result. The differential diagnosis is defined by the patient's history. If there is progressive dysphagia for solids such that only purreed food can be successfully ingested, then a structural lesion should be suspected. Acute symptoms of complete esophageal obstruction while ingesting solids are also indicative of a persistent narrowing in the esophagus. On the other hand, if the dysphagia is for both liquids and solids and/or there is an association with chest discomfort, then a motor abnormality may be more likely.
 1. Structural (obstructive) causes of esophageal dysphagia
   a. Esophageal and gastric carcinomas
   b. Mucosal rings (Schatzki's), muscular rings, esophageal webs, and peptic strictures.
   c. Vascular and mediastinal compression.

    d. Hiatal hernia.

  2. Motor (nonobstructive) causes of esophageal dysphagia

    a. Achalasia.

    b. Diffuse esophageal spasm.

    c. Nutcracker esophagus.

    d. Esophagitis.

IV. Approach to Workup

In a patient with dysphagia, a thorough history and physical exam evaluating for neurologic, myopathic, or rheumatologic disease is essential. The level at which the bolus is not advancing in patients with oropharyngeal dysphagia is very accurate; however, in a patient with esophageal dysphagia, localization of the problem is inexact. A good method to use in starting the diagnostic workup is radiology. A swallowing video-fluoroscopy is better than an upper gastrointestinal series or a barium esophagogram in a patient with oropharyngeal dysphagia because of the complex events taking place. Within 1 sec, the video playback allows careful analysis of the relationship of the oropharyngeal structures during the course of the swallow. If a patient describes the dysphagia as a sticking sensation in the suprasternal notch or chest, a barium esophagogram is a good first test because this will provide information not only on structural abnormalities but on motor abnormalities as well (the latter are often discovered during the fluoroscopic part of the test). The information obtained radiographically will dictate the next step. Upper endoscopy will be needed if there is a structural abnormality such as a benign stricture or suggestion of a tumor. Even if achalasia is suspected by the barium esophagogram, upper endoscopy is indicated to rule out a malignancy at the gastroesophageal junction. The gold standard with regard to motility disorders is an esophageal manometry study. This is indicated if the dysphagia appears to be nonobstructive.

Bibliography (Heartburn)

Cohen S, Harris LD. Does hiatus hernia affect competence of the gastroesophageal sphincter? *N Engl J Med* 284:1053–1056, 1971.

Dodds WJ. The pathogenesis reflux disease. *AJR* 151:49–56, 1988.

Dodds WJ, Dent J, Hogan WJ, et al. Mechanisms of gastroesophageal reflux in patients with reflux esophagitis. *N Engl J Med* 308:1547–1552, 1982.

Sloan, S, Kahrilas PJ. Impairment of esophageal emptying with heated hernia. *Gastroenterology* 100:596–605, 1991.

Sloan S, Rademaker AW, Kahrilas PJ. Determinants of gastroesophageal junction competence: hiatus hernia, lower esophageal sphincter or both? *Ann Int Med* 117:977–982, 1992.

Bibliography (Dysphagia)

Kahrilas PJ, Kishk SM, Helm JF, et al. Comparison of pseudoachalasia and achalasia. *Am J Med* 82:439–446, 1987.

Marshall JB, Dysphagia: Diagnostic pitfalls and how to avoid them. *Postgrad Med* 85:243–260, 1989.

Marshall JB, Diagnosis of esophageal motility disorders. *Postgrad Med* 87:81–94, 1990.

Stuart RC, Hennessy TPJ. Primary disorders of oesophageal motility. *Br J Surg* 76:1111–1120, 1989.

Approach to the Patient with Vomiting

Bennett Plotnick, M.D.

I. Problem and Differential Diagnosis
Vomiting may be a manifestation of a wide variety of conditions.
A. Gastrointestinal obstruction
B. Gastroparesis
C. Pregnancy
D. Motion sickness
E. Radiation sickness
F. Drug toxicity
G. Hepatitis
H. Myocardial infarction
I. Renal failure
J. Increased intracranial pressure
K. Asthma
L. Zollinger-Ellison syndrome
M. Diabetes mellitus
N. Thyrotoxicosis
O. Epilepsy
Serious complications of vomiting include:
A. Aspiration pneumonia
B. Mallory-Weiss syndrome
C. Esophageal rupture
D. Volume and electrolyte depletion
E. Acid-base imbalance
F. Malnutrition

II. Focus of History and Physical Examination
A. Relation to meals
1. Early (soon after eating)
a. Psychogenic vomiting
b. Peptic ulcer disease
c. Acute gastritis
2. Delayed (more than 1 hr after meals)
a. Gastric outlet obstruction
b. Motility disorder such as diabetic or postvagotomy gastroparesis
c. Succussion splash present on physical exam.
3. Early morning
a. Pregnancy
b. Bilious vomiting in patients with prior gastrectomy
c. Uremia
d. Alcoholism
e. Postnasal drip
f. Increased intracranial pressure
B. Vomitus content
1. Old food
a. Gastric outlet obstruction
b. High small bowel obstruction
c. Gastroparesis

2. Undigested food
  a. Esophageal disease such as achalasia or Zenker's diverticulum
3. Blood
4. Bile
  a. Excludes gastric or proximal duodenal obstruction.
  b. Common after gastric surgery.
C. Vomitus odor
  1. Feculent
    a. Intestinal obstruction
    b. Ileus
    c. Gastrocolic fistula
    d. Ischemia
    e. Bacterial overgrowth
D. Significant other features obtained from the history and physical exam include:
  1. Duration of vomiting
  2. Patient's age
  3. Presence or absence of weight loss
  4. Presence of an abdominal mass
  5. Dysphagia
  6. Chest pain
  7. Jaundice
  8. Abdominal distention and character of bowel sounds
  9. Presence of cardiovascular disease suggesting intestinal ischemia.

III. **Diagnostic Approach**
A. Careful history and physical exam, with particular attention to the preceding discussion.
B. Upper gastrointestinal (GI) x-ray with small bowel follow-through, as well as air contrast lower GI and upper endoscopy, to exlude the presence of an anatomic obstruction.
C. Radionuclear gastric emptying study to determine the presence of gastroparesis if no evidence of obstruction is found and the history is suggestive of a motility disorder.
D. Computed tomography (CT) scan of the head if the history suggests increased intracranial pressure
E. CT scan of the abdomen if the history and physical exam suggest a hepatic, pancreatic, or biliary source or if an abdominal mass is suspected.
F. Mesenteric angiography if intestinal ischemia is suspected.

Bibliography

Feldman M. Nausea and vomiting, in Sleisenger MH (ed): *Gastrointestinal Disease*, ed 4. Philadelphia, Saunders, 1989, pp 222–235.

Hanson JS, McCallum RW. The diagnosis and management of nausea and vomiting: A review. *Am J Gastroenterol* 80:210–218, 1985.

Malagalada JR, Camilleri M. Unexplained vomiting. A diagnostic challenge. *Ann Intern Med* 101:211–218, 1984.

Approach to the Patient with Abdominal Pain

Bennett Plotnick, M.D.

I. Problem

Acute abdominal pain is an important symptom in many diseases of the surgical and nonsurgical abdomen. The assessment of acute abdominal pain is one of the most challenging problems in medicine. A careful history and physical examination are required to separate conditions that require surgery from those pain syndromes that occur daily.

II. Differential Diagnosis of the Problem

A. Intra-abdominal
   1. Generalized peritonitis
      a. Perforated viscus
      b. Primary bacterial peritonitis
      c. Nonbacterial peritonitis
      d. Familial Mediterranean fever
   2. Localized peritonitis
      a. Appendicitis
      b. Cholecystitis
      c. Peptic ulcer
      d. Meckel's diverticulitis
      e. Regional enteritis
      f. Colonic diverticulitis
      g. Colitis
      h. Abdominal abscess
      i. Gastroenteritis
      j. Pancreatitis
      k. Acute hepatitis
      l. Pelvic inflammatory disease
      m. Endometritis
      n. Lymphadenitis
   3. Pain from increased visceral tension
      a. Intestinal obstruction
      b. Intestinal hypermotility
      c. Biliary obstruction
      d. Ureteral obstruction
      e. Hepatic capsule obstruction
      f. Renal capsule obstruction
      g. Uterine obstruction
      h. Ruptured ectopic pregnancy
      i. Aortic aneurysm
   4. Ischmia
      a. Intestinal angina or infarction
      b. Splenic infarction
      c. Torsion
      d. Hepatic infarction
      e. Tumor necrosis
   5. Retroperitoneal neoplasms
B. Extra-abdominal
   1. Thoracic
      a. Pneumonitis
      b. Pulmonary embolism

    c. Pneumothorax
    d. Empyema
    e. Myocardial infarction
    f. Myocarditis, endocarditis
    g. Esophagitis, esophageal spasm
    h. Esophageal rupture
2. Neurogenic
    a. Radiculitis
    b. Tabes dorsalis
    c. Abdominal epilepsy
3. Metabolic
    a. Uremia
    b. Diabetes Mellitus
    c. Porphyria
    d. Acute adrenal insufficiency
4. Toxins
    a. Hypersensitivity reactions
    b. Drugs
5. Miscellaneous
    a. Muscular contusion, hematoma, or tumor

III. Focus of History and Physical Examination
A. Pattern of pain
  1. Location
    a. Visceral pain is poorly localized, whereas parietal pain is localized to the area of disease. Radiation of pain often occurs, as seen in shoulder pain from diaphragmatic irritation and back pain from biliary, duodenal, and pancreatic diseases.
  2. Intensity and character
    a. Burning or gnawing pain of a duodenal ulcer.
    b. Tearing pain of a ruptured aneurysm.
    c. Excruciating pain of mesenteic infarction or perforated ulcer.
  3. Relation to time
    a. Pain persisting for more than 6 hr usually suggests a surgical abdomen.
    b. Colicky pain of intestinal obstruction.
    c. Steady pain of ischemia or strangulation.
  4. Associated signs and symptoms
    a. Anorexia, nausea, vomiting.
    b. Diarrhea, constipation.
    c. Renal function.
    d. Gynecologic history.
B. Physical exam
  1. Inspection
    a. Tachycardia, fever, and diaphoresis suggest sepsis and toxemia.
    b. Frequent patient movements and changing of position are seen with visceral pain, whereas movement is avoided in the patient with parietal pain.
    c. Distention, as seen in obstruction and ascites.
  2. Auscultation
    a. Hyperperistalsis in obstruction and enteritis.
    b. Hypoperistalsis in ileus and peritonitis.
    c. Bruits seen in aortic or splenic artery aneurysm.
  3. Palpation
    a. Rigidity and guarding in adjacent peritonitis.
    b. Palpable mass may be produced by inflammation, tumors, hematomas, or an enlarged viscus.
    c. Rebound tenderness.
    d. Hyperesthesia may be seen corresponding to the dermatome of the parietal pain.
    e. Mandatory genital rectal and pelvic exams with stool for occult blood.

IV. Diagnostic Approach
A. Complete blood count
  1. Important for evaluating blood loss and infection.
B. Urinalysis
  1. Microscopic exam may suggest infection or stone disease.
C. Electrolytes
  1. Necessary to estimate the extent of fluid losses. Blood sugar and urine acetone analyses to rule out ketoacidosis.
D. Serum amylase
  1. Not specific for pancreatitis, as in perforation and other inflammatory diseases of the abdomen.
E. Paracentesis
  1. Mandatory in the presence of ascites.
F. Chest roentgenogram
  1. Important in determining the presence of free intraperitoneal air, pneumonitis, or a subdiaphragmatic process.
G. Plain abdominal roentgenogram
  1. Calcification in an aortic aneurysm.
  2. Obliteration of the psoas shadow, indicating retroperitoneal fluid.
  3. Gas pattern indicating areas of obstruction.
  4. Bowel wall gas indicating infarction.
  5. Kidney or ureteral stones.
  6. Air in the gallbladder or biliary tree.
  7. Stones in the gallbladder or pancreas.
H. Ultrasound or computed tomography scanning

    1. Important in diagnosis of pancreatobiliary disease, presence of aortic aneurysm, abdominal abscess, and pelvic diseases such as pelvic inflammatory disease and ectopic pregnancy.

I. Exploratory laparotomy is mandatory in:
    1. Severe generalized pain unresponsive to treatment.
    2. Generalized peritonitis.
    3. Free intraperitoneal air.
    4. Free intraperitoneal blood.
    5. Posttraumatic peritonitis.
    6. Clinical diagnosis of:
      a. Ruptured aortic aneury.
      b. Mesenteric infarction.
      c. Intestinal obstruction.

Bibliography

Cope Z: *Cope's Early Diagnosis of the Acute Abdomen*, ed 16, New York, Oxford University Press, 1983.

Fields HL. *Pain*. New York, McGraw-Hill, 1987.

Sarfeh IJ. Abdominal pain of unknown etiology. *Am J Surg* 132:22, 1976.

Way W. Abdominal pain, in Sleisenger MH (ed): *Gastrointestinal Disease*. ed 4. Philadelphia, Saunders, 1989, p 238.

Chapter 54-D

Malabsorption and Maldigestion

Michael D. Brown, M.D.

I. Definition

The decreased intestinal absorption of protein, fat, carbohydrates, and vitamins. *Malabsorption* refers to loss of mucosal absorptive function, while *maldigestion* refers to loss of intraluminal digestive function.

A. Intraluminal maldigestion

Loss of luminally active enzymes and bile salts necessary for the early processes of digestion. Examples include pancreatic insufficiency and bacterial overgrowth.

B. Mucosal malabsorption

Loss of the ability to further hydrolyze and absorb nutrients from the lumen secondary to loss or damage of the small bowel epithelium. Examples include celiac sprue and Crohn's disease.

C. Lymphatic obstruction

Obstruction of draining lymphatics leads to an inability to transport chylomicrons into the serum and when severe, leads to a protein-losing enteropathy. Examples are congenital lymphangiectasia and tuberculosis.

II. Etiology

There are many disease states associated with malabsorption and/or maldigestion.

A. Intraluminal maldigestion

1. Bacterial overgrowth

Bacterial overgrowth may occur in conditions leading to small bowel stasis (obstruction/dysmotility), loss of gut immunocompetence, and achlorhydria. This results in bacterial growth in the small intestine exceeding 10^5 organisms. There are three proposed mechanisms for maldigestion secondary to bacterial overgrowth:

a. Conversion of conjugated bile salts to free bile acids by bacterial enzymes.

b. Binding and uptake of vitamin B_{12} by bacteria.

c. Direct mucosal damage by bacterial endotoxins and proteases.

2. Pancreatic exocrine deficiency

Destruction of the pancreatic parenchyma and/or pancreatic duct obstruction may lead to loss of intraluminal proteases, bicarbonate, and lipases. A 90% loss of pancreatic function is necessary to achieve steatorrhea secondary to pancreatic insufficiency. Chronic pancreatitis may result from chronic alcohol ingestion, hypercalcemia, congenital malformations (pancreas divisum, annular pancreas), and idiopathic pancreatitis. Other pancreatopathies associated with malabsorption include pancreatic carcinoma, cystic fibrosis, and pancreatic fistula. Diabetes is a frequent complication. Fat malabsorption is usually marked, and protein malabsorption with resulting azatorrhea can be significant in severe cases of pancreatic insufficiency. Vitamin and carbohydrate malabsorption does not occur, with the exception of vitamin B_{12}, the absorption of which is impaired by loss of protease cleavage and dissociation of the R protein–vitamin B_{12} complex.

3. Hepatobiliary dysfunction
   Liver failure and/or biliary duct obstruction can lead to a deficiency of intraluminally active bile salts and fat malabsorption.

B. Mucosal malabsorption
   1. Celiac sprue
      Celiac sprue is characterized by nonspecific destruction of the proximal small bowel mucosa secondary to an immune response to the protein portion of certain cereal grains (gluten). α-Gliadin appears to be the portion of gluten that is most culpable. A genetic predisposition is suggested by the increased incidence in patient's families and by the distribution of genetic markers. Human leukocyte antigen (HLA)-B8 and HLA-DR3 are found in 60–90% of all sprue patients. Histologically, the typical columnar mucosa is cuboidal or flat. Patients develop marked steatorrhea and azatorrhea, with resultant weight loss. The mainstay of therapy is a gluten-free diet. Patients must fastidiously avoid foods containing wheat, rye, barley, and probably oat brans. Rice, corn, soybeans, and potatoes are allowed. Dairy products may also be limited initially. Rare cases of refractory sprue require steroid therapy. Complications include strictures and lymphoma.
   2. Tropical sprue
      This disorder is seen in tropical climates or in patients returning to temperate zones from these areas. It is characterized by mild to moderate fat and protein malabsorption, with destruction of the mucosal surface. The surface villi are coalesced into clumps, unlike the flat mucosa seen in celiac sprue. The proposed etiol-

ogy is chronic intestinal contamination with enteric pathogens including *Klebsiella*, *Escherichia coli*, and *Enterobacter*. The permissive events allowing bacterial overgrowth of the proximal small bowel in these patients are not clear. Therapy includes folic acid (5 mg/day) and antibacterials, typically tetracycline (250 mg four times per day). Treatment may be necessary for several months, and cessation is based on the clinical response.

3. Crohn's disease
   Malabsorption secondary to this transmural inflammatory process may be caused by:
   a. Small bowel bypass secondary to fistulas or surgery.
   b. Bacterial overgrowth secondary to stasis from obstruction.
   c. Loss of small bowel mucosal surface area secondary to inflammation and/or surgical resection.

4. Lymphoma
   Bowel lymphomas may be associated with mucosal malabsorption secondary to infiltration and destruction of small bowel mucosa.

5. Whipple's disease
   This is a multisystem disease characterized by a thickened and edematous small bowel mucosa with flattening of the villi, as in celiac sprue. The characteristic histologic findings include the presence of periodic acid-Schiff (PAS)-positive staining macrophages and small bacilli in the lamina propria. These lesions result in marked malabsorption with diarrhea secondary to a severe steatorrhea. In addition, these patients may present with a variety of extraintestinal manifestations, including:
   a. Neurologic (10%): Manifests as dementia, lethargy, convulsions, and cranial neuropathies.
   b. Cardiac: Pericarditis, valvulopathy, and congestive heart failure secondary to invasion of the cardiac tissues by the causative bacilli.
   c. Joint: Arthritis is the most common extraintestinal manifestation and may be present for years prior to the onset of bowel disease. The arthritis is typically migratory, affecting small and large joints. Permanent joint deformity does not occur.

Therapy is aimed at eradication of the offending but as yet unidentified microorganism. First-line therapy includes 6 months to 1 year of trimethoprim-sulfamethoxazole. For patients unable to tolerate this medication, chloramphenicol or penicillin are alternatives. From 30% to 40% of patients may relapse and are treated with the same antibacterials.

6. Amyloidosis
Both primary and secondary types of amyloidosis have been associated with malabsorption. Possible mechanisms include ischemia from arteriolar infiltration, amyloid infiltration of the lamina propria, and intestinal dysmotility with stasis and secondary bacterial overgrowth.

7. Abetalipoproteinemia
This is a rare hereditary condition characterized by the inability of the enterocyte to synthesize apoprotein B, which is necessary for chylomicron formation. Fat cannot leave the enterocytes, and the mucosal biopsy demonstrates large fat globules in the enterocytes. Patients present with fat malabsorption, acanthocytic red blood cells, and neurologic signs which include ataxia, retinitis pigmentosa, tremors, and nystagmus. Treatment includes medium-chain substitutes for long-chain triglycerides and fat-soluble vitamin supplements.

8. Radiation enteritis
Acute radiation injury can lead to loss of mucosal absorptive surface but is usually self-limited. More important, chronic radiation injury can lead to malabsorption secondary to ischemia from fibrosis of the mucosal arterioles and bacterial overgrowth from bowel stasis secondary to strictures.

9. Eosinophilic gastroenteritis
This is a rare disorder of middle age associated with a variety of food allergies, eczema, and allergic rhinitis. It is characterized by various depths of a patchy eosinophilic infiltrate. The serosa, submucosa, and mucosa of the stomach, small bowel, or colon may be involved. A peripheral eosinophilia is always seen. The mucosal type presents with typical symptoms of malabsorption, including diarrhea, weight loss, and abdominal pain.

The submucosal process presents with symptoms of obstruction and gut dysmotility, which may lead to stasis and bacterial overgrowth. The serosal process presents with ascites. Diagnosis is typically made by biopsy of the affected portion of the digestive tract but requires full-thickness biopsy in the subserosal variant. Serosal disease is diagnosed by ascitic eosinophilia and peritoneal biopsy. Therapy includes corticosteroids and, rarely, surgery in case of obstruction.

10. Hypogammaglobulinemia
Secondary hypogammaglobulinemia may occur in malabsorptive states accompanied by a protein-losing enteropathy such as Crohn's disease and Whipple's disease, acquired immunodeficiency syndrome (AIDS) enteropathy, and celiac sprue. Primary hypogammaglobulinemia is rarely associated with malabsorption, and investigation of steatorrhea in these patients may reveal giardiasis.

11. Parasitic infections
A wide variety of parasites have been associated with malabsorption secondary to loss of enterocytes or coating of the mucosal surface by organisms or competition for intraluminal nutrients

12. Disaccharidase deficiency
Lactose intolerance is the most common inherited or acquired disaccharidase deficiency but is not associated with steatorrhea. Symptoms include bloating, diarrhea, and abdominal cramping after ingestion of lactose-containing foods. The diagnosis of typically made by the response to therapeutic measures. Small bowel biopsy with lactase measurements or screening with the oral lactose tolerance test or lactose breath test are required for a definite diagnosis. Therapy includes avoidance of dairy products and lactase supplementation.

13. Endocrinopathies
Hyper- and hypothyroidism are associated with altered gut motility and can be associated with a mild to moderate malabsorption syndrome. Mild steatorrhea is seen in Addison's disease and hypoparathyroidism.

14. Drug-associated
Antibiotics may be associated a mild malabsorption secondary to changes in bacte-

rial flora. Colchicine, methotrexate and laxatives may directly damage the intestinal mucosa. Cholestyramine binds bile salts and can lead to a mild malabsorption of fat and fat-soluble vitamins. Octreotide acetate, the synthetic somatostatin analogue, can be associated with diminished fat absorption secondary to a direct reduction in small intestinal absorptive capacity, diminished pancreatic secretions and altered gut motility.

15. AIDS enteropathy

The severe wasting syndrome seen in AIDS patients is often accompanied by the onset of chronic diarrhea, anorexia, and severe weight loss. Malabsorption in these cases may be secondary to chronic opportunistic infections of the small bowel such as *Mycobacterium avium-intracellulare, Giardia, Cryptosporidium,* or cytomegalovirus. Human immuno-deficiency virus (HIV) itself may directly damage small bowel mucosa and lead to malabsorption. Therapy is directed at the organism but is often unsuccessful.

16. Short bowel syndrome

Obviously, loss of significant amounts of the small bowel may lead to severe steatorrhea and may require lifelong parenteral nutritional support. Parenteral supplementation is necessary in patients with less than 2 ft of remaining jejunum or ileum. Loss of the distal ileum results in specific malabsorption of fat, bile salts, and vitamin B_{12}. If more than 100 cm of distal ileum is resected, fat malabsorption is severe. Over time some intestinal adaptation occurs, with hypertrophy of remaining villi and enlargement and elongation of unresected small bowel. Therapy includes parenteral or refined enteral nutrition and antidiarrheals. Some enteral intake appears to be crucial for adaptation.

C. Lymphatic obstruction

Tuberculosis, lymphoma, metastatic carcinoma, retroperitoneal fibrosis, and primary lymphangiectasia are associated with lymphatic obstruction, moderate to severe fat malabsorption, and, in some cases, protein-losing enteropathy. Biopsy shows dilated lymphatic lacteals. Therapy is aimed at the underlying disease. Dietary supplementation with medium-chain triglycerides may help.

III. **Diagnostic Tests for Malabsorption** (Figure 54D-1)

A. Serum tests

Low levels of total protein, albumin, carotene, cholesterol, calcium, phosphorus, and magnesium and prolongation of the prothrombin time suggest fat and protein malabsorption. Low folate, vitamin B_{12}, and iron levels suggest malabsorption of water-soluble substances. Abnormalities in these serum markers of malabsorption coupled with clinical findings should prompt further workup, starting with fecal fat evaluation.

B. Stool tests

A 24-hr stool collection for volume and fat should be obtained in all patients with suspected steatorrhea. The 72-hr fecal fat measurement is the gold standard but is very cumbersome to obtain. The 24-hr exam appears to be sensitive enough to use as a screen. Stool fat in excess of 6 g in 24 hr is abnormal, however this degree of fecal fat loss may be seen in diarrheal states unassociated with malabsorption. Stool fat exceeding 12 g in 24 hr is a more discriminate indicator of malabsorption. Sudan staining of the stool for fat is neither sensitive nor specific; quantitative testing is required. Stool levels of α-1-antitrypsin are used to assess bowel protein losses and diagnose protein-losing enteropathies.

C. D-Xylose absorption test

This is the best test for identifying mucosal malabsorption. It involves ingestion of 25 g of D-xylose followed by measurement of blood xylose levels at 2 hr and of urine xylose levels at 5 hr. Abnormal mucosal absorption is likely when urine excretion is less than 4 g in 5 hr and blood serum levels are less than 20 mg/dl. Sensitivity exceeds 90% and specificity exceeds 98%. Urine D-xylose excretion may be falsely lowered by renal insufficiency, delayed gastric emptying, and medications such as glipizide, neomycin, and aspirin. Serum measurements are usually accurate in these situations; however, delayed gastric emptying, aspirin, glipizide, portal hypertension, and ascites may falsely decrease the serum rise of D-xylose.

D. Hydrogen breath test

Bacterial breakdown of nonabsorbed carbohydrates leads to production of breath hydrogen. Patients with mucosal absorptive disorders will malabsorb the selected test carbohydrate (lactose, lactulose, sucrose), allowing the colonic

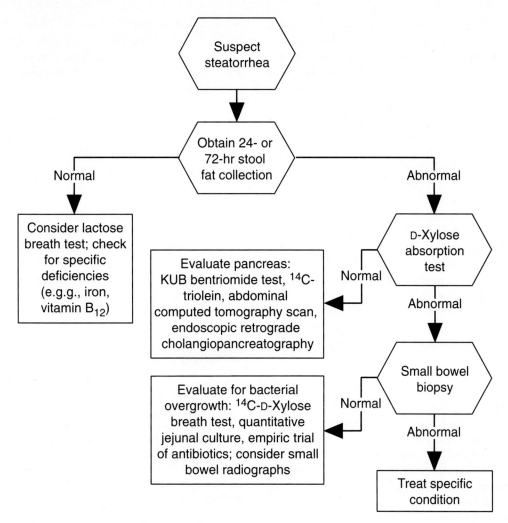

Figure 54D-1. Decision Analysis Flow Chart for Steatorrhea

bacteria to create a peak in breath hydrogen. Bacterial overgrowth leads to a similar but earlier peak. Patients with pancreatic disease can have abnormal hydrogen breath tests.

E. Small bowel biopsy

The small bowel mucosal biopsy is obtained with either a capsule device or endoscopic biopsy forceps. Flattening of the villi is seen in a variety of conditions and is a nonspecific injury. Celiac sprue, tropical sprue, bacterial overgrowth, lymphoma, *Giardia* infections, and radiation injury may all demonstrate flattening of villi. Specific characteristics of the small bowel biopsy in a variety of conditions are as follows:

1. Celiac and tropical sprue: Increased lymphocytes and plasma cells in the lamina propria.
2. Crohn's disease: Noncaseating granulomas.

3. Lymphoma: Malignant lymphocytes in the lamina propria.
4. Amyloidosis: Amyloid deposits in blood vessels.
5. Abetalipoproteinemia: Lipid-filled epithelial cells.
6. Lymphangiectasia: Dilated lymphatic lacteals in the lamina propria.
7. Giardiasis: Presence of trophozooites.
8. Whipple's disease: PAS-positive macrophages in the lamina propria and gram-negative bacilli.

F. Breath tests

1. ^{14}C D-Xylose

This is best test for bacterial overgrowth. Although the gold standard is quantitative anaerobic culture this is difficult both to obtain and to reproduce. The ^{14}C-D-xylose breath test measures the amount of $^{14}CO_2$ exhaled 1 hr after a 1-g oral dose. Bacteria break down the labeled xylose to labeled CO_2, and in patients with bacterial overgrowth an early marked increase in exhaled $^{14}CO_2$ is measured. Xylose offers the advantage of being completely absorbed in the proximal small bowel. This avoids the false-positives due to colonic breakdown of substrate in patients with increased small bowel transit time.

2. Cholyl-^{14}C-glycine

   Cholyl-^{14}C-Glycine is a bile salt which enters the enterohepatic circulation upon ingestion. In bacterial overgrowth, the bile salt is broken down, with release of glycine. The glycine is then converted to $^{14}CO_2$ after absorption and is exhaled and measured in increased amounts. The test is limited by small bowel disease or resection, which can result in decreased absorption of the labeled bile salt with subsequent colonic breakdown, leading to a false-positive result.

3. ^{14}C-Triolein

   ^{14}C-Triolein is a labeled triglyceride. It is typically broken down by pancreatic lipases, a with resultant release of $^{14}CO_2$. In patients with pancreatic insufficiency, the amount of exhaled $^{14}CO_2$ in 6 hr is reduced. Unfortunately, pancreatic insufficiency must be moderate to severe to be detected by this breath test.

G. ^{75}SeHCAT test

   ^{75}SeHCAT is a radioactive taurocholic acid analog which enters the enterohepatic circulation. In patients with bile salt malabsorption due to idiopathic bile salt malabsorption or ileal resection, retention of the radioactive label is diminished due to breakdown or stool losses. After ingestion, patients are scanned with a gamma camera. Those with less than 34% of the dose remaining after 3 days have evidence of bile salt malabsorption.

IV. **Therapy of Patients with Maldigestion and Malabsorption**

   A. Pancreatic insufficiency

      Pancreatic replacement therapy: Enzyme replacements, supplementation of the diet with medium-chain triglycerides, and bicarbonate therapy are the cornerstones of therapy for chronic pancreatitis.

   B. Small bowel injury

      Supplementation of the diet with fat- and water-soluble vitamins, medium-chain triglycerides, elemental diets, divalent cations (magnesium, calcium), and antidiarrheals are nonspecific approaches. Therapy is usually aimed at the underlying disease.

Bibliography

Brasitus TA, Sitrin MD. Intestinal malabsorption syndromes. *Annu Rev Med* 41:339–347, 1990.

Fisher RL (ed). Malabsorption and nutritional status support. *Gastroenterol Clin North Am* 18:467–666, 1989.

Merrick MV. Bile acid malabsorption. Clinical presentations and diagnosis. *Dig Dis* 6:159–169, 1988.

Saavedra JM, Perman JA. Current concepts in lactose malabsorption and intolerance. *Annu Rev Nutr* 9:475–502, 1989.

Trier JS. Intestinal malabsorption: Differentiation of cause. *Hosp Pract [Off]* 23:195–211, 1988.

Riley SA, Turnberg LA. Maldigestion and malabsorption, in Sleisenger MH, Fordtran, JS (eds): *Gastrointestinal Disease*, ed 5. Philadelphia, Saunders, 1993 p. 1009–1027.

Casellas F, Chicharro L, Malagelada JR. Potential usefulness of hydrogen breath test with D-xylose in clinical management of intestinal malabsorption. *Dig Dis Sci* 38:321–327, 1993.

Chapter 54-E

Diarrhea

Michael D. Brown, M.D.

I. **Definition**

Diarrhea is more than 250 ml stool per day.

A. Typically associated with an increase in stool liquidity and frequency, as well as volume.

II. **Differential Diagnosis**

An increase in the frequency of bowel movements or change in stool liquidity may not be secondary to diarrhea per se. Stool volumes must exceed 250 ml/day. Hyperdefecation may be associated with hyperthyroidism and anorectal incontinence and should not be misinterpreted as diarrhea.

A. The differential diagnosis of acute and chronic diarrhea is lengthy (Tables 54E-1 and 54E-2).

III. **Focus of the History and Physical Examination**

A. Description of symptoms

1. Stool appearance

Watery stools or a high volume suggest a secretory diarrhea. Semiformed, malodorous stools suggest steatorrhea. The presence of blood suggests inflammatory bowel disease or an infectious diarrhea with mucosal destruction. Mucus is suggestive of irritable bowel syndrome.

2. Duration

The vast majority of episodes of diarrhea are acute, self-limited processes lasting for no more than 4 to 5 days and requiring no diagnostic or therapeutic intervention. Diarrhea persisting for more than 3 weeks is considered chronic and requires investigation.

3. Associated symptoms

The patient should be queried about complaints of fever, chills, and diaphoresis. Presence of these symptoms suggests a more severe inflammatory process typically requiring more immediate attention. Abdominal pain, its location, and its association with the onset and offset of diarrhea are important, although most patients note some crampy abdominal pain in the lower quadrants. The physican should ask about symptoms of the extraintestinal involvement seen in inflammatory bowel disease, such as arthritis, eye pain, rash, or jaundice. Complaints of incontinence (anorectal disorders), nocturnal diarrhea (secretory diarrheas, diabetic diarrhea), and intermittent constipation (irritable bowel syndrome) should be noted. Weight loss is suggestive of laxative abuse or malabsorptive disorders such as Crohns' disease.

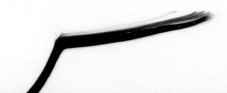

Table 54E-1.   Causes of Acute Diarrhea

Viral	Rotavirus, Norwalk agent, adenoviruses
Bacterial	*Campylobacter, Aeromonas, Pleisomonas, Salmonella, Shingella, Vibrio cholerae,* invasive *Escherichia coli, Yersinia enterocolitica.* Toxin-mediated: *Staphylococcus aureus, Clostridium difficile, C. perfringens, C. botulinum, Bacillus cereus, Vibrio parahemolyticus*
Parasitic	*Giardia lamblia, Entamoeba histolytica, Cryptosporidium, Isospora belli*
Medications	Magnesium based antacids, quinidine, laxatives, colchicine, digitalis, propranolol, theophylline, nonsteroidal anti-inflammatory drugs, antibiotics, chemotherapeutic agents, diuretics
Idiopathic	Ulcerative colitis, Crohn's disease
Miscellaneous	Postobstructive conditions (impaction, stricture, carcinoma), diverticulitis, radiation injury
Vascular	Ischemic bowel disease, vasculitis

4. Additional history

The physician should ask about recent travel, particularly out of the country. Check for contact with others with similar complaints, especially contact with preschool children in whom fecal-oral contact is frequent. Inquire about pets and their health. Sexual preference and promiscuity must be noted. Recent emotional stress may result in a self-limited diarrhea or exacerbation of irritable bowel syndrome.

B. Physical examination

In severe secretory diarrheas, patients may present with hypotension, tachycardia, and/or orthostatic changes. Fever may be present. Temporal wasting may be prominent. Thyromegaly, lymphadenopathy, oral aphthous ulcers, abdominal pain or mass, hepatomegaly, perianal disease, bruits, skin lesions, red eye, abdominal distention, and a peripheral neuropathy are some of the physical findings that should be sought when examining a patient with diarrhea.

C. Screening laboratory abnormalities

In severe secretory diarrhea, electrolyte abnormalities may be marked, with hypokalemia, hypo- or hypernatremia, and metabolic acidosis. Steatorrhea may be accompanied by hypophosphatemia, hypocalcemia, and hypomagnesemia. Hypoalbuminemia and other findings of malnutrition may be prominent. Anemias, either micro- or macrocytic, are often seen. Liver function tests may be abnormal.

IV. **Diagnostic Approach** (see Figure 54E-1)

Initial evaluation should include the following:

A. Stool volume collection. It is important to ensure that diarrhea actually exists by demonstrating output exceeding 250 ml/day.

B. Stool electrolytes: Can be helpful in a few cases. Measure stool sodium and potassium levels. $[(Na^+ + K^+) \times 2] - serum$ osmolarity

Table 54E-2.   Causes of Chronic Diarrhea

Infectious	Entamoeba histolytica, *Giardia lamblia, Mycobacterium, Clostridium difficile, Cryptosporidium, Isospora belli,* human immunodeficiency virus
Neoplastic	Neuroendocrine tumors (VIPoma, gastrinoma, somatostatinoma, Pancreatic-polypeptideoma (PPoma), carcinoid), pancreatic adenocarcinoma, small and large bowel adenocarcinomas, lymphoma, villous adenomas
Endocrine	Hyperthyroidism, diabetes mellitus, Addison's disease
Autoimmune	Vasculitis, scleroderma
Malabsorption	Disccharidase deficiency, celiac sprue, tropical sprue, Whipple's disease, pancreatic insufficiency, abetalipoproteinemia, short bowel syndrome, bacterial overgrowth syndrome
Inflammation	Ulcerative colitis, Crohn's disease, collagenous colitis, lymphocytic colitis, ischemic bowel disease, radiation injury, diverticulitis, solitary rectal ulcer
Motility	Irritable bowel syndrome, dumping syndrome, narcotic bowel, chronic idiopathic intestinal pseudo-obstruction

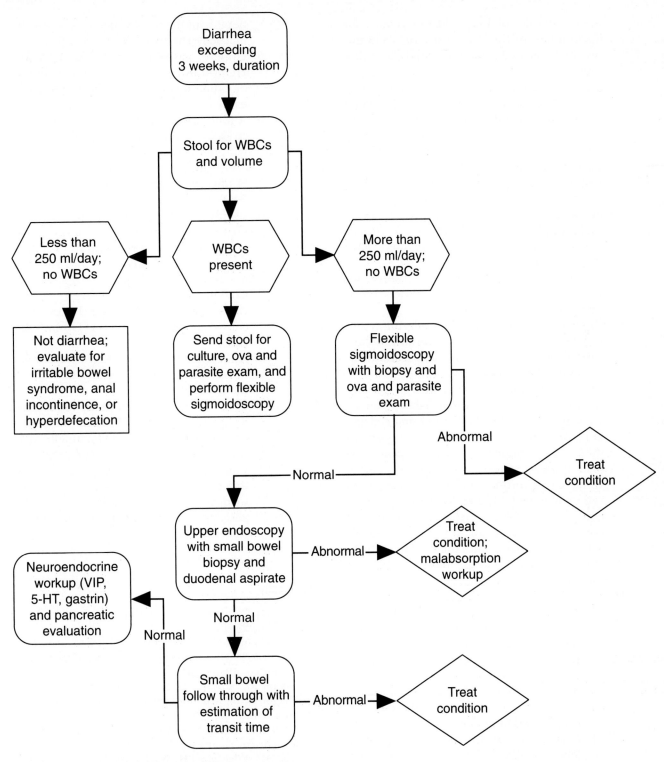

Figure 54E-1. Algorithm for evaluation of chronic diarrhea.

= stool osmole gap. Gap values exceeding 100 are strongly suggestive of secretory diarrhea. A value of 50 suggests secretory diarrhea. Note that the measured osmolarity used is

that of serum; stool osmolarity is *not* used, as it can be artificially elevated by bacterial action on the stool.

C. Stool cultures and smear for ova and parasites: Typically of low yield but remain an integral part of the initial workup. Yield improves if obtained in patients with fecal leukocytes.

D. Alkalinization of stool: Stool containing phenolthalein laxatives will turn bright pink when mixed with 1N sodium hydroxide. This is an essential examination in the evaluation of chronic diarrhea. The physician may also wish to check the stool for magnesium, sulfate, and phosphate to rule out laxative abuse.

E. Examination of stool for blood (guaiac testing) and white blood cells (smear): Very helpful in the initial evaluation, as the presence of blood and/or white blood cells suggests a more severe process.

F. Sudan fat stain: Not particularly sensitive, but specific for steatorrhea and a better screen than a 72-hr fecal fat collection.

G. Flexible sigmoidoscopy: Very helpful in ruling out disorders such as ulcerative colitis, Crohn's disease, melanosis coli, pseudomembranous colitis, other types of infectious colitis, and ischemic colitis, as well as diseases where gross mucosal abnormalities can be seen. It is also helpful in diagnosing collagenous and microscopic colitis by biopsy. In these two conditions the mucosa appears normal; however, there are diagnostic microscopic characteristics. Fresh stool specimens can be obtained and are particularly important in diagnosing amebiasis. The use of cleansing enemas prior to the exam is to be avoided, as it may reduce the yield of cultures and can alter the microscopic appearance of the mucosa.

H. Further diagnostic testing may include:

1. Thyroid function tests: Hyperthyroidism can be associated with both hyperdefecation and steatorrhea.

2. Erythrocyte sedimentation rate and C-reactive protein: Elevated in inflammatory bowel disease.

3. Cortisol level: Addisons' disease can present with diarrhea.

4. Gastrin and vasoactive intestinal peptide levels: Zollinger-Ellison syndrome may present with diarrhea. Vasoactive intestinal polypeptide levels are elevated in patients with the watery diarrhea hypokalemia achlorhydria (WDHA) syndrome.

5. Upper gastrointestinal radiographs: Helpful in patients with Crohn's disease or other small bowel malabsorptive diseases.

6. Abdominal computed tomography or ulstrasound scan: May be helpful in cases of lymphoma or in the search neuroendocrine tumors.

7. Studies for malabsorption (see Chapter 54D).

8. Esophagogastroduodenoscopy: Allows direct visual examination of a small portion of the small bowel, aspiration of duodenal contents for *Giardia*, and bacterial quantitation and biopsy.

9. Colonoscopy: May be necessary in diseases characterized by patchy or right colonic involvement, such as Crohn's disease.

10. Anorectal manometry: May be necessary to rule out incontinence and to evaluate the cause of diarrhea.

11. Urine tests: Useful tests include 5-hydroxyindoleacetic acid (carcinoids), metanephrines, and vanillylmandelic acid (pheochromocytoma) and narcotics.

12. Empiric trails: Occasionally, empiric therapy based on a reasonable diagnostic suspicion is useful (e.g., broad-spectrum antibiotics in a patient with presumed bacterial overgrowth).

Bibliography

Binder HJ. Pathophysiology of acute diarrhea. *Am J Med* 88(Suppl 6A):2S–4S, 1990.

Fine K, Guenter JK, Fordtran JS. Diarrhea, in Sleisenger MH, Fordtran JS (eds): *Gastrointestinal Disease,* ed 5. Philadelphia, Saunders, 1993 p 1043–1072.

Guerrant RL, Shields DS, Thorson SM, et al. Evaluation and diagnosis of acute infectious diarrhea. *Am J Med* 78(Suppl 6B):91–98, 1985.

Read NW, Krejs GJ, Read MG, et al. Chronic diarrhea of unknown origin. *Gastroenterology* 78:264–271, 1980.

Siegel DL, Edelstein PH, Nachamkin I. Inappropriate testing for diarrheal diseases in the hospital. *JAMA* 263:979–982, 1990.

CHAPTER **54-F**

Constipation

Sheldon Sloan, M.D.

I. Definition

Constipation is difficult to define because, as a symptom, it remains very subjective. When surveying a population, self-definitions of constipation range from straining to defecate, a feeling of incomplete evacuation, long periods between bowel movements, and the need to take laxatives to defecate. Traditional definitions include undefined self-reported symptoms, and stool frequency (fewer than three times per week in adults), and the most objective definition is whole gut transit time (the upper limit of normal mouth-to-anus transit time is 68 hr in adults).

A. Epidemiology and contributing factors
1. Gender differences: In children, boys are affected more often than girls; however, in older subjects, this pattern is reversed. Self-reported constipation is about three times greater in women than men.
2. Age, race, and socioeconomic differences: Self-reporting of constipation increases greatly after age 65. A slightly greater percentage of Caucasians than non-Caucasians report constipation in the United States. Lower socioeconomic status and ed-

ucation are also correlated with higher self-reported rates of constipation.
3. Exercise: Level of physical activity is correlated with self-reports of constipation and stool frequency. People who exercise regularly tend to have higher stool frequencies and fewer reports of constipation than those with a sedentary lifestyle.
4. Diet: Although a treatment for constipation is a diet high in fiber and liquids, in population samples of self-reported constipation, there is no significant correlation with either fiber or liquid intake. The mode of action of fiber is probably due to the breakdown of undigested complex carbohydrates by colonic bacteria, which increases the osmolality as well as the production of irritating short chain fatty acids that promote bowel motility.

B. Risks of constipation
1. Urinary tract infections may be associated with constipation.
2. Stercoral ulcers and perforation are caused by pressure necrosis from prolonged contact with hard stool.

3. Colon cancer has been linked to constipation, especially in women. The magnitude of the increased risk is not known.

4. Fecal incontinence may result from chronic straining, which stretches the pelvic floor and damages the pudendal nerve.

5. Surgery is performed more frequently in patients with constipation, particularly young women.

II. Mechanisms of Constipation

A. Decreased peristaltic activity of the colon is seen in patients who are chronically constipated. This condition does not seem to be correlated with delayed transit time in the colon.

B. Increased nonperistaltic segmental contractions in the colon: These contractions retard the movement of stool toward the anus and are reported to be more common in patients with constipation.

C. Decreased rectal tone is associated with megarectum and is seen in association with chronic constipation especially in children. Megarectum reduces the ability to perceive rectal distention or the urge to defecate. Because it allows a larger stool to develop in the rectum, defecation becomes more painful.

D. Decreased rectal sensitivity occurs in persons with constipation. The threshold for the first sensation of rectal distention, as well as for the urge to defecate, are elevated. This could perpetuate or exacerbate constipation by reducing the frequency of attempts and the motivation to defecate. Decreased rectal sensitivity is often seen in patients with megarectum.

E. Pelvic floor dyssynergia is a condition in which, instead of relaxation of the puborectalis sling fibers encircling the rectum when straining to defecate, there is a paradoxical contraction, preventing passage of stool through the anus.

III. Diagnostic Approach

A. History: Important information includes stool frequency and consistency, the longest period between bowel movements, fiber content of the diet, surgical history, blood in stool, pain while defecating, concurrent medications, and use of laxatives.

B. A physical examination should be done, evaluating for any other systemic illness (e.g., hypothyroidism), with particular attention paid to the rectal exam. The rectum should be carefully examined for evidence of perianal disease, including hemorrhoids, rectal pro-lapse, tenderness with careful digital rectal exam, fecaloma, and anal sphincter tone.

C. Diagnostic studies should be directed first at ruling out an obstruction, which can be accomplished with a flexible sigmoidoscopy and barium enema or a colonoscopy. Once an obstruction is ruled out, colonic motility and anorectal function can be assessed.

1. Whole gut and segmental transit time can be measured by the use of radiopaque markers that assess the mouth-to-anus transit time. This is accomplished by having the patient ingest a known quantity of small markers and obtaining serial abdominal films.

2. Anorectal manometry is done in the gastrointestinal motility laboratory. This test measures sphincter tone, ability to augment the tone voluntarily (anal squeeze), the reflexive response to rectal distention (a normal response being a relanation of the internal and sphincter and a slight increase in the tone of the external anal sphincter), and the subjective perception of rectal distention.

3. Defecography is a radiologic assessment of the anatomy and function of the pelvic floor during the act of defecation. It consists of instilling a barium/fiber enema and then using videofluoroscopy and taking serial radiographs during defecation.

IV. Differential Diagnosis

A. Mechanical lesions in the colon include tumors, volvulus, hernias, strictures, diverticulitis, infectious causes (chronic amebiasis, lymphogranuloma venereum, syphilis, tuberculosis), ischemic colitis, corrosive enemas, previous surgery, and endometriosis.

B. Muscular abnormalities include diverticular disease, segmental dilatation of the colon, myotonic dystrophy, systemic sclerosis, and dermatomyositis.

C. Lesions specific to the rectum include tumors, rectocele, internal rectal prolapse, and surgical stricture.

D. Descending perineum syndrome.

E. Anal lesions include stenosis, anterior ectopic anus, anal fissure, and mucosal prolapse.

F. Neurogenic causes

1. Peripheral causes include Hirschsprung's disease (ananglionosis), hypoganglionosis, hyperganglionosis, ganglioneuromatosis, autonomic neuropathy, and Chagas' disease.

2. Central nervous system causes include Parkinson's disease, intracerebral tumors, cerebrovascular accidents, and disorders localized to the medulla and spinal cord, including meningocele, Shy-Drager syndrome, multiple sclerosis, and trauma.

G. Medications include narcotics, iron, bismuth, calcium- and aluminum-containing antacids, anticholinergics, Parkinson's disease medications, monoamine oxidase inhibitors, heavy metals (arsenic, lead, mercury), and antidepressants.

H. Metabolic disorders include amyloid, uremia, hypokalemia, diabetic neuropathy, diabetic acidosis, and porphyria.

I. Endocrine disorders include hypothyroidism, hypercalcemia, panhypopituitarism, and hyperparathyroidism.

J. Irritable bowel syndrome.

V. Treatment

Treatment for constipation should be individualized and aimed at the specific defect (e.g., megarectum). Lifestyle modifications, including taking time out of a busy schedule to defecate, increasing the amount of exercise, and increasing the amount of dietary fiber may be all that is needed to relieve constipation.

A. Laxatives: Patients are usually familiar with the various forms of laxatives before seeking medical attention for constipation, and it is important to recognize the pathophysiology to recommend the correct agent. In general, use of nonbulking laxatives as a long-term treatment for constipation should be avoided except when clearly indicated.

1. Bulk laxatives include poorly digestible polysaccharides which are broken down in the colon by bacteria. This increases the stool bulk primarily by promoting bacterial growth.

2. Stool softeners include docusate sodium, docusate calcium, and docusate potassium, which work by binding water and softening the stools.

3. Lubricants such as mineral oil can reduce absorption of fat-soluble vitamins and should be avoided in patients prone to aspiration.

4. Hyperosmolar agents such as magnesium citrate, magnesium hydroxide, magnesium sulfate, and sodium phosphate cause a net secretion of water into the small intestine and colon which then acts as a volume stimulus to defecation. Caution must be used since the chronic use of these agents can cause electrolyte imbalances. Lactulose is indigestible and is broken down by the colonic bacteria, which also produces a large amount of gas.

5. Stimulants such as bisacodyl, cascara, senna, and phenolphthalein can lead to dependency and electrolyte imbalance if used on a chronic basis.

B. Habit training is used for the treatment of slow rectal transit associated with megarectum.

C. Biofeedback may be helpful in patients with slow rectal transit secondary to pelvic floor dyssynergia.

D. Sphincter myectomy for outlet delay constipation is not effective except for patients with Hirschsprung's disease.

E. Subtotal colectomy appears to be ineffective in patients with idiopathic constipation. Most patients are satisfied with the outcome. However, the complication rate is high, including recurrence of constipation, small bowel obstruction, diarrhea, and incontinence. This form of treatment is irreversible and should be performed only when colonic transit is significantly delayed.

Bibliography

Burkitt DP, Walker ARP, Painter NS. Effect of dietary fiber on stools and transit times, and its role in the causation of disease. *Lancet* 2:1408–1411, 1972.

Camilleri M, Neri M. Motility disorders and stress. *Dig Dis Sci* 34:1777–1786, 1989.

Lennard-Jones JE, Constipation: Pathophysiology, clinical features and treatment, in Henry MM, Nd Swash M (eds): *Coloproctology and the Pelvic Floor. Pathophysiology and Management.* London, Butterworth, 1985, pp 350–375.

Turnball GK, Bartram CI, Lennard-Jones JE. Radiolgic studies of rectal evacuation in adults with idiopathic constipation. *Dis Col Rectum* 31;190–197, 1988.

Approach to the Patient with Intestinal Obstruction

Bennett Plotnick, M.D.

I. Problem

Intestinal obstruction is present when there is lack of progression of intestinal contents. It may be caused by occlusion, as in mechanical obstruction, or by lack of peristalsis, as in paralytic ileus.

II. Differential Diagnosis

A. Mechanical intestinal obstruction
  1. Obsturation obstruction
    a. Polypoid tumors
    b. Intussusception
    c. Gallstones
    d. Foreign bodies
    e. Bezoars
    f. Feces
  2. Intrinsic bowel lesions
    a. Atresia
    b. Stenosis
    c. Strictures
      (1) Neoplastic
      (2) Inflammatory
      (3) Chemical
      (4) Anastomotic
    d. Vascular abnormalities
      (1) Arterial occlusion
      (2) Venous occlusion
  3. Extrinsic bowel lesions
    a. Adhesions
      (1) Previous surgery
      (2) Previous peritonitis
    b. Hernias
      (1) Internal
      (2) External
    c. Neoplastic
    d. Abscesses
    e. Volvulus
    f. Congenital bands
B. Ileus
  1. Surgical operations
  2. Peritonitis
  3. Unrelieved mechanical obstruction
  4. Gram-negative sepsis
  5. Electrolyte imbalance
  6. Retroperitoneal hemorrhage
  7. Spinal or pelvic fractures
C. Secondary intestinal pseudo-obstruction
  1. Intestinal smooth muscle
    a. Collagen vascular disease
    b. Amyloidosis
    c. Primary muscle disease
  2. Endocrine disorders
    a. Myxedema
    b. Diabetes mellitus

    c. Hypoparathyroidism
    d. Pheocromocytoma
  3. Neurologic diseases
    a. Parkinson's disease
    b. Hirschsprung's disease
    c. Chagas' disease
    d. Familial autonomic dysfunction
  4. Drugs
    a. Phenothiazines
    b. Tricyclic antidepressants
    c. Antiparkinson medications
    d. Ganglionic blockers
    e. Clonidine
    f. Mushroom poisoning

III. Focus of the History and Physical Examination

A. History: Intestinal obstruction is characterized by typical symptoms of cramping abdominal pain, obstipation, abdominal distention, and vomiting. Proximal obstruction produces less distention and more vomiting, while distal obstruction typically produces more distention and less vomiting, which may be fecalent. Other important historical features include prior abdominal surgery, the presence of intestinal bleeding, medications, and constitutional complaints such as fever, weight loss, and early satiety.

B. Physical exam: Important aspects of the physical exam are the presence of fever, dehydration, peritonitis, and ascites. One should look carefully for hernias, abdominal scars, the presence or absence of stool in the rectum, and the presence of occult blood. Bowel sounds tend to be high-pitched, musical rushes in mechanical obstruction unless late in impending infarction and decreased or absent in ileus and pseudo-obstruction.

IV. Diagnostic Approach

A. An obstructive series is mandatory in any patient suspected of having intestinal obstruction. The typical small bowel obstruction pattern usually includes minimal or no colonic air, with multiple gas-filled, distended small bowel loops resembling an inverted U. In colonic obstruction there may be colonic distention and no small bowel distention if the ileocecal valve is competent or both small and large bowel distention if the ileocecal valve is incompetent. Uniform gaseous distention throughout the stomach, small intestine, colon, and rectum is seen in patients with paralytic ileus.

B. Barium x-ray: A careful, unprepared barium enema may be useful in patients with an inconclusive obstructive series to delineate the site of obstruction or to differentiate obstruction from ileus. Barium by mouth should be avoided if colonic obstruction cannot be excluded.

C. Sigmoidoscopy or colonoscopy may be useful diagnostically in cases of large bowel obstruction to evaluate the area of obstruction and to look for synchronous neoplasms, and may be therapeutic in cases of suspected volvulus.

Bibliography

Colemont LJ, Camilleri M. Chronic intestinal pseudo-obstruction diagnosis and treatment. *Mayo Clin Proc* 64:60–70, 1989.

Jones RS, Schiemer BD. Intestinal obstruction, pseudo-obstruction, and deus, in Sleisenger MH (ed): *Gastrointestinal Disease*, ed 4. Philadelphia, Saunders. pp 369–381, 1989.

Miller LD, Mackie JA. The pathophysiology and management of intestinal obstruction. *Surg Clin North Am* 42:1285–1962.

CHAPTER **54-H**

Gastrointestinal Bleeding

John Schaffner, M.D.

I. Problem

Gastrointestinal (GI) bleeding can occur anywhere between the mouth and the anus. Many different lesions can present as a source of hemorrhage. The presentation can be divided into acute and chronic bleeding.

A. Acute GI bleeding is rapid loss of blood that is evident by the passage of blood from the mouth or the anus.

1. Upper GI (UGI) bleeding may present as vomiting blood or "coffee-ground" material, the passage of melena or bright red blood per rectum, hypotension, or syncope.

   a. Melena is black, tarry stool that is usually caused by a UGI source. Approximately 200–500 ml of blood is necessary to cause melena.

   b. Bright red blood per rectum from a UGI source usually requires 500–1000 ml of blood moving rapidly through the GI tract. Any UGI source can cause bright red rectal bleeding. Twenty percent of patients who pass large amounts of bright red blood per rectum are bleeding from a UGI source.

2. Lower GI (LGI) bleeding is usually any

bleeding that occurs beyond the ligament of Treitz. Patients may pass bright red blood, dark blood, maroon stools, or even black stools. The appearance of bleeding does not point specifically to the location of bleeding.

B. Chronic GI bleeding is present when patients present with either occult blood–positive stools and/or iron deficiency anemia. The amount of blood loss can vary from microscopic to recurrent episodes of acute hemorrhage.

1. The UGI tract may be a source of chronic GI bleeding, with or without associated GI symptoms. More frequently, however, patients with a UGI source have associated symptoms.

2. The LGI tract is the usual source of occult blood–positive stools or iron deficiency anemia. Patients often have no other associated symptoms related to the GI tract problem.

II. Differential Diagnosis

A. UGI bleeding can occur from the esophagus, stomach, duodenum, or biliary tree. On occasion, oropharyngeal sources can mimic UGI bleeding. OL3

707

1. Esophagus: peptic esophagitis, esophageal ulcer, esophageal varices, Mallory-Weiss tear, esophageal carcinoma, foreign body, infectious esophagitis (cytomegalovirus, herpes, *Candida*).
2. Stomach: gastric ulcer, gastric cancer, gastritis, leiomyoma, lymphoma, gastric varices, telangiectasias, stomal ulcers.
3. Duodenum: duodenal ulcer, duodenitis, neoplasms, diverticulum, aortoenteric fistula.
4. Biliary tract and pancreas: neoplasms of the pancreas, cholangiocarcinoma, hepatocellular carcinoma, fistula.

B. LGI bleeding can be divided by age groups. It can occur from the ligament of Treitz to the anal canal. As much as 20% of massive LGI bleeds may be from UGI source.
   1. Age 0–20 years: Meckel's diverticulum, polyps, inflammatory bowel disease.
   2. Age 20–60 years: diverticulosis, carcinoma, hemorrhoids/fissures, polyps, inflammatory bowel disease.
   3. Age >60 years: diverticulosis, carcinoma, angiodysplasia, polyps, ischemic bowel disease.

III. **Focus of the History and Physical Examination** (see Figures 54H-1 and 65H-2)
   A. Relevant immediate history
      1. Description of the bleeding: melena, hematemesis, hematochezia.
      2. Symptoms of volume depletion: lightheadedness, syncope.
      3. History of bleeding disorders or use of anticoagulants.
      4. Intensive care unit, burn, and head trauma patients.
   B. Relevant past history
      1. History of peptic ulcer disease: only 50% of patients bleed from recurrent ulcer.
      2. History of liver disease: up to 70% bleed from varices.
      3. History of aortic graft: necessary to look for aortoenteric fistula.
      4. History of acetylsalicylic acid or nonsteroidal anti-inflammatory drug use.
      5. History of anemia.
   C. Focus of the examination
      1. Assessment of volume status
         a. Orthostasis: 10–15% of patients are depleted
         b. Hypotensive: 25% of patients are depleted.
         c. Shock: 40% of patients are depleted.

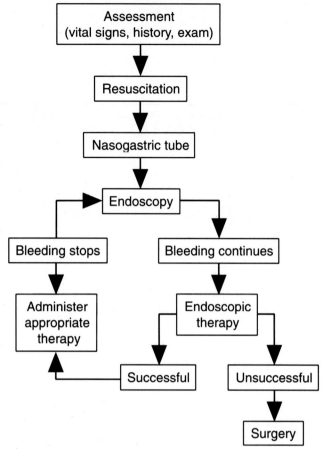

Figure 54H-1.   Acute UGI bleeding.

      2. Assessment of active bleeding
         a. Stability of vital signs.
         b. Nasogastric tube
            (1) Bright red blood indicates active bleeding.
            (2) Absence of coffee grounds does not necessarily mean that bleeding has stopped.
            (3) Clear return does not exclude active bleeding.
   D. Frequency of defecation may indicate continued bleeding.
      1. Visualization of the bleeding site
         a. Endoscopy is the most accurate diagnostic method.
            (1) Best assessment of active bleeding.
            (2) Helps to determine further therapy.
            (3) Allows for endoscopic therapy.
         b. Barium studies not advised for active bleeding.
         c. Arteriography may reveal the site of bleeding.

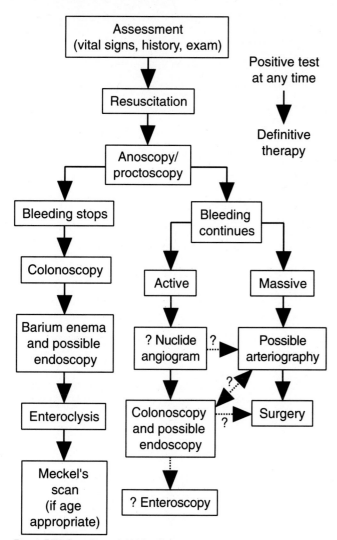

Figure 54H-2. Acute LGI bleeding.

should be directed by the nature of the bleeding.

1. UGI bleeding
   a. Endoscopy is the procedure of choice.
   b. For bleeding beyond the reach of the endoscope, enteroclysis is more sensitive than standard small bowel x-ray.
   c. Small bowel enteroscopy is available in some centers for endoscopic examination of the small bowel.
   d. Radionuclide-tagged red blood cell studies may be useful in identifying the location of the bleeding.
   e. Arteriography can find some occult lesions throughout the GI tract.
   f. For chronic bleeding, enteroclysis may reveal an abnormality in the small intestine.
2. LGI bleeding
   a. Colonoscopy is the procedure of choice.
   b. Anoscopic exam should be done in patients with intermittent rectal bleeding.
   c. Barium enema may be helpful in occasional cases when colonoscopy is negative. These exams often provide supplemental information.
   d. Arteriography may reveal vascular abnormalities that were not detected by colonoscopy.

Bibliography

Fleischer D. Endoscopic therapy of upper gastrointestinal bleeding in humans. *Gastroenterology* 90:217–234, 1986.

Schaffner JA. Acute upper gastrointestinal bleeding. *Drugs* 37:97–104, 1989.

Schrock TR. Colonoscopic diagnosis and treatment of lower gastrointestinal bleeding. *Surg Clin North Am* 69:1309–1325, 1989.

Silverstein FE, Gilbert DA, Tedesco FJ, et al. The National ASGE Survey on upper gastrointestinal bleeding: Clinical prognostic factors. *Gastrointest Endosc* 27:80–93, 1981.

   d. Radioactive nuclide studies may be helpful for localizing LGI or occult bleeding.
E. Chronic GI bleeding
   In patients with chronic bleeding, evaluation

Jaundice

Howard Rosenblate, M.D.

I. **Definition**
  A. Jaundice, or icterus, is defined as the yellow coloration of sclera and skin when bilirubin accumulates in these tissues, reflecting an increase in serum levels above 2 mg/dl. The diagnostic challenge is determined by the initial distinction between obstructive and nonobstructive causes. A basic knowledge of bilirubin metabolism and the concepts of jaundice and cholestasis are necessary to establish a rational and cost-effective workup.
  B. Cholestasis is clinically manifested as the retention in blood of substances such as bile acids, alkaline phosphatase (an enzyme localized in the hepatocyte canalicular membrane,) and bilirubin that are normally excreted in bile. Cholestasis can also be defined functionally as a decrease in canalicular bile flow. The morphologic description of cholestasis is provided by a pathologist when bile accumulates in liver cells and biliary structures (bile plugs).

II. **Differential Diagnosis**
  A. The first step should be to establish if the hyperbilirubinemia is conjugated (direct reacting) or unconjugated (indirect reacting). In normal persons, serum bilirubin is unconjugated, but the diazo reaction overestimates the direct fraction. A direct reaction over 30% of the total bilirubin suggests that hepatobiliary disease is present.
  B. Unconjugated hyperbilirubinemia results from bile overproduction or deficient hepatic uptake and conjugation (see Table 54I-1).
  C. Elevated serum conjugated bilirubin is more common and is seen in hepatocellular disease, as well as in intra- and extrahepatic cholestasis (see Table 54I-2).

III. **Focus of the History and Physical Examination**
  It is important to state that a good history, physical examination, and routine and basic laboratory tests are able to predict the cause of jaundice correctly in 80–90% of cases.
  A. History: The events that surround the onset of jaundice, other symptoms, and the pertinent past medical, social, and family histories are summarized in Table 54I-3.
  B. Physical examination: A careful physical examination may elicit clues to the diagnosis and, with the help of the history and routine laboratory work, serve as a guide to additional diagnostic procedures or tests that will confirm the diagnosis (see Table 54I-4).

Table 541-1. Common Causes of Unconjugated Hyperbilirubinemia

Disorder	Mechanism
Hemolysis	Production
Ineffective erythropoiesis	Production
Hematomas	Production
Gilbert's syndrome	Glucuronil transferase
	Hepatic uptake
	Associated hemolysis
Physiologic jaundice (newborn)	Production
	Glucuronyl transferase
	Enhanced intestinal absorption

C. Laboratory evaluation
  1. Tests of hepatic function
    a. Bilirubin: In severe hemolytic disorders and Gilbert's syndrome, the unconguated bilirubin level rarely exceeds 5–6 mg/dl. In cases of impaired intrahepatic excretion or extrahepatic cholestasis, conjugated hyperbilirubinemia is observed, and more than 50% is in the direct-reacting form. When jaundice is chronic, bilirubin can bind to albumin (will not be filtered well by the kidney) and persist in plasma even though the cause of obstruction has been removed or the hepatocellular injury has resolved.
      (1) Urine bilirubin is present with elevated direct or conjugated bilirubin.
    b. Urobilinogen: When bacteria act on conjugated bilirubin, urobilinogen will form and enter the enterhepatic circulation. Urobilinogen can filter through the glomerulus, and a level exceeding 4 mg/dl may be seen in bilirubin overproduction and hepatocellular disease. Its mere presence also means that bile duct obstruction is not complete.
    c. Serum bile acids: Normal serum bile acid levels support the diagnosis of Gilbert's disease. Their elevation in moderate and severe liver disease does not contribute significantly to the diagnostic yield, so they need not be obtained routinely.

    d. Clotting: In cases of advanced hepatocellular dysfunction, the prothrombin time will be prolonged, and the partial thromboplastin time may be normal or prolonged. It is not necessary to obtain the levels of individual factors. In cases of extrahepatic cholestasis, particularly when antibiotics are used, vitamin K may be deficient and the prothrombin time will be prolonged. However, the patient will respond to parenteral administration of vitamin K.
    e. Albumin: A low level is helpful in chronic conditions and indicates decreased synthesis. After acute injuries,

Table 541-2. Causes of Conjugated Hyperbilirubinemia

Disease	Diagnostic Approach
Hepatocellular Disease	
Alcholic liver disease (alcoholic hepatitis)	History, chemistry
Viral hepatitis (A, B, C, or non-B, non-C)	Serology
Autoimmune hepatitis	Autoimmune markers
End-stage cirrhosis	History, physical exam
Storage diseases (Wilson's disease, hemochromatosis)	Chemistry, liver biopsy
Intrahepatic Cholestasis	
Primary biliary cirrhosis	Chemistry, liver biopsy
Drugs	
Chlorpromazine	
Clavulanic acid	
Rifampin, others	History, exclusion
Sepsis	Clinical
Congenital hyperbilirubinemia	Liver biopsy
Extrahepatic Cholestasis	
Cholelithiasis	History, US, ERCP
Malignancy	
Ampullary	
Head of pancreas	
Cholangiocarcinoma	ERCP, PTC
Primary sclerosing cholangitis	
Large ducts	
Intrahepatic ducts	ERCP, PTC

Abbreviations: US, ultrasound scan; ERCP, endoscopic retrigrade cholangiopancreatography; PTC, percutaneous transhepatic cholangiogram.

Table 541-3. Significance of the History in Patients with Jaundice

Factor	Significance
Onset	
Acute, flu-like	Viral hepatitis
Subacute	Choledocholithiasis
Slow	Malignancy
Age	Other than 55, > malignancy
Systemic Symptoms	
Fever	Viral hepatitis, cholangitis
Fatigue	Hepatitis, malignancy
Weight loss	Malignancy
Pruritus	PBC, malignancy, cholestasis
Pain	
Cholic	Cholelithiasis
Continuous, dull	Malignancy
GI Symptoms	
Nausea, vomiting	Hepatitis, cholangitis
Anorexia	Hepatitis, malignancy
Light-colored stools	Hepatitis, malignancy
History of dyspepsia	Cholelithiasis
Risk Factors	
Promiscuity	Hepatitis
Homosexuality	Hepatitis B
IV drug use	Hepatitis B, C
Blood transfusion	Hepatitis C
Health care	Hepatitis B, C (less common)
Nurseries, schools	Hepatitis A
Alcohol	Alcoholic hepatitis, cirrhosis
Family History	
Far East, Mediterranean	Hepatitis B
Afro-American	Sickle cell disease
Medications	
Acetaminophen	Toxicity
Neuroleptics	Toxicity
Chemotherapy	Toxicity, veno-occlussive disease
Systemic Conditions	
Severe congestive heart failure	Passive congestion
Sepsis	Cytokine-induced cholestasis
Inflammatory blood disease	Sclerosing cholangitis
Pregnancy	Cholestasis, acute fatty liver
Past Surgical History	
Cholecystectomy	Retained common bile duct stone
Common bile duct	Duct stricture, duct stone
Recent surgery	Benign postoperative surgery

problems such as sepsis may influence catabolism more than synthesis. In volume overload, a dilution factor becomes important.

2. Tests of hepatocellular injury
   a. Transaminases (alanine and aspartate aminotransferase [ALT, AST]) are ele-

Table 541-4. Physical Examination Findings and Possible Implications

Findings	Posible Implication
General	
Malnutrition	End-stage cirrhosis, malignancy
Enlarged lymph nodes	Malignancy
Skin	
Deep or greenish jaundice	Prolonged cholestasis
Bronze yellow	Hemochromatosis, cirrhosis
Excoriations	Cholestasis
Xanthomas, xanthelasmas	PBC
Spider angiomas	Cirrhosis
Eyes	
Kayser Fleischer rings	Wilson's disease
Neck	
Jugular vein distention	Right-sided heart failure
Chest	
Gynecomastia	Cirrhosis
Abdomen	
Ascites	Cirrhosis, malignancy, congestive heart failure
Tender hepatomegaly	Hepatitis, cholangitis
Firm, small liver	Cirrhosis
Splenomegaly	Cirrhosis, portal hypertension
Palpable gallbladder	Malignancy, duct obstruction
Distended abdominal veins	Cirrhosis, portal hypertension
Genitalia	
Testicular atrophy	Cirrhosis
Feminine pubic hair	Cirrhosis
Extremities	
Peripheral edema	Cirrhosis, congestive heart failure
Palmar erythema	Cirrhosis
Neurologic Exam	
Asterixis	Liver failure
Confusional stage	Liver failure
Coma	Liver failure

vated, ALT being more liver specific. The higest levels (>300 IU) are seen in viral, ischemic, and drug-induced diseases. Rapid changes are characteristic of ischemic events or temporary injury when a stone is passed. An AST:ALT ratio above 2 is suggestive of alcoholic hepatitis.

b. A lactic dehydrogenase (LDH) test is available and LDH-5 isoenzyme is of hepatic origin, but this information rarely adds to the information given by transaminases.

c. Cholestasis indicators: Elevation of the bile canalicular enzyme alkaline phosphatase is typically observed. The level can be normal or low even in the presence of cholestasis, as well as in patients with zinc deficiency, hypophosphatasia, hypothyroidism, pernicious anemia, and acute hemolysis complicating Wilson's disease. A striking increase in the level of alkaline phosphatase may be seen without a significant elevation of bilirubin. This enzyme may originate in other sites (bone, intestine, placenta), and it may be necessary to obtain other enzymes that rise with cholestasis, such as 5'nucleotidase and γ-glutamil-transpeptidase (GGTP).

d. Other tests: Viral serologies, antimitochondrial antibody, antinuclear antibody, anti-smooth muscle antibody, ceruloplasmin, α-1-antitrypsin, and ferritin.

IV. Diagnosis

After the history, physical exam and laboratory tests, in imaging procedure may be required to continue the evaluation. The tests should be sensitive, specific, and cost effective and should provide a rapid diagnosis. The following algorithm is suggested:

A. Ultrasound to screen for dilation of extrahepatic and/or intrahepatic ducts.

B. Dilated intra- and/or extrahepatic ducts
1. Endoscopic retrograde cholangiopancreatography (ERCP)
   a. Risks: Pancreatitis related to endoscopy, technical difficulty.
   b. Advantage: Therapeutic capability: sphincterotomy, stents, removal of stones, samples for diagnosis.
      or
2. Percutaneous transhepatic or cholangiography (PTC)
   a. Risks: Biliary leak, bleeding, infection.
   b. Advantage: Therapeutic capability.
      or
3. Computed tomography (CT)
   a. Risks: Minor (reaction to contrast).
   b. Advantage: Better definition than ultrasound (US), detection of mass, biopsy capability.
      or
4. Endoscopic ultrasound (EUS)
   a. Risks: New technology, endoscopy related.
   b. Advantage: No contrast, excellent staging.

C. No dilation of ducts.
1. Observation: When benign condition is suspected.
2. CT: When malignancy is strongly suspected.
3. Liver Biopsy
   a. guided (US, CT, or laparoscopy).
   b. Unguided: Percutaneous or transvenous jugular.

Bibliography

Frank B. Clinical evaluation of jaundice. *JAMA* 262:3031–3034, 1989.

Kozarek RA, Sanowski RA. Nonsurgical management of extrahepatic obstructive jaundice. *Ann Intern Med* 96:743–745, 1982.

Lyche KD, Brenner DA. A logical approach to the patient with jaundice. *Contemp Intern Med* 4:43–58, 1992.

Chapter 54-J

Noncardiac Chest Pain

Sheldon Sloan, M.D.

I. Definition

Noncardiac chest pain is a diagnosis relating to chest pain of esophageal origin. Historically, patients with chest pain have undergone a cardiac diagnostic workup. Patients with a normal or insignificant lesion on coronary angiogram have an excellent prognosis; however, many of them still have a compromised lifestyle and continue to have anxiety regarding their chest pain. Over the past 15 years, new information about these patients has come to light. Esophageal motility disorders, primarily "nutcracker" esophagus, as well as gastroesophageal reflux disease, afflict one-third to one-half of these patients. Recent studies, using rapid atrial pacing with and without ergonovine, have uncovered a subset of patients with normal coronary arteries and chest pain who have an abnormal coronary artery vasodilator reserve.

II. Differential Diagnosis

One confounding factor is the possible presence of coexistent esophageal and cardiac disease. It is therefore imperative to rule out a cardiac source.

A. Gastroesophageal reflux disease: Up to 75% of patients with chest pain and a normal cardiac workup have either an abnormal 24-hr pH study or a significant number of reflux episodes correlated with their chest pain. One of the easiest tests to perform is a Bernstein test (see Chapter 55D). Although the sensitivity and specificity of this test are around 80%, if the test is positive, then the treatment is specific. The workup for noncardiac chest pain should include upper endoscopy, which will detect even mild changes at the gastroesophageal junction, as well as structural abnormalities such as a stricture, tumor, or hiatal hernia.

B. Esophageal motility disorders: Of the motility disorders, the one most commonly reported in noncardiac chest pain patients is nutcracker esophagus. Diffuse esophageal spasm may cause chest pain; however, the number of patients with this disorder is significantly less than those with nutcracker esophagus. Diffuse esophageal spasm (DES) has been described in patients with coronary artery spasm, making the differentiation between the two conditions difficult. Achalasia patients may also complain of chest pain with accompanying dysphagia. Hypertensive lower esophageal sphincter patients have also been described as having chest pain.

715

III. History and Physical Examination

A good history, focusing on onset of the chest pain in relation to meals, may be a clue to the etiology of the pain. Typically, patients with reflux-induced chest pain will have postprandial onset or when supine. Exertional reflux has also been described and may be confused with exertional angina. Chest pain during a meal may be more indicative of a motility abnormality such as nutcracker esophagus, DES, or achalasia. Physical exam should rule out a costochondral component of the patient's chest pain.

IV. Diagnostic Approach

A. Rule out cardiac disease appropriate for age, symptoms, and risk factors. This may entail only an electocardiogram, a treadmill stress test, or a cardiac catheterization.

B. Esophageal workup may start with either an upper endoscopy or a barium esophagogram. The advantage of an upper endoscopy is the detection of mild esophagitis, which may not be detected on a barium study. If esophagitis is present, then treatment for reflux disease should be instituted.

C. An esophageal motility study should be performed if the endoscopy or the barium study is inconclusive. This will allow for diagnosis of a motility disorder, as well as testing of the patient for acid-sensitive esophagus using a Bernstein test.

D. If the diagnosis is not obtained by the above tests, then a 24-hr ambulatory pH study is useful in correlating chest pain episodes with reflux events.

Bibliography

Benjamin SB, Gerhardt DC, Castell DO. High amplitude, peristaltic esophageal contractions associated with chest pain and/or dysphagia. *Gastroenterology* 77:478–483, 1979.

Cannon RO, Cattau EL, Yakshe PN, et al. Coronary flow reserve, esophageal motility, and chest pain in patients with angiographically normal coronary arteries. *Am J Med* 88:217–222, 1990.

Hewson EG, Sinclair JW, Dalton CB, et al. Twenty-four hour esophageal pH monitoring: The most useful test for evaluating non-cardiac chest pain. *Am J Med* 90:576–583, 1991.

Richter JE, Bradley LA, Castell DO. Esophageal chest pain: Current controversies in pathogenesis, diagnosis, and therapy. *Ann Intern Med* 110:66–78, 1989.

Upper Gastrointestinal Endoscopy

John Schaffner, M.D.

I. Introduction

Upper gastrointestinal endoscopy allows direct inspection of the esophagus, stomach, and duodenum to the third portion. Special instruments can visualize the entire small intestine. Images are transmitted through fiberoptics or by computer generation. The endoscope gives the user numerous therapeutic modalities as well as diagnostic capabilities.

II. Indications

  A. Diagnostic indications
    1. Dyspepsia
    2. Dysphagia
    3. Odynophagia
    4. Vomiting
    5. Abdominal pain
    6. Anemia
    7. Abnormal upper gastrointestinal (GI) tract
    8. Hematemesis/melena
    9. Suspected infection in an immunocompromised host
    10. Biopsy and/or collection of a specimen from the duodenum
    11. Cancer screening for high-risk individuals (Barrett's esophagus, pernicious anemia)—controversial
    12. Evaluation of caustic injury
  B. Therapeutic indications
    1. Esophageal or pyloric dilation
    2. Ablation of tumors with a laser or cautery
    3. Foreign body removal
    4. Gastrointestinal bleeding
      a. Monopolar or bipolar electrocoagulation
      b. Injection therapy for variceal and nonvariceal bleeding
      c. Laser therapy
      d. Mechanical therapy including hemoclips and banding
      e. Topical therapy (e.g., tissue adhesives)
    5. Polypectomy
    6. Placement of feeding tubes
    7. Manipulations through the ampulla of Vater
    8. Esophageal stent placement

III. Potential Findings

  A. Inflammatory diseases
    1. Esophagitis, gastritis, and duodenitis
    2. Infectious esophagitis caused by herpes virus, *Candida*, and cytomegalovirus

3. Radiation- and chemotherapy-induced changes
4. Pill esophagitis
5. Alkali injuries

B. Ulcer disease
1. Esophageal ulcers usually secondary to reflux, with concomitant Barrett's esophagus
2. Gastric ulcer
3. Duodenal ulcer

C. Neoplastic diseases
1. Adenocarcinoma of the esophagus, stomach, and duodenum
2. Squamous cell carcinoma of the esophagus
3. Lymphoma of the GI tract
4. Metastatic disease, particularly of the breast, lung, and pancreas, as well as melanoma
5. Kaposi's sarcoma
6. Benign tumors, particularly leiomyomas and lipomas

D. Miscellaneous conditions
1. Pyloric obstruction secondary to previous ulcer scarring
2. Gastric bezoar

IV. Limitations of the Study

The procedure requires a relatively cooperative patient with an empty stomach. Therapeutic maneuvers may be affected by the location, as well as by specific circumstances (e.g., excessive bleeding, retained food, retching patient). Another potential limitation is the cost, endoscopy being considerably more expensive than an upper GI series.

V. Contraindications

A. Absolute
1. Uncooperative patient
2. Profound coagulopathy
3. Known or suspected perforation
4. Lack of adequate technical support

B. Relative
1. Urgency of the procedure must be weighed against instability of the patient
2. Massive bleeding without a protected airway

VI. Complications

Complications of upper endoscopy are rare. Fatal complications are reported at a rate of 3 per 10,000 cases, and morbid complications total approximately 0.2%.

A. Medication related—respiratory depression, hypoxemia
B. Procedure related—arrhythmias, perforation, bleeding, aspiration

VII. Risks and Benefits

The risks are low, and the benefits are usually significant in terms of diagnostic yield and directing of appropriate medical care. Continuing additions of diagnostic and therapeutic modalities will increase the benefits without significantly increasing the risk.

Bibliography

Fleischer D. Endoscopic therapy of upper gastrointestinal bleeding in humans. *Gastroenterology* 90:217–234, 1986.

Kahn KL, Kosecoff J, Chassin MR, et al. The use and misuse of upper gastrointestinal endoscopy. *Ann Intern Med* 109:664–670, 1988.

Lower Gastrointestinal Endoscopy

John Schaffner, M.D.

I. Introduction

Flexible sigmoidoscopy and colonoscopy permit direct inspection of the colon to the ileoceal valve and, in some instances, into the ileum. Images are transmitted through fiberoptics or by computer generation. The flexible sigmoidoscope usually allows inspection to the area of the splenic flexure, although this is both operator and patient dependent. Colonoscopy enables a much more extensive view beyond the splenic flexure

II. Indications

A. Flexible sigmoidoscopy is a much more limited exam than colonoscopy. It is primarily a screening tool, though it can be used for other purposes. It is often used in conjunction with air-contrast barium enema. Two lengths of flexible sigmoidoscope are available (35 and 60 cm). Although the shorter instrument is easier to use, a small percentage of lesions will be missed.

  1. Diagnostic indications for flexible sigmoidoscopy

    a. Colon cancer screening

    b. Evaluation of left colon abnormalities seen on lower GI studies.

    c. Evaluation of bright red rectal bleeding

    d. Evaluation of an abnormal digital rectal exam

    e. Evaluation of acute and chronic diarrhea

    f. To obtain rectal biopsy and/or stool specimens

    g. Evaluation of changes in bowel habits

    h. Evaluation of ischemic colitis

    i. Evaluation of known left colon disease

B. Colonoscopy can be performed with several different types of instruments. Advanced training is required for colonoscopy that is not needed for flexible sigmoidoscopy. The colonoscope is used as both a diagnostic and a therapeutic tool.

  1. Diagnostic indications for colonoscopy

    a. Evaluation of occult blood in stool

    b. Evaluation of anemia

    c. Evaluation for inflammatory bowel disease

    d. Colon cancer screening in high-risk patients

    e. Evaluation of acute and chronic diarrhea

    f. Evaluation of rectal bleeding

    g. Postpolypectomy surveillance

    h. Evaluation of an abnormal barium en-
       ema
  2. Therapeutic indications
    a. Polypectomy
    b. Cauterization of bleeding sites, includ-
       ing angiodysplasia
    c. Laser therapy of obstructing tumors
    d. Decompression of a volvulus or pseudo-
       obstruction
    e. Removal of a foreign body

III. Potential Findings
A. Inflammation
  1. Acute infectious colitis
  2. Idiopathic ulcerative proctitis
  3. Ulcerative colitis
  4. Crohn's disease
  5. Rectal ulcers
  6. Ischemic colitis
  7. Radiation proctitis
  8. Diverticulitis
B. Sources of bleeding
  1. Colon cancer
  2. Colon polyps
  3. Diverticulosis
  4. Angiodysplasia
  5. Hemorrhoids
  6. Anal fissure
  7. Varices
  8. Active inflammation
  9. Endometriosis
  10. Meckel's diverticulum
  11. Upper GI bleeding
C. Miscellaneous
  1. Melanosis coli
  2. Condyloma
  3. Foreign bodies

IV. Limitations of the Study
The procedure is limited by the patient's anatomy, the preparation of the patient, and the skill
of the operator.
A. Flexible sigmoidoscopy: The only preparation required in most patients is one or two
enemas prior to the procedure. In skilled
hands, the text takes less than 5 min. Difficulties in passing the scope can occur with extensive diverticular disease and in some women
after hysterectomy.
B. Colonoscopy: Colonoscopy requires a full
bowel preparation. Adhesions, large hernias,
diverticular disease, colon redundancy, and
difficult anatomy may not allow complete examination to the cecum. Because of the anatomy of the colon, some blind spots may occur
(e.g., in the sigmoid colon, at the flexures, or

behind the haustra). In some cases, barium
enema is a complementary exam to colonoscopy. In studies, 85% of colonoscopic exams
could not reach the cecum.

V. Contraindications
The contraindications to flexible sigmoidoscopy
are similar to those of colonoscopy. Many of these
relate to the overall state of health of the patient.
The judgment of the physician is necessary to
weigh the risks against the benefits to be derived
from the examination.
A. Severe colitis because of the increased risk of
colon perforation or precipitation of toxic
megacolon.
B. Suspected colonic perforation, including
acute diverticulitis.
C. Medically unstable patients
D. Uncooperative patients
E. Recent colonic anastomosis
F. Large abdominal aortic aneurysm
G. Profound coagulopathy

VI. Complications
A. Diagnostic procedures
  1. Adverse reactions to premedication
    a. Respiratory depression
    b. Nausea and vomiting
    c. Arrhythmia
    d. Thrombophlebitis at the injection site
  2. Hemorrhage
  3. Perforation
  4. Vasovagal reflex
  5. Arrhythmias
  6. Abdominal distention
B. Therapeutic procedures
  1. Hemorrhage usually occuring after poly-
    pectomy. Most bleeding occurs immedi-
    ately but may be delayed up to 2–3 weeks.
    Bleeding may occur in about 1% of poly-
    pectomies.
  2. Perforation occurs in less than 0.5% of
    colonoscopies and less frequently in sig-
    moidoscopy.
  3. Explosion of colonic gases during electro-
    cautery is rare. Elimination of nonabsorb-
    able carbohydrate from colon prepara-
    tions (i.e., mannitol or lactulose) should
    minimize the risk of this complication.

VII. Risks and Benefits
The risks are low, and the benefits are usually
significant in terms of diagnostic yield and directing of appropriate medical care. As with any
procedure, the risk/benefit ratio must be examined for each individual patient.
A. The value of screening flexible sigmoidos-

copy is still unclear. Current recommendations differ, and definitive studies of benefit are ongoing. Medical costs are an integral part of screening exams. Although no data have demonstrated that lives will be saved by screening flexible sigmoidoscopy, this may be only a statistical problem.

B. The benefits of colonoscopy may be great for many patients. The proper utilization of colonoscopy in some situations remains to be determined. The cost, increased risk, and availability are factors that may help determine the future role of colonoscopy in certain settings.

Bibliography

Irvine EJ, O'Connor JO, Frost RA, et al. Prospective comparison of double contrast barium enema plus flexible sigmoidoscopy vs. colonoscopy in rectal bleeding: Barium enema vs. colonoscopy in rectal bleeding. *Gut* 29:1188–1193, 1988.

Neugut AI, Pita S. Role of sigmoidoscopy in screening for colorectal cancer: A critical review. *Gastroenterology* 95:492–499, 1988.

Selby JV, Freidman GD. Sigmoidscopy in the periodic health examination of asymptomatic adults. *JAMA* 261:595–601, 1989.

Endoscopic Retrograde Cholangiopancreatography: Diagnosis and Therapy

Syed Zaidi, M.D.

I. Procedure

The procedure involves the passage of a side-viewing, flexible upper endoscope into the second portion of the duodenum, where the ampulla of Vater is cannulated, contrast is injected into the biliary and pancreatic ducts under fluoroscopic guidance, and images are obtained. A variety of therapeutic modalities can also be performed, including sphincterotomy, biliary stone extraction, stent placement, and balloon dilatation of biliary strictures.

II. Indication

A. Jaundice: Workup for either cholestasis or extrahepatic biliary obstruction secondary to the presence of stones, strictures, or tumor.

B. Gallstone pancreatitis.

C. Recurrent or chronic pancreatitis when preoperative mapping may be helpful.

D. Evaluation of suspected pancreatic malignancy.

E. Sphincter of Oddi manometry in cases of suspected sphincter of Oddi spasm.

F. Evaluation of unexplained chronic abdominal pain, weight loss, and steatorrhea.

III. Potential Findings

A. Normal anatomic variants.

B. Ampullary stenoses and benign or malignant ampullary tumors.

C. Biliary and pancreatic fistulas.

D. Pancreatic duct dilatation, strictures, intraductal stones, or pseudocysts suggestive of chronic pancreatitis.

E. Pancreatic tumors.

F. Choledocholithiasis.

G. Benign and malignant strictures of the bile ducts.

H. Benign and malignant tumors of the bile ducts.

IV. Limitations of the Study

A. Requires skilled personnel with specialized training in both diagnostic and therapeutic endoscopic retrograde cholangiopancreatography.

B. Requires surgical and radiologic backup in case of inability to drain the common bile duct adequately.

C. Complements other diagnostic modalities and should not be considered a substitute test.

V. Contraindications

There are usually relative contraindications, which include the following:

A. Severe and uncorrectable coagulation disorders.

B. Uncooperative patient.

C. Acute myocardial infarction or other severe cardiopulmonary or systemic illnesses in which the risk of the procedure may outweigh the benefit resulting from it.

VI. **Complications**

A. Respiratory depression and hypotension related to premedication.

B. Pancreatitis. The incidence is usually 1–3%, but it has been reported as being as high as 17%.

C. Cholangitis. This usually occurs in cases of inadequate drainage.

D. Bleeding. The incidence is up to 2.5% postsphincterotomy.

E. Perforation. Incidence of retroperitoneal perforation postsphincterotomy is reported to be around 0.5%.

F. Impaction of the stone basket in the common bile duct.

Bibliography

Borsch G, Wegner M, Wedmann B, et al. Clinical evaluation, ultrasound, cholescintigraphy and ERCP in cholestasis. A prospective clinical study. *J Clin Gastroenterol* 10:185–190, 1988.

Jacobson IM. *ERCP: Diagnostic and Therapeutic Applications*. New York: Elsevier, 1989.

Siegel JH. *ERCP: Technique, Diagnosis and Therapy*. New York: Raven Press, 1992.

Siegel JH, Yatto RP. Approach to cholestasis—an update. *Arch Intern Med* 142:1877–1879, 1982.

CHAPTER 55-D

Esophageal Motility

Sheldon Sloan, M.D.

I. Introduction

Esophageal motility testing involves the use of a manometric catheter within the upper stomach and esophagus. The indication of the test is primarily for the evaluation of dysphagia, severe gastroesophageal reflux disease, and noncardiac chest pain.

II. Equipment Used in Esophageal Motility Testing

A. Basically, two catheters are used in evaluating esophageal motility. The more commonly used type is a multilumen, water-perfused catheter with three to eight side ports. The other type is a nonperfused catheter with three solid-state, strain-gauge sensing ports. The advantage of the perfused catheter is its cost. Both catheters are multiuse, but the initial cost of the solid-state strain-gauge catheter is 10 times greater. Both catheters are connected through a transducer to the polygraph machine such that a continuous tracing is obtained. Computer analysis of the motility tracing is now available, with the instantaneous pressure tracing visualized on a monitor screen, similar to bedside electrocardiographic and hemodynamic monitoring. The catheter is passed transnasally so that the pressure sensing ports are within the upper stomach, across the lower esophageal sphincter, and within the body of the esophagus.

B. Protocols vary with regard to the number of swallows obtained and the maneuvers applied during esophageal motility testing; however, the basic information obtained is the same.

III. Evaluation of the Lower Esophageal Sphincter (LES)

LES function is assessed in two ways during esophageal motility testing. Resting pressure is important to evaluate in assessing whether the sphincter is hypo-, normo-, or hypertensive. The pressures for each range vary among laboratories. LES pressure is relative to gastric pressure. In general, a resting pressure less than 10 mmHg is considered hypotensive, a resting pressure of 10–35 mmHg is normotensive, and a resting pressure greater than 35 mmHg is hypertensive. The other piece of important information about the LES is the degree of relaxation in relation to swallowing. A normal sphincter should relax close to the gastric pressure shortly after the initiation of swallowing. Three different techniques are used to assess LES function.

A. Rapid pull-through technique: The catheter

is passed so that all sensing ports are in the stomach. With the patient suspending respiration, the catheter is pulled out at a steady rate so that all ports are passed through the LESS into the esophagus. This provides the tone as well as the level of the LES. The rapid pull-through technique does not give information about LES relaxation.

B. Station pull-through technique: All pressure sensing ports are placed in the stomach, and the catheter is pulled back 0.5 to 1.0 cm at a time. This allows each port to be pulled through the sphincter, andLES relaxations can be assessed by having the patient swallow with each lead in the LES. This technique also allows measurement of resting LES tone.

C. Dent sleeve: This is a 6-cm membrane positioned at the distal end of the catheter that measures the highest pressure anywhere along its length. This catheter is stationed such that the Dent sleeve is positioned within the LES, and a distal port measures gastric pressure and proximal ports measure esophageal pressure.

IV. **Esophageal Function**

Esophageal function is measured by placing two or more pressure-sensing ports within the body of the esophagus. This method detects primary peristalsis, peristaltic amplitude, peristaltic wave duration, and peristaltic wave velocity. This aspect of the exam is done with water swallows, since a larger percentage of dry swallows are not propagated to the distal esophagus.

V. **Evaluation of the Upper Esophageal Sphincter (UES)**

UES testing is done by positioning one pressure sensor within the oral pharynx, one within the UES, and the remaining sensors within the body fo the esophagus. UES relaxation is noted, as well as the timing to pharyngeal contraction during the swallow. In certain conditions, such as cricopharyngeal achalasia, the UES will not relax completely in association with the pharyngeal phase of swallowing.

VI. **Provocative Tests**

Provocative tests of the esophagus are used to elicit motor abnormalities or symptoms that may not be evident during routine manometry. These include the following:

A. Bernstein test: With the manometry catheter or nagogastric tube in place, a midesophageal port is used to instill 0.1 N HCl or saline at a set rate, with the patient blinded to which is being infused. A positive test is one in which the patient describes symptoms that are similar to the presenting complaint (e.g., chest pain, heartburn, nausea, dyspepsia). The overall sensitivity and specificity in patients with gastroesophageal reflux disease is about 80%.

B. Edrophonium test: This test is performed with the manometry catheter in place while 80 μg/kg edrophonium is rapidly infused intravenously. The patient is asked to swallow water, and the manometry tracing as well as the patient's symptoms are monitored. Although there is no consensus on what constitutes a positive test, it is safe to say that reproduction of symptoms (e.g., chest pain or dysphagia) with concurrent motility tracing abnormalities is strongly suggestive. Motor disorders such as diffuse esophageal spasm or nutcracker esophagus may be accentuated with the edrophonium infusion.

C. Bethanachol is generally no longer used as a provocative test, primarily due to the side effects of the infusion and the fact that the information can be obtained with edrophonium.

Bibliography

Castell DO, Richter JE, Boag Dalton C (eds). *Esophageal Motility Testing*. New York, Elsevier, 1987.

Dent J, Chir B. A new technique for continuous sphincter pressure measurement. *Gastroenterology* 71:263–267, 1976.

Dodds WJ, Stef JJ, Hogan WF. Factors determining pressure measurement accuracy by intraluminal manometry. *Gastroenterology* 70:117–123, 1976.

Gerhardt DE, Castell DO. Anatomy and physiology of the esophageal sphincters, in Castell DO, Johnson LF (eds): *Esophageal Function in Health and Disease*. New York, Elsevier Biomedical, 1983, pp 17–29.

CHAPTER 55-E

Liver Biopsy

Donald M. Jensen, M.D.

I. **Procedure: Technical Description**
Percutaneous liver biopsy utilizes a 16- or 18-gauge needle to obtain a core of liver tissue for histologic analysis. Specimens may be obtained percutaneously, after percussing hepatic dullness, or with the use of ultrasound or computed tomography guidance. In the presence of coagulopathy, a transvenous approach may be used.

II. **Indications**
A. To diagnose suspected hepatic disease, including space-occupying lesions.
B. To monitor the course of liver disease, such as chronic hepatitis or primary biliary cirrhosis.
C. To obtain liver tissue for metabolic analysis or culture.
D. To stage lymphomas.
E. To assess drug hepatotoxicity, such as in methotrexate therapy for rheumatoid arthritis.

III. **Potential Findings**
A. Primary liver disease, including acute and chronic hepatitis, drug hepatotoxicity, primary biliary cirrhosis, hemochromatotis, α-1-antitrypsin deficiency, alcoholic hepatitis, and cirrhosis.
B. Cholestatic disorders, including sclerosing cholangitis, large duct obstruction, granulomatous liver disease, and liver abscesses.
C. Tumors, both primary and metastatic.

IV. **Limitations of the Study**
A. Core size may be inadequate to document certain focal lesions (sampling variability).
B. Space-occupying lesions may not be within reach of the biopsy needle.
C. Fragmentation of the specimen may preclude a histologic diagnosis of cirrhosis.

V. **Contraindications**
A. Absolute
1. Uncooperative patient
2. Abnormal coagulation studies
a. Prothrombin time >2–3 sec prolonged or <50%
b. Partial thromboplastin time >20 sec of control
c. Platelet count <75,000
d. Bleeding time >10 min
3. Infected pleural effusion or peritonitis
B. Relative
1. Ascites
2. Extrahepatic biliary obstruction
3. Uremia
4. Suspected vascular tumors

VI. Complications
  A. Intra-abdominal bleeding or subcapsular hematoma
  B. Pneumothorax
  C. Gallbladder or bile duct perforation
  D. Infection
  E. Vasovagal reaction
VII. Risks and Benefits
  A. Although percutaneous liver biopsy, when properly performed, is a safe procedure with less than a 1% risk of serious intraperitoneal bleeding, it is still an invasive procedure that should be undertaken only if the information cannot be obtained by less invasive means.

  B. In certain high-risk patients, alternative means of obtaining liver tissue should be considered, including open (surgical), laparoscopic, and transvenous biopsy.

Bibliography

Ishak KG, Schiff ER, Schiff L: Needle biopsy of the liver. In: Schiff L, Schiff ER, eds. Diseases of the liver, ed 6. Philadelphia, JB Lippincott, 1987:339.

Lebrec D, Goldfarb G, Degott C, et al: Transvenous liver biopsy—an experience based on 1000 hepatic tissue samplings with this procedure. *Gastroenterology* 83:338, 1982.

CHAPTER 56

Esophageal Diseases

Sheldon Sloan, M.D.

Esophageal Motility Disorders

I. Problem

There has been a great deal of interest in esophageal motility disorders over the past decade, particularly as it relates to noncardiac chest pain. The presence of abnormal manometric findings (e.g., high peristaltic amplitude) must correlate with symptoms; otherwise, the condition may be just a variant of normal. At least four motility disorders have been described, including primary achalasia, diffuse esophageal spasm, nutcracker esophagus, and hypertensive lower esophageal sphincter. All of these disorders carry relatively specific manometric criteria. The suspicion of a motility disorder is hightened with symptoms of dysphagia, chest pain (without a cardiac cause), and regurgitation. Symptoms may be incapacitating to the point where the patient loses weight (e.g., achalasia) or is limited in activity because of the belief that the chest pain is related to the heart (e.g., nutcracker esophagus). The following is a description of the motility disorders, with the attendant workup and treatment approaches.

Primary Achalasia

I. Definition

II. Manometric Criteria

The primary defect is at the level of the lower esophageal sphincter so that relaxation in response to a swallow is nonexistent or incomplete. The resting pressure of the lower esophageal sphincter is usually elevated (>35 mmHg); however, this is not a necessary criterion. In addition, the esophageal body usually has little or no peristalsis. Contractile waves in the esophagus are simultaneous and of relatively low amplitude (20–30 mmHg), consistent with a common cavity phenomenon. Patients with achalasia and a predominant chest pain complaint may have higher-amplitude simultaneous contractions (>60 mmHg) and are classified as having vigorous achalasia.

III. Etiology

There is no consensus as to what causes achalasia. In certain areas of the world (e.g., Ireland) the prevalence is higher, suggesting an infectious or genetic cause.

IV. Pathophysiology

The primary defect is the loss of ganglion at the level of the myenteric plexus. Some investigators feel that this defect occurs first at the lower esophageal sphincter and secondarily within the esophageal body.

V. Diagnosis

Progressive dysphagia for solids and liquids is almost always present in patients with achalasia. Weight loss, chest pain, regurgitation of undigested food without a sour or bitter taste, and chronic cough are also reported, although to a lesser extent. Physical findings are nonspecific and are usually related to weight loss. There may be loss of the gastric air bubble and, therefore, less tympany in the left upper quadrant. Diagnostic tests include the following:

A. Radiography: A chest x-ray may show an air-fluid level in the esophagus, as well as loss of the gastric air bubble. A barium esophagogram will demonstrate loss of peristaltic activity, a dilated esophagus, and tapering at the level of the gastroesophageal (GE) junction (bird's beak). It may also provide clues to a tumor that is clinically mimicking achalasia (pseudoachalsia). In general, the barium esophagogram is an excellent first test in the workup of dysphagia. Lastly, in a patient with suspected pseudoachalasia, a computed tomography (CT) scan at the level of the GE junction should be done to rule out infiltrating gastric carcinoma originating in the cardia of the stomach.

B. Endoscopy: This is necessary to rule out cancer at the level of the cardia in the stomach. An infiltrative gastric carcinoma may not be evident on a barium esophagogram. It is also important to rule out esophageal carcinoma in a patient with long-standing achalasia. Biopsies can be obtained at the level of the GE junction to rule out cancer. The endoscopist can also develop a sense of the nature of the narrowing at the GE junction because the resistance encountered while going through may be a clue (greater resistance is suggestive of a fixed lesion such as a malignancy).

C. Esophageal manometry: This study is essential in making the diagnosis of achalasia. Manometric criteria should be met as discussed above. In addition, there are clues from the motility study that will direct the therapy. If the lower esophageal sphincter

pressure is less than 10 mmHg, a pneumatic dilatation may not be indicated. If high-amplitude, simultaneous contractions are seen within the body of the esophagus (i.e., vigorous achalasia), then a trial of calcium channel blockers or nitrates may temporize the patient's symptoms.

VI. Differential Diagnosis

Because a malignancy can mimic primary achalasia, one of the most important diseases to rule out is pseudoachalasia. Chagas' disease, chronic idiopathic intestinal pseudo-obstruction, amyloidosis, and other esophageal motility disorders must also be included in the differential diagnosis.

VII. Treatment

Treatment includes medical therapy, dilatation with a balloon, and surgical myotomy.

A. Medical therapy is directed at lowering smooth muscle tone. This is accomplished primarily with calcium channel blockers such as nifedipine or nitrates. Either agent should probably be administered sublingually to ensure absorption. Caution must be used with respect to the peripheral vasodilation that takes place with these agents. The patients should either take a test dose in an office setting, with blood pressure monitoring, or be warned of the possible hypotensive side effects.

B. Pneumatic dilatation of the lower esophageal sphincter is the most common form of treatment. The success rate of forceful dilatation ranges from 70% to 90%, and the risk of perforation ranges from 2% to 5%. Some patients will need more than one dilatation; however, if results are not achieved after two dilatations, surgical therapy should strongly be considered.

C. Heller myotomy is the surgery of choice for achalasia. It involves making an incision at the level of the GE junction and, if limited, will decrease the incidence of postoperative gastroesophageal reflex.

VIII. Monitoring

Patient monitoring is basically done clinically by assessing the return of symptoms of dysphagia, weight loss, or chest pain. Because gastroesophageal refulx disease can be a problem after forceful dilatation or surgery, antireflux therapy may need to be initiated.

IX. Prognosis

Prognosis is excellent with a successful dilatation or surgical manipulation of the lower esophageal sphincter in achalasia patients. Because there is a sevenfold increased risk of squamous cell carcinoma in patients with long-standing achalasia, return of symptoms should be thoroughly investigated to ensure the absence of a malignancy.

Diffuse Esophageal Spasm

I. Definition

Diffuse esophageal spasm is a rare disorder of the esophagus characterized by a motility pattern showing simultaneous high-amplitude, prolonged esophageal body contractions. Patients with this disorder typically complain of chest pain and dysphagia.

II. Etiology

There is some evidence that the abnormal contractions may result from a neuropathic disorder, with some common pathophysiologic mechanisms between diffuse esophageal spasm and achalasia.

III. Pathophysiology

There is an exaggerated response to cholinergic agents similar to that seen in other denervated states such as achalasia. Simultaneous contractions may be due to an impaired balance between the excitatory and inhibitory innervation of the smooth muscle.

IV. Diagnosis

Diagnosis of diffuse esophageal spasm is suspected in patients with dysphagia to liquids or solids. These patients may also complain of chest pain and may have already had a workup for cardiac causes of chest pain. The workup for diffuse esophageal spasm is very similar to that for achalasia (see above), which includes a barium esophagogram, an upper endoscopy, and an esophageal motility study.

A. Radiography: The barium esophagogram in diffuse esophageal spasm reveals a pattern described as *corkscrew esophagus, rosary bead esophagus, pseudodiverticulosis, segmental spasm, elevator esophagus, functional diverticula, curling,* and *knuckle-buster.*

B. Endoscopy: This test is done to rule out a constricting lesion at the level of the lower esophageal sphincter which can cause proximal spasm.

C. Manometry: The diagnosis of diffuse esophageal spasm is confirmed by the motility pattern of the esophagus. Although criteria vary, most investigators agree that si-

multaneous contractions in response to a water swallow in the presence of normal lower esophageal sphincter function must exist. Simultaneous contractions should be present during at least 30% of the water swallows, which are usually but not always accompanied by high-amplitude, prolonged pressure waves.

V. Differential Diagnosis

Other primary esophageal motility disorders must be ruled out, as well as gastroesophageal reflux disease, which in some instances can precipitate spasm. The workup, as outlined above, should be adequate to rule out a malignancy.

VI. Treatment

As with achalasia, the primary pathophysiology is related to smooth muscle dysfunction; therefore, medications that affect the smooth muscle may relieve the symptoms. Calcium channel blockers, either sublingual or oral, as well as nitrates, have been successful in treating this disorder. Because many of these patients have chest pain, it is imperative to reassure them that they have a motility disorder and that the long-term prognosis is excellent. Esophageal dilatation and surgical therapy (long esophageal myotomy) are controversial forms of treatment for this disorder and should be used cautiously in only the most severe cases.

VII. Patient Monitoring

Clinical follow-up regarding symptom improvement or worsening should be all that is needed. Repeated reassurance is also important. If symptoms worsen over time, repeat manometry studies should be done to rule out progression to achalasia.

VIII. Prognosis

The long-term outlook is good. There have been reports of Prinzmetal's angina in patients with diffuse esophageal spasm, suggesting a widespread smooth muscle disorder. This should be ruled out during coronary angiography in patients with suspected diffuse esophageal spasm.

Nutcracker Esophagus

I. Definition

Nutcracker esophagus is a recently described motility disorder characterized by high-amplitude peristaltic contractions. It accounts for up to 45% of the motor disorders in patients with noncardiac, angina-like chest pain.

II. Diagnosis

Diagnosis of nutcracker esophagus is suspected in patients with noncardiac chest pain. The symptom typically described by the patient is central chest pain, which may radiate to the epigastric area and occasionally to the neck, arms, and back. Dysphagia is also a frequent complaint (up to 70%) in patients with nutcracker esophagus. Because the motility pattern in the esophagus is peristaltic, a barium esophagogram may not detect this abnormality. Esophageal manometry is required to confirm the diagnosis. Although the amplitude varies between reports, in general the esophageal body will exhibit high-amplitude ($\geq$150 mmHg) and usually prolonged peristaltic contractions. Symptoms should be present during these contractions. Edrophonium will augment the contractions and will either elicit symptoms or exacerbate preexisting symptoms. One of the more convincing manometric finding is the onset of symptoms with the onset of the peristaltic contraction and the resolution of symptoms once the peristaltic wave front has passed.

III. Treatment

As with diffuse esophageal spasm, calcium channel blockers and nitrates are the mainstay of medical therapy. Again, probably more important than medical therapy is reassurance that the patient has an esophageal motility disorder and not angina. Patients who understand their diagnosis are less likely to feel disabled by their pain even though the pain does not always resolve. Esophageal dilatation and surgery are not currently recommended.

Hypertensive Lower Esophageal Sphincter

This is a controversial motility disorder of the esophagus. The manometric criteria vary between laboratories, with values greater than three standard deviations greater than the mean (>40 mmHg) used as the cutoff. Dysphagia and chest pain are frequently described by patients. Delayed bolus transit at the level of the GE junction has been described. These patients respond clinically to calcium channel blockers and nitrates. Hypertensive lower esophageal sphincter is probably part of a continuum of esophageal motility abnormalities that ultimately result in achalasia.

Esophageal Narrowing

I. Problem

Esophageal narrowing may result from a congen-ital condition, as well as from an acquired focal or diffuse decrease in the caliber of the esophagus due to benign or malignant causes. Congenital abnormalities of the esophagus causing narrowing usually present in childhood; however, in some cases, these conditions are not diagnosed until adulthood. The converse is true with acquired causes of esophageal narrowing; however, conditions such as reflux disease may become manifest, resulting in peptic strictures early in life.

II. Diagnosis

Diagnosis of esophageal narrowing in infants is suspected by regurgitation, aspiration, apnea, and failure to thrive. In adults, the symptom that predominates is dysphagia for solids and acute esophageal obstruction. Esophageal obstruction is characterized by severe chest discomfort and inability to swallow, including oral secretions. Radiography (barium esophagogram) plays a frontline role in diagnosing esophageal narrowing, and the workup follows that outlined in Chapter 54B.

III. Differential Diagnosis

A. Congenital conditions
   1. Esophageal atresia: There are four variants of esophageal atresia, with a reported incidence of 1:1,000 to 1:4,500 live births. The most common variant consists of an incompletely developed esophagus with a proximal pouch and a tracheoesophageal fistula connected to the distal esophagus. Symptoms are manifested almost immediately after birth and include fluid nasal and oral regurgitation, coughing, cyanosis, and apnea during feeding. Esophageal narrowing is seen after surgical correction of the esophageal atresia and is secondary to a short surgical stricture.
   2. Congenital esophageal stenosis: This is a rare condition characterized by a short focal narrowing usually located around the junction of the middle and distal thirds of the esophagus. It may result from remnants of tracheobronchial structures. Most cases involve narrowing of 1–2 cm in length. A recent report in a young adult involved narrowing over the entire esophagus; this observation has also been made in our laboratory in a young adult. Therefore, esophageal stenosis may present after childhood.
   3. Muscular hypertrophy of the esophagus: This consists of hypertrophy of the circular smooth muscle, with rare involvement of the longitudinal and/or muscularis mucosa. It has been associated with motor

abnormalities, specifically spasm of the esophagus. In spite of the hypertrophy, the lumen is generally well preserved. The most common site of involvement is in the distal esophagus, with rare involvement of the entire esophagus.

4. Esophageal rings: These tend to be asymptomatic unless the luminal diameter is <13mm. A Schatzki's ring at the level of the GE junction is comprised of mucosa and submucosa. A muscular ring may also occur in a similar location; however, there is some controversy as to the true existence of this entity.

B. Acquired conditions: The symptoms usually present in acquired focal and diffuse narrowing of the esophagus can occur with caustic injury, GE reflux diseases, severe infection involving the mucosa, or malignancy.

1. Physical injury: This includes peptic strictures from reflux esophagitis, annular strictures from caustic ingestion, strictures from radiation, and scarring secondary to sclerotherapy.

2. Infections may cause strictures, particularly chronic cytomegalovirus, candida, or tuberculosis esophagits.

3. Miscellaneous benign causes include narrowing from pemphigus, epidermolysis bullosa, eosinophilic infiltration, intramural hematoma, and ulcers due to Barrett's esophagus.

C. Neoplastic causes: These include squamous esophageal carcinoma, adenocarcinoma arising from Barrett's esophagus or from the cardia of the stomach; metastatic cancer to the esophagus, particularly from the lung; and circumferential leiomyoma.

IV. Treatment

Treatment varies, depending on the diagnosis. In general, with benign narrowing such as a peptic stricture or a Schatzki's ring, esophageal dilatation with an orally passed bougienage is most effective. Surgical correction of congenital anomalies or neoplastic causes of esophageal narrowing may be needed. There is little role for medications in a symptomatic individual with a benign cause of esophageal narrowing.

Gastroesophagel Reflux Disease

I. Definition

Gastroesophageal esophageal reflux disease (GERD) is a common disorder, with heartburn being the most common presenting symptom. Up to 44% of the adult population complains of heartburn at least once a month, and 7% complain of heartburn daily. The end result from varying pathophysiologic components is acid reflux from the stomach into the esophagus. Typically the onset is in adulthood, and except for a high incidence during pregnancy, there is little sexual difference. The mechanisms of reflux are varied and involve defects or alterations in the normal defenses to combat reflux. These include normal motor function (peristalsis of the esophagus), quantity of saliva, mucosal resistance to acid, normal lower esophageal sphincter tone, normal gastric emptying, normal acid and pepsin components of gastric secretion, and the absence of a hiatal hernia.

II. Manifestations

Symptoms can occur without gross injury to the esophageal mucosa. Severe injury can occur without seemingly significant symptoms.

A. Typical symptoms

1. Heartburn: This is a subjective symptom that is interpreted differently by each patient. It is usually localized to the midepigastrium as a burning sensation with radiation up the substernum. Most often, it occurs postprandially within 2 hr, but occasionally it awakens the patient at night (nocturnal heartburn).

2. Regurgitation: Associated with the heartburn is regurgitation of gastric contents into the mouth with either a sour or a bitter taste. The nature of the regurgitation depends on the gastric contents (gastric acid, pepsin, bile).

3. Belching.

4. Reflux dyspareunia: Reflux symptoms during sexual intercourse occur frequently (77% in one study). They are attributed to a weak antireflux barrier and increased abdominal pressure.

B. Atypical symptoms

1. Noncardiac chest pain: Because reflux symptoms can be confused with angina, it is important to rule this out for the patients age and history (e.g., with an electrocardiogram, treadmill stress test, cardiac catheterization). Pain fibers from the heart and the esophagus seem to be closely linked. Reflux can increase with exertion, making the diagnosis more difficult. Studies using a 24-hr pH probe have identified approxi-

mately 75% of noncardiac chest pain patients as having gastroesophageal reflux, a definite or probably cause of their chest pain.

2. Pulmonary manifestations
   a. Asthma-two mechanisms have been proposed as a reason why GERD can cause asthma.
      (1) Microaspiration of reflux contents from the esophagus into the upper airway.
      (2) Vagally mediated reflux arc triggered by acid in the midesophagus.
   b. Bronchitis.
   c. Bronchiectasis.
   d. Aspiration pneumonia.
   e. Pulmonary fibrosis.
3. Ear, nose, and throat manifestations
   a. Hoarseness due to reflux laryngitis.
   b. Vocal cord granulomas.
   c. Halitosis.
   d. Dental enamel loss.
C. Esophageal manifestations
   1. Esophagitis: Ranges from erythema of the squamous mucosa of the distal esophagus to ulcerations (erosive esophagitis).
   2. Strictures: Caused by repeated injury and scarring.
   3. Bleeding: Can occur from erosions in the esophagus.
   4. Barrett's epithelium: Metaplasia of the squamous mucosa to columnar mucosa. This is usually seen in patients with long-standing GERD; however, the symptoms of patients with Barrett's esophagus may be no different from those of patients without esophagitis. There is a potential for malignancy (adenocarcinoma of the esophagus) in patients with Barrett's esophagus (up to 19% in some series).

III. Mechanisms

The pathophysiology of GERD is multifactorial. Offensive as well as defensive forces balance each other to limit gastric acid exposure of the distal esophagus.

A. The lower esophageal sphincter (LES) has been implicated as the main line of defense in preventing the entrance of gastric contents into the distal esophagus. The premise of this argument is that unless the resting LES tone is less than 10 mmHg, reflux generally does not occur. The most common LES profile in subjects with and without GERD is called *transient lower esophageal sphincter relaxation (tLESRs)*.

Two other LES profiles have been described in patients with reflux disease. Those with a low resting LES pressure (<10 mmHg) but above the resting gastric pressure can reflux with increased intra-abdominal pressure, a condition called *stress reflux*. In the other LES profile, the resting pressure is close to the gastric pressure, thereby allowing free reflux of gastric contents into the esophagus even without increased intra-abdominal pressure. As noted in Chapter 54A, many substances can decrease the resting LES tone, including chocolate, alcohol, spearmint, peppermint, fatty foods, and medications.

B. The presence of a hiatal hernia is not synonymous with GERD; however, almost all patients with severe mucosal disease (i.e., esophagitis) have a hiatal hernia. Historically, hiatal hernias were thought to be the sole cause of reflux disease; however, with improved manometric technique, the LES became the focus of GERD research. More recently, there has developed a more balanced view of the relationship of hiatal hernias to GERD. Studies have shown that there is decreased eophageal volume clearance as well as esophageal acid clearance in patients with large axial hiatal hernias. Larger hernias also seem to be more susceptible to increases in abdominal pressure.

C. Delayed gastric emptying can increase reflux. With gastric distention, the LES relaxes so that venting can occur (i.e., belching). With the LES relaxed, gastric contents can reflux (sour belching), especially if the gastric pressure is elevated.

D. Hypersecretory states such as Zollinger-Ellison syndrome can cause reflux by increased gastric distention from increased fluid, as well as a consistently low pH of the stomach.

IV. Treatment

A. Lifestyle modifications
   1. Cessation of smoking.
   2. Avoiding a supine position for 2–3 hr after eating.
   3. Avoiding refluxigenic foods (e.g., fatty foods, chocolate, spearmint, peppermint, wine).
   4. Losing weight.
   5. Avoiding tight clothing.
   6. Elevating the head of the bed >30 degrees.
B. Medications
   1. Antacids for occasional symptoms.
   2. Alginic acid for occasional symptoms.
   3. H-2 blockers for occasional symptoms or for the treatment of esophagitis.

4. Promotility agents such as metoclopramide or bethanacol in conjunction with H-2 blockers.

5. Omeprazole for refractory symptoms or severe erosive esophagitis.

C. Surgery is reserved for patients with refractory disease in spite of therapeutic or super-therapeutic doses of H-2 blockers or omeprazole. The most common procedure is a fundoplication (Nissen). The results are good; however, with time the stomach wrap may loosen or migrate.

Bibliography

Esophageal Diseases

Reynolds JC, Parkman HP. Achalasia. *Gastroenterol Clin North Am* 18:223–255, 1989.

Rothstein RD, Ouyang A. Chest pain of esophageal origin. *Gastroenterol Clin North Am* 18:257–273, 1989.

Stuart RC, Hennessy TPJ. Primary disorders of oesophageal motility. *Br J Surg* 76:1111–1120, 1989.

Esophageal Narrowing

Aprigliano F. Esophageal stenosis in children. *Ann Otol* 89:391–396, 1980.

Ein SH, Friedberg J. Esophageal atresia and tracheoesophageal fistula: Review and update. *Otolaryngol Clin North Am* 14:219–246, 1981.

Fonkalsrud EW. Esophageal stenosis due to tracheobronchial remnants. *Am J Surg* 124:101–103, 1972.

Sloper JC. Idiopathic diffuse muscular hypertrophy of the lower oesophagus. *Thorax* 9:136–146, 1954.

Gastroesophageal Reflux Disease

Cohen S, Harris LD. Does hiatus hernia affect competence of the gastroesophageal sphincter? *N Engl J Med* 284:1053–1056, 1971.

Dodds WJ. The pathogenesis of gastroesophageal reflux disease. *AJR* 151:49–56, 1988.

Dodds WJ, Dent J, Hogan WJ, et al. Mechanisms of gastroesophageal reflux in patients with reflux esophagitis. *N Engl J Med* 308:1547–1552, 1982.

Sloan S, Kahrilas PJ. Impairment of esophageal emptying with hiatal hernia. *Gastroenterology* 100:596–605, 1991.

Sloan S, Rademaker AW, Kahrilas PJ. Determinants of gastroesophageal junction incompetence: hiatus hernia, lower esophageal sphincter, or both? *Annals of Internal Medicine* 117:977–982, 1992.

Gastric Motility Disorders

Sheldon Sloan, M.D.

I. Gastric Physiology

Once a bolus has successfully traversed the esophagus into the stomach, a complex, well-orchestrated sequence of events takes place. The stomach receives the food and reduces it to manageable particle size so that it can continue the digestion process into the small intestine. The fundus, antrum, and pylorus each have separate roles in this process. The fundus acts as a reservoir and relaxes to accept an ingested bolus, a process thought to be mediated by nonadrenergic, noncholinergic vagal efferent fibers. The fundus then regains tone, which displaces the meal toward the antrum. The antrum acts on the meal, grinding it up into smaller particles. Depolarization begins in the pacemaker zone in the body of the stomach and progresses down the antrum toward the pylorus at a rate of 3 waves per minute. The pylorus acts as the regulator for particles exiting the stomach. The pylorus is thought to alter its size, depending on the luminal contents, and closes off completely as the antral contraction progresses toward it.

A. Control of liquid emptying is dependent in part on the reservoir capacity of the fundus. With a vagotomy, the intragastric pressure is increased and accelerated emptying of liquids is seen. Liquids empty in gushes associated with coordinated contractions of the antrum, pylorus, and duodenum. Nutrients are delivered to the small intestine by way of a feedback loop to the fundus, which slows down gastric emptying. Receptors in the small intestine sensitive to lipids, osmolality, and amino acids are also thought to exist, playing a role in regulating gastric emptying. Receptors in the duodenum sensitive to a drop in pH may delay gastric emptying for liquids.

B. Control of solid emptying is primarily due to the forces in the antrum, which break up solids into small particles (1 mm) which are then emptied as a suspension.

C. During the fasting state, four phases of interdigestive motor activity are seen. Phase I starts 2–3 hr after a meal and is a quiescent period lasting for about 1 hr. Phase II is characterized by more electrical activity with some mechanical coupling and lasts for about 30 mins. Phase III is a period that sweeps particles as large as 2 cm in diameter down from the fundus to the pylorus, which is open and relaxed, thus allowing remaining particles in the stomach that were not previously reduced to a small enough size to pass into the small intestine. Phase III lasts for about 10 min followed by decreased activity, which constitutes phase IV.

II. Methods Used in Measuring Gastric Emptying

A. Radiographic studies including a barium-hamburger meal are cumbersome and require numerous x-rays of the abdomen for a complete study.

B. The most common method for measuring gastric emptying is the use of radioisotopes. Technetium-99 sulfur coloid bound to chicken livers is used to measure solid phase emptying. Together with Indium-111, a liquid phase of emptying can be simultaneously measured because the gamma phase peak differs from that of technetium. The total radiation exposure with this method is approximately that of one chest x-ray. Gastric emptying of solid foods is probably the best indicator of gastric function in regard to stasis. In order to obtain an optimal gastric emptying study, patients must be off any medications that may influence gastric motility, including anticholinergics, narcotics, levodopa, progesterone, and metoclopramide.

C. Manometry using solid-state or perfused sensor technologies placed within the antrum, duodenum, and upper small bowel can determine fed and fasting patterns of phasic pressure activity.

D. Electrogastrography: This involves placement of cutaneous electrodes on the skin over the stomach to measure the slow wave activity of the stomach. The main purpose of this test is to detect gastric dysrhythmias such as tachygastria, characterized by increased slow wave activity, and bradygastria, characterized by decreased slow wave activity.

III. Disorders of Gastric Motility

A. Rapid gastric emptying can be seen in peptic ulcer disease and Zollinger-Ellison syndrome, as well as after vagotomy and antrectomy.

B. *Gastroparesis* is the term used for disorders causing gastric stasis. Nausea, bloating, fullness, and early satiety may be more sensitive indicators of gastroparesis than vomiting. Essential in the workup of these symptoms is the ruling out of mechanical obstruction, either with an upper endoscopy or an upper gastrointestinal radiographic series.

1. Gastric ulcers and gastritis are associated with delayed gastric emptying.

2. Infections including Norwalk virus, herpes-varicella-zoster, botulinum toxin, Epstein-Barr virus, and possibly *Helicobacter pylori* may cause gastroparesis. Viral infections have been implicated in idiopathic gastroparesis, which can be prolonged.

3. Diabetes mellitus is one of the more classic disease states associated with gastroparesis. A high percentage of patients with peripheral neuropathy will have abnormal gastric emptying studies; however, only a small portion are symptomatic.

4. Systemic conditions affecting the visceral autonomic nervous system and causing gastroparesis include amyloidosis, Riley-Day syndrome, Shy-Drager syndrome, irradiation, paraneoplastic syndromes, peripheral labyrinthine disorders causing vertigo, abdominal migraine variant, and "cardiac vomiting" seen in patients with an acute myocardial infarction.

5. Central nervous system disorders affecting gastric motility include lesions of the vagal nerve and vestibular nuclei, increased intracranial pressure (central vomiting), visceral epilepsy, and high spinal cord transection.

6. Medications affecting gastric motility include calcium channel blockers, β-agonists, bromocriptine, levodopa, anticholinergic agents, and opiates.

7. Psychogenic vomiting may be a voluntary act, as seen in certain eating disorders.

8. Metabolic states such as hypothyroidism or pregnancy may be associated with gastroparesis. Hyperthyroid disease may cause rapid gastric emptying.

IV. Treatment

Treatment for gastroparesis varies, depending on the cause. A careful history, including all medicatons, may be the key to alleviating gastroparesis (e.g., the anticholinergic effect of antidepressants). Tighter control of blood glucose levels in diabetics has been associated with improvement in gastric motility.

A. Metoclopramide: This is a dopamine agonist which acts centrally as an antiemetic and peripherally as a prokinetic agent on gastrointestinal smooth muscle. In the stomach, the drug increases the frequency and amplitude of antral contractions. Metoclopramide has been shown to be effective in diabetic gastroparesis as well as in postgastric resection gastroparesis. The usual dosage is 10 mg 15–30 min before meals and at bedtime; however, the dose should be reduced (to 5 mg) in older patients until its tolerance is known. Subcutaneous administration in the range of 1–5 mg may be needed in patients with severe gastroparesis. The major disadvantage to this medication is the side effects. Drowsiness, restlessness, and anxiety are the most common side effects. Extrapyramidal reactions including oculogyric crisis, opisthotonos, trismus, and torticollis occur in about 1% of patients. Metoclopramide should not be used when there is evidence of a mechanical obstruction, or with simultaneous use of phenothiazines (these augment the side effects) or anticholinergic medications (antagonize prokinetic actions), or in patients with pheochromocytoma or Parkinson's disease.

B. Erythromycin: In spite of its well-known properties as an antibiotic, the role of erythromycin as a prokinetic agent used for gastroparesis has recently been described. Erythromycin has been reported to significantly improve gastric emptying in diabetics when used intravenously and, to a lesser extent, orally. It acts by virtue of it similarity to a gut hormone called *motilin* that stimulates motility. In part, because of this observation pharmaceutical investigation is now focusing on erythromycin like drugs that are agonists of motilin. The dosages used were 200 mg intravenously or 250 mg orally before meals.

C. Domperidone: This promising agent is a dopamine antagonist similar to metoclopramide that stimulates gut motility without affecting the central nervous system, since it does not cross the blood-brain barrier. Unfortunately, at the time of this writing, it is has not been approved for use in the United States. It increases peristaltic activity and the amplitude of contraction of the antrum and duodenum. Side effects are mainly related to its effect on prolactin secretion and include breast enlargement, nipple tenderness, galactorrhea, and amenorrhea. Extrapyramidal and dystonic reactions are generally not seen.

D. Cisapride: This is another prokinetic agent now commercially available. It does not have antidopaminergic properties and acts by facilitating acetylcholine release at the level of the myenteric plexus. Intravenous cisapride accelerates gastric emptying in patients with diabetic, postgastric surgery, and idiopathic gastroparesis states. Oral cisapride has also been shown to improve gastric emptying.

Bibliography

Camilleri M, Malagelada JR, Abell TL, et al. Effect of six weeks of treatment with cisapride in gastroparesis and intestinal pseudoobstruction. *Gastroenterology* 96:704–712, 1989.

Janssens J, Peeters TL, Vantrappen G, et al. Improvement of gastric emptying in diabetic gastroparesis by erythromycin: Preliminary studies. *N Engl J Med* 322:1028–1031, 1990.

McCallum RW. Motor function of the stomach in health and disease, in Sleisinger MH, Fordtran JS (eds.). Gastroinestinal Disease. Pathophysiology and Management, ed. 4 Philadelphia, Saunders, 1989, pp 675–713.

Read NW, Houghton LA. Physiology of gastric emptying and pathophysiology of gastroparesis. *Gastroenterol Clin North Am* 18:359–373, 1989.

CHAPTER 57-B

Gastritis

Syed Zaidi, M.D.

I. Definition

Gastritis is a very broad term referring to a variety of acute and chronic inflammatory conditions of the stomach which may be localized or present throughout the stomach. These conditions may be divided into the following types:
A. Acute erosive or hemorrhagic gastritis.
B. Chronic erosive (Varioliform) gastritis.
C. Chronic nonerosive gastritis (types A & B).
D. Specific Gastritides
   1. Granulomatous.
   2. Hypertrophic gastropathy.
   3. Eosinophilic gastritis.
   4. Infectious gastritis.

II. Etiology and Pathogenesis

A variety of agents and conditions have been implicated in the lesions resulting from the various forms of gastritis.
A. Acute erosive gastritis: Etiology
   1. Stress erosions occurring in a setting of severe trauma, burns, head injury, or overwhelming medical or surgical illnesses.
   2. Aspirin and nonsteroidal anti-inflammatory drugs.
   3. Ethanol use.
   4. Reflux of bile acid.
   5. Radiation therapy.
   6. Mechanical trauma: Use of nasogastric tube or secondary to retching (prolapse gastropathy).
      a. The pathogenesis of acute mucosal injury involves several factors which result in disruption of the mucosal barrier to back diffusion of gastric acid. Hypersecretion of acid, however, is seen only in cases of head injury. Usually in an acute care condition there is hyposecretion of acid. The factors contributing to the defense of the mucosal lining include:
      (1) Mucosal blood flow.
      (2) Epithelial cell renewal.
      (3) Mucus production.
      (4) Bicarbonate secretion.
      (5) Prostaglandin secretion.
      b. Ischemia is probably the most important factor which plays a major role in the clinical settings of acute mucosal injury by disrupting all the protective mechanisms and allowing back diffusion of acid.

B. Chronic erosive (varioliform) gastritis. The etiology is unknown, though in some cases the antrum is infected with *Helicobacter pylori*. The condition is also called *lymphocytic gastritis* and may represent gastric manifestations of celiac disease or other spruelike illnesses. It is characterized by thickened gastric folds with multiple small nodules accompanied by central erosions.

C. Chronic nonerosive gastritis
1. Type A: Involves the body and fundus of the stomach, usually with sparing of the antrum. The etiology of this form of gastritis is in most cases thought to be autoimmune and results in atrophic-appearing gastric mucosa. It is the usual cause of pernicious anemia.
2. Type B: Predominantly involves the antrum but may extend proximally; the causative agent is usually *H. pylori*. Other possible etiologies include reflux of bile and pancreatic juices.

D. Specific forms of gastritis
1. Hypertrophic gastropathy (Menetrier's disease): The etiology is unknown. The condition is characterized by enlarged gastric folds and hypertrophy of the gastric mucosa. A similar condition known as *hypertrophic hypersecretory gastropathy* is associated with hypersecretion of acid.
2. Eosinophilic gastritis: This condition, which is usually limited to the antrum, is a rare gastritis of unknown etiology characterized by eosinophilic infiltration of the stomach. Peripheral eosinophilia commonly accompanies it.
3. Granulomatous gastritis: A variety of conditions are associated with granulomatous infiltration of the stomach, including Crohn's disease, sarcoidosis, tuberculosis, syphilis, and fungal infections. In certain cases, however, no etiologic agent can be found, and the condition is termed *idopathic*.
4. Infectious gastritis
   a. Phlegmonous gastritis is a rare but extremely serious condition usually caused by α-hemolytic streptococci and occasionally by other bacteria such as pneumococci, staphylococci, *Escherichia coli*, and *Clostridium perfringens*. It usually occurs in the setting of severe malnutrition, systemic illness or infection, and trauma. It is a life-threaten-

ing illness, and even with early diagnosis and surgery, mortality can be up to 20%.
   b. Other infections causing gastritis include cytomegalovirus (CMV), herpes virus, and various parasitic infestations.

III. **Diagnosis**
A. History: The patient may be completely asymptomatic. However, a history should be obtained regarding predisposing conditions such as nonsteroidal anti-inflammatory drug use, ethanol use, and underlying medical or surgical illnesses. The usual symptoms are as follows:
1. Abdominal pain, nausea, and vomiting.
2. Gastrointestinal bleeding. This is the most common manifestation of erosive gastritis and may present as melena or hematemesis.
3. Gastritis may present with symptoms of gastric outlet obstruction such as early satiety, especially in cases of granulomatous and eosinophilic gastritis.
4. In cases of phlegmonous gastritis, an acute abdomen may be present.

B. Clinical signs and physical findings: The gastrointestinal physical exam is usually normal unless patient has signs of bleeding or other concomitant illnesses.

C. Diagnostic tests
1. A complete blood count may reflect anemia, macrocytosis, or eosinophilia.
2. Double-contrast barium studies may detect gastric erosions, however, endoscopy is more sensitive for both erosive and nonerosive gastritis.
3. Endoscopic biopsy may be very helpful in elucidating the diagnosis in cases of *H. pylori*; in granulomatous, eosinophilic, and CMV-associated gastritis; and in some cases of hypertrophic gastropathy which may require a full-thickness surgical biopsy.
4. Gastric acid secretion studies may be helpful for evaluation of hypo- or hyersecretors and associated conditions such as pernicious anemia and hypertrophic gastropathy.
5. Additional tests such as chest x-ray and small bowel follow-up may be indicated to determine the presence of systemic disease such as tuberculosis, sarcoidosis, and Crohn's disease.

IV. Differential Diagnosis

The differential diagnosis mainly involves differentiating one form of gastritis from another and excluding an underlying malignancy such as gastric adenocarcinoma or lymphoma. The latter question usually arises in the case of thickened gastric folds and may be extremely difficult to answer. In some cases, a full-thickness gastric biopsy preceded by a computed tomography scan or endoscopic ultrasound scan may be indicated.

V. Treatment

A. Acute nonhemorrhagic gastritis will usually resolve with elimination of etiologic factors such as nonsteroidals and ethanol. Symptomatic patients may be treated with antacids and H-2 receptor antagonists. Prostaglandin analogs may be used for prophylaxis in high-risk patients on nonsteroidals.

B. Stress erosions may be prevented by proyhlaxis with either antacids or continuous H-2 receptor blocker infusions to maintain an intragastric pH above 4.0. Sucralfate and misoprostol have also been shown to prevent stress erosions.

C. Acute hemorrhagic gastritis is treated mainly by supportive measures, with emphasis on correction of underlying and precipitating factors such as sepsis. Endoscopic therapy with the use of electrocoagulation and laser coagulation is usually precluded or limited by widespread diffuse gastric bleeding.

D. Specific treatment should be directed toward the etiology of specific gastritides and may involve the use of steroids, antituberculous medications, and antifungal therapy.

E. As a last resort, surgery may be required for acute or chronic complications of gastritis.

VI. Patient Monitoring

A. Patients with predisposing conditions which may lead to the development of acute gastritis should be monitored closely for the development of complications which may be life-threatening. Stress prophylaxis is the key, and major emphasis is placed on it to reduce the incidence of stress erosions.

B. Routine surveillance of patients with chronic atrophic gastritis or *H. pylori*–associated gastritis for the development of carcinoma is controversial. Until more definite data and guidelines are available, routine monitoring is not warranted.

VII. Prognosis

Gastritis is usually self-limited and the overall prognosis is good. However, acute hemorrhagic or *phlegmonous gastritis* may be life-threatening. Other gastritides, if not diagnosed and treated appropriately, may lead to significant morbidity and mortality.

Bibliography

Haot J, Jouret A, Willette M, et al. Lymphocytic gastritis—Prospective study of its relationship with varioloform gastritis. *Gut* 31:282, 1990.

Isenberg JI, McQuaid KR, Laine L, et al. Gastritis, in Yamada T (ed), *Textbook of Gastroenterology*. Philadelphia, Lippincott, 1991, p. 1298.

Klieman RL, Adair CG, Ephgrave KS. Stress ulcers: Current understanding of pathogenesis and prophylaxis. *Drug Intell Clin Pharm* 22:452, 1988.

Kaufman G. Aspirin induced mucosal injury: Lessons learned from animal models. *Gastroenterology* 96:606, 1989.

Weinstien WM. Gastritis, in Sleisenger MH, Fordtran JS (eds), *Gastrointestinal Disease*. Philadelphia, Saunders, 1989, p. 792.

Gastric Ulcer

Seymour M. Sabesin, M.D.

I. **Definition**
   Gastric ulcers penetrate through the muscularis mucosae and are distinguished from gastric erosions by their depth. They vary in size, ranging from a few millimeters to 2 cm or greater.

II. **Epidemiology**
   A. In contrast to duodenal ulcers, there has been no decrease in hospitalizations for gastric ulcers over the past 20 years. Gastric ulcers occur about equally in men and women, and their peak incidence is between ages 55 and 65.
   B. About 87,500 new cases of gastric ulcer are diagnosed each year.

III. **Etiology and Pathophysiology**
   Many of the factors leading to the development of duodenal ulcers are also thought to be important for the formation of gastric ulcers. Details of these pathophysiologic events are included in Chapter 57D. Although acid and pepsin secretion may be lower in patients with gastric ulcers than in those with duodenal ulcers, it is thought that an impairment in the gastric mucosal defense barrier is most important in the pathogenesis of gastric ulcer disease.
   A. Pathophysiologic factors

   1. Impaired gastric mucosal barrier.
   2. Motility abnormalities such as reflux of duodenal contents (acid, pepsin, bile acids) into the stomach.
   3. Gastritis (perhaps caused by *Helicobacter pylori*).
   4. Aspirin and other nonsteroidal anti-inflammatory drugs.
   5. Smoking.
   6. Stress; there is no evidence that emotional stress is a direct cause of gastric ulcers.
   7. Genetic factors. See Chapter 57D for a discussion of genetic factors in peptic ulcer disease.

IV. **Diagnosis**
   A. History: As is true for duodenal ulcers, it is not possible to make a definitive diagnosis of a gastric ulcer on the basis of the patient's history of abdominal pain. Asymptomatic gastric ulcers are common. Thus, there is a poor correlation between pain and the presence of an ulcer. The nonspecific nature of the abdominal pain and its variable relationship to meals make it difficult to differentiate gastric ulcers from other acid-peptic disorders and from many other diseases.

B. Clinical signs and physical findings
   1. Epigastric pain, reported as severe, is described in two-thirds of patients. Radiation of pain to the back may occur in one-third of patients.
   2. The pain may be relieved by food or antacids or may be increased by food. There is so much variability in the response to food that this factor is not helpful in making the diagnosis of gastric ulcer.
   3. One-third to two-thirds of patients complain of anorexia, weight loss, nausea, vomiting, or other symptoms of dyspepsia such as excessive bloating or belching.
   4. Physical examination is usually normal unless there is pyloric channel obstruction.
C. Diagnostic tests
   1. X-ray studies can be quite accurate in diagnosing gastric ulcers if they are more than 5 mm in diameter. The major problem is in distinguishing benign from malignant ulcers. Despite the development of radiologic criteria to differentiate gastric neoplasms from benign ulcers, 7% of previously diagnosed benign ulcers have been found to be malignant at surgery. Therefore, endoscopy is recommended in all patients in whom an x-ray diagnosis of a benign ulcer is made.
   2. Endoscopy permits direct visualization of the stomach, and biopsy specimens of ulcers and other lesions can be obtained. Endoscopy should be performed on all patients with x-ray diagnosis of a benign ulcer, multiple biopsy specimens and cytologic specimens obtained to exclude malignancy, and repeat endoscopy performed to document complete healing. Endoscopy, rather than x-ray, should be the first diagnostic test in patients complaining of abdominal pain; however, if an x-ray study was performed and the patient treated with antisecretory medication, an endoscopy should be performed 8 weeks later to document complete healing and exclude malignancy if the ulcer is not completely healed.
   3. Laboratory testing to measure acid secretion is not helpful in making a diagnosis of a gastric ulcer or in differentiating a benign from a malignant lesion.

V. **Differential Diagnosis**
   The differential diagnosis includes a variety of upper gastrointestinal acid-peptic disorders (e.g., duodenal ulcer, gastroesophageal reflux disease, nonulcer dyspepsia), pancreatic diseases, and biliary tract diseases. Most important is the differentiation of benign from malignant gastric ulcers.

VI. **Treatment**
   Chapter 57D contains a comprehensive discussion of the types, mode of action, and safety of various drugs used for ulcer therapy. The only major difference between the treatment of duodenal and gastric ulcers is related to the duration of therapy. Specifics of concern to gastric ulcer are as follows:
   A. Histamine H_2-receptor antagonists (H_2-RA) are the major class of drugs for the treatment of benign gastric ulcers.
   B. Therapy with any one of the four H_2-RAs should be continued until the ulcer heals completely. Healing of most gastric ulcers occurs in 8–12 weeks with standard twice-daily or even single doses of the H_2-RAs.
   C. Neither omeprazole nor sucralfate has been approved for the treatment of gastric ulcers.
   D. Antacids can heal gastric ulcers, but the exact dosing regimens are not known. The large and frequent doses required to approximate the healing obtained with H_2-RAs limits the usefulness of antacids for gastric ulcer therapy.
   E. The prostaglandin analog misoprostil has been approved only for the prophylaxis of nonsteroidal anti-inflammatory drug (NSAID)-induced gastric ulcers.
   F. General measures: No dietary restrictions are required. NSAIDs and salicylates should not be taken by patients with gastric ulcers, and cigarette smoking should be discontinued.

VII. **Patient Monitoring**
   A. Patients should be followed closely to ascertain whether complete healing of gastric ulcers has occurred. Monitoring involves endoscopic confirmation of healing to exclude malignancy.
   B. Nonhealed gastric ulcers after 12 weeks of therapy should be treated for an additional 4 weeks. After 16 weeks of therapy, if the ulcers have not healed, surgery may be required. Factors related to nonhealing include poor compliance with therapy, concomitant use of NSAIDs or salicylates, and

smoking. These factors should be evaluated before patients are referred for surgery. Increasing the dose of an H_2-RA using omeprazole or initiating combination therapy (e.g., H_2-RA and sucralfate) may be considered in patients with nonhealed ulcers, particularly elderly patients who may be poor surgical risks.

VIII. Prognosis

A. Most gastric ulcers heal after 8–12 weeks of therapy.

B. Recurrent ulcers can be treated with a full course of therapy with an H_2-RA.

C. Although none of the H_2-RAs have been approved for long-term maintenance therapy of gastric ulcers, elderly patients, particularly those with concomitant serious illness, multiple recurrences, and previous bleeding or perforation, should be considered for maintenance therapy.

Bibliography

Alexander-Williams J, Wolverson RL. Pathogenesis and pathophysiology of gastric ulcer, in Isenberg JI, Johansson C (eds), *Clinics in Gastroenterology*. London, Saunders, pp 601–619, 1984.

Feldman M, Burton ME. Histamine$_2$-receptor antagonists: Standard therapy for acid-peptic disease. *N Engl J Med* 323:1749–1755, 1990.

Flemstrom G, Turnberg LA. Gastroduodenal defense mechanisms, in Isenberg JI, Johansson C (eds), *Clinics in Gastroenterology*. London, Saunders, pp 327–354, 1984.

Freston JW. Mechanisms of relapse in peptic ulcer disease. *J Clin Gastroenterol* 11(Suppl 1):534–538, 1989.

Peters MN, Richardson CT. Stressful life situations, acid hypersecretion, and ulcer disease. *Gastroenterology* 84:114–119, 1983.

Soil AH. Pathogenesis of peptic ulcer disease and implications for therapy. *N Engl J Med* 322:909–916, 1990.

Susser M. Causes of peptic ulcers: A selected epidemiologic view. *J Chronic Dis* 20:435–438, 1967.

CHAPTER 57-D

Duodenal Ulcer

Seymour M. Sabesin, M.D.

I. Definition

Duodenal ulcers (DU) are defects in the mucosa which penetrate through the muscularis mucosae. The ulcers vary greatly in size and depth, and the clinical significance of mucosal erosions less than 3 mm in diameter is problematic. DU occur most commonly in the first part of the duodenum. They may be either single or multiple. Recurrent ulcers tend to attack areas of previous mucosal injury, eventually leading to scarring and distortion of the duodenum because of the intense inflammatory response surrounding the ulceration.

II. Epidemiology

A. It is difficult to design accurate epidemiologic studies because detection of ulcers based on clinical symptoms is inaccurate and because endoscopic studies in large populations cannot be performed. In addition, ulcers recur frequently, often without producing symptoms; therefore, accurate detection is extremely difficult. The following data provide an estimate of DU epidemiology based on published studies.

B. Prevalence

1. The point prevalence of DU in endoscopic studies is 1.4%.
2. In a 12-month period, the prevalence is 1.8% in men and 1.7% in women (1981) and 1.8% in men and 2.0% in women (1984).
3. The lifetime prevalence is about 10% in men and about 4% in women.

C. Incidence

1. Yearly incidence: 0.15% in men and 0.03% in women.
2. The age-specific incidence increases with age, becoming as high as 0.3% in men at the age of 75–79.
3. It has been estimated that 200,000 to 400,000 new cases of DU occur in the United States each year.

III. Etiology and Pathophysiology

Present evidence indicates that peptic ulcer is a disease of genetic heterogeneity. Thus, ulcers in different patients have in common the presence of gastric acid but differ in their mechanisms of mucosal damage. Both genetic and nongenetic factors are involved.

A. Genetic influences

1. Genetic factors are important in the pathogenesis of ulcers in some patients. Familial aggregation of peptic ulcer has been noted for nearly a century. A positive family history of ulcer is obtained in 5–15% of control subjects compared with 20–50% of patients with ulcers. Ulcer prevalence is two to three times greater in first-degree relatives of ulcer patients than in similar relatives of controls. The concordance for ulcers in monozygotic twins consistently exceeds that of dizygotic twins but is less than 100%. This indicates that an interaction between a genetic predisposition and an environmental agent occurs in twins with ulcers.

2. Effect of ABO antigens: People who secrete ABO antigens in saliva and gastric juice (secretors) are 40–50% less likely than nonsecretors to develop a DU, whereas the presence of blood group 0 is associated with a 30–40% increased incidence of DU. The relative risks of DU in nonsecretors and those with blood group 0 are 1.5 and 1.3, respectively. Individuals who are both nonsecretors and of blood group 0 have a relative risk of 2.5, suggesting that these risk factors are multiplicative rather than additive.

3. Effect of pepsinogens: Nearly 50% of patients with DU have high serum pepsinogen I levels. Individuals with this trait are five times more likely to develop DU than those without it. Since individuals with high serum pepsinogen I levels have high maximum gastric acid outputs, they have a pathophysiologic link between the pepsinogen level and peptic ulceration.

4. Inherited syndromes: Some inherited syndromes give rise to ulcers, including multiple endocrine neoplasia syndrome type 1, sporadic gastrinoma, and systemic mastocytosis.

5. Polygenic inheritance: Polygenic inheritance was believed to explain the genetics of ulcer disease. Recently the concept of genetic heterogeneity has been viewed as more consistent with the varying physiologic disturbances and clinical manifestations. This hypothesis holds that a disease is actually a group of disorders with both genetic and nongenetic etiologies, which by a variety of pathogenetic mechanisms result in a similar clinical expression. Thus DU is viewed not as one but as a host of disorders having in common a crater in the lining of the gastrointestinal tract. Thus, peptic ulcer patients with a strong family history of ulcer disease, high serum pepsinogen I levels, and high maximum acid secretory outputs may have a different basis for their ulcers than those with no apparent genetic predisposition.

B. Nongenetic factors

1. Cigarette smoking: Cigarette smokers have an increased incidence of ulcers, a high relapse rate, and relative resistance to therapy. Nicotine reduces gastric mucus secretion, pancreatic bicarbonate secretion, pyloric sphincter pressure, and duodenal mucosal bicarbonate secretion. Cigarette smoking reduces gastric mucosal prostaglandin synthesis and gastric mucosal blood flow.

2. Nonsteroidal anti-inflammatory drugs (NSAIDs): The use of NSAIDs is strongly linked to duodenal and gastric ulcers. People who use aspirin 4 or more days weekly for 3 months have an increased incidence of ulcers, and the daily use of aspirin to prevent myocardial infarction increases the prevalence of gastric ulcer sixfold. Aspirin injures the gastric mucosa in two ways. First, aspirin is directly toxic to surface mucosal cells at a pH of 3.5 or less. The injury fosters influx of H^+ into the cells, which sets in motion a cascade of events that severely damages the mucosa. Second, a systemic effect of aspirin and all other NSAIDs reduces gastric mucosal prostaglandin synthesis by inhibiting cyclooxygenase activity.

3. Role of psychological factors: There is no evidence that people in stressful jobs have more or fewer ulcers than do those in less stressful jobs. People with ulcers may encounter more stressors than those without ulcers, and they perceive stressful life events more negatively. As a group, they cope less well with stress and exhibit more personality disturbances. Contrary to common belief, ulcers are not more likely to occur in hard-driving individuals and no "ulcer personality" has been found. The mechanisms by which psychological factors might cause ulcers is unclear. Gastric acid hypersecretion and ulcers may occur during periods of severe emotional

stress; however, cause-and-effect relationships have not been clearly established.

4. Role of dietary factors: There is no evidence that diet causes ulcers. Beverages containing alcohol or caffeine, as well as decaffeinated colas, stimulate gastric acid secretion, but the ingestion of such beverages is unlikely to be ulcerogenic.

C. Factors affecting the gastroduodenal mucosa: The integrity of the gastroduodenal mucosa depends on achieving a balance between aggressive (acid, pepsin) and defensive forces (gastric mucosal barrier) operating at or in the mucosa. Peptic ulcers result from an imbalance between aggressive forces and factors responsible for maintaining mucosal defense (e.g., mucus and bicarbonate secretion, mucosal blood flow). Ulcers are caused by an increase in aggressive forces, a decrease in defensive forces, or both. Acid secretion in DU patients is increased or normal. Thus, excessive aggressive forces in the form of gastric acid are thought to be of great importance in DU.

D. Increased aggressive forces

1. There are geographical differences in the frequency of acid secretory or delivery defects. An increased parietal cell mass is found in 50% of DU patients in Scotland and Wales and in as few as 20% of DU patients in the United States.

2. Enhanced secretory drive due to high serum gastrin levels occurs in the Zollinger-Ellison syndrome, retained gastric antrum, and hyperfunction of antral G cells.

3. Increased vagal drive of acid secretion occurs in about 30% of DU patients. Approximately 25–60% of DU patients have parietal cells that are unusually sensitive to gastrin stimulation.

4. The frequency of accelerated gastric emptying and defects in the negative feedback inhibition of acid secretion are unknown.

5. Some physiologic defects may have a genetic basis (e.g., increased parietal cell mass, enhanced gastrin response to a protein meal, and rapid gastric emptying).

6. Other aggressive factors are pepsin, bile acids, pancreatic juice, and lysolecithin. Pepsin's proteolytic activity may be injurious to the mucosa, but such an effect is difficult to separate from that of acid. Persons with high serum pepsinogen levels also have increased gastric acid and pepsinogen secretion. Bile refluxed into the stomach may be injurious to the gastric mucosa. Ionized bile acids disrupt the mucosal barrier to hydrogen ions by dissolving membrane lipids; bile acids may also have other injurious effects on the gastric mucosal barrier.

E. Impaired mucosal defense: Gastroduodenal defense is a complex, dynamic, and integrated process involving several factors.

1. Mucus: The first line of defense is a layer of mucus which adheres to the surface epithelium. Mucus forms an unstirred water layer through which acid diffuses slowly. Within and beneath the mucous gel, hydrogen ions from the gastric lumen are neutralized by bicarbonate ions secreted from the epithelial cells. This process eliminates significant contact of acid with epithelial cells, thereby preventing back diffusion of acid into the cells.

2. Bicarbonate: Bicarbonate secretion by gastric and duodenal epithelia appears to be essential for mucosal protection. The most obvious role is in neutralizing hydrogen ions before they can damage the epithelia.

3. Prostaglandins: Prostaglandin-mediated mucosal defense involves several mechanisms and varies with the prostaglandin employed. Mucus and bicarbonate secretion are stimulated by E prostaglandins, which also stimulate or preserve cell restitution of a disrupted epithelial surface. Prostaglandins and some lipoxygenase products enhance gastric mucosal blood flow. Relative or absolute decreases in mucosal prostaglandin synthesis occur in some ulcer patients. The efficacy of exogenous prostaglandin E compounds (e.g., misoprostil) in healing ulcers provide only circumstantial evidence that mucosal prostaglandin deficiency is involved in the pathogenesis of peptic ulcers. Prostaglandins inhibit acid secretion at doses that heal ulcers; however, they are important in maintaining mucosal integrity and, therefore, play a role in ulcer disease.

4. Epithelial restitution: This process enhances defense by the rapid and continuous replacement of surface cells. The gastroduodenal mucosa turns over in 2–4 days. Epithelial restitution is underway constantly; it is not known if the rate of this process is disturbed in ulcer disease.

5. Mucosal blood flow: This is important for delivering oxygen and nutrients to the epithelium and for carrying away toxic metabolic products and back-diffused hydrogen ions.

6. *Helicobacter pylori*:

    a. *H. pylori* infection of the gastroduodenal mucosa may undermine mucosal defense and contribute to ulcer disease. *H. pylori* has only recently been cultured from the stomach of ulcer patients. It causes chronic gastritis, a condition that is present in most adults throughout the world. *H. pylori* infection has been increasingly implicated in the etiology of peptic ulcers.

    b. *H. pylori* is present in chronically inflamed mucosa in most patients with peptic ulcers, and the association is closer with DU than with gastric ulcers. The organism occupies a protected niche in mucus at the surface of mucosal epithelial cells. Virulence is enhanced by the ability of *H. pylori* to survive the acidic environment of the stomach. Tissue injury probably is induced by harmful enzymes released by *H. pylori*, including urease, lipases, and catalase. *H. pylori* infects metaplastic gastric mucosa that is found in the duodenum of nearly all patients with DU. Thus, the sequence of events appears to be gastric infection and induction of gastritis. Once gastric metaplasia develops in the duodenum, presumably in response to an increased acid load in patients prone to develop DU, the organism infects the metaplastic tissue, induces duodenitis, and fosters tissue breakdown and ulceration. This sequence is presently hypothetical, but it is likely that *H. pylori* is involved in the pathogenesis of ulcers in at least a subset of patients with duodenal ulcer disease.

IV. **Diagnosis**

A. History

   1. It is almost impossible to diagnose a DU on the basis of the patient's history.

B. Clinical signs and physical findings

   1. Epigastric pain: May be relieved by food or alkali. It occurs episodically and frequently during the night.

   2. In some patients, the pain is not relieved by food and may actually be increased by it.

3. Variable percentages of patients may have one or more of the following symptoms: anorexia, weight loss, nausea, vomiting, heartburn, fatty food intolerance, bloating, and belching.

4. DU may be asymptomatic in many patients. Bleeding ulcers may be asymptomatic and may be detected only by weakness, dizziness, postural syncope, and other symptoms indicating severe anemia or rapid blood loss.

5. Posterior perforation may be associated with a change in the pain pattern (back pain) and in some patients may cause pancreatitis. Free perforation produces a rapid onset of severe, diffuse abdominal pain.

6. Early satiety and postprandial vomiting suggest pyloric outlet obstruction.

7. Physical examination is not helpful unless the patient has anemia, evidence of gastrointestinal bleeding, or signs indicative of pyloric channel obstruction.

C. Diagnostic tests

   1. Routine laboratory studies are not helpful in making a specific diagnosis of DU disease.

   2. Radiologic studies (upper gastrointestinal series) are being largely replaced by gastrointestinal endoscopy, which is much more sensitive and specific. In addition, with endoscopy, lesions can be biopsied, cytologic specimens obtained, and superficial lesions detected much more easily than with x-ray studies.

V. **Differential Diagnosis**

The differential diagnosis includes a number of other acid-peptic disorders, including gastric ulcer, gastroesophageal reflux disease, nonulcer dyspepsia, gastric cancer, Crohn's disease, pancreatic diseases, and biliary tract disease.

VI. **Medical Treatment**

A. General measures: Prior to the advent of the H_2-receptor antagonists (H_2-RAs) in the mid-1970s, ulcer patients were treated with a combination of dietary restrictions and antacids. It is now recognized that such measures are not required. Patients have prompt relief from symptoms and experience ulcer healing without the implementation of dietary regimens which do not influence the healing process. The best dietary advice is to avoid foods that the patient knows will cause abdominal distress. Frequently this distress is related to nonspecific dyspepsia or gastroesophageal reflux completely and thus is unrelated to the peptic ulcer disease.

B. Drug treatment: Drugs heal ulcers by reducing gastric acid secretion, bolstering mucosal defense, or both.

1. Drugs that decrease acidity: Drugs inhibit acid secretion either by blocking receptors on parietal cells or by inhibiting intracellular processes of acid secretion. The basolateral surface of parietal cells contains receptors for the major physiologic stimulants of acid secretion: histamine, gastrin, and acetylcholine. Histamine activation of H_2 receptors results in formation of cyclic AMP. Cyclic AMP provides energy for the final step in acid secretion: activation of the proton pump, H^+/K^+ APTase, to exchange H^+ for K^+ at the luminal surface. Gastrin and cholinergic agents act through calcium-dependent mechanisms. Calcium-dependent kinases are activated, followed by increased activity of the proton pump, the H^+/K^+ ATPase. H_2 antagonists inhibit the cyclic AMP pathway, whereas antimuscarinic and antigastrin agents block calcium-mediated acid secretion. Prostaglandins inhibit acid secretion by blocking histamine-induced increases in cyclic AMP. Omeprazole, the most potent inhibitor of acid secretion, binds irreversibly to this proton pump, thereby preventing hydrogen ion secretion, the final common pathway for acid secretion. Antacids neutralize acid secreted into the gastric lumen.

2. H_2-RAs

a. Since the introduction of the first H_2-RA, cimetidine, three others—ranitidine, famotidine, and nizatidine—have become available in the United States. The H_2-RAs relieve ulcer symptoms, heal ulcers, and reduce their recurrence rate. Healing rates and the control of daytime and nocturnal pain are comparable with twice-daily and at-bedtime single-dose regimens. Symptoms typically improve within 5–7 days and disappear in most cases within 2–4 weeks. Symptoms typically disappear before the ulcer has completely healed.

b. The ideal duration of therapy is unknown. Treatment for 4–6 weeks is usually recommended because symptoms often have disappeared by then and most ulcers have healed. An additional 4–6 weeks of treatment is commonly recommended for elderly patients and those who continue to smoke cigarettes.

(1) Cimetidine

(a) Cimetidine efficacy is well established in DU and in preventing DU recurrence. Several dosage forms are used, including twice-daily or single at-bedtime doses. Although several side effects have been reported, it appears, from extensive studies, that cimetidine is a very safe drug, with a frequency of side effects below 5%. Gastrointestinal symptoms, particularly diarrhea, nausea, and vomiting are the most frequent adverse reactions. No increase in side effects was found in patients treated continuously for 4 years, and no different adverse reactions were found. The frequency of central nervous system (CNS) effects has been documented in hospitalized patients. There is no evidence that the incidence of CNS reactions is higher with cimetidine than with other H_2-RAs, and there have been no comparative studies.

(b) Gynecomastia and impotence have been reported rarely due to an antiandrogenic effect. Most of these occurrences have been reported in patients with Zollinger-Ellison syndrome treated with very high doses of cimetidine for prolonged periods. Drug interactions occur with cimetidine due to binding of the drug to the hepatic cytochrome P-450 microsomal enzyme system. Most drug interactions result in pharmacokinetic changes that have little clinical significance. Three drugs with narrow therapeutic indices that interact with cimetidine are phenytoin, theophylline, and warfarin. Patients taking these drugs should have appropriate monitoring for toxicity. Serum theophylline levels should be determined and prothrombin time ratios obtained, particularly when the dose is increased or another drug is added or deleted. Subsequent dosage adjustments can be made if necessary.

(2) Ranitidine: Twice-daily doses of 150 mg and an at-bedtime dose of 300 mg are effective in healing DU. A 150-mg at-bedtime dose significantly reduces the frequency of ulcer recurrence. Ranitidine is very safe; headache and dizziness are among the most frequent side effects. CNS reactions appear to be similar qualitatively to those reported with cimetidine. As with cimetidine, very rare idiosyncratic reactions have been reported, including fever, nephritis, various hematologic abnormalities, and hepatitis. Some drug interactions have been reported, but the mechanisms are obscure. Ranitidine binds weakly to the cytochrome P-450 system.

(3) Famotidine: This drug has a longer elimination half-life than cimetidine or ranitidine (2.5–3.5 vs. 2 hr), and its duration of antisecretory action is about 30% longer. Its efficacy is comparable to that of the other H_2-RAs. At the 20-mg at-bedtime dose, its efficacy is comparable to that of the other H_2-RAs in preventing ulcer recurrence. Relatively few side effects have been reported. Headache is the most frequent reaction, and mental confusion has been reported.

(4) Nizatidine: This agent has no known unique features. Its efficacy is similar to that of the other H_2-RAs. No comprehensive studies of its safety have been reported, but the drug appears to be safe based on efficacy trials. No drug-drug interactions have been documented.

(5) Proton pump inhibitors
  (a) Inhibition of the proton pump, a H^+/K^+ ATPase, profoundly reduces acid secretion. Omeprazole, the only proton pump inhibitor available, is a prodrug requiring acid for activation. Omeprazole diffuses from plasma into the parietal cells and then into the acid space of the secretory canaliculus. The compound then converts to the active agent, cationic sulfenamide, which covalently binds sulhydryl groups on the luminal surface of the proton pump. The irreversible reaction causes prolonged acid inhibition because new ATPase must be synthesized before acid secretion resumes.
  (b) Omeprazole in doses of 20 mg or more inhibits acid secretion in most patients. The 20-mg dose results in DU healing rates comparable to those produced by cimetidine, 600 mg twice daily, or ranitidine, 150 mg twice daily. The drug is highly effective in Zollinger-Ellison syndrome. The safety profile of omeprazole is evolving. The primary concern is with prolonged treatment because of the observation that lifelong treatment in rats produced gastric carcinoids. Gastric carcinoids occur in human patients in a setting of hypergastrinemia such as occurs in chronic atrophic gastritis and Zollinger-Ellison syndrome. The magnitude of hypergastrinemia in these conditions greatly exceeds that associated with omeprazole treatment in humans. No gastric carcinoids or other lesions have been described in humans treated chronically with omeprazole. Prolonged acid suppression theoretically fosters enteric infections, but these have not been described in patients treated with ome-

prazole. Omeprazole inhibits cytochrome P-450 enzymes, thereby influencing the disposition of drugs using this metabolic system; however, clinically significant drug interactions are uncommon.

    (c) Antacids: Despite the fact that nonabsorbable antacids have been used for decades in treating peptic ulcers, it is only recently that the efficacy of antacids in DU was established. A regimen of 1,007 mmol/liter daily in seven divided doses was designed to provide maximum buffering of gastric acid during the daytime. Diarrhea due to the magnesium-containing agents and constipation due to those containing aluminum are the most common side effects. The ease of administration, efficacy, and safety of the H_2-RAs have resulted in little utilization of antacids for DU therapy.

  3. Enhancement of mucosal defense

    a. Sucralfate: This sulfated disaccharide complex with aluminum hydroxide apparently heals ulcers by bolstering mucosal defense, although its precise mode of action is uncertain. The drug binds to the base of ulcers, presumably affording local protection against further acid-pepsin attack. The drug also forms complexes with pepsin, and the drug may stimulate prostaglandin synthesis. Sucralfate, 1 g four times daily, heals DU at a rate comparable to that of conventional doses of H_2-RAs. The drug reduces the frequency of ulcer recurrences when given in doses of 1 and 2 g daily. Sucralfate therapy is safe. Although some aluminum is absorbed from the compound, this is not known to be clinically significant. Constipation and large tablet size are annoying to some patients, particularly the elderly.

VII. Patient Monitoring and Prognosis

  A. Treating the initial ulcer

    1. The H_2-RAs are used most frequently as first-line treatment because of their well-established efficacy, safety, and convenience. For DU, a single nighttime-only dose should be used initially. If patients continue to have epigastric pain after 2 weeks, the dose should be divided and given twice daily. Treatment should be continued for 4–6 weeks in most patients; elderly patients with serious concomitant disease and those who continue to smoke cigarettes probably should be treated for 8 weeks.

    2. Sucralfate is also an excellent choice for first-line therapy. Antacids are inconvenient as they must be taken at least 4 times daily and large doses are frequently associated with gastrointestinal side effects.

    3. Omeprazole is an effective although relatively expensive choice for first-line DU therapy. It seems best to reserve this drug for patients with severe or recurrent ulcers.

  B. Treating recurrences

    1. The majority of patients will experience relapse within a year of healing of the initial ulcer. Patients should be told this and a strategy developed for dealing with the problem. Two strategies are available: intermittent or maintenance therapy. Maintenance therapy with half doses of H_2-RAs taken at bedtime is appropriate for patients with aggressive ulcer disease. These include patients with more than two recurrences per year, those who have suffered a significant hemorrhage, and those with serious underlying diseases. Such conditions as pulmonary insufficiency, heart failure, and cirrhosis increase the mortality if surgery must be performed to deal with a complicated ulcer recurrence. The elderly often are candidates for maintenance therapy because of their concomitant illnesses, as are patients who will not discontinue cigarette smoking. Intermittent therapy is appropriate for patients who have infrequent ulcer recurrences and no identifiable risk factors, such as cigarette smoking.

    2. Maintenance therapy reduces the frequency of recurrences to about 25% per year. The duration of maintenance therapy is unknown, but it should be continued for at least 2 years if the beneficial effects are to be realized. In some patients, particularly the elderly with concomitant illnesses, maintenance should be continued for life.

C. Resistant ulcers. Resistant ulcers have been defined as those that fail to heal on therapy for 8 weeks. Less than 10% of ulcers are resistant by this criterion. The reasons for failure to heal vary. Some patients are non-compilant with therapy. Others have unusually high acid secretory rates, and a few are relatively resistant to H_2-RAs. Patients who continue to smoke are more likely to have resistant ulcers. Large ulcers heal at the same rate as small ulcers. Because they are large, however, a longer period of treatment is required for complete healing. Thus, a higher percentage of large ulcers are more likely to be unhealed at a given time—8 weeks, for example. Most resistant ulcers can be managed by treatment with the same agent for an additional period of time, typically 1 month. Increasing the dose of an H_2-RA is effective in some cases but may be less effective than switching to another therapeutic class. Omeprazole is effective in many resistant ulcers, although twice the usual daily dose may be necessary. Antibiotic treatment intended to eradicate *H. pylori* has also been associated with healing of some resistant ulcers. Two weeks of therapy with a combination of bismuth subsalicylate plus two antibiotics is the most effective regimen for eradicating *H. pylori*.

D. Bleeding ulcers: Management of acute upper gastrointestinal hemorrhage due to ulcers should be directed at resuscitation rather than ulcer healing. Up to 85% of lesions stop bleeding spontaneously. The minority of patients with rapid, ongoing hemorrhage should undergo diagnostic and therapeutic endoscopy. If active bleeding is present, it should be treated by intervention with some modality of therapeutic endoscopy such as the heater probe. If bleeding has stopped but a visible vessel is seen in the ulcer base, it too should be treated with thermal intervention because the risk of rebleeding in such patients is increased.

E. Surgical treatment: The frequency of surgical operations for peptic ulcer disease has decreased dramatically in the past two decades. The decline antedated the availability of H_2-RAs. The indications for surgery are uncontrollable hemorrhage, perforation, and gastric outlet obstruction. Intractability, the most frequent indication for surgery a decade ago, is rarely an indication now. Such patients are generally managed successfully with current medical treatment. The surgical procedures result in a reduction of the acid-producing capacity by the stomach. The frequency of complications is proportional to the amount of tissue removed. For example, a subtotal gastrectomy is followed by the highest incidence of complications such as diarrhea, weight loss, and the "dumping syndrome." The rate of ulcer recurrence is, however, less than 5%. A vagotomy and pyloroplasty has a low frequency of surgical complications but a recurrence rate similar to that of patients treated continuously with an H_2-RA. An antrectomy and vagotomy is a reasonable compromise between these extreme operations and has a low frequency of side effects and recurrences. A superselective vagotomy (parietal cell vagotomy, partial gastric vagotomy) results in denervation of the corpus of the stomach containing parietal cells, while vagal fibers innervating the distal stomach and profoundly influencing gastric emptying are retained. The ulcer recurrence rate may be as high as 20% in 5 years, depending on the skill of the surgeon in performing the parietal cell vagotomy.

Bibliography

Feldman M, Burton ME. Histamine$_2$-receptor antagonists: Standard therapy for acid-peptic diseases. *N Engl J Med* 323:1749–1755, 1990.

Freston JW. Mechanisms of relapse in peptic ulcer disease. *J Clin Gastroenterol* 11(Suppl 1):534–538, 1989.

Kurata JH, Corboy ED. Current peptic ulcer time trends: An epidemiological profile. *J Clin Gastroenterol* 10(3):259–268, 1988.

Maton PN. Omeprazole. *N Engl J Med* 324:965–975, 1991.

Penston JG, Wormsley KG. Review article: Maintenance treatment with H_2-receptor antagonists for peptic ulcer disease. *Aliment Pharmacol Ther* 6:3–29, 1992.

Peterson WL. *Hellcobacter pylori* and peptic ulcer disease. *N Engl J Med* 324:1043–1048, 1991.

Soil AH. Pathogenesis of peptic ulcer disease and implications for therapy. *N Engl J Med* 322:909–916, 1990.

Celiac Disease

John Schaffner, M.D.

I. **Definition**

Celiac disease, also known as *celiac sprue*, *nontropical sprue*, and *gluten-sensitive enteropathy*, can be defined as a small intestinal disorder with characteristic mucosal changes that results in malabsorption of nutrients and improvement following gluten withdrawal.

II. **Etiology**

The etiology is unknown. The disease affects both children and adults.

A. There is no certain explanation for the time of onset of the disease.

B. Intestinal adenovirus protein could be a trigger.

   1. There is a similar gene sequence among gliadin, an alcohol extract of gluten, and adenovirus 12.
   2. Eighty-nine percent of untreated celiacs have neutralizing antibody to adenovirus 12 versus 17% of controls.

III. **Pathophysiology**

The pathogenesis of celiac disease is unknown. The disease results from the ingestion of gluten, a water-insoluble protein fraction of certain grains, notably wheat, rye, oats, and barley. By means of unknown mechanisms, the gluten interacts with the small intestinal mucosa, resulting in loss of the villus surface. Different hypotheses have been proposed to explain the disease.

A. Immune and genetic theory

   1. Definite genetic component, but the exact role is uncertain.
   2. High incidence of human leukocyte antigen (HLA)-B8, HLA-DR3, and HLA-DQw2.
   3. Strong association with dermatitis herpetiformis.
   4. B-cell alloantigens and Gm allotype markers on the IgG heavy chain are also found with higher frequency in celiac patients.
   5. Anti-gliadin and anti-reticulin antibodies found with higher frequency in celiacs.

B. Enzyme deficiency

   1. No definitive evidence.
   2. Some peptidase levels are reduced in active disease but return to normal with gluten withdrawal.

C. Lectin hypothesis

   1. No definitive evidence.
   2. Some plant lectins do damage surface epithelium; no link to gliadin established.

IV. Diagnosis

    A. History: There is great variation in the presentation of patients with celiac disease.

       1. Gastrointestinal symptoms

          a. Diarrhea and steatorrhea.

          b. Weight loss and flatulence.

       2. Extraintestinal symptoms related to malabsorption.

          a. Vitamin deficiencies: A, B complex, B_{12}, D, K, folate, pyridoxine.

             (1) Dermatitis, osteopenia, hypoprothrombinemia, anemia, ecchymoses, neuropathy.

          b. Mineral deficiencies: iron, calcium, magnesium, hypokalemia.

             (1) Anemia, osteopenia, tetany.

          c. Symptoms related to vitamin or mineral deficiency may be the only manifestation of disease.

          d. Approximately 5% of celiacs have diabetes mellitus.

          e. Dermatitis herpetiformis is more common in celiacs.

    B. Clinical signs and physical findings

       1. General findings may vary considerably, depending upon the severity and duration of disease.

          a. Emaciation and signs of weight loss.

          b. Clubbing in severe cases.

          c. Peripheral edema secondary to hypoalbuminemia.

       2. Findings related to specific deficiencies

          a. Pallor secondary to anemia, which may be iron, folate, or vitamin B_{12} deficiency.

          b. Cheilosis and glossitis.

          c. Hperkeratosis follicularis secondary to vitamin A deficiency.

          d. Chvostek or Trousseau's signs due to hypocalcemia.

          e. Findings of peripheral neuropathy.

    C. Diagnostic tests

       1. Stool examination demonstrates excessive fat.

          a. Qualitative or quantitative exam.

          b. C14 triolein breath test will also detect steatorrhea.

       2. Hematologic tests

          a. Anemia may be microcytic or macrocytic.

          b. Howell-Jolly bodies may be present secondary to functional hyposplenism.

          c. Hypoprothrombinemia.

       3. Biochemical tests

          a. Diarrhea may cause altered electrolyte levels.

          b. Calcium, magnesium, and zinc levels may be low.

          c. Serum albumin level may be reduced.

          d. Cholesterol may be reduced.

       4. Immunologic tests

          a. Anti-gliadin antibody is present in over 90% of celiacs.

          b. Anti-reticulin antibody is present in 75% of celiacs.

          c. Anti-endomysial antibodies are present in 70% of celiacs.

          d. In other gut disorders, these antibodies may be present much less frequently.

       5. Oral tolerance tests

          a. Xylose is the most commonly used screening test to determine the small intestinal cause of steatorrhea.

          b. Lactose intolerance is common among active celiacs but is not useful in diagnosis.

       6. Radiologic evaluation

          a. Small bowel x-ray may show dilation and a distorted mucosal pattern.

          b. Excessive fluid is often present in the small intestine.

          c. The small bowel study may be normal.

       7. Endoscopic evaluation

          a. There is an abnormal-appearing duodenum in some patients.

          b. In other patients, the duodenum may be normal.

       8. The key to the diagnosis of celiac disease is a small bowel biopsy. The biopsy is not pathognomonic for celiac disease, but the loss of normal villus architecture is needed for the diagnosis. Because of the lifelong therapy required for the disorder, the diagnosis should not be made without histologic confirmation.

          a. Repeat biopsy after therapy is advocated by some to ensure a response to the diet.

          b. In the past, a third biopsy after gluten challenge was recommended for confirmation.

V. Differential Diagnosis

    A. Celiac disease is included in the differential diagnosis of steatorrhea. Steatorrhea can be caused by numerous diseases that can be divided into three categories:

       1. Abnormal intraluminal digestion

          a. Pancreatic insufficiency

b. Cholestasis
c. Bacterial overgrowth
d. Loss of bile salts
2. Abnormal mucosal absorptive surface
   a. Celiac disease
   b. Tropical sprue
   c. Parasitic infection
   d. Lymphoma, Whipple's disease
   e. Eosinophilic gastroenteritis
   f. Zollinger-Ellison syndrome
   g. Viral gastroenteritis
   h. Hypogammaglobulinemia
3. Inadequate absorptive surface
   a. Short bowel syndrome
B. Celiac disease may also be part of the differential diagnosis of isolated vitamin or mineral deficiencies, as well as of general signs such as growth failure or weight loss.

VI. Treatment

The treatment of celiac sprue consists of complete withdrawal of gluten from the diet. This includes all wheat, rye, barley, and oat products, as well as foods derived from them. Gluten-containing products may be included as thickeners or fillers. Many processed foods have gluten-containing ingredients. In addition, alcohols derived from the fermentation of grains are not tolerated by celiacs.

A. The response to gluten withdrawal is usually prompt.
   1. Clinical improvement is often seen within 1 week.
   2. Biochemical improvement may also be rapid.
   3. Histologic improvement may not be complete, particularly in adults.
B. Reasons for failure to respond to the diet
   1. Incomplete removal of gluten from the diet (most common)
   2. Wrong diagnosis
   3. Lymphoma
   4. Refractory sprue
C. Supplemental therapy
   1. Patients found deficient in any substance should be replenished until their health is restored.

2. Steroids may be used for refractory sprue.

VII. Patient Monitoring

No standards are available for monitoring patients with celiac disease. Follow-up for symptoms is adequate for most patients. Standard medical care with a yearly blood count and blood chemistries is adequate for the well patient. Patients who have recurrent symptoms should have their diet reviewed. Repeat biopsy may be necessary for recurrent symptoms.

VIII. Prognosis

The vast majority of patients with celiac disease who maintain a gluten-free diet will have a normal life span. The complications of the disease are poorly understood. Potential complications, particularly lymphoma, may be preventable by strict dietary adherence.

A. Lymphoma of the small intestine occurs with greater frequency in celiac patients.
   1. It occurs in a small percentage of these patients.
   2. Recent evidence shows that adherence to a gluten-free diet for >5 years reduces the risk of lymphoma to that of the normal population.
B. Refractory sprue is a rare occurrence in which the patients no longer responds to a gluten-free diet alone.
   1. Some patients may respond to immunosuppressive therapy.
   2. A different disease entity may be present.

Bibliography

Classic reviews
Cole SG, Kagnoff MF. Celiac disease. *Ann Rev Nutr* 5:241–266, 1985.
Stokes PL, Ferguson R, Holmes GKT, et al: Familial aspects of coeliac disease. *QJ Med* 45:567–582, 1976.

Recent citations
Kagnoff MF. Understanding the molecular basis of coeliac disease. *Gut* 31:497–499, 1990.
Logan RF, Rifkind EA, Turner ID, et al. Mortality in celiac disease. *Gastroenterology* 97:265–271, 1989.

Chapter 58-B

Infectious Diarrhea

Michael D. Brown, M.D.

I. Definition

Diarrhea secondary to infectious organisms is one of the leading causes of worldwide morbidity and mortality. Adults living in the United States can expect 1.5 episodes of infectious diarrhea per year. These are typically viral in etiology and are life-threatening only in the elderly and the very young. In the Third World, however, children suffer five to six episodes of infectious diarrhea per year and the condition remains the leading cause of childhood mortality, resulting in 12,600 deaths per day. Because of the viral etiology of most diarrheas in the United States, winter is the most likely time of year for infections to occur. Most bacterial diarrheas can occur year round.

II. Pathophysiology

Infectious diarrheas are divided into two categories based on the mechanism of bowel injury.

A. Toxigenic diarrheas

Diarrheas caused by toxins (e.g., cholera toxin) are typically large in volume, watery, and nonbloody. The cytotoxins alter the absorptive capacity of the villi in the upper small bowel, and the excess volume exceeds the colon's absorptive capability. There is no invasion, and therefore there are no white blood cells in the stool. Volume loss can be life-threatening. The organisms adhere to the bowel but do not invade.

B. Invasive diarrheas

These diarrheas are usually colon-based infections caused by organisms which penetrate the mucosa and disrupt the absorptive surface via ulceration (e.g., *Shigella*). Diarrhea may be secondary to enterotoxin production, reactive inflammatory responses in the lamina propria, or disruption of the luminal surface, with a resultant decrease in absorption and an increase in exudation. Fecal leukocytes are a hallmark of invasive diarrheas, which are typically bloody. Diarrheal volumes tend to be less than those seen in toxigenic diarrheas.

III. Etiology

A general diagnostic approach to infectious diarrhea is shown in Figure 58B-1.

A. Viral

1. Rotavirus: An RNA virus causing secretory diarrhea in children. It spreads via fecal-oral contamination and is frequent in children in day-care settings. Infection leads to flattening of the villi of the small bowel and a decrease in absorptive capability. Stool

Table 58B-1.   Clinical Features of Diarrhea

Site of Infection	Small Bowel	Large Bowel
Organisms	*Vibrios*, ETEC, rotavirus, Norwalk agent, *Staph. aureus, B. cerus, Aeromonas, Plesiomonas, Giradia,*	*Campylobacter, Shigella,* EIEC, EHEC, *Entamoeba histolytica*
Location of pain	Midabdomen	Lower abdomen, rectum
Volume of stool	Large	Small
Type of stool	Watery	Exudative, bloody, mucoid
Blood in stool	Rare	Common
White blood cells in stool	Rare	Common (except amoeba)
Flexible sigmoidoscopy	Normal	Ulcers, friability, granularity, hemorrhage

Source: Sleisenger MH, Fordtran JS (eds). *Gastrointestinal Disease,* ed. 5. Phildelphia, Saunders, 1993, p 1154.

detection is usually unnecessary but can be achieved with radioimmunoassay. Therapy consists of volume repletion.

2. Norwalk agent: A DNA virus that is a common vector of viral diarrhea in adults. Infections are usually accompanied by a typical viral prodrome and a marked watery diarrhea. The upper small bowel is affected, with flattening of the villi and decreased absorptive capability. Transmission is fecal-oral. Detection of the virus in stool is not necessary for therapy, although a radioimmunoassay is available. Therapy is aimed at rehydration.

3. Miscellaneous viral agents: Adenoviruses, calicivirus, echovirus, and coxsackievirus have been associated epidemiologically with diarrheal outbreaks. Cytomegalovirus and herpesvirus are associated with diarrhea in immunocompromised patients.

B. Bacterial (endotoxin-producing and invasive)

1. *Vibrio cholera:* The prototypical toxigenic diarrhea. The organism is a gram-negative, short, curved rod. It secretes a toxin which increases adenylate cyclase activity in the upper small bowel mucosa. This results in increased cellular levels of cyclic adenosine monophosphate. Both a decrease in absorption and an increase in secretion occur. Diarrheas can approach 20 liters/day. In addition to diarrhea, vomiting, abdominal pain, and distention are common. Cholera is mainly a problem of Third World countries, where it is spread by water and food contamination and occurs after ingestion of a large inoculum. This problem occurs particularly after natural disasters. Human-to-human

transmission can also occur, and there is a 5% carrier rate. Therapy is aimed at aggressive volume support, with antibiotics (tetracycline) and public health measures used to ensure contaminate-free water and food sources. Mortality rates can be as low as 1% with this therapy.

2. *Vibrio parahaemolyticus:* A common etiologic agent in diarrheas associated with the ingestion of seafood, particularly shellfish. It occurs mostly in Asia and Australia and in coastal areas of the United States. The various strains produce a wide variety of enterotoxins. Diarrhea is moderate in volume and rarely hemorrhagic. The diarrhea usually lasts for 24 to 48 hr. Patients may also complain of nausea, vomiting, abdominal cramping, and headaches. Therapy is usually symptomatic, and antibiotics are rarely indicated. Mortality is unusual.

3. *Aeromonas:* The *Aeromonas* species contain some pathogenic strains, which result in a watery, enterotoxin-mediated diarrhea. Symptoms may also include nausea, vomiting, and crampy abdominal pain. Most patients give a history of ingestion of untreated well or spring water. A recent study of men in a Veterans Administration hospital revealed *Aeromonas* species as the most frequently recovered fecal pathogen. The actual incidence of this organism in both acute and chronic diarrhea is unknown, but it may be very common. Diagnosis is made with stool cultures, but growth requires a specific oxidase medium.

4. *Escherichia coli:* A few of subtypes of this

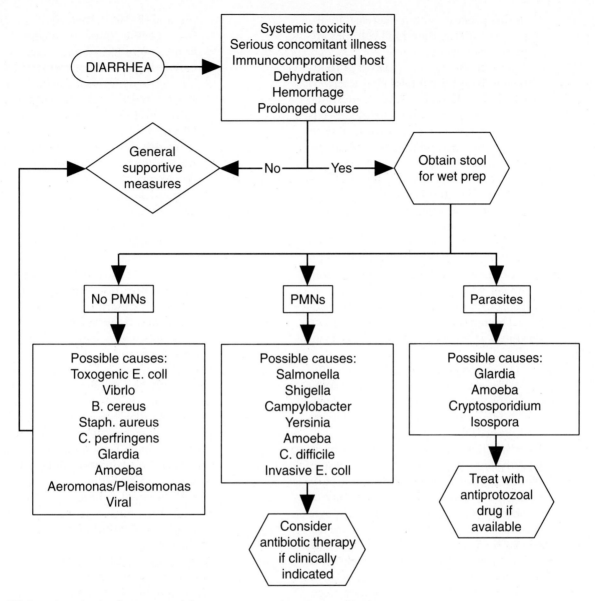

Figure 58B-1. Algorithm for diagnostic and therapeutic options for infectious diarrhea.

typical gut commensal are pathogenic. They may lead to diarrhea via toxigenic, invasive, or adherent mechanisms.

a. Enteropathogenic *E. coli* (EPEC): Associated with outbreaks of diarrhea in neonates. Pathogenicity is related to both adherence to epithelial cells and toxin production.

b. Enterotoxigenic *E. coli* (ETEC): Secondary to ingestion of contaminated foodstuffs or water. All pathogenicity is related to two toxins (heat labile and heat stable) produced in the upper small bowel. No structural damage to the epithelium is seen. The presentation is typically with watery diarrhea, which can be voluminous or minimal. This organism is one of the most frequent causes of travelers' diarrhea.

c. Enteroadherent *E. coli* (EAEC): Causative organism in a diarrhea seen in neonates and travelers. Pathogenicity appears to be secondary to the ability of the organism to form an adherent layer overlying the small bowel mucosa. The enterocyte villus is damaged in this process, with a decrease in absorptive ability. Diarrheal volumes are not excessive.

d. Enteroinvasive *E. coli* (EIEC): A foodborne dysenteric illness characterized by bloody diarrhea, fever, tenesmus, abdominal pain, and white blood cells in the stool. The organism is able to invade the mucosa and secrete an enterotoxin.

e. Enterohemorrhagic *E. coli* (EHEC): Caused by the best-known of the pathogenic *E. coli* subtypes, 0157:H7. It is responsible for outbreaks of hemolytic-uremic syndrome in children and hemorrhagic diarrhea in two episodes related to hamburger ingestion. Bowel wall inflammation can be severe, with marked lower gastrointestinal hemorrhage and even perforation. Injury is secondary to a potent cytotoxin.

(1) Diagnosis is difficult due to the general lack of appropriate typing procedures in most hospitals. Samples must be sent to regional reference laboratories.

5. *Shigella:* Characterized by the classic bacillary dysentery picture of low volume, bloody diarrhea, fever, abdominal pain, rectal pain, and leukocytosis. It may be associated with arthritis (Reiter's syndrome). Four different species are responsible: *S. dysenteriae, S. boydii, S. sonnei,* and *S. flexneri.* Pathogenicity is related to invasion of the colonic mucosa, with ulceration, exudation, and hemorrhage. Despite this penetration, bacteremia is rare. An endotoxin-mediated injury also occurs, and may cause a watery diarrhea and enhance cell death after invasion. *Shigella* is transmitted via the fecal-oral route and requires relatively low numbers of organisms for infectivity. Diagnosis is made by stool culture.

6. *Salmonella*

a. Nontyphoidal salmonellosis: *S. enteritidis* consists of nearly 2,000 subspecies. They can present with either a bloody or nonbloody diarrhea. The organisms appear to cause injury by invasion of the large or small bowel mucosa. There are five clinical pictures associated with *S. enteritidis:* gastroenteritis (75%), ty-

phoidal (5–10%), bacteremia (5–10%), site specific (5%; involving bones, joints, meninges, bone marrow, and gallbladder), and a carrier state (<1%). The gastroenteritis is associated with a self-limited, bloody diarrhea that resolves in 4–5 days. Bloody stool with leukocytes is usual, but a nonbloody secretory diarrhea can be seen. Diagnosis is made by stool culture. Longer, more serious courses are seen with salmonella colitis. Patients with sickle cell disease, acquired immunodeficiency syndrome, malignancy, achlorhydria, and ulcerative colitis are at increased risk of salmonellosis. The organism requires a fairly large inoculum for infection. The mode of transmission is described as "food, flies, fomites, and fingers" (the four Fs). Dairy products, eggs, and chickens are the most common food vectors.

7. *Campylobacter jejuni:* The most common form of bacterial diarrhea in the United States. The clinical picture is typically that of a watery diarrhea, although one-half of patients may have bloody diarrhea and 90% may have fecal leukocytes. Patients may also complain of myalgia, arthralgia, nausea, and vomiting. The colon is the site of mucosal invasion. The disease is usually transmitted from contaminated poultry. Stool culture is the best method of diagnosis.

8. *Bacillus cerus:* Characterized by a syndrome of nausea and vomiting or diarrhea mediated by an endotoxin. It is associated with ingestion of Chinese foods. It isd a cause of "food poisoning," as the toxin is produced in the food prior to ingestion. There is essentially no incubation period; symptoms occur within minutes to hours after ingestion of contaminated food. The syndrome is self-limited, as the toxin clears the gastrointestinal tract. The organism cannot be diagnosed with stool culture.

9. *Staphylococcus aureus:* Similar to *B. cerus* in clinical picture and pathogenesis. A preformed toxin in food leads to a secretory diarrhea, without evidence of invasion. The small bowel is the site of injury.

10. *Yersinia:* Seventy percent of patients present with an enterocolitis induced by

consumption of contaminated water or food. This organism can cause a syndrome reminiscent of Crohn's ileitis. The injury is mediated by both an enterotoxin and the invasiveness of the organism. Diarrhea can therefore be either bloody or watery. Diagnosis is made by culture on a specific oxidase medium. Bacteremia with seeding of distant organs can occur in immunocompromised patients.

C. Protozoal

1. Amebiasis: The dysentery secondary to amebiasis may be a mild, watery diarrhea or a fulminant, invasive, and occasionally fatal process. Symptoms include tenesmus, abdominal cramping, bloody diarrhea, fever, and orthostasis. Laboratory testing reveals a mild to moderate leukocytosis, mild anemia, and evidence of volume depletion. Ulcerations may be deep enough to cause colonic perforation. Endoscopic exam may demonstrate "volcano" ulcers which are raised, discrete, erythematous lesions. Unusual intestinal manifestations include amebomas (firm nodules filled with trophozoites and necrotic tissue) and strictures. Extraintestinal manifestations include liver abscesses (occurring in association with colitis in only 20%) and cutaneous amebiasis. Diagnosis is based on the finding of trophozoites in a wet preparation of stool. The sample must be examined within 2 hr of recovery, as the trophozoites autolyze quickly. Evidence of erythrophagocytosis confers pathogenicity. Serologic tests are particularly helpful in patients from nonendemic areas. Indirect hemagglutination and indirect immunofluorescence are reported to be 95% sensitive, with a high negative predictive value.

2. *Giardia:* The most common protozoal cause of diarrhea in the United States. The organism is consumed in contaminated water or foodstuffs. High attack rates are reported in the western United States and parts of the former Soviet Union. The organism appears to cause diarrhea by coating the small bowel mucosa, enhancing mucus secretion, mucosal invasion, competition for host nutrients, and altered gut motility. The infections appear more frequently and are more severe in patients with dysgammaglobulinemias. Patients complain of chronic, persistent, or intermittent diarrhea. The symptoms may be very similar to those of irritable bowel syndrome. The diarrhea may be accompanied by nausea, vomiting, and abdominal pain. The physical exam and laboratory tests are nonspecific, and stools do not contain white blood cells. Diagnosis is made with small bowel mucosal biopsy, duodenal aspirate, or stool exam for trophozoites. The stool exam is the easiest to obtain but is positive in only 50%. An enzyme-linked immunosorbent assay of the stool for trophozoite fragments is becoming more widely available and greatly exceeds the sensitivity of the stool exam.

3. Cryptosporidia and microsporidia: Clinically important in the immunocompromised (see Chapter 58C).

IV. Treatment

General measures: The vast majority of infectious diarrheas require only supportive measures for treatment. This includes intravenous or oral hydration and temporary avoidance of oral intake, particularly lactose-containing foods. Antidiarrheals should be used only in those without fecal leukocytes. Inhibition of colonic motility in patients with severe inflammation can lead to toxic dilatation. Antibiotics are reserved for those who are immunocompromised, toxic, or suffering a complicating concomitant illness. Doxycycline, trimethoprim-sulfamethoxazole, and ciprofloxacin are effective in almost all bacterial infections. Metronidazole is effective in amebiasis and giardiasis.

Bibliography

Cheney CP, Wong RK. Acute infectious diarrhea. *Med Clin North Am* 77:1169–1196, 1993.

Gorbach SL. Infectious diarrhea and bacterial food poisoning, in Sleisenger MH, Fordtran JS (eds): *Gastrointestinal Disease,* ed 5. Philadelphia, Saunders, 1993 p 1128–1173.

Gurrant RL, Bobak DA. Medical progress: Bacterial and protozoal gastroenteritis. *N Engl J Med* 325:327–340, 1991.

Holmberg SD, Schell WL, et al: *Aeromonas* intestinal infections in the United States. *Ann Intern Med* 105:683–689, 1986.

Owen RL. Parasitic diseases, in Sleisenger MH, Fordtran JS (eds): *Gastrointestinal Disease,* ed 5. Philadelphia, Saunders, 1993 p 1190–1222.

CHAPTER 58-C

AIDS and the Gastrointestinal Tract

Michael D. Brown, M.D.

I. **Definition**

The gastrointestinal (GI) tract is frequently involved in AIDS patients. The disorders are typically infectious or neoplastic and reflect the deficit in immune surveillance. Symptoms are typically distressing and include diarrhea, incontinence, hematochezia, hematemesis, nausea and vomiting, weight loss/wasting, odynophagia, dysphagia, and abdominal pain. In general, GI tract disorders associated with AIDS are difficult to treat and have a high recurrence rate. They often herald a rapidly progressive downhill course in the disease.

II. **The Oral Cavity**

A. Signs and symptoms

Odynophagia is the main presenting complaint. Dysgeusia may be a problem as well. Bleeding is unusual.

B. Etiologies

1. Oral candidiasis: This is secondary to invasive oral candidal infections. It is the most commonly found GI tract lesion. It presents as an adherent white plaque which demonstrates pseudohyphal and yeast forms on histologic exam. The most frequent complaint is odynophagia. When it is associated with dysphagia, the esophagus is also involved in >85%. Therapy should be initiated with fluconazole (200 mg on day 1 followed by 100 mg/day for 21 days) and followed by amphotericin B if the patient is unresponsive. Ketoconazole should be avoided, as it requires an acid environment for conversion to an absorbable compound and many AIDS patients are hypo- or achlohydric.

2. Oral hairy leukoplakia: This oral lesion is characterized by a grayish-white membrane with a rough or hairy surface. Histologically, it appears as an epithelial cell hyperplasia with small keratin projections, giving the lesion a rough appearance. It is associated with human papilomavirus and Epstein-Barr virus.

3. Herpes simplex virus (HSV) and cytomegalovirus (CMV): HSV is often a coinfection with *Candida*. Typical lesions of both HSV and CMV oral infectionsw are small groups of painful vesicles or discrete ulcerations. Odynophagia and dysphagia

can be very severe. Therapy includes acyclovir for HSV, ganciclovir for CMV, and topical anesthetics for both.

C. Neoplastic diseases

Kaposi's sarcoma and lymphoma: Rarely, the oral mucosa may be involved by these tumors. The lesions of Kaposi's sarcoma can be found in the oral cavity in 5–10% of patients with skin lesions.

III. The Esophagus

A. Signs and symptoms: dysphagia, odynophagia and chest pain are the most common presenting complaints. Regurgitation and heartburn may also occur.

B. Etiologies

1. Candidiasis: The lesions are similar to those seen in the oral cavity. This disease occurs in ≤50% of AIDS patients (less frequently in homosexuals) at some point and is a common presenting infection. Upper GI radiographs may demonstrate a shaggy mucosa. Endoscopy is the best exam for diagnosis, as it allows for brush cytology and biopsy, which will demonstrate pseudohyphae. Bleeding is a rare complication but can be clinically significant. It is often associated with a herpes coinfection in ~50%. When herpetic vesicles rupture, *Candida* may invade the denuded mucosa. Initial therapy with fluconazole is effective in most cases. Patients who do not respond may require amphotericin B.

2. HSV: This infection creates a diffuse ulcerative process characterized by severe odynophagia. Bleeding from coalesced ulcers may be marked. Vesicles are rarely seen, as the disorder is typically diagnosed late in its course. Diagnosis can be made with endoscopic biopsy of the ulcer rim and histologic examination or epithelial cells for nuclear inclusions. Multinucleated giant cells may also be seen and are characteristic. HSV I and II are seen in AIDS patients. Acyclovir is the drug of choice.

3. CMV: This is a less common esophageal pathogen than HSV. Typically, it presents with odynophagia and dysphagia. Endoscopically, it is seen as a distal esophagitis or a single large, deep, linear ulcer. It is diagnosed via endoscopic biopsy when cytoplasmic inclusions are seen in stromal or vascular endothelial cells. Treatment with ganciclovir is the only widely available therapy; the response is incomplete at best. Treatment with the investigational drug foscarnet, a pyrophosphate analogue, appears to offer a slightly better clinical response.

4. Miscellaneous infections: *Mycobacterium avium-intracellulare* (MAI) can involve the esophagus but is typically asymptomatic. *Pneumocystis* has also been found in the esophageal mucosa, but its clinical significance is unclear.

IV. The Stomach

A. Signs and symptoms: Early satiety, abdominal pain, nausea, vomiting, and hematemesis are typical presenting complaints of AIDS patients with gastric disorders. Patients may show evidence of epigastric tenderness and occasionally gastric outlet obstruction, with abdominal distention and a succussion splash.

B. Etiologies

CMV presents as abdominal pain, nausea/vomiting, and/or bleeding. It is characterized by punctate erosions and ulcerations, thickened mucosal folds, and diminished gastric distensibility during endoscopy or air-contrast studies. Diagnosis is made with endoscopic biopsy and the demonstration of typical intracytoplasmic inclusions. The endoscopic findings include gastritis, gastric outlet obstruction, and focal ulceration with bleeding. The response to ganciclovir is poor.

C. *Cryptosporidium* can present with a distal gastritis or outlet obstruction. Diagnosis is made by endoscopic biopsy. There is no commercially available therapy; however, spiramycin is variably reported as effective. Balloon dilatation of the gastric outlet may be helpful in selected cases.

D. *Mycobacterium tuberculosis* can present with either a diffuse nodular, ulcerative, or ulceronodular gastric process. MAI may also be present in the gastric mucosa. Therapy includes standard antituberculosis mediations, typically triple therapy with isoniazid, pyrazinamide, and rifampin. MAI is poorly responsive to most antituberculosis medications.

V. The Small Intestine

A. Sign and symptoms: Diarrhea is a common symptom in AIDS. It is present at diagnosis in 30% of patients and occurs at some time in 80%. Its onset is associated with a progressive wasting syndrome and a marked drop in the

Table 58C-1. Approach to AIDS Patients with Diarrhea

1. Stool volume measurement, stool examination for white blood cells and acid-fast bacilli.
2. Stool culture for enteric pathogens such as *Salmonella, Shigella, Campylobacter,* and *Yersinia.* Viral cultures for HSV and CMV may also be obtained.
3. Stool for ova and parasites such as *Cryptosporidium, Amoeba,* and *Giardia.*
4. Flexible sigmoidoscopy with biopsy* and stool aspirate for *Amoeba.*
5. Upper endoscopy with duodenal aspirate for *Giardia* and small bowel biopsy.*

*Colonic and duodenal biopsy specimen should be examined for histopathologic changes, acid-fast bacilli, viral inclusions, and parasites. Electron microscopy may be necessary for microsporidia.

patient's activity level. The malnutrition associated with the diarrhea further compromises the immune system, with a rapid downhill course.

B. Evaluation of diarrhea in AIDS patients: The need for aggressive evaluation of diarrhea in these patients is controversial; however, upon initial presentation, a through workup is reasonable. Table 58C-1 lists the appropriate tests.

C. Etiologies
1. Altered gut immunosurveillance systems: Patients with AIDS have reduced numbers of IgA-producing plasma cells in the gut mucosa. Other changes in the gut wall which enhance infectious complications include a breakdown in the gut-associated lymphoid tissue (GALT) and loss of intramucosal activated T cells.
2. Infections (opportunistic)
   a. Viral
      (1) CMV: Although more commonly associated with colonic pathology, CMV is seen throughout the small bowel and is characterized by punctate erosions. Diagnosis may be difficult antemortem, but the virus may be found in biopsy specimens obtained during upper endoscopy. Effective therapy for small bowel CMV is lacking; however, ganciclovir may be used. Follow-up of the patient's response is difficult.
      (2) Human immunodeficiency virus (HIV) enteropathy: Although diminishing as identification tech-

niques improve, there remains a persistent group of patients with a secretory diarrhea and associated wasting in whom no pathogens are identified. There is support for the theory of direct invasion of enterocytes by HIV, with resultant villous atrophy and malabsorption. Whether the minimal changes seen in villous architecture with HIV infection are solely responsible for the diarrhea in this subgroup remains debatable. Loss of the ability to absorb micronutrients may occur with these minimal changes and may further reduce the gut's ability to protect itself from infection.
   b. Bacterial
      (1) MAI: Diarrhea is a unique feature of the MAI infections in AIDS patients. MAI can be found in 10–20% of small bowel biopsy specimens in patients with AIDS-related diarrhea. It is characterized by the appearance of a curved, acid-fast organism found in abundance in the mucosa. Active infection is more likely than colonization when systemic features such as fever, malaise, and disphoresis are reported. Whether colonization alone is a pathogenetic cause of diarrhea is unclear. Unfortunately, effective therapy for gut MAI is not available.
   c. Protozoal
      (1) *Cryptosporidium:* This single-cell protozoan is a fairly common cause of traveler's diarrhea, as well as an opportunistic infection found in 50% of patients with AIDS-related diarrhea. In immunocompetent hosts, infestations rapidly resolve; however, AIDS patients develop a severe, watery, nonbloody diarrhea with marked weight loss, occasional crampy abdominal pain, and dehydration. Fecal-oral transmission is the mechanism of infection. The organism appears to adhere to the small bowel mucosa and invaginate into the wall of individual enterocytes. How this condition leads

to diarrhea remains speculative. Microscopic damage is negligible. *Cryptosporidium* is capable of damaging the autonomic innervation of the gut, leading to disordered motility and diarrhea. A secretory component of the diarrhea must also exist, given the typically high stool outputs (1 to 3 liters/day). The organism has been found in the stomach, colon, and biliary tract. The last is the site most closely associated with the development of abdominal pain, and infection appears to occur as a coninfection with CMV. Diagnosis is typically by stool examination for the organism. *Cryptosporidium* can also be found on mucosal biopsy in patients with negative stools. There is currently no effective therapy, although spontaneous resolution has been reported in a few patients in whom good nutritional status (and hence some degree of immunocompetence) was restored.

d. *Isospora belli:* A single-cell protozoan, *Isospora* causes a syndrome very similar to that of *Cryptosporidium*, with profuse watery diarrhea, weight loss, abdominal pain, and occasional vomiting. It is found in 1–5% of patients with AIDS-related diarrhea. It occurs in small bowel and colonic mucosa but not in the biliary tract. Diagnosis is by stool examination or small bowel biopsy, but electron microscopic examination is necessary to confirm it. Patients typically respond well to treatment with trimethoprim-sulfamethoxazole.

e. *Microsporidia:* This has recently been identified as a cause of pathogen-negative AIDS diarrhea in 33% of those so diagnosed. It is not currently known how this organism produces diarrhea, as it is not associated with a tissue response. It has been found in the small and large bowels via electron microscopy of biopsy specimens. To date, there is no widely available, effective therapy.

3. Fungi: *Candida* can be cultured and identified in smears from small bowel aspirates in AIDS patients. Its significance as a small bowel pathogen is questionable.

4. Bacterial infections (nonopportunistic): AIDS patients are at increased risk for developing a variety of nonopportunistic gut infections, including *Shigella*, *Salmonella* (20-fold increased risk), *Campylobacter* (with a high relapse rate), *Giardia*, and *Amoeba* (rare). The clinical appearance of and diagnostic approach to these infections are similar to those in immunocompetent patients and are described elsewhere in this text.

D. Neoplasms

1. Kaposi's sarcoma involves the GI tract in 50% of patients with visceral lesions. This neoplasm appears to arise from lymphatic epithelial cells and is usually found in the bowel submucosa. Its frequency is now declining, occurring in 30% of all homosexuals with AIDS. The homosexual population is the only group routinely found to develop Kaposi's sarcoma. The small bowel is a frequent location of lesions; however, antemortem identification is difficult. The lesions can present as nodules with central ulcerations, polyps, or flat hemorrhagic lesions. Bleeding, obstruction, perforation, and abdominal pain may be presenting symptoms, although most patients are asymptomatic. Treatment of asymptomatic enteric Kaposi's sarcoma does not alter the outcome and is not currently warranted. Symptomatic disease is responsive to chemotherapy and radiation therapy. Single-drug regimens offer the best risk-benefit ratio and typically consist of vincristine, vinblastine or etoposide (VP-16).

2. Lymphoma: AIDS patients have an increased risk of developing non-Hodgkin's lymphoma. The majority of the lesions are of B-cell origin. Chronic viral infections may be the etiologic agents. Most patients present with weight loss, abdominal pain, fever, and malaise. Enteric involvement occurs in 27–36% of patients with AIDS-associated lymphoma. Small bowel lesions are typically exophytic lesions which can lead to obstruction, pain, perforation, and bleeding. Diagnosis is typically made by the characteristic X-ray appearance and/or biopsy. Gallium scanning may be helpful. Median survival for all AIDS patients with lymphoma is 6 months and is typically not

altered by therapy. The most widely used chemotherapy regimen consists of methotrexate, bleomycin, adriamycin, cyclophosphamide, vincristine, and dexamethasone (M-BACOD), with reported complete response rates of 54–67%. Problems remain with aggressive immunosuppression in these patients, and therapy may shorten survival in some patients. Large-cell lymphomas respond poorly. Surgery may be necessary for perforations and obstruction.

VI. The Colon

A. Signs and symptoms: Diseases involving the colon in AIDS patients present with rectal bleeding, low-volume (proctitic) diarrhea, and crampy abdominal pain. Constipation, rectal pain, and tenesmus may also be presenting findings.

B. Etiologies
1. Infectious diseases
   a. Viral
      (1) CMV is the most frequently encountered colonic pathogen. Patients can present with abdominal pain, diarrhea, and rectal bleeding. The mucosal damage can vary from mild erythema and low-grade inflammation to marked ulceration and necrosis of the bowel wall with perforation. The diagnosis is made by endoscopic biopsy, which demonstrates the typical enlarged mucosal cells and intranuclear inclusions. Red to purple granules found in the cytoplasm help separate this infection from HSV. Therapy includes antidiarrheals and ganciclovir. The response of CMV colitis to antiviral therapy has been disappointing.
      (2) HSV is associated with a proctitis characterized by ulcerations of the rectal mucosa. Perianal ulcerations are common, but pancolitis is distinctly unusual. Symptoms typically include rectal pain, bleeding, and tenesmus. Diagnosis is made with endoscopic biopsy and the finding of typical intracytoplasmic inclusions. Therapy includes acyclovir and antidiarrheals.
   b. Bacterial
      (1) *Salmonella*, *Shigella*, and *Campylo-*

bacter can cause acute colitis in AIDS patients. The symptoms, risk of systemic toxicity, and chronicity of these diseases are increased in patients with AIDS. Therapy is similar in AIDS and immunocompetent patients with systemic signs.
      (2) MAI is associated with a moderately severe chronic diarrhea and weight loss. Diagnosis is made with colonic mucosal biopsy. There is no currently effective therapy.
   c. Protozoal
      (1) Amebiasis is seen as a more severe pancolitis in AIDS patients. The characteristic lesions are diffusely spread punctate ulcers, although a more confluent ulceration can be noted in the immunocompromised. Perforation is a risk. The risk of amebic liver abscess does not appear to be increased. Diagnosis is made by demonstrating the presence of trophozoites in stool aspirates. Trophozoites showing erythrophagocytosis are pathognomonic but are rarely seen on biopsy. Serology is probably of little use in the AIDS population. Therapy includes metronidazole for tissue-invasive organisms and luminally active diiodohydroxyquin for cyst eradication.
2. Neoplasms
   a. Kaposi's sarcoma and, rarely, lymphoma have been reported in the colon in patients with AIDS. Patients may present with abdominal pain, bleeding, obstruction, or perforation. The approach to diagnosis and treatment is similar to that for small bowel neoplasms.

VII. The Pancreas

CMV infections, Kaposi's sarcoma, and non-Hodgkin's lymphoma involving the pancreas have been reported to occur in AIDS patients.

Bibliography

Bartlett JG, Belitsos PC, Sears CL. AIDS enteropathy. *Clin Infect Dis.* 15:726–735, 1992.

Cello JP. Gastrointestinal manifestations of HIV infection. *Infect Dis Clin North Am* 2:387–396, 1988.

Dieterich DT, Kotler DP, Busch DF, et al: Ganciclovir treatment of cytomegalovirus colitis in AIDS: a randomized, double-blind, placebo-controlled multicenter study. *J Infect Dis* 167:278–82, 1993.

Erskine D. The use of drugs in patients with gastrointestinal manifestations of AIDS. *Baillieres Clin Gastroenterol* 4:563–585, 1990.

Friedman SI. Gastrointestinal manifestations of AIDS. *Gastroenterol Clin North Am* 17:451–648, 1988.

Kotler DP. *Gastrointestinal and Nutritional Manifestations of the Acquired Immunodeficiency Syndrome.* New York, Raven Press, 1991.

Molina JM, Sarfati C, Beauvais B, et al. Intestinal microsporidiosis in human immunodeficiency virus-infected patients with chronic unexplained diarrhea: prevalence and clinical and biologic features. *J Infect Dis* 167:217–221, 1993.

Moroni M, Esposito R, Cernuschi M, et al. Treatment of AIDS-related refractory diarrhoea with octreotide. *Digestion* 54(Suppl 1):30–32, 1993.

Santangelo WC, Krejs GJ. Gastrointestinal manifestations of the acquired immunodeficiency syndrome. *Am J Med Sci* 292:328–334, 1986.

CHAPTER 58-D

Pseudomembranous Colitis

Michael D. Brown, M.D.

I. **Definition**

Pseudomembranous colitis is a toxin-mediated inflammatory lesion of the colon occurring in about 10% of patients with antibiotic-associated diarrhea. *Clostridium difficile* is the causative organism in 99% of cases.

II. **Etiology**

C. difficile is a spore-forming, gram-positive obligate anaerobe. It can be found in 5% of normal persons but is reported to be present in 50% of hospitalized patients. Antibiotic therapy is presumed to diminish the populations of gut bacteria that suppress *C. difficile* growth and toxin production. The typical pseudomembranous lesion may appear at any time after initiation of antibiotic therapy or up to 6 weeks after its discontinuation. Upon cessation of antibiotic therapy gut flora remains altered, providing a permissive environment for *C. difficile* growth.

III. **Pathophysiology**

A. Antibiotics: Every antibiotic except vancomycin, including metronidazole, has been associated with the development of pseudomembranous colitis.

B. Spread of the organism: Infective spores may persist on room furnishings for months. The major route of transmission, however, is person-to-person cross-infection via hand transmission. The dose of organisms necessary for infection is small.

C. Mechanism of injury: *C. difficile* is not enteroinvasive but secretes toxins which mediate the injury. Two toxins have been characterized to date:

1. Toxin A: enterotoxin.

2. Toxin B: cytotoxin.

Both toxins appear to attack membranes and epithelial cell microfilaments. Toxin A stimulates neutrophil chemotaxis and fluid flux, and toxin B interferes with mucosal protein synthesis and is the more potent cytopathogen. Other still uncharacterized toxins may participate in the injury process. Identification of the toxin, not culture of the organism, is the basis for diagnosis, as there are nontoxigenic forms of *C. difficile*.

D. Diagnosis

1. History: The patient will typically complain of a nonbloody diarrhea characterized by greenish, watery stool and crampy abdominal pain. The patient will have

started taking antibiotics 5–7 day earlier or will have recently discontinued them. There may be a history of exposure to fomites from other persons with diarrhea or recent hospitalization. There may be a history of a predisposing condition, such as cystic fibrosis, AIDS, or malignancy.

2. Physical examination: There are no specific findings. There may be evidence of volume depletion, fever, and tachycardia. The abdominal exam may show distention and diffuse abdominal pain. A more severe picture may emerge with signs of toxicity, including high fever, hypotension, marked stomach distention, absent bowel sounds, lack of diarrhea, and peritoneal signs. This picture is most commonly seen in patients with colonic inertia induced by antidiarrheal therapy or the postpartum period. Occasionally pseudomembranous colitis is complicated by a diffuse arthritis.

3. Diagnostic tests
   a. Blood tests: Leukocytosis, hypoalbuminemia, elevated erythrocyte sedimentation rate, and azotemia may be seen.
   b. Stool leukocytes: Stool leukocytes are seen in 50% of cases and are helpful in differentiating pseudomembranous colitis from the more benign forms of antibiotic-associated diarrhea.
   c. Radiographs: The kidney, ureter, and bladder may show a dilated colon and the thumbprinting seen with bowel wall edema. Computed tomography scans of the abdomen may demonstrate thickening of the colonic wall and pericolic regions along with distention, particularly in severe cases.
   d. Endoscopic appearance: Pseudomembranes appear as dirty white to yellow plaques which bleed upon biopsy. The intervening mucosa is erythematous, ulcerated, and friable. The mucosa appears exudative. The typical lesions are usually best seen in the left colon.
   e. Histologic appearance: Pseudomembranes appear as collections of necrotic debris, fibrin, mucus, and neutrophils. The inflammatory process is mucosa based but may become transmural. From 10% to 20% of patients with toxin-positive stool and colitis fail to demonstrate classic pseudomembranes.

f. Specific stool analysis: Toxin detection is essential in establishing a diagnosis of *C. difficile* pseudomembranous colitis. Stool cultures are not believed to offer the clinical correlation of toxin assays and are therefore not routinely done. The standard toxin assay is a tissue culture–based analysis which is 95–100% sensitive and specific. Toxin is not found in the stool of carriers, although 2–8% of those shedding toxin may be asymptomatic. Assay results are typically not cytotoxin A or B specific. More rapid assays for cytotoxin are now available using counterimmunoelectrophoresis (CIE) and enzyme-linked immunosorbent assays (ELISA) techniques.

E. Therapy
   1. Initial measures
      a. Stop the use of the offending antibiotic if feasible. If an antibiotic is needed, consider changing to one which is infrequently associated with antibiotic-associated pseudomembranous colitis (AAPMC).
      b. Provide volume support.
      c. Discontinue antidiarrheals.
      d. Take enteric isolation precautions.
   2. Antibiotics that are necessary in severe or persistent cases should be administered orally if at all possible.
      a. Oral metronidazole (250 mg orally three times per day for 7–10 days) is considered the best first-line therapy. It is far less expensive than vancomycin but is a very rare cause of AAPMC. Use IV metronidazole only in those cases in which oral administration is impossible.
      b. Oral vancomycin (125–500 mg orally four times per day for 7–14 days) should be reserved for the seriously ill or for those who fail metronidazole therapy.
      c. Bacitracin (25,000 units four times per day for 7–14 days) is effective but is rarely used.
   3. Toxin binders
      a. Cholestyramine (4 g orally three times per day for 5–10 days) is reserved for those with mild disease who are able to discontinue antibiotics. It is often used in combination with metronidazole or

vancomycin. Relapse rates are high without the addition of an antibiotic.
4. Alteration of fecal flora
   a. *Lactobacillus* preparations (1 g orally four times per day for 7–14 days).
   b. Fecal enema (fresh feces via enema twice three days apart).
F. Relapse: Relapses occur in 5–50% and can be multiple (10–15). They are typically milder than the initial occurrence. Therapy ranges from observation to a repeat 7- to 10-day course of an antibiotic followed by 3 weeks of toxin binders or *Lactobacillus* preparations.

Bibliography

Bartlett JG. Pseudomembranous enterocolitis and antibiotic-associated colitis, in Sleisenger MH, Fordtran JS (eds): *Gastrointestinal Disease*, ed 5. Philadelphia, Saunders, 1993 p 1174–1189.

Bartlett JG. *Clostridium difficile:* Clinical considerations. *Rev Infect Dis* 12(Suppl 2):S243–251, 1990.

Lyerly DM, Krivan HC, Wilkins TD, et al. *Clostridium difficile:* Its disease and toxins. *Clin Microbiol Rev* 1:1–18, 1988.

Shellito PC. Pseudomembranous colitis. *New Engl J Med* 326:1059, 1992

Tedesco FJ. Pseudomembranous colitis: Pathogenesis and therapy. *Med Clin North Am* 66:655–664, 1982.

CHAPTER 58-E

Short-Bowel Syndrome

Bennett Plotnick, M.D.

I. **Definition**

Short bowel syndrome is present when the absorptive surface provided by the small intestine is inadequate to maintain nutrition. The severity of symptoms is related to two factors.

A. Extent of resection

Resection of up to 40% of the small intestine is generally well tolerated.

B. Level of resection

The duodenum, proximal jejunum, distal ileum, and ileocecal valve are the most important levels for small bowel absorption.

II. **Etiology**

Conditions that require massive small bowel resection are generally those in which the intestinal blood supply is threatened or large areas of intestine are involved in a disease process.

A. Thromboses or emboli of the superior mesenteric artery.

B. Low-flow ischemia of the superior mesenteric arterial bed.

C. Superior mesenteric vein thromboses.

D. Volvulus of the small intestine.

E. Strangulated hernia.

F. Crohn's disease.

G. Neoplasm.

H. Trauma.

I. Jejunoileal bypass for obesity.

III. **Pathophysiology**

The specific features of short bowel syndrome are a reflection of the length of resection, level of resection, and length of time after surgery for small bowel adaptation.

A. Immediate postoperative period

1. Reduction of absorption of all nutrients, including water, electrolytes, fat, protein, carbohydrates, vitamins, and trace elements.

2. Large fluid losses (in excess of 5 liters/ day) be seen.

3. Gastric hypersecretion predisposing the patient to complications of peptic ulcer disease and compromising absorption by causing mucosal damage and impaired lipid digestion. This condition reverts to normal in patients who survive the immediate postoperative period.

B. Duodenal resection or bypass

1. Anemia secondary to iron and folate deficiency.

2. Osteopenia secondary to calcium malabsorption.

C. Ileocecal valve resection
   1. Predisposes to overgrowth of colonic flora.
D. Ileal resection
   1. Vitamin B_{12} malabsorption.
   2. Resection of less than 100 cm of the distal ileum.
      a. Cholerrheic diarrhea secondary to bile salt malabsorption without steatorrhea as hepatic synthesis compensates to maintain adequate concentrations of intraluminal bile salts.
   3. Resection of more than 100 cm of the distal ileum.
      a. Steatorrhea develops, as the loss of the bile salt pool is too large to be replaced by maximum hepatic synthesis.

IV. Diagnosis

Short bowel syndrome should be suspected in any patient after small bowel resection and confirmed by a history, physical exam, and laboratory data.

A. Historical data: prior intestinal resection, with specific details of malnutrition.
   1. Prolonged diarrhea.
   2. Weight loss, fatigue, and weakness from calorie deprivation.
   3. Symptoms of vitamin deficiency such as bleeding, neuropathy, osteopenia, and anemia.
B. Physical findings depend on the severity and duration of malabsorption.
   1. Early: Signs of dehydration, hypocalcemia and hypomagnesemia
   2. Late: Signs of malabsorption such as cachexia, purpura, increased skin pigmentation, multiple vitamin deficiencies, trace element deficiencies, anemia, osteopenia, and peripheral neuropathies.
C. Laboratory data to confirm the clinical diagnosis.
   1. Early
      a. Sodium and water depletion, as well as hypokalemia secondary to massive fecal fluid losses.
      b. Elevated serum gastrin level.
      c. Hypocalcemia and hypomagnesemia.
   2. Late
      a. Laboratory data seen in typical panmalabsorption syndromes.
      b. Abnormal Schilling's test, suggestive of vitamin B_{12} malabsorption or bacterial overgrowth.
      c. Elevated quantitative fecal fat level.

d. ^{14}C-xylose absorptive test to exclude bacterial overgrowth.
e. Decreased prothrombin time and reduced cholesterol, carotene, zinc, and albumin levels are common. Anemia secondary to iron, folate, and vitamin B_{12} deficiencies, as well as low levels of calcium and magnesium, should be specifically sought.

V. Differential Diagnosis

Short bowel syndrome may be confused with other causes of malabsorption and diarrhea not related to small bowel resection.
A. Bacterial overgrowth.
B. Crohn's disease.
C. Pancreatic insufficiency.
D. Primary small bowel disease.
   1. Lymphoma
   2. Sprue
   3. Whipple's disease
   4. Giardiasis
   5. Radiation enteritis

VI. Treatment

Management of short bowel syndrome is aimed at replacing electrolyte and water losses early and maintaining nutritional support long term.
A. Early fluid and electrolyte management to replace the massive fluid losses.
B. Early recognition, treatment, and prevention of elevated gastric secretion and resultant ulcer complications.
C. Early oral feedings in the form of elemental diets and medium chain tryglycerides are important to stimulate adaptive mucosal hyperplasia of the remaining intestine.
D. Antidiarrheal agents may facilitate absorption by increasing luminal contact time.
E. Replacement of specific vitamins, especially calcium, vitamin D, folic acid, iron, parenteral vitamin B_{12} as the clinical condition dictates.
F. Cholestyramine is useful for controlling diarrhea in patients with less than 100 cm of ileal resection by binding unabsorbed bile salts.
G. Hyperalimentation may be needed in patients whose nutrition cannot be maintained despite intensive nutritional support with elemental diets, medium chain tryglycerides, polycose, and multivitamin replacement.
H. Broad-spectrum antibiotic therapy is needed if bacterial overgrowth is suspected.
I. Small bowel transplantation may ultimately

be an option for these patients, but at present it must be considered experimental.

VII. Patient Monitering

Patients with short bowel syndrome must be followed carefully for signs of electrolyte imbalance and nutritional depletion.

VIII. Prognosis

The prognosis in patients with short bowel syndrome varies directly with the length and location of the remaining intestine and the ability of the remaining viable intestine to adapt.

A. Patients with more than 25% of functional small intestine remaining after resection have a good prognosis, especially if the remaining intestine includes the duodenum, proximal jejunum, and distal ileum.

B. Patients with less than 25% of functional small intestine remaining have a poor prognosis and generally will need parenteral hyperalimentation to survive.

Bibliography

Cortot A, Fleming CR, Malagelada JR. Improved nutritional absorption after cimetidine in short-bowel syndrome with gastric hypersecretion. *N Engl J Med* 300:79, 1979.

Pritchard TJ, Kirkman RL. Small bowel transplantation. *World J Surg* 9:860, 1985.

Weser E. Nutritional aspects of malabsorption. Short gut adaptation. *Am J Med* 67:1014, 1979.

Williams SJ, Evans P, King RFGJ. Gastric acid secretion and gastrin production in the short bowel syndrome. *Gut* 26:914, 1985.

Trier JS, Lipsky M. The short bowel syndrome, in Sleisenger MH (ed): *Gastrointestinal Disease,* ed 4. Philadelphia, Saunders, 1989, p 1106.

Chapter 58-F

Vascular Diseases of the Intestinal Tract

Bennett Plotnick, M.D.

I. **Definition**
   Vascular diseases of the intestine encompass a group of disorders in which visceral ischemia is a common abnormality. These diseases can be divided into the following six major categories:
   A. Intestinal angina
   B. Acute mesenteric arterial occlusion
   C. Mesenteric arterial embolization
   D. Nonocclusive intestinal infarction
   E. Colonic ischemia
   F. Mesenteric venous thrombosis
II. **Etiology**
   A. Intestinal angina: Occlusive vascular disease atherosclerotic in origin, affecting at least two of the three major splanchnic vessels.
   B. Acute mesenteric arterial occlusion: This occurs when the intestinal blood flow reaches a critical level, resulting in intestinal infarction. Etiologies inclue atherosclerosis (most common), embolism, dissecting aortic aneurysm, fibromuscular hyperplasia, vasculitis, and the use of oral contraceptives.
   C. Mesenteric arterial embolization: Emboli most commonly lodge in the superior mesenteric artery. The most common etiology arises from mural thrombi in the heart.

Other etiologies include vegetations from endocarditis, valvular prostheses, atrial myxomas, and atherosclerotic plaques in the thoracic or upper abdominal aorta.
   D. Nonocclusive intestinal infarction: This occurs when infarction is present without demonstrable occlusion, usually in low-flow mesenteric states such as congestive heart failure, shock, and anoxia. The use of α-adrenergic vasoconstrictors and digitalis is common.
   E. Colonic ischemia: This results from localized occlusive disease in the inferior mesenteric artery or its collaterals. It may be due to atherosclerosis or abdominal and vascular surgery and may be seen less commonly in hypercoagulable states, amyloid, vasculitis, aortic aneurysm, obstructing colorectal cancers, renal transplantation, and vasopressin or oral contraceptive use.
   F. Mesenteric venous obstruction: This occurs in the superior mesenteric vein in 95% of cases. It is associated with a variety of etiologies, including portal hypertension, congestive heart failure, abdominal neoplasms, intra-abdominal inflammation, abdominal

surgery or trauma, hypercoagulable states, and oral contraceptive use.

III. Pathophysiology

A. Intestinal ischemia: The superior mesenteric artery and collaterals are partially or completely occluded, resulting in postprandial pain analogous to that of angina pectoris.

B. Acute mesenteric arterial occlusion: Complete occlusion due to atherosclerotic changes affecting at least two of the major splanchnic vessels, leading to infarction with resulting peritonitis.

C. Mesenteric arterial embolization: Acute occlusion of the superior mesenteric artery, if not recognized, will result in infarction and resulting peritonitis.

D. Nonocclusive intestinal infarction: The presence of inadequate tissue perfusion results in shunting of blood away from the mesentery, a condition aggravated by the use of digitalis and other mesenteric vasoconstrictors, resulting in intestinal ischemia and infarction.

E. Colonic ischemia: Localized ischemia of the inferior mesenteric artery and critical collaterals results in localized colonic ischemia and infarction in the "watershed" area of the colon (splenic flexure), which lacks adequate collaterals between the inferior and superior mesenteric arteries.

F. Mesenteric venous thombosis: Stasis in the mesenteric venous bed leads to stasis and resultant infarction.

IV. Diagnosis

The diagnosis of diseases affecting the intestinal blood supply depends on a high index of suspicion, along with a thorough history and physical exam.

A. Intestinal angina

1. History: Postprandial pain occurring 15 to 30 minutes after eating and lasting for several hours in an older patient with evidence of widespread atherosclerosis should alert one to the diagnosis. This pain results in fear of eating and weight loss. Steatorrhea may be present.

2. Physical exam: Weight loss and the presence of atherosclerosis. An abdominal bruit is nonspecific but may be present.

3. Tests: Laboratory tests are nonspecific. Steatorrhea is mild. Angiography shows >50% narrowing in two of the three major vessels.

B. Acute mesenteric arterial occlusion.

1. History and physical exam: The diagnosis should be suspected in a patient with severe abdominal pain that is out of proportion to the physical and laboratory findings. If the condition is undiagnosed after 8 hr, signs of infarction with peritonitis and leukocytosis develop. The patient may pass blood per rectum.

2. X-ray findings: Ileus with air-fluid levels or gas in the bowel wall or portal vein may be seen. Ultrasound or computed tomography (CT) scanning may help exclude other entities.

C. Nonocclusive intestinal infarction

1. The diagnosis should be suspected in a patient with recent myocardial infarction, congestive heart failure, shock, or anoxia who develops signs of intestinal infarction. Angiography excludes the presence of emboli and thrombosis. Findings include narrowed or irregular branches of the superior mesenteric artery, spasm of the arcades, and impaired filling of the intramural vessels.

D. Colonic ischemia

1. History and physical exam: Most patients are over age 50 and have evidence of atherosclerosis. They typically present with abrupt onset of lower abdominal cramping, rectal bleeding with fever, and vomiting. The physical exam suggests left-sided colitis.

2. Tests: The kidney, ureters, and bladder (KUB) may show thumbprinting, suggesting ischemia or intramural hemorrhage. Endoscopic findings such as ulceration, hemorrhage, or pseudomembranes are nonspecific. Biopsies may show ischemic changes. Follow-up barium enema may show intramural hemorrhage, stricture, and sawtooth irregularity. These changes generally occur in the splenic flexure and rectosigmoid. Angiography is rarely helpful due to the occlusions localized to the smaller vessels.

E. Mesenteric venous thrombosis

1. History and physical exam: The patient may present with an acute abdomen, but in many cases the process may be more gradual, with the development of abdominal discomfort over several weeks. Physical findings are nonspecific, but the

patients appear sicker than their physical findings warrant.

   2. Tests: Bloody peritoneal fluid is typical. Small bowel thickening and irregularity are commonly seen on KUB testing, CT scanning, and ultrasound. Angiography shows intense arterial spasm without venous drainage.

V. Differential Diagnosis

A. Intestinal angina
   1. Peptic ulcer disease
   2. Chronic pancreatitis
   3. Biliary tract disease
   4. Irritable bowel syndrome
   5. Occult carcinoma
B. Acute mesenteric arterial occlusion
   1. Perforated viscus
   2. Pancreatitis
   3. Acute cholecystitis
   4. Ruptured aortic aneurysm
   5. Renal colic
C. Mesenteric arterial embolization
   1. Acute surgical abdomen
   2. Similar to (B) above
D. Nonocclusive intestinal infarction
   1. Similar to (B) above
E. Colonic ischemia
   1. Nonspecific ulcerative colitis or proctitis
   2. Infectious colitis
   3. Crohn's colitis
   4. Diverticulitis

VI. Treatment

Management of intestinal ischemia depends on prompt diagnoses.

A. Intestinal angina: Reconstructive surgery should be attempted only if other abdominal disease is excluded and at least two major vessels are involved. Bypass, endarterectomy, and reimplantation are all effective.
B. Acute mesenteric arterial occlusion: Initial supportive measures include fluids, antibiotics, and electrolyte replacement. The usefulness of intra-arterial infused vasodilators (papaverine) has not been conclusively established. At surgery, revascularization of viable bowel or resection of necrotic bowel is the primary goal.
C. Mesenteric arterial embolization: As soon as the diagnosis is established and the patient stabilized, laparotomy and embolectomy are performed.
D. Nonocclusive intestinal infarction: The primary goal is to avoid surgery in this population unless peritonitis is present. Medical management includes improving cardiac output and avoiding the use of digitalis and vasoconstricting agents. The use of potent intra-arterial vasoconstrictors should be considered, although their effectiveness is not established.
E. Colonic ischemia: Initial management includes rescuscitation with fluids, broad-spectrum antibiotics, and bowel rest. Surgery is reserved for those patients suspected of developing perforation or significant colonic stricture.
F. Mesenteric venous thrombosis: The diagnosis is confirmed at surgery by the presence of arterial pulsation and a venous thrombosis. Infarcted bowel is resected. Postoperative anticoagulation is recommended except in patients at high risk, such as those with portal hypertension, severe trauma, polycythemia vera, and underlying neoplasm.

VII. Patient Monitering

Patients with intestinal ischemic syndromes may be at risk for recurrence. This is especially important in patients with embolization, venous occlusion, and nonocclusive infarction. Potentially treatable or reversible etiologies should be addressed.

VIII. Prognosis

A. Intestinal angina: Corrective surgery in a select population has been useful in providing relief of pain and correction of malabsorption.
B. Acute mesenteric arterial occlusion: Prognosis depends on the amount of viable intestine salvaged and the degree of resulting malabsorption.
C. Mesenteric arterial embolization: Because the patients are younger and the diagnosis is suspected sooner, these patients generally have a more favorable prognosis.
D. Nonocclusive intestinal infarction: These patients generally have a poor prognosis due to their underlying disease.
E. Colonic ischemia: Most patients respond to medical management and do not require surgical intervention. A small percentage progress to colonic perforation or develop subsequent colonic stricture.
F. Mesenteric venous thrombosis: In general, the overall prognosis is better than that of arterial disease. The mortality rate, formerly as high as 80%, may currently be as low as 20%.

Bibliography

Gillespie IE. Intestinal ischemia. *Gut* 26:653, 1985.

Grendell JH, Ockner RK. Mesenteric venous thrombosis. *Gastroenterology* 82:358, 1982.

Grendell JH, Ockner RK. Vascular diseases of the bowel, in Sleisenger MH (ed): *Gastrointestinal Disease*, ed 4. Philadelphia, Saunders, 1989, p 1903.

Marston, A. *Vascular Disease of the Gastrointestinal Tract. Pathophysiology. Recognition and Management.* Baltimore, Williams and Wilkins, 1986.

Rosen A, Korobkin M, Silverman PM, et al. Mesenteric vein thrombosis. CT identification. *Am J Radiol* 143:83, 1984.

CHAPTER 58-G

Crohn's Disease

John Schaffner, M.D.

I. **Definition**

Crohn's disease is a chronic inflammatory disease of the gastrointestinal tract that can affect any part of the gastrointestinal system from the mouth to the anus.

II. **Etiology**

The etiology of Crohn's disease is unknown. Numerous potential etiologies including infections, host abnormality, immune-mediated damage, and environmental factors have not been shown to play a role.

A. Infections: Because of the granulomatous reaction, an infectious etiology has been most strongly suspected. Atypical mycobacteria have been found in a proportion of patients with Crohn's disease, though it is unclear if they are causative.

III. **Pathophysiology**

The pathophysiology of the disease is unknown. The cause of the symptoms is much clearer.

A. Diarrhea: There are multiple potential causes of diarrhea in Crohn's disease, depending in part on the location of the disease.

1. With terminal ileal disease

a. Bile salt malabsorption leading to choleretic diarrhea.
b. Partial bowel obstruction.
c. Bacterial overgrowth.
d. Malabsorption with extensive small bowel involvement.
e. Short bowel after surgical resection.
f. Malabsorption after ileal resection secondary to a decreased bile salt pool.

2. With colonic disease

a. Protein-losing enteropathy with extensive inflammation.
b. Loss of absorptive surface for water.
c. Inflammatory diarrhea.

3. Other conditions

a. Associated disaccharidase deficiency.
b. Zinc deficiency.
c. Enteric fistulas leading to short circuits.

B. Abdominal pain

1. Usually secondary to partial bowel obstruction.
2. Pain may have an origin outside the luminal gastrointestinal tract.

a. Gallstones
b. Kidney stones

IV. Diagnosis

The clinical picture of Crohn's disease depends in part on the area of involvement.

A. History
   1. The most common symptoms are abdominal pain and diarrhea. Symptoms are usually insidious in onset.
   2. Fever usually below 102°F.
   3. Weight loss common, usually due to decreased intake.
   4. Peak incidence in young adulthood.
   5. May present like acute appendicitis.
   6. Perirectal disease common (fissures, fistula) and may precede other symptoms.
   7. May present with growth failure in children.
   8. May present with extraintestinal manifestation before significant gut symptoms appear.
      a. Arthritis or arthralgia.
      b. Blurred vision secondary to iritis or uveitis.
      c. Skin lesions like erythema nodosum or pyoderma gangrenosum.
      d. Liver disease.
      e. Perirectal disease.

B. Clinical signs and physical findings
   1. Abdominal pain frequent, most commonly in the right lower quadrant.
   2. Possible palpable, tender mass in the right lower quadrant.
   3. Depending upon the degree of obstruction, abdomen may be distended.
   4. Rushes of fluid may be elicited by palpation.
   5. Inspection of perirectal area may reveal fistula or fissures.
   6. Possible signs of any of the extraintestinal manifestations (same as for ulcerative colitis; see ulcerative colitis IV-B-2).
   7. Possible finding of anemia.
   8. Increased incidence of gallstones.

C. Diagnostic tests: The diagnosis can be made with the clinical picture and compatible findings on x-ray or at endoscopy. At times, the diagnosis is made at laparotomy.
   1. Laboratory data may reveal anemia or signs of malnutrition.
      a. Anemia secondary to iron, vitamin B_{12}, or folate deficiency.
      b. Albumin and cholesterol levels may be low.
      c. Erythrocyte sedimentation rate may be elevated, though this finding is not reliable.
      d. Multiple "activity indices" have little clinical utility in assessing disease activity.
   2. Endoscopically, the colon may reveal nonspecific erythema.
      a. Earliest lesion is apthoid ulcer.
      b. Asymmetric, spotty mucosal involvement.
      c. Rectum usually spared, except for perirectal disease.
      d. Long linear ulcers.
      e. Usually worse in the right colon.
   3. In some patients, x-ray may be the best way to make the diagnosis, particularly when the colon is normal.
      a. Apthous ulcers seen on air-contrast studies.
      b. Same asymmetry and "skip" areas as seen on colonoscopy.
      c. Rectal sparing.
      d. Terminal ileal disease with ulcerated mucosa and luminal narrowing—"string sign."
      e. Possible duodenal or antral narrowing.
      f. Strictures.
      g. Fistulas from bowel to bowel, bladder, vagina, or skin.

V. Differential Diagnosis

A. Other inflammatory bowel disease, including ulcerative colitis and Behcet's colitis.
B. Infectious enteritides
   1. Parasitic diseases, including giardiasis, strongyloidiasis, and schistosomiasis.
   2. *Yersinia enterocolitica*—Other bacteria are less likely because of the chronic nature of Crohn's disease.
C. Irritable bowel syndrome—Abdominal pain and diarrhea in young people are a common presentation for this diarrhea, as well as for Crohn's disease, and are more common in the former.
D. Carbohydrate intolerance (lactose, sorbitol) can mimic symptoms of Crohn's disease.

VI. Treatment

Treatment is aimed at decreasing inflammation and providing symptomatic relief.

A. Treatment of inflammation
   1. Sulfasalazine is used in Crohn's disease, as well as in ulcerative colitis. More effective with colon involvement. Efficacy in treating small bowel disease is uncertain.

Ulcerative Colitis

John Schaffner, M.D.

I. **Definition**
Ulcerative colitis (UC) is an inflammatory disease of the colonic mucosa. The disease begins in the rectum and may extend as far as the cecum, but it is limited to the colon.

II. **Etiology**
The cause of UC is unknown. Several potential etiologies have been proposed.
A. Infectious: No convincing evidence exists.
B. Genetic: Although there is some genetic association with human leukocyte antigen (HLA) phenotypes and familial tendencies, no convincing evidence is available.
C. Psychologic: There is no convincing evidence that psychologic factors are causative.
D. Immunologic: Although there are some abnormalities in the immunologic status of individuals with UC, a causal relationship has not been confirmed.

III. **Pathophysiology**
The initial insult to the colon mucosa is unknown. The role of different immunologic mediators is also unknown.
A. The arachidonic acid pathway appears to be responsible for the inflammatory response.
1. The cyclooxygenase pathway may be important.
   a. Increased levels of prostaglandins and metabolites have been found in inflamed tissue.
   b. Prostaglandins may be responsible for diarrhea secondary to altered electrolye transport.
2. The lipoxygenase pathway also appears to be important.
   a. Leukotrienes, part of this pathway, may be important mediators of the inflammatory response.
   b. Leukotriene inhibitors may be effective therapy.

IV. **Diagnosis**
A. History: Typically, patients with UC present with bloody diarrhea.
1. The disease affects primarily young adults over age 20. There is a second incidence peak in the fifth decade.
2. Mild disease presents in 60% of patients.
   a. Diarrhea and bleeding are not severe.
   b. There are less frequent complaints of extraintestinal manifestations.

3. Moderate disease affects about 25% of individuals with UC.

4. Severe disease affects about 15% of individuals with UC. It usually presents with more abrupt onset of symptoms. Fulminant disease can result in death.

B. Clinical signs: UC has many clinical patterns. The most common one is a relapsing pattern, with bouts of diarrhea interspersed with normal periods. Disease may be chronic with long-standing diarrhea. It may also be fulminant, with severe symptoms occurring abruptly in the absence of prior symptoms.

1. GI signs and symptoms
   a. Rectal bleeding is the most common symptom.
   b. Diarrhea may vary considerably in severity.
   c. Abdominal pain may be present in patients with moderate and severe disease. Pain is frequently related to bowel movements.
   d. Weight loss correlates with the severity of disease.
   e. Fever may be present when disease is active.

2. Extraintestinal manifestations: UC can affect numerous organ systems. Although these symptoms and signs frequently accompany active disease, they may be the sole manifestation or presenting complaint in UC patients.
   a. Bone and joint (15–20%): Arthritis may accompany UC.
      (1) Peripheral arthritis usually coincides with disease activity.
      (2) Larger joints usually affected.
      (3) Spondylitis also occurs, with no relationship to disease activity.
      (4) Usually associated with presence of HLA-B27.
   b. Skin (5–15%): Erythema nodosum and pyoderma gangrenosum occur with about equal frequency in UC. Both lesions are usually associated with extensive colitis and active disease.
   c. Eye (3–10%): Several abnormalities may be seen in UC.
      (1) Uveitis is the most common lesion.
      (2) Episcleritis, keratitis, and neuritis are seen less frequently.
      (3) Cataract as a complication of therapy is also important.

d. Renal: Two primary disorders occur in UC.
   (1) Renal stones occur in 5% of patients and are usually composed of urate. They are caused by dehydration, calcium mobilization, and altered urine composition.
   (2) Pyelonephritis occurs with increased frequency.
e. Liver (5–10%): Multiple hepatic abnormalities may be present in patients with UC.
   (1) Pericholangitis may be a form of sclerosing cholangitis.
   (2) Sclerosing cholangitis (PSC) has a more variable course than was initially thought.
   (3) Cholangiocarcinoma may be a complication of PSC.
   (4) Fatty liver, chronic hepatitis, and cirrhosis may also be seen.
f. Hematologic: Several abnormalities may be present.
   (1) Anemia usually occurs secondary to iron deficiency. However, hemolytic anemia may also occur.
   (2) Coagulation abnormalities may occur. Hypoprothrombinemia is seen in more severe disease. Thromboembolic disease occurs with increased frequency in patients with UC.
g. Other conditions
   (1) Growth failure may occur in children secondary to poor caloric intake.
   (2) Numerous nutritional deficiencies can arise in patients with active disease.

3. GI complications
   a. Toxic megacolon, that is, toxic dilatation of the colon, usually involving the transverse colon. Patients are usually ill and require intensive therapy. This condition may be precipitated by antidiarrheal medication, narcotics, or diagnostic tests.
   b. Bowel perforation can occur, usually during severe disease.
   c. Colon cancer: The risk is associated with the extent and duration of disease. After 8–10 years, the risk is approximately 1% per year, although the exact incidence is unclear.

4. Physical findings: Examination is generally nonspecific. Findings of extraintestinal manifestations may be helpful in the diagnosis. Otherwise, the severity of the illness, as well as the presence of GI complications (toxic megacolon, bowel perforation), may be discerned from the exam.

C. Diagnostic tests: The diagnosis is made by visualization of the colon. Findings by radiography or direct visualization are most often nonspecific. Biopsy is also relatively nonspecific. Confirmation of negative microbiologic tests, a compatible history, visualization, and pathologic analysis, taken together, provide the diagnosis.

1. Endoscopic findings: The rectum involved with inflammation appears granular, hyperemic, and friable. There may be small, punctate erosions to larger, more discrete ulcers. An extensive exudate can be present. Pseudopolyps may also occur. Chronic disease can result in loss of submucosal vascularity and a short, tubular colon.

2. Radiographic findings: The colon may have a diffuse, granular appearance. Haustral markings may be lost and the colon shortened. Pseudopolyps may also be seen, as well as areas of luminal narrowing. Chronic disease may lead to increased distance in the presacral space secondary to fibrosis.

3. Pathologic features: Crypt abscesses, distorted crypt architecture, and inflammation may vary, depending on disease activity. The disease is confined to the mucosa on gross specimens.

V. Differential Diagnosis

A. Crohn's disease: The primary disorder in the differential diagnosis of UC is Crohn's disease. Although after diagnostic testing a diagnosis can usually be made, a small percentage of patients may be defined as "indeterminate," with disease not typical of either UC or Crohn's disease.

B. Infectious colitis: Numerous organisms can produce a disease that looks similar to UC.
1. Bacteria: *Salmonella, Shigella, Campylobacter, Escherichia coli, Clostridium difficile.*
2. Parasites: *Amoeba, Schistosoma, Strongyloides.*

C. Ischemic colitis, radiation enteritis, graft-versus-host disease, and Behcet's disease can potentially mimic UC.

VI. Treatment

Management is aimed at decreasing the inflammation and treating the symptoms.

A. Treatment of inflammation
1. Sulfasalazine is now known to act by delivering 5-aminosalicylic acid (5-ASA) directly to the colon. Bacterial degradation of sulfapyridine-5 ASA releases the 5-ASA in the colon. This therapy is useful for mild to moderate disease and for maintaining remission. It works in the arachidonic acid pathway.
   a. Primary side effects are nausea and vomiting, though reactions to sulfa can occur.
   b. Oral preparations of 5-ASA without sulfa are available. Additional compounds with more proximal action may soon be available.
   c. Rectal 5-ASA is also useful as bedtime treatment for 2–6 weeks.
   d. Maintenance: 2 g/day sulfasalazine; treatment = up to 6 g/day.
2. Steroids: Hydrocortisone, prednisone, and adrenocorticotropic hormone (ACTH) are used for more severe disease. They have no proven ability to maintain remission.
   a. ACTH may be more effective for severe exacerbation in patients never treated with steroids.
   b. Steroid treatment with prednisone is started at doses ranging from 40 to 60 mg.
   c. Once the patient in remission, steroid is tapered.
   d. Rectal steroids may alleviate rectal bleeding, tenesmus, and urgency.
3. Immunosuppressants
   a. Azathioprine and 6-mercaptopurine
      (1) No proven effect when used alone.
      (2) Steroid sparing.
      (3) Used in low doses; monitor the white blood cell count.
   b. No other agents are commonly used at this time.
4. Antibiotics
   a. No antibiotic has proven efficacy.
   b. Metronidazole is not effective.

B. Diet therapy: No proven link exists between diet and UC. Disease activity may dictate the diet, which must be individualized.
1. No specific restrictions for patients with mild to moderate disease.

a. Be aware of lactose or other food intolerances.

b. Altering the fiber content of the diet may affect diarrhea.

2. An elemental diet may be of therapeutic benefit for some patients.

3. Parenteral nutrition is indicated for more severe disease, particularly in malnourished patients.

C. Symptomatic treatment: Disease activity should be considered when offering symptomatic therapy. The best therapy is still aimed at controlling inflammation.

1. Antidiarrheal and antispasmodic medications should be avoided in patients with moderate to severe disease; they may precipitate toxic megacolon.

2. Narcotics: Use with caution, as they can also precipitate toxic megacolon.

3. Bulk agents: May be used in the absence of active disease to help control diarrhea.

D. Surgery: Removal of the colon is curative, through occasionally extraintestinal manifestations are reported after colectomy.

1. Indications for surgery include colon cancer, bleeding, perforation, toxic megacolon, and severe disease resistant to treatment.

2. Total colectomy is the procedure of choice.

a. Ileostomy is the standard operation for patients with UC.

b. Continent ileostomy may be used.

c. Ileoanal anastomosis offers patients the opportunity of continence with maintenance of sexual function.

VII. Patient Monitoring

The extent and activity of the disease determine the degree of monitoring required.

A. Patients with active disease need close follow-up to change medical regimens as needed.

1. Blood count and erythrocyte sedimentation rate can be followed.

2. Examination of the rectal mucosa can give a good indication of disease activity if symptoms persist.

B. Patients with inactive disease need periodic blood counts to check for anemia.

C. Patients with UC that has affected the colon to the splenic flexure or more proximally and that has existed for more than 8 years need close follow-up.

1. The risk of colon cancer in these individuals is significantly increased, though the amount of increase controversial.

2. There is debate about how frequently colonoscopic exams should be performed. The current recommendation is yearly colonoscopy with biopsy to look for dysplasia.

3. At present, the existence of disease activity does not alter these recommendations, though the screening exam should preferably not be done during a flare-up because of the difficulty of interpreting dysplasia in active inflammation.

VIII. Prognosis

The majority of patients will function well with periods of relapse; those with sustained remissions have a normal life expectancy. A small group presents with fulminant disease. The majority of deaths from UC occur in this group. The other major cause of death is colon cancer. Morbidity is due to chronic diarrhea and blood loss. Colectomy cures the disease, though there is significant morbidity associated with the surgery. Newer surgical techniques are aimed at reducing postoperative morbidity.

Bibliography

Greenstein AJ, Janowitz HD, Sacher DB. The extraintestinal complications of Crohn's disease and ulcerative colitis: A study of 700 patients. *Medicine* 55:401–412, 1976.

Nugent FW, Haggitt RC, Gilpin PA. Cancer surveillance in ulcerative colitis. *Gastroenterology* 100:1241–1248, 1991.

Peppercorn MA. Advances in drug therapy for inflammatory bowel disease. *Ann Intern Med* 112:50–60, 1990.

Chapter 58-I

Colon Polyps

John Schaffner, M.D.

I. Definition
A polyp is defined as any visible tissue that protrudes into the lumen of the gastrointestinal tract. The term *polyp* does not define the histology. Polyps can be pedunculated (on a stalk) or sessile (adherent and flat). The size of polyps can range from minuscule to very large (>5 cm).

II. Etiology
The etiology of adenomatous polyps is unknown. Genetics, diet, and environmental and geographic factors may all play a role. The etiology of hyperplastic and hamartomatous polyps is also unknown. Several familial polyposis syndromes are well characterized.

A. Familial adenomatous polyposis
1. Autosomal dominant.
2. More than 100 adenomas.
3. Primarily found in the colon and rectume, though the small intestine and stomach can also be affected.
4. Very high malignant potential by age 40.
5. Treatment is colectomy.
B. Gardner's syndrome
1. Similar to familial polyposis.
2. Extracolonic lesions including osteomas, epidermal cysts, and soft tissue tumors.
C. Turcot's syndrome
1. Familial polyposis plus brain tumors.
D. Peutz-Jeghers syndrome
1. Autosomal dominant with incomplete penetrance.
2. Multiple hamartomas throughout the gastrointestinal tract.
3. Mucocutaneous pigmentation.
4. Slightly increased risk of cancer.
E. Cronkhite-Canada syndrome
1. Multiple hamartomatous polyps different from those in Peutz-Jeghers syndrome.
2. Protein-losing enteropathy and malabsorption.
3. Alopecia, hyperpigmentation, and onycholysis.

III. Pathophysiology
A. Adenomas have abnormal cellular proliferation and maturation patterns. The cause of this abnormality is unknown.

B. Five percent of adenomatous polyps may undergo malignant transformation.

C. The more villous features a polyp has and the larger a polyp is, the more likely malignant change will occur.

IV. Diagnosis

A. History: Polyps generally have no signs or symptoms.

1. When larger, polyps may cause visible rectal bleeding.

2. Polyps may also cause occult bleeding, detected by a screening examination, though the sensitivity and specificity of screening tests for detecting polyps are low.

3. Very large polyps, particularly small bowel hamartomas, can cause intussusception.

B. Polyps are almost always detected by sigmoidoscopic or colon examination performed either for screening or for an unrelated problem. The pathology of polyps cannot be determined by radiologic testing. Therefore, polyps identified by x-ray require direct visualization and removal.

C. Diagnostic testing for colon polyps includes endoscopic examination of the colon or air-contrast barium enema.

1. Full-column barium enema is too insensitive for detecting smaller polyps.

2. The sensitivity of air-contrast barium enema for the detection of polyps varies.

3. Colonoscopy is the most sensitive method for detecting polyps. It also allows removal and pathologic evaluation.

4. Flexible sigmoidoscopy to 60 cm is the method presently used to screen populations for colon cancer and polyps.

   a. Patients found to have adenomatous polyps on flexible sigmoidoscopy should have colonoscopy because of the presence of multiple polyps in 30% of patients.

   b. The follow-up of patients with hyperplastic polyps is controversial because of the debate over the association of hyperplastic and adenomatous polyps.

   c. The pathology of diminutive polyps seen on screening examination can be determined only by microscopic evaluation.

V. Differential Diagnosis

The differential diagnosis of polyps depends on their pathologic appearance. The concern about polyps focuses on the risk of malignancy arising in these tissues.

A. Adenomatous polyps are benign glandular neoplasms occurring in three patterns: tubular, villous, and tubulovillous. The risk of malignancy in adenomatous polyps relates to the size and number of villous features.

B. Hyperplastic or metaplastic polyps are not true neoplasms. They are mucosal excrescences representing epithelial hyperplasia. These polyps have no malignant potential.

C. Hamartomatous polyps are conglomerations of tissue normally present in the intestine. The risk of malignancy is slightly increased.

D. Inflammatory polyps or pseudopolyps are associated with inflammatory bowel disease. They are not neoplastic and represent regenerated or residual tissue from the extensive inflammatory process. There is no malignant potential.

E. The presence of more than 100 adenomatous polyps is required for a diagnosis of familial polyposis and Gardner's syndrome. Other syndromes require extraintestinal findings.

VI. Treatment

The treatment of polyps is removal by either endoscopic or surgical techniques. The size, number, and location will of the polyps determine the most appropriate approach.

VII. Patient Monitoring

A. Adenomatous polyps require follow-up examination. Up to 30% of patients with these polyps will be found to have them 1 year later.

1. Current recommendations for screening patients at low risk for cancer include flexible sigmoidoscopy for 2 consecutive years starting at age 50, with subsequent exams every 3–5 years. There is no consensus about the efficacy of this approach.

2. Patients with more than one polyp are at greater risk of developing polyps in the future.

3. Once polyps are identified, they should be removed unless the patient's circumstances dictate otherwise.

4. The long-term follow-up of patients with polyps is not well defined. Repeat

colonoscopy every 3 years after a second examination 1 year after the initial polyp is identified is one of the current recommendations.

B. There is controversy regarding follow-up for nonadenomatous polyps.

VIII. Prognosis

The prognosis for patients with colon polyps is excellent. Most colon cancers could probably be prevented if patients with polyps were identified early.

Bibliography

Bronner MP, Haggitt RC. The polyp-cancer sequence: Do all colorectal cancers arise from benign adenomas. *Gastrointest Endoscopy Clin NA* 3:611–622, 1993.

Burt RW, Samowitz WS. The adenomatous polyp and the hereditary polyposis syndromes. *Gastrointest Clin North Am* 17:657–678, 1988.

O'Brien MJ, Winawer SJ, Zauber AG, et al. The National Polyp Study. Patient and polyp characteristics associated with high-grade dysplasia in colorectal adenomas. *Gastroenterology* 98:371, 1990.

CHAPTER 58-J

Carcinoid Syndrome

Jack Ohringer, M.D.
Michael D. Brown, M.D.

I. **Definition**

Carcinoid syndrome is a rare syndrome associated with diarrhea, abdominal cramping, flushing, telangiectasia, cyanosis, skin lesions, bronchospasm, and heart murmurs caused by humoral factors secreted by tumors originating in the digestive or pulmonary tract.

II. **Etiology**

A. Carcinoid tumors arise from enterochromaffin or enterochromaffin-like cells.

B. The characteristic features of the tumors are determined by their site of origin. The enterochromaffin cell is characterized biochemically by the characteristics of its *amine content*, *precursor uptake*, and *decarboxylation*, and is therefore known by the acronym *APUD*. More than 90% of carcinoid tumors originate in the gastrointestinal (GI) tract.

C. The most frequent sites in the GI tract, in descending order, are the appendix, terminal ileum, and rectum. Rarely, the colon, stomach, and duodenum may also harbor carcinoid tumors.

III. **Pathophysiology**

A. The syndrome is due to the increased production of a variety of substances, principally 5-hydroxytryptamine (serotonin), 5-hydroxytryptophan, histamine, kinins, catecholamines, and prostaglandins.

B. Peptide hormones have also been reported to be secreted excessively in this syndrome.

C. Although carcinoid tumors may differ widely in their ability to produce these substances, the most characteristic abnormality is the production of serotonin and its subsequent metabolite, 5-hydroxyindoleacetic acid (5-HIAA).

D. In patients with carcinoid syndrome, dietary tryptophan is hydroxylated to 5-hydroxytryptophan and is subsequently decarboxylated to serotonin.

E. The pharmacologic effects of serotonin mediate the production of symptoms including diarrhea, intestinal hypermotility, nausea, vomiting, and abdominal pain.

F. Serotonin may also be responsible for the fibrosis observed within the heart due to the stimulation of fibroblasts.

G. Serotonin may also be responsible for the bronchospasm observed in the syndrome.

H. Kinins produced, specifically bradykinin, lysyl-bradykinin, and tachykinins, are likely to be responsible for the flushing episodes observed.

IV. **Diagnosis**

The diagnosis of carcinoid tumors is based upon special studies on tissue obtained at biopsy. Often suspicion exists in regard to patients with clinical or biochemical evidence of the syndrome.

A. History

Patients with a history of the classic carcinoid syndrome, including diarrhea, abdominal cramping, flushing, nausea and vomiting, telangiectasia, weight loss, and bronchospasm, should be evaluated biochemically. Not all patients with carcinoid tumors will exhibit features of the syndrome. Some will complain of abdominal obstruction, rectal bleeding, or cough.

B. Clinical signs and physical diagnosis

The finding of telangiectasia may alert the clinician to the possibility of carcinoid tumors. New onset of wheezing, flushing episodes, or psychosis may be associated with the carcinoid syndrome. Crampy abdominal pain, rectal bleeding, or isolated hepatomegaly are nonspecific signs which may occur due to the tumor burden.

C. Tests

1. Routine laboratory tests are generally useless. Liver metastases may cause an increase in alkaline phosphatase and gamma glutamyl transferase. Fat malabsorption may occur and may be quantified in the stool. Chest x-ray may reveal a carcinoid lesion in the lung. Upper GI exam may demonstrate carcinoid lesions in the esophagus, stomach, duodenum, and jejunum. Endoscopic procedures are useful in confirming this diagnosis and obtaining tissue for histologic confirmation. Approximately 50% of patients with carcinoid tumors have other areas of involvement, and these tumors should be sought. Computed tomography (CT) scanning is extremely useful in evaluating the location and extent of disease. If disease is identified in the liver, it can be biopsied under CT guidance to obtain a tissue specimen. Metastatic deposits to the liver tend to be highly vascular, and angiography may be useful.

2. The biochemical marker most useful in diagnosing carcinoid syndrome is increased urinary 5-HIAA. Although the range is wide, most patients excrete 60–1,000 mg/day. A variety of medications can falsely elevate or decrease the urinary 5-HIAA level. Certain foods rich in serotonin such as bananas, pineapples, avocados, tomatoes, red plums, eggplant, and walnuts should be avoided. Gastric and bronchial carcinoids secrete 5-hydroxytryptophan, which is converted to serotonin in the kidney. In such cases, 5-hydroxytryptophan may be excreted in the urine. Serotonin can be measured in the blood. Because ectopic production of hormones occurs, particularly from tumors derived from the pancreas and bronchus, measurement of adrenocorticotropic hormone, melanocyte-stimulating hormone, insulin, gastrin, glucagon, 17-hydroxysteroids, and ketosteroids is indicated in the appropriate clinical setting suggesting overproduction.

V. **Differential Diagnosis**

A. Without metastases (depending on the location of the primary tumor)

1. Lung
   a. Carcinoma of the lung
2. Stomach and small bowel
   a. Carcinoma of stomach or the small bowel
   b. Acute appendicitis
   c. Crohn's disease
   d. Leiomyoma
   e. Lymphoma
3. Colon
   a. Carcinoma of the colon
   b. Lymphoma
   c. Leiomyoma

B. With metastases (carcinoid syndrome)

1. Menopause
2. Cirrhosis
3. Idiopathic flushing
4. Systemic mastocytosis

VI. **Treatment**

Treatment depends on the location of the primary tumor. Appendiceal carcinoids seldom mestastasize, but they do so commonly when of extra-appendiceal origin. Carcinoid tumors originating in the abdomen grow slowly. Even after they metastasize to the liver, survival for 5 to 10 years is not uncommon. Bronchial carcinoids tend to be more aggressive.

A. Surgical treatment

1. Patients with carcinoid syndrome generally have metastatic disease and cannot be

cured with surgery except in the very rare cases of primary ovarian or bronchial tumor causing the symptoms.

2. Indicated for GI tumors causing obstructive symptoms.

3. Risk of surgery is increased due to the possibility of anesthesia or surgical manipulation causing carcinoid crisis.

4. A long-acting somatostatin analogue, octreotide acetate (Sandostatin™) is indicated for the treatment of diarrhea and the symptoms of the carcinoid syndrome. It may also result in some slowing of tumor growth.

B. Medical treatment

1. Methysergide maleate (serotonin antagonist), in a dose of 6–24 mg/day, controls flushing, asthma, and diarrhea.

2. Cyproheptadine, another serotonin antagonist (6–30 mg/day), can also control attacks with fewer side effects. It can be used in acute attacks in a dose of 50–75 mg infused over 1 to 2 hr.

3. A combination of H1 and H2 receptor antagonists: Diphenhydramine hydrochloride, 50 mg every 6 hr, with cimetidine, 300 mg every 6 hr, can block the flushing.

4. Corticosteroids may help patients with bronchial carcinoids.

5. Prochlorperazine, 10 mg three times per day, is occasionally helpful.

6. Phenoxybenzamine, 10–30 mg daily, may help prevent kallikrein release.

7. Methyldopa, 250–500 mg every 6 hr, may help diarrhea.

8. Somatostatin analogues suppress flushing, hypotension, and diarrhea.

C. Chemotherapy

1. Responses seen with a combination of 5-fluorouracil and streptotocin.

VII. Patient Monitoring

A. Assess the nutritional state.

B. Search for signs of heart failure.

C. Assess the hydrational status.

D. Search for signs of intestinal obstruction.

E. Assess for possible jaundice.

F. Treat diarrhea with loperimide, diphenoxylate or octreotide acetate.

VIII. Prognosis

This depends on the location of the primary tumor. Patients with ileal carcinoids with metastases to the liver may live for as long as 23 years. Patients with bronchial carcinoids have a much poorer prognosis, similar to that of carcinoma.

Bibliography

Basser RL, Green MD. Recent advances in carcinoids and gastrointestinal neuroendocrine tumors. *Curr Opin Oncol* 3:109–120, 1991.

Kvols LK, Reubi JC. Metastatic carcinoid tumors and the malignant carcinoid syndrome. *Acta Oncol* 32:197–201, 1993.

Marshall JB, Bodnarchuk G. Carcinoid tumors of the gut. Our experience over three decades and review of the literature. *J Clin Gastroenterol* 16:123–129, 1993.

Vinik AI, Thompson N, Eckhauser F, et al: Clinical features of carcinoid syndrome and the use of somatostatin analogue in its management. *Acta Oncol* 28:389–402, 1989.

Vinik AI, McLeod MK, Fig LM, et al: Clinical features, diagnosis, and localization of carcinoid tumors and their management. *Gastroenterol Clin North Am* 18:865–896, 1989.

Chapter 58-K

Irritable Bowel Syndrome

Bennett Plotnick, M.D.

I. Definition

Irritable bowel syndrome is a functional disorder of the gastrointestinal system characterized by abdominal pain, bloating, and altered stool frequency and consistency. Symptoms of disturbed defecation are also frequently present.

II. Etiology

A. Occurs in 15–20% of adults.

B. Females are more likely to see a physician.

C. Occurrence of personality and emotional disorders or threatening life events are probably important in distinguishing patients with irritable bowel syndrome from those who do not seek medical advice.

III. Pathophysiology

The actual mechanism is unknown, but several theories are based on epidemiologic, physiologic, and psychopathologic data.

A. Epidemiology

1. Low frequency of irritable bowel syndrome in African countries may be related to their relatively high intake of dietary fiber.

2. Patients with irritable bowel syndrome may be more likely to have other somatic symptoms.

3. The onset of irritable bowel syndrome may follow symptoms of viral gastroenteritis.

B. Physiology

1. While evidence is far from conclusive, some studies have shown abnormal gut motility and a lowered threshold to maneuvers which simulate luminal distention.

C. Psychopathology

1. From 40% to 50% of patients meet criteria for psychiatric disease.

2. Patients with irritable bowel syndrome are more likely to experience stressful life events prior to developing symptoms.

3. Patients with irritable bowel syndrome tend to seek health care and exhibit illness behavior more frequently than normal people.

4. Patients with irritable bowel syndrome may have a high incidence of previous physical or sexual abuse.

IV. Diagnosis

A. History: frequently useful

1. Abdominal pain that is relieved or altered by defecation, or altered stool frequency or consistency in relation to the pain.

2. Abdominal distention or bloating.

3. Sensation of rectal fullness or incomplete evacuation.
4. Mucous stools.
5. Important to exclude organic etiologies such as lactose intolerance, drug side effects, laxative abuse, and artificial sweeteners.

B. Clinical signs and physical findings
1. With the exception of multiple abdominal scars, there are no agreed-upon signs of irritable bowel syndrome.

C. Diagnostic tests
1. Complete blood count and erythrocyte sedimentation rate may suggest organic pathology.
2. Sigmoidoscopy may reveal proctitis or melanosis coli, indicating laxative abuse.
3. Barium enema useful for patients older than 40.
4. Stool exam for giardiasis and fecal fat.
5. Lactose exclusion diet.
6. Gallbladder ultrasound scan and upper gastrointestinal x-ray for patients with dyspepsia.

V. **Differential Diagnosis**
Specific diagnostic alternatives depend on the prominence of certain symptoms.
A. Pain
1. Gallbladder disease.
2. Intestinal obstruction.
3. Intermittent porphyria.
4. Angina pectoris.
5. Lead poisoning.
B. Diarrhea
1. Lactose intolerance or laxative abuse.
2. Secretory diarrhea: carcinoid, gastrinoma, VIPoma, and choleretic diarrhea in short bowel patients.
3. Inflammatory bowel disease.
4. Hyperthyroidism or Addison's disease.
C. Constipation
1. Medication side effects.

2. Laxative dependence.
3. Factitious.
4. Hypothyroidism or hypoparathyroidism.

VI. **Treatment**
A. The patient should be assured that organic pathology has been excluded.
B. Recognizable causes should be sought and avoided.
C. Psychologic management should focus on reassurance and support. Sedatives and antidepressants should be avoided.
D. High-fiber diets, especially for those with constipation. Psyllium preparations are useful adjuncts.
E. Antidiarrheal agents such as lomotil or loperamide are beneficial when diarrhea is severe.
F. Antispasmodics are given in anticipation of painful cramping.
G. Treatment of excessive gas is rarely successful.

VII. **Patient Monitering**
Patients with irritable bowel syndrome should be followed and monitered on a regular basis. Development of symptoms or signs of organic disease needs to be sought and evaluated appropriately.

VIII. **Prognosis**
Although irritable bowel syndrome is associated with severe pain and discomfort, there is no predisposition to offer life-threatening or chronic conditions. There is also no evidence that it affects longevity.

Bibliography

Friedman G. The irritable bowel syndrome. Realities and trends, *Gastroenterol Clin North Am* 25, 1991.

Schuster M. Irritable bowel syndrome, in Sleisenger MH (ed): *Gastrointestinal Disease*, ed 4. Philadelphia, Saunders, 1989, p 1402.

Sleisenger MH, Fordtran JS. The irritable bowel syndrome. *Semin Gastrointest Dis* 1:1, 1990.

CHAPTER 58-L

Small Intestine Motility Disorders

Sheldon Sloan, M.D.

I. **Introduction**
   A. To understand the disease states within the small intestine, it is important to understand the normal motility patterns that exist. Normal gastrointestinal motility is characterized by a cyclical motor activity during the fasting state known as the *interdigestive motor complex* (see Chapter 57A). This motor complex originates in the gastroduodenal region and propagates caudally for various distances down the small bowel. Phase I of the interdigestive motor complex is a quiescent period with minimal contractle activity. Phase II is a period of intermittent phasic pressure activity. Phase III, also called the *migrating motor complex (MMC)* or *housekeeper complex*, is characterized by regular, repetitive contractions propagated to the distal small bowel with a frequency of up to 12/min and lasting approximately for 10 min. Phase IV is a return to less organized and less frequent contractile activity.
   B. Disorders of small intestinal motility can be subdivided into structural, myopathic, and neuropathic etiologies.
   C. Small intestine motility is measured using manometric techniques involving a catheter with multiple pressure measuring ports spaced approximately 10 cm apart that is fluoroscopically positioned after nasogastric tube insertion.

II. **Structural Disorders Leading to Abnormal Small Bowel Motility**
   A. Gastric surgery may disrupt small bowel motility. Tonic contractile activity of the gastric remnant may be abnormal after vagotomy.
   B. Partial bowel obstruction has been shown to have abnormal contractile patterns. They consist of bursts of activity after eating which last for about 1 min and occur every 1 to 2 min.
   C. Superior mesenteric artery syndrome in young, active women who have recurrent vomiting and abdominal pain may have an abnormal proximal small bowel motility pattern explaining the duodenal dilatation and hypoactivity rather than a mechanical cause.

III. **Myopathic Disorders**
   A. Amyloidosis causes dysfunction by infiltration of the muscle layers.
   B. Progressive systemic sclerosis (scleroderma) involves the smooth muscle, causing fibrosis and atrophy.
   C. Dystrophia myotonica is associated with ab-

normal motility throughout the gastrointestinal tract. Pathologically, there are degenerative changes, with fatty infiltration and collagen deposition among the smooth muscle.

D. Hollow visceral myopathy is a generalized disorder of the gastrointestinal smooth muscle which is characterized histologically by degeneration and fibrosis of the circular and longitudinal muscle layers. Patients may also have involvement of the genitourinary tract. They may have limited or extensive disease of the gut. This disorder may be transmitted genetically, as either an autosomal dominant or recessive trait, or may occur sporadically.

IV. Neuropathic Disorders

A. Peripheral neuropathy
1. Acute causes secondary to viral infections such as Epstein-Barr virus, herpes zoster, and Guillain-Barré syndrome are associated with persistent gut motility abnormalities.
2. Diabetes mellitus is associated with a decrease in distal antral contractions during phase III of the interdigestive motor complex. There are also reduced postprandial phasic pressures in the duodenum, nonpropagated uncoordinated bursts of contraction in the proximal small bowel, and pylorospasm.
3. Amyloid neuropathy may cause a syndrome similar to pseudo-obstruction. Uncoordinated, nonpropagated phasic pressure bursts in the small bowel are seen manometrically.
4. Other conditions associated with a chronic peripheral neuropathy include:
    a. Chronic autonomic neuropathy with neuronal intranuclear inclusions.
    b. Chronic sensory and autonomic neuropathy of unknown etiology.
    c. Neurofibromatosis.
    d. Paraneoplastic neuropathy.
    e. Drug-induced neuropathy.
B. Pandysautonomia.
C. Idiopathic orthostatic hypotension.
D. Spinal cord injury.
E. Parkinson's disease.
F. Epilepsy.
G. Multiple sclerosis.
H. Brain stem lesions.
I. Chronic intestinal pseudo-obstruction.

V. Irritable Bowel Syndrome

Abnormal interdigestive motor complexes ranging from a decreased to an increased number of MMCs have been described.

Bibliography

Camilleri M, Phillips SF. Disorders of small intestinal motility. *Gastroenterol Clin North Am* 18:405–424, 1989.

Sarna SK, Otterson MF. Small intestinal physiology and pathophysiology. *Gastroenterol Clin North Am* 18:375–404, 1989.

Acute Pancreatitis

Donald M. Jensen, M.D.

I. Definition

A single episode of pancreatic inflammation resulting from the intrapancreatic activation of proteolytic and lipolytic enzymes.

A. Acute edematous pancreatitis. A self-limited episode of mild to moderate severity characterized by interstitial edema of the pancreas.

B. Acute hemorrhagic pancreatitis. Moderate to severe pancreatic inflammation leading to coagulative necrosis and focal hemorrhage. This may spread to surrounding tissue.

II. Etiology

A. Alcohol consumption.

B. Biliary tract disease and gallstones.

C. Metabolic disorders

1. Hypertriglyceridemia (usually >1,000 mg/dl).

2. Hypercalcemia.

D. Endoscopic retrograde cholangiopancreatography (ERCP) (less than 1% of cases).

E. Postoperative—usually abdominal procedures.

F. Medications—including thiazides, estrogens, sulfonamides, azathioprine, tetracycline, valproic acid, and furosemide.

G. Infections—mumps, viral hepatitis, coxsackie virus, and mycoplasma.

H. Duodenal ulcer—penetrating posteriorly.

I. Pancreas divisum.

J. Collagen-vascular diseases, particularly systemic lupus erythematosus.

K. Renal failure and postrenal transplantation.

L. Blunt abdominal trauma.

M. Hereditary pancreatitis.

N. Scorpion bites.

O. Parasites—flukes and worms.

P. Ischemia/hypotension.

III. Pathophysiology

Although the exact mechanism(s) is largely unknown, intrapancreatic activation of digestive enzymes occurs, leading to a cascade of secondary phenomena including release of histamine, bradykinin, and other vasoactive substances. Recent evidence suggests that zymogen granules may fuse with lysosomes, resulting in cathepsin-mediated conversion of trypsinogen to trypsin.

IV. Diagnosis

A. History: In the appropriate etiologic setting, a history of abdominal pain, with or without

nausea, vomiting, and abdominal distention, should suggest the diagnosis. The pain
is typically epigastric in location but may be
periumbilical or located in the right or left
upper quadrant. The pain is usually described as boring and dull, with radiation to
the back or flank.
  B. Clinical signs and physical findings: Tachycardia, fever, and hypotension may occur,
associated with third-space fluid sequestration in the retroperitoneum. Abdominal
tenderness, with decreased or absent bowel
sounds, is often present. Jaundice may occur
if there is associated bile duct obstruction.
  C. Diagnostic tests
    1. Laboratory studies: Acute pancreatitis is
typically associated with an increase in
serum and urinary amylase activity. An
increased serum lipase level confirms the
pancreatic origin of the amylase. Anemia, leukocytosis, hyperglycemia, hypocalcemia, and elevated aminotransferase
and lactic dehydrogenase levels (LDH)
may also occur and may have prognostic
value. Hypoxemia and metabolic acidosis
may be present in severe cases.
    2. Radiographic studies: A plain x-ray of
the abdomen may disclose an ileus, bowel
perforation, or intestinal ischemia. Computed tomography (CT) scanning is very
useful in severe or unresolved cases to
detect areas of necrosis, secondary bacterial infection, hemorrhage, and pseudocysts. ERCP may prove useful in some
patients with suspected gallstone pancreatitis. Ultrasonography may detect gallstones.
  V. **Differential Diagnosis**
The differential diagnosis of acute pancreatitis
is lengthy but can be divided into biliary tract,
intestinal, vascular, and miscellaneous categories.
  A. Biliary tract disease
    1. Acute cholecystitis
    2. Choledocholithiasis with biliary colic
    3. Ascending cholangitis
  B. Intestinal disorders
    1. Peptic ulcer disease (penetrating)
    2. Perforated viscus
    3. Acute intestinal obstruction
    4. Mesenteric ischemia/infarction
    5. Appendicitis
  C. Vascular disorders
    1. Myocardial infarction

    2. Dissecting aneurysm
    3. Vasculitis
  D. Miscellaneousa conditions
    1. Viral hepatitis
    2. Alcohol hepatitis
    3. Pneumonia
    4. Renal colic
    5. Diabetic ketoacidosis
  VI. **Treatment**
Since episodes of acute pancreatitis resolve
without sequelae in 85–90% of patients, good
supportive care is all that is necessary.
  A. Fluid resuscitation: Volume depletion should
be corrected promptly with intravenous fluids and electrolytes. In some cases, as much
as 4–6 liters may be necessary during the
first 24 hr.
  B. Pain control: Meperidine (Demerol), 50–
100 mg every 4–6 hr IV or IM, is the preferred agent.
  C. Resting the pancreas: Patients should remain NPO until pain improves and inflammation subsides. Patients with ileus, nausea,
or vomiting should have nasogastric suction.
  D. Nutritional support may become necessary in
patients whose disease is particularly severe or
protracted (NPO more than 3–5 days). Oral
refeeding should proceed slowly with a high-
carbohydrate, low-protein, low-fat diet.
  E. Approach to complications
    1. Hemorrhagic pancreatitis, infected pan-
creatic necrosis, abscess, and infected acute
pseudocysts usually require surgical drainage. CT scanning may be particularly useful in recognizing these complications.
    2. Systemic complications such as Adult
Respiratory Distress Syndrome (ARDS),
pleural effusions, and renal insufficiency
should be aggressively treated.
  VII. **Patient Monitoring**
  A. Fluid and electrolytes: Urine output should
be carefully recorded. Serum electrolytes,
blood urea nitrogen, creatinine, glucose,
and calcium should be monitored at least
daily. Magnesium and zinc deficiencies
should be assessed and replaced as needed.
  B. Amylase, lipase, and liver enzymes should
be measured and followed closely over the
initial 48 hr.
  C. Arterial blood gases should be assessed at
admission and at 48 hr, more often if necessary.
  D. Clinical examination may be the most useful
monitoring tool to detect deterioration.

VIII. Prognosis

Prognostic factors have been well described from acute pancreatitis.

A. On admission:
   Age >55 years
   WBC >16,000/mm^3
   Glucose >300 mg/dl
   LDH >350 U/liter
   SGOT >250 SF U

B. During initial 48 hr:
   Hematocrit fall >10%
   BUN rise >5 mg/dl
   Calcium <8 mg/dl

   PaO$_2$ <60 mm Hg
   Base deficit >4 mEq/liter

C. Interpretation of results

No. of positive signs:	0–2	3–4	5–6	7–8
Mortality rate:	0.9%	16%	40%	100%

Bibliography

Balthazar E, Ranson JHC, Naidich D, et al: Acute pancreatitis: prognostic value of computed tomography. *Radiology* 156:767, 1985.

Ranson JHC: Etiologic and prognostic factors in human acute pancreatitis. *Am J Gastroenterol* 77:633, 1982.

Chronic Pancreatitis

Donald M. Jensen, M.D.

I. Definition

Chronic pancreatitis is characterized by persistent or recurrent abdominal pain, with or without pancreatic insufficiency, and histologic evidence of fibrosis and destruction of acinar cells.

II. Etiology

A. Alcohol is the most important contributing factor to the development of chronic pancreatitis, accounting for more that 60% of all cases and 90% of cases of calcific pancreatitis. In general, consumption of at least 50 g of alcohol daily for 5 to 20 years is necessary before the first attack.

B. Metabolic disorders
1. Hypercalcemia
2. Hyperlipidemia
3. Porphyria
4. Hemochromatosis

C. Congenital conditions
1. Pancreas divisum
2. Cystic fibrosis
3. Schwachman syndrome
4. Hereditary pancreatitis

D. Trauma

E. Tropic chronic pancreatitis

F. Idiopathic

III. Pathophysiology

The pathogenesis of acute and chronic pancreatitis is unknown. However, in alcohol-induced chronic pancreatitis there may be precipitation of an alcohol "stone" protein in the pancreatic ducts which has an affinity for calcium, leading to the calcific changes observed.

IV. Diagnosis

A. Clinical presentation
1. Abdominal pain occurs in over 90% of individuals and is indistinguishable from that seen in acute pancreatitis. Typically, the pain is epigastric in location but may be periumbilical or in the right or left upper quadrant, and is steady and boring in nature.
2. Weight loss is common. It may be due to several factors, including the following:
   a. Malabsorption of fat and protein secondary to insufficient lipase and proteolytic enzyme activity.
   b. Anorexia due to chronic abdominal pain and long-term use of narcotic analgesics.
   c. Glycosuria secondary to diabetes mellitus due to islet cell loss.

B. Physical examination: There are no physical findings specific for chronic pancreatitis. Cachexia and abdominal tenderness in the midepigastrium may suggest the diagnosis.

C. Laboratory investigations
1. Serum amylase levels during an acute attack, but these are often normal and may be depressed.
2. Macrocytic anemia may occur in up to 50% of patients due to vitamin B_{12} malabsorption.
3. Steatorrhea in excess of 10 g/day on a 100-g fat diet.
4. Tests of exocrine pancreatic function
   a. Secretin test: An orally passed triple-lumen tube (Dreiling tube) is positioned fluoroscopically at the ligament of Treitz, and 1 U of secretin per kilogram is given intravenously over 1 min. Duodenal fluid is collected and analyzed for HCO_3^-. A level below 90 mEq/liter suggests the diagnosis.
   b. Bentironide test: Patients ingest orally 500 mg of bentironide, a synthetic peptide, which is cleaved by pancreatic proteolytic enzymes (chyneotrypsin) to release para-aminobenzoic acid (PABA). PABA is absorbed from the proximal small intestine, conjugated by the liver, and excreted in the urine. Recovery of less than 60% of the liberated PABA in a 6-hr urine collection suggests pancreatic insufficiency.
5. Radiologic studies
   a. Plain x-ray of the abdomen may demonstrate pancreatic calcifications (in one-third of patients).
   b. Malabsorption syndromes: Small intestinal diseases such as sprue, Crohn's disease, and lymphoma should be considered in the differential diagnosis of weight loss and steatorrhea.

V. **Treatment**
A. Pain management
1. Discontinue alcohol ingestion.
2. Small feedings and analgesics.
3. Pancreatic enzyme replacement: Even in the absence of significant steatorrhea, the abdominal pain in some individuals may improve after a trial of pancreatic enzymes.
4. Obliteration of the celiac ganglion: Percutaneous injection of alcohol into the ganglion has been associated with pain relief for as long as 6 months.

5. Surgery
   a. Longitudinal pancreaticojujunostomy (Puestow procedure).
   b. Caudal pancreaticojejunostomy (Duval procedure).
   c. Sphincteroplasty.
   d. Pancreatic resection.
6. Therapeutic endoscopic retrograde cholangiopancreatography.
   a. Sphincterotomy.
   b. Pancreatic duct stents.
B. Malabsorption (maldigestion)
1. Pancreatic enzyme replacement: To eliminate malabsorption of fats, at least 30,000 IU of lipase must be delivered to the duodenum with each meal. Since pancreatic enzyme is inactivated by a pH less than 4.0, H_2 blockers are administered concomitantly.
C. Diabetes mellitus: Insulin therapy is often required, but patients are also prone to develop hypoglycemia secondary to glucagon deficiency.
D. Nutritional support: Small, frequent feedings high in protein are better tolerated. Oral medium chain triglycerides may be substituted for long chain triglycerides to improve fat intake.

VI. **Patient Monitoring**
A. Analgesic requirements: Analgesic use may eventually decrease with progressive destruction of the pancreas. Unfortunately, many patients become addicted to the narcotic.
B. Nutritional requirements
1. Weight loss: Periodic measurements of weight are important.
2. Fecal fat: Persistent steatorrhea may indicate inadequate pancreatic enzyme replacement or overindulgence.
3. Vitamin supplementation.
4. Blood sugar and ketones.

VII. **Prognosis**
The mortality rate is approximately 3–4% per year, but less than half of the deaths are directly attributable to the pancreatic disease. Pancreatic carcinoma is unusual except in hereditary pancreatitis.

Bibliography

DiMagno EP. Medical treatment of pancreatic insufficiency. *Mayo Clin Proc* 54:435, 1979.

Singer MV, Gyr K, Sarles H. Revised classification of pancreatitis. *Gastroenterology* 89:683, 1985.

CHAPTER 60

Acute Cholecystitis

Michael Uzer, M.D.

I. Definition
An acute inflammation of the gallbladder wall.

II. Etiology
A. Calculous: Transient obstruction of the cystic duct by gallstones. Accounts for more than 90% of cases.
B. Acalculous: Less common; occurs in critically ill, hospitalized patients.

III. Pathophysiology
A. Cystic duct obstruction in the presence of saturated bile triggers a prostaglandin-mediated inflammatory response. The gallbladder mucosa secretes water, resulting in distention, increased luminal pressure, and impaired gallbladder perfusion, which can lead to necrosis and perforation.
B. Bacterial infection plays a secondary role, and bile cultures are positive in one-half of patients with acute cholecystitis.
C. Bile stasis and increased lithogenicity of bile are believed to be important in the pathogenesis of acalculous cholecystitis.

IV. Diagnosis
A. History
   1. Most common in older women.
   2. Pain is typically constant and localizes to the right subcostal region. Pain does not usually radiate.
B. Clinical signs and physical findings
   1. Right upper quadrant tenderness, involuntary guarding, and fever.
   2. Peritoneal signs uncommon unless perforation has occurred.
   3. A tender, palpable gallbladder is pathognomonic but is present in only 20% of patients.
C. Diagnostic tests
   1. Laboratory: Leukocytosis, mild transaminase and alkaline phosphatase elevations; mild bilirubin and amylase elevations not uncommon.
   2. Radiology
      A. Plain film: May show calcified gallstones, biliary air, or free peritoneal air.
      B. Ultrasound: Thickened gallbladder wall, pericholecystic fluid, gallbladder distention.
      C. Scintigraphy HIDA, PIPIDA, DISIDA
         1. Test of choice.

2. Failure of gallbladder to visualize at 45 min.
3. False-positive: Severe hepatocellular disease hyperalimentation.
4. Severe jaundice may not allow adequate excretion of dye to evaluate gallbladder filling and cystic duct patency.

V. Differential Diagnosis

A. Acute pancreatitis.
B. Perforated gastroduodenal ulcers.
C. Right-sided nephrolithiasis.
D. Acute hepatitis.
E. Hepatic congestion due to right heart failure.
F. Hepatic abscess, primary or metastatic tumors.
G. Myocardial infarction of the inferior wall.
H. Acute appendicitis.
I. Cholangitis.

VI. Treatment

A. Antibiotics: against coliforms, enterococci, *Pseudomonas*.
B. Surgery
   1. Early surgery (by 48 hr) preferable unless a serious contraindication exists.
   2. Late: 6–8 weeks after successful medical management.
   3. Laparoscopic technique feasible even in the acute setting.
C. Nonsurgical intervention

1. Percutaneous cholecystostomy for drainage.
2. Newer techniques for extracting or pulverizing stones percutaneously.

VII. Patient Monitoring

Acute cholecystitis may be complicated by a number of processes for which the clinician must be alert:

A. Choledocholithiasis: 15–20%
B. Empyema of the gallbladder.
C. Ischemia/infarction of the gallbladder.
D. Perforation.
E. Biliary-enteric fistula leading to gallstone ileus or cholangitis.

VIII. Prognosis

A. Depends on the presence of concomitant complicating illness and suppurative complications.
B. Overall mortality for calculous cholecystitis is 5%.
C. Mortality for acalculous cholecystitis approaches 40%.

Bibliography

Jivegard L, Thornell E, Svanvik J. Pathophysiology of acute obstructive cholecystitis: implications for non-operative management. *Br J Surg* 74:1084–1086, 1987.

Sievert W, Vakil NB. Emergencies of the biliary tract. *Gastroenterol Clin North Am* 17:245–265, 1988.

CHAPTER 61-A

Cirrhosis

Daniel R. Ganger, M.D.

I. Definition

Cirrhosis is a diffuse process characterized by fibrosis and the conversion of normal liver architecture into abnormal nodules. It is the end result of different chronic liver diseases following hepatocellular necrosis. Fibrosis alone or nodular formation without fibrosis is not sufficient to establish the diagnosis of cirrhosis. It can be subdividred according to morphology, etiology, stage of development, and speed of progression.

The morphologic classification is based on the size of the nodules:

A. *Micronodular:* Thick, regular septa, nodules of almost equal size, 0.5 to 1 cm in diameter, involving every lobule.

B. *Macronodular:* Septa and nodules of variable size, 1 to 5 cm in diameter, with collapse and regeneration reflected by large cells and plates of cells of different thickness. This usually represents a later stage.

C. *Mixed:* The process of regeneration in a micronodular pattern results in a macronodular or mixed type.

This classification may be of limited clinical value, although traditionally morphology has been associated with etiology, that is, a micronodular pattern and alcoholism.

II. Etiology

A. The etiology of cirrhosis is usually a single entity, although genetic, environmental, and metabolic factors may add to the development and speed of progression of the disease.

B. The following etiologies have been associated with cirrhosis:

1. Viral: Following hepatitis B, B and D, C, and non-B, non-C types.

2. Alcohol abuse.

3. Metabolic: Iron overload (hemochromatosis), Wilson's disease, α-1-antitrypsin deficiency, type IV glycogenesis, congenital tyrosinosis, galactosemia, cystic fibrosis, prolonged malnutrition, and long-term parenteral hyperalimentation, particularly with short bowel syndrome and after jejunoileal bypass surgery.

4. Biliary: Primary or secondary to biliary obstruction.

5. Autoimmune (formerly known as *lupoid*).

6. Hepatic venous outflow: Chronic Budd-Chiari syndrome, severe right-sided heart failure.
7. Drugs and toxins: Amiodarone, methotrexate (in combination with alcohol abuse), isoniazid, vitamin A used in excess, carbon tetrachloride
8. Indian childhood cirrhosis.
9. Syphilis (in neonates).
10. Cryptogenic causes.

III. Pathophysiology

The architectural changes may lead to portal hypertension and its consequences, as well as the destruction of liver parenchyma which results in hepatic cell failure. Inflammatory destructive processes and metabolic disorders will eventually alter hepatocyte function and will often result in the total destruction of functional hepatic cells. The multiple functions of the hepatocyte will therefore be severely impaired, resulting in some of the following conditions:

A. Decrease synthesis of proteins (e.g., albumin, transferrin, retinol-binding protein). Decreased synthesis of vitamin K–dependent plasma proteins (factors II, IX, X, and VII, protein C, protein S), fibrinogen, and factor V but only in cases of advanced cirrhosis.
B. Alteration in energy metabolism: Inability to export fuels (glucose and acetoacetate) to peripheral tissues due to problems with gluconeogenesis, glycolysis, glycogen, and fatty acid metabolism).
C. Failure to convert ammonia to urea.
D. Fat metabolism: Impaired triglycerides and cholesterol synthesis, depending on the etiology of the liver disease. In hepatocellular injury (alcoholic, viral hepatitis, and drug induced) there may be transient hypertriglyceridemia. Lipoproteins may be abnormal (decrease in the α band and absence of pre-β). In chronic cholestasis there is hypercholesterolemia (and elevated levels of lipoprotein X). In end-stage cirrhosis, the low cholesterol level reflects a severely impaired synthetic capacity.
E. Impaired detoxification of drugs and toxins: Impaired conjugation (glutathione system) and function of other enzymes that catalyze oxidation.
F. Impaired clearance of plasminogen activators, resulting in enhanced fibrinolysis.
G. Impaired storage and alteration in the canalicular excretion of bilirubin, resulting in jaundice.
H. Decreased synthesis and excretion of bile acids: Results in maldigestion and malabsorption of fat and liposoluble vitamins (A, D, E, K). Vitamin D–impaired activation to 25-hydroxy vitamin D (25-OH-D).
I. Impaired function of the vitamin B complex.
J. Impaired metabolism of hormones: Results in estrogenization and feminization of males. Alteration in insulin metabolism (insulin resistance and diabetes).

IV. Diagnosis

A. History
1. Symptoms are dependent on the stage at presentation.
a. Latent: Cirrhosis may be discovered after an abnormal examination for other reasons, with abnormal biochemistry, as an incidental finding at the time of abdominal surgery, or on sophisticated imaging of the liver (computed tomography).
b. Clinical: There are symptoms and features related to the particular cause. In general, fatigue, anorexia, dyspepsia, abdominal pain or jaundice, loss of libido, abdominal distention, gastrointestinal hemorrhage, or swelling of the lower extremities may be presenting symptoms.
c. End stage: Wasting and weight loss, extreme fatigue, jaundice and ascites. Indistinguishable from the symptoms of any advanced malignancy. Hepatocellular carcinoma often appears in patients with cirrhosis and must be considered.
2. Past history of jaundice, hepatitis, blood product transfusion, medications, toxins, family history of chronic liver disease, travel.
3. Social: Excessive alcohol consumption, intravenous drug use.
B. Clinical signs and physical findings
1. Hepatomegaly may be the first manifestation that will lead the clinician to suspect cirrhosis. A small, shrunken liver is found in end-stage cirrhosis. The normal liver span, as measured in the midclavicular line, is 9–12 cm. A space measuring two finger breadths under the costal margin usually indicates hepatomegaly, ex-

cept in cases of emphysema. The liver feels firm, with round edges initially and then more firm. Auscultation should be performed. A bruit suggests arteriovenous communication, as seen in hepatoma complicating cirrhosis.

2. Splenomegaly: Can be detected on physical exam initially in a minority of patients, although the spleen is usually enlarged on imaging tests (ultrasound, computed tomography). When portal hypertension is present, a spleen tip is often palpable.

3. Stigmata of chronic liver disease: Palmar erythema; vascular spider angiomas on the face, chest, back, and upper extremities; parotid gland enlargement (in alcoholics); gynecomastia and testicular atrophy; feminine pubic hair distribution; Dupuytren's contraction (in alcoholics); and white nails.

4. Fluid overload, hyperdynamic circulation, portal hypertension: Tachycardia, low blood pressure (systolic, 90–110 mmHg), warm skin.

5. Prominent abdominal wall veins, ascites, lower extremity edema, large hemorrhoids, hypertrophic pulmonary osteoarthropathy.

6. Liver cell failure: Jaundice, muscle wasting, fetor hepaticus, asterixis.

7. Epistaxis, gum bleeding, hematomas.

C. Diagnostic tests

1. Liver biopsy: The diagnosis of cirrhosis can be suspected clinically and considered even more strongly when varices are found on endoscopy, but it is confirmed only by the gold standard: liver biopsy. When there are no contraindications, such as ascites or coagulopathy, this test can be performed through the traditional intercostal route, via percutaneous needle biopsy, under ultrasound or laparoscopic guidance (which may help avoid the sampling error) for further safety. In the rare cases in which liver biopsy is essential and a coagulopathy exists, transvenous jugular needle biopsy has been found to be safe. The tissue examination is helpful in establishing the diagnosis and may add to etiology and activity of the process. Serial biopsies are used to assess the progress of the disease, particularly when evaluating a treatment

that might alter the natural course of the disease and when other parameters, such as biochemical tests, are not helpful.

2. Laboratory data: The laboratory presentation of cirrhosis is variable and depends on the stage of the disease.

a. Asymptomatic (latent) cirrhosis: Serum chemistries may be normal, with the exception of a slight increase in transaminase, alkaline phosphatase, or gamma glutamyl transpeptidase levels.

b. Clinical cirrhosis: Serum transaminase elevation represents necrosis or inflammation if the disease process leading to cirrhosis is still active. Alkaline phosphatase may be elevated, particularly when a biliary process is the main cause of cirrhosis. Elevation of unconjugated bilirubin could result from decreased hepatic uptake when there is a significant collateral circulation. Elevation of conjugated bilirubin is seen with cholestasis.

c. Serum albumin levels are below normal as a result of a decreased synthetic function. Elevation of the globulin fraction of the serum total protein may occur concomitantly with the abnormally low serum albumin level, usually as a result of a polycloncal response.

d. The prothrombin time may be prolonged (or depressed if expressed as a percentage of normal) and does not respond to vitamin K therapy. Platelets levels may be lower as an expression of hypersplenism.

e. Virologic (hepatitis B surface antigen, hepatitis B core antibody, hepatitis B e antigen and antibody, hepatitis delta antibody, hepatitis C antibody), immunologic (antinuclear antibody, anti–smooth muscle antibody, anti–liver kidney microsomal antibody), ceruloplasmin, urine copper levels, ferritin, iron, total iron-binding capacity, and α-1-antitrypsin studies are helpful for etiologic classification.

f. Decompensated cirrhosis: In addition to the conditions mentioned above, albumin levels are lower and serum cholesterol may be depressed. Anemia may be present; it is usually macrocytic and rarely hypochromic.

3. Radiologic Examinations
   a. Ultrasound: Cirrhosis is suggested when areas of liver parenchyma appear with different attenuation. The borders may appear irregular, and the caudate lobe may seem enlarged. Ultrasound is not reliable, unless other findings, such as ascites or an enlarged spleen, are apparent.
   b. Computed tomography: In addition to the above findings on ultrasound, computed tomography may demonstrate some helpful vascular structures (varices, collateral vessels). Focal lesions are seen more clearly.
   c. Magnetic resonance imaging: Has no significant advantage over the above modalities.
   d. Scintiscanning (liver spleen scan): Suggests cirrhosis and portal hypertension when there is an irregular distribution of colloid in the liver and an increased uptake by the spleen and vertebrae. It may give an estimate of parenchymal cell function.
   e. Angiography: Not indicated. Abnormal biliary structures can be seen when percutaneous cholangiograms are obtained in cirrhotic patients for other indications.
4. Other tests: Serum test to assess increased fibrosis in the liver is still a research tool. More specific liver function tests, such as the galactose elimination test, aminopyrine breath test, indocyanine green test, and so on are rarely needed in clinical practice.

V. **Differential Diagnosis**
   A. Asymptomatic (latent) cirrhosis may be confused with benign entities such as steatosis or mild hepatitis.
   B. Clinical cirrhosis: Alcoholic or viral hepatitis, Budd-Chiari syndrome, congestive heart failure, congenital hepatic fibrosis, or causes of presinusoidal portal hypertension may present with similar biochemical or radiologic abnormalities.
   C. End-stage cirrhosis: Malignancy should be suspected and hepatocellular carcinoma may complicate long-standing cirrhosis of any etiology. Portal vein thrombosis or bacterial peritonitis may decompensate an otherwise stable cirrhotic.

VI. **Treatment**
   A. The treatment of complications of portal hypertension and of diseases that lead to cirrhosis is discussed elsewhere. Current therapies of viral hepatitis, primary biliary cirrhosis, and sclerosing cholangitis are moderately effective, and it is still unknown if the progression of cirrhosis will be significantly modified. The use of colchicine to prevent fibrosis, ursodeoxycholic acid in cholestasis, propranolol for prevention of first variceal bleeding, or norfloxacin in patients with ascites to prevent spontaneous bacterial peritonitis cannot be widely recommended until larger controlled studies demonstrate their value.
   B. The diet should be low in salt (2 g or less when ascites is present), and the patient may require restricted fluid intake and protein. Protein may need to be restricted when there is a history of hepatic encephalopathy precipitated only by food intake. One gram of protein per kilogram (of dry weight) is adequate for most patients with latent or early cirrhosis. In advanced or end-stage cirrhosis, use the maximum amount of protein (40 to 60 g) that will keep the patient free from encephalopathy. Use of branched chain amino acids is controversial. End-stage cirrhosis is better treated (selected cases) with orthotopic liver transplantaton.
   C. Patients with cirrhosis should be cautioned to avoid the use of nonsteroidal anti-inflammatory agents, aspirin, acetaminophen, aminoglycosides, sedatives, and, obviously, alcohol.

VII. **Patient Monitoring**
   Patients should be carefully watched for complications of portal hypertension. The development of hepatocellular carcinoma is not uncommon. Serial ultrasound scans and measurement of α-fetoprotein have been found to be helpful only in a selected group of patients with chronic hepatitis B in the Far East.

VIII. **Prognosis**
   Although the lesion in cirrhosis is considered irreversible, active inflammation and fibrosis deposition can be stopped and the progression of disease arrested. The need to predict the progression and prognosis is extremely important today, since liver transplantation has become a successful method of treatment, although donor availability remains scarce. The Child's Pugh classification (A, B, C), which de-

pends on jaundice, ascites, encephalopathy (nutritional state in the original classification), serum albumin concentration, and prothrombin time, is helpful. Other prognostic formulas use mainly these parameters to predict more accurately who will decompensate. The following conditions are considered to augur a poor prognosis:

A. Persistent jaundice.
B. Ascites refractory to conventional diuretics.
C. Persistent hypotension.
D. Small liver.
E. Encephalopathy.
F. Persistent hypoprothrombinemia.
G. Bleeding esophageal varices.
H. Hyponatremia, hypocholesterolemia, and hypoalbuminemia.
I. Episodes of infections, particularly spontaneous bacterial peritonitis.

Bibliography

Bonsel GJ, Klompmaker IJ, Van't Veer F, et al. Use of prognostic models for assessment of value of liver transplantation in primary biliary cirrhosis. *Lancet* 335:493–497, 1990.

Sherlock S. *Diseases of the Liver and Biliary System.* Blackwell Scientific Publications, Cambridge, MA, 1989, pp 410–424.

Viral Hepatitis

Donald M. Jensen, M.D.

I. **Definition**
Acute inflammation of the liver of less than 6 months' duration caused by hepatitis A, B, C, D, or E viruses.

II. **Etiology**
A. Hepatitis A virus (HAV)
1. Enterovirus type 72.
2. A 27-nm, single-stranded RNA, nonenveloped virus with cubic symmetry.
3. Inactivation
a. Boiling for 5 min.
b. Formalin (1:4000).
c. Chlorine (1 mg/liter for 30 min).
4. Worldwide distribution, but endemic in many tropical and subtropical areas.
5. Seasonal pattern—in temperate zones: late autumn; in tropical zones: rainy seasons.
B. Hepatitis B virus (HBV)
1. Hepadnavirus type 1.
2. A 42-nm, double-stranded DNA virus with a single-stranded segment.
3. Three morphologic forms of the virus.
a. Complete virion (Dane particle).
b. Surface antigen particles 22 nm in diameter.

c. Tubular forms of surface antigen 22 nm in diameter.
4. The complete virion contains the following:
a. An outer surface glycolipoprotein coat: hepatitis B surface antigen (HBsAg).
b. A nucleocapsid (core) composed of a 19,000-MW hepatitis B core antigen (HBcAg). This protein does not circulate freely.
c. Within the virus core is the double-stranded DNA. This viral DNA replicates through an RNA intermediate which completes the plus strand of the DNA within the virion.
d. An RNA-dependent DNA polymerase enzyme is capable of directing the synthesis of viral DNA and is also detected within the viral core.
C. Hepatitis C virus (HCV)
1. Unclassified RNA virus similar to the flaviviridae.
2. A 30- to 60-nm virus with a 10,000-kD, single-stranded RNA coding for a single polypeptide.
D. Hepatitis D virus (HDV) (delta hepatitis)

1. An incomplete RNA virus which requires the presence of HB_sA_g for replication and transmission.
2. Nucleic acid studies suggest that HDV may be more closely related to plant viroids than human viruses are.

E. Hepatitis E virus (HEV)
   1. A 27- to 30-nm RNA virus of unclassified taxonomy.
   2. Similar morphologically to HAV but distinct serologically.

III. **Pathophysiology**
Liver infection with the hepatitis virus may result in cell injury by one of two basic mechanisms: a viral cytopathic effect or immune-mediated cytolysis. For most hepatitis viruses, the exact mechanism is unclear. However, evidence favors an immune (cytolytic T-cell)-mediated effector mechanism for hepatitis B. The target antigen appears to be a hepatitis B core peptide on the liver cell surface in close proximity to histocompatibility locus antigens.

IV. **Diagnosis**
A. Hepatitis A: IgM anti-HAV is positive during acute hepatitis. Positive anti-HAV (total) with a negative IgM anti-HAV is seen in the serum of patients with previous hepatitis A infections.
B. Hepatitis B: During acute hepatitis B infections, HBsAg, HBcAg, and IgM anti-HBc antibody are positive. With recovery, anti-HBs antibody appears, with loss of HBsAg.
C. Hepatitis C: Anti-HCV antibody is present in the sera of only 20% of patients with acute non-A, non-B hepatitis. No other test is available at present.
D. Hepatitis D: IgM anti-HDV and total anti-HDV are present in acute HDV infection (either coinfection or superinfection). However, antibody may not appear until 1 or 2 weeks after the onset of the hepatitis.
E. Hepatitis E: No commercial test is yet available. Electron microscopy (immune) of the stool filtrate may reveal 27- to 30-nm viral particles.

V. **Differential Diagnosis**
A. Acute drug hepatotoxicity, cardiac failure/shock liver, hepatic steatosis, granulomatous liver disease, opportunistic infections (e.g., cytomegalovirus, herpes simplex virus, toxoplasmosis, listeriosis, etc.).
B. Secondary syphilis.
C. Chronic hepatitis.
D. Sickle cell hepatopathy.
E. Alcoholic liver disease.

F. Hepatic malignancy.
G. Biliary tract obstruction (acute).

VI. **Treatment**
Treatment is generally symptomatic.
A. Diet: A high-carbohydrate, low-fat diet may be better tolerated and may cause less nausea. Fluid intake should be encouraged.
B. Rest: Although absolute bed rest is not necessary, vigorous physical activity should be avoided.
C. Isolation: Blood and body fluid precautions should be instituted for hepatitis B, C, and D and stool precautions for hepatitis A and E.
D. Treatment and contacts
   1. Hepatitis A: All household members should receive immune serum globulin, 0.02 ml/kg, within 2 weeks.
   2. Hepatitis B: Intimate contacts should receive hepatitis B immune globulin, 0.06 ml/kg, followed by the hepatitis B vaccine sequence.
   3. Hepatitis C: Barrier precautions of sexual contacts (10% risk).
   4. Hepatitis D: Same as for hepatitis B.
   5. Hepatitis E: No published recommendations.

VII. **Patient Monitoring**
A. Clinical symptoms: A sense of well-being and return of appetite often signify clinical improvement.
B. Laboratory studies: Serum aminotransferase, bilirubin level, and prothrombin time together are the most useful parameters. Serologic studies are generally not very helpful unless aminotransferases fail to normalize completely.

VIII. **Prognosis**
The magnitude of the aminotransferase elevation does not predict survival. In severe (fulminant) cases, age <11 or >40 years, a prothrombin time >50 sec, and total bilirubin >18 mg/dl signify a poor prognosis. In nonfulminant acute hepatitis, declining aminotransferase levels in conjunction with a rising serum bilirubin level and an increasing prothrombin time (in seconds) are considered bad prognostic signs.

Bibliography

Kuo G, Choo Q-L, Alter HJ, et al: An assay for circulating antibodies to a major etiologic virus of human non-A, non-B hepatitis. *Science* 244:362, 1989.

Robinson WS. Biology of human hepatitis viruses. In Zakim D, Boyer TD, (eds). Hepatology: A Textbook Of Liver Disease, ed 2. Philadelphia, WB Saunders Company, 1990, p 890.

Alcoholic Liver Disease

Donald M. Jensen, M.D.
Seymour Sabesin, M.D.

I. **Definition**
   Acute or chronic liver disease, with typical histologic patterns, in association with excessive alcohol consumption.
   A. Fatty liver: May develop after days to weeks of heavy alcohol consumption and is reversible upon cessation of drinking.
   B. Alcoholic hepatitis: Acute inflammation of the liver usually associated with 6–10 years of heavy alcohol consumption (80–120 g/day). May or may not be reversible.
   C. Cirrhosis (Laennec's or micronodular): Irreversible consequence of alcohol liver injury. Alcoholic hepatitis may be an intermediate stage.

II. **Etiology**
   Although excessive alcohol consumption is necessary for the development of the liver injury, there is considerable variability in the amount and duration of alcohol ingestion which is required to produce the liver disease.
   A. Epidemiologic data suggest a linear relationship between the amount of alcohol ingested and the incidence of alcoholic cirrhosis.
   B. The incidence of cirrhosis increases markedly when consumption of alcohol exceeds 160 g/day.
   C. Women seem to be much more susceptible to the hepatic effects of alcohol and may demonstrate liver injury with less alcohol ingestion over shorter periods of time.
   D. A statistically increased incidence of cirrhosis can be demonstrated with as little as 20 g/day of alcohol in women and 40 g/day in men.
   E. The co-occurrence of hepatitis C infection may aggravate the liver injury caused by alcohol.
   F. Alcoholic liver injury may occur even in the presence of adequate nutritional intake.

III. **Pathophysiology**
   Over 90% of ingested alcohol is metabolized by the liver, with the subsequent formation of acetaldehyde and hydrogen via three enzyme pathways: alcohol dehydrogenase, catalase, and the microsomal ethanol oxidizing system (MEOS). Most toxic effects of alcohol can be related to the generation of excessive amounts of hydrogen and acetaldehyde.
   A. Consequences of increased hydrogen: This

leads to an increase in the ratio of nicotina-mide-adenine dinucleotide (reduced form) to nicotinamide-adenine dinucleotide, with an altered redox state.

1. Increases oxygen consumption by hepatocytes and may leave centilobular hepatocytes relatively hypoxic.
2. Increases production of ketones from fatty acids.
3. Increases lactate production, with development of hyperlactacidemia and hyperuricemia.

B. Consequences of acetaldehyde production
1. Decreases hepatic protein synthesis and secretion, leading to hepatocyte swelling.
2. Damages mitochondria.
3. May promote lipid peroxidation.
4. Depresses glutathione production.
5. Chronic alcohol ingestion is associated with a proliferation of the microsomes and induction of the MEOS, leading to increased production of acetaldehyde.

IV. Diagnosis

A. History: Signs or symptoms of liver disease in association with heavy alcohol consumption should be present. However, the history may underestimate the patient's alcohol consumption by up to 40%. Likewise, mild to moderate chronic alcohol ingestion may be associated with severe liver injury in women; with the use of acetaminophen, carbon tetrachloride, and methotrexate; and with the occurrence of hepatitis C.

B. Clinical signs and physical findings.
1. Early: Hepatomegaly secondary to fatty infiltration and hepatocyte swelling. May or may not be associated with ascites, gynecomastia, jaundice, and cachexia.
2. Later: The development of alcoholic hepatitis may be asymptomatic or associated with jaundice, fever (occasionally to 101°–102°F), tender hepatomegaly, splenomegaly, variceal hemorrhage, ascites, confusion (encephalopathy), gynecomastia, testicular atrophy, palmar erythema, parotid enlargement, and leukonychia.
3. Late: Alcoholic cirrhosis may be asymptomatic or associated with jaundice, cachexia, ascites, encephalopathy, variceal hemorrhage, spontaneous bacterial peritonitis, hepatorenal syndrome, and cutaneous manifestations of cirrhosis.

C. Diagnostic tests: Laboratory, radiographic, and histologic features are not, by them-

selves, diagnostic and must be interpreted in the context of the case as a whole. For example, up to 17% of alcoholics with a characteristic aminotransferase enzyme pattern may have nonalcoholic liver disease when biopsied. Furthermore, typical histologic lesions of alcoholic hepatitis may occasionally be observed in nonalcoholic, obese women with hyperlipidemia (nonalcoholic steatonecrosis), as well as in patients following jejunoileal bypass procedures.

1. Laboratory tests
a. Aminotransferases: In patients with alcoholic hepatitis, the aspartate aminotransferase (AST) (serum glutamic-oxaloacetic transaminase) level is elevated more than the alanine aminotransferase (ALT) (serum glutamic-pyruvic transaminase). The ALT may even be normal. It is rare for the AST level to exceed a 10-fold elevation in the absence of a concomitant liver disease.
b. Alkaline phosphatase: This activity may be normal or mildly increased. Marked increases (greater than threefold) suggest biliary tract disease, intrahepatic mass lesions, or alcoholic cholestasis.
c. Gamma glutamyl transferase (GGT): GGT levels are frequently elevated in alcoholics, even in the absence of significant liver disease. Alcohol ingestion presumably induces the synthesis of this enzyme.

2. Radiographic studies: Plain radiographs of the abdomen are rarely useful diagnostically in suspected alcoholic liver disease. Ultrasonography may be useful to exclude biliary obstruction, cholelithiasis, and space-occupying lesions. Technetium liver-spleen scans may demonstrate poor hepatic Kupffer cell uptake of the radiopharmaceutical, with increased uptake in the lungs, skeleton, and spleen.

3. Histologic studies: Liver biopsy is an important diagnostic tool, not only for differentiating alcoholic from nonalcoholic liver disease, but also for determining the type of liver injury (fatty liver, alcoholic hepatitis, or cirrhosis). These are not distinct entities but may occur together in the same patient.
a. Fatty liver: Significant alcohol consumption for 2 to 8 days may be suffi-

cient to induce fatty liver. The fat seen on biopsy may be diffuse and is mostly macrovesicular. Pericentral sclerosis may also be seen and is thought to be a marker for the subsequent development of cirrhosis.

b. Alcoholic hepatitis: Typical lesions consist of steatosis, hydropic degeneration of hepatocytes, Mallory bodies (alcoholic hyaline), and an inflammatory infiltrate consisting largely of polymorphonuclear leukocytes. Centrilobular deposition of collagen may be seen extending along the sinusoids.

c. Cirrhosis: The end stage of alcoholic liver injury is cirrhosis. This is typically micronodular, with a generally uniform appearance.

V. Differential Diagnosis

A. Fatty liver and hepatomegaly: The differential diagnosis includes nonalcoholic steatonecrosis, diabetes mellitus, morbid obesity, postileojejunal bypass surgery, starvation, and drug use.

B. Alcoholic hepatitis: Diagnostic considerations include acute cholangitis, liver abscess, metastatic disease, viral hepatitis, autoimmune chronic active hepatitis, Q fever, leptospirosis, and drug hepatotoxicity, especially with amiodarone.

C. Cirrhosis: Other causes of cirrhosis in nonalcoholic patients are possible. In particularly, hemochromatosis, α-1-antitrypsin deficiency, viral hepatitis, Wilson's disease, and autoimmune chronic active hepatitis should be considered.

VI. Treatment

A. Abstinence from alcohol: Many studies have demonstrated improved survival, even in alcoholic cirrhotics, if alcohol consumption is stopped.

B. Improved nutrition: Nutritional supplementation (or support) should be considered in malnourished patients. Those with alcoholic hepatitis may benefit particularly from an increased caloric intake and may tolerate 3,000 kcal/day with up to 100 g of protein without developing encephalopathy.

C. Corticosteroids: Patients with severe alcoholic hepatitis and encephalopathy may benefit from a 28-day course of methylprednisolone in a dose of 32 mg/day. The severity of the disease is determined by the pro-

thrombin time and serum bilirubin level. A meta-analysis of all studies investigating corticosteroid use in alcoholic hepatitis discovered that hepatic encephalopathy was an additional independent variable.

D. Other therapies of potential benefit
1. Propylthiouracil.
2. Colchicine.
3. Anabolic steroids.
4. Hepatic transplantation.

VII. Patient Monitoring

A. Encephalopathy: Patients with severe alcoholic hepatitis may develop confusion and agitation. Although this is likely to be hepatic encephalopathy, alcohol withdrawal syndrome, subdural hematomas, hypoglycemia, and sepsis should all be considered in the differential diagnosis.

B. Bilirubin level and prothrombin time: These laboratory parameters are much more useful in monitoring the functional state of the liver than are the serum aminotransferases. Aminotransferase activity does not accurately reflect liver damage and offers no useful prognostic information.

C. Electrolytes and renal function: These should be monitored closely in patients hospitalized with alcoholic hepatitis or with complications of cirrhosis. Magnesium and zinc deficiencies are also not uncommon and should be assessed initially.

D. Nutritional status: Biochemical indices of nutrition (albumin, transferrin, lymphocyte count) may be misleading due to liver injury or marrow suppression. Physical signs of malnutrition must be sought.

VIII. Prognosis

A. Alcoholic hepatitis: Mild and moderately severe cases often improve with abstinence and improved nutrition. In severe cases, up to 35% will die within 28 days, and 47% of those with severe alcoholic hepatitis and encephalopathy will die during the same period. Corticosteroid treatment may significantly reduce this mortality rate at 28 days.

B. Cirrhosis: The 5-year survival rate for patients with alcoholic cirrhosis *without* ascites, jaundice, or hematemesis is 68% in those who continue to drink and 89% in abstainers. Cirrhosis complicated by ascites, jaundice, or hematemesis is associated with a 34% 5-year survival rate in those who continue to drink and with a 60% survival rate in abstainers.

Bibliography

Imperiale TF, McCullough AJ. Do corticosteroids reduce mortality from alcoholic hepatitis? A meta-analysis of the randomized trials. *Ann Intern Med* 113:299, 1990.

Levin DM, Baker AL, Rochman H, et al. Nonalcoholic liver disease: Overlooked causes of liver injury in patients with heavy alcohol consumption. *Am J Med* 66:429, 1979.

Powell W, Klatskin G. Duration of survival in patients with Laennec's cirrhosis. *Am J Med* 44:406, 1968.

Chronic Hepatitis

Donald M. Jensen, M.D.

I. **Definition**
Hepatic inflammation persisting for more than 6 months in association with a characteristic histologic pattern (see below).

II. **Etiology**
  A. Autoimmune
     1. Classic type (antinuclear antibody positive)
     2. Liver-kidney-microsome (LKM) antibody positive
  B. Hepatitis B virus (with or without delta)
  C. Hepatitis C virus
  D. Drugs/medications
     1. α-Methyldopa
     2. Isoniazid
     3. Oxyphenisitin
     4. Dantrolene
     5. Nitrofurantoin
  E. Wilson's disease
  F. α-1-Antitrypsin deficiency

III. **Pathophysiology**
Presumably results from interaction of immunoreactive lymphocytes with antigens expressed on the hepatocyte plasma membrane. Liver cell membrane autoantibodies may also play a role. The mechanism for drug-induced and metabolic chronic hepatitis (e.g., Wilson's disease) is not well understood.

IV. **Diagnosis**
  A. History
     1. Persistent fatigue or jaundice may be the only symptom.
     2. Amenorrhea, arthralgias, skin rash.
  B. Clinical signs and physical findings
     1. Jaundice
     2. Spider telangiectasias
     3. Ascites
     4. Hepatomegaly
     5. Splenomegaly
  C. Diagnostic tests
     1. Liver biopsy: Demonstrates one of four basic histologic lesions. This classification may not pertain to chronic hepatitis type C.
        a. Chronic persistent hepatitis (CPH)
        b. Chronic lobular hepatitis (CLH)
        c. Chronic active hepatitis (CAH)
           (i) With bridging necrosis/fibrosis
           (ii) With multilobular collapse
        d. CAH and cirrhosis (active cirrhosis)

2. Serologic studies
   a. Autoimmune type
      (i) Antinuclear autoantibody (ANA)
      (ii) Anti-smooth muscle autoantibody (ASMA)
      (iii) LKM autoantibody
   b. Hepatitis B type
      (i) Hepatitis B surface antigen (HbsAg)
      (ii) Anti-HBc antibody (IgM negative)
   c. Hepatitis C type
      (i) Anti-hepatitis C virus antibody positive (80%)
   d. Wilson's disease
      (i) Low or low-normal ceruloplasmin
      (ii) Increased urinary copper excretion
      (iii) Kayser-Fleischer rings
      (iv) Increased hepatic copper content
   e. α-1-Antitrypsin deficiency
      (i) Low α-1-antitrypsin serum level
3. Radiologic studies
   a. Ultrasound: May demonstrate other causes of persistently elevated liver enzyme levels such as gallstones, mass lesions, or dilated bile ducts.
   b. Liver scan: May demonstrate redistribution of the isotope with decreased liver uptake and increased bone and splenic uptake in advanced cases.

V. Differential Diagnosis
A. Alcoholic liver disease
B. Granulomatous liver disease
C. Primary biliary cirrhosis
D. Primary sclerosing cholangitis
E. Primary or metastatic cancer
F. Steatosis

VI. Treatment
A. Autoimmune
   1. Prednisone alone or a combination of prednisone and azathioprine.
B. Hepatitis B: symptomatic or α-interferon 5 megaunits daily for 16 weeks or 10 megaunits thrice weekly for 16 weeks.
C. Hepatitis C: interferon, 3 megaunits thrice weekly (mu TIW) for 24 weeks for symptomatic cases.
D. Drug-induced: Discontinue using the offending agent.
E. Wilson's disease: Penicillamine, 250 mg three or four times per day.
F. α-1-Antitrypsin deficiency: Symptomatic.

VII. Patient Monitoring
A. Aminotransferase activity is most useful, especially if monitored in conjunction with tests of hepatocellular function such as the prothrombin time and the serum bilirubin, cholesterol, and albumin levels.
B. Liver biopsy: Occasionally useful to establish the response to therapy.
C. Clinical response: Increased sense of well-being and improved appetite may be early predictors of the response to treatment.

VIII. Prognosis
A. Untreated autoimmune CAH and Wilson's disease are progressive disorders, with subsequent development of cirrhosis and death.
B. Chronic hepatitis B and C are more indolent, with only 20–40% of cases progressing to cirrhosis. Hepatocellular carcinoma may be a late complication.

Bibliography

Czaja AJ: Natural history, clinical features, and treatment of autoimmune hepatitis. *Sem Liv Dis* 4:1, 1984.

Perrillo RP, Schiff ER, Davis GL, et al: A randomized, controlled trial of interferon alfa-2b alone and after prednisone withdrawal, in the treatment of chronic hepatitis B. *N Engl J Med* 323:295, 1990.

Chapter 61-E

Primary Biliary Cirrhosis

Howard Rosenblate, M.D.

I. **Definition**
Chronic, progressive (granulomatous) inflammatory destruction of the intrahepatic bile ducts.

II. **Etiology and Pathophysiology**
A. Exact etiology is still unknown, but many features point to a profound immunologic disturbance.
1. Can be found in more than one family member, but there is no clear-cut pattern of inheritance and no consistent genetic markers.
2. Increased display of class II histocompatibility antigen (HLA) on bile duct epithelium.
3. Cytotoxic T cells are seen surrounding and infiltrating the bile duct epithelium.
4. Suppressor T cells are reduced in number and function.
5. Similar structural changes seen in graft-versus-host disease following bone marrow transplantation.
6. Other ducts with a high concentration of human leukocyte antigen class II antigens on their epithelium (lacrimal, salivary, pancreatic) are involved, hence the term *dry gland syndrome*.
B. Associated diseases

1. Scleroderma
2. Rheumatoid arthritis
3. Thyroiditis
4. Interstitial pneumonitis
5. Systemic lupus erythematosus
6. Renal tubular acidosis
7. Sjögren's syndrome
8. Breast carcinoma
9. Celiac disease

III. **Diagnosis**
A. History
1. Middle-aged female (90%)
2. Pruritus
3. Fatigue
B. Clinical signs and physical findings
1. Well-nourished woman.
2. Jaundice may or may not be present.
3. Skin xanthomas, xanthelasma, and hyperpigmentation may or may not be present.
4. Excoriations occur if pruritus is severe.
5. Hepatomegaly is often present.
C. Stages in the natural history
1. Preclinical phase with normal biochemical tests—2 to 10 years.
2. Asymptomatic phase with abnormal biochemical tests.

  3. Symptomatic anicteric.
  4. Symptomatic icteric.
  D. Diagnostic tests
    1. Elevated alkaline phosphatase and gamma-glutamyl transpeptidase.
    2. Cholesterol often increased.
    3. Modest elevation in transaminases.
    4. Mild increase in bilirubin (in the icteric phase).
    5. Increased IgM (80%).
    6. Circulating antibodies against mitochondria (>95%).
       a. The anti-mitochondrial antibody (AMA) is directed against M2, a specific antigen of the inner mitochondrial membrane.
    7. Antinuclear antibody (anticentromere antibody) is occasionally present.
    8. Liver biopsy
       a. Stage I: Florid bile duct lesions, often with noncaseating granulomas.
       b. Stage II: Ductal proliferation.
       c. Stage III: Bridging necrosis and fibrosis; paucity of bile ducts; cholestasis.
       d. Stage IV: Cirrhosis.
       e. Increased hepatic copper and copper-associated protein. Mallory bodies (in about 25%). Stages can overlap.

IV. **Differential Diagnosis**
  A. Primary sclerosing cholangitis
  B. Large bile duct obstruction
  C. Chronic active hepatitis
  D. Drug-induced cholestatic liver disease
  E. Cholestatic viral hepatitis
  F. Cholangiocarcinoma
  G. Sarcoidosis

V. **Treatment**
  A. General measures
    1. Control of itching
       a. Antihistamines
       b. Phenobarbital
       c. Cholestyramine
       d. Rifampin
       e. Plasmapheresis
    2. Fat-soluble vitamins (A, D, E, K) and calcium.
  B. Corticosteroids: Good for the liver, bad for the bones.
  C. Colchicine.
    1. Anti-inflammatory and antifibrotic.
       a. Interferes with collagen synthesis.
       b. Activates hepatic collagenase.
       c. Interferes with intracellular transport of collagen.

    2. Three controlled trials have shown improvement in biochemical tests but no change in liver biopsy.
  D. Ursodeoxycholic acid
    1. Rationale: Replacement of toxic or detergent (hydrophobic) bile acids (deoxycholic, chenodeoxycholic, and lithocholic acids) which accumulate during the course of the disease with nondetergent or hydrophilic bile acids.
    2. Six studies have shown improvement in hepatic tests, and two studies have shown improvement in histology.
  E. Methotrexate
    1. Oral pulse methotrexate (15 mg/week) resulted in improvement in symptoms and hepatic tests in nine women with precirrhotic symptomatic primary biliary cirrhosis.
    2. Liver histology improved in four of the women and did not worsen in the other five.
    3. Double-blind, controlled study of methotrexate versus colchicine now in progress.
  F. Hepatic transplantation
    1. Timing can be based on various prognostic indicators or survival numbers.
    2. However, when intractable pruritus, marked jaundice, fatigue interfering with previous lifestyle, bleeding esophageal varices, ascites, or encephalopathy occurs, hepatic transplantation must be considered.
    3. One-year survival in primary biliary cirrhosis is 70–90%, post transplantation.

VI. **Patient Monitoring**
Blood chemistries and physical examination every 4 to 6 months.
  A. If two successive 6-month bilirubin tests show a level above 2 mg%, survival is about 49 months.
  B. When the bilirubin level exceeds 6 mg%, the patient is unlikely to survive for more than 2 years.
  C. Mayo prognostic index: Variables are bilirubin, albumin, age, prothrombin time, and peripheral edema.

Bibliography

  Kaplan MM, Knox TA. Treatment of primary biliary cirrhosis with low-dose weekly methotrexate. *Gastroenterology* 101:1332–1338, 1991.

Chapter 61-F

Primary Sclerosing Cholangitis

Donald M. Jensen, M.D.

I. Definition

Primary sclerosing cholangitis (PSC) is a chronic cholestatic liver disease associated with fibrosis and inflammation of the intra- and extrahepatic bile ducts. Secondary biliary cirrhosis is a late feature.

II. Etiology

Although no specific etiologic agent has been identified, the following diseases are associated:

A. Inflammatory bowel disease (70%)
B. Others
   1. Thyroiditis (Reidel's struma)
   2. Retroperitoneal fibrosis
   3. Histiocytosis X
   4. Mediastinal fibrosis
   5. Vasculitis

III. Pathophysiology

Strictures of the biliary tree lead to intrahepatic cholestasis and occasionally to jaundice. Unresolved cholestasis eventually leads to a secondary biliary cirrhosis and portal hypertension. Liver failure and death follow in this progressive disorder.

IV. Diagnosis

A. History: The average age of onset is 40 years, but PSC may occur at any time from infancy through adulthood. The male:female ratio is 2:1. Patients are frequently detected because of the discovery of an asymptomatic elevation of alkaline phosphatase. Pruritus, jaundice, fatigue, or pain may also be initial symptoms.

B. Clinical signs and physical findings: Normal physical exams occur in about one-half of the patients. Jaundice, hepatomegaly, and splenomegaly may be observed.

C. Diagnostic tests
   1. Laboratory studies
      a. Increased alkaline phosphatase, gamma glutamyl transferase, and 5-nucleotidase.
      b. Increased bilirubin in 50%.
      c. Mild to moderate elevation in serum aminotransferases.
      d. Hypergammaglobulinemia (30%).
   2. Radiographic studies
      a. Endoscopic retrograde cholangiopancreatography: The diagnostic study of choice to demonstrate strictures and focal dilatation of intra- and extrahepatic bile ducts.
   3. Liver biopsy: Of limited value and rarely demonstrates diagnostic features.

V. Treatment
A. Management of chronic cholestasis
1. Pruritus: cholestyramine, 4–16 g/day, with or without phenobarbital, may be useful.
2. Fat-soluble vitamin deficiencies: Vitamins A, D, and K may be supplemented if deficiencies are documented.
B. Management of complications
1. Dominant strictures may be dilated by endoscopic or percutaneous routes.
2. Suppurative cholangitis is treated with antibiotics.
3. Portal hypertension is managed as in other cirrhotic individuals.
C. Treatment of primary disease
1. Liver transplantation offers the best results for end-stage PSC.
2. Colectomy does not influence the natural history of PSC.
3. Medical therapy is of unproven benefit, but currently evaluated treatments include the following:
   a. Methotrexate.
   b. Ursodeoxycholic acid.
   c. Immunosuppressive agents.

VI. Patient Monitoring
A. Cholangiocarcinoma develops in 10–15% of PSC patients. A sudden deterioration in the clinical course should suggest this possibility.
B. Clinical symptoms and routine liver chemistries are the most useful means of assessing the disease activity. Computed tomography scanning and cholangiography may prove useful in evaluating changes in biliary excretion.

VII. Prognosis
PSC is a progressive and uniformly fatal disease for symptomatic patients, with a 33% mortality rate over a 5- to 108-month follow-up period.

Bibliography

LaRusso NF, Weisner RH, Ludwig J, et al: Primary sclerosing cholangitis. *N Engl J Med* 310:899, 1984.

Chapter 61-G

Portal Hypertension

Howard Rosenblate, M.D.

I. **Definition and Classification**
   A. Normal portal pressure is 5–10 mmHg (7–14 cm of water). A wedged hepatic venous pressure more than 5 mmHg greater than the inferior vena cava pressure (wedged hepatic gradient) equals portal hypertension.
   B. Increased resistance and increased portal flow result in portal hypertension (portal pressure = portal flow × vascular resistance). The increased resistance is the result of cirrhosis or other factors mentioned below. The increased portal flow occurs as a result of "the hyperdynamic circulation of cirrhosis." Vasodilatory substances originating from the pancreas or intestines (Glucagon, prostacyclin, prostaglandios, bile salts, and endotoxin mediated activation of nitric oxide) and usually metabolized by the liver are not degraded by the sick hepatocytes and now bypass the liver through portalsystemic collaterals. There exists a generalized peripheral vasodilation that results in increased cardiac output and heart rate as well as decreased systemic vascular resistance (SVR). Sodium retention by the kidney adds to the hyperdy-

namic state. This process is mediated by activation of carotid barroreceptors.
   C. The block can be presinusoidal, sinusoidal, or postsinusoidal.
   D. Presinusoidal causes of portal hypertension
      1. Portal vein thrombosis
      2. Cavernous transformation of the portal vein
      3. Splenic vein thrombosis
      4. Schistosomiasis
      5. Congenital hepatic fibrosis
      6. Sarcoidosis
      7. Toxins
         a. Vinyl chloride
         b. Arsenic
         c. Copper
      8. Idiopathic portal hypertension
   E. Sinusoidal causes of portal hypertension
      1. Cirrhosis—any cause
      2. Acute liver disease
         a. Alcoholic hepatitis
         b. Alcoholic fatty liver
         c. Fulminant hepatitis
      3. Metastatic carcinoma
   F. Postsinusoidal causes of hypertension

1. Hepatic vein thrombosis (Budd-Chiari syndrome)
2. Veno-occlusive disease
3. Inferior vena cava thrombosis or webs
4. Alcoholic central hyalone sclerosis
5. Cardiac disease
   a. Constrictive pericarditis
   b. Valvular heart disease
   c. Cardiomyopathy
G. Increased portal venous blood flow
   1. Arterial venous fistula
   2. Splenomegaly, that is, myelofibrosis with extramedullary hematopoiesis, polycythemia rubra vera, Gaucher's disease, leukemia, lymphoma

II. Collateral Circulation

A. Gastric and esophageal varices (in which the left gastric and short gastric veins of the portal system anastomose with the intracostal, diaphragmatic-esophageal, and azygous veins of the caval system).

B. Rectal varices (anastomosis of the superior hemorrhoidal veins of the portal system with the middle and inferior hemorrhoidal veins of the caval system).

C. Collaterals in the falciform ligament through the periumbilical veins (relics of the obliterated fetal circulation).

D. Collaterals develop where the abdominal organs are in contact with the retroperitoneal tissues (veins in the splenorenal ligament or between the spleen and adrenal gland and in veins developing in scars of previous laparotomies).

E. Blood from the gastroesophageal collaterals, and from the retroperitoneal and abdominal venous systems, reach the superior vena cava via the azygous systems.

F. Pathophysiology
1. The increased resistance to portal blood flow leads to the development of these collaterals, which deviate portal blood into the systemic veins.
2. There is increased blood flow in the portal system because of a rise in cardiac output and splanchnic vasodilatation.
3. The increased total portal flow increases the variceal transmural pressure, and rupture can occur.

III. Clinical Diagnosis

A. History
1. Diagnosis or etiology of cirrhosis.
2. History of gastroesophageal bleeding episodes.

B. Physical examination
1. Splenomegaly (most important sign).
2. Ascites.
3. Dilated superficial abdominal wall veins.
4. Stigmata of cirrhosis.
5. Liver may be large or small.

C. Laboratory tests
1. Pancytopenia or parts thereof.
2. Blood chemistries compatible with liver disease.

D. Imaging studies
1. Doppler ultrasound to assay the patency and flow in the portal vein, hepatic vein, and hepatic artery.
2. Liver-spleen scan.
3. Computed tomography scan. Besides assessing the visceral organs, the collateral circulation may be defined.
4. Magnetic resonance imaging.

E. Special tests
1. Endoscopy.
2. Measurement of azygous vein blood flow.
3. Abdominal angiography with measurement of hepatic artery flow, portal venous blood flow, and, most important, wedged hepatic vein pressure, and portal systemic gradient.

IV. Complications

A. Bleeding esophageal varices
1. Tension in the variceal wall is related to transmural pressure (TP), wall thickness (W), and the radius (r) of the varix. When $T = P \times r/W$ is greater than the tension in the wall, rupture occurs.
2. Esophagitis and reflux play little if any part in rupture.
3. Endoscopy is the gold standard, as it will establish the presence or absence of varices and, if present, determine whether or not they are bleeding. Cirrhotics can bleed from ulcers, gastritis, or Mallory Weiss tears (i.e., not all upper gastrointestinal bleeding in patients with cirrhosis and varices has to come from the varices).
4. Treatment of bleeding esophageal varices
   a. Check for postural hypotension.
   b. Restore blood volume.
   c. Avoid excessive use of saline solutions.
   d. Gastric lavage.
   e. Administer plasma if clotting factors needed.
   f. Vasopressin: Bolus of 20 units over 20 min followed by infusion at a rate of 0.4 units/min.

(1) Lowers portal pressure by constricting arteriolar smooth muscles in the splanchnic vascular bed. This reduces blood flow and pressure in the portal vein.

(2) Also constricts coronary arteries and smooth muscles in the esophagus and causes increased peristalsis.

(3) Addition of nitroglycerin reduces adverse hemodynamic side effects.

(4) Somatostatin not yet shown to have a definite advantage over vasopressin.

g. Balloon tamponade

(1) Sengstaken-Blakemore tube.

(2) Minnesota tube.

(3) Linton Nicholas tube.

All are generally successful in providing temporary control of bleeding esophageal varices.

h. Endoscopic sclerotherapy (sclerosing solution injected either into the varix or adjacent to it).

(1) Results similar regardless of what agent is used or method of injection.

(2) Success in control of acute bleeding varies from 73% to 95%.

(3) Once bleeding is controlled, several sessions of sclerotherapy at intervals of 1 to 3 weeks are performed until varices are obliterated.

(4) Frequency of rebleeding is reduced.

(5) Gastric varices may increase in size, and congestive gastropathy may occur. Colonic varices may enlarge.

(6) Long-term survival has not yet been shown to be unequivocally increased in controlled trials of sclerotherapy.

(7) Complications includes fever, chest pain, aspiration pneumonia, pleural effusions, mediastinitis, esophageal ulcers, esophageal stricture, and esophageal perforation.

i. Portal systemic shunts

(1) Decrease portal pressure and stop bleeding from esophageal varices. Portal pressure falls, hepatic venous pressure falls, and hepatic artery pressure increases.

(2) However, there is an increased incidence of hepatic encephalopathy, and liver function often deteriorates after shunting.

(3) Portacaval shunt (end-to-site): The end of the portal vein is anastomosed to the side of the inferior vena cava, allowing marked decompression of a portal venous system. All of the portal flow is diverted into the systemic circulation.

(4) Side-to-side portacaval shunt: The side of the portal vein is anastomosed to the side of the inferior vena cava and is the most effective shunt for relieving ascites. Continued portal perfusion of the liver may occur.

(5) Mesocaval shunt: A Dacron graft or vein graft is placed between the superior mesenteric vein and the inferior vena cava or the superior mesenteric vein is anastomosed to the proximal end of a divided inferior vena cava and the distal end is ligated. This shunt is, in effect, a side-to-side shunt, but shunt occlusion is common.

(6) Distal splenorenal shunt: Veins feeding the esophageal varices are ligated (coronary, right gastric, and right gastroepiploic), and a splenorenal shunt is constructed (the proximal end of the splenic vein is anastomosed to the left renal vein). The spleen is preserved, and retrograde flow in the short gastric veins is possible. The hope is that portal flow will be preserved and post-shunt encephalopathy decreased.

(7) Nonoperative decompression (transjugular intrahepatic portosystemic shunt): Can be done in the radiology suite. Some reports indicate a 50% decrease in portal pressure. The goal is to decrease gradient below 12 mm Hg.

(8) General results of portosystemic shunts

(a) Elective shunts stop bleeding from esophageal varices and prevent this mode of death.

(b) However, death from hepatic failure is increased, and post-shunt encephalopathy varies from 25% to 75%.

(c) Emergency portacaval shunts have a mortality of 41–58%, and survival depends on Child's classification.

B. Medical therapy to prevent variceal rebleeding
   1. Propranolol and nadolol
      a. Decrease portal pressure when given in doses to decrease the resting pulse 25%.
      b. Block β-1 receptors to decrease cardiac output.
      c. Block β-2 receptors, causing splanchnic vasoconstriction by preventing vasodilatation.
   2. Six studies have focused on prevention of the first variceal hemorrhage. Overall bleeding in the propranolol-treated groups was approximately one-half that of the control group.
   3. Recent analysis of individual patients from four randomized, controlled trials suggests that propranolol and nadolol are effective in preventing the first bleeding episode and reducing the mortality rate associated with gastrointestinal bleeding in cirrhotics.

Bibliography

Cello JP, Grendell JH, Crass RA, et al. Endoscopic sclerotherapy versus portacaval shunts in patients with severe cirrhosis and acute variceal hemorrhage. *N Engl J Med* 316:11, 1987.

Ring EJ, Lake JR, Roberts JP, et al. Using transjugular intrahepatic portosystemic shunts to control variceal bleeding before liver transplantation. *Ann Intern Med* 116:304, 1992.

Westaby D, MacDougall BRD, Williams R. Improved survival following injection sclerotherapy for esophageal varices: Final analysis of a controlled trial. *Hepatology* 5:827, 1985.

Hepatorenal Syndrome

Howard Rosenblate, M.D.

I. **Definition**
Unexplained renal failure in a patient with hepatic failure in the absence of identifiable renal disease.
   A. Ascites almost always present.
   B. Common in alcoholic cirrhosis.
   C. Kidneys are anatomically and physiologically normal if transplanted into a patient with renal failure.

II. **Etiology**
The etiology is unknown, but the syndrome can be precipitated by events that decrease effective blood volume.
   A. Diuretic therapy.
   B. Gastrointestinal bleeding.
   C. Large-volume paracentesis.

III. **Pathophysiology**
   A. Significant reduction in renal perfusion, especially renal cortical perfusion.
   B. Decrease in glomerular filtration rate.
   C. Decrease in arterial pressure.
   D. Increase in plasma renin activity and activation of the renin-angiotensin system.
   E. Increase in the plasma norepinephrine concentration.
   F. Possibly altered ratio of vasodilator prostaglandin E_2 (PGE_2) to vasoconstrictor prostaglandin thromboxane A_2 (TxA_2).
   G. Possible decrease in prekallikrein, leading to diminished kinin formation in the kidney.
      1. Bradykinin is a renovasodilator.
   H. Possible role of the hepatorenal reflex.
      1. Infusion of glutamine in the rat superior mesenteric vein cause hepatocyte swelling, which leads to marked decrease in the glomerular filtration rate and urinary flow.
      2. Similar infusion into the jugular vein has no effect.
      3. Spinal transection or renal denervation of a section of the vagal hepatic nerves abolishes the effect noted with superior mesenteric vein infusion.

IV. **Diagnosis**
Prerenal failure and acute renal failure must be excluded.
   A. History and physical findings
      1. Chronic liver disease with ascites.
   B. Diagnostic tests
      1. Increasing azotemia and decreasing urine output.

2. Urine sodium concentration less than 10 mEq/liter and urine:plasma osmolality ratio greater than 1.

3. Expanding the intravascular volume is not helpful.

V. Differential Diagnosis

A. Acute renal failure from other causes
   1. Urine sodium greater than 30 mEq/liter.
   2. Urine osmolality equal to plasma osmolality.

B. Iatrogenic hepatorenal syndrome
   1. Nephrotoxic drugs (aminoglycosides or cyclosporine).
   2. Diuretics.
   3. Lactulose (can lead to severe diarrhea).
   4. Prostaglandin inhibition secondary to the use of nonsteroidal anti-inflammatory drugs.

C. Prerenal failure.

VI. Treatment

A. No effective conservative treatment; "treatment" consists of *prevention*.

B. Dialysis not helpful in true hepatorenal syndrome but can be used in acute liver failure while waiting to see if recovery will occur.

C. Hepatic transplantation.

VII. Prognosis

Uniformly fatal without hepatic transplantation.

Bibliography

Gines P, Gines A, Salmeron JM, et al. Sequential changes of arterial pressure and endogenous vasoconstrictor systems and cirrhosis with ascites. Relationship with hepatorenal syndrome (abstract). *Hepatology* 14(4):86A, 1991.

Koppel MH, Koburn JW, Mims MM, et al. Transplantation of cadaveric kidneys from patients with hepatorenal syndrome. *N Engl J Med* 280:1367, 1969.

Lang F, Tschernko E, Schulze E, et al. Hepatorenal reflex regulating kidney function. *Hepatology* 14(4):590, 1991.

O'Connor DT, Stone RA. The renal kallikrein-kinin system: Description and relationship to liver disease, in Epstein M (ed): *The Kidney and Liver Disease*, ed 2. New York. Elsevier Biomedical, 1983, p 469.

Zipser RD, Radvan GH, Kronberg I, et al. Urinary thromboxane B_2 and prostaglandin E_2 in the hepatorenal syndrome: Evidence for increased vasoconstrictor and decreased vasodilator factors. *Gastroenterology* 84:697, 1983.

CHAPTER 61-I

Hepatic Encephalopathy

Donald M. Jensen, M.D.

I. Definition

A neuropsychiatric syndrome occurring in conjunction with hepatic dysfunction and portal-systemic shunting.

II. Etiology

Precipitating factors for hepatic encephalopathy in cirrhotic patients include:

A. Gastrointestinal bleeding
B. Azotemia
C. Infection
   1. Spontaneous bacterial peritonitis
   2. Other causes
D. Tranquilizer or sedative drug use
E. Hypokalemic alkalosis
F. Excessive dietary protein ingestion
G. Constipation
H. Hepatic parenchymal injury

III. Pathophysiology

Although the exact pathophysiologic mechanism of hepatic encephalopathy is unknown, severeal theories have some basis of support.

A. Ammonia theory: Ammonia as a cause of hepatic encephalopathy is supported predominantly by clinical observations. Blood ammonia levels are frequently elevated in patients with hepatic encephalopathy, although the magnitude of the elevation correlates poorly with the degree of encephalopathy. Finally, therapies to reduce blood ammonia concentrations have generally been associated with improvements in encephalopathy.

B. Amino acid/false neurotransmitter theory: Plasma levels of aromatic amino acids, methionine, and octopamine have been described in hepatic encephalopathy. False neurotransmitters such as octopamine and phenylethanolamine could compete with endogenous dopamine and noradrenaline, resulting in disordered neuronal communication.

C. Gamma-aminobutyric acid (GABA)/endogenous benzodiazepine theory: Stimulation of brain GABA receptor by GABA-like compounds or endogenous benzodiazepine compounds could lead to central nervous system (CNS) depression.

All three major theories have proponents and are supported by laboratory and clinical observation.

IV. Diagnosis

Clinical signs and symptoms vary in severity

from mild alterations in mood, sleep-wake disturbances, and poor judgment to lethargy, confusion, and coma.

A. Clinical signs and physical findings

Stage 0   Normal state of consciousness and personality; no neuromuscular abnormalities

Stage I   Hypersomnia, insomnia, or sleep-wake inversion; irritability, shortened attention span; euphoria or depression; impaired handwriting, tremor.

Stage II   Lethargy; inappropriate behavior; ataxia; amnesia for the past; slurred speech; hypoactive reflexes.

Stage III Somnolence, confusion; semi-stupor; loss of place; bizarre behavior; inability to compute; hyperactive reflexes; nystagmus; clonus; rigidity.

Stage IV   Stupor; unconsciousness; loss of self; dilated pupils; opisthotones.

B. Diagnostic tests

1. Blood ammonia: Levels are elevated in most patients with the syndrome but correlate poorly with the stage of encephalopathy.

2. Cerebrospinal fluid glutamine: Levels are increased and tend to correlate better with stage of encephalopathy.

3. Electroencephalogram: Triphasic ("slow") waves are typical but neither sensitive nor specific.

4. Number Connection Test: A sensitive and semiquantitative test of cerebral dysfunction.

V. Differential Diagnosis

A. Causes of cerebral dysfunction in patients with liver disease

1. Subdural hematomas (bilateral)
2. Cerebral edema (fulminant hepatic failure)
3. Hypoglycemia
4. Hyponatremia (severe)

B. Causes of cerebral dysfunction in any patient

1. Cerebrovascular accident
2. Drug overdose
3. Meningitis/encephalitis
4. Uremia
5. Hyperglycemia
6. Postictal state

VI. Treatment

A. Identify and remove the precipitating insult (see Section II).

B. Decrease gut absorption of toxic nitrogenous compounds.

1. Lactulose syrup, 15–30 ml orally or via nasogastric tube every 4–6 hr. Titrate the dosage to two or three bowel movements daily. *Avoid inducing diarrhea.*

2. Neomycin, 500 mg p.o. every 4–6 hr, may be used in patients intolerant to lactulose. Care should be taken, however, to avoid nephro- and ototoxicity by monitoring serum levels.

C. Diet

1. A low-protein (<40 g) diet may be instituted *temporarily* but should not be a long term treatment Cirrhotic patients require *at least* 50 g of protein daily to avoid catabolism. Restricting the intake of red meat is often helpful.

2. Supplemental branch chain amino acids (Hepaticaid, Hepatamine) may be useful in selected cases. These are supplements, not total nutritional sources.

D. Liver transplantation may be necessary in particularly refractory cases. Remember that some forms of CNS dysfunction may be irreversible, such as non-Wilsonian hepatolenticular degeneration and some alcohol-induced CNS lesions.

VII. Patient Monitoring

A. Clinical signs and symptoms, along with the Number Connection Test, are most effective.

B. Blood ammonia level correlates poorly with the stage of disease, but in some patients it may be useful.

VIII. Prognosis

The prognosis for complete recovery from the initial episode is generally good, particularly if an identified precipitating cause is discovered. Repeated episodes in patients with large portal-systemic shunts are more difficult to treat and may require other intervention.

Bibliography

Conn HO, Lieberthal MM. The Hepatic Coma syndromes and Lactulose. Baltimore, Williams & Wilkins, 1979.

Jensen DM. Portal-systemic encephalopathy and hepatic coma. *Med Clin North Am* 70:1081–1092, 1986.

Hemochromatosis

Howard Rosenblate, M.D.

I. **Definition**

Hemochromatosis is a human leukocyte antigen (HLA)-linked, autosomal recessive condition that often results in accumulation of excess iron stores in the body.

II. **Etiology**

A. The H-gene is located on the short arm of chromosome 6 close to the HLA-A3 locus.

B. Studies indicate that 72% of patients with hemochromatosis possess the HLA-A3 antigen compared with 28% of the normal population.

C. Studies indicate that 10% of Caucasians are heterozygous for this gene and 0.3% of Caucasians are homozygous.

III. **Pathophysiology**

A. Dietary iron is absorbed from the intestine in the ferrous form to a level of 1 mg/day (normal men) and 2 mg/day (normal menstruating women).

1. Iron links with a glycoprotein called *transferrin*, by which it is carried in the serum.

a. The serum iron-binding capacity (transferrin) is about 250 ng/dl and is about one-third saturated.

2. *Ferritin* is a combination of the protein apoferritin and iron and is the major cellular iron storage protein present in normal serum. Its concentration is proportional to body iron stores.

3. *Hemosiderin* is made up of aggregates of ferritin molecules.

B. The normal total body content of iron is 4 g.

1. About 3 g is present in hemoglobin, myoglobin, catalase, and other respiratory pigments.

2. Storage iron comprises 0.5 g, and 0.3 g is found in the liver (the predominant storage site for iron absorbed from the gut).

3. When the liver's storage capacity for iron is exceeded, iron is deposited in other parenchymal tissues (pancreas, adrenals, pituitary, gonads, heart, and skeletal muscle).

4. The body has no excretory mechanism for iron; it cannot be eliminated in urine, feces, or sweat.

a. The normal iron burden is meticulously balanced (the amount absorbed offsets the amount shed by blood loss and by exfoliation of epithelial cells).

b. Patients with hemochromatosis absorb

2–5 mg iron per day, even though they are iron overloaded.

c. By the time symptoms appear, patients may have accumulated 20–60 g of iron in storage organs.

5. The excess iron is toxic to the hepatocytes.

a. Hemosiderin is deposited in the peribiliary lysosomes, where release of iron causes membrane fragility and rupture, with release of hydrolytic enzymes into the cytosol, resulting in fibrosis.

IV. Diagnosis

A. History

1. The patient may be asymptomatic or lethargic, with bronze or slate gray skin pigmentation, diminished sexual activity, diabetes mellitus, joint pain, congestive heart failure, cardiac arrhythmias, or menstrual irregularities.

B. Clinical signs and physical findings

1. Hepatomegaly, pigmented skin, loss of body hair, testicular atrophy, arthropathy of metacarpal phalangeal joints and larger joints (hips and knees).

2. Hepatoma risk

a. Primary liver cancer develops in about 14% of patients with hemochromatosis.

b. The risk is 200 times greater than normal.

C. Diagnostic tests

1. Elevated serum iron

2. Elevated transferrin saturation

3. Elevated serum ferritin

4. Liver biopsy

a. Iron is found in hepatocytes, Kupffer cells, bile duct epithelium, and connective tissue.

b. Increased quantitative hepatic iron.

5. Imaging.

a. Magnetic resonance imaging

(1) Iron is a naturally occurring paramagnetic contrast agent. In hemochromatosis there is a marked decrease in P2 relaxation time.

6. Diagnosis is not complete until the physician screens the patient's first-degree relatives.

a. If saturation if greater than 50% or if the ferritin level is greater than 800 mcg/L, liver biopsy is suggested.

V. Differential Diagnosis

A. Other types of cirrhosis (especially alcoholic) with iron overload.

B. Iatrogenic (blood transfusions).

C. Massive dietary iron intake (Bantu siderosis).

D. Porphyria cutaneous tarda.

VI. Treatment and Patient Monitoring

A. Phlebotomy (The extraction of 500 ml blood removes 250 mg of iron and 130 mg of iron from tissue stores).

1. Weekly or even twice-weekly phlebotomy for about 2 years.

2. Check iron parameters and do repeat liver biopsy to check that removal of iron is complete.

3. Iron stores should be depleted completely and rapidly, as the body can increase the rate of iron absorption six to seven times normal.

4. Once iron stores are depleted, phlebotomy should be performed every 3 or 4 months.

VII. Prognosis

A. If diagnosis is made before cirrhosis and diabetes mellitus occur, the prognosis is excellent, with a normal life expectancy.

B. Five-year mortality in treated patients with hemochromatosis is 11% versus 67% in untreated patients.

C. Two patients had apparent reversal of established cirrhosis with phlebotomies.

D. Primary liver cancer is not prevented by adequate venesection therapy unless the diagnosis is made and treatment is begun before cirrhosis develops.

E. Arthropathy is unaffected by treatment.

F. Cardiac failure may decrease.

G. Hypogonadism may lessen.

Bibliography

Edwards CQ, Griffen LM, Goldgar D et al. Prevalence of hemochromatosis among 11,068 presumably healthy blood donors. *N Engl J Med* 318:1355, 1988.

Chapter 61-K

The Liver in Pregnancy

Howard Rosenblate, M.D.

I. Normal Physiologic Changes
  A. Hemodynamic
   1. A 40–50% increase in blood volume.
     a. Plasma: 1.5 liters
     b. Red blood cells: 0.5 liter
   2. Increase in cardiac output, stroke volume, and heart rate.
   3. Decrease in peripheral vascular resistance.
   4. Increase in renal blood flow.
   5. Hepatic blood flow unaltered but is now a smaller fraction of cardiac output (decreased from 35% to 29%).
   6. Azygous vein flow is increased and esophageal varices can develop.
  B. Blood chemistries
   1. Plasma proteins
     a. Decrease in albumin (10–60%) reflects hemodilution and possibly decreased synthesis.
     b. Increase in ceruloplasmin, fibrinogen, thyroxine-binding globulin, α-1, α-2, β-globulins, and transferrin.
     c. Normal prothrombin time.
   2. Plasma lipids
     a. Increase in peripheral lipolysis and synthesis of triglycerides results in a 300% increase in triglycerides.

     b. Increased cholesterol (25–60%).
   3. Bile acids are unchanged or can be increased two- to threefold, but increased lithogenicity of bile occurs.
   4. Hepatic tests
     a. Rising alkaline phosphatase as pregnancy continues due to the heat-stable placental fraction.
     b. Normal gamma-glutamyl transpeptidase (GGTP)-5′ nucleotidase.
     c. Increased serum leucine aminopeptidase (placental fraction).
     d. *Unchanged* transaminases.
     e. Decreased urea nitrogen and uric acid.
  C. Physical exam
   1. Cutaneous vascular changes
     a. Development of spider angiomas.
     b. Development of palmar erythema.
   2. Decreased blood pressure, especially in the second trimester.

II. Liver Disease Unique to Pregnancy
  A. Hyperemesis gravidarum
   1. Can be associated with a mild increase in bilirubin and transaminases.
   2. No liver sequelae.
  B. Intrahepatic cholestasis of pregnancy
   1. Characterized by pruritus and jaundice,

commencing usually in late pregnancy and disappearing after delivery.

2. Frequently recurrent.
3. High incidence in Chile and Scandinavia.
4. Probably an inherited sensitivity to the cholestatic effects of estrogens.
5. Cholestatic enzymes elevated, but occasionally very high transaminase levels occur.
6. Prothrombin time can become prolonged.
7. Liver failure and hepatic encephalopathy do *not* occur.
8. Liver biopsy shows cholestasis.
9. The prognosis for the fetus is not as benign as for the mother.
   a. Increased rate of prematurity.
   b. Increased rate of stillbirths.
10. Careful monitoring of the mother and fetus during the third trimester recommended.
11. Therapy includes cholestyramine and/or phenobarbital and vitamin K, if needed. All are safe to use.

C. Liver diseases associated with the spectrum of preeclampsia/eclampsia

1. Preeclampsia: Develops in 5–10% of all pregnancies, but most women with preeclampsia exhibit no clinical or laboratory evidence of liver disease. Liver involvement in eclampsia may be the primary cause of death.
   a. Hepatic pathology reveals diffuse deposition of fibrin.
   b. Periportal and portal tract hemorrhage.
   c. Ischemic necrosis.

2. HELLP syndrome (microangiopathic hemolytic anemia, elevated liver enzymes, and low platelets)
   a. Probably the middle of the spectrum of liver disease of preeclampsia.
   b. Occurs in 10–12% of all women with preeclampsia.
   c. Onset may be sudden.
   d. Hepatocellular necrosis present in all patients but to a variable extent.
   e. Hyperbilirubinemia secondary to hemolysis and hepatic dysfunction.
   f. Prothrombin time may be prolonged, but true disseminated intravascular coagulation (DIC) is uncommon.
   g. Renal dysfunction universal.
   h. Treatment includes close monitoring of the mother, liver function tests, platelet count, fetal monitoring, and assessment of fetal lung maturity. Treat hypertension with magnesium sulfate and volume expansion.
   i. If the fetal or maternal condition deteriorates, perform immediate delivery (cesarean section).
   j. Steroids can be used to gain time for fetal lung maturity to take place.
   k. Sudden fetal death can occur.
   l. Maternal mortality is low (2–3%).
   m. Liver necrosis heals, without evidence of chronic liver disease.
   n. HELLP syndrome almost never recurs with subsequent pregnancies.

3. Hepatic rupture
   a. Due to confluent periportal hemorrhage and necrosis from preeclampsia.
   b. Can occur in 1% of preeclamptics.
   c. More common in older multiparous women.
   d. Sudden onset of right upper quadrant pain, liver tenderness, diffuse abdominal pain with peritonitis. Shock often present.
   e. Best diagnostic test is the computed tomography scan.
   f. Prompt laparotomy is the most effective treatment.

4. Acute fatty liver of pregnancy
   a. Rare and often fatal (to the mother and fetus) disorder occurring in the third trimester.
   b. Characterized pathologically by microvesicular fat in the centrilobular region (similar to Reyes syndrome).
   c. More common in prima gravidas, in twin pregnancies, and in women with a male fetus.
   d. Etiology unknown, but the marked increase in hepatic triglycerides and free fatty acids suggests abnormality in lipid metabolism. Free fatty acids interfere with mitochondrial function and adversely affect protein synthesis.
   e. Clinical features include signs of preeclampsia plus epigastric pain, nausea, vomiting, headache, restlessness, and malaise. Hypertension and proteinuria are seen in 21%.
   f. Laboratory test abnormalities include leukocytosis, fragmented erythrocytes, decreased platelets, decreased clotting factors, and DIC. Transaminases are

only modestly elevated, but hyperbilirubinemia is usually present.

g. Hypoglycemia is often present, and hepatic encephalopathy can develop rapidly.

h. Some renal insufficiency occurs in the majority of women.

i. Viral hepatitis in preeclampsia-related liver disease must be ruled out to establish the diagnosis.

j. Historically, maternal mortality (usually secondary to complications of liver failure) is 50% and infant mortality is also 50%. However, more recent studies indicate a maternal mortality of 22%.

k. Treatment is urgent delivery.

l. The disease does *not* recur in subsequent pregnancies, and no chronic liver disease occurs.

III. Viral Hepatitis Complicating Pregnancy

A. Clinical features of hepatitis A, B, and C no different from those in the nonpregnant state.

B. Hepatitis E is epidemic non-A, non-B hepatitis.

1. Unique feature is fulminant hepatitis with an unusually high mortality among pregnant women (approximately in the third trimester) (20%).

Bibliography

Bradley DW, Krawczynski K, Cook EH, et al. Enterically transmitted non-A, non-B hepatitis: Etiology of disease in laboratory studies in nonhuman primates, in Zuckerman AJ (ed): *Viral Hepatitis and Liver Disease*. New York, Alan R Liss, 1988, pp 138–147.

Hibbard LT. Maternal mortality due to acute toxemia. *Obstet Gynecol* 42:263, 1973.

Kenopp RH, Warth MR, Carrol CJ. Lipid metabolism in pregnancy. *J Reprod Med* 10:95, 1973.

Larrey D, et al. Recurrent jaundice caused by recurrent hyperemesis gravidarum. *Gut* 25:1414, 1984.

MacKenna J, Dover NL, Brame RG, et al. Preeclampsia associated with hemolysis, elevated liver enzymes and low platelets: An obstetrical emergency? *J Obstet Gynecol* 62:751, 1983.

Potter JM, Nestle PJ. The hyperlipidemia of pregnancy in normal and complicated pregnancies. *Am J Obstet Gynecol* 153:165, 1979.

Riely CA, Latham PS, Romero R, et al. Acute fatty liver of pregnancy: A reassessment based on observations in nine patients. *Ann Intern Med* 106:703, 1987.

Weinstein L. Syndrome of hemolysis, elevated liver enzymes and low platelet count: A severe consequence of hypertension in pregnancy. *Am J Obstet Gynecol* 142:159, 1982.

Hepatic Transplantation

Donald M. Jensen, M.D.

I. Procedure: Technical Description

Orthotopic liver transplantation (OLT) involves removal of the native diseased liver, including the intrahepatic portion of the inferior vena cava, and replacement with a cadaveric donor liver of similar or smaller size and of the same ABO blood type. Venovenous bypass is occasionally used to prevent intestinal and renal congestion and to maintain blood flow to the right atrium.

II. Indications

A. End-stage cirrhosis with less than a 1- to 2-year life expectancy.

B. Fulminant hepatic failure unresponsive to conservative measures.

C. Certain genetic metabolic disorders, such as homozygous hypercholesterolemia, tyrosinemia, and primary hyperoxaluria for which OLT corrects the metabolic defect even in the absence of structural liver disease.

D. Poor quality of life or intractable symptoms related to liver disease which is not associated with an immediate threat to life, such as intractable pruritus or hepatic encephalopathy.

E. Carcinoma (primary) of the liver without evidence of extrahepatic spread.

III. Contraindications

A. Absolute

1. Sepsis or other serious infection outside the hepatobiliary system

2. Metastatic cancer

3. Significant cardiopulmonary disease

B. Relative

1. Age above 65 years

2. Portal vein thrombosis

3. Previous biliary tract surgery

4. Chronic renal insufficiency

5. Active alcoholism or intravenous drug use

6. Human immunodeficiency virus positivity

7. Prior side-to-side portocaval shunt

IV. Complications

A. Perioperative

1. Acute graft dysfunction

2. Graft infarction

3. Graft rejection

4. Infection

   a. Bacterial

   b. Viral

5. Renal failure

6. Biliary Leak

B. Late
   1. Graft rejection
   2. Infection
   3. Biliary stricture
   4. Cancer recurrence
   5. Hypertension
   6. Renal insufficiency
   7. Hepatitis
V. **Risks and Benefits**
   A. Results
      1. One-year survival = 75%.
      2. Five-year survival = 60–70%.

3. Results are better if the recipient is not hospitalbound or in the intensive care unit and has a serum creatinine level below 1.8 mg/dl.

Bibliography

Maddrey WC, Vanthiel DH: Liver transplantation: an overview. *Hepatology* 8:948, 1988.

Williams JR, Vera SR, Peters TG, et al: Survival following hepatic transplantation in the cyclosporine era. *Am Surg* 52:291, 1986.

CHAPTER 62

Granulomatous Diseases

Donald M. Jensen, M.D.

I. **Definition**
A focal, well-circumscribed, microscopic collection of inflammatory cells, consisting predominantly of mononuclear phagocytes, that is clearly distinct from the surrounding uninvolved liver parenchyma.

II. **Etiology**
  A. Infectious causes
    1. Bacterial
        a. Tuberculosis
        b. Leprosy
        c. Brucellosis
    2. Mycotic
        a. Histoplasmosis
        b. Coccidiomycosis
    3. Parasitic
        a. Schistosomiasis
        b. Toxocariasis
    4. Viral
        a. Cytomegalovirus
    5. Rickettsial
        a. Q fever
    6. Spirochetal
        a. Secondary syphilis
  B. Drugs and compounds
    1. Beryllium

    2. Phenylbutazone
    3. Allopurinol
    4. Sulfonamides
    5. Quinidine
    6. Chlorpropamide
    7. Carbamazepine
  C. Others
    1. Sarcoidosis
    2. Primary biliary cirrhosis
    3. Crohn's disease
    4. Hodgkin's disease
    5. Jujunoileal bypass
    6. Wegener's granulomatosis
    7. Polymyalgia rheumatic
    8. Hypogammaglobulinemia
    9. Carcinoma

III. **Pathophysiology**
The presence of hepatic granulomas implies that the liver is actively destroying or isolating foreign antigenic substances or microorganisms by means of phagocytic and cellular immune mechanisms.

IV. **Diagnosis**
  A. History
    1. Fever—most common symptom
    2. Weight loss

3. Night sweats
4. Malaise

B. Clinical signs and physical findings
1. Hepatomegaly
2. Splenomegaly
3. Lymphadenopathy
4. Skin lesions

C. Diagnostic tests
1. Alkaline phosphatase elevation is frequent.
2. Bilirubin is normal or only mildly elevated.
3. Aminotransferase levels are usually elevated but less than 10-fold.
4. Liver biopsy is very useful in establishing the diagnosis of hepatic granuloma, but less helpful in delineating the etiology. Special stains may demonstrate infectious organisms. Culture of the biopsy specimen should also be obtained if infectious causes are likely.
5. Serologic tests may prove useful, especially for primary biliary cirrhosis (mitochondrial autoantibody) and certain infections (brucellosis, Q fever, cytomegalovirus, Epstein-Barr virus, toxoplasmosis, syphilis, and fungi).

V. Differential Diagnosis

Typically, the differential diagnosis involves other disorders associated with high alkaline phosphatase levels, hepatomegaly, and minimal or absent jaundice. These disorders include extrahepatic biliary obstruction, primary sclerosing cholangitis, primary or metastatic neoplasms, amyloidosis, passive congestion, and intrahepatic cholestasis due to drugs or viral hepatitis.

VI. Treatment

Treatment depends upon the correct identification of the cause of the garanulomas. Since tuberculosis and sarcoidosis are the most common causes, a therapeutic trial of antituberculous therapy is occasionally warranted.

VII. Patient Monitoring

Follow-up and management are dependent upon the etiology of the granulomas. In general, there should be a gradual improvement in clinical symptoms, along with a decrease in alkaline phosphatase activity.

VIII. Prognosis

With the exception of primary biliary cirrhosis, AIDS-related lesions and lymphomas, the prognosis is generally good following the institution of specific automicrobial therapy or withdrawal of offending agents.

Bibliography

Alexander JF, Galambos JT: Granulomatous hepatitis. *Am J Gastroenterol* 59:23, 1973.

Simon HB, Wolff SM: Granulomatous hepatitis and prolonged fever of unknown origin: a study of 13 patients *Medicine (Balt)* 52:1, 1973.

SECTION 8

Hematology

CHAPTER 63

Hematopoiesis

Solomon S. Adler, M.D., F.A.C.P.

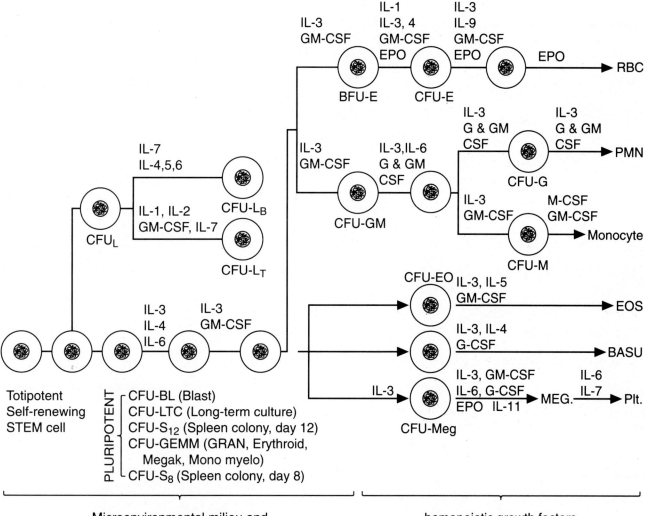

Figure 63-1   Hemopoietic stem cell hierarchy and growth factors.

Abbreviations: L$_B$, B-Lymphocyte; L$_T$, T-lymphocyte; MEG, megakaryocytes; $_L$, lymphoid; IL, interleukin; CSF, colony-stimulating factor; CFU, colony-forming unit (i.e., in vitro assayable hemopoietic precursor cells); BL, blasts; GEMM, granulocyte, erythroid, monocyte, macrophage; GM, granulocyte-macrophage; G, granulocyte; M, macrophage; E, erythroid; BFU-E, burst-forming unit (early erythroid precursor); CFU-E, colony-forming unit erythroid (late erythroid precursor); EO, eosinophil. Recently discovered factors, including IL-11 for megakaryocytes and stem cell factor or kit ligand, which synergize with many other factors, add to the complexity of progenitor cell regulation.

851

CHAPTER 64

Approach to the Patient with Anemia

Walter Fried, M.D.

I. Problem
Everyone, regardless of age, must be considered to be anemic if the hematocrit is less than the lower limit of the normal range in the laboratory.

II. Differential Diagnosis
A low hematocrit or hemoglobin is almost always diagnostic of anemia. Exceptions are as follows:
A. Plasma volume is expanded due to fluid overload, congestive heart failure, or paraproteinemia.
B. There is evidence that occasional persons older than 80 may have a reduced hematocrit due to no identifiable cause other than their age. However, it is unwise to attribute anemia to aging unless a thorough search for an etiology was first conducted.

III. History and Physical Examination
A. Signs and symptoms referable to anemia per se
  1. Pallor
  2. Easy fatigability
  3. Exacerbation of congestive heart failure
  4. Exacerbation of ischemic cardiac and/or cerebral disease
B. Anemias that progress slowly are less symptomatic than those of rapid onset.

C. Most anemias are secondary to other conditions, and the presenting symptoms are often determined by the primary disease.

IV. Diagnostic Approach
The following procedure can be used to investigate the etiology of anemias.
A. Determine the reticulocyte index as follows:
  Patient's hematocrit/45 × percentage of reticulocytes
  1. If high:
    a. It may be due to recovery from anemia. If so, the hematocrit should be rising.
    b. If the hematocrit is stable or falling, then the anemia is most likely due to hemolysis.
  2. If it is normal or low, the anemia is hyporegenerative.
B. In the case of hyporegenerative anemias, look next at the mean corpuscular volume (MCV).
  1. Normocytic
    a. If there is also a reduction in the white blood cell (WBC) count and/or the platelet count, then the abnormality is probably located in the multipotential stem cell or in the hematopoietic mi-

croenvironment. The diagnosis will almost always be based on the marrow biopsy.

   b. If the WBC and platelet counts are normal, then consider the following:

     (1) Disease of the erythroid committed progenitors

     (2) Decreased erythropoietin production

     (3) Mild iron deficiency anemia

     (4) Anemia of chronic disease

     (5) Sideroblastic anemia

     (6) Combined macro- and microcytic anemia

2. Microcytic: microcytic anemias are always the result of a defect in hemoglobin synthesis and include:

   a. Moderate and severe iron deficiency

   b. Some anemias of chronic disease

   c. Thalassemia

   d. Some sideroblastic anemias

3. Macrocytic: macrocytic anemias are the result of impaired DNA synthesis and include:

   a. Vitamin B_{12} deficiency

   b. Folic acid deficiency

   c. Liver disease

   d. Primary marrow dyscrasias

   e. Use of antimctabolites, alkylating agents, mitotic poisons, and other drugs that interfere with DNA synthesis.

CHAPTER 65

Anemia

Walter Fried, M.D.

Normocytic Anemia—Aplastic Anemia

I. Definition
Aplastic anemia is a hematopoietic disorder characterized by pancytopenia and hypoplasia of the hematopoietic cells in the bone marrow.

II. Etiology
Although the cause of aplastic anemia cannot be determined in most cases, a variety of conditions have been implicated.
  A. Radiation exposure
  B. Pharmaceutical agents
    1. That cause dose-related aplasia
      a. Alkylating agents
      b. Antimetabolites
    2. That cause aplasia idiosyncratically
      a. Chloramphenicol
      b. Phenylbutazone
      c. Sulfa drugs
      d. Others
  C. Occupational exposure, particularly to petroleum-derived hydrocarbons such as benzene, TNT, and Stoddard reagents.
  D. Viral infections
    1. Hepatitis B
    2. Human immunodeficiency virus (HIV)
    3. Epstein-Barr virus (EBV)
  E. Congenital—Fanconi's anemia
  F. Aplastic anemia of pregnancy
  G. Idiopathic

III. Pathophysiology
Aplastic anemia is the consequence of processes which either result in the destruction of hematopoietic stem cells or interfere with their ability to replicate and/or differentiate. These defects may result from:
  A. Destruction of the hematopoietic stem cells.
  B. Somatic mutations that result in defects in their ability to replicate or differentiate.
  C. Accessory cell dysfunction
    1. Presence of T lymphocytes that suppress hematopoiesis.
    2. Imbalance in the production or concentration of stimulatory and inhibitory growth factors in the microenvironment.

IV. Diagnosis
  A. History
    1. Presenting complaints include dyspnea, fatigue, fever, and/or bleeding.
    2. Symptoms of preexisting cardiac or cerebral ischemia may be exacerbated.
    3. It is important to determine if there was

exposure to potentially causative occupational, pharmaceutical, or infectious conditions.

B. Physical findings
   1. Signs of congestive heart failure may occur if the anemia is severe and/or if there was preexisting heart disease.
   2. Petechia or ecchymoses.
   3. Splenomegaly is usually absent.
C. Diagnostic procedures and laboratory tests
   1. The blood smear contins no abnormal cells.
   2. The complete blood count (CBC) shows pancytopenia.
   3. The bone marrow biopsy and aspirate show:
      a. Hypocellular marrow.
      b. Decreased cell:fat ratio.
      c. Absence of abnormal cells.

V. **Differential Diagnosis**
Aplastic anemia must be differentiated from other conditions that cause pancytopenia, such as aleukemic leukemia and myelodysplastic syndromes. These conditions are almost always definitively diagnosed on the bone marrow biopsy.

VI. **Therapy**
A. Severe aplastic anemia (reticulocyte index <1.0, absolute neutrophil level <500/mm, and platelet, level <20,000/mm).
   1. Allogeneic bone marrow transplantation is the treatment of choice if:
      a. The patient has a human leukocyte antigen (HLA)-identical sibling (use of matched marrow from an unrelated donor is under investigation as an alternative).
      b. The patient is <50 years old.
   2. In patients ineligible for marrow transplantation, antithymocyte globulin (ATG), cyclosporine, or both may be effective.
   3. Other treatments that are occasionally effective in refractory cases include:
      a. High-dose steroids.
      b. Splenectomy.
      c. Plasmapheresis.
B. Nonsevere aplastic anemia
   1. ATG and/or cyclosporine.
   2. Androgenic-anabolic steroids.
   3. Supportive care.
      a. Transfusions
      b. Trial of erythropoietin, GM-CSF, or G-CSF.

VII. **Patient Monitoring**
The patient should be monitored closely for fever, bleeding, and severity of the anemia.

VIII. **Prognosis**
Severe aplastic anemia treated with:
A. Supportive care only—less than 20% survive for 1 year.
B. Bone marrow transplantation—70% cured.
C. ATG and/or cyclosporine
   1. Forty percent respond and become transfusion independent.
   2. Twenty percent or more of these patients are at risk of recurrence of aplasia or of developing paroxysmal nocturnal hemoglobinuria, myelodysplasia, or acute leukemia.

Normocytic Anemia—Pure Red Cell Aplasia

I. **Definition**
Red cell aplasia is an anemia associated with almost total absence of erythropoiesis, along with normal or near-normal myelopoiesis and thrombopoiesis.

II. **Etiology**
A. Inherited Blackfan-Diamond syndrome (will not be discussed)
B. Acute red cell aplasia
   1. Viral infections
      a. Parvovirus
      b. EBV
   2. Pharmaceutical agents
      a. Diphenylhydantoin
      b. Chloramphenicol
      c. Sulfa drugs
C. Chronic acquired red cell aplasia
   1. Thymoma—found in 50% of cases
   2. Lymphoproliferative disorders
      a. Chronic lymphocytic leukemia
      b. Large granular lymphocytosis
   3. Autoimmune disorders
   4. Idiopathic

III. **Pathogenesis**
A. In cases associated with parvovirus infection, the virus has been shown to enter and destroy erythroid cells.
B. Most other acquired cases are believed to be the result of antibodies directed against antigens on erythroid precursors.
C. In the Blackfan-Diamond syndrome, the defect is in the erythroid progenitors.

IV. **Diagnosis**
A. History: Presenting symptoms are the result

of the anemia. Other data that should be elicited include:

1. Medications
2. Recent infections
3. Present and past autoimmune disorders
4. Neoplasms

B. Physical findings
1. Signs attributable to severe anemia, including exacerbation of congestive heart failure.
2. Splenomegaly and adenopathy are not present.

C. Laboratory and x-ray studies
1. CBC—normocytic anemia with normal red cell morphology, white blood cell (WBC) count, and platelet count.
2. Absolute reticulocytopenia.
3. Bone marrow aspirate and biopsy.
   a. Normal cellularity with absent erythropoiesis.
   b. Although myeloid and megakaryocytic cells are usually normal, they may occasionally be atypical.
4. Computed tomography (CT) scan of the mediastinum should be done in all cases to exclude the presence of a thymoma.
5. Blood tests for:
   a. Antinuclear antibodies.
   b. Rheumatoid factor.
   c. Immune complexes.
   d. Liver and renal function.
6. Urinalysis.
7. A few specialized laboratories are capable of detecting autoantibodies directed to erythroid precursors.

V. Differential Diagnosis

Red cell aplasia must be differentiated from other causes of normocytic anemia. The near-total absence of erythropoiesis in a severely anemia patient with normal myelopoiesis and megakaryopoiesis is de facto proof of this condition.

VI. Therapy

A. Supportive—transfusions.
B. Treatment of the primary condition.
C. Discontinue the use of any suspected medication.
D. Removal of the thymoma, if present (this does not always correct the anemia).
E. The specific therapy for primary cases is immunosuppression using the following agents, either in sequence or in combination:
1. Prednisone
2. Cyclophosphamide
3. ATG
4. Cyclosporine
5. In cases refractory to these medications, one may try the following:
   a. High-dose intravenous immunoglobulins (effective in cases secondary to parvovirus)
   b. Plasmapheresis
   c. Splenectomy

VII. Patient Monitoring

This consists of monitoring the severity of the anemia and the reticulocyte count.

VIII. Prognosis

A. In cases secondary to an identified condition, the prognosis is determined by the responsiveness of the primary condition to therapy.
B. In acute cases, patients recover when the offending medication is discontinued or the viral infection subsides.
C. Primary cases—60% of patients have a complete remission after immunosuppression, and about 50% of these remain in remission after discontinuation of medication.

Normocytic Anemia—Anemia of Chronic Renal Failure

I. Definition

A normocytic, nonregenerative, mild hemolytic anemia that occurs in persons with impaired renal function.

II. Etioloty

Renal failure, regardless of the cause.

III. Pathogenesis

A. Decreased erythropoietin production due to:
1. Damage to the site of erythropoietin production.
2. Decreased hemoglobin oxygen affinity, resulting in more efficient oxygen delivery.
B. Mild hemolysis

IV. Diagnosis

A. History: The prominent features of the history are those related to the renal disease.
B. Physical examination: No specific findings.
C. Diagnostic tests
1. CBC: normocytic anemia with normal WBC and platelet counts.
2. Blood smear: contains burr cells in proportion to the severity of the uremia.

3. Decreased reticulocyte index relative to the severity of the anemia.
4. Decreased serum erythropoietin level relative to the severity of the anemia.
5. High serum iron and ferritin levels.
6. Marrow aspirate is normally cellular, with normal maturation, and the erythroid series is relatively reduced.

V. Differential Diagnosis

All patients with renal failure are anemic. It is important to determine whether the anemia is due to renal failure alone or is complicated by conditions that occur in association with renal failure and its treatment, such as:

A. Iron deficiency which is differentiated by the presence of low serum iron and ferritin levels.
B. The anemia of chronic disease which is also associated with a low serum iron level.
C. Microcytosis, which suggests iron deficiency or aluminum toxicity.
D. Increased hemolysis, which may result from:
   1. Hypersplenism.
   2. Pentose phosphate shunt dysfunction.
   3. Microangiopathic hemolysis.
   4. Abnormal dialysate.

VI. Treatment

A. Adequate dialysis.
B. Administration of erythropoietin to maintain the hematocrit between 35% and 40%.

VII. Patient Monitoring

A. CBCs to detect worsening of the anemia and a change in the MCV.
B. Serum iron and ferritin levels.

VIII. Prognosis

The natural history of the anemia is to progress as the severity of the renal failure increases until end-stage renal failure occurs, at which time the anemia usually remains constant unless it is complicated by another condition. The severity of the anemia varies from patient to patient and is in general not related to the etiology of the renal failure except in the case of polycystic disease, in which the anemia is slower to develop and is generally less severe. Almost all patients respond to the administration of erythropoietin with amelioration of the anemia.

Normocytic Anemia—Anemia of Hypothyroidism and/or Hypopituitarism

I. Definition

A normocytic and hyporegenerative anemia associated with these endocrinopathies.

II. Etiology

Hypothyroidism and/or hypopituitarism.

III. Pathophysiology

The hypometabolic state that accompanies the decreased function of these endocrine organs results in decreased oxygen requirements and, consequently, decreased erythropoietin production.

IV. Diagnosis

A. The anemia is normocytic.
B. The reticulocyte index is normal.
C. The serum iron, ferritin, and creatinine levels are normal.

V. Differential Diagnosis

A mild normocytic anemia associated with normal serum iron, ferritin, and creatinine levels in a patient with hypothyroidism or hypopituitarism is presumably secondary to the endocrinopathy.

VI. Treatment

The treatment is directed to correction of the primary condition.

VII. Patient Monitoring

It is important to follow the course of the anemia as the endocrine deficiency is corrected. If the anemia persists after correction of the endocrinopathy, then other causes for the anemia should be sought.

VIII. Prognosis

Anemia should be corrected within several weeks after correction of the endocrine deficiency.

Microcytic Anemia—Iron Deficiency Anemia

I. Definition

An anemia resulting from depletion of the body's iron stores.

II. Etiology

A. Blood loss due to:
   1. Gastrointestinal bleeding.
   2. Vaginal bleeding.
   3. Hematuria (very rare cause).
B. Nutritional—only in association with conditions that result in increased requirements for iron.
   1. During infancy.
   2. During pregnancy.
C. Malabsorption
   1. Due to chelation of iron in the gastrointestinal (GI) tract by substances such as clay and starch.
   2. Postgastrectomy: The absorption of fer-

ric iron is impaired (this is usually not the sole cause of iron deficiency).

3. Severe diffuse disease of the duodenum (where most iron is absorbed).

III. Pathophysiology

Iron deficiency anemia occurs when there is insufficient iron available from the stores and from the daily diet to produce sufficient hemoglobin to replace that lost daily by senescence of red cells (about 0.8% daily) plus that lost by bleeding.

IV. Diagnosis

A. History: The presenting symptoms may be related to the anemia or to the cause of the bleeding. The clinician should ask specifically about:

1. GI symptoms such as:
   a. Change in bowel habits
   b. Pain
   c. Vomiting
   d. Weight loss
   e. Bleeding
2. In females of childbearing age
   a. Description of menses
   b. Pregnancies

B. Physical examination

1. Signs of congestive heart failure.
2. Orthostatic hypotension or tachycardia, which suggest that the blood loss was rapid and large.

C. Laboratory findings

1. Decreased serum iron
2. Increased total iron-binding capacity (TIBC) (this occurs only if the anemia is not associated with malignant, infectious, or inflammatory disease).
3. Decreased serum ferritin level.
4. Absent stainable iron in the bone marrow.

V. Differential Diagnosis (see Table 65-1)

VI. Therapy

Once the diagnosis of iron deficiency is estab-

lished, a search for a source of blood loss is required.

A. In males and postmenopausal females, this includes indoscopic and, if needed, radiologic investigations of the GI tract.

B. In females of childbearing age, this includes an examination of the reproductive tract.

C. Replenishment of iron stores

1. Ferrous sulfate or comparable oral iron compounds should be taken until the anemia is corrected and then for an additional 6 months to restore the iron stores.
2. Iron dextran may be given parenterally (either IV or IM) if the patient is unwilling to take oral iron or is unreliable. If parenteral iron replacement is used, then the dose must be carefully calculated to provide the amount required for synthesis of the hemoglobin needed to correct the anemia and to replenish the iron stores, and no more.

VII. Patient Monitoring

The CBC must be monitored at frequent intervals until the anemia has been corrected and then at increasingly longer intervals.

VIII. Prognosis

The prognosis is dependent on the ability to correct the condition responsible for the blood loss.

Microcytic Anemia—The Anemia of Chronic Disease

I. Definition

A mild to moderate nonprogressive anemia that accompanies inflammatory, infectious, and neoplastic diseases.

II. Etiology

Inflammatory, infectious, and/or neoplastic disease.

Table 65-1.   Differential Diagnosis of Microcytic Anemia

Anemia	Serum Fe	TIBC	Serum Ferritin	MCV	Bone Marrow
Mild iron deficiency	Low	High	Low	Normal or low	Absent iron stores
Severe iron deficiency	Low	High	Low	Low	Absent iron stores
Chronic disease	Low	Low	High	Normal or low	Normal or high iron stores
Iron deficiency and chronic disease	Low	Low	Low or low normal	Normal or low	Absent iron stores
Sideroblastic anemia	Normal or high	Normal	High	Normal or low	Ringed sideroblasts
Thallassemia	High	Normal	High	Low	High iron stores

III. **Pathophysiology**
   A. Inability of the reticuloendothelial system to process iron derived from senescent erythrocytes. Therefore there is insufficient iron available to the erythroid precursors to maintain a normal rate of erythropoiesis.
   B. The erythrocyte life span is often modestly reduced.
   C. The serum erythropoietin titer is sometimes lower than expected for the reduced red cell mass.

IV. **Diagnosis**
   A. The primary disease causing the anemia is rarely subtle and usually determines the patient's symptoms.
   B. The anemia is rarely severe (hemoglobin is seldom lower than 9.0g/dl).
   C. The MCV is either normal or low.
   D. Both the serum iron and the TIBC are always low.
   E. The serum ferritin level is high unless the patient is also iron deficient.

V. **Differential Diagnosis** (see Table 65-1)

VI. **Treatment**
   A. Therapy should be directed toward correcting the primary condition.
   B. Occasionally the primary condition is not readily correctable and the anemia is sufficiently severe to cause symptoms. Erythropoietin may then be tried. It should be noted that relatively large doses may be required and at considerable expense.

VII. **Patient Monitoring**
   The CBC should be monitored as the primary condition is treated to be sure that the anemia, as well as the primary condition, is corrected.

VIII. **Prognosis**
   The prognosis is related to the primary condition.

Microcytic Anemia—Sideroblastic

I. **Definition**
   An anemia characterized by the presence of ringed sideroblasts in the bone marrow and by ineffective erythropoiesis.

II. **Etiology**
   A. Congenital
      1. Sex-linked
      2. Other
   B. Acquired (primary)
      1. Benign
      2. Myelodysplastic
   C. Secondary: toxic exposure to lead, alcohol, alkylating agents, antituberculous drugs, and other drugs.

III. **Pathogenesis**
   The ringed sideroblasts which characterize this disorder consist of erythroid progenitors in which the mitochondria are distended with nonferritin iron, which accumulates because of inability to be incorporated into heme.

IV. **Diagnosis**
   A. History: Should emphasize familial incidence, exposure to toxins in the workplace, and alcohol and drug use.
   B. Physical examination: Aside from the signs attributable to anemia in general, splenomegaly is sometimes present.
   C. Laboratory findings
      1. CBC: Except for the primary acquired cases, the WBC and platelet counts are normal. The MCV may be normal or low (if there is also folate deficiency, it may even be high).
      2. The peripheral blood smear contains anisocytosis and always a population of microcytes (even if the MCV is not low). In cases secondary to lead toxicity, the erthrocytes show prominent basophilic stippling.
      3. The reticulocyte index is usually normal.
      4. The marrow aspirate is hypercellular, with an increased erythroid:myeloid ratio. Prussian blue stain shows numerous ringed sideroblasts.
      5. The serum iron and ferritin levels are high.
      6. The indirect bilirubin may be high if there is much ineffective erythropoiesis.

V. **Differential Diagnosis**
   A. Any anemia associated with the presence of a large number of ringed sideroblasts in the marrow is a sideroblastic anemia.
   B. Primary acquired sideroblastic anemia cannot always be distinguished from the preleukemic variety (myelodysplastic), but the following information may be helpful:
      1. It occurs predominantly in elderly patients.
      2. WBC and platelet abnormalities are uncommon.
      3. Karyotypic abnormalities are less common.

VI. **Therapy**
   A. Discontinue exposure to potentially causative agents and conditions.
   B. A trial of high-dose pyridoxine is always indicated.
   C. Transfusions.
   D. Androgenic-anabolic steroids are sometimes effective.

E. In chronic cases with iron overload, chelation therapy may be required.

VII. Patient Monitoring

The serum ferritin level as well as the CBC should be monitored in chronic cases to detect the inception of iron overload.

VIII. Prognosis

A. Congenital: A lifelong, often transfusion-dependent anemia with a high risk of causing hemochromatosis.

B. Primary: Usually a mild to moderate chronic anemia of elderly persons. It is often difficult to distinguish this from the preleukemic variety.

C. Secondary: The prognosis is dependent on the ability to correct the offending condition.

Macrocytic Anemia—Vitamin B_{12} Deficiency

I. Definition

The anemia caused by deficiency of vitamin B_{12}.

II. Etiology

A. Malabsorption caused by:
  1. Lack of intrinsic factor
     a. Postgastrectomy
     b. Pernicious anemia
  2. Chronic pancreatitis
  3. "Blind loop" syndrome
  4. Tapeworm Diphyllobothrium (D. *latum*)
  5. Disease or removal of the terminal ileum
B. Nutritional deficiency is extremely rare and occurs only in vegans.

III. Pathophysiology

A. Megaloblastic changes are the result of defective DNA synthesis. In the hematopoietic cells, this results in an imbalance between maturation and proliferation. Vitamin B_{12} is a cofactor in an important reaction involved in endogenous thymidine synthesis.

B. Neurologic changes result from the accumulation of methylmalonic acid, a toxic metabolite of propionic acid. Vitamin B_{12} is an essential cofactor for its metabolism.

IV. Diagnosis

A. History
  1. A family history of pernicious anemia or autoimmune disease is frequently present in patients with pernicious anemia.
  2. Query the patient about stomach or bowel surgery.
  3. In addition to the symptoms of anemia, GI disturbances may occur.
  4. Numbness and tingling of the extremities are the earliest signs of neurologic damage.
B. Physical examination
  1. Pallor and mild jaundice are common.
  2. Smooth, depapillated tongue.
  3. Neurologic abnormalities may include:
     a. Posterolateral column degeneration.
     b. Peripheral neuropathies.
     c. Abnormalities in mentation (particularly in elderly patients).
C. Laboratory studies:
  1. CBC shows a macrocytic anemia, with or without neutropenia and thrombocytopenia.
  2. Peripheral blood smear shows macro-ovalocytes and hypersegmented "polys."
  3. The serum vitamin B_{12} level is reduced.
  4. Shilling test shows reduced vitamin B_{12} absorption in all cases. This is corrected by addition of intrinsic factor in patients with pernicious anemia and gastrectomy.
  5. Serum lactic dehydrogenase and indirect bilirubin levels may be elevated.
  6. The bone marrow is hypercellular. Usually there is erythroid hyperplasia and megaloblastic maturation in all three cell lines.
  7. Antibodies to intrinsic factor are found in about 20% of cases of pernicious anemia.
  8. Because of the high incidence of gastric carcinoma, patients with pernicious anemia should have GI endoscopy for any suspicious symptoms.

V. Differential Diagnosis

Vitamin B_{12} deficiency is distinguished from other macrocytic anemias by a low serum vitamin B_{12} level and an abnormal Shilling test.

VI. Therapy

A. Vitamin B_{12}, 1,000 μg given IM daily for at least 7 days (longer in patients with severe neurologic defects), then weekly for 1 month, then monthly for life.

B. Treatment of etiologic conditions, such as bacterial overgrowth in a "blind loop" of bowel, tapeworms, or inflammatory disease of the terminal ileum.

VII. Patient Monitoring

A. The CBC should be followed until the anemia is completely corrected.

B. The serum potassium level must be closely monitored during the early phases of therapy to avoid severe hypokalemia.

C. Patients with pernicious anemia should be monitored for early signs and symptoms of gastric carcinoma.

VIII. Prognosis

A. Reticulocytosis should begin within 3 days of initiating therapy, and the anemia should improve steadily and resolve completely.

B. The neurologic abnormalities are likely to improve with therapy but are rarely corrected completely.

Macrocytic Anemia—Folate Deficiency

I. Definition

The anemia associated with folic acid deficiency.

II. Etiology

A. Nutritional: daily requirement is 100–200 μg. Folic acid is found in most leafy vegetables, yeast, and, to a lesser extent, in most meats. It is, however, heat labile and may be destroyed if the food is overcooked.

B. Dietary deficiency occurs commonly in alcoholics, elderly persons with poor dentition, and impoverished populations.

C. Increased folate requirements occur during pregnancy, as well as in patients with hemolytic anemia and rapidly growing neoplasms.

D. Some medications impair the absorption and utilization of folic acid. These include:
1. Diphenylhydantoin.
2. Phenobarbital.
3. Estrogens used in contraceptive pills.

E. Malabsorption of folic acid occurs in diffuse inflammatory bowel diseases such as sprue.

III. Pathogenesis

Folic acid is required as a donor of methyl groups in the conversion of uridine to thymidine. Deficiency results in decreased DNA synthesis and megaloblastic maturation disturbances in the hematopoietic cells, as well as in other proliferating cells in the body.

IV. Diagnosis

A. History: The history should include a compete listing of medications and dietary components.

B. Laboratory studies
1. MCV: Macrocytic indices are always present unless a cause of microcytic anemia also exists.
2. Leukopenia and thrombocytopenia are common.
3. Blood smear shows macro-ovalocytes and hypersegmented "polys."

4. Low serum folate levels are almost always diagnostic. However, in occasional instances, one may also want to determine the red cell folate level, which is less labile and less likely to be falsely depressed.

V. Differential Diagnosis

A. Folate deficiency must be differentiated from vitamin B_{12} deficiency, since administration of folic acid alone to a patient with vitamin B_{12} deficiency can exacerbate the neurologic defects. Therefore, the serum vitamin B_{12} level should always be determined.

B. A low serum folate level should be sufficient to distinguish folate deficiency from other macrocytic anemias, such as those associated with liver disease, use of antimetabolites and alkylating agents, and primary marrow dyscrasia.

VI. Therapy

A. Correction of all associated conditions that are correctable.

B. Administration of folic acid—1 mg daily p.o.

VII. Patient Monitoring

Blood counts must be monitored until they are completely corrected.

VIII. Prognosis

Folic acid deficiency is always correctable. The patient's prognosis is dependent on the primary condition.

Bibliography

Camitta BM, Storb R, Thomas ED: Aplastic anemia pathogenesis, diagnosis, treatment, and prognosis. *N Engl J Med* 306:645–652 & 712–718, 1982.

Colon-Otero G, Hook CC, Menke D: A practical approach to the differential diagnosis and evaluation of the adult patient with macrocytic anemia. *Med Clin North Am* 76:581–597, 1992.

Cook JD, Lynch SR: The liabilities of iron deficiency. *Am J Hematol* 68:803–809, 1986.

Cook JD, Lynch SR, Reusser ME, et al: Estimates of iron sufficiency in the US population. *Blood* 68:726–731, 1986.

Cook JD, Skikne BS: Iron deficiency: definition and diagnosis. *J Int Med* 226:349–355, 1989.

Dainiak N, Dewey MC, Hoffman R: Mechanisms of abnormal erythropoiesis in malignancy. *Cancer* 51:1101–1106, 1983.

Krantz SB, Means RT: Progress in understanding the pathogenesis of the anemia of chronic disease. *Blood* 80:1639–1647, 1992.

Lindenbaum J: Status of laboratory testing in the diagnosis of megaloblastic anemia. *Blood* 61:624–626, 1983.

Rubins JM: The role of myelofibrosis in malignant leukoerythroblastosis. *Cancer* 51:308–311, 1983.

Storb R, Tginas ED: Acquired severe aplastic anemia: progress and perplexity. *Blood* 64:325–328, 1984.

CHAPTER 66-A

Hemoglobinopathies

Henri Frischer, M.D. Ph.D.

I. **Definition**
Autosomally inherited abnormalities of the structure or synthesis of globin.
  A. Structural hemoglobinopathies: almost 400 mutations have been identified.
  B. Thalassemias: heterogeneous inherited anemias with defective globin synthesis.
II. **Etiology**
  A. Biology
    1. Hemoglobin (Hb) contains two pairs of globin chains and four molecules of heme.
    2. The globin chains can be alpha, beta, gamma, delta, epsilon, or zeta.
    3. A separate gene controls the synthesis of each globin chain.
    4. Normal persons inherit:
       a. Four alpha-chain genes (two from each parent, on chromosome 16).
       b. Two beta-chain genes (one from each parent, on chromosome 11).
       c. Two delta-chain genes (closely linked to the beta locus).
       d. Four gamma-chain genes (chromosome 11).
    5. At birth, cord blood contains 75% Hb F (alpha-2–gamma-2).

  a. The balance is mainly Hb A1 (alpha-2–beta-2).
    6. In the first months of life, fetal Hb decreases gradually.
    7. Adult blood contains:
       a. More than 97% Hb A1.
       b. Less than 1% Hb F.
       c. Hb A2 (alpha-2–delta-2), between 2% and 3.5%.
  B. Sickle Syndromes
  Disorders with sickle Hb (alpha-2–beta-2$^{glu6 \rightarrow val}$) include:
    1. Homozygous SS disease or sickle cell anemia.
    2. Heterozygous Hb AS or sickle cell trait.
    3. Compound heterozygosity with Hb S (e.g., SC, S/beta-thalassemia).
  C. Thalassemias
    1. Beta-thalassemia: Most beta-thalassemias are point mutations that interfere with mRNA splicing and transcription. Globin-chain synthesis is absent in null-thalassemia and depressed in plus-thalassemia.
       a. Beta-thalassemia minor or beta-thalassemia trait: Heterozygous beta-thalassemia; mild microcytic anemia.

b. Beta-thalassemia major (Cooley's anemia): Homozygosity for two beta-thalassemia alleles; severe anemia.

c. Beta-thalassemia intermedia: Genetically heterogeneous; moderately severe anemia.

2. Alpha-thalassemias: Most alpha-thalassemias are caused by gene deletions.

a. Alpha-thalassemia-2 trait: One alpha gene is missing; asymptomatic silent carrier state.

b. Alpha-thalassemia-1 trait: Deletion or inactivation of two alpha-globin genes; mild microcytic anemia.

c. Hb H disease: Triple deletion of alpha-globin genes; hemolytic disease of variable severity.

d. Hydrops fetalis with Hb Barts: Total absence of alpha genes; gamma 4 tetramers (Hb Bart's); intrauterine death.

D. Other hemoglobinopathies

1. Hb C (alpha-2–beta-2$^{\text{Glu6}\rightarrow\text{Lys}}$)

a. Common in people of West African origin.

2. HbE (alpha-2–beta-2$^{\text{Glu26}\rightarrow\text{Lys}}$)

a. Second most common Hb variant in the world.

b. Mostly concentrated in South East Asia.

3. Hb D and G

a. No uncommon.

b. Hb D can interact with and be confused with HbS.

c. Hb G-Philadelphia, an alpha-chain mutant, is the most common Hb D-like variant in the United States.

4. Unstable hemoglobins: A very heterogeneous group of mutations causing:

a. Introduction of a charged residue in the Hb core.

b. Introduction of a charged residue in the alpha-1–beta-1 interface.

c. Disruption of the alpha helix.

d. Deletions of multiple residues.

e. Subunit elongation.

f. Exposure of globin sulfhydryl groups.

g. Heme loss.

5. Hemoglobinopathies with aberrant oxygen transport

a. Abnormally high or low oxygen affinity.

b. About 45 mutations associated with erythrocytosis, more than 12 with low oxygen affinity.

6. Hbs M

a. Various mutations that permanently oxidize Hb iron (ferric HbMs).

7. Hereditary persistence of Hb F (HPHF): Defective switch from gamma chain to delta-beta chain synthesis.

III. **Pathophysiology**

A. Sickle syndromes

1. Deoxygenated Hb S polymerizes into fibers.

2. Rate of sickling is modulated by intracellular content.

3. Hb F retards sickling; acidosis accelerates sickling.

4. Fibers deform the cells; cell deformation is reversible at first.

5. Development of cell dehydration, increased viscosity, loss of elasticity, irreversible cell sickling.

6. Adherence to endothelium, cell clumping, aggregates of rigid sickle cells obstruct the microcirculation.

7. Tissue hypoxia leads to further sickling and larger infarcts.

8. Painful crisis, anemia, organ damage.

B. Thalassemias

Globin-chain suppression leads to hypochromia and microcytosis. In the thalassemic traits, microcytosis is out of proportion to the degree of anemia. Unbalanced excess of the unaffected globins dominates pathophysiology.

1. Beta-thalassemia major

a. Alpha-chain excess precipitates in the bone marrow.

b. Compensatory hypersecretion of erythropoietin, ineffective extramedullary erythropoiesis.

c. Severe anemia results from:

(1) Decreased and ineffective erythropoiesis.

(2) Shortened red blood cell (RBC) survival.

(3) Hypochromic microcytosis.

d. Iron overload develops as a consequence of increased gastrointestinal absorption and transfusions.

2. Alpha thalassemia

a. Excess non-alpha chains (gamma or beta) accumulate.

(1) Circulating Hb Bart's (gamma-4) is seen in younger children.

(2) Circulating Hb H (beta-4) is seen in older persons.

b. Hb H is thermally and oxidatively unstable and has a high oxygen affinity.

C. Other hemoglobinopathies

1. Hb C and Hb S/C
   a. Hb C is less soluble than Hb A.
   b. Hyperactive K:Cl cotransport and cell dehydration.
   c. Globin crystallization and spherocytosis.
2. Hb E
   a. Amino acid substitution leads to alternative splicing of beta mRNA.
   b. Mutation acts like a mild beta-thalassemia allele for HbE.
   c. Moreover, the Hb E protein is itself unstable to oxidants and thermal stress.
3. Unstable Hbs
   a. Heme loss, thiol oxidation, globin precipitation.
   b. Hemolytic crisis can be triggered by oxidant drugs.
   c. Denatured globin forms Heinz bodies.
   d. Heinz bodies attach to the membrane.
   e. Rigid RBCs are trapped in the spleen.
   f. Hemolytic anemia.
4. Hemoglobinopathies with high oxygen affinity
   a. Left shift of the oxygen affinity curve (low p50).
   b. Compensation by increased erythropoietin.
   c. Synthesis of 2,3-diphosphoglycerate (2,3-DPG) not increased.
   d. Erythrocytosis.
5. Hemoglobinopathies with low oxygen affinity
   a. Right-shifted oxygen saturation curve (high p50).
   b. Decreased erythropoietin production.
   c. The Hb level is adjusted slightly downward (about 12.0 g/dl).
   d. The increased fraction of deoxyhemoglobin may result in mild cyanosis.
6. Hbs M
   a. Permanent autooxidation of heme iron.
   b. Lifelong cyanosis.

IV. **Diagnosis**

A. Sickle syndromes
1. Sickle trait
   a. In the United States about 8% of African-Americans are heterozygous (Hb AS).
   b. Persons with the sickle trait are almost always asymptomatic.

c. An occasional carrier may sustain a splenic infarct or have painless hematuria.
d. Individuals with the sickle trait have between 35 and 45% Hb S and about 60% Hb A.
2. Homozygous sickle cell anemia: In the United States about 0.15% of African-Americans are homozygous (Hb SS).
   a. Clinical onset
      (1) Patients become symptomatic after the sixth month of life.
      (2) By then most of the Hb F has been replaced by Hb S.
   b. Systemic manifestations
      (1) Impaired growth and development.
      (2) Increased susceptibility to infections.
   c. Anemia
      (1) Invariably present; hematocrit between 18% and 30%.
      (2) Hemolytic crises: exacerbation of anemia with increased reticulocytosis; uncommon except with coexisting glucose-6-phosphate dehydrogenase (G-6-PD) deficiency.
      (3) Aplastic crises: increased anemia without reticulocytosis.
          (a) Viral or bacterial infection.
          (b) Folic acid deficiency.
   d. Vaso-occlusive episodes
      (1) Microinfarcts (painful crises).
      (2) Macroinfarcts (organ damage).
   e. Chronic organ damage: cardiovascular, hepatobiliary, genitourinary, skeletal (avascular necrosis of the femoral head), visual, central nervous system.
   f. Laboratory
      (1) Peripheral smear: irreversibly sickled forms (2–50% of RBCs).
      (2) Reticulocytosis (5–25%); nucleated RBCs, Howell-Jolly bodies.
      (3) Leukocytosis (12,000–15,000/μl).
      (4) Sickling under anoxia: positive solubility test or sickle preparation slide.
      (5) Hb electrophoresis: needed for confirmation.
      (6) In homozygous sickle cell anemia:
          (a) Hb S (80–98%).
          (b) No Hb A on electrophoresis (unless there has been a recent transfusion).
          (c) Hb F is 2–20%.

(d) Hb A2 is not increased.
3. Combined syndromes with Hb S
   a. Sickle-beta-thalassemia (S/beta-Thal): See Section IV, B, 1, d).
   b. Sickle/C disease (Hb SC)
      (1) Mild to moderate anemia (hematocrit: 30–38%).
      (2) Adult splenomegaly not rare.
      (3) Prone to develop retinopathy, hematuria, complications of pregnancy.
      (4) Peripheral smear shows spherocytes, target cells, occasional sickle cells.
      (5) Intracellular clumps of crystalloid Hb are best seen in RBCs exposed to hypertonic sodium chloride.
      (6) Hb electrophoresis: approximately 50% Hb S, 50% Hb C, no increase in Hb F.
   c. Sickle cell/D disease (Hb S/D)
      (1) Hb D interacts unfavorably with Hb S during deoxygenation.
      (2) Clinically, Hb S/D disease can resemble Hb S/beta thalassemia or Hb SS disease.
      (3) See Section V, A, 4.
   d. Hb S/HPHF (hereditary persistance of hemoglobin F).
      (1) Benign condition.
      (2) Hemoglobin pattern: Hb S, 70–80%; Hb F, 20–30%, homogeneously distributed.
B. Thalassemias
   1. Beta-thalassemia
      a. Beta-thalassemia minor
         (1) Usually affects persons of Mediterranean, Asian, or African ancestry.
         (2) Mild microcytic anemia; mean corpuscular volume (MCV) is less than 75 fl.
         (3) Often lifelong personal or family history of microcytic anemia unresponsive to iron therapy.
         (4) Low MCV can be masked by reticulocytosis or megaloblastosis.
         (5) Peripheral smear shows target cells and microcytes.
         (6) Hb A2 is diagnostically elevated (usually 3.5–8%).
         (7) Pathognomonic elevation of A2 can be masked by iron or folate deficiency.
         (8) Hb F is often elevated (1–5%).
      b. Beta-thalassemia major
         (1) Severe anemia, onset after 6 months, Hb can fall to 3 g/dl or lower.
         (2) Growth retardation, skeletal abnormalities.
         (3) Jaundice, cholelithiasis, hepatosplenomegaly.
         (4) Postpuberty hypogonadism, endocrine dysfunctions.
         (5) Myocardial hemosiderosis.
         (6) High-output congestive heart failure.
         (7) Untreated victims die, usually from heart failure, before age 30.
         (8) The smear shows severe microcytosis and targeting.
         (9) Hb F remains predominant even in the older child.
         (10) Prenatal diagnosis by amniocentesis and chorionic villous biopsy is available.
             (a) Abnormal gene identified by direct analysis of fetal DNA.
             (b) Diagnosis possible before the 18th week of gestation.
      c. Beta-thalassemia intermedia
         (1) Clinically defined thalassemic syndrome with chronic hemolytic anemia.
         (2) Patient may require transfusions during periods of stress.
         (3) Hepatosplenomegaly; iron overload is often present in adults.
         (4) Clinical beta-thalassemia intermedia is genetically heterogeneous and can represent:
             (a) Compound heterozygosity for two beta-thalassemia alleles ameliorated by alpha-thalassemia
                 (i) Concomitant deletion of one or two alpha genes (alpha-beta-thalassemia)
             (b) Heterozygous beta-thalassemia complicated by concomitant intrinsic or acquired RBC disorder.
                 (i) Hereditary spherocytosis, G-6-PD deficiency, other enzymopathies, immune hemolysis.
      d. Combined thalassemic states
         (1) Sickle cell–beta-thalassemia

    (a) Painful crises less frequent and severe than in SS disease.

    (b) Hemolytic anemia of variable severity.

    (c) Adult splenomegaly is not rare.

    (d) Hypochromic, microcytic RBCs.

    (e) Electrophoresis shows Hb S, 60–90%; Hb A, 0–30%; Hb A2 greater than 3.5%; Hb F, 10–30%.

    (f) Hb F is heterogeneously distributed among RBCs.

(2) Hb S delta–beta-thalassemia

    (a) Clinically benign, with few or no crises.

    (b) Most of the Hb is S.

    (c) Hb F is increased 20–40%.

    (d) Hb A is absent.

    (e) Hb A2 is decreased.

(3) Hb S/Hb Lepore

    (a) Moderate hemolytic anemia and splenomegaly.

    (b) Most of the Hb is S without A.

    (c) Hb Lepore constitutes 10% and Hb F 10–25% of the total.

2. Alpha-thalassemia

  a. Silent alpha-thalassemia-2 trait

    (1) Very common in persons of Southeast Asian, Chinese, and African ancestry.

    (2) Frequency of more than 20% in some populations (e.g., African-Americans).

    (3) No hematologic manifestations.

    (4) Usually detected when:

      (a) A carrier becomes the parent of a child with Hb H disease.

      (b) The other parent has alpha-thalassemia-1 trait.

    (5) Hb Barts (gamma 4) can be increased (up to 3%) in cord blood.

  b. Alpha-thalassemia-1 trait

    (1) Common in certain populations (e.g., 3–4% in Taiwan).

    (2) Resembles beta-thalassemia minor but there is no elevation of Hb A2.

    (3) Hb Barts in cord blood: 3–8%.

    (4) Screening for RBCs with Hb H inclusions is possible by special staining tests.

  c. Hb H disease (beta 4)

    (1) Clinically an alpha-thalassemia intermedia.

    (2) Seen mostly in Orientals.

    (3) Transfusions may be required.

    (4) Blood smears incubated with brilliant cresyl blue can reveal multiple small intraerythrocytic precipitates of Hb H.

    (5) In fresh blood, alkaline electrophoresis shows a fast-moving component; this comprises up to 30% of the total Hb.

    (6) Hb H is oxidatively unstable.

    (7) Positive dichlorophenolindophenol (DCIP) precipitation test.

  d. Fetal hydrops syndrome

    (1) Disease seen mostly in Southeast Asians.

    (2) Absence of alpha genes.

    (3) Severe Coombs'-negative anemia (Hb, 3–10 g/dl).

    (4) Stillbirth.

    (5) Mothers of affected children are often toxemic.

    (6) Ultrasound studies can reveal fetal hydrops.

    (7) Amniocentesis can yield fetal fibroblasts without alpha genes.

    (8) Hb electrophoresis of fetal blood shows mostly Hb Barts, some Hb H, traces of Hb Portland (masquerading as a trace of Hb A1), and lack of normal Hb A and F.

3. Hb Lepore (delta-beta fusion thalassemia)

  a. Found mainly in Greece and Italy.

  b. Comprises 5–10% of cases with beta-thalassemia.

  c. Clinically resembles beta-thalassemia or alpha-thalassemia-1 trait.

  d. Abnormal Hb Lepore: about 6% of the total.

  e. Hb Lepore migrates in the area of Hb S.

  f. Solubility test for Hb S is negative.

4. Hb switching disorders

  a. Pancellular hereditary persistence of Hb F (HPHF)

    (1) Asymptomatic condition.

    (2) Very high Hb F with uniform distribution in homozygotes.

    (3) Hb F is 10–35% in heterozygotes.

  b. HPHF-beta-thalassemia

    (1) Resembles beta-thalassemia trait.

    (2) Unusually high Hb F.

  c. HPHF-delta-beta-thalassemia

    (1) Presents rarely as thalassemia intermedia.

C. Other hemoglobinopathies
  1. Hb C syndromes
    a. Hb C trait (Hb AC)
      (1) About 2.4% African-Americans are heterozygotes.
      (2) About 0.02% are CC homozygotes.
      (3) Trait is clinically harmless.
      (4) Blood film shows target cells.
      (5) By electrophoresis: Hb C is 30–40% of the total.
    b. Homozygous Hb C disease
      (1) Mild hemolytic anemia with splenomegaly.
      (2) Hematocrit averages 33%.
      (3) MCV is microcytic (72 fl).
      (4) Many target cells and spherocytes.
      (5) Hb crystallizes within RBCs (forming rectangular blocks staining dark red).
      (6) Positive hypertonic saline crystallization test.
      (7) By electrophoresis:
        (a) Hb C accounts for most of the RBC's hemoglobin.
        (b) Hb A is absent.
        (c) Hb F is slightly elevated.
    c. Hb CC/beta-thalassemia-null
      (1) Variable microcytic anemia.
      (2) Splenomegaly.
      (3) Electrophoresis:
        (a) Hb CF pattern with more than 90% Hb C.
    d. Hb CC/beta-thalassemia-plus
      (1) Anemia is less severe than in the null type.
      (2) Electrophoresis pattern is Hb C > Hb F > Hb A.
        (a) Hb C, 65–80% (on top of Hb A2).
        (b) Hb A, 20–30%.
        (c) Hb F, about 5%.
    e. Alpha-thalassemia/Hb C trait
      (1) Microcytic RBCs.
      (2) Hb C is less than 30%.
    f. Alpha-thalassemia trait/homozygous CC
      (1) Hb F increases up to 20%.
  2. Hb E syndromes
    a. Hb E trait
      (1) No anemia, often microcytosis (about 75 MCV in AE, below 70 in EE).
      (2) Standard alkaline electrophoresis: 30–35% Hb E, with the remainder being Hb A.
    b. Hb EE homozygous
      (1) Variable, ranging from compensated mild anemia to thalassemia intermedia.
      (2) Hb E accounts for 95% of the total; the balance is Hb F.
    c. HbE/beta-thalassemia
      (1) Clinically severe; resembles beta-thalassemia intermedia or major.
      (2) In Hb E/beta-thalassemia-null, Hb A is missing. From 60% to 90% of the Hb is Hb E; the remainder is fetal Hb and Hb A2.
      (3) In Hb E/beta-thalassemia-plus, about 10% of the Hb is A.
  3. Unstable Hb variants
    a. Moderate to very severe hemolysis.
    b. Splenomegaly and hypersplenism (with moderate thrombocytopenia).
    c. Oxidative hemolysis after drug therapy or infections, as in G-6-PD deficiency (e.g., Hb Zurich, beta[63 His-Arg]).
    d. Dipyrroluria with dark urine can occur; pigmenturia is produced from catabolized heme.
    e. In blood films stained with supravital stains (methyl or crystal violet), precipitated globin appears as Heinz bodies (dark blue particles, 0.5–2 μm, near cell membrane).
    f. Unstable Hb
      (1) Are rarely detected by routine electrophoresis.
      (2) Are very vulnerable to denaturation by heat or isopropanol.
      (3) Show no deficiency of G-6-PD.
      (4) Show positive ascorbate-cyanide or Heinz body tests.
  4. Hemoglobinopathies with high oxygen affinity
    a. Increased RBC with increased RBC mass
      (1) Hb can increase up to 20 g/dl.
      (2) Ruddiness but no hyperviscosity symptoms.
    b. White blood cell (WBC) counts, platelet counts and the peripheral smear are normal.
    c. Electrophoresis is rarely helpful diagnostically.
    d. Most high-affinity HBs can be diagnosed by a combination of:
      (1) Whole blood p50.
      (2) Whole blood oxygen dissociation curve.

(3) Red cell 2.3-DPG.

(4) Hb spectroscopy.

(5) Serum erythropoietin levels.

5. Hbs with low oxygen affinity

a. Usually there is mild familial cyanosis.

b. Transmission is autosomal dominant.

c. Some decrease in Hb concentration.

6. Hb M

a. Frank cyanosis.

b. No associated symptoms.

c. Autosomal dominant.

d. Hb M blood is brown.

e. Electrophoresis is rarely helpful; neutral or acid agar gel electrophoresis may show a brown band of Hb M.

f. Special detection tests for Hb Ms:

(1) Aberrant spectroscopic peak located anywhere between 575–610 nm.

(2) Aberrant kinetics of complexation with cyanide.

V. Differential Diagnosis

A. Syndromes with Hbs S, C, D, E, and O

1. SS disease

a. SS chest pain with rib infarction versus pneumonitis and pulmonary infarction.

(1) Infiltrate on the chest x-ray is diagnostically useful. Rib films can help.

(2) Sputum culture and Gram stain may help.

b. Abdominal sickle crises versus surgical abdomen.

(1) In SS: usually normal bowel sounds, no rebound tenderness.

c. SS joint pain versus osteomyelytis, gout, or rheumatoid arthritis

(1) Effusions due to sickling:

(a) Clear fluid, no crystals, no bacteria.

(b) Low white blood cell count (<1,000 mononuclear cells per cubic millimeter).

2. Sickle cell-beta thalassemia

a. Splenomegaly in adults is more common than in Hb SS; the MCV is low in S/beta-thalassemia.

b. S/beta-thalassemia shows an increased level of HbA2 that is not seen in Hb SS.

c. Hb S/beta-thalassemia null versus HbS/ beta-thalassemia plus:

(1) The null type is clinically more severe (hematocrit can be less than 30%).

(2) S/beta-thalassemia-null has an Hb SF pattern on alkaline electrophoresis.

(3) S/beta-thalassemia-plus has an Hb SFA pattern.

3. Sickle/C disease

a. Can be confused with Hb S/O Arab.

b. Hb S/O Arab (alpha-2–beta-2$^{121\ \text{Glu-Lys}}$ is more severe).

4. Sickle/D disease must be distinguished from milder Hb SS states.

a. Hb D and S can be confused because they comigrate on alkaline electrophoresis.

b. Hb D is separated from Hb S by acid citrate agar electrophoresis.

c. Hb D does not sickle.

d. In Hb S/D a positive sickle cell preparation is found in only one of the patient's parents.

e. Hb S/D double heterozygotes have a moderately severe sickling syndrome.

5. Hb E syndromes

a. Hb E does not separate well from other slow bands (Hb A2, C, or O).

(1) Hb A2 is less abundant than Hb E.

(2) Hb C separates from Hb E by acid citrate agar electrophoresis.

(3) Hb E is distinguished from Hb O and other variants by oxidative instability.

(4) Positive dichlorophenolindophenol precipitation test with Hb E.

6. Hb S/O Arab syndrome

a. Hb O Arab (alpha-2–beta-2$^{\text{Glu}121\ \text{Lys}}$) is slow-moving on alkaline electrophoresis (in the A2, C, and E regions).

b. Hb S/O Arab is more severe than Hb S/C disease.

B. Thalassemia and Hb switching disturbances

1. Beta-thalassemia minor versus iron deficiency anemia

a. In favor of iron deficiency

(1) Decreased iron and ferritin levels.

(2) Elevated free erythrocyte porphyrin (FEP) levels.

b. In favor of beta-thalassemia trait

(1) History of repeated administration of iron.

(2) Refractory microcytic anemia without bleeding.

(3) Normal iron parameters.

(4) Elevated Hb A2.

(5) Microcytosis with elevated Hb A2 in a first-degree relative.

(6) Normal FEP levels.
2. Alpha-thalassemia-1 trait
  a. Familial hypochromic microcytosis.
  b. No evidence of iron deficiency.
  c. Low or normal levels of Hb A2.
  d. Presence of RBC inclusions by specialized tests.
  e. Precise definition requires demonstration of the missing alpha genes.
3. Hereditary persistence of Hb F (HPHF)
  a. Homogeneous distribution of high Hb F.
  b. Differs from the heterogeneous increases of Hb F found in other hemoglobinopathies, aplastic anemia, and myeloproliferative states.
C. Other Hemoglobinopathies
1. Hemoglobinopathies with high oxygen affinity and erythrocytosis
  a. The p50 level is low.
  b. No leukocytosis or thrombocytosis (differs from myeloproliferative disorders).
  c. If the family study is not informative, diagnosis must exclude:
    (1) Polycythemia.
    (2) Renal disease.
    (3) Erythropoietin-generating tumors.
    (4) Response to chronic hypoxemia.
    (5) 2,3 Diphosphoglyceromutase-phosphatase deficiency.
2. Hemoglobinopathies with decreased oxygen affinity
  a. Blood p50 is high.
  b. Mild cyanosis.
  c. The Hb is deoxygenated but not oxidized.
  d. Deoxygenated Hb must be distinguished from oxidized ferric ($Fe3^+$) methemoglobin seen in:
    (1) Acquired or hereditary methemoglobinemias A.
    (2) Methemoglobinemias M.
3. Unstable hemoglobinopathies versus G-6-PD deficiency
  a. Oxidative hemolytic crises can be seen as in G-6-PD deficiency (drugs, infections, acidosis).
  b. Unstable Hbs are transmitted in an autosomal dominant manner; G-6-PD deficiency is X-linked.
  c. Splenomegaly is more common in unstable hemoglobinopathies than in G-6-PD deficiency.
  d. Unstable Hbs produce a markedly ab-

normal peripheral smear; G-6-PD deficiency does not.
4. Hemoglobinopathies with cyanosis versus hereditary enzymatic cyanosis
  a. In favor of hemoglobinopathy:
    (1) Autosomal dominant inheritance.
    (2) No consanguinity.
    (3) No RBC NADH methemoglobin diaphorase deficiency.
    (4) No RBC NADPH methemoglobin reductase.
5. Hb M's versus low oxygen affinity mutations
  a. Hbs with low oxygen affinity have decreased blood p50.
  b. In alpha-chain Hb Ms, cyanosis is present at birth.
  c. In beta-chain Hb Ms, cyanosis begins after 6 months.

VI. Treatment and Patient Monitoring
A. Sickle cell disease syndromes (e.g., Hb SS, S/beta-thalassemia, S/D)
No treatment is necessary for the person with the sickle cell trait. Currently, management of the patient with sickle cell anemia is primarily supportive.
1. Infections
  a. Prevention, early detection, and treatment of intercurrent infections are important.
  b. Pneumococcal sepsis can be prevented by administration of the polyvalent vaccine.
  c. Prophylactic treatment with penicillin is indicated, particularly in children.
2. Crises
  a. Painful crises require effective and prompt analgesia and hydration.
  b. Oxygen is indicated during acute crises with arterial hypoxemia.
  c. It is important to search for and identify underlying infections.
3. Prevention of nutritional anemia
  a. Oral folic acid can support bone marrow function.
4. Transfusions or exchange transfusions
  a. Indicated for life-threatening problems and intractable crises
    (1) Central nervous system complications (stroke)
    (2) Severe chest syndrome
    (3) Extreme anemia
    (4) Splenic sequestration, hypovolemic shock
    (5) Priapism

(6) Therapeutically unresponsive chronic leg ulcers

(7) Major surgery requiring prolonged general anesthesia

(8) Complicated pregnancy (third trimester); Hb < 6 gm/dl

b. Untoward effects of transfusions

(1) Transmission of hepatitis and other viral diseases

(2) Alloimmunization

(3) Delayed transfusion reactions

(4) Iron overload

(5) Lack of clear-cut efficacy (during pregnancy for instance)

5. Genetic counseling can play an important role in prevention; antenatal diagnosis of sickle cell anemia is possible. Molecular genetic techniques can provide timely intrauterine diagnosis.

6. Experimental treatments: Hydroxyurea and other agents to increase Hb F have not yet been shown to be effective. Bone marrow transplantation is under study.

B. Thalassemias

1. Beta- or alpha-thalassemia-1 trait

a. No treatment is needed.

b. The differential diagnosis of thalassemia trait versus iron deficiency is important to prevent:

(1) Inappropriate administration of iron if thalassemia is mistaken for iron deficiency.

(2) Failure to investigate the underlying cause if iron deficiency is mistaken for thalassemia.

2. Silent alpha-thalassemia trait

(1) Asymptomatic state.

(2) May be clinically relevant for genetic counseling.

3. Beta-thalassemia major or intermedia

a. Transfusions

(1) Benefits are associated with major risks.

(2) Risk of hepatitis diminished by immunization for hepatitis B.

(3) Hypertransfusion programs aim to maintain Hb levels above 9–10 g/dl.

(4) Supertransfusion programs (to keep Hb above 12 g/dl) are under investigation.

(5) Effectiveness of transfusing younger RBCs (neocytes) is under study.

b. Chelation therapy for hemosiderosis

(1) Iron overload by age 40 is the rule.

(2) Deferoxamine mesylate can be given subcutaneously by pump.

(3) Deferoxamine begun before 8–10 years of age decreases iron after 3–5 years of use.

(4) Therapy may include tea with meals to chelate intestinal iron.

(5) Oral iron chelating agents are under investigation.

c. Other measures

(1) Folic acid supplementation is useful; avoid iron supplementation.

(2) Splenectomy may be required for:

(a) Increased transfusion needs.

(b) Massive splenomegaly.

(c) Clinically significant functional hypersplenism.

(3) Plastic surgery may reduce facial distortion caused by extramedullary hematopoiesis.

d. Experimental therapies under consideration

(1) Bone marrow transplantation.

(2) Gene manipulation (hypomethylation of gamma genes by 5-azacytidine).

(3) Successful gene replacement in thalassemia remains a goal for the future.

4. Hb H disease

a. Avoid oxidant drugs, as in G-6-PD deficiency; avoid iron supplementation.

b. Patients do not usually require transfusions or splenectomy.

5. Fetal hydrops syndrome

a. No treatment is available.

b. Genetic counselling.

C. Other hemoglobinopathies

1. Unstable hemoglobinopathies

a. Avoid drugs that cause oxidative hemolysis (see Chapter 66C; V1, 6A2)

b. Folate supplementation (1–2 mg/day).

c. Polyvalent antipneumococcal vaccination and prophylactic penicillin may help.

d. Splenectomy is useful in a minority of selected patients.

2. Hemoglobinopathies with erythrocytosis

a. Do not usually require phlebotomy.

b. Treatment with drugs used in polycythemia rubra vera is contraindicated.

3. Hemoglobinopathies with low oxygen affinity

a. Require reassurance.

b. Other medical interventions are contraindicated.

4. Methemoglobinemias caused by Hbs M
   a. Require reassurance.
   b. The greatest dangers to cyanotic patients with HbM are iatrogenic:
      (1) Inappropriate investigation (e.g., cardiac catheterization).
      (2) Misguided treatment for enzymopathy (e.g., ascorbate or methylene blue).

VII. Prognosis

A. Benign to grave, depending on genetic factors and effectiveness of supportive care.
B. More patients with sickle cell syndromes survive into adulthood in the United States.
C. Factors that may improve the prognosis in sickling disorders include:
   1. A higher level of Hb F (Hbs S and F copolymerize poorly in RBCs).
   2. Milder abnormalities in whole blood rheology.
   3. Coexisting mild alpha-thalassemia (effect still under investigation).

4. Vigorous prevention of infection in childhood.
5. Avoidance of unnecessary transfusions.
6. Immunization against hepatitis B.
7. Judicious prevention and/or management of iron overload.

Bibliography

Bunn HF, Forget GB. *Hemoglobin: Molecular, Genetic and Clinical Aspects*. Philadelphia, Saunders, 1986.

Frischer H, Bowman J. Hemoglobin E, an oxidatively unstable mutation. *J Lab Clin Med* 85:531, 1975.

Karlsson K. Review: Treatment of genetic defects in hematopoietic cell function by gene transfer. *Blood* 78(10):2481–2492, 1991.

Lin CK, Lee SH, Wang CC, et al. Alpha-thalassemic traits are common in the Taiwanese population: Usefulness of a modified hemoglobin H preparation for prevalence studies. *J Lab Clin Med* 118(6):599–603, 1991.

Stamatoyannopoulos G, Nienhuis AW, Majerus PW, Varmus H. (Eds). The Molecular Basis of Blood Diseases, ed 2. WB Saunders Co, Philadelphia pp 107–244, 1994.

Weatherall DJ, Clegg JB. *The Thalassaemia Syndromes*. New York, Blackwell, 1983.

CHAPTER 66-B

Red Blood Cell Membrane Disorders

Henri Frischer M.D., Ph.D.

I. **Definition**
Heterogeneous group of inherited disorders with deformed red blood cells (RBCs), that can be associated with changes in membrane stability and function. The types of aberrant RBC shapes include:
A. Spherocytes.
B. Elliptocytes.
C. Pyropoikilocytes.
D. Stomatocytes.
E. Xerocytes (crenated, dark desiccated cells).
F. Acanthocytes (spur cells).

II. **Etiology**
A. Hereditary spherocytosis (HS)
   1. Multiple causes
      a. Autosomal dominant trait is relatively common (about 1 per 5,000 persons).
      b. A rare form of severe autosomal recessive HS exists.
   2. Heterogeneous primary defects may affect:
      a. Ankyrin (protein 2.1), a common defect linked to chromosome 8 (8p11.2).
      b. Alpha-spectrin (on chromosome 1), decreased synthesis in severe recessive HS.

B. Beta-spectrin (on chromosome 14), oxidative instability.
C. Band 3 anion exchange protein.
D. Protein 4.2.
E. Hereditary elliptocytosis (HE)
   1. Multiple causes
      a. Autosomal dominant transmission with variable clinical severity is most common.
      b. Autosomal recessive HE is rare.
   2. Heterogeneous primary defects may affect:
      a. Alpha- or beta-spectrin; alpha mutants predominate (codon 28 is a "hot spot"); mutations usually interfere with the association of spectrin dimers into tetramers.
      b. Protein 4.1 (partial deficiency).
      c. Glycophorin C (deficiency of the Gerbich blood group produces the elliptocytic "Leach" phenotype).
      d. Abnormal band 3 (deletion of codons 400–408 produces malaria-resistant Southeast Asian ovalocytosis).
F. Hereditary pyropoikilocytosis (HPP)
   1. Multiple causes

a. Most patients are compound heterozygotes for two mutations affecting
alpha-spectrin.
2. Primary defects may alter:
a. Spectrin structure or synthesis.
b. The thermal stability of the protein is
usually markedly decreased (also
found in homozygous HE).
D. Hereditary stomatocytosis (Hydrocytosis)
E. Hereditary xerocytosis (HX)
1. Autosomal dominant RBC membrane
transport disorders; the responsible mutations have not yet been defined.
2. Some instances of hereditary hydrocytosis with hemolysis have high membrane
phosphatidylcholine.
F. Acanthocytosis
1. Definition: Hereditary or acquired RBC
abnormalities of the membrane lipid bilayer. RBCs have multiple medium-sized
irregularly distributed thorns (spur
cells).
2. Syndromes
a. Acanthocytosis-abetalipoproteinemia
(1) Autosomal recessive deficiency of
apolipoprotein B.
b. Chorea-acanthocytosis
(1) Autosomal recessive chorea of
adult onset.
(2) Acanthocytosis of unknown
mechanism.
c. Spur cell hemolytic anemia of severe
liver disease
(1) Acquired depression of lecithin
cholesterol acyl transferase
(LCAT).
(2) Elevated unesterified cholesterol
in RBC membranes.
(3) Additional membrane lesions may
contribute to the formation of
spur cells.
d. Miscellaneous types
(1) McLeod blood group, malnutrition.

III. Pathophysiology
A. Hereditary spherocytosis
1. The underlying mutation results in a
secondary or primary loss of spectrin.
2. Primary loss of ankyrin disconnects beta-
spectrin from the anion exchange protein.
3. Spectrin loss correlates with disease severity and triggers a complex chain of
events:

a. Weakened lipid–cytoskeleton bonds.
b. Exposure of normally buried phos-
phatidylserine.
c. Loss of surface area, decreased surface: volume ratio.
d. Decreased resistance to shear stress.
e. Increased osmotic fragility.
f. Diminished barrier to sodium entry.
4. Compensatory activation of $Na^+ K^+$ AT-
Pase leads to:
a. Extrusion of $3Na^+$ for every $2K^+$ imported.
b. Red cell dehydration with high mean
corpuscular hemoglobin concentration (MCHC).
5. Dehydrated, rigid spherocytes are
trapped in the spleen.
a. Exhaustion of RBC adenosine
triphosphate (ATP).
b. Pump failures, first for sodium later
for calcium.
c. Entry of Na^+ and water becomes unopposed.
d. K^+ is lost.
e. Intracellular Ca^{+2} increases.
6. Intrasplenic hemolysis.
B. Hereditary elliptocytosis and pyropoikilocytosis
1. The spleen traps elliptocytes and py-
ropoikylocytes, as well as spherocytes.
2. The increased disease severity in neonates may reflect the excess of 2,3-
diphosphoglycerate (2,3-DPG) that fails
to bind to Hb F.
C. Hereditary stomatocytosis (hydrocytosis)
1. Sodium and water leak into the RBCs.
2. This cannot be completely compensated
for by increased $Na^+ K^+$ ATPase.
3. The entry of Na^+ and water exceeds the
loss of K^+.
4. The RBCs swell and are destroyed in the
spleen.
D. Hereditary xerocytosis (HX)
1. In HX (also in acquired oxidative damage with elevation of RBC Ca^{+2}):
a. Potassium is lost without equivalent
entry of sodium.
b. RBCs become dehydrated (xerocytosis or dessicocytosis).
c. The RBC 2,3-DPG level falls.
E. Acanthocytosis
1. Alterations of membrane lipids in acanthocytosis
a. Excess of free cholesterol or sphingo-

myelin within the outer leaflet of the RBC's membrane bilayer.
b. Deficit of lipids within the inner leaflet of the membrane (McLeod blood group anomaly).
c. Unbalanced membrane lipids with relative excess of outer leaflet produces irregular extrusions (spurs).

2. Alterations of lipid bilayer that can mimic acanthocytosis (see also Section V, E)
   a. Echinocytosis
      (1) Membrane projections (like those of acanthocytosis) reflect an excess of outer leaflet lipids.
      (2) The cell extrusions are more uniformly distributed and smaller than the spurs of acanthocytes.
   b. Drug-induced stomatocytosis
      (1) Chlorpromazine, amiodarone, or calcium channel blockers interact with the RBC membrane.
      (2) The inner leaflet of the lipid bilayer expands (e.g., through drug intercalation).
      (3) Relative excess of inner leaflet lipids produces RBCs with a transverse slit (stomatocytes).

IV. Diagnosis
A. Hereditary spherocytosis (HS)
   1. Clinical presentations
      a. Typical mild HS
         (1) Diagnosis in the autosomal dominant or sporadic form is suggested by:
            (a) Unexplained splenomegaly.
            (b) Unconjugated jaundice and reticulocytosis, with or without anemia.
            (c) Early gallstones.
            (d) Anemic exacerbations during pregnancy or with infectious mononucleosis or parvovirus infections.
      b. Severe forms of HS
         (1) Autosomal recessive form.
         (2) Can present in early childhood.
         (3) Severe hemolysis may require transfusions.
      c. Complications of HS
         (1) Anemic crises (aplastic, hemolytic, or megaloblastic).
         (2) Bilirubin gallstones.
         (3) Rarely, leg ulcers, paravertebral hematopoiesis, hemochromatosis,

mental retardation, and skeletal anomalies.
   2. Laboratory tests
      a. Blood film and routine laboratory tests
         (1) Microspherocytes (small cells without central pallor).
         (2) Reticulocytosis, usually less than 15%, may be as high as 80%.
         (3) MCHC increased in about half of the patients.
         (4) Elevated unconjugated bilirubin, negative Coombs' test.
         (5) Increased lactate dehydrogenase, decreased haptoglobin (hemolytic bouts).
      b. Osmotic fragility is increased.
      c. Autohemolysis in HS
         (1) Characteristically increased (2–50%).
         (2) Completely corrected with glucose.
         (3) Incompletely corrected with ATP.
   3. Screening of family members (spherocytes, MCHC, reticulocytosis).
B. Hereditary elliptocytosis (HE)
   1. Clinical presentations
      a. Mild HE
         (1) Asymptomatic trait or variable hemolysis.
         (2) Usually detected when more than 20% elliptocytes found on blood smear.
         (3) Splenomegaly.
      b. Severe HE
         (1) Seen in homozygotes or double heterozygotes.
         (2) Marked to severe hemolytic anemia.
         (3) Can present as neonatal hemolytic poikilocytosis.
         (4) After the first year of life, the disease becomes milder.
   2. Laboratory tests
      a. Peripheral smear
         (1) Many elliptocytes but also poikilocytes, spherocytes, and fragments.
      b. Osmotic fragility
         (1) Normal in common HE.
         (2) Increased in severe HE and HPP.
      c. Special studies
         (1) Spectrin extracts show an increased dimer:tetramer ratio.
C. Hereditary pyropoikilocytosis (HPP)
   1. Clinical presentations

a. Variable hemolysis and splenomegaly.
2. Laboratory tests
   a. Severe poikilocytosis, cell fragments, spherocytes, elliptocytes.
   b. Mean corpuscular volume (MCV) less than 74.
   c. Osmotic fragility increased.
   d. Markedly increased autohemolysis incompletely corrected by glucose (unlike HS).
   e. Thermal instability of RBCs
      (1) Normal red cells fragment at 50°C.
      (2) HPP red cells usually fragment at 46°C.
D. Hereditary stomatocytosis (hydrocytosis)
   1. Hemolytic process; more than 20% of the RBCs contain slits (stomatocytes).
   2. The cup-shaped cells can often best be seen in wet blood film preparations.
   3. Osmotic fragility and autohemolysis increased; incompletely corrected by glucose.
E. Hereditary xerocytosis (HX)
   1. Variable hemolysis, splenomegaly.
   2. The smear shows a mixture of stomatocytes, echinocytes, and target cells.
   3. MCHC is increased.
   4. Decreased red cell 2,3-DPG level (useful diagnostically).
   5. Increased thermal stability of RBC's.
F. Acanthocytosis
   1. Abetalipoproteinemia
      a. Autosomal recessive.
      b. Malabsorption, blindness, ataxia, and mental retardation.
      c. Peripheral smear can show up to 90% acanthocytes.
      d. Plasma cholesterol is less than 50 mg/dl; absence of apoprotein B.
   2. Spur cell hemolytic anemia in liver disease
      a. Severe hemolysis and underlying liver failure.
   3. Chorea-acanthocytosis
      a. Neurologic disease (late-onset chorea, ticks, hypotonia) with variable RBC acanthocytosis.
      b. Palmitic acid (C16) is increased and stearic acid (C18) decreased in RBC membranes.
   4. Acanthocytosis of the McLeod blood group
      a. X-linked (Xp21) defect with compensated hemolysis.

b. Kx antigen is missing; Kx protein is a precursor component of the autosomal Kell antigen.
   c. Patients can sometimes develop late-onset muscular dystrophy and movement disorder.
   d. The muscle and neurologic disease may reflect conjoint deletion of Kx and closely linked genes.
5. Acanthocytosis of hypothyroidism
   a. The RBC findings may lead to correct investigation and diagnosis of the endocrine disease.
6. Other syndromes with acanthocytosis
   a. Malnutrition (anorexia), myelodysplastic syndromes.

V. **Differential Diagnosis**
   A. Hereditary spherocytosis (HS)
      1. HS versus ordinary HE
         a. Osmotic fragility is increased in HS but not in ordinary HE.
      2. HS versus spherocytic hereditary elliptocytosis
         a. In spherocytic HE the osmotic fragility is increased, as in HS.
         b. However, spherocytic HE shows elliptocytes plus spherocytes (unlike HS).
         c. In spherocytic HE cell fragmentation is:
            (1) More prominent than in HS.
            (2) Less prominent than in HPP
      3. HS versus RBC fragmentation hemolysis with spherocytes
         a. Schistocytes are prominent in syndromes with fragmentation hemolysis.
      4. HS versus Hb C with spherocytosis
         a. Hb electrophoresis distinguishes Hb C from HS.
      5. HS versus unstable hemoglobinopathies with Heinz bodies and spherocytosis
         a. Heat, isopropanol, and dichlorophenol-indophenol (DCIP) stability tests are positive in the globin disorders.
      6. HS versus enzymopathies associated with occasional spherocytosis
         a. Phosphoglucose isomerase or hexokinase deficiencies can show spherocytes.
         b. Enzymopathies (but not common HS) are transmitted in an autosomal recessive manner.
         c. Specific enzyme assays are needed for diagnosis.

7. HS versus autoimmune hemolysis with spherocytosis
   a. Warm IgG autoantibodies with positive Coombs' test found in autoimmune spherocytosis.
8. HS versus neonatal isoimmune hemolysis with spherocytosis
   a. The Coombs' test may be negative.
   b. The infant's RBCs elute anti-A or anti-B IgG antibodies.
   c. ABO incompatibility between mother and child.
9. HS versus unconjugated hyperbilirubinemia of Gilbert's syndrome.
   a. Gilbert's syndrome lacks spherocytes or reticulocytosis.

B. Hereditary elliptocytosis (HE)
1. Elliptocytosis is seen as part of poikilocytosis in many conditions other than HE
   a. The most reliable differentiation of HE is based on a positive family history.
   b. Elliptocytes as part of poikilocytosis are seen in:
      (1) Iron deficiency.
      (2) Thalassemia.
      (3) Megaloblastic anemia.
      (4) Sickle cell syndromes.
      (5) Myelofibrosis.
      (6) Leukoerythroblastic reactions.
      (7) Pyruvate kinase deficiency.
      (8) Myelodysplasia.
      (9) Absence of glycophorin C (Gerbich blood group).
2. Severe elliptocytosis with fragmented poikilocytes versus schistocytes
   a. In HE the fragmented RBCs are usually rounder.
   b. Sharp, bizarre schistocytes are seen in syndromes with fragmentation hemolysis:
      (1) Thrombotic thrombocytopenic purpura.
      (2) Microangiopathic hemolysis.
      (3) Disseminated intravascular coagulation.
      (4) Vasculitis.
      (5) Heart prosthesis, valve hemolysis.
      (6) Hemolytic-uremic syndrome.
      (7) Eclampsia, hepatic disease, thrombocytopenia.
      (8) Metastatic carcinoma.
   c. In fragmentation hemolysis there is increased excretion of iron in the urine.

C. HPP versus ordinary HE
1. HPP shows a complex mixture of morphological abnormalities.
2. In HPP elliptocytes are not the most prominent abnormality.
3. In HPP the red cell thermal stability is markedly decreased.

D. Hereditary versus acquired stomatocytosis
1. Acquired stomatocytosis is seen in:
   a. Acute alcoholism.
   b. Exposure to chlorpromazine, calcium channel blockers, amiodarone.
   c. Rh antigen deficiency (Rh null phenotype) with stomatocytes and hemolysis.

E. Acanthocytes (spur cells) must be differentiated from echinocytes (burr cells).
1. Echinocytes have more uniform, smaller spikes.
2. Echinocytes are seen in states with low erythrocyte ATP.
   a. Hypomagnesemia
   b. Hypophosphatemia
   c. Pyruvate kinase deficiency
   d. Blood storage artefacts (at alkaline pH)
   e. Uremia
   f. Long-distance runners

VI. **Treatment**
A. Hereditary spherocytosis (HS)
1. Supportive measures until definitive therapy is provided
   a. Prophylactic folate supplementation (1 or 2 mg/day).
   b. In rare cases, blood transfusions may be necessary during aplastic crisis.
2. Splenectomy
   a. Curative: reticulocytosis disappears but spherocytosis persists.
   b. Indications:
      (1) Growth retardation.
      (2) Symptomatic hemolytic disease.
      (3) Gallstones in the patient or in relatives with the disease.
   c. Splenectomy may not be needed in mild adult-onset HS.
   d. Even when indicated, splenectomy should be delayed until the age of 5 years.
   e. Screening for gallstones should precede splenectomy.
   f. Combined cholecystectomy/splenectomy in HS patients with cholelithiasis.

g. Antipneumococcal polyvalent vaccination should precede surgery.

h. Treatment failure or recurrence of anemia suggests:

(1) Misdiagnosis of HS instead of

(a) Pyruvate kinase or other enzymopathies.

(b) Unresponsive membrane disorder (e.g., hereditary xerocytosis or stomatocytosis).

(2) Failure to remove (or regrowth of) accessory spleen.

(a) Disappearance of postsplenectomy Howell-Jolly bodies is suggestive.

(b) Ectopic splenic tissue can be located by radionuclide scanning.

B. Hereditary elliptocytosis (HE)

1. Common heterozygous HE

a. Usually requires no treatment.

b. Some patients with hemolysis may benefit from folate support.

c. Splenectomy is rarely needed.

2. Homozygous HE

a. Most patients benefit from splenectomy.

C. Hereditary pyropoikilocytosis (HPP)

1. Splenectomy can be useful in transfusion-dependent patients.

2. Severe neonatal HPP may improve as the child ages.

D. Hereditary stomatocytosis

1. Most patients do not require splenectomy.

2. The operation may benefit some patients with severe hemolysis.

3. In stomatocytosis with high phosphatidylcholine, splenectomy is contraindicated.

E. Hereditary xerocytosis (HX)

1. Splenectomy is ineffective.

2. Fortunately, in HX the Hb is rarely below 9 g/dl.

F. Acanthocytosis

1. Abetalipoproteinemia

a. Dietary restriction of long-chain fatty acids.

b. Supplementation with vitamins A, K, and E and folate.

2. Spur cell hemolytic anemia

a. Supportive care.

b. Splenectomy may improve hemolysis.

c. Surgery is rarely performed given the severe liver failure.

3. Rh-null disease

a. Transfusions must be avoided or minimized.

b. Patients will form antibodies to all D RBCs.

VII. **Patient Monitoring**

The patient with hereditary spherocytosis should be monitored before and after surgery.

A. Ultrasound scan for gallstones is indicated after early childhood.

B. Postsurgical monitoring is needed to detect:

1. Gallstones (a minority of patients with HS develop gallstones after splenectomy).

2. Postsplenectomy infections.

3. Inadequate therapeutic response to splenectomy (see Section VI, A, 2h).

4. Persisting hyperbilirubinemia (may point to Gilbert's syndrome).

VIII. **Prognosis**

A. Prognosis is favorable in most cases of HS.

B. Life-threatening autosomal recessive HS is fortunately very rare.

C. HS with central nervous system or cardiac disease is uncommon.

D. HS patients with very low spectrin have a more severe disease.

E. Prognosis is grave in hepatic spur cell anemia.

Bibliography

Chilcote RR, LeBeau MM, Dampier C, et al. Association of red cell spherocytosis with deletion of the short arm of chromosome 8. *Blood* 69:156–159, 1987.

Floyd PB, Gallagher PG, Valentino LA, et al. Heterogeneity of the molecular basis of hereditary pyropoikilocytosis and hereditary elliptocytosis associated with increased levels of the spectrin alpha I/74-kilodalton tryptic peptide. *Blood* 78(5):1364–1372, 1991.

Lux SE, Becker PS. Disorders of the red cell membrane skeleton: Hereditary spherocytosis and hereditary elliptocytosis, in Scriver CR, Beaudet AL, Sly WS et al. (eds) *The Metabolic Basis of Inherited Disease*, ed 6. New York, McGraw-Hill, 1989, pp 2367–2408.

Palek J. (Guest Editor). Cellular & Molecular Biology of Red Blood Cell Membrane Proteins in Health and Disease. IV: Structure-Function Relationships and Disorders. *Seminars Hematol* 30(3), 169–247, 1993

Red Cell Enzymopathies

Henri Frischer M.D., Ph.D.

I. Definition

Inherited disorders of red blood cell (RBC) enzymes with hemolytic or nonhemolytic manifestations.

II. Etiology

A. Hexose monophosphate shunt (HMS) and glutathione pathway
  1. Glucose-6-phosphate dehydrogenase (G-6-PD) deficiency
    a. The most common RBC enzymopathy:
      (1) Affects more than 100 million people.
      (2) Has a geographic distribution resembling that of malaria.
      (3) Is X-linked.
    b. There are more than 400 G-6-PD variants.
      (1) Gd A occurs in about 10% of Afro-Americans males.
      (2) Gd B$^-$ is seen mostly in Mediterraneans and Asians.
      (3) Gd Canton is common in the Orient.
      (4) Many "private" G-6-PD variants exist.
    c. Mutations within the nicotinamide-adenine dinucleotide phosphate (NADP) domain lead to congenital nonspherocytic hemolytic anemia (CNSHA).
  2. Other conditions with oxidative hemolysis
    a. Glutathione reductase deficiency (severe).
    b. Gamma-glutamylcysteine synthetase deficiency.
    c. Glutathione synthetase deficiency.

B. Anaerobic red cell glycolysis
  1. Pyruvate kinase (PK) deficiency
    a. The least uncommon disorder of glycolysis.
    b. At least three genetic PK loci.
      (1) Leukocyte PK is coded on chromosome 15.
      (2) Kidney PK is coded on chromosome 9.
      (3) Red cell PK gene remains unmapped.
  2. Glucose phosphate isomerase deficiency (GPI)
    a. Less prevalent than pyruvate kinase deficiency.
    b. GPI is a single dimeric enzyme.
    c. Gene mapped to chromosome 19.
  3. Rare glycolytic enzymopathies

a. Autosomal recessive deficiencies
   (1) Hexokinase (HK)
   (2) Phosphofructokinase (PFK)
   (3) Fructosediphosphate aldolase (FA)
   (4) Triosephosphate isomerase (TPI)
b. X-linked glycolytic deficiency
   (1) Phosphoglycerate kinase (PGK)

C. Nucleotide salvage system (with clinical manifestations)
1. Pyrimidine 5′-nucleotidase deficiency
2. Adenylate kinase deficiency
3. Adenosine deaminase excess

III. Pathophysiology

A. Hexose monophosphate shunt (HMS) and glutathione (GSH)
1. Glucose-6-phosphate dehydrogenase (G-6-PD) and 6-phosphogluconic dehydrogenase (6-PGD)
   a. X-linked G-6-PD, the first enzyme of the HMS, generates NADPH from glucose-6-P (G-6P) and NADP.
      (1) G-6-PD functions normally at a fraction of its maximal capacity (HMS restraint).
      (2) Normally, some G-6-PD molecules remain in the monomeric, submaximally active, configuration.
      (3) NADP binds G-6-PD monomers into multimers that are catalytically more active.
      (4) NADPH oxidation raises the level of NADP, thus lifting HMS restraint by activating G-6-PD.
      (5) If G-6-PD is active, NADPH can also be produced by 6-PGD as its substrate becomes available.
   b. Autosomal 6-PGD, while producing NADPH, also removes 6-PG, a regulatory molecule (see below).
      (1) Homozygous 6-PGD deficiency is an extremely rare cause of oxidative hemolysis.
2. Oxidant stress and related defensive HMS enzymes
   a. Oxidant stress produces activated oxygen species (e.g., radicals) that can damage tissue.
   b. Superoxide dismutase rapidly converts superoxide anion O_2^- into metabolizable peroxide.
   c. Glutathione disulfide (GSSG) and NADP are produced as GSH and NADPH trap active oxygen.
   d. HMS activates up to 30-fold as NADP

rises; NADPH production increases massively. Increased NADPH stabilizes catalase and supports glutathione reductase (GSSG-R).
   e. Catalase removes some peroxides but less effectively than glutathione peroxidase (GSH-Pxase).
   f. GSH-Pxase depends totally on GSH to detoxify organic and inorganic peroxides.
   g. GSH-S-transferase also depends on GSH to generate drug–GSH conjugates.
   h. GSH is renewed from GSSG/NADPH by GSSG-R, a flavoenzyme physiologically modulated by 6-PG.
   i. GSSG-R activity is essential for defensive HMS mobilization in response to most hemolytic drugs.
3. Failure of antioxidant defenses in G6PD deficient RBCs
   a. Witout G-6-PD, NADPH and 6-PG fall, 6-PGD is ineffective, and GSSG-R is metabolically activated.
   b. Under oxidant stress (infections, drugs, acidosis), the demand for NADPH and GSH escalates.
   c. Despite increased GSSG-R cycling, the GSH supply cannot keep up with increasing peroxide levels.
   d. Oxidants are poorly inactivated, hemoglobin is destabilized with heme loss and Heinz bodies.
   e. Proteins cross-link, lipids lose unsaturated bonds, cytosol Ca^{+2} rises, oxidative RBC lysis ensues.
4. Special features accompanying the loss of GSH in GSH synthetase deficiency
   a. Decreased GSH fosters oxidative hemolysis and also activates gamma-glutamyl-cysteine synthetase.
   b. Trapped gamma-glutamylcysteine accumulates and is diverted into 5-oxoproline.
   c. Indirect severe 5-oxoprolinemia leads to metabolic acidosis.

B. Anaerobic glycolysis
1. Adenosine triphosphate (ATP) primes glycolysis by supporting rate-limiting HK and PFK.
2. HK and glucose-6-phosphate isomerase alter G6P, fructose-6-phosphate (F6P), and HMS function.
3. PFK uses ATP to produce fructose 1,6-

diphosphate (F1,6-DP): F1,6-DP activates pyruvate kinase (PK) downstream, and thereby helps repay the ATP debt.

4. Fructose-diphosphate-aldolase, triose-phosphate isomerase, glyceraldehyde-3-phosphate dehydrogenase: These activities are needed to produce NADH and 1,3-diphosphoglycerate (1,3-DPG).

5. NADH supports methemoglobin diaphorase and preserves the functional capacity of hemoglobin.

6. 1,3-DPG is the precursor substrate for the synthesis of 2,3-diphosphoglycerate (2,3,-DPG). 1,3-DPG is used by the diphosphoglyceromutase component of diphosphoglyceromutase-phosphatase.

7. 2,3-DPG: Very abundant intraerythrocytic compound (1 mole 2,3-DPG/mole Hb).

   a. Regulates the oxygenation-deoxygenation of hemoglobin (2,3-DPG favors oxygen release).

   b. Increases with chronic hypoxemia; decreases with acidosis and with increased demand for ATP.

      (1) H$^+$ decreases 2,3-DPG by inhibiting DPGmutase while stimulating DPG phosphatase.

      (2) Falling 2,3-DPG increases ATP produced by phosphoglycerokinase (PGK) and PK.

      (3) Absence of 2,3-DPG in homozygous 2,3-DPG-mutase-phosphatase deficiency causes erythrocytosis.

C. Erythrocytic nucleotide salvage

   1. Function

      To maintain normal flexible equilibrium of ATP (about 88%), adenosine diphosphate (ADP) (10%), and adenosine monophosphate (AMP) (about 2%).

   2. Importance

      a. Nucleotide salvage is important because RBCs:

         (1) Depend heavily on ATP.

         (2) Cannot synthesize nucleotides de novo.

         (3) Are at constant risk of losing AMP.

         (4) Contain very little nonadenine nucleotides.

   3. Disorders

      a. Adenylate kinase (AK) deficiency

         (1) Results in hemolysis by disturbing the ATP/ADP/AMP equilibrium.

      b. Genetic excess of adenosine deaminase (ADA)

         (1) AMP is dephosphorylated to diffusible adenosine.

         (2) RBC AMP loss must be replenished from plasma adenosine.

         (3) This is accomplished by adenosine kinase (AdK).

         (4) In ADA excess:

            (a) An mRNA defect raises ADA up to 100-fold.

            (b) Defect is manifested in RBCs only.

            (c) Adenosine (from plasma) is deaminated too rapidly.

            (d) Adenosine kinase fails to salvage AMP.

            (e) As AMP becomes depleted, ATP and other adenine nucleotides fall.

            (f) Hemolysis ensues when about one half of normal ATP has disappeared.

      c. Deficiency of ADA (as opposed to ADA excess)

         (1) Does not interfere with nucleotide salvage.

         (2) Does not decrease RBC survival.

         (3) However, ADA-deficient lymphocytes accumulate deoxyadenine nucleotides.

         (4) Dysfunction results in combined immunodeficiency.

      d. Pyrimidine 5′ nucleotidase (Pyr-5′Nase) deficiency

         (1) Normally maturing RBCs degrade DNA and RNA.

         (2) RNA breakdown produces pyrimidine-nucleotide monophosphates.

         (3) Pyrimidine-nucleotide monophosphates are nondiffusable and toxic to the RBCs.

         (4) Pyr-5′Nase removes pyrimidine-nucleotide monophosphates without degrading AMP and guanosine monophosphate (GMP).

         (5) The products of Pyr-5′Nase (cytidine or uridine) can diffuse ouside the RBCs.

         (6) Pyr-5′Nase deficit produces hemolytic anemia.

IV. **Diagnosis**

   A. Disorders of the hexose monophosphate shunt and glutathione

1. G-6-PD deficiency
   a. Genotypes at risk
      (1) Hemizygous deficient males
      (2) Homozygous deficient females
      (3) Some heterozygous females
   b. Clinical manifestations
      (1) Hemolysis crises with infections or acidosis
      (2) Drug-induced oxidative hemolysis
      (3) Favism
      (4) Congenital nonspherocytic hemolytic anemia (CNSHA)
      (5) Neonatal hyperbilirubinemia
      (6) Transfusion accidents (particularly in young children).
   c. Course of hemolysis in African-American Gd A⁻ variety
      (1) Latent phase
      (2) Phase of acute hemolysis.
      (3) Spontaneous recovery with compensated hemolysis
          (a) Younger RBC's have more active G6PD activity.
          (b) Younger cells can replace destroyed older cells.
   d. Clinical course in variants other than Gd A⁻: Spontaneous recovery may not occur in more severe types (e.g., (GdB⁻, Bd Canton).
      (1) The mutant enzyme is very unstable.
      (2) Bone marrow may not be able to compensate.
      (3) Transfusions may be needed for survival.
   e. Laboratory tests
      (1) Usually the RBC smear is not informative (rarely, bite or blister cells occur in severe hemolysis).
      (2) Definitive diagnosis must rely on assays (10–15% residual activity in Gd A⁻ RBCs).
      (3) To document decreased RBC G-6-PD, it may be necessary to:
          (a) Separate the RBCs by cell age (to detect the deficiency in older cells).
          (b) Use the ratio of G-6-PD to other cell age-sensitive enzyme activities (e.g., 6-phosphogluconic dehydrogenase, PK, or HK).
          (c) Measure glutathione reductase with and without flavin-adenine dinucleotide (FAD); in G-6-PD deficiency, GSSG-R is elevated and resists further activation by FAD.
          (d) Assay G-6-PD activity in first-degree relatives, taking account of X-linkage.
          (e) Repeat assays later when the RBCs are older and transfusion effects have subsided.
2. Deficiencies of gamma-glutamylcysteine synthetase or of glutathione synthetase
   a. GSH in RBCs is reduced to less than 10% of normal.
   b. Homozygotes with hemolysis may have also neurologic disease.
3. Glutathione reductase deficiency
   a. Isolated GSSG-R deficiency must be severe (<10% of normal activity) to have clinical manifestations.
   b. Clinically significant deficiency is seen:
      (1) In homozygous genetic GSSG-R deficiency, a very rare condition.
      (2) After antitumor chemotherapy with bischloronitrosourea (BCNU or carmustine), a much more common occurrence.
   c. Severe GSSG-R deficiency results in:
      (1) Increased susceptibility to oxidative hemolysis (particularly if G-6-PD deficiency is also present).
      (2) Life-threatening pulmonary and hepatic complications after high-dose BCNU chemotherapy.
B. Disorders of anaerobic glycolysis with hemolysis
   1. PK deficiency
      a. The most prevalent disorder of anaerobic glycolysis.
      b. Produces CNSHA of variable severity.
      c. Most affected individuals are compound heterozygotes.
      d. RBCs contain mixture of two PK variants.
      e. RBC 2,3-DPG is characteristically elevated, and the final diagnosis depends on specific assays.
   2. Glucose phosphate isomerase deficiency
      a. The second most prevalent disorder of anaerobic glycolysis, produces CNSHA of variable severity.
   3. Hexokinase (HK) deficiency
      a. Variable hemolysis.
      b. HK activity is markedly higher in younger than in older RBCs.

c. RBC age effects are diagnostically important.
4. PFK deficiency
   a. RBCs contain PFK-M and PFK-L (liver); muscle contains only PFK-M.
   b. Homozygous deficiency of the muscle subtype (PFK-M) is primarily a myopathy.
   c. RBC PFK is half-normal, with compensated hemolysis.
   d. Exertional muscle weakness and rhabdomyolysis with reticulocytosis strongly suggest PFK deficiency.
5. Fructosediphosphate aldolase
   a. Rare cause of congenital nonspherocytic hemolytic anemia (CNSHA).
6. Triosephosphate isomerase (TPI) deficiency
   a. Clinical aspects
      (1) Neuromuscular dysfunction.
      (2) Increased propensity for infections.
      (3) Cardiac arrhythmias and increased risk of sudden death.
   b. Laboratory tests
      (1) Dihydroxyacetone phosphate reaches cytotoxic levels.
      (2) Red cell TPI activity is 5–20% of normal.
      (3) Electrophoretic TPI band is decreased to absent.
7. Phosphoglycerate kinase (PGK) deficiency
   a. X-linked disorder with CNSHA in PGK-deficient hemizygotes.
   b. Hemolysis can be associated with myopathy or progressive central nervous system manifestations.
C. Nucleotide salvage pathway
   1. Pyrimidine-5′-nucleotidase (Pyr-5′Nase) deficiency
      a. Autosomal recessive disorder about as prevalent as pyruvate kinase deficiency.
      b. CNSHA is quite variable ranging from moderate to severe.
      c. RBCs show marked basophilic stippling.
         (1) Stippling is best seen in smears prepared from blood unexposed to ethylenediaminetetraacetic acid (EDTA).
      d. Acid RBC extracts reveals an ultraviolet absorption peak.
         (1) Maximum at 265–270 nm.

(2) The normal adenine peak is at 258 nm.
      e. Other diagnostic epiphenomena include:
         (1) Elevation of RBC GSH to twice the normal value
         (2) Ribosephosphate pyrophosphokinase (RPPK) <50% of normal.
   2. Excess RBC adenosine deaminase
      a. Compensated hemolysis.
      b. May be transmitted in an autosomal dominant manner.
   3. AK deficiency
      a. RBCs have less than half normal AK activity.
      b. Variable CNSHA, sometimes with psychomotor disturbance.
D. RBC enzymopathies without primary hemolysis
   1. 2,3-Diphosphoglyceromutase-phosphatase deficiency
      a. Autosomal recessive erythrocytosis
   2. NADH-methemoglobin diaphorase deficiency
      a. Autosomal recessive cyanosis
   3. Adenosine deaminase deficiency
      a. Combined immunodeficiency
   4. Hypoxanthine-guanine P-ribosyl transferase deficiency
      a. Neurologic dysfunction and megaloblastic changes.
   5. Porphobilinogen deaminase (PBG-deaminase)
      a. Acute intermittent porphyria

V. **Differential Diagnosis**
   A. G-6-PD deficiency and disorders of glutathione
      1. Consider common G-6-PD deficiency in the differential diagnosis of Coombs' test-negative hemolysis.
      2. Suspect G-6-PD deficiency particularly if the patient with hemolysis:
         a. Is of African-American, African, Mediterranean, East Indian, or Oriental ancestry.
         b. Is infected, febrile, or acidotic.
         c. Has been exposed to substances incriminated in oxidative hemolysis (see Section VI).
         d. Has unusually high bilirubinemia during hepatitis.
         e. Is a neonate with hyperbilirubinemia unexplained by fetomaternal incompatibility.

f. Has a family history of anemia or gall-stones.

g. Gives a family history with an X-linked transmission pattern (e.g., maternal uncles, sister's sons).

h. Has a peripheral blood smear that is not particularly remarkable.

3. Periodic hemolytic crises suggest a defect of HMS or GSH synthesis.

4. More chronic hemolysis suggests a defect in glycolytic or nucleotide metabolism.

   a. However, there are many exceptions.

     (1) HMS disorders can present as chronic CNSHA.

     (2) Many glycolytic and nucleotide metabolic defects have hemolytic crises punctuating CNSHA.

5. Early hemolytic crisis cannot be ruled out for lack of reticulocytosis, a delayed response to RBC destruction.

B. Other disorders

1. Special syndromes with CNSHA

   a. With recurrent infections or cardiac arrythmias, consider triosephosphate isomerase deficiency.

   b. With myopathy consider PFK deficiency (or glycogenosis VII).

   c. With neurological dysfunction consider PGK deficiency.

2. Genetic considerations

   a. RBC enzymopathies are transmitted either in an autosomal recessive or an X-linked manner. There may be some rare exceptions (excess adenosine deaminase, instances of AK deficiency).

   b. Most other hereditary hemolytic disorders are transmitted in an autosomal dominant manner (hemoglobinopathies and membrane disorders).

   c. In the differential diagnosis of unexplained hemolysis, consanguinity strongly favors an autosomal enzymopathy.

   d. X-linkage with CNSHA, without G-6-PD deficiency, suggests PGK deficiency, particularly if the patient has neuropsychiatric disturbances.

   e. In autosomal familial erythrocytosis:

     (1) Recessive transmission suggests 2,3-DPG deficiency.

     (2) Dominant transmission suggests high-affinity hemoglobins or unresponsiveness to erythropoietin.

3. The peripheral blood smear in the differential diagnosis of congenital hemolysis

   a. A smear with prominent, multiple RBC abnormalities favors a hemoglobinopathy or membrane disorder rather than an RBC enzymopathy.

   b. Some noteworthy exceptions include:

     (1) Basophilic stippling in Pyr-5'Nase deficiency.

     (2) Bite cells in rare instances of severe G-6-PD deficiency (splenic pitting of aggregates of Hb).

     (3) Dehydrated, spiculated cells in some patients with PK deficiency.

     (4) Occasional spherocytes in PGI deficiency.

4. Screening tests and direct assays for specific enzyme

   a. Useful screening tests exist for G-6-PD and some other RBC enzymopathies.

   b. Final diagnosis requires specific assay.

5. Evaluation of RBC substrates: 2,3-DPG content is very valuable in the differential diagnosis of CNSHA and familial erythrocytosis.

   a. Markedly elevated in PK deficiency.

   b. Partially decreased in HK or glucose phosphate isomerase deficiencies.

   c. Severely decreased in DPG-mutase-phosphatase deficiency.

6. Other studies

   a. Separation of older and younger red cells.

     (1) Diagnostically important during acute hemolysis or when HK deficiency is suspected.

   b. Lead levels in the differential diagnosis of pyrimidine-5'-Nase deficiency.

     (1) Lead poisoning (with Pb > 200 μg/dl) mimics genetic pyrimidine-5'-Nase deficiency.

   c. Copper and ceruloplasmin studies

     (1) Needed to diagnose Wilson's disease as the underlying cause of oxidative hemolysis.

   d. Severe hypophosphatemia may rarely lead to hemolysis akin to PK deficiency (ATP loss).

VI. **Monitoring, treatment, and prevention**

A. G-6-PD deficiency

1. Importance of detection: The correct diagnosis of G-6-PD deficiency often permits one to:

   a. Remove an offending agent.

b. Prevent unnecessary testing.

c. Avoid transfusions, particularly in Afro-American (GdA⁻) G-6-PD deficiency.

d. Avert inappropriate splenectomy.

2. Prevention of oxidative hemolysis

a. G-6-PD-deficient persons should avoid exposure to substances capable of triggering hemolysis.

b. Potentially hemolytic agents include:

  (1) 8-Aminoquinoline antimalarials (primaquine).

  (2) Sulfonamides (e.g., sulfamethoxazole).

  (3) Sulfones (diamino-diphenyl-disulfone or dapsone).

  (4) Nitrofurantoin, furazolidone.

  (5) Naphthalene.

  (6) High doses of vitamin K.

  (7) Carmustine (BCNU).

  (8) Doxorubicin.

  (9) Phenazopyridine.

  (10) Nalidix acid, acetanilid.

  (11) Methylene blue.

  (12) Isosorbide dinitrate.

  (13) Raw fava beans and unripe peaches.

3. Treatment

a. Indications for transfusion

  (1) Severe CNSHA.

  (2) Acute life-threatening hemolysis.

  (3) Aplastic crisis.

  (4) Exchange transfusions may be necessary to prevent neonatal kernicterus.

b. Folate

  (1) Support of erythroid bone marrow is useful in managing the hemolytic process.

c. Splenectomy

  (1) Ineffective and contraindicated in G-6-PD deficiency and other disorders of the HMS.

d. Vitamin E

  (1) A beneficial role for tocopherol in G-6-PD deficiency with CNSHA remains uncertain.

B. Other disorders

1. Supportive management of the hemolytic process

a. Folate supplementation.

b. Transfusions as required.

c. Splenectomy.

  (1) Can be useful in severe forms of some RBC enzyme deficiencies:

    (a) PK

    (b) PGI

    (c) TPI

    (d) PGK

    (e) Pyrimidine-5′ Nase.

  (2) Unfortunately, response to splenectomy is often variable and poorly predictable.

2. Some special considerations

a. Glutathione synthetase deficiency and 5-oxoprolinemia

  (1) Require management of hemolysis as well as of severe metabolic acidosis (sodium bicarbonate).

b. PFK deficiency

  (1) The hemolysis is usually well compensated.

  (2) Myopathy may benefit from increased carbohydrate diet.

c. TPI deficiency

  (1) Anti-infection monitoring, prevention and early intervention.

d. 2,3,-DPG-mutase-phosphatase deficiency

  (1) Avoidance of inappropriate treatment for polycythemia rubra vera.

e. NADH-methemoglobin diaphorase deficiency

  (1) Ascorbate or methylene blue can be used to treat cyanosis.

  (2) Provided that the patient is proven *not* to have concomitant G-6-PD deficiency.

VII. Prognosis

A. Prognosis varies widely with the specific diagnosis.

B. Outlook is excellent in conditions like the common milder forms of G-6-PD deficiency with a self-limited course.

C. Prognosis is guarded in some disorders with transfusion-dependent CNSHA and severe systemic manifestations (e.g., TPI deficiency).

Bibliography

Frischer H, Ahmad T. Consequences of erythrocytic glutathione reductase deficiency. *J Lab Clin Med* 109(5):583–588, 1987.

Hohl RJ, Kennedy EJ, Frischer H. Defenses against oxidation in human erythrocytes: Role of glutathione reductase in the activation of glucose decarboxylation by hemolytic drugs. *J Lab Clin Med*, 117(4):325–331, 1991.

Luzzatto L, Mehta A. Glucose-6-phosphate-dehydrogenase deficiency, in Scriver CR, *The Metabolic Basis of Inherited Disease*, ed 6, Vol II, chap 91. New York, McGraw-Hill, 1991, pp 2237–2265

Valentine WN, Paglia DE. Erythroenzymopathies and hemolytic anemia: The many faces of inherited variant enzymes. *J Lab Clin Med* 115(1):12–20, 1990.

Valentine WN, Tanaka KR, Paglia DE. Pyruvate kinase and other enzyme deficiency disorders of the erythrocyte, in Scriver CR *The Metabolic Basis of Inherited Disease*, ed 6, Vol II, chap 94. New York, McGraw-Hill, 1991, pp 2341–2365.

CHAPTER 67

Immune Hemolysis

Richard J. Sassetti, M.D.

I. **Definition**

Immune hemolysis is accelerated destruction of red blood cells with adherent antibodies directed to antigens either intrinsic to the red blood cell surface or adsorbed onto it.

II. **Etiology**

A. Hemolysis occurs when the humoral immune system recognizes antigenic substances carried on the surface of the red blood cell. Substances such as drugs and bacterial, viral, or cellular degradation products need not be on the surface of the cell at the time they are processed by the antigen recognition cells. Hemolysis can be:
   1. Alloimmune in transfusion or hemolytic disease of the newborn.
   2. Xenoimmune in infections.
   3. Autoimmune in connective tissue diseases or malignancy.

B. Immune hemolysis secondary to infections may have two components.
   1. Cross-reactivity between the constituents of the invading organism and cell surface constituents of the infected individual (e.g., cold agglutinins associated with *Mycoplasma pneumoniae* or Epstein-Barr virus

infections). Organisms carry polysaccharide surface structures which may be identical to red blood cell antigens in the Ii blood group system. Response to the infectious agent stimulates production of antibodies which bind to the host red blood cells, shortening red blood cell survival.
   2. The other component (less well characterized) is due to the binding of degradation products of infectious agents to the red blood cell surface and attachment of antibodies elicited in the xenoimmune response.

III. **Pathophysiology**

A. Binding of antibody can result in either of two outcomes or a combination of both:
   1. Intravascular hemolysis.
   2. Extravascular hemolysis.

B. The sole or predominent route depends on:
   1. The class and subclass of the immunoglobulin.
   2. Blood group antigen system.
   3. Degree of involvement of the complement system.
   4. Macrophage Fc and complement receptors.

C. The nature of the antibody elicited will depend on the nature of the antigenic material. Polysaccharide antigens of xenogeneic origin tend to elicit antibodies of the IgM class. Polypeptide antigens tend to elicit antibodies of the IgG class. Details of the humoral immune response are covered elsewhere.

1. IgM antibodies (cold reacting) bind most strongly below body temperature. In spite of relatively poor binding to red blood cells at body temperature, IgM can bind sufficient amounts of complement to form the membrane attack complex, membrane rupture, and spilling of hemoglobin in the vascular space. The reticuloendothelial system (RES) receptors for the Fc portion of the IgM molecule are inefficient, so any entrapment by the RES is due to largely reversible binding to macrophage receptors for complement (sequestration).

2. IgG antibodies bind most strongly at 37.5°C and are warm reacting. IgG is an inefficient activator of complement. However, the RES has strong, efficient IgG Fc receptors. Except in rare circumstances, IgG induces extravascular hemolysis. The pathogenesis of hemolysis secondary to alloimmunization is discussed in Chapter 75A, Section IV.4.

IV. **Diagnosis**

A. Immune hemolysis is a secondary process in at least two-thirds of cases and appears to be idiopathic in the remainder. The diagnosis of immune hemolysis is based on the demonstration of immunoglobulin or complement on the patient's red blood cells; that is, the direct antiglobulin test (DAT) (direct Coombs' test) is positive.

B. There are rare occasions when the hemolytic efficiency of the antibody is so great that amounts below the level of sensitivity of the test are sufficient to produce significant hemolysis while the DAT is negative, making immune hemolysis a "rule-out" diagnosis. Antiglobulin tests use two reagent antisera: one with specificity for IgG, the other for complement.

C. The possible patterns of positivity are as follows:

	I	II	III
Anti-IgG	+	−	+
Anticomplement	−	+	+

D. Pattern I is seen in:
1. Idiopathic autoimmune hemolysis.
2. Treatment with α-methyldopa.
3. Lymphoproliferative disorders or other forms of cancer.
4. Delayed hemolytic transfusion reactions.
5. Occasionally in patients being treated with penicillin.

E. Pattern II is seen in:
1. Cold agglutinin disease.
2. Infections associated with the production of cold agglutinins.
3. Lymphoproliferative disorders or other forms of cancer.
4. Immediate hemolytic transfusion reactions due to ABO blood group incompatibility.

F. Pattern III is seen in:
1. Immune complex diseases.
2. Drug-related immune hemolysis.
3. Autoimmune diseases which produce circulating immune complexes.

G. The hemolysis of allogeneic cells may be brisk enough to initiate hypersplenism or a secondary autoimmune hemolysis in which the hemolytic process is more severe and/or prolonged than can be accounted for by the number of allogeneic cells present at the initiation of the process.

H. Table 67-1 lists the general categories of disease associated with the various types of hemolysis.

V. **Differential Diagnosis**

The diseases with which immune hemolysis can be confused are:

Table 67-1. Diseases Associated with Hemolysis

Warm reactive antibody
  Idiopathic
  Secondary
    Collagen vascular diseases
    Lymphoproliferative diseases
    Carcinomas
    Drugs
    Miscellaneous
Cold reactive antibody
  Idiopathic
  Secondary
  Lymphoproliferative diseases
  Infections
  Miscellaneous
Combined Reactivity
  Paroxysmal cold hemoglobinuria

A. Hereditary membrane abnormalities.

B. Red blood cell enzymopathies whose clinical syndromes are induced by drugs.

C. Hemolysis induced by infectious agents such as *Clostridium* or *Malaria* species.

VI. Treatment (see Table 67-2)

A. Treatment of secondary immune hemolysis is unnecessary unless the process is contributing significantly to morbidity. In most cases, secondary immune hemolysis will improve as the primary disease is successfully treated. If therapeutic intervention is necessary, it is the same as that of the idiopathic varieties.

B. The first line of treatment of warm antibody hemolysis is intervention in the erythrophagocytic process taking place largely in the spleen. This can be achieved with:

1. Conventional therapies

    a. Glucocorticoids.

    b. Modified androgens such as danazol.

    c. Intravenous immunoglobulins.

    d. Splenectomy may be necessary and is successful in about 70% of cases resistant to the conventional nonsurgical interventions listed above. It should be considered after an adequate trial of the more conventional treatments.

2. Unconventional therapies

    a. Treatment with vinblastine-loaded, IgG-sensitized platelets.

    b. Transfusion of Rh-positive blood into Rh-negative patients, with simultaneous administration of anti-Rh immunoglobulin.

    c. Immunosuppressive drugs.

    d. Plasmapheresis should be considered only as a temporizing measure.

C. In cold antibody hemolysis (IgM), Fc blockade or ablation are ineffective since the primary mechanism does not involve Fc receptors.

D. Treatment consists of:

1. Immunosuppressive chemotherapy.

2. Reduction of the patient's exposure to cold may provide significant relief of symptoms and slow the process remarkably.

3. Penicillamine can be used as an interim therapy to reduce IgM to the monomeric form, eliminating intravascular hemolysis. This is a poorly tolerated treatment.

4. Plasmapheresis is theoretically attractive but impractical.

VII. Prognosis

Generally the prognosis is good. Most secondary immune hemolysis abates as the primary disease is controlled or spontaneously abates. Stopping the use of implicated drugs will reverse drug-induced hemolysis.

Table 67-2. Laboratory Findings

Findings	Antibody Reactivity	
	Warm	**Cold**
Anemia*	+	+
Reticulocytosis†	+	+
Morphology		
Red blood cell polychromasia†	+	+
Spherocytosis	+	±
Erythrophagocytosis	+	0
Plasma hemoglobin	0	↑
Plasma lactic dehydrogenase	N–↑	↑↑
Plasma haptoglobin	↓	↓↓↓
Urine hemoglobin	0	0–↑↑↑
Urine hemosiderin	0	↑
Plasma complement	N	N–↓
Red blood cell survival	↓	↓
DAT reactivity pattern	I, II	II, III

*Absent if the rate of cell production equals the rate of destruction. This is called the *hemolytic state*.

†Absent or disproportionately low if the bone marrow is suppressed.

Bibliography

Rosse WF. *Clinical Immunohematology: Basic Concepts and Clinical Applications*. Boston, Blackwell, 1986, p 427.

CHAPTER 68

Mechanically Induced Hemolytic Anemias

Richard J. Sassetti, M.D.

I. **Definition**
   Mechanically induced hemolysis is the accelerated destruction of red blood cell secondary to disruption of the normal vascular endothelium–red blood cell interface.

II. **Etiology**
   Disruption of the red blood cell–vascular interface has three main causes:
   A. Disruption or interruption of the normal vascular endothelial surface.
   B. Highly turbulent blood flow (beating).
   C. Activation of the coagulation system.
   The diseases are listed in Table 68-1.

III. **Pathophysiology**
   A. As biconcave disks, red blood cells are highly deformable and capable of withstanding shear stresses higher than those normally encountered. Through heterogeneous mechanisms, the abnormalities listed in Table 68-1 create circumstances in which red blood cells are exposed to inordinately high shear stresses.
      1. In microangiopathic processes, high shear rates are generated by turbulent flow or passage through meshes of fibrin strands in vessels with high flow rates.

   2. In macroangiopathic processes, high shear rates are generated by:
      a. Narrow orifices.
      b. Turbulent flow.
      c. Interface with foreign (usually plastic) surfaces.
   3. In both processes, the red blood cells are deformed by the high shear rates beyond their elastic ability to recover and are torn into fragments. During fragmentation, hemoglobin is spilled in the vascular space and red blood cell fragments anneal their membrane, take hydrodynamically unstable forms, and lose much of their normal deformability. These fragments are removed from the circulation by the sieving function of the spleen.
   4. In the combined form, fragmentation of red blood cells is produced by repeated pulsatile, high-pressure compression of blood vessels, both large and small, in the soles of the feet of runners with improper footwear or in those whose gait results in unusually heavy footfalls.
   B. In arterial abnormalities, the hemolysis may start insidiously and remain asymptomatic

Table 68-1. Diseases Caused by Mechanically Induced Hemolysis

---

Macroangiopathic (arterial)
  Ruptured sinus of Valsalva
  Ruptured chordae tendineae
  Coarctation of the aorta
  Aortic aneurysm
  Mural patches
  Arterial graft, hemodialysis shunt
  Valvular aortic stenosis, artificial valves with
    cloth-covered struts, improper seating, exposed
    plastic surface, or small outlet
Microangiopathic (arteriolar)
  Kassabach-Merritt syndrome
  Thrombotic thromocytopenic purpura (TTP)
  Hemolytic-uremic syndrome (HUS)
  Eclampsia and preeclampsia
  Autoimmune diseases
  Allograft rejection
  Chemotherapy or radiotherapy
  Disseminated intravascular coagulation
Combined macrovascular and microvascular
  March or "jogger's" hemolysis

---

for a prolonged period during which there is steady, undetectable loss of hemoglobin in the urine until the patient becomes iron deficient. At that point the hematocrit decreases and the rheologic properties change, with an increase in blood turbulence and shear stresses that accelerate the hemolytic process.

IV. **Diagnosis**
  A. The history is particularly helpful. Macroangiopathic (arterial) forms secondary to aortic stenosis may be the only ones without a clear, unequivocal history. Changes in cardiovascular dynamics together with changes in auscultatory findings may signal problems with replacement valves. Except for the Kassabach-Merritt syndrome, in which the hemangioma may not be readily apparent, and the hemolytic uremic syndromes (HUS and TTP), which may not have typical presentations, the microangiopathic forms are secondary to other disease processes whose symptoms, signs, and acuity may obscure the diagnosis.
  B. Essential for diagnosis
    1. Anemia.
    2. Significant numbers of schistocytes (fragmented red blood cells), as well as other abnormal red blood cell forms.
    3. Microcytosis detected visually on the peripheral smear, along with polychromatophilia or reticulocytosis.
    4. Evidence of hemolysis (increased indirect bilirubin and serum lactic acid dehydrogenase, as well as decreased or absent haptoglobin).
  C. The mean corpuscular volume may be increased or normal in the early acute phase, with an active bone marrow erythroid response, but decreased in the late, chronic, iron-deficient, bone marrow-unresponsive stage. In severe cases, hemoglobinemia may be visually detectable in plasma. In milder cases, plasma hemoglobin may not be detectable but urine hemoglobin may be present. In mild chronic cases, increased urinary hemosiderin may be the only indicator of hemoglobin loss.

V. **Differential Diagnosis**
  A. In the acute hemoglobinuric form the differential diagnosis includes myoglobinuria, clostridial infections, paroxysmal cold and paroxysmal nocturnal hemoglobinuria, cold agglutinin syndrome, and acute hemolytic transfusion reaction.
  B. In the chronic form the differential diagnosis includes all other causes of hemolysis, such as
    1. Hemoglobinopathies and red blood cell enzymopathies.
    2. Delayed transfusion reactions.
    3. Infections.
    4. Autoimmune and drug-induced hemolysis.

VI. **Treatment**
Treatment is directed to the underlying cause. Valve-induced hemolysis may be reduced by increasing the hematocrit by transfusion to reduce turbulence or by valve replacement.

VII. **Prognosis**
The prognosis for the hemolytic component is generally good. Correction of the causative anatomical abnormalities or treatment of the underlying disease will reverse or at least reduce the hemolysis.

Bibliography

Erslev AJ, Martinez J. Erythrocyte disorders: Anemia related to mechanical damages to erythrocytes. In Williams W, Beutler E, Erslev A, et al (eds). *Hematology*, ed 4. New York, McGraw Hill, 1991, p 653.

CHAPTER 69

Hypersplenism

Richard J. Sassetti, M.D.

I. **Definition**

Removal of the formed elements of the blood at an accelerated rate by the spleen.

II. **Etiology**

A. The vascular sinuses of the spleen have exit lumina with diameters less than that of the transiting cell. The blood circulates through the sinus at low velocity, bringing the formed elements into prolonged, close contact with the macrophages, which remove senescent cells. Successful passage is dependent on the traversing cell's having maximum deformability and little or no immunoglobulin fixed to its surface for which the macrophages have receptors.

B. Hypersplenism may be secondary to disease processes which enlarge the spleen (see Table 69-1).

III. **Pathogenesis**

A. Two interrelated pathogenetic factors are responsible for shortened blood cell survival:

1. Sequestration of a larger than normal portion of the circulating cell mass.

2. Phagocytosis by macrophages lining the sinuses with which the cells are in intimate contact.

B. Primary immune processes may induce hypersplenism and serve to worsen the accelerated immune destruction of the blood cells (see Chapter 67). The binding of antibody-coated cells by the macrophages induces proliferation of the functional cells of the spleen, resulting in sequestration of a greater volume of cells.

C. The superimposed hypersplenic engorgement adds sequestration to the immunity-induced phagocytosis.

D. Hypersplenism resulting from a chronic process related to splenic hypertrophy induced by one cell line may result in the sequestration of other cell lines, producing bilineal cytopenia or pancytopenia.

IV. **Diagnosis**

A. The diagnosis of hypersplenism has four components:

1. Enlargement of the spleen.

2. Reduction in the number of one or more of the circulating blood elements.

3. Normal to hyperactive marrow in all three cell lineages.

4. Improvement or return to normal of the circulating blood elements only after splenectomy.

Table 69-1. Hypersplenism Secondary to Diseases Enlarging the Spleen

Category	Cause
Congestion	Compression of the portal vein (including cirrhosis of the liver)
Congenital processes	Red blood cell abnormalities
	Red blood cell enzymopathies
	Hemoglobinopathies
	Storage diseases
Inflammatory processes	Infections
	Collagen vascular diseases
Myeloproliferative disorders	Chronic myelogenous leukemia
	Myelofibrosis with myeloid metaplasia, polycythemia
Lymphoproliferative disorders	Chronic lymphocytic leukemia, lymphoma

B. The signs and symptoms of hypersplenism may merge with or be overshadowed by those of the primary disease.
1. In the pure form of the disease, patients may have symptoms related to the most profound cytopenia, which may be anemia, infection, or evidence of impaired blood coagulation.
2. Mechanical impairments related to the spleen enlargement may produce early satiety or anorexia, left upper quadrant discomfort, or abdominal or pleuritic pain secondary to splenic infarcts.
3. Physical signs include a readily palpable spleen or one shown to be enlarged by imaging techniques. A splenic rub secondary to a splenic infarct or a vascular bruit secondary to altered hemodynamics in the enlarged organ may be detected.
4. Laboratory findings include the cytopenia in one or more cell lines and, very likely, evidence of marrow hyperactivity such as polychromatophilia, mild macrocytosis, or reticulocytosis in the red blood cells. Giant platelets or left-shifted granulocytes may be seen if the cytopenia is in the platelet or granulocyte lines.

V. **Treatment**
Treatment consists of management of the underlying disorder. Splenectomy may be necessary if cytopenias create a large transfusion demand or are life-threatening.

VI. **Prognosis**
The prognosis of hypersplenism is related to the degree of resulting cytopenias. Thrombocytopenia may reach levels which predispose to bleeding. Granulocytopenia may reach levels predisposing to infection.

Bibliography

Erslev AJ. Hypersplenism and hyposplenism, in William W, Beutler E, Erslev A, et al (eds). *Hematology*, ed 4. New York, McGraw Hill, 1991, p 700.

Chapter 70-A

Hemochromatosis

Walter Fried, M.D.

I. Definition
Hemochromatosis is a condition characterized by excessive deposition of iron in the parenchymal cells of the liver and other tissues.

II. Etiology
A. Hereditary hemochromatosis is an autosomal recessive disorder caused by a mutation in an unidentified region of chromosome 6.
1. The abnormal gene occurs in 5–10% of the population, and the disease occurs in about 0.3%.
2. Heterozygotes are asymptomatic.
B. Erythropoietic hemochromatosis is due to iron overload associated with severe chronic, ineffective erythropoiesis:
1. In thalassemia major.
2. In chronic sideroblastic anemia.
C. African siderosis is caused by chronic increased intake of dietary iron due to consumption of beer brewed in iron pots (among the Bantu tribesmen of South Africa).
D. Hypertransfusional states: characterized by deposition of iron in the reticuloendothelial cells. However, iron overflow may be deposited in the parenchymal cells and cause organ dysfunction.

E. Iron overload may be due to liver disease; rarely is enough iron deposited to cause significant organ damage.

III. Pathogenesis
When iron is deposited in parenchymal cells in excess of the cells' ability to package it into ferritin, it may catalyze the formation of free radicals that cause cell injury.
A. In hereditary hemochromatosis there is a defect in the ability of intestinal epithelium to block physiologically the entry of dietary iron in response to excessive iron stores.
B. In cases secondary to chronic ineffective erythropoiesis and to liver disease, iron absorption is physiologically increased but intestinal cell function is normal.
C. In African siderosis, the intestinal cells function normally to limit the percentage of dietary iron that is absorbed, but the total amount ingested is excessive.

IV. Diagnosis
A. Physical examination
1. The skin shows a bronze discoloration.
2. There may be arthritis due to iron deposition in the synovia.
3. The liver is enlarged and firm.

4. Cardiac arrhythmias and a constrictive cardiopathy may occur.
5. Endocrine abnormalities may include:
   a. Hypopituitarism.
   b. Hypogonadism.
   c. Hypoadrenalism.
   d. Diabetes mellitus.
B. Laboratory studies
   1. High serum iron level, with transferrin saturation of >55%.
   2. High serum ferritin level.
   3. Abnormalities on liver function tests.
   4. Magnetic resonance imaging (MRI) of the liver can detect excessive iron deposition.
   5. Quantitation of the iron stores in liver biopsy specimens usually shows more than 20 g when significant organ damage is present.
   6. Abnormal glucose tolerance.
   7. Serum assays of endocrine function.
   8. Echocardiogram to demonstrate abnormality of myocardial function.
   9. Serum iron and transferrin saturation is the most sensitive way of detecting early disease in family members of patients with hemochromatosis.
   10. Human leukocyte antigen typing can be used to detect homozygosity.
   11. Although liver iron stores and the serum ferritin level may be excessive, the marrow iron stores may be normal or only slightly increased.

V. Differential Diagnosis

The most difficult differentiation is between hemochromatosis, with its resultant liver disease, from iron overload secondary to liver disease. In the latter condition the liver iron content rarely exceeds 5 g, whereas in the former it is usually in excess of 20 g before liver dysfunction occurs.

VI. Therapy

A. Hereditary: phlebotomy weekly, without decreasing the hemoglobin level below 10.5 g/100 ml until the iron stores are normal, then as needed to maintain the serum ferritin at about 100 pg/ml. Erythropoietin may increase the ability to phlebotomize patients with very high iron stores.
B. In hemochromatosis associated with anemia, it is often impossible to phlebotomize patients; chelation therapy, using continuous subcutaneous infusion of desferrioxamine, is the treatment of choice.

VII. Patient Monitoring

During therapy, the serum iron is monitored frequently. A fall in serum iron level indicates depletion of the iron stores, barring an intercurrent infection. Hepatic iron may be monitored by MRI of the liver if the serum iron is an unreliable indicator because of complicating conditions.

VIII. Prognosis

A. Beginning therapy prior to the development of organ damage will prevent it from occurring.
B. If therapy is initiated after organ damage has occurred, reduction of the iron content will halt disease progression and improve function in most organs, although joint damage, impotence, and, in most cases, diabetes are not corrected.

Bibliography

Amos DB, Cartwright GE, Edwards CQ, et al: Homozygosity for hemochromatosis: clinical manifestations. *Ann Intern Med* 93:519–525, 1980.

Bunn HF, Cheron RG, Cooper B, et al: Clinical consequences of acquired transfusional iron overload in adults. *N Engl J Med* 304:319–324, 1981.

Mier WA, McLaren GD, Braun W, et al: Evidence of heterogeneity in hereditary hemochromatosis: Evaluation of 174 persons in nine families. *Am J Med* 76:806–814, 1984.

Shafer AI, Cheron RG, Dluhy R, et al: Clinical consequences of acquired transfusional overload in adults. *N Engl J Med* 304:319–334, 1981.

Chapter 70-B

Erythrocytosis

Walter Fried, M.D.

I. Definition

A variety of disorders characterized by an increased red blood cell mass.

II. Etiology

A. Primary
1. Polycythemia rubra vera.
2. Familial erythrocytosis with a normal or low serum erythropoietin level.

B. Secondary
1. Decreased oxygen delivery to the kidneys due to:
   a. General hypoxia
   (1) High altitude.
   (2) Pulmonary disease with chronic hypoxia.
   (3) Heart disease with right-to-left shunting.
   (4) Increase in hemoglobin-oxygen affinity.
   b. Regional hypoxia in the kidney
   (1) Renovascular disease.
   (2) Hypertension.
   (3) Renal cysts.
   c. Intermittent hypoxia during sleep.
   d. Paraneoplastic erythropoietin production with:

(1) Hypernephroma.
(2) Hepatoma.
(3) Cerebellar hemangioblastoma.
(4) Leiomyoma.
(5) Others.
   e. Miscellaneous
   (1) Postrenal transplant.
   (2) Familial with high serum erythropoietin levels.

III. Pathogenesis

A. Primary: Results from abnormalities in the hematopoietic stem cell and normal or low serum erythropoietin levels.

B. Secondary: Is due to an increase in the serum erythropoietin level that may result from any of the causes listed above.

IV. Diagnosis

A. History
1. Is there a history of familial incidence?
2. Is there a history of renal disease or hypertension?
3. Are there symptoms of heart or lung disease?
4. Does the patient smoke cigars or cigarettes?
5. Is there a history of pruritus after bath-

ing? (This occurs in polycythemia rubra vera.)

6. Is there a history of thrombotic or bleeding episodes? (This occurs in polycythemia rubra vera.)

7. Do headaches occur?

B. Physical examination: Look for the following:
   1. Hypertension
   2. Splenomegaly
   3. Plethora
   4. Cyanosis
   5. Clubbing of the fingers
   6. Cardiac and pulmonary abnormalities
   7. Excessive obesity ("Pickwickian syndrome")

C. Laboratory and x-ray studies: Suggested sequence (until a cause is found)
   1. Complete blood count.
   2. Cr51 red cell mass determination.
   3. Serum creatinine, uric acid, erythropoietin, and liver enzymes.
   4. Arterial blood gases.
   5. Times intravenous pyelogram.
   6. Hemoglobin-oxygen dissociation curve (to screen for the existence of abnormal hemoglobins with a high oxygen affinity).
   7. Sleep study to detect nocturnal hypoxia.

D. Differential diagnosis
   1. First, distinguish true from spurious erythrocytosis by a red blood cell mass determination.
   2. Then distinguish patients with polycythemia rubra vera from those with secondary erythrocytosis by determining if they meet the criteria for the former.
      a. Category A criteria:
         (1) Increased red blood cell mass.
         (2) Arterial oxygen saturation >92%.
         (3) Splenomegaly.
      b. Category B criteria:
         (1) >400,000 platelets.
         (2) White blood cell count >20,000/ml^3.
         (3) Leukocyte alkaline phosphatase score >100.
         (4) High serum vitamin B_{12} or unsaturated vitamin B_{12} binding capacity.
      c. The diagnosis of polycythemia rubra vera is made if:
         (1) All three category A criteria are met, or if
         (2) The first two category A criteria and any two category B criteria are met.

   3. The patients with erythrocytosis who do not meet the above criteria probably have secondary erythrocytosis, and the workup should continue as described in the previous section.

V. Therapy

A. Therapy for polycythemia rubra vera is discussed in Chapter 72-A.

B. Patients with secondary polycythemia should be cautiously phlebotomized to a hematocrit of 42–45%.

VI. Patient Monitoring

The hematocrit is the best monitor.

VII. Prognosis

The prognosis is determined by the primary condition.

Bibliography

Berlin NI: Diagnosis and classification of the polycythemias. *Sem Hematol* 12:239, 1975.

Caro J, Cobbs E, Erslev AJ, et al: Plasma erythropoietin in polycythemia. *Am J Med* 66:243–247, 1979.

Caro J, Erslev AJ: Pathophysiology and Classification of Polycythemia. *Scand J Hematol* 31:287–292, 1983.

Caro J, Erslev AJ: Pure erythrocytosis classified according to erythropoietin titers. *Am J Med* 76:57–61, 1984.

Wasserman LR: Polycythemia vera study group: a historical perspective. *Sem Hematol* 23:183–187, 1986.

Chapter 70-C

Porphyrias

Henri Frischer, M.D., Ph.D.

I. **Definition**
Hereditary enzymatic defects of heme biosynthesis with excessive production and excretion of porphyrins and precursors.

II. **Etiology and Pathophysiology**
   A. Sites of Heme Synthesis
      1. Heme is synthesized mainly in bone marrow and liver.
      2. About 85% of heme is in hemoglobin, and 15% is in P-450 and catalase.
      3. Hepatic porphyrias have excessive amounts of porphyrins in liver.
      4. Erythropoietic porphyrias have excess porphyrins in erythroid tissues and plasma.
   B. Enzymes of heme synthesis and corresponding porphyrias: Eight enzymes participate sequentially in the biosynthesis of heme. Mutations at each step cause a different type of porphyria.
      1. Delta amino-levulinic acid synthetase (ALA-S)
         a. Properties
            (1) First enzyme of heme biosynthesis.
            (2) Condenses glycine and succinyl-CoA into *d*-aminolevulinic acid.
            (3) Mitochondrial pyridoxal phosphate-dependent proteins.
               (a) Hepatic ALA-S
                  i) Coded by an autosomal gene on chromosome 3.
                  ii) Relatively hypoactive, rate-limiting, short-lived.
                  iii) Strongly induced when free heme decreases (as in acute intermittent porphyria).
               (b) Erythroid ALA-S
                  i) Coded by an X-linked gene.
                  ii) Not rate-limiting.
                  iii) Not incuded when free heme falls.
         b. Disturbances
            (1) Autosomal hepatic ALA-S
               (a) No clinical syndrome has been associated with a deficiency.
            (2) X-linked erythroid ALA-S
               (a) Hemizygous deficiency of erythroid ALA-S probably causes sideroblastic X-linked, pyridoxine-responsive anemia.
      2. Amino-levulinic acid dehydratase (ALA-D)

a. Properties
  (1) Converts *d*-ALA into porphobilinogen (PBG).
  (2) Cytoplasmic enzyme contains zinc.
  (3) Zinc protects sulfhydryl groups and can be displaced by lead.
b. Disturbances
  (1) Hereditary autosomal recessive ALA-D deficiency
    (a) Early onset of visceral crises, rare.
  (2) Hereditary autosomal dominant ALA-D deficiency
    (a) Late onset of visceral crises or neuropathy, rare.
  (3) Acquired ALA-D deficiency in lead poisoning is common.
3. Porphobilinogen deaminase (PBG-deaminase)
  a. Properties
    (1) Condenses four PBG into a linear tetrapyrrole.
    (2) Product is hydroxymethylbilane (HMB).
  b. Disturbances
    (1) Heterogeneous, autosomal dominant PBG deaminase deficiencies.
    (2) Causes acute intermittent porphyria (AIP).
    (3) Patients with one-half of the normal PBG deaminase in liver and red blood cells.
      (a) Accumulate and excrete PBG and ALA.
      (b) Porphyrin precursors trigger neurotoxic and visceral attacks.
      (c) Mechanism of the crisis remains unclear.
4. Uroporphyrinogen III synthase (UPS-III)
  a. Properties
    (1) Cytoplasmic enzyme in bone marrow normoblasts.
    (2) Converts HMB into reduced uroporphyrinogen III.
  b. Disturbances
    (1) Rare autosomal recessive UPS-III deficiency causes congenital erythropoietic porphyria (CEP or Gunther's disease).
      (a) The enzyme is markedly decreased in erythroid cells.
      (b) URO-III is low and URO-I derivatives are very high.
      (c) Accumulation of URO-I is toxic.
        i) Hemolytic anemia.

    ii) Splenomegaly and sometimes hypersplenism.
5. Uroporphyrinogen decarboxylase (UPD)
  a. Properties
    (1) Cytoplasmic enzyme.
    (2) Converts uroporphyrinogen into coproporphyrinogen III.
  b. Disturbances
    (1) Relatively common heterogeneous, autosomal dominant deficiencies.
      (a) Deletion of mRNA exon 6 in at least five unrelated families.
    (2) Affected heterozygotes have porphyria cutanea tarda (PCT)
      (a) Cutaneous and hepatic disorder.
      (b) No neurologic manifestations.
      (c) Fifty percent enzyme activity in liver and red blood cells.
    (3) In many patients with sporadic PCT,
      (a) UDP is depreassed in the liver but not in red blood cells.
      (b) Liver enzyme inhibited with increases of:
        i) Tissue iron.
        ii) A particular cytochrome P-450 isozyme.
    (4) Excess of hepatic uroporphyrinogen is excreted in urine.
    (5) Urine products are oxidized uroporphyrins.
    (6) There is very little excess porphyrin in stool.
6. Coproporphyrinogen oxidase (CO)
  a. Properties
    (1) Mitochondrial protein.
    (2) Converts coproporphyrinogen III into protoporphyrinogen IX.
  b. Disturbances
    (1) Autosomal dominant CO deficiency causes hereditary coproporphyria (HCP).
      (a) Fifty percent enzyme activity in liver, lymphocytes, and leukocytes.
7. Protoporphyrinogen oxidase (PO)
  a. Properties
    (1) Mitochondrial protein.
    (2) Converts reduced protoporphyrinogen IX into oxidized proto-gen IX.
  b. Disturbances
    (1) Autosomal dominant lack of PO causes variegate porphyria (VP).

(a) Disorder with skin and neurologic manifestations.

(b) Affected persons have half-normal enzyme activity.

  (2) Acquired PO deficiency in Gilbert's disease

(a) Fifty percent of normal enzyme activity.

(b) Inhibition by elevated bilirubin is the most probable mechanism.

    8. Ferrochelatase (FC),

      a. Properties

(1) Terminal enzyme of heme biosynthesis.

(2) Mitochondrial protein.

(3) Incorporates ferrous iron into protoporphyrin IX to generate heme.

      b. Disturbances

  (1) Autosomal dominant FC deficiency of FC causes:

(a) Erythropoietic protoporphyria (EPP).

(b) A not uncommon disorder with cutaneous photosensitivity.

(c) Occasional liver disease.

(d) Fifty percent normal FC activity in erythrocytes, reticulocytes, and liver.

(e) Excess of free protoporphyrins diffuses into plasma.

(f) Plasma protoporphyrins are taken up by skin and liver.

(g) In the skin

  i) Light (around 400 nm) excites protoporphyrins.

  ii) Fluorescent products activate oxygen.

  iii) Reactive oxygen species damage the tissue.

  iv) Lesions trigger an inflammatory response.

(h) In the liver

  i) Biliary excretion of protoporphyrins.

  ii) Fluorescent gallstones.

III. Diagnosis and Differential Diagnosis of Porphyrias

  A. General prevalence and clinical presentations

    1. In the United States, the most prevalent porphyrias are:

      a. Porphyria cutanea tarda (PCT).

      b. Erythropoietic protoporphyria (EPP).

      c. Acute intermittent porphyria (AIP)

(more prevalent in people of Swedish ancestry).

    2. AIP affects the nervous system but not the skin.

    3. PCT, EPP and congenital erythropoietic porphyria (CEP) affect the skin but not the nervous system.

    4. Variegate porphyria (VP) and hereditary coproporphyria (HCP) affect the skin and the nervous system.

  B. Specific porphyrias

    1. Acute intermittent porphyria (AIP)

      a. Diagnosis of AIP is based on:

(1) Abdominal and neurologic clinical findings without skin lesions.

(2) Increased PBG and ALA in urine.

(3) Absence of stool porphyrin abnormalities.

(4) Decreased PBG deaminase in red blood cells.

(5) Autosomal dominant family pattern (genetic aspects are also important for management).

      b. Clinical aspects: AIP is clinically latent in the large majority of the heterozygous carriers.

  (1) Precipitating factors

(a) Acute attacks of AIP usually begin after puberty.

(b) Crises can be triggered by many factors (see Section IV).

  i) Low caloric intake (e.g., voluntary dieting).

  ii) Premenstruation.

  iii) Oral contraceptive steroids.

  iv) Infections.

  v) Surgical stress.

  vi) Alcohol, barbiturates.

  vii) Many other inducers of liver ALA-synthase and P-450.

  (2) Abdominal pain

(a) Steady or cramping.

(b) Nausea and ileus are common.

(c) No fever, leukocytosis, or rigidity.

(d) There may be multiple abdominal surgical scars.

  (3) Neurological manifestations

(a) Acute peripheral neuropathies.

(b) Seizures and psychiatric disturbances.

      c. Laboratory tests

  (1) Urine: During a crisis: high levels of PBG and ALA (colorless porphyrin precursors).

(a) No primary excess of urinary porphyrins.
  i) Nevertheless, red or brown by-products occur upon oxidation.
  ii) Suspect AIP if urine darkens when left standing in the light.
(b) Between crises, PBG and ALA remain usually slightly elevated.
(2) Stool: No abnormalities in AIP (stool abnormalities found in HCP and VP).
(3) Red cells: Decreased PBG deaminase in red blood cells (about 50% of normal). Found in most but not all disease variants.

2. Porphyria cutanea tarda (PCT)
  a. Clinical aspects of common autosomal dominant heterozygous PCT: Skin disorder with hepatic complications but no neurologic manifestations. The differential diagnosis includes other cutaneous porphyrias or hemochromatosis.
  (1) Skin
    (a) Skin fragility in areas exposed to light or to mechanical trauma.
    (b) Small white plaques often precede bullous lesions.
    (c) Hypertrichosis, hyperpigmentation, and pseudoscleroderma can follow.
  (2) Liver
    (a) Liver damage (uroporphyrin toxicity) is common in untreated PCT.
    (b) Liver diseases include cirrhosis, hemosiderosis, and carcinoma.
    (c) Exposure to alcohol, iron, or estrogens enhances the danger.
    (d) Hemosiderin found in periportal hepatocytes with portal inflammation.
  b. Laboratory tests
  (1) Urine
    (a) High uroporphyrin-I and 7-carboxylate porphyrin-III.
    (b) Uroporphyrins > coproporphyrins favors PCT.
    (c) Coproporphyrins > uroporphyrins favors VP or HCP.
  (2) Stool: The characteristic abnormality is increased isocoproporphyrins.
  (3) Plasma: Plasma porphyrin mea-

surements may help monitor treatment.
(4) Erythrocytes: Increased PBG deaminase is common.
  (a) Decreased uroporphyrinogen decarboxylase is uncommon.

3. Variegate porphyria (VP)
  a. Clinical aspects
  (1) Seen particularly in South African Africaaners and people of Swedish ancestry.
  (2) Combined skin and abdominal manifestations, as in HCP; VP is more severe.
    (a) The skin lesions resemble those of PCT.
    (b) The neurovisceral crises resemble those of AIP.
  (3) Between attacks, the diagnosis of HC (or VP) is helped by finding:
    (a) Skin changes with increased porphyrins in stool.
    (b) Gallstones contain protoporphyrins.
  b. Laboratory tests
  (1) Stools
    (a) Fecal protoporphyrin is characteristically and continuously high.
    (b) Stool coproporphyrin is also increased.
    (c) The interpretation of fecal porphyrin patterns can be difficult (bacterial metabolism and dietary variation introduce artifacts).
    (d) Direct measurements of copro and protoporphyrins in bile may:
      i) Facilitate the diagnosis of VP (and of HCP).
      ii) Prevent attacks in affected relatives.

4. Hereditary coproporphyria (HCP)
  a. Clinical aspects
  (1) HCP resembles VP, although HCP is usually milder.
  (2) Autosomal dominant transmission with skin and visceral manifestations.
  (3) Between attacks, the diagnosis of HC (or VP) is helped by finding: skin changes with increased porphyrins in stool.

b. Laboratory tests
  (1) Stools
    (a) Stool porphyrins are elevated in HCP (and in VP) but not in AIP.
    (b) The main fecal (and urinary) porphyrin is coproporphyrin III.
    (c) Protoporphyrin is not increased.
  (2) Urine
    (a) Urinary PBG and ALA are increased in HCP (as in VP and AIP).

5. Erythropoietic porphyria (EPP, ferrochelatase deficiency or protoporphyria)
  a. Clinical aspects: A not uncommon disorder with autosomal dominant transmission.
    (1) Skin
      (a) Cutaneous photosensitivity with burning, erythema, and swelling.
      (b) Intolerance to the sun is usually noted in childhood.
    (2) Liver
      (a) A minority of patients with EPP develop hepatic damage.
      (b) Liver disease can range from mild to fetal.
    (3) Other manifestations
      (a) Significant hemolysis is rare.
      (b) There is no neurologic involvement.
  b. Laboratory tests
    (1) Urine
      (a) Can fluoresce after ultraviolet irradiation.
      (b) Does not contain porphyrin precursors (D-ALA or PBG).
    (2) Stools, erythrocytes, plasma, bile
      (a) Diagnostic elevation of free nonzinc protoporphyrins.

6. Congenital erythropoietic porphyria (CEP)
  a. Clinical aspects
    (1) Very rare autosomal recessive disorder.
    (2) CEP is likely when a young child has a combination of:
      (a) Severe mutilating cutaneous photosensitivity.
      (b) Hemolytic anemia.
      (c) Reddish teeth and red-brown urine.

    (3) The skin disease of homozygous CEP is much more severe than in heterozygous PCT, EPP, VP, or HCP.
  b. Laboratory tests
    (1) Type I porphyrin derivatives are characteristically elevated in:
      (a) Urine and plasma (uroporphyrin I).
      (b) Stools (mainly coproporphyrin I).
      (c) Erythroid cells.

IV. **Treatment, Prevention, and Monitoring of Porphyria**
  A. Acute intermittent porphyria
    1. Treatment of the acute attack: Patients with an acute attack of AIP must be usually hospitalized.
      a. Symptomatic relief
        (1) Severe pain requires frequent doses of a narcotic analgesic (e.g., meperidine).
        (2) Nausea and anxiety can be alleviated by phenothiazines.
        (3) Persistent sinus tachycardia may yield to propanolol.
        (4) Insomnia can respond to chloral hydrate.
        (5) Treatment of seizures can be very difficult.
          (a) Phenytoin, mephytoin, valproate, and barbiturates are dangerous.
          (b) Bromides will not induce ALA-S and P-450.
          (c) Clonazepam may be less dangerous than phenytoin or barbiturates.
      b. Antiporphyria measures
        (1) Parenteral glucose (10% dextrose to provide 300–500 g carbohydrate per day).
        (2) Intravenous hematin (panhematin).
          (a) Up to 4 mg/kg IV over a 30-min period once a day for 3 to 14 days.
          (b) Heme-arginate (3 mg/kg IV) or albumin-bound hematin may be more stable than hematin and less prone to induce phlebitis.
          (c) Response to hematin can be noted within 48 hr.

(3) The role of colchicine in aborting or mitigating abdominal pain is uncertain.

  c. Monitoring: Close, continuous observation is needed to monitor for:

    (1) Respiratory paralysis and the need for respiratory assistance.

    (2) Neurologic or myocardial failure.

    (3) Severe tachycardia or hypertensive crisis.

    (4) Electrolyte imbalance (hyponatremia, excess antidiuretic hormone).

2. Prevention: AIP (and other neurovisceral porphyrias) are major pharmacogenetic entities. Death due to respiratory paralysis may occur in 25% of patients with an acute attack. Patients should be provided with a medical warning bracelet and written information.

  a. Circumstances or agents that must be avoided to prevent acute attacks:

    (1) Crash dieting and long intervals between meals.

    (2) Ingestion of alcohol.

    (3) Barbiturates and many anticonvulsants (see above).

    (4) Chlordiazepoxide, meprobamate, pentazocine (Talwin).

    (5) Sulfonamides, chlorpropamide.

    (6) Griseofulvin.

    (7) Exogenous estrogens, progesterones.

    (8) Chloroquine, imipramine.

    (9) Many other compounds activating P-450.

  b. Agents that are relatively safe in AIP and can be administered when needed:

    (1) Morphine, buprenorphine (Temgesic), aspirin, acetaminophen.

    (2) Phenothiazines.

    (3) Glucocorticoids.

    (4) Bromides.

    (5) Vitamin K.

    (6) Clonidine, nifedipine.

    (7) Penicillin, vancomycin.

  c. Luteinizing hormone-releasing hormone (LHRH)

    (1) Antiovulatory LHRH agonists may prevent repeated premenstrual AIP crises.

B. Variegate porphyria and hereditary coproporphyria: The prevention and treatment of acute attacks in variegate porphyria and he-

reditary coproporphyria are similar to those for AIP.

C. Other porphyrias

1. Porphyria cutanea tarda

  a. Significant risk of liver disease including hepatoma (greater than 15% in some series).

  b. Hepatoma risk correlates with length of untreated disease and presence of cirrhosis.

  c. Baseline imaging studies of the liver are needed.

  d. Alcohol, iron, exogenous estrogen, and barbiturates must be rigorously avoided.

  e. Repeated phlebotomies to bring ferritin to low normal levels and abate porphyrinuria.

  f. Chloroquine phosphate in low doses (e.g., 125 mg biweekly).

    (1) Consider particularly if phlebotomy is unwise (with anemia or heart disease).

    (2) Chloroquine may promote excretion of excess hepatic porphyrins.

  g. Phlebotomies combined with low-dose chloroquine may provide fastest remission.

  h. Desferrioxamine treatment is ineffective in PCT.

2. Erythropoietic protoporphyria (EPP)

  a. Skin photosensitivity

    (1) Beta-carotene (60 to 180 mg p.o. daily in adults).

    (2) Effective in minimizing cutaneous photosensitivity.

    (3) Topical light blockers may be useful.

  b. Liver failure

    (1) Liver failure in EPP is difficult to treat.

    (2) Cholestyramine can promote increased biliary excretion of protoporphyrins.

    (3) Liver transplantation may be needed in life-threatening disease.

3. Congenital erythropoietic porphyria (CEP)

  a. Hemolytic disease in homozygous children with severe CEP

    (1) May require multiple transfusions.

    (2) Deferoxamine to decrease iron burden.

    (3) Splenectomy may decrease the need for transfusion.

(4) Oral charcoal (25 g daily or twice daily) may help deplete excessive uroporphyrin I.

(5) Metabolic alkalinization may facilitate porphyrin excretion.

b. Prevention of mutilating cutaneous scars

(1) Sunscreen lotions.

(2) Prompt attention to skin infections.

V. Prognosis

A. The prognosis depends greatly on the type of porphyria and on its management.

B. In acute attacks of neurovisceral porphyrias the outlook is favorable if:

1. The diagnosis is recognized and precipitants are removed.

2. Treatment is begun before severe neurologic damage or respiratory insufficiency occurs.

C. Under unfavorable circumstances, acute porphyrias can be fatal or crippling, with irreversible quadriplegia, blindness, and other neurologic sequelae.

D. In PCT the long-term prognosis is greatly improved by measures to prevent or reverse liver damage.

Bibliography

Bonkovsky HL, Healey JF, Lourie AN, et al. Intravenous heme-albumin in acute intermittent porphyria: Evidence for repletion of hepatic hemoproteins and regulatory heme pools. *Am J Gastroenterol* 86(8):1050–1056, 1991.

Desnick RJ, Anderson KE. Heme biosynthesis and its disorders: The porphyrias and sideroblastic anemias, in Hoffman R, Benz Jr EJ, Shattil SJ, et al. (eds). *Hematology: Basic Principles and Practice*. New York, Churchill Livingstone, 1991, pp 350–367.

Elder GH. The cutaneous porphyrias. *Semin Dermatol* 9(1):63–69, 1990.

Kappas A, Sassa S, Galbraith RA, et al. Porphyrins and heme, in Scriver CR, Beaudet AL, Sly WS, et al (eds). *The Metabolic Basis of Inherited Disease*, ed 6, Vol I, part 8, chap 52. New York, McGraw-Hill, 1989, pp 1305–1365.

Logan GM, Weimer MK, Ellefson M, et al. Bile porphyrin analysis in the evaluation of variegate porphyria. *N Engl J Med* 324(20):1408–1411, 1991.

Siersema PD, ten-Kate FJ, Mulder PG. Hepatocellular carcinoma in porphyria cutanea tarda: frequency and factors related to its occurrence. *Liver* 12(2):56–61, 1992.

CHAPTER 71

Non-Neoplastic White Blood Cell Disorders

Thomas F. Lint, Ph.D.
William H. Knospe, M.D.

Neutropenia

I. Definition

Less than 1,000 neutrophils per cubic millimeter. When the level of neutrophils is less than 500/mm³, the risk of acute bacterial or fungal infection is markedly increased.

II. Etiology and Pathophysiology

A. Congenital: genetically mediated (e.g., Kostmann's syndrome, constitutional leukopenia in blacks).

B. Cyclic: genetically mediated (autosomal dominant) disorder due to cyclic failure of stem cells and/or growth factor production; fever and infection at nadirs of neutropenia.

C. Drugs often invoke a variety of mechanisms: idiosyncratic, immune, direct or indirect injury. (Table 71-1)

  1. Immunologic: Drug-stimulated antibodies injure mature or immature precursors in bone marrow (e.g., aminopyrine, phenytoin).

  2. Drug toxicity: Direct injury to hematopoietic stem cells (e.g., chloramphenicol, gold salts, chlorpromazine, cytotoxic drugs).

  3. Accumulation of toxic metabolites.

D. Autoimmune and alloimmune reactions: Antibodies directly injure polymorphonuclear leukocytes or mature precursors (e.g., systemic lupus erythematosus, transfusion reaction). (Table 71-2)

E. Myelodysplasia and neoplasia: Leukopenia results from abnormal maturation or cell differentiation.

F. Hypersplenism: Almost any form of splenomegaly may result in sequestrational neutropenia.

G. Acquired immune deficiency syndrome (AIDS).

III. Diagnosis

A. Fever, chills, sore throat, pneumonia or other localized infections, septic shock.

B. Blood: Leukopenia with reduction in absolute granulocyte level (less than 500 neutrophils per cubic millimeter of blood markedly increases the risk of infection).

C. Bone marrow

  1. Drug associated: Usually hypocellular, with decreased to absent later members of granulocytic series (myelocytes, metamyelocytes, and mature polymorphonuclear leukocytes). Early granulocytic cells may

Table 71-1. Drugs Associated with Agranulocytosis

Anticonvulsants	**Antihypertensives**	**Diuretics**
Carbamazepine	Captopril	Acetazolamide
Ethosuximide	Diazoxide	Bumetanide
Mephenytoin	Hydralazine	Chlorthalidone
Phenytoin	Methyldopa	Chlorothiazide
Trimethadione	Propranolol	Ethacrynic acid
		Hydrochlorothiazide
Antidepressants	**Analgesics and**	Mercurials
Desipramine	**Anti-inflammatory Agents**	Methazolamide
Imipramine	Acetylsalicylic acid	
	Aminopyrine	**Anti-infectives**
Antipsychotics	Antipyrine	Ampicillin
Butyrophenones	Colchicine	Carbenicillin
Clozapine	Fenoprofen	Cephalexin
Loxapine	Gold salts	Cephalothin
Molindone	Ibuprofen	Chloramphenicol
Phenothiazines	Indomethacin	Clindamycin
Thioxanthenes	Oxyphenylbutazone	Cloxacillin
	Phenylbutazone	Doxycycline
Anxiolytics		Gentamicin
Chlordiazepoxide	**Others**	
Diazepam	Allopurinol	**Anti-Infectives**
Meprobamate	Levamisole	Griseofulvin
	Penicillamine	Isoniazide
Antiparkinsonian agents		Lincomycin
Levodopa	**Antithyroid Agents**	Methicillin
	Carbimazole	Metronidazole
Antihistamines	Methimazole	Nafcillin
Brompheniramine	Methylthiouracil	Nitrofurantoin
Promethazine	Propylthiouracil	Novobiocin
	Thiouracil	Oxacillin
Sulfonamides		Penicillin
Sulfadiazine	**Hypoglycemic Agents**	Rifampin
Sulfamethoxazole-trimethoprim	Chlorpropamide	Streptomycin
Sulfapyridine	Tolbutamide	
Sulfasalazine		**Antimalarials**
Sulfathiazole	**H₂ antagonists**	Dapsone
Sulfisoxazole	Cimetidine	Hydroxychloroquine
		Quinine
Antiarrhythmics		Pyrimethamine
Procainamide		
Propranolol		
Quinidine		

be present, with a maturation arrest at the progranulocyte or myelocyte level.

2. In immunogenic agranulocytosis, lymphocytes may be increased and plasma cells may be present.

3. When the drug-related antibody is directed at mature neutrophils, the marrow

may be hyperplastic and granulocytic hyperplasia may exist, and all stages of granulocyte maturation may be present.

4. Hypersplenism is characterized by neutropenia in blood, granulocytic hyperplasia in marrow, and an enlarged spleen.

5. Cyclic neutropenia may show alternating

Table 71-2. Drugs Associated with Antileukocyte Antibodies

Aminopyrine
Ampicillin
Chlorpropamide
Chlorpromazine
Clozapine
Dicloxacillin
Lidocaine
Methimazole
Nafcillin
Phenytoin
Procainamide
Propylthiouracil
Sulfasalazine

aplasia, maturation arrest, or granulocytic hyperplasia.

IV. **Therapy**
   A. Withdrawal of drug(s).
   B. Persistent neutropenia due to precursor cell injury and/or myelodysplasia may be improved with growth factors such as granulocyte colony-stimulating factor (G-CSF) or granulocyte-macrophage colony-stimulating factor (GM-CSF). Cyclic neutropenia may also be improved.
   C. Hypersplenism is treated by splenectomy; transient improvement can occur following splenic irradiation or corticosteroid administration.
   D. Treatment of agranulocytosis
      1. Hospitalize the patient and stop the drug or drugs or the offending agent.
      2. Obtain hematologic consultation.
      3. Provide reverse isolation.
      4. Monitor vital signs and urinary output; observe for signs of septic shock.
      5. Complete fever workup: urinalysis, routine and culture, sputum culture, blood cultures, chest x-ray, careful examination of skin for infectious lesions.
      6. Institute empiric antibiotic therapy if the clinical condition warrants it.

V. **Prognosis**
   Patients whose neutrophil level exceeds 1,000/mm^3 following therapy or stopping of drugs have an excellent prognosis.

VI. **Patient Monitoring**
   Complete blood counts should be done at least every 2 days until recovery of normal blood counts is observed. The patient should have weekly blood counts for 4 weeks afterward.

Neutrophilia

I. **Definition**
   Leukocyte counts exceeding 12,000/mm^3 with more than 50% neutrophils.
   A. Pool shifts (from marrow or marginating pools) secondary to infection, stress, corticosteroid use, endotoxin, hypoxia, and adrenalin.
   B. Increased proliferation in infections, neoplasms, and myeloproliferative disorders including chronic granulocytic leukemia and inflammation.
   C. Leukemoid reactions: When any of the above are markedly immature granulocytes, nucleated red blood cells and thrombocytosis may be present in the blood, although usually these changes are transient. If they persist, marker studies such as a cytogenetic study of the bone marrow, leukocyte alkaline phosphatase histochemistry of blood, and monoclonal antibodies (flow cytometry) may reveal the neoplastic or benign character of the neutrophilia and/or leukemoid reaction.

Qualitative Disorders of Phagocytic Cell Function

I. **Definition**
   Adequate host defense against extracellular bacterial and fungal pathogens requires normal phagocyte (neutrophil, macrophage, monocyte and eosinophil) function. Defects in chemotaxis, opsonization, ingestion, degranulation, or metabolic stimulation result in a greatly increased risk of infection. The leukocyte count is usually normal, but the leukocytes are intrinsically defective in function.

II. **Specific Defects (Table 71-3)**

Bibliography

Clark RA, Malech HL, Gallin JI, et al. Genetic variants of chronic granulomatous disease: Prevalence of deficiencies of two cytosolic components of the NADPH oxidase system. *N Engl J Med* 321:647–652, 1989.

Rotrosen D, Gallin JI: Disorders of phagocyte function. *Ann Rev Immunol* 5:127–150, 1987.

Table 71-3. Qualitative Disorders of Phagocytic Cell Function

Abnormality	Etiology	Abnormality of Neutrophil Function	Clinical Effects
Chemotactic defects Cellular defects may also be present in Chediak-Higashi syndrome and lazy leukocyte syndrome. Inhibition of chemotaxis identified in alcoholic liver disease. Wiskott-Aldrich syndrome, neoplasms, and thermal injury.	Genetically mediated C5 absence. Membrane maturation defect.	Defective response to chemotactic stimuli.	Recurrent infections.
Opsonization (adherence defects) *Opsonin deficiencies* (IgG) in some combined immunodeficiencies; X-linked hypogamma-globulinemias; common variable immunodeficiency (acquired) and selective IgG subclass deficiency.		Failure of phagocytes to bind microorganisms.	Recurrent pyogenic infections.
Degranulation defects: 1. Chediak-Higashi syndrome most important defect.	Autosomal recessive.	Failure to release contents of lysosomal granules is first step in killing of ingested microorganisms or release of granules with defective structure or reduced enzyme content.	Associated with pancytopenia, albinism; defective natural killer cells; recurrent pyogenic infections.
2. Specific granule deficiencies have also been identified.	Genetic.		

Intracellular killing defects:			
1. Chronic granulomatous disease (CGD) in which defects of reduced nicotinamide-adenine dinucleotide phosphate oxidase are present (most important intracellular killing defect).	X-linked (60% of cases) autosomal recessive (33% of cases).	Abnormal cytochrome b 558 subunit (x-linked); absent 47-kd phospho-protein essential to activation of NADPH oxidase.	Wide variety of infections with catalase positive organisms which do not produce H_2O_2 such as *Staphylococcus aureus*, *Serratia marcescens*, *Klebsiella*, *Candida* species, *Aspergillus*.
2. Severe glucose-6-phosphate dehydrogenase deficiency associated with a defect in hexose monophosphate shunt stimulation, resulting in a spectrum of infections similar to that of CGD.		Failure to regenerate cytoplasmic NADPH via glucose oxidation through the hexose monophosphate shunt.	
3. Myeloperoxidase deficiency associated with only a slightly increased risk of infection with *Staphylococcus* or *Candida* species.	Autosomal recessive.	Mild deficit in microbial killing of ingested organisms secondary to defective utilization of peroxide.	

Myeloproliferative and Myelodysplastic Disorders: Introduction

Solomon S. Adler, M.D., F.A.C.P.

Myeloproliferative Disorders (Definition)

I. **Group of clonal hemopoietic stem cell disorders involving:**
   A. Totipotent stem cells.
   B. Multipotent stem cells.
II. **Excessive production of at least one blood cell line.**
   A. Always in marrow.
   B. Usually also in blood.
III. **Maturation in the chronic phase is not substantially dysplastic**
IV. **Entities included by Dameshek in the *myeloproliferative disorders*, (*MPD*), a term he coined in the 1950s:**
   A. Chronic granulocytic leukemia (CGL).
   B. Polycythemia vera (PV).
   C. Essential (idiopathic) thrombocytosis (ET).
   D. Agnogenic myeloid metaplasia (AMM or myelofibrosis with myeloid metaplasia, MMM).
   E. Paroxysmal nocturnal hemoglobinuria (PNH).
   F. DiGuglielmo's disease (DiGug).
V. **Revision of Dameshek's classification**
   A. Remove from MPD and include under the myelodysplasias.

1. Digug: This usually is classified with one of the refractory anemias.
2. Ph chromosome-negative CGL.
   a. Usually has dysplastic features.
   b. More aggressive than Ph-positive CGL.
   B. PNH: difficult to classify as MPD or myelodysplastic disorder.
      1. Not a typical MPD.
         a. The only proliferative element in PNH is the erythroid series, and this is in response to the hemolytic anemia, not spontaneous.
         b. PNH is the only MPD that evolves either to
            (1) Acute leukemia or to
            (2) Aplastic anemia.
      2. Not a typical myelodysplastic disorder.
         a. Morphologic maturational abnormalities are usually mild or absent.
         b. However, severe functional dysplasia of cell membranes is present.

Chronic Granulocytic Leukemia (CGL)

I. **Definition**
   Uncommon (~20% of all adult leukemias)

clonal totipotent or multipotent stem cell disorder with:

A. Granulocytic hyperplasia of marrow and blood (<5% blasts in marrow, chronic phase).
B. Hyperplasia of other cell lines (often).
   1. Basophilia and/or eosinophilia.
   2. Thrombocytosis.
C. Philadelphia (Ph) chromosome (i.e., reciprocal translocation of a portion of 9q and 22q).
D. Extramedullary hemotopoiesis, especially in the spleen.

II. Etiology

A. Ionizing radiation: Latent period about 4–11 years.
B. Associated with human leukocyte antigen (HLA) types CW3 and CW4.
C. Unknown (vast majority).

III. Pathophysiology

A. Ph chromosome
   1. Translocation of C-Abelson (C-abl) oncogene on chromosome 9 to the breakpoint cluster region (bcr) of chromosome 22.
   2. Production of aberrant tyrosine kinase (usually p210) product of C-abl-bcr fusion gene.
B. Unchecked granulocytic proliferation
   1. Organ infiltration and mass effects.
   2. Hyperleukocytosis syndrome (rare in the chronic phase).
   3. Hypermetabolism.
C. Disturbed stem cell differentiation
   1. Cytopenias.
   2. Clonal progression to a blastic disorder.

IV. Diagnosis

A. History: Search for symptoms related to the following:
   1. Anemia
      a. Fatigue
      b. Malaise
      c. Splenomegaly
      d. Early satiety
      e. Abdominal discomfort
      f. Weight loss
   2. Hypermetabolism
      a. Fever
      b. Sweats
      c. Weight loss
      d. Gout
   3. Marrow expansion
      a. Bone pain
   4. Severe Hyperleukocytosis: ~10%
      a. Central nervous system abnormalities

      b. Pulmonary impairment
      c. Priapism
   5. Organ infiltration
      a. Local tumors (granulocytic sarcomas)
      b. Arthritis
B. Clinical signs and physical findings
   1. Pallor
   2. Splenomegaly
   3. Hepatomegaly
   4. Lymphadenopathy (uncommon)
   5. Gouty arthritis
   6. Signs of hyperviscosity (if present)
      a. Tachypnea
      b. Lethargy, stupor
   7. Signs of thrombocytopenia
      a. Petechiae
      b. Ecchymosis
C. Diagnostic tests
   1. Complete blood count (CBC), with special attention to the differential count
      a. Granulocytosis with a left shift through blasts.
      b. Basophilia and/or eosinophilia and/or circulating megakaryocytes or their fragments.
      c. Thrombocytosis or thrombocytopenia.
      d. Leukocyte alkaline phosphatase score very reduced.
   2. Blood chemistries, etc.
      a. Elevated lactic dehydrogenase (LDH).
      b. Hyperuricemia.
      c. Pseudohyperkalemia, pseudohypoglycemia, spurious hypoxemia.
      d. Elevated vitamin B_{12} level and increased B_{12} binding capacity (especially transcobalamin I (TCI)).
   3. Bone marrow
      a. Hypercellular—especially myeloid.
         (1) Often megakaryocytic hyperplasia.
         (2) Pseudo-Gaucher cells.
      b. Stainable iron: often decreased-absent.
      c. Cytogenetics
         (1) Ph chromosome: in ~90% of CGL.
         (2) Atypical or masked Ph chromosome
            (a) Not detectable cytogenetically as a Ph chromosome but bcr-Abl rearrangement is present.
            (b) Detected by molecular genetic techniques.

(3) Other chromosomal abnormalities
  (a) Double Ph chromosome.
  (b) Chromosomes seen in progressive disease (see Section VII, B,3) may be present at diagnosis in some patients.

V. Differential Diagnosis
A. Other myeloproliferative disorders
  1. PV, AMM, ET (these generally have less left-shifted granulocyte series in blood; usually do not have a low leukocyte alkaline phosphatase [LAP] score and are, with very rare exceptions, Ph chromosome negative).
B. Leukemoid reaction
  1. A cause such as inflammaton, infection, or cancer is usually detectable.
  2. White blood cell count usually $<5 \times 10^4/\text{mm}^3$; usually little left shift.
  3. Ph chromosome negative.
  4. LAP score usually elevated or normal.
  5. Splenomegaly usually absent.

VI. Treatment
A. Bone marrow transplantation for patients <55–60 years old.
  1. Allogeneic or syngeneic.
  2. Preferably within the first year of diagnosis.
B. Interferon-α (IFN-α)
  1. Often results in temporary reduction of Ph-positive population of cells; not known if IFN therapy prolongs survival more than chemotherapy with hydroxyurea.
C. Chemotherapy
  1. Hydroxyurea: 500 μg–5 g/day as needed prolongs survivorship compared to busulfan.
  2. Busulfan: 2 mg qod–6 μg/day.
    a. Start with a low dose; some patients are extremely sensitive and become aplastic with a very small dose; check blood counts frequently.
D. Adjunctive treatments
  1. Splenectomy.
  2. Radiotherapy—to spleen or to a mass (if present).
  3. Leukapheresis.
    a. Emergent therapy for hyperleukocytosis syndrome.

VII. Patient Monitoring
A. Symptoms and signs
  1. New or worsening systemic complaints, increasing spleen size, masses.

B. Tests
  1. Blood count: Progressive leukocytosis, left shift, worsening cytopenias.
  2. LAP
    a. Increasing values suggest progressive disease.
  3. Chromosomes
    a. Stable or a decrease in the percentage of Ph chromosome-positive cells versus new abnormalities (e.g., additional Ph chromosome, loss of chromosome 22 q; trisomy 8 or 19; iso 17 q).

VIII. Course of the Disease Prognosis
A. Prognostic indicators at presentation
  1. Percentage of blood blasts (higher—poorer prognosis).
  2. Liver and spleen size (larger—poorer prognosis).
  3. Basophil/eosinophil percentage (higher—poor prognosis).
B. Course
  1. Clinical progression
    a. Progressively more refractory phase (accelerated phase) eventuating in fully blastic leukemia: ~50–70%.
    b. Sudden blastic transformation: ~15%.
    c. Progressive disease without blastic transformation, with death due to complication of cytopenias.
  2. Types of blastic transformations
    a. Acute nonlymphoblasic myeloblastic (M_1 or M_2) or myelomonocytic (M_4).
    b. Acute nonlymphoblastic-erythroblastic (M_6): 10–20%; other-rare.
    c. Acute lymphoblastic: 20–30%.
C. Prognosis
  1. With appropriate standard chemotherapy or:
    a. Chronic phase
      (1) Median survival with busulfan ~40–47 months; 5-year survival is ~25–35%. With hydroxyurea, median survival is about 1 year longer, with 5-year survival being ~60%. With interferon, 5-year survival is ~60%.
    b. Blastic phase: <6 months.
  2. With bone marrow transplantation: long-term survival
    a. In the chronic phase
      (1) Overall, 40–60%.
      (2) Within 1 year of diagnosis, up to 80%.

b. In the accelerated phase, ~30%.

c. In the blastic phase, ~10%.

Polycythemia Vera (PV)

I. Definition

Uncommon (0.4–1.6/10^5 population) clonal hemopoietic stem cell disorder, with a peak incidence in 50- to 60-year-old persons with

A. Marrow panmyelosis.

B. Peripheral increase in the red blood cell mass.

1. Colony-forming unit-erythroid (CFU-E) grow in culture without addition of erythropoietin.

C. Frequent accompanying leukocytosis and/or thrombocytosis.

II. Etiology

A. Unknown—vast majority.

B. Ionizing radiation—weak association.

C. Familial tendency—rare.

III. Pathophysiology

A. Excessive red blood cell mass results in increased blood viscosity and hypervolemia, leading to:

1. Tissue hypoxia.

2. Thrombotic tendency.

3. Erythromelalgia.

B. Thrombocytosis

1. Thrombotic tendency.

C. Platelet dysfunction

1. Hemorrhagic phenomena.

D. Extramedullary hematopoiesis

1. Organomegaly—especially splenomegaly.

IV. Diagnosis

A. History

1. Ruddy complexion.

2. Thrombotic phenomena: ~30%.

a. Peripheral arterial occlusion.

b. Deep venous thrombosis with or without pulmonary embolism.

c. Abdominal thromboses.

(1) Hepatic portal vein.

(a) About 50% of all Budd-Chiari syndrome cases are related to PV.

(2) Mesenteric veins.

(3) Splenic vein.

d. Coronary artery disease.

e. Cerebrovascular accident.

3. Other symptoms

a. Pruritus, especially after a warm bath: ~40%.

b. Peptic ulcer disease.

c. Symptoms of splenomegaly (abdominal discomfort, early satiety).

d. Hemorrhagic phenomena

(1) Minor: epistaxis, gingival bleeding, ecchymoses.

(2) Serious or life-threatening: rare (major gastrointestinal, etc.).

e. Neurologic (red blood cell mass and thrombocytosis related).

(1) Headache, dizziness, tinnitus, vertigo.

(2) Visual disturbances.

B. Clinical signs

1. Red blood cell hypervolemic signs.

a. Facial plethora.

b. Congestion of conjunctiva and mucous membranes.

c. Retinal vein engorgement.

2. Splenomegaly: ~75% at diagnosis (mild-moderate).

3. Neurologic signs.

4. Erythromelalgia.

C. Diagnostic tests

1. CBC

a. Hematocrit >60% nearly always indicates an elevated red blood cell mass.

b. Elevated red blood cell count, often with decreased mean corpuscular volume (MCV).

c. Leukocytosis (12–25 × 10^3/mm³): about two-thirds of patients.

d. Basophilia (>3%): about two-thirds of patients.

e. Thrombocytosis at diagnosis: ~50% of patients.

2. Bone marrow

a. Panmyelosis, often with striking megakaryocytosis.

b. Stainable iron: absent-markedly decreased.

3. Other tests

a. Platelet aggregation—abnormal in ~50%.

b. Oxygen saturation.

(1) ≥92% in ~90% of patients.

(2) Slightly reduced (88–92%) saturation in 10% of patients.

c. LAP—often elevated.

d. Vitamin B_{12} often >900 pg/ml.

e. Unbound vitamin B_{12} binding capacity often >2,200 pg/ml.

f. Erythropoietin level—not elevated.

g. P_{50} and oxygen saturation curve—normal.

h. Cloning of late erythroid progenitor cells (CFU-E)

　　(1) Growth without additional erythropoietin; probably is a very reliable diagnostic test for PV.

i. Chromosomal analysis

　　(1) Abnormalities found in ~20% of patients with uncomplicated PV; frequency increases with duration.

　　(2) 20q-, +8, and +9 are most common; likely not related to therapy.

V. Differential Diagnosis

A. Relative (stress, spurious) erythrocytosis

　1. Decreased plasma volume; normal red blood cell mass.

　2. Usually occurs in overweight male smokers.

B. Inappropriate elevation of erythopoietin

　1. Neoplasia

　　a. Hypernephroma—1–3%.

　　b. Hepatocellular carcinoma—up to 10%.

　　c. Cerebellar hemangioblastoma—up to 15%.

　　d. Miscellaneous tumors: uterine tumors, pheochromocytoma, aldosteronoma.

　2. Nonneoplastic

　　a. Bartter's syndrome.

　　b. Hydronephrosis.

　　c. Ovarian cysts, renal cysts.

C. Appropriate erythropoietin elevation

　1. Elevated carboxyhemoglobin usually occurs as a result of smoking.

　　a. Assess level after a regular day of smoking, not the next morning i.e., after overnight smoking "holiday"; $T_{1/2}$ of carboxyhemoglobin is 6–10 hr.

　　b. Carboxyhemoglobin does not alter routine blood gas values.

　2. Hemoglobin abnormalities that shift the oxygen dissociation curve to the left

　　a. P_{50} not always diagnostic; the full oxygen dissociation curve may be needed.

　　b. Hemoglobin electrophoresis is often normal.

　3. Pulmonary insufficiency

　　a. Must exclude intermittent disorders such as sleep apnea.

　4. Right-to-left cardiac shunts.

D. Isolated primary erythrocytosis (may evolve into PV)

　1. Diagnosis of exclusion.

VI. Treatment

A. Maintain red blood cell mass at the lower limit of normal.

　1. Perform phlebotomies for control of the red blood cell mass.

　2. Drug therapy

　　a. Hydroxyurea

　　　(1) May decrease the number of phlebotomies needed.

　　　(2) Useful in older patients who may have difficulty tolerating phlebotomies.

　　　(3) Requires both frequent blood counts initially to regulate the dose and daily medication.

　　　(4) Leukemogenic potential unclear.

　　b. ^{32}P

　　　(1) May control the red blood cell volume and thrombocytosis.

　　　(2) Requires less intensive monitoring than for hydroxyurea.

　　　(3) One or two doses may control the disorder for long periods.

　　　(4) Leukemia

　　　　(a) Ten percent of patients will develop leukemia; thus, reserve ^{32}P therapy for older patients who need it.

　　c. Chlorambucil—contraindicated because of (2) below

　　　(1) Requires frequent blood counts.

　　　(2) Leukemogenic (up to 15–20% of patients will develop acute nonlymphoblastic leukemia).

B. Control thrombocytosis, especially in patients with neurologic symptoms and relatively normal platelet function.

　1. Anagrelide

　2. Hydroxyurea

　3. IFN-α

　4. ^{32}P

　5. Alkylating agents

C. Inhibit platelet function instead of controlling thrombocytosis.

　1. May be an alternative in young patients who cannot be treated with or do not respond to anagrelide; watch for bleeding problems.

　2. A PV study group showed no benefit from acetylsalicylic acid (ASA) usage, but that study did not *rigidly* keep the red blood cell mass at the *lower* limit of normal.

D. Control of pruritus

　1. Try aspirin, cyproheptadine, choles-

tyramine, or cimetidine if not controlled with phlebotomy.

VII. Patient Monitoring

A. CBC and platelet counts; assess red blood cell mass if needed—use initially to correlate hematocrit with desired red blood cell mass (low normal) to define desired hematocrit level.

B. Interval history and physical exam, especially to evaluate for neurologic symptoms and progressive splenomegaly.

VIII. Course of the Disease and Prognosis

A. Causes of death and relative frequencies
   1. Thrombosis: 30%
      a. Risk of abdominal surgery with high red blood cell mass is extremely high; use emergent phlebotomy.
   2. Evolution to acute nonlymphoblastic leukemia: 10–20%.
      a. Highest incidence in patients treated with alkylating agents; intrinisic risk probably 1–2%.
   3. Other neoplasms: ~15%.
   4. Hemorrhagic phenomena: ~5%.
      a. Incidence of complications is higher, but usually they are mild.
   5. Evolution to secondary myelofibrosis (spent phase): ~15%.
      a. Lag period: 2–15 years.
      b. Death due to complications of cytopenias or intercurrent illness.

B. Duration of survival (median)
   1. Untreated: ~2–3 years.
   2. Appropriately treated: 9–12 years. Survivorship of up to ~20 years has been reported.

Agnogenic Myeloid Metaplasia (AMM) (Myelofibrosis with Myeloid Metaplasia, MMM)

I. Definition

Chronic clonal MPD with the following characteristics:

A. Extramedullary hemopoiesis (ineffective), especially splenic and hepatic.

B. Marrow fibrosis or at least a marked increase in reticulin.

II. Etiology

A. Vast majority—unknown.

B. Toxins (e.g., benzene).

C. Ionizing radiation.

III. Pathophysiology

A. Disturbed clonal hemopoiesis results in:
   1. Extramedullary hematopoiesis and organ enlargement.

B. Increased megakaryocyte mass in marrow may liberate large amounts of growth factors. Platelet derived growth factor (PDGF) and transforming growth factor (TGF-β) (and possibly interleukin-1 and tumor necrosis factor-α) cause secondary fibrosis of the marrow

IV. Diagnosis

A. History
   1. Median age: ~60 years.
   2. Asymptomatic at diagnosis: ~25%.
   3. Symptoms
      a. General constitutional: fatigue weakness, weight loss, fever (uncommon).
      b. Symptoms of splenomegaly and hepatomegaly: abdominal discomfort, early satiety.
      c. Bone pain.
      d. Thrombocytopenia-related symptoms.

B. Signs and physical manifestations
   1. Splenomegaly: ~100%: one-third mild, one-third moderate, one-third massive (>15 cm).
   2. Hepatomegaly: ~65%.
      a. Signs of portal hypertension may exist.
   3. General signs of systemic illness or cytopenias: fever, edema, pallor, bruising, petechiae.
   4. Other abnormalities
      a. Extramedullary masses, adenopathy: ~15%.
      b. Sweet's syndrome—neutrophilic dermatosis.
      c. Effusions containing hemopoietic cells.

C. Diagnostic tests
   1. CBC
      a. Teardrop-shaped red blood cells, circulating normoblasts.
      b. Evidence of hemolysis (hypersplenism, etc.).
         (1) Reticulocytosis, red blood cell survival (reduced) with ^{51}Cr therapy.
      c. Leukocytosis with immature elements (usually <5% blasts), circulating megakaryocytes or their fragments, hyper- or hyposegmentation of neutrophils.
      d. Platelets—one-third elevated, one-third decreased.

e. Pancytopenia: ~10%.
2. Bone marrow
   a. Often inaspirable.
   b. Moderate-marked increase in reticulin.
   c. Mild-marked fibrosis.
   d. Patchy hypercellularity with maturational abnormalities (mild).
   e. Megakaryocytosis.
   f. Cytogenetics: ~50% nonrandom abnormalities; chromosomes 5, 7, 8, 9, and 20 most commonly involved.
3. Other tests
   a. Immunology tests—abnormalities in up to 50% of patients: positive antinuclear antibodies, red blood cell antibodies, immune complexes, etc.
   b. PNH-related tests (Ham's etc.) occasionally positive.
   c. LAP not helpful.
      (1) Elevated in ~25% and decreased in ~25%.
   d. Characteristic changes may be seen on bone x-rays.

V. Differential Diagnosis
A. CGL has Ph chromosome; AMM does not.
B. Hairy cell leukemia—marrow is inaspirable but the biopsy is characteristic, and cells stain with acid phosphatase, which is tartrate fast and tartrate resistant acid phosphatase (TRAP) positive.
C. Secondary marrow fibrosis
   1. Neoplastic related: lymphomas, breast cancer, myeloma, prostate cancer, angioimmunoblastic lymphadenopathy with dysgammaglobulinemia, giant lymph node hyperplasia, lymphocytic myelofibrosis, etc.
   2. Nonneoplastic: systemic lupus erythematosus, polyarteritis nodosa, tuberculosis, rickets, histiocytosis, sarcoidosis, sickle cell anemias, vitamin B_{12} or folate-reversible fibrosis (very rare).

VI. Treatment
A. Supportive.
B. Bone marrow transplantation—younger patients.
   1. Problem: long pre-engraftment phase.
C. Reversal of cytopenias
   1. Anemia—erythropoietin ± G-CSF (?).
   2. Granulocytopenia—granulocyte—colony-stimulating factor (G-CSF) or granulocyte-macrophage colony-stimulating factor (GM-CSF).

D. Control organomegaly and thrombocytosis, if present.
   1. IFN.
   2. Chemotherapy (hydroxyurea, busulfan, etc.).
E. Uncontrollable spleen-related symptoms
   1. Splenectomy or low-dose radiation therapy.

VII. Patient Monitoring
A. Physical
   1. Organ size.
   2. Signs of liver dysfunction.
B. CBC, platelet count, blood chemistries, and liver function tests.

VIII. Course of the Disease and Prognosis
A. Death is related to complications of the following:
   1. Cytopenias.
   2. Portal hypertension plus hepatic dysfunction.
   3. Evolution to blastic leukemia.
   4. Complications of surgery
      a. Thrombotic
      b. Hemorrhagic
      c. Infectious
B. Survivorship without marrow transplantation
   1. Median: ~5 years.
   2. Range: <1 year to ~15 years.

Essential Thrombocytosis (ET) (Primary Thrombocythemia)

I. Definition
Chronic clonal MPD with thrombocytosis >6–10^5/mm³ (usually ≥10^6/mm³), without abnormalities diagnostic of CGL, PV, or AMM.

II. Etiology
Unknown.

III. Pathophysiology
Related to:
A. Increased to platelet mass—thrombosis.
B. Dysfunctional platelets—bleeding.

IV. Diagnosis
A. History
   1. Asymptomatic: About one-half to two-thirds of patients (depending on study).
   2. Symptomatic: About one-half to two-thirds of patients.
      a. Hemorrhagic or thrombotic
         (1) Hemorrhagic
            (a) Usually mild mucosal
            (b) Severe
               i. Surgery related.
               ii. Aspirin related.

(2) Thrombotic
    (a) Headache, dizziness, transient ischemic episodes, visual disturbances, erythromelalgia, priapism.
    (b) Myocardial infarcts and completed strokes.
b. Other symptoms
    (1) Pruritus: 10–15%.
    (2) Recurrent abortion.
    (3) Pyoderma gangrenosum (rare).
B. Signs and physical manifestations
  1. Signs of bleeding
  2. Signs of thrombosis
    a. Erythromelalgia, priapism, etc.
  3. Splenomegaly
    a. Physical: about one-third.
    b. On scan: about two-thirds.
C. Diagnostic tests
  1. CBC
    a. Leukocytosis (to ~40,000/mm^3): ~50%.
    b. Anemia: absent-mild.
    (1) May be iron deficiency related.
  2. Other blood tests
    a. Iron decreased; total iron-binding capacity (TIBC) elevated, especially with gastrointestinal bleeding.
    b. LAP—not helpful (usually normal).
    c. LDH—often mildly elevated.
  3. Bone marrow
    a. Megakaryocytic hyperplasia and atypia.

V. Differential Diagnosis
A. Chronic reactive thrombocytosis related to:
  1. Inflammation (e.g. Crohn's disease, rheumatoid arthritis, colitis, polyarteritis nodosa).
  2. Chronic infections (e.g., tuberculosis, fungal infections).
  3. Iron deficiency.
  4. Splenectomy.
  5. Malignancy.
B. Other myeloproliferative disorders.
C. 5 q—myelodysplastic disorder.

VI. Treatment
A. Asymptomatic patients, especially if young, may not need therapy.
B. Give aspirin if the bleeding time is not prolonged.
C. For older or symptomatic patients, even if young, give:
  1. Anagrelide.
  2. Hydroxyurea.

3. IFN-α.
4. Other forms of chemotherapy (e.g., alkylating agents).
D. Plateletpheresis for emergent treatment (e.g., preoperatively or for a vascular occlusive episode in progress).

VII. Patient Monitoring
A. History and physical exam: for bleeding or thrombotic symptoms or signs of progressive splenomegaly (uncommon).
B. CBC and platelet counts.

VIII. Course of the Disease and Prognosis
A. Episodes of thromboses or bleeding.
  1. Platelet count not predictive of thrombotic events.
B. Progression to leukemia
  1. Rare (<5%) with alkylating agent therapy.
C. Survivorship
  1. Median: ~10 years (longer for young, asymptomatic patients).
  2. Eighty percent of patients survive for ~5 years.

Paroxysmol Nocturmal Hemoglobinemia (PNH)

I. Definition
Clonal hemopoietic stem cell disorder, classified by some as a myeloproliferative disorder and by others as a myelodysplastic disorder.
A. Myeloid elements (red blood cells, white blood cells, megakaryocytes) which are supersensitive to complement (C)-mediated lysis, as manifested clinically by:
  1. Chronic intravascular hemolysis and hemosiderinuria.
  2. Possible evolution to asplastic anemic or leukemia.

II. Etiology
Unknown; presumably somatic mutation.

III. Pathogenesis
A. Membrane defect
  1. Defective membrane phosphatidylinositol glycan (PIG) linkage leads to deficiency of membrane-bound proteins, including:
    a. Decay-accelerating factor (DAF, CD55).
    (1) Increases the rate of inactivation of C3Bb complement activity.
    (2) Leads to mildly C-sensitive blood cells, primarily red blood cells (de-

fects also found on white blood cells and platelets).

   b. Membrane inhibitor of reactive lysis (MIRL, CD59)

     (1) Inactivates the later portion of the C pathway.

     (2) Leads to more profound lysis than does the lack of DAF.

   c. Acetylcholinesterase—no known pathogenetic importance.

   d. FCγ RIII on neutrophils.

B. Consequences of the membrane defect

  1. Mild-severe chronic hemolysis.

  2. Severity depends on the degree of DAF and MIRL defects.

C. Consequences of intravascular hemolysis

  1. Anemia

    a. Symptomatically mild-severe.

  2. Urinary iron loss

    a. Hemosiderinuria with secondary iron deficiency anemia.

    b. Hemoglobinuria—not in all patients.

D. Consequences of hemolysis, platelet abnormalities, and possibly other factors

  1. Thrombosis

    a. Deep vein.

    b. Portal vein—Budd-Chiari syndrome.

    c. Mesenteric (abdominal pain).

    d. Central nervous system (headaches, strokes).

  2. Renal

    a. Hyposthenuria.

    b. Tubular dysfunction.

    c. Insufficiency.

    d. Proteinuria.

  3. Fetomaternal disorders

    a. Excess fetal loss.

    b. Excess maternal death.

    c. Excess nonfatal maternal complications

     (1) Thrombotic

     (2) Hemorrhagic

IV. Diagnosis

A. History

  1. Symptoms of anemia

    a. Symptoms of hypoxemia.

    b. Pagophogia due to iron deficiency.

  2. Jaundice

  3. Unexplained pain

    a. Head.

    b. Eye.

    c. Abdominal.

  4. Deep vein thrombosis, possibly with pulmonary embolism.

  5. Intermittent red urine (hemoglobinuria).

  6. Spontaneous abortions.

  7. Neurologic abnormalities.

B. Physical manifestations

  1. Jaundice.

  2. Signs of thrombosis, if present.

  3. Signs of thrombocytopenia, if present.

  4. Splenomegaly—when present, usually mild.

C. Diagnostic tests

  1. General blood tests

    a. Decreased hemoglobin.

    b. Microcytosis if iron deficiency has supervened.

    c. Reticulocytosis (unless severe iron deficiency exists).

    d. Haptoglobin reduced-absent.

    e. Other cytopenias.

     (1) Leukopenia.

     (2) Thrombocytopenia.

  2. Bone marrow in nonaplastic/leukemia phase

    a. Erythroid hyperplasia.

    b. Decreased-absent iron.

    c. Mild dyshematopoiesis.

  3. Special tests

    a. Red blood cell complement sensitivity.

     (1) Ham's acidified serum test.

     (2) Sucrose lysis tests.

     (3) Others (e.g., thrombin test, inulin test).

    b. Red blood cell membrane defects

     (1) Acetylcholinesterase.

     (2) DAF.

     (3) MIRL.

  4. Urine hemosiderin: almost always present.

V. Differential Diagnosis

A. Other hemolytic anemias

  1. Immune.

  2. Microangiopathic.

B. Aplastic anemia

  1. PNH may be transformed into or present as full-blown aplastic anemia.

C. Hereditary erythroblastic multinuclearity with positive acidified serum test (HEMP AS)

  1. May give false-positive Ham's test.

  2. Different mechanism for C-mediated lysis.

  3. Red blood cell precursors are multinucleated.

VI. Treatment

A. Supportive

1. Iron therapy.
   a. May increase hemosiderinuria, which is of little clinical consequence.
2. Transfusions if needed.
   a. A recent study suggests that washed red blood cells are not required.
3. Anticoagulation
   a. For thrombotic events—not prophylactic.
B. Ameliorative
   1. Glucocorticoids.
      a. May decrease hemolysis.
      b. Daily steroids are not advised.
         (1) Every other day (QOD) regime preferable.
   2. Androgens.
      a. Some patients benefit; mechanism has not been defined.
C. Bone marrow transplantation
   1. For severe disease.
   2. After evolution to aplastic anemia.
D. Splenectomy
   1. Generally not indicated.
   2. May be hazardous.

VII. Prognosis
A. Variable, depending on severity of disease.
   1. Disease may decrease in severity with time in some.
   2. Death frequently due to complications of the disease.
B. Evolution to aplastic anemia.
C. Evolution to acute nonlymphoblastic leukemia (rare).

Myelodysplastic Disorders (MDD) or Preleukemic Disorders

I. Definition
Clonal preleukemic or oligoleukemic disorders are characterized by
A. Refractory anemia.
B. Additional cytopenias (often).
C. Abnormal differential counts (often).
D. Overt marrow maturational abnormalities.
E. Progression to overt leukemia or to increasingly severe cytopenias and refractoriness to all hematinics.

II. Etiology
Similar to that of acute leukemia.
A. Toxins such as benzene.
B. Ionizing radiation.
C. Chemotherapy and/or radiotherapy for previous malignancies such as lymphoma, breast cancer, ovarian cancer, myeloma (development of MDD or leukemia in myeloma may be a de novo phenomenon as well), and testicular cancer.

III. Pathogenesis
A. Oncogene-related abnormalities
   1. Disturbed cell maturation.
   2. Disturbed cell proliferation.
   3. Increased apoptosis (programmed cell death)
B. Abnormal or insufficient numbers of normal formed blood elements leads to:
   1. Anemia and its signs and symptoms.
   2. Infections.
C. Clonal progression of stem cell abnormality
   1. Overt leukemia.
   2. Severe cytopenias and marrow hyperplasia or hypoplasia (less common).

IV. Diagnosis
A. History and symptoms
   1. General systemic complaints
      a. Malaise, fatigue, fevers.
   2. Symptoms of cytopenias
      a. Shortness of breath.
      b. Symptoms of infections.
      c. Bleeding.
   3. Other symptoms
      a. Arthralgias.
      b. Bone pain.
      c. Skin lesions consistent with Sweet's syndrome (neutrophilic dermatosis).
         (1) Eczematous patches beginning on the face and legs.
         (2) Neutrophil infiltration.
         (3) Usually occur in women.
         (4) Last for 6–10 weeks.
B. Physical manifestations
   1. Pallor.
   2. Petechiae.
   3. Splenomegaly: ~10% (especially in CMMOL).
   4. Hepatomegaly: ~5%.
C. Diagnostic tests (figures 72A-2 gives blast percentage criteria.)
   1. CBC
      a. Red blood cell abnormalities
         (1) Anemia: ~90%.
         (2) MCV often elevated.
         (3) Anisocytosis and poikilocytosis.
         (4) Nucleated red blood cells: ~10%.
         (5) Reticulocytosis even without hemolysis.
      b. White blood cell abnormalities
         (1) Neutropenia: ~50%.

Table 72A-1.   French-American-British (FAB) Classification of Myelodysplastic Disorder (Modified)

	Blood Blasts	BM Percentage of Blasts	Percentage of Transformation of ANLL	Survival
Refractory anemia (RA)	<1	<5	15–20+	~2–4+ years (median)
RA with ringed siberoblasts (RARS)*	a) <1	<5	0–2	70%: 5 years (median: up to 76 months)
	b) <1	5	>20	20% 5 years (median: ~2 years)
RA with excess blasts (RAEB)	<5	5–20	45–50	9–18 months (median)
RA in transformation (RAEBIT)	>5 and/or	20–30	60	2.5–6.5 months (median)
Chronic myelomonocytic leukemia (CMML)†	a) 1	<5	20	~2–3 years (median)
	b) —	5–20	20	1 year

*RARS is not officially subcategorized. Patients with acquired RARS and no other telltale signs of MDS (i.e., no dysgranyulocytopoiesis or dysmegakaryocytopenias) have, in all likelihood, a benign disorder (category a). Patients with RARS and other abnormalities are very similar to those with RA, or RAEB or RAEB-T, depending on the number of blasts in the marrow. To fall under the RS rubric, ≥15% of all marrow nucleate cells must be ringed sideroblasts. The overall median survival of RARS patients in the literature ranges from ~14 months to ~5 years.

†CMML is not officially subcaterogized. Patients with CMML who have >5% marrow blasts have a much shorter median survival than those without such blasts. Overall survival ranges from 5 to 17 months; a few studies report substantially longer survivals.

According to some authorities, Ph chromosome-negative, CGL, and PNH should be considered myelodysplastic disorders as well.

(2) Left shift.
(3) Hypogranulation of neutrophils.
(4) Monocytosis.
(5) Neutrophil nuclear abnormalities.
   (a) Hypolobulation (Pelger-Huet anomaly).
   (b) Ringed nuclei.
   (c) Sigma-shaped nuclei.
c. Platelet abnormalities
   (1) Thrombocytopenia: ~25%
   (2) Thrombocytosis: ~5%.
   (3) Abnormal platelet forms.
d. Marrow abnormalities
   (1) Cellularity
      (a) Increased.
      (b) Decreased: ~10–15%.
   (2) Dyserythropoiesis
      (a) Megaloblastoid maturation.
      (b) Nuclear budding, karyorrhexis.
      (c) Poor hemoglobinization.
      (d) Multinuclearity.
      (e) Increased stainable iron.
      (f) Ringed sideroblasts.
   (3) Dysgranulocytopoiesis
      (a) Hypogranulation.
      (b) Hyposegmentation of neutrophils.

      (c) Left shift (up to 30% blasts).
   (4) Monocytosis
   (5) Megakaryocyte abnormalities
      (a) Micomegakaryocytes.
      (b) Hypolobulated nuclei.
e. Cytogenetic abnormalities
   (1) Chromosomes 5q−, 7q−, +7, −7, +8, 9q−, 10q−, and 20q−.
   (2) In seconday dysplastic syndromes, chromosomes −5, 5q−, and −7 are especially common.
f. In vitro granulocyte culture abnormalities
   (1) Reduced numbers of colonies.
   (2) Excess clusters (aggregates of small numbers of cells).
g. Miscellaneous blood abnormalities
   (1) Increased red blood cell fetal hemoglobin (Hgb F).
   (2) Alteration of red blood cell antigens.
   (3) Elevation of serum LDH.
   (4) Hypergammaglobulinemia (~50% of CMML).
h. Specific types of myelodysplastic disorders
   (1) Five FAB types (Table 72A-1)
   (2) 5q-syndrome
      (a) Thrombocytosis.

(b) Megaloblastic changes.
(c) 5q chromosomal abnormality often resulting in loss of chromosomal material coding for IL-3, GM-CSF, M-CSF, C-fms oncogene (M-CSF receptor), interferon regulatory factor I, and others.
    (3) Ph chromosome-negative CGL.
    (4) PNH (according to some experts).

V. Differential Diagnosis

A. Benign sideroblastic anemias.
  1. Idiopathic.
  2. Drug related.
B. Aplastic anemia.
C. Myeloproliferative disorders.
D. Acute leukemia.
E. Toxic marrow effects (e.g., lead poisoning).

VI. Treatment

A. Bone marrow transplant in patients 55 years old: ~40–50% disease-free survival for 2–3 years in patients with a median age of ~35.
  1. Syngeneic
  2. Allogeneic
B. Acute leukemia-type chemotherapy—complete remission (CR) in 50% of selected patients; duration of CR is ~5–11 months. Consider such therapy in:
  1. Older patients with RAEBIT.
  2. Younger patients with progressive disease or with RAEB or RAEBIT who have no suitable marrow donor.
C. Supportive care
  1. Red blood cell transfusions.
  2. Platelet transfusions.
  3. Antibiotics.
D. Hematopoietic growth factors
  1. GM-CSF
    a. Use with caution in patients with >15% blasts in the marrow.
    b. May protect patients from infections even if neutrophils do not increase in number (due to improvement in PMN function).
  2. G-CSF
    a. May improve PMN function and white cell count.
    b. Recent study suggests that G-CSF should not be given to patients with high risk RAEB.
  3. Other cytokines (e.g., IL-3, IL-6) used in clinical trials.
  4. Erythropoietin

    a. In patients with moderate-severe anemia with an inappropriate erythropoietin response.
E. Antithymocyte globulin
  1. In hypoplastic myelodysplastic disorders; an occasional response occurs.
F. Treatments found not to prolong survival and is not advised except in a formal study setting:
  1. Low-dose Ara-C.
  2. Retinoic acid.
  3. Vitamin D.

VII. Patient Monitoring

A. Physical examination
  1. Splenomegaly.
  2. Signs of bleeding.
B. Diagnostic tests
  1. Blood CBC, platelet count, and differential.
  2. Bone marrow aspirate and biopsy.
  3. Increase in blasts.
  4. Progressive cytogenetic alterations.

VIII. Prognosis (Table 72A-2)

A. Progression from less severe refractory anemia to a more ominous type is common.

Bibliography

Myeloproliferative Disorders

Polycythemia Vera

Diez-Martin JL, Graham DL, Petitt RM, et al. Chromosome studies in 104 patients with polycythemia vera. *Mayo Clin Proc* 66:287–299, 1991.

Golde DW, Cline MJ. Pathogenesis of polycythemia vera—new concepts. *Am J Hematol* 1:351–355, 1976.

Hoffman R, Wasserman LR. *Natural History and Management of Polycythemia Vera*. Chicago, Year Book Medical Publishers, 1979, pp 255–283.

Lofvenberg E, Wahlin A. Management of polycythemia vera, essential thrombocytopenia and myelofibrosis with hydroxyurea. *Eur J Hematol* 41:375–381, 1988.

Nand S, Messmore H, Fisher SG, et alo. Leukemic transformation in polycythemia vera: Analysis of risk factors. *Am J Hematol* 34:P32–36, 1990.

Newton LK. Neurologic complications of polycythemia and their impact on therapy. *Oncology* 4:59–66, 1990.

Silver RT: A new treatment for polycythemia vera: Recombinant interferon alfa. *Blood* 76:664–665, 1990.

Agnogenic Myeloid Metaplasia

Manoharan A. Myelofibrosis. Prognostic factors and treatment. *Br J Hematol* 69:295–298, 1988.

Ward HP, Block MH. The natural history of agnogenic myeloidf metaplasia (AMM) and a critical evaluation of its relationship with the myeloproliferative syndrome. *Medicine* 50:357–420, 1971.

Essential Thrombocytopenia

Cortelazzo S, Viero P, Finazzi G, et al. Incidence and risk for thrombotic complications in a historical cohort of 100 patients with essential thrombocythemia. *J Clin Oncol* 8:556–562, 1990.

Hehlmann R, Jahn M, Baumann B, et al. Essential thrombocytopenia. Clinical characteristics and course of 61 cases. *Cancer* 61:2487–2496, 1988.

McIntyre KJ, Hoagland CH, Silverstein MN, et al. Essential thrombocytopenia in young adults. *Mayo Clin Proc* 66:149–154, 1991.

Silverstein MN, Petitt RM, Solberg LA, et al. Anagrelide: A new drug for treating thrombocytosis. *N Engl J Med* 318:1292–1294, 1988.

Myelodysplastic Disorders

Bennett JM, Catovsky D, Daniel MT, et al. Proposals for the classification of the myelodysplastic syndromes. *Br J Hematol* 51:189–199, 1982.

Block M, Jacobson LO, Bethard WF. Preleukemic acute human leukemia. *JAMA* 152:1018–1028, 1953.

Koeffler PH. Myelodysplastic syndromes (preleukemia). *Semin Hematol* 23:284–299, 1986.

List AF, Garewal HS, Sandberg AA. The myelodysplastic syndromes: Biology and implications for management. *J Clin Oncol* 8:1424–1441, 1990.

Rowley JD, Golomb HM, Vardiman JW. Nonrandom chromosome abnormalities in acute leukemia and dysmyelopoietic syndromes in patients with previously treated malignant disease. *Blood* 58:759–767, 1981.

Saarni MI, Linman JW. Preleukemia: The hematologic syndrome preceding acute leukemia. *Am J Med* 55:38–48, 1973.

Acute Leukemias

Stephanie A. Gregory, M.D.

I. Definition

Acute leukemia is a malignant clonal disorder originating from an abnormal stem cell. It is a self-perpetuating proliferation of one or more of the white cell elements in the bone marrow and blood, eventually leading to progressive cytopenias and death. Acute leukemias are characterized by large numbers of primitive hematopoietic cells called blasts.

II. Classification

A. Acute leukemias may be classified into acute lymphocytic leukemia (ALL) or acute non-lymphocytic leukemia (ANLL).
1. ALL: 80% children, 20% adults.
2. ANLL: 80% adults, 20% children.

B. Classification of acute leukemia is made using several laboratory techniques, including light microscopy, histochemistry, enzymes, cell surface markers, and chromosomal studies.

C. The French-American-British (FAB) classification is as follows:
1. ALL
L1—Childhood—usually homogeneous cell type common adult lymphocytic leukemia antigen (CALLA) + usually—can be B cell or T cell.
L2—Adult—can be CALLA+, B cell or T cell (usually heterogeneous).
L3—Burkitt's lymphoma.
2. ANLL
M_1—Myeloblastic without maturation.
M_2—Myeloblastic with maturation.
M_3—Promyelocytic.
M_4—Myelomonocytic.
M_5—Monocytic.
M_6—Erythroleukemia (DiGuglielmo syndrome).
M_7—Megakaryocytic leukemia.

III. Etiology

A. Still not clearly understood

B. Predisposing factors
1. Inherited host susceptibility.
2. Exposure to physical or chemical agents causing chromosomal damage (e.g., radiation, benzene, cytotoxic drugs).
3. Virally induced transformation of susceptible stem cells.

IV. Pathophysiology

Leukemias are clonal in origin (arise from a single transformed cell). This transformation results in abnormal proliferation and differentiation of this cell and its progeny.

A. The evidence for clonality comes from chromosome studies and from the presence of only one glucose-6-phosphate dehydrogenase (G-6-PD) type in tumor cells of a patient whose normal cells are heterozygous for G-6-PD types.

B. In vitro cultures of leukemic bone marrows show abnormal growth patterns.

C. The crucial problem is the failure to mature normally and produce functional terminal cells.

D. Leukemic cells, since they are immature, tend to stay in the marrow and remain capable of dividing, producing more and more dysfunctional cells that give them a growth advantage over normal cells; eventually, they "pack" the marrow. They may inhibit the growth of normal cells.

E. The leukemic cell cycle is longer than normal due to a prolonged S-phase, but the cell death rate is high. However, the tumor doubling time may be as short as 4 days. When the number of leukemic cells exceeds 10^{12}, the acute leukemias rapidly lead to death. Diagnosis is made when the tumor burden is 10^9. Complete clinical remission occurs when the number of leukemic cells is less than 10^9 (usually 10^6). Cure occurs only when the last leukemic cell is gone.

F. Because of large cell turnover and ineffective hematopoiesis, there is a high nucleic acid turnover and hyperuricemia occurs. Toxic levels may accumulate, especially after chemotherapy (tumor lysis), and may be associated with hyperkalemia and renal failure.

G. Marrow replacement causes anemia, thrombocytopenia, and granulocytopenia. Bleeding is a major problem, but infection is the usual cause of death.

V. Diagnosis

A. History
1. The patient may be asymptomatic.
2. Usually there is a history of upper respiratory infection, fever, petechiae, bruising or bleeding. Fatigue is common.
3. The onset is usually abrupt, with signs and symptoms of a few weeks' duration.

B. Clinical signs
1. Pallor, petechiae.
2. Occasional splenomegaly or lymphadenopathy (especially in ALL).
3. Occasionally, tissue infiltration can be found in acute leukemia.

a. Skin, bone, lymph nodes, and gums are often affected in ANLL of the monocytic leukemia (M5) variety.
b. Central nervous system (CNS) infiltration is more common in ALL.
c. Severe symptoms occur in patients with circulating blast counts greater than 100,000 (hyperleukocytosis syndrome). Headaches, confusion, lethargy, pulmonary and renal problems, cranial nerve palsies, seizures, and coma may occur.

C. Diagnostic test
1. Light microscopy
a. Examination of the peripheral blood and bone marrow confirms the presence of blasts.
b. ALL blasts are small, with a dark, thin rim of cytoplasm, faint nucleoli, and no Auer rods (rod-like, primitive granules).
c. ANLL blasts are larger, with a more irregular shape and paler blue cytoplasm with more prominent nucleoli. Auer rods are present in 50% of cases of ANLL.

2. Histochemistry: Histochemical staining is useful in differentiating ALL from ANLL.
a. The common histochemical stains performed are the myeloperoxidase, Sudan black, esterase, and periodic acid–Schiff (PAS) stains.
(1) The PAS stain is often positive in ALL, especially if it occurs in a "blocking" pattern.
(2) The other stains are positive to varying degrees in the different types of ANLL.
(a) Myeloperoxidase stain
i) Often negative in ALL and usually positive in ANLL.
(b) The nonspecific esterase stain is negative in ALL and often positive in ANLL.

3. Enzymes: Terminal deoxynucleotidyl transferase (Tdt) is positive in approximately 95% of ALL patients.

4. Cell surface markers: Immunologic methods reveal different surface antigens that are dependent on cell lineages.
a. The leukemic cells are studied for surface immunoglobulin (SIg), which is characteristic of B cells.

b. The CALLA is positive in many patients with ALL.

c. T-cell antigens are found in T-cell ALL, and myeloid antigens are positive in ANLL.

5. Chromosomes: Leukemias are thought to arise from chromosomal aberrations that cause malignant transformation.

a. The following chromosome abnormalities are commonly found:
APL—(M_3) translocation t(15–17).
AML—(M_2) translocation t8, 21.
Burkitt's lymphoma/leukemia—t(8,14).
AML—16 inversion with abnormal eosinophils.
Therapy-related acute leukemias 5q-, 7q-.
CML, occasionally ALL $^+$Ph t(9;22).

b. ALL: Clonal chromosomal abnormalities have been found in more than 90% of patients.

(1) Three types of translocation have been reported in about one-third of adults and one-fifth of childhood cases: t(4;11), t(8;14), t(9;22).

(2) Patients with these abnormalities have a shorter survival (less than 12 months or 50% long-term remission in those without these translocations).

(3) Hyperdiploidy with more than 50 chromosomes is a favorable prognostic indicator in children with B-cell ALL.

VI. Differential Diagnosis

A. Myelodysplastic syndromes

1. Preleukemic syndromes can mimic acute leukemias by presenting with pancytopenia and occasional blasts in the peripheral smear.

2. Myelodysplastic syndrome includes the following:

a. Refractory anemia with ringed sideroblasts.

b. Refractory anemia without ringed sideroblasts.

c. Chronic myelomonocytic leukemia.

d. Refractory anemia with excess blasts.

e. Refractory anemia in transformation.

B. Aplastic anemia

1. Pancytopenia can be a presenting laboratory finding in acute leukemia and can be confused with aplastic anemia.

C. Megaloblastic anemia

1. Vitamin B_{12} and folic acid deficiency can present with pancytopenia.

VII. Therapy

Therapy for ALL and ANLL differs. Therefore, each will be discussed separately.

A. ALL therapy: Can be divided into remission induction consolidation and maintenance; CNS prophylaxis; and bone marrow transplantation.

1. Remission induction consolidation and maintenance:

a. Induction therapy is aimed at destroying as many leukemic cells as quickly as possible.

b. Vincristine, prednisone, asparaginase, and anthracyclines are used.

c. Induction therapy produces a complete remission (CR) in about 95% of children and 75% of adults.

d. A CR is defined as a normocellular marrow with less than 5% blasts.

e. After remission additional therapy called *consolidation* or *intensification* is given, which often includes drugs similar to those used in induction with the addition of cyclophosphamide, methotrexate, and occasionally cytosine arabinoside.

f. Maintenance therapy: Given for 2–3 years in an attempt to reduce the number of leukemic cells to zero. Methotrexate and 6-mercaptopurine are the most commonly used drugs for maintenance.

2. CNS prophylaxis

a. The CNS is a sanctuary for ALL cells, and some leukemic cells have entered the CNS in 70% of patients at the time of diagnosis. Meningeal leukemia may occur months after a bone marrow CR of the CNS if not treated prophylactically soon after diagnosis.

b. The main therapies for CNS prophylaxis include intrathecal methotrexate and cranial irradiation, which are occasionally given as combined modality therapy over 2½ weeks following induction remission therapy.

3. Bone marrow transplantation

a. Children with CALLA+ ALL and standard risk factors have a good prognosis with chemotherapy and need not be considered for marrow transplantation in first remission.

b. In patients of any age with refractory leukemia, those who relapse while receiving maintenance chemotherapy and those in high-risk categories (white blood cell count greater than 750,000, age greater than 35, unfavorable chromosome abnormalities) should be transplanted as soon as a CR is obtained.

c. Marrow transplants can be done from
   (1) A human leukocyte antigen (HLA)-matched sibling.
   (2) An HLA-matched unrelated donor.
   (3) Autotransplantation with the patient's remission marrow after "purging" with chemotherapy or monoclonal antibodies.
   (4) Long-term survival with bone marrow transplantation from any source approaches only 20–30% at the present time.

B. ANLL therapy: As with ALL, ANLL therapy includes induction-remission and consolidation therapy. Long-term maintenance (2–3 years) therapy in ANLL has not been proven to affect survival. CNS prophylaxis is not routinely added in ANLL.

1. Induction remission: Unlike ALL, marrow ablation must occur in order to induce a CR. An exception is the use of a vitamin A derivative (Trentoin) which has been shown to induce maturation of leukemic blasts in acute promyelocytic leukemia (M_3).

   a. Current induction regimens include cytosine arabinoside and daunorubicin (or idarubicin) given aggressively to induce marrow aplasia.
      (1) In 60–80% of patients, normal marrow regenerates in 4–6 weeks.
      (2) Intensive supportive care with blood products and multiple antibiotics must be given during the time of marrow aplasia.
      (3) Hematopoietic growth factor (granulocyte colony-stimulating factor [G-CSF], granulocyte-macrophage colony-stimulating factor [GM-CSF]) can shorten the period of cytopenias if given following therapy.
      (4) Approximately 30% of patients may require a second induction therapy in order to achieve a CR.

2. Consolidation: Therapy may be given within 4–8 weeks following a CR and often is as intense as induction therapy.
   a. Consolidation therapy may include bone marrow transplantation with an HLA-matched sibling. If this is done in the first remission and in patients less than 30 years of age, there is a 50% long-term survival.
   b. If a patient is too old or does not have an HLA-matched donor, consolidation therapy often includes more intense chemotherapy with the same drugs used to induce a CR or with high-dose cytosine arabinoside. The long-term survival of adult ANLL patients using this form of therapy approaches 25%.

VIII. **Prognosis**
A. ALL
   1. Remission rates are determined by age, leukemic cell count, phenotype, and karyotype.
   2. Adults with ALL do not have the same long-term, continuous remission rates as children.
      a. In patients older than 16 years, the overall survival is only 20%, with cure rates decreasing rapidly after age 50.
      b. In patients younger than 16 years, the 10-year disease-free survival is 40–50%.
   3. Poor prognostic factors for survival in ALL in addition to age include the following:
      a. White blood cell counts greater than 30,000/mm^3—adverse factor; less than 15,000/mm^3—favorable factor.
      b. Adults with CALLA+ ALL do better than adults with null-cell ALL. T-cell ALL adult patients with aggressive therapy respond surprisingly well.
      c. Biphenotypic patients (ALL patients may express myeloid as well as lymphoid surface antigens) have a poor prognosis.
      d. The prognosis is poorest in patients with translocation of chromosomes t(9;22) (Philadelphia chromosome) and t(8;14).
      e. Children with hyperdiploidy have a more favorable prognosis.
      f. Marrow transplantation in ALL carries only 20–30% long-term survival.

B. ANLL
   1. Of the 60–80% of patients who obtain a

CR following induction therapy, must relapse within 24 months and only 20–25% survive disease-free beyond 5 years.

2. Bone marrow transplantation in ANLL has produced up to a 40–50% long-term disease-free survival, but it can be offered to only a select group of patients.

3. Certain variants of ANLL are more difficult to treat and carry a poorer prognosis.

   a. Acute monocytic leukemia (M_4) is often associated with tissue infiltration (gum hypertrophy, skin infiltration, CNS leukemia).

   b. Acute megakaryocytic leukemia (M_7) is associated with an inaspirable bone marrow and marked fibrosis, and is more difficult to treat than the M_4 variety.

   c. Biphenotypic ANLL: Certain leukemias have surface antigens that are both myeloid and lymphoid and are less responsive to chemotherapy.

   d. Therapy-related leukemias or acute leukemias following myelodysplastic syndromes carry a poor prognosis.

   e. Certain chromosome abnormalities are poor prognostic indicators (e.g., 7q- or 5q- syndrome often seen in myelodysplastic syndromes or therapy-related leukemias).

Bibliography

Lukens JN: Classification and differentiation of the acute leukemias. In Lee GR, Bithell TC, Foerster J, et al (eds.): *Wintrobe's Clinical Hematology,* ed 9., vol. 2 Philadelphia, Lea & Febiger, 1993, p 1873–1891.

Lukens JN: Acute lymphocytic leukemia. In Lee GR, Bithell TC, Foerster J, et al (eds): *Wintrobe's Clinical Hematology,* ed. 9., vol. 2 Philadelphia, Lea & Febiger, 1993, p 1892–1919.

Greer JP, Kinney MC: Acute Nonlymphocytic Leukemia. In Lee GR, Bithell TC, Foerster J, et al (eds.): *Wintrobe's Clinical Hematology,* ed. 9., vol. 2, Philadelphia, Lea & Febiger, 1993, p 1920–1945.

Henderson ES: Acute leukemia: General considerations. In Williams WJ, Beutler E, Erslev AJ, Lichtman MA (eds.): *Hematology,* ed. 4, New York, McGraw-Hill Publishing Co, 1990, p 236–250.

Lichtman MA, Henderson ES: Acute myelogenous leukemia. In Williams WJ, Beutler E, Erslev AJ, Lichtman MA (eds.): *Hematology,* ed. 4, New York, McGraw-Hill Publishing Co., 1990, p 251–272.

Chapter 72-C

Chronic Lymphocytic Leukemia and Variants

William H. Knospe, M.D.

I. **Definition**
   Neoplastic proliferation of differentiated lymphocytic cells with lymphocytosis of blood and bone marrow. Survival is usually greater than 1 year.
II. **Etiology**
   Unknown.
III. **Pathophysiology**
   A. Lymphocytosis of blood and bone marrow with a white blood count (WBC) varying from 14,000/mm³ to 100,000/mm³ or greater due to accumulation of long-lived, hypoproliferative lymphocytes.
   B. Variable infiltration and enlargement of lymph nodes and spleen by lymphocytes.
   C. Immune deficiency is progressive and is associated with increasing infection.
   D. Increased incidence of associated ("second") neoplasms is attributed to a weakening of cellular immunity.
IV. **Diagnosis**
   A. History: B-cell chronic lymphocytic leukemia (CLL) is usually asymptomatic at diagnosis. Blood count abnormalities are often noted at routine examination or when the patient is hospitalized with another disorder.

B. Clinical signs and physical findings: Lymphadenopathy and splenomegaly are variable.
   C. Diagnostic tests
      1. Monoclonal markers of lymphocytes: surface immunoglobulins, usually IgM or IgD; CD5; CD19, and CD20, and HLA-DR.
      2. Hypogammaglobulinemia.
      3. Autoimmune manifestation in 10–15% of patients: idiopathic thrombocytopenic purpura (ITP), autoimmune hemolytic anemia, Sjögren's syndrome.
      4. Chromosome changes: trisomy 12; tr14q⁺:6q.
V. **Treatment**
   A. Biweekly chlorambucil/prednisone.
   B. Fludarabine for relapsed or resistant CLL; COP (Cytoxan, Oncovin, prednisone) or CHOP (Cytoxan, hydroxydaunorubicin [Adriamycin], Oncovin, and prednisone) for resistant CLL.
   C. Immunoglobulin infusions as prophylaxis for the propensity for infection.
VI. **Patient Monitoring**
   A. History and physical examination.

933

B. Complete blood counts monthly to yearly, depending on the stage of disease.

VII. **Prognostication—Rai Schema** (Table 72C-1)

VIII. **Differential Diagnosis**

A. Hairy cell leukemia
1. Atypical lymphocytosis of large, atypical lymphocytes with villous, cytoplasmic processes.
2. Typical presentation with leukopenia, anemia, and splenomegaly; leukemic phase rare; inaspirable bone marrow with characteristic biopsy.
3. Usually atypical B cells, rarely T cells; histochemical marker by tartrate-resistant acid phosphatase (TRAP).
4. Infections common.
5. Vasculitis and atypical mycobacterial infection may occur.
6. Therapy
   a. Splenectomy has been the standard initial therapy.
   b. Interferon-α is now an appropriate first-line therapy, with a 70–80% response rate; pentostatin also has a 70–80% response rate but has a much higher complete remission rate and may become the treatment of choice.

B. Wäldenstrom's macroglobulinemia
1. A hybrid disorder falling between CLL and multiple myeloma.
2. Increased numbers of plasmacytoid, pleomorphic lymphocytes in blood and bone marrow; leukopenia.
3. Splenomegaly is common, and lymphadenopathy may be present.
4. Marker studies show monoclonal serum IgM.
   a. A hyperviscosity syndrome may result from an increased IgM level in plasma

with heart failure, capillary and retinal hemorrhages, and characteristic venoconstriction of retinal veins.
5. There is a high proportion of associated neoplasms, particularly of the gastrointestinal tract.
6. Therapy
   a. Chlorambucil and/or prednisone, cyclophosphamide, and/or prednisone; melphalan/prednisone; plasmapheresis of the hyperviscosity syndrome is present.

C. Prolymphocytic leukemia
1. Very similar in its clinical characteristics of CLL, except that primitive, blast-like B lymphocytes represent the predominant cell type. This disorder may be misdiagnosed as acute leukemia.
2. Splenomegaly is common; platelets are usually normal.
3. Markers show surface immunoglobulin and CD5 lymphocytes, as in CLL, and are crucial in differentiating prolymphocytic leukemia from acute leukemia or lymphoma.
4. Therapy: similar to that of CLL; biweekly chlorambucil/prednisone; fludarabine is said to be highly effective and may become the treatment of choice.

D. T-cell CLL
1. Clinical features similar to those of B-cell CLL, except that monoclonal antibodies identify lymphocytes as the T cell type. The course is variable, usually with a shorter survival and a poor response to therapy.

E. Human T-cell lymphotropic virus-1 (HTLV-1)
1. Has features of CLL but is characterized

Table 72C-1. Staging of CLL According to Rai et al.

Clinical Stage	Characteristics	Median Survival (Months)
Stage 0	Absolute lymphocytosis >15,000/mm^3	>150
Stage 1	Absolute lymphocytosis plus lymphadenopathy	105
Stage 2	Absolute lymphocytosis and lymphadenopathy plus enlarged liver and/or spleen	71
Stage 3	Absolute lymphocytosis and lymphadenopathy plus anemia (hemoglobin <11 g/dl)	19
Stage 4	Absolute lymphocytosis and lymphadenopathy plus thrombocytopenia (platelet count <100,000/mm^3)	19

Source: Liepman MK. The chronic leukemias. *Med Clin North Am* 64:715, 1980.

by large, atypical T lymphocytes in blood and bone marrow identified by monoclonal antibodies.
2. Cutaneous lesions, marked lymphadenopathy, and hepatosplenomegaly are common.
3. Hypercalcemia and lytic bone lesions are common.
4. There is a variable course but the period of survival is usually short (1–2 years).
5. Therapy: More aggressive chemotherapy indicated with regimens such as CHOP or induction therapies appropriate for ALL.

F. Sézary syndrome (mycosis fungoides)
1. The Sézary syndrome is characterized by erythroderma (diffusely red and thickened desquamating skin).
2. Lymphocytosis of blood and skin is present, with large, atypical T lymphocytes of the helper-inducer type which have characteristic cerebriform nuclei on electron microscopic examination. The bone marrow is usually spared, at least early in the course.

3. Skin changes form a continuum ranging from erythroderma to plaque formation to tumor formation. Eventually, systemic progression occurs, with lymph node, spleen, liver, lung, bone marrow, gastrointestinal tract, kidney, heart, and CNS involvement.
4. Survival is variable; median survival is 8–9 years after diagnosis.
5. Therapy: Topical therapy of skin with mechlor ethamine (nitrogen mustard); photochemotherapy with psoiden and ultraviolet A light; whole body electron beam therapy; systemic combination chemotherapy such as CHOP.

Bibliography

Dighiero G, Travade P, Chevret S, et al. B-cell chronic lymphocytic leukemia; Present status and future directions. *Blood* 78:1901–1914, 1991.

Foon KA, Rai KR, Gale RP. Chronic lymphocytic leukemia: New insights into biology and therapy. *Ann Intern Med* 113:525–539, 1990.

Plasma Cell Disorders

Richard J. Sassetti, M.D.

I. **Definition**

Plasma cell disorders (PCD) (monoclonal gammopathies) consist of clonal proliferation of pre-B-cell lymphocytes which have differentiated sufficiently to produce and secrete all or parts of the immunoglobulin molecule (monoclonal paraprotein).

A. Disordered clonal proliferation may range from slow and small to clinically large and fatal.

B. Progression which is slow or undetectable and asymptomatic is considered benign or essential.

II. **Etiology**

The mechanism of the transforming event is unknown. Epidemiologic evidence suggests a variety of factors associated with other malignancies:

A. Genetic predisposition.

B. Radiation exposure.

C. Chronic antigenic stimulation.

D. Exposure to a variety of organic chemicals, including pesticides.

III. **Pathophysiology**

A. General: The abnormal clone originates in the bone marrow, where it usually proliferates in clusters (multiple myeloma) or, less frequently, maintains its diffuse single-cell characteristics.

1. Plasma cell–derived osteoclast-activating factor produces bone resorption in the area immediately surrounding the myeloma or plasma cell.

a. In multiple myeloma, this produces lytic bone lesions. In the case of the single cell, diffuse osteoporosis results.

b. The increased clearance of solubilized calcium results in kidney failure and the metabolic abnormalities of hypercalcemia.

2. Rarely, the abnormal cells arise in or migrate to extramedullary sites and proliferate as extramedullary plasmacytomas.

B. The immunoglobulin product of the abnormal clone can be detected as a homogeneous band with a narrow electrophoretic mobility in serum or urine.

1. The nature of the product is dependent on the immunoglobulin synthetic capability of the clone.

a. Synchronous synthesis of both heavy and light chains produces whole molecules.

b. Imbalanced synthesis occurs, with excess production of free light chains (whole molecules and free light chains).

c. Light chain disease: failure to synthesize heavy chains.

d. Heavy chain disease: Fc pieces only.

e. Nonsecretory myeloma: In about 1% of cases, there is a complete failure to synthesize or secrete an intact or fragmentary monoclonal protein. Such cases are remarkable for the absence of all the consequent pathophysiologic effects that derive from these proteins.

2. The immunoglobulin products associated with the advanced stages of disease are clearly abnormal, but many of those associated with the benign forms have normal functions and may be antibodies with well-defined antigenic specificity.

3. The spectrum of early disease has given rise to the following nomenclature: *essential* or *benign monoclonal gammopathy, secondary monoclonal gammopathy, plasma cell disorder of undetermined significance (PCDUS)*, and *monoclonal gammopathy of unknown significance (MGUS)*.

IV. **Diagnosis** (Table 72D-1)

A. Diagnostic efforts must differentiate:

1. Primary from secondary disease.

2. Malignant from benign disease.

a. History: The classic triad of bone pain, anemia, and renal failure characteristic of advanced multiple myeloma is no longer commonly seen. The most frequent diagnostic problem is the determination of the significance of a mono-

clonal protein on serum electrophoresis (often found as the patient is being evaluated for nonspecific symptoms).

(1) Frequent infections, bone pain, and anemia are common. In secondary PCD the symptoms and signs of the primary disease will dominate. Patients with macroglobulinemia or myeloma with IgG3 paraprotein may present with Raynaud's syndrome or hyperviscosity syndrome.

b. Physical findings restricted to areas of pain or extramedullary plasmacytomas.

c. Laboratory tests

(1) Blood: Normocytic or slightly macrocytic anemia. Hemoglobin levels less than 12 g/dl are associated with multiple myeloma, while higher levels indicate a benign process. The peripheral smear will demonstrate rouleau formation. The erythrocyte sedimentation rate will be rapid.

(a) In more advanced cases there may be a leukopenia or thrombocytopenia reflecting a myelophthisic effect.

(b) In macroglobulinemia there may be a preponderance of lymphocytes with plasmacytoid characteristics. In the case of a lymphoma, the picture may include cells with the lymphoma-specific morphologic characteristics. If there is an associated cold agglutinin syndrome, there may be a spurious macrocytosis

Table 72D-1.   Categories of Plasma Cell Disorders and the Associated Immunoglobulin Abnormality

Category	Name	Molecular Product
Malignant	Multiple myeloma	IgG, IgA, IgD, IgE; nonsecretory
	Light chain disease	κ, λ chains
	Waldenström's macroglobulinemia	IgM
	Miscellaneous diseases†	IgG, IgA, IgM
	Lymphoreticular malignancies	IgG, IgM
	Carcinomas*	IgG, IgA, IgM
	Amyloidosis	Light chains; occasional whole immunoglobulin as well
	Heavy chain disease	Fc portions of the α, γ, δ, μ chains
Unknown	Asymptomatic healthy individual	IgG, IgM, IgA

*Colon, biliary tree, breast, prostate, etc.

† Acquired von Willebrand's disease, cryoglobulinemia, angioedema, rheumatoid arthritis, systemic lupus erythematosus, lichen myxedematosis, thyroid disease, infections, myeloproliferative disorders, etc.

confirmed by the presence of high-titer-significant red cell agglutination and cold agglutinins.

(2) Plasma studies will reveal a monoclonal protein on immunoelectrophoresis which defines the immunoglobulin class. Quantification will determine the status of the remaining immunoglobulins.

(a) In 80% of cases there will be a monoclonal protein of the IgG, IgA, IgE, IgM, or IgD classes, but in 1% of cases there will be no detectable monoclonal protein and all the immunoglobulins will be decreased or absent. In macroglobulinemia the protein will be IgM. In benign forms the level of protein will be less than 4 g/dl, and the quantity of other immunoglobulins may be normal or only slightly depressed.

(b) β-2-Microglobulin is a marker which is elevated in proportion to the tumor mass. Levels less than 3 mg/liter suggest a benign process.

(c) Creatinine and calcium elevations suggest the renal failure of multiple myeloma.

(d) Coagulation is often impaired by large amounts of paraprotein (especially IgA). This may be severe enough to cause a bleeding diathesis.

(e) Hyperviscosity occurs secondary to increased IgM, IgA, or IgG3 levels.

(3) Urine studies reflect the degree of renal failure. Monoclonal light chains (either κ or λ) occur in 20% of cases. This proportion increases with disease progression. The benign forms show no evidence of renal failure with the levels of monoclonal light chain usually present.

(4) Bone marrow examination will show increased numbers of plasma cells. In macroglobulinemia these cells will have the appearance of plasmacytoid lymphocytes. In myeloma their appearance may vary from single mature plasma cells to a syncytium of plasmablasts with multinuclearity and other cytologic markers of dysplastic maturation. Less than 10% plasmacytosis is associated with a benign process, while higher levels are associated with multiple myeloma.

(5) X-ray examination includes:
(a) Punched-out lesions.
(b) Diffuse osteoporosis.

(6) Radionuclide scans are seldom of value.

(7) It is unusual for the benign forms and macroglobulinemia to have visible bone lesions.

B. Since macroglobulinemia represents a lymphoproliferative disorder distinguishable only by the presence of paraprotein, patients most frequently present with the full spectrum of findings of the lymphoid malignancies and may have symptoms of hyperviscosity, cryoglobulinemia, or cold agglutinin syndrome.

1. Associated malignancies are found in 10–25% of cases of paraprotein. Patients with multiple myeloma, macroglobulinemia, or benign monoclonal gammopathy merit study for it.

2. Primary systemic amyloidosis may have an accompanying monoclonal gammopathy in the serum and light chains in the urine. Appropriate biopsies for amyloid will differentiate amyloidosis from other diseases.

V. Treatment

A. Benign monoclonal gammopathy often cannot be differentiated from nascent multiple myeloma or from a process secondary to some other disease in a nascent state. While no treatment is necessary as long as the process appears benign, it is mandatory that these patients be followed indefinitely or until changes in findings suggest progression.

B. "Smoldering," indolent, or stable multiple myelomas do not require immediate treatment. The patient is asymptomatic, with a normal serum calcium level, normal renal function, and a stable serum paraprotein level but has lytic bone lesions and a hemoglobin level less than 12 g/dl. Since there is no evidence of benefit from early therapy, and since there is a dose-related potential for alkylating agent–induced acute leukemia, treatment should be withheld until signs of progression appear.

1. The mainstay of treatment consists of alkylating agents and glucocorticoids.
2. The alkylating agents used are BCNU, chlorambucil, cyclophosphamide, and melphelan.
3. Other agents include vincristine, doxorubicin, and α-interferon.
4. No single agent has produced a fully satisfactory remission rate. Agents are used in various combinations, dosage cycles, and treatment cycles.

Bibliography

Bergsagel DE. Plasma cell neoplasms—general consideration, in Williams W, Beulter E, Erslev A, et al (eds), *Hematology*, ed 4. New York, McGraw Hill, 1991, p 1101.

Chapter 72-E

Hodgkin's Disease

John L. Showel, M.D.

I. **Definition**
   A. A malignant neoplasm of unknown etiology usually arising in lymph nodes.
   B. Bimodal age distribution with peak incidences in late adolescence and after age 45.
   C. Extent of involvement divided into easily defined stages.

II. **Pathophysiology**
   A. The disease pursues a chronic or subacute course.
   B. It appears to spread in a predictable way via the lymphatics from node group to node group, with hematogenous spread only in the late stages.
   C. It often mimics an inflammatory illness with fevers, chills, malaise, low-grade anemia, mildly elevated white blood cell count, and eosinophilia.
   D. Pathology
      1. Reed-Sternberg cell: Must be present for diagnosis.
         a. Large, single or multinucleated cell with a bean-shaped nucleus containing a large, eosinophilic nucleoli.
         b. Essential for diagnosis of Hodgkin's disease, but similar cells may be seen in

infectious mononucleosis, other viral disorders, and other malignancies.
         c. Origin of the Reed-Sternberg cell is uncertain; appears to be of macrophage-monocyte lineage; perhaps derived from dendritic reticulum cells (antigen-presenting cells) of lymph nodes.
      2. Histologic subtypes
         a. Rye classification
            (1) Lymphocyte predominant: 10–15% of all cases of Hodgkin's disease; many normal lymphocytes, few Reed-Sternberg cells, little fibrosis.
            (2) Nodular sclerosis: 35–40% of all cases of Hodgkin's disease; much fibrosis; lacunar cells, background of normal cells.
            (3) Mixed cellularity: 35–40% of all cases of Hodgkin's disease; plentiful Reed-Sternberg cells, few lymphocytes, little fibrosis.
            (4) Lymphocyte depleted: 5–10% of all cases of Hodgkin's disease; many Reed-Sternberg cells, few lymphocytes, some difuse fibrosis and necrosis.

b. Clinical-pathologic correlates
  (1) Lymphocyte-predominant Hodgkin's disease: Occurs in young males and presents with localized cervical adenopathy in a low stage; excellent prognosis.
  (2) Nodular sclerosis Hodgkin's disease: Typically occurs in young females and presents with a large mediastinal mass; relatively good prognosis but a high probability of mediastinal and pulmonary relapse
  (3) Mixed cellularity Hodgkin's disease: Occurs in all age groups and tends to present in an advanced stage: relatively good prognosis with aggressive treatment.
  (4) Lymphocyte-depleted Hodgkin's disease: Oftens occurs in elderly patients and presents with constitutional symptoms, liver involvement, and bone marrow involvement; often without peripheral adenopathy; poor prognosis even with aggressive therapy; recent National Cancer Institute data suggest that 25–30% of these patients may actually have large cell non-Hodgkin's lymphoma and account for the apparently poor prognosis of the lymphocyte-depleted subgroup of patients with Hodgkin's disease.

III. Diagnosis
A. Clinical signs and physical findings
  1. Presentation
    a. Cervical, supraclavicular, and mediastinal nodes most commonly involved.
      (1) Superficial nodes enlarged in more than 70% of cases.
      (2) Mediastinal adenopathy in 50–60% of cases.
  2. Spleen and para-aortic nodes involved in 25–40% of cases.
  3. Infradiaphragmatic presentations uncommon (about 15% of cases).
  4. Liver and bone marrow involvement rate is 5–15%.
  5. Waldeyer's ring, mesenteric nodes, and extranodal sites involved very rarely and suggest a diagnosis other than Hodgkin's disease.
  6. Constitutional symptoms (See table 72E-1,B).

a. Fever greater than 38°C for 3 consecutive days.
b. Night sweats.
c. Unexplained weight loss of more than 10% of usual body weight.
  7. Other symptoms: cough, chest pain, superior vena cava syndrome (SVC syndrome) (rare), edema, ascites (? nephrotic), pruritus (10–15% of cases), alcohol-induced pain (1–10% of cases).
B. Laboratory findings
  1. Blood counts
    a. Granulocytosis in 25% of cases at diagnosis; eosinophilia, monocytosis, or leukemoid reaction occasionally seen.
    b. Lymphocytopenia in 20% of cases at presentation, especially in the late stage.
    c. Anemia in 10% of cases at presentation; usually underproduction, rarely hemolytic.
    d. Thrombocytosis in about 10% of cases at presentation.
  2. Leukocyte alkaline phosphatase often elevated.
  3. Elevated erythrocyte sedimentation rate (ESR) in 50% of cases at presentation, especially with constitutional symptoms.
  4. Acute-phase reactants: serum copper, haptoglobin, etc.; usually parallel ESR.
  5. Mild elevations of liver function tests, particularly alkaline phosphatase; these do not correlate with histologic involvement by Hodgkin's disease.
C. Disease workup or staging must be carefully performed.
  1. Careful physical examination.
  2. Laboratory evaluation (see Section III, B).
  3. Chest x-ray.
  4. Computed tomography (CT) scan with contrast of the chest, abdomen, and pelvis.
  5. ^{67}Ga scan.
  6. Marrow biopsy (bilateral posterior iliac) in the presence of "constitutional" symptoms or stage III or IV disease (up to 15% of patients show bone marrow involvement).
  7. Lymphangiogram if CT scan is negative or equivocal.
  8. Laparotomy in selected patients with splenectomy and biopsies of liver, celiac, mesenteric, para-aortic, and iliac nodes.
D. Immunologic abnormalities in Hodgkin's disease
  1. Ewing (1928): "Tuberculosis follows Hodgkin's disease like a shadow."

2. Abnormal cellular immunity in Hodgkin's disease; correlates with stage of disease
   a. Decreased skin test reactivity: purified protein derivative, candida.
   b. Lympyocyte response to phylohemagglutinin diminished; E-rosette formation diminished
   c. Skin test reactivity often returns to normal following successful therapy, but defects in T-cell function, as measured by the in vitro response to mitogens, may persist for many years following remission.
   d. Hodgkin's disease patients have an increased risk of infection with tuberculosis, viruses, and parasites, particularly *Pneumocystis carinii*.
3. Humoral immunity normal in Hodgkin's disease patients.
   a. Immunoglobulin levels decreased during treatment and after splenectomy.
   b. Increased risk of pneumococcal and *Haemophilus influenzae* sepsis after splenectomy.
   c. Patients should receive pneumococcal vaccine prior to splenectomy.
E. Staging classification (Table 72E-1)

IV. Differential Diagnosis
A. Any disease with nodal enlargement may be confused with Hodgkin's disease.
B. Persistently enlarged (more than 6 weeks) node with enlargement greater than 2 cm should be biopsied.

V. Patient Monitoring
A. History and physical exam required every few weeks or more often.
B. Serial chest films, CT scan, or ^{67}Ga scan, depending on involvement.

VI. Treatment
A. General principles
   1. Therapy should be of sufficient intensity to be curative while seeking to minimize the acute and chronic toxicities of treatment.
   2. Choice of therapy is based primarily on the stage of disease.
   3. Radiotherapy planning must be meticulous, and chemotherapy must be given intensively.
B. Radiation therapy
   1. Dose-response effect: Local control approaches 100% for doses in excess of 4,000 rads. Usual clinical dose is 4,000–4,400 rads, given as 200–250 rads/day, 5 days/week.
C. Chemotherapy
   1. Single agents: No role in initial management of Hodgkin's disease; may be considered for palliative therapy in patients with far advanced disease; complete remission (CR) rates are low, and remission are of short duration.
   2. Combination chemotherapy
      a. MOPP still the gold standard; complete remission obtained in 60–80% of patients with stages III and IV Hodgkin's disease, with 50–60% long-term disease-free survival.
         (1) Usual treatment plan is two additional cycles after achieving CR, with a minimum of six cycles for most patients.
         (2) Careful restaging should be done to confirm the CR prior to stopping therapy.
      b. Alternating non-cross-resistant regimens

Table 72E-1. Clinical Characteristics of Hodgkin's Disease

Stage	Disease Location	Treatment	Cure Rate
I	Single node group	Radiation	80–90%
II	Two or more regions on one side of diaphragm	Radiation therapy ± chemotherapy	75–90%
III	Disease on both sides of diaphragm	Chemotherapy ± radiation therapy	60%
IV	Disseminated disease with extranodal sites involved	Chemotherapy	20–50%

Notes: Letters A or B are added to the Roman numeral to denote the absence (A) or presence (B) of fever, night sweats, or weight loss (10% or more of body weight).

The subscript E is used to denote disease confined to a single localized extranodal site or a localized nodal site adjacent to an area of nodal involvement.

Chemotherapy refers to combinations of drugs, such as Mustargen, Oncovin, procarbazine, and prednisone (MOPP) or Adriamycin, bleomycin, vinblastine, and dacarbazine (ABVD).

(1) MOPP/ABVD
  (a) ABVD equivalent to MOPP in newly diagnosed patients.
  (b) ABVD produces CR in 50% of MOPP failures with prolonged disease free survival (DFS) in 25–30%, hence the concept *non-cross-resistant.*
  (c) Eight-year results of Milan MOPP versus MOPP/ABVD study in patients with stage IV Hodgkin's disease:

	% CR	% RFS	Overall Survival (%)
MOPP	74.4	45.1	63.9
MOPP/ABVD	88.9	72.6	83.9

(2) Chemotherapy for relapsed Hodgkin's disease
  (a) Relapse following radiation therapy: Restage→MOPP→60–80% CR→40–60% cure rate.
  (b) Relapse following MOPP therapy
    i) If more than 1 year since initial remission, retreat with MOPP→50% CR→25% cure rate.
    ii) If less than 1 year since initial remission, treat with salvage chemotherapy
      • ABVD produces a 40–60% CR rate and a 25–30% cure rate in this group of patients.

      • Other salvage regimens available; none are superior to ABVD.
  (c) Relapse following MOPP + ABVD therapy
    i) Consider high-dose chemotherapy with autologous marrow reinfusion.
      • Seattle regimen: High-dose chemotherapy + total body irradiation + allogeneic marrow transplant; some long-term survivors posttransplant.

D. Treatment summary
  1. Stages IA and IIA disease are usually treated by radiation therapy, using a mantle or extended-mantle field.
  2. Bulky mediastinal disease should be treated with chemotherapy, regardless of the stage. Radiation therapy is often added.
  3. Stage IB, stage IIB, or extranodal disease should receive primary chemotherapy followed by radiation therapy.
  4. Stages III and IV disease are usually treated with chemotherapy (stage III A_1, upper abdominal disease with involvement of fewer than five splenic nodules, may be treated with radiation therapy using an extended-mantle field).

Bibliography

DeVita VT Jr, Hellman S, Rosenberg SA. *Lymphoma and Hodgkin's Disease. Cancer Principles and Practice of Oncology,* ed 2. Philadelphia, Lippincott, 1985.

Kaplan HS. *Hodgkin's Disease,* ed 2. Cambridge, Mass, Harvard University Press, 1980.

Chapter 72-F

Non-Hodgkin's Lymphomas

John L. Showel, M.D.

I. Definition

A diverse group of diseases representing malignant neoplastic proliferations of lymphocytes or cells which in their normal state are mediators of immune function. Lymphomas arise in or may invade every organ system and anatomic region. They may remain localized or spread via lymphatic channels or blood vessels. Non-Hodgkin's lymphomas are grouped into three major categories defined by clinical behavior and histology.

A. Low-grade lymphomas: These are indolent but eventually progresive neoplasms which are readily treated but rarely cured. They are frequently widespread at presentation and involve the bone marrow about one-half of the time. They include:
   1. Diffuse, well-differentiated (closely related to chronic lymphocytic leukemia). Waldenström's macroglobulinemia is a variant.
   2. Nodular small cell cleaved.
   3. Nodular mixed.
   4. Diffuse small cell cleaved.

B. Intermediate-grade lymphomas: These are more rapidly progressive, involve the bone marrow less often, and are curable in up to one-half of the cases by combination chemotherapy using a regimen such as CHOP (Cytoxan, Adriamycin or hydroxydaunorubicin, Oncovin, and prednisone) given monthly for six to eight cycles. They include:
   1. Nodular large cell.
   2. Diffuse large cell.
   3. Diffuse immunoblastic.

C. High-grade lymphomas: These are extremely fast-growing tumors with a strong tendency to involve the marrow and invade the central nervous system. They are less common in adults than in children. They include:
   1. Diffuse lymphoblastic.
   2. Diffuse small cell noncleaved.
   3. Burkitt's lymphoma.
   4. Diffuse immunoblastic in acquired immunodeficiency syndrome (AIDS).

II. Etiology

Generally unknown. These lymphomas are seen with increased frequency when major perturbations of the immune systems have occurred (e.g., in AIDS, common variable immune deficiency, allograft recipients).

III. Pathophysiology

Like other neoplasms, lymphomas are space-occupying tumors and invade organ systems. These features give rise to their clinical, radiographic, and laboratory features.

A. Examples directly related to lymphoma involvement include:
1. Node and splenic enlargement.
2. Effusions.
3. Bleeding.
4. Bone pain.
5. Spinal cord compression.
6. Elevated uric acid
7. Elevated lactic dehydrogenase.

B. Remote effects may include:
1. Anemia.
2. Thrombocytopenia.
3. Fever, sweats, weight loss.
4. Rash.

IV. Diagnosis

A. Clinical presentation
1. Node enlargement.
2. Unexplained fever, malaise, weight loss.

B. Generous tissue sample for biopsy.

C. Staging or extent of disease workup. The stages are those used in Hodgkin's disease.
1. Physical examination.
2. X-rays, computed tomography, gallium scans. Lymphangiograms are less frequently used than in Hodgkin's disease.
3. Marrow biopsies from each posterior iliac crest.
4. Spinal tap in selected cases.

V. Differential Diagnosis

A. Other tumors.

B. Collagen vascular diseases.

C. Clonal or nonclonal lymphoid expansions.
1. Infectious mononucleosis.
2. Lymphoid tumors in immunosuppressed allograft recipients. These may disappear with reduction of immunosuppressing drugs and may not recur. They are often related to Epstein-Barr virus.
3. Pseudolymphomas of the lung or stomach often are lymphomas.
4. Angioimmunoblastic lymphadenopathy (AILD).
5. Castlemann's disease.
6. Lymphoid vasculitis.
7. Histiocytic medullary reticulosis.

VI. Treatment

A. Early disease
1. Indolent lymphomas (stages I and II)
   a. Local radiation.
2. Aggressive lymphomas (stage I)
   a. Extended-field radiation therapy after negative-staging laparotomy.
   b. Combination chemotherapy after clinical staging.

B. Advanced disease
1. Indolent lymphomas (none are curative)
   a. Single-agent alkylators.
   b. Cyclophosphamide, vincristine, prednisone (CVP) or cyclophosphamide, nitrogen mustard, vincristine (Oncovin), procarbazine, prednisone (CMOPP) combination chemotherapy.
   c. Total body or total nodal radiation.
   d. Watching and waiting.
2. Aggressive lymphomas (curative for some patients)
   a. CMOPP, (BACOD), CHOP, (COMLA): older combination chemotherapy regimens; 30–40% cure rate.
   b. ProMACE-MOPP, M-BACOD, COP-BLAM, MACOP-B, ProMACE-CytaBOM: newer combination chemotherapy regimens; probably more than 40% cure rate.

VII. Patient Monitoring

A. Periodic clinical evaluations including x-rays or scans of areas with previously known disease.

B. Patients are usually immunocompromised, and close attention must be paid to fever and other symptoms of infection.

VIII. Prognosis

A. Inversely related to disease volume.

B. Marrow and central nervous system spread usually means incurable disease.

C. Disseminated high-grade tumors are usually lethal.

Bibliography

Devita VT Jr, Hellman S, Rosenberg SA. *Lymphoma and Hodgkin's Disease. Cancer Principles and Practice of Oncology*, ed 2. Philadelphia, Lippincott, 1985.

Chapter 73-A

Physiology of Hemostasis

Edmond Ray Cole, Ph.D.

I. Definition

Blood vessel injury is a common event provoking a spectrum of physiologic responses which, to a large degree, are dependent on the extent of injury and which lead to the arrest of bleeding.

II. Formation of the Platelet Plug

The sequence of events in the formation of the platelet plug in response to blood vessel injury includes:

A. Initial vasoconstriction.

B. Platelet shape change.

C. Adhesion of platelets to the exposed subendothelial components (collagen, microfibrils, basement membrane), involving several adhesive ligands which interact with receptors on the platelet surface.

   1. Von Willebrand factor (vWF) is the bridge between the specific platelet glycoprotein (GP) receptor 1b•IX and exposed subendothelium.

   2. GP 1a acts as a bridge between the activated platelet and collagen.

D. Platelet aggregation is the process whereby platelets adhere to each other to form the hemostatic platelet plug.

   1. Platelets are activated from their resting state by a number of chemical stimuli such as thrombin, epinephrine, adenosine diphosphate (ADP), and collagen.

   2. Membrane-associated and cytoplasmic enzymes are activated, resulting in adhesion, aggregation, and secretion of the contents of platelet granules, as well as providing a procoagulant surface on which coagulation reactions take place.

   3. Thrombin binds to its receptor GP V and stimulates the expression of the fibrinogen receptor GP 11b•111a. Fibrinogen is necessary for platelet aggregation by acting as an adhesive ligand. Thrombin stimulates membrane-associated phosphoinositide hydrolysis and activation of protein kinase C.

   4. Collagen activates platelets via the prostaglandin pathway.

   5. ADP is involved in the exposure of the fibrinogen receptor GP 11b•111a complex on the platelet surface.

   6. Arachidonic acid released from membrane phospholipids by phospholipase A_2 is converted to cyclic endoperoxides prostaglandin G_2 (PGG_2) and prostaglandin H_2

(PGH$_2$) by fatty acid cycloxygenase and to thromboxane A$_2$ (TXA$_2$) by platelet thromboxane synthetase.

   a. Activation of the prostaglandin pathway in endothelial cells is similar to that in platelets, except that the product, prostacyclin (PGI$_2$), has an effect opposite to that of TXA$_2$.

   b. TXA$_2$ and PGI$_2$ are hydrolyzed to their inactive derivatives, TXB$_2$ and 6-keto-PGF$_{1\alpha}$, respectively.

  7. Cyclic adenosine monophosphate (cAMP) participates in the regulation of platelet aggregation and release reactions.

E. Platelet secretion is a process whereby contents of the α-granules and dense granules become available to potentiate the adhesion and aggregation aspects of primary hemostasis.

  1. α-Granules contain a number of proteins which are secreted in response to agonists—fibrinogen, vWF, coagulation factor V, thrombospondin (TSP), β-thromboglobulin, platelet factor 4 (antiheparin factor), and platelet-derived growth factor.

  2. Dense granules contain ADP, adenosine triphosphate (ATP), serotonin, and the divalent cations, Ca^{+2} and Mg^{+2}.

F. Other adhesive proteins serve as ligand to anchor the platelet to other cell surfaces or to facilitate platelet–platelet interactions.

  1. TSP is a thrombin-sensitive protein secreted from the α-granules that binds to a platelet surface receptor GP IV.

  2. Fibronectin and vitronectin are involved in platelet–platelet interactions and bind to platelet surface receptors GP 1c and GP 11b•111a (fibrinogen receptor), respectively.

G. Ca^{+2} is necessary for most platelet reactions. Ca^{+2} mobilization is the central event, and the source of Ca^{+2} is thought to be the dense tubular system.

  1. Ca^{+2} Is thought to initiate hydrolysis of phospholipids by phospholipase A$_2$.

  2. Ca^{+2} activates the myosin light chain kinase necessary for platelet contraction.

  3. Protein phosphorylation is stimulated by Ca^{+2}-dependent protein kinase C.

H. Procoagulant aspects of platelet activation

  1. Activated vitamin K–dependent factors of the coagulation pathways bind to negatively charged phospholipids via Ca^{+2}.

  2. Platelet activation makes phosphatidyl serine and phosphatidyl inositol accessible on the platelet surface and available for coagulation reactions.

III. **Secondary hemostasis (coagulation)**

This is the series of reactions leading to the formation of firbin, which reinforces and stabilizes the platelet plug. Coagulation may be achieved by either or both of two pathways.

A. The intrinsic pathway is initiated by contact of Factor XII (Hageman factor) with a foreign surface.

  1. Factor XII, upon contact with a negatively charged foreign surface, undergoes a conformational change to yield Factor XII$_a$.

  2. Factor XII$_a$ and XII fragments (XII$_f$), by proteolytic cleavage, activate plasma prekallikrein (Fletcher factor) to yield plasma kallikrein (PK).

  3. PK proteolytically cleaves high molecular weight kininogen (HMWK) (Fitzgerald factor) to produce bradykinin.

  4. HMWK also serves as a promoter function, increasing the surface-dependent activation of Factor XII, supporting the cleavage of Factor XII by kallikrein, and accelerating the initial rate of prekallikrein activation by Factor XII$_f$.

  5. Factor XI is converted to factor XI$_a$ by activated factor XII by limited proteolysis, a process accelerated by HMWK.

B. Vitamin K–dependent coagulation factors and the formation of membrane-bound enzyme complexes

  1. Prothrombin (factor II), Factors VII, IX, and X, and proteins C and S, all depend on vitamin K for postribosomal modification of the polypeptide structure, involving formation of γ-carboxyglutamic acid residues in the N-terminal region of the molecule.

  2. The γ-carboxyglutamate resides chelate calcium, which binds the four vitamin K–dependent procoagulant Factors II, VII, IX, and X to negatively charged membrane phospholipids.

C. Factors VIII-C and V are considered to be regulatory factors which greatly influence the procoagulant activity of the activated factors IX and X.

  1. Factor VIII complex is now known to contain two activities required for normal hemostasis: vWF, necessary for platelet adhesion reactions, and Factor VIII-coagulant activity (factor VIII-C).

   a. Factor VIII-C, a product of a gene of

the X chromosome, is sensitive to the presence of proteolytic enzymes. Thrombin changes the protein to a form with high procoagulant activity, and further proteolytic action by activated protein C inactivates Factor VIII-C.

b. vWF is synthesized by endothelial cells and megakaryocytes. In plasma, the vWF part of the Factor VIII complex is present as polymers of subunit polypeptides. These polymers range in size from dimers of 500,000 daltons to large multimers of over 10 million, with the function of vWF in support of platelet adhesion at the site of vascular injury related to multimer size.

c. Factor V circulates as a large protein in plasma and bears some structural relationship to factor VIII:C. Like Factor VIII-C, factor V is very sensitive to the presence of proteolytic enzymes. Thrombin alters the native form of Factor V to yield a higher procoagulant activity; activated protein C degrades both forms of Factor V, with the loss of procoagulant activity.

D. Amplification of procoagulant activity is largely a function of complex formation between the activated vitamin K–dependent factor, Ca^{+2}, membrane phospholipids, and the regulatory factor (factor V or VIII-C).

1. Factor IX (Christmas factor) circulates in plasma as an inactive zymogen.

   a. It is activated by Factor XI_a or by a complex of tissue Factor (thromboplastin) and Factor VII_a.

   b. Factor IX_a forms a complex with calcium ion, the phospholipid surface, and the regulatory factor, Factor VIII-C, which results in an increase in activity by several degrees of magnitude.

2. Factor X (Stuart-Prower factor) may be activated in either of two ways: by components of the intrinsic pathway or by components of the extrinsic pathway.

   a. By the Factor IX_a–Ca^{+2}–phospholipid– factor VIII-C complex.

   b. By a complex of Factor VII_a, phospholipids, and tissue factor, a membrane protein expressing receptor activity for Factor VII or Factor VII_a.

E. Prothrombin activation

1. Due to its γ-carboxyglutamic acid residues, prothrombin readily binds to the Factor X_a–Ca^{+2}–phospholipid–Factor V complex and undergoes activation to produce thrombin.

2. Amplification of the coagulation cascade is due particularly to thrombin's effect on Factors VIII-C and V.

3. Thrombin converts fibrinogen to fibrin; activates protein C and Factor XIII; is an important activator of platelets, which release substances involved in vasoconstriction, platelet adhesion reactions, platelet aggregation, and clot retraction; and provides membrane phospholipids.

F. Fibrinogen is a soluble plasma protein with a molecular weight of 340,000, composed of two monomeric units, each containing an Aα, a Bβ, and a γ-chain. Disulfide bonds not only connect the two halves of the molecule but also link the Aα and Bβ chains, as well as the Bβ and γ-chains.

1. Thrombin has great substrate specificity with regard to fibrinogen, hydrolyzing arginine-glycine bonds of the Aα and Bβ chains and exposing charged polymerization sites in fibrin monomer.

2. Polymerization of fibrin monomers results in the formation of long polymers (fibrin).

3. Fibrin clot stabilization is brought about by the formation of covalent bonds between adjacent γ-chains, catalyzed by thrombin-activated, calcium-dependent Factor XIII_a.

G. Regulation of coagulation reactions

1. Clearance of activated coagulation factors

   a. Dilution by rapid blood flow.

   b. Degradation by the liver.

   c. Absorption of active factors on fibrin and other surfaces.

2. Inhibition by antithrombin III (heparin cofactor).

   a. The major protease inhibitor in plasma, antithrombin III, in the absence of heparin slowly neutralizes thrombin, as well as most other serine proteases of the coagulation pathway.

   b. Heparin, a highly negatively charged glycosaminoglycan, binds at a positively charged lysine site on antithrombin, inducing a conformational change in antithrombin structure, making more accessible an arginine reactive center.

   c. Inhibition by the heparin–antithrombin complex is very rapid compared to inhibition of antithrombin alone.

3. Inhibition of the coagulation pathways by protein C is due to proteolytic degradation of the activated forms of Factors VIII-C and V.
   a. Protein C, a vitamin K–dependent Gp in plasma, is activated to protein C_a by the thrombin–thrombomodulin complex.
   b. Protein C_a in the presence of its cofactor, protein S, and a phospholipid surface degrades activated Factors VIII-C and V.
   c. Protein S is present in plasma in two forms—as a complex in which protein C is bound to C4b binding protein and as the unbound form. Only the free form is active as the cofactor of protein C.

IV. Fibrinolysis

Fibrinolysis is the major defense mechanism against permanent occlusion of blood vessels as the result of hemostasis.

A. Fibrinolysis is brought about by the conversion of the zymogen, plasminogen, to plasmin, a serine protease. Plasminogen contains five triple-loop structures (kringles) with a high-affinity lysine-binding site on kringle 1.
   1. Lysine-binding sites bind plasminogen to fibrin, to α_2-antiplasmin, and to TSP.
   2. Plasminogen adsorbed to fibrin is rapidly activated.
B. Conversion of plasminogen to plasmin is achieved by a number of activators: intrinsic, extrinsic, and exogenous.
   1. The intrinsic system of activation involves conversion of plasminogen to plasmin by kallikrein generated by the contact phase of caogulation.
   2. The intrinsic system of activation involves the activators from the endothelium and possibly other sources: Tissue-type plasminogen activator (t-PA) and single-chain urokinase-type plasminogen activator (scu-PA).
      a. t-PA has two kringle structures having considerable homology to those of plasminogen, in addition to epidermal growth factor and finger domains. The second kringle and finger domains are involved in the binding of t-PA to fibrin and are responsible for the fibrin specificity of t-PA.
      b. scu-PA is cleaved by plasmin to the two-chain form, identical to urinary urokinase (UK).
      c. Both t-PA and UK are serine proteases and are direct activators of plasminogen.
   3. The exogenous activator, streptokinase, must form a 1:1 complex with plasminogen, and it is this complex that activates plasminogen.
C. Plasmin cleaves fibrinogen and fibrin at a number of lysyl and arginyl bonds in an ordered sequence.
   1. Small peptide sequences are removed from the α- and β-chains near the C-terminus of each to produce fragment X.
   2. Plasmin digestion of fragment X releases a D-fragment to yield fragment Y. Fragment Y is further cleaved to yield a second D-fragment and an E-fragment.
   3. If crosslinking of fibrin has occurred between the γ-chains, then fibrin proteolysis by plasmin yields D-D (D-dimer) fragments.
   4. The Y-, D-, and E-fragments may modulate the hemostatic process by inhibiting fibrin monomer polymerization or platelet adhesion, aggregation, and release reactions.
D. Regulation of fibrinolysis
   1. Plasmin is inhibited by several plasma protease inhibitors. The primary plasmin inhibitor is α_2-antiplasmin.
   2. α_2-Macroglobulin, α_1-antitrypsin, antithrombin III, inter-α-trypsin inhibitor, and C-1-esterase inhibitor have a lesser role in plasmin inhibition.
   3. Plasminogen activator inhibitors (PAI) help regulate the fibrinolytic system. PAI-1 from endothelial cells is the primary inhibitor of t-PA. PAI-2 from the placenta reacts with both t-PA and two-chain UK-PA and is found in elevated amounts in plasma during pregnancy. PAI-3 is considered to be identical to the inhibitor of activated protein C.

Bibliography

Collen D, Lijmen HR. Fibrinolysis and the control of hemostasis, in Stamatoyannopoulos G, Nienhuis A, Leder P, et al (eds), *The Molecular Basis of Blood Diseases*. Philadelphia, Saunders, 1987, p 662.

Esmon NL. Thrombomodulin, in Coller BS (ed), *Prog Hemost Thromb* 9:29–55, 1989.

Handin RI, Wagner DD. Molecular and cellular biology of von Willebrand factor, in Coller BS (ed), *Prog Hemost Thromb* 9:233–259, 1989.

Ratnoff OD. Evolution of knowledge about hemostasis, in Ratnoff OD, Forbes CD (eds), *Disorders of Hemostasis*, ed 2. Philadelphia, Saunders, 1991, p 1.

Rosenberg RD. Regulation of the hemostatic mechanism, in Stamatoyannopoulos G, Nienhuis A, Leder P, et al (eds), *The Molecular Basis of Blood Diseases*. Philadelphia, Saunders, 1987, p 534.

Saito H. Normal hemostatic mechanisms, in Ratnoff OD, Forbes CD (eds), *Disorders of Hemostatis*, ed 2. Philadelphia, Saunders, 1991, p 18.

Wiman B, Hamsten A. The fibrinolytic enzyme system and its role in the etiology of the thromboembolic disease, in Kwaan HC, Kazama M (eds), Clinical aspects of fibrinolysis. *Semin Thromb Hemost* 16:207–216, 1990.

Chapter 73-B

Plasma Coagulation Disorders

Rajalaxmi McKenna, M.D.

Inherited Bleeding Disorders

A. Genetic mutation(s) are responsible for the inherited disorders of hemostasis, causing a deficiency of specific coagulation factors important for hemostasis.
B. The physiologic importance of these factors is evident from the pattern of bleeding associated with inherited deficiencies of each of these factors.
C. The pattern of bleeding is different with defects of plasma coagulation factors versus defects in primary hemostasis.

Hemophilias

I. Definition
  A. Bleeding disorder due to a deficiency or a defect of coagulation Factor VIII-C (hemophilia A) or Factor IX (hemophilia B or Christmas disease).
  B. The frequency of Factor VIII-C deficiency is 1:10,000 male births; that of Factor IX deficiency is 1:25,000–1:30,000 male births.

II. Etiology
  A. Transmitted as an X-linked disorder with excessive bleeding in males.

B. Point mutations, deletions, and stop codons have been described in the respective genes.
C. These mutations result in a reduced or altered coagulation factor.
D. Carriers with reduced levels of Factor VIII-C or Factor IX can have a bleeding disorder.
E. Factor VIII-C is the product of a locus on chromosome X, while Factor VIII von Willebrand Factor antigen is the product of an autosomal gene.
F. Identifying the specific genetic defect(s) is the best approach to determining the carrier status.
G. The level of Factor VIII-C can rise with exercise, pregnancy, and estrogens.

III. Pathophysiology
Formation of a fibrin clot is delayed, and the clot formed is small and friable, resulting in delayed onset of bleeding after injury.

IV. Diagnosis
  A. Clinical features
    1. Excessive bleeding into joints, muscles, and deep tissues is characteristic of plasma coagulation defects.
    2. In severe cases of hemophilia A, the basal

Factor VIII-C level is <1%; patients bleed at circumcision; have spontaneous bleeds into joints, muscles, and the abdomen; and develop crippling joint deformities.

3. Moderately severe cases of hemophilia A have basal levels of Factor VIII-C between 2% and 5%; they escape crippling joint deformities but bleed after minor trauma.

4. Mild cases of hemophilia A have basal levels of Factor VIII-C between 6% and 30%; bleeding occurs after injury, surgical procedures, and ingestion of antiplatelet drugs.

5. Delayed onset of bleeding after injury is characteristic.

B. Laboratory findings
1. Prolonged activated partial thromboplastin time (aPTT), correction of prolonged aPTT by the addition of normal plasma, normal prothrombin time (PT), and normal primary hemostasis.
2. Assays of Factor VIII-C or Factor IX will determine the reduced basal level and establish the specific diagnosis.

V. Differential Diagnosis
Can be confused with any bleeding disorder.
A. Factor VIII-C– or Factor IX–related bleeding disorders are identical by history and physical examination. Specific factor assays are essential to differentiate between them.
B. Von Willebrand's disease includes abnormalities of Factor VIII and must be excluded by appropriate studies.
C. Acquired inhibitors, particularly to Factor VIII, must be differentiated from the inherited disorder.
D. Other plasma coagulation defects should be excluded.
E. Combined plasma coagulation defects may also exist.

VI. Treatment
A. 1-Deamino-8-D-arginine vasopressin (DDAVP), 0.3 μg/kg, for mild hemophilia A; check pre- and post-DDAVP Factor VIII-C levels to confirm that an adequate response has occurred.
B. Cryoprecipitate obtained from one donor is excellent to minimize exposure to blood-borne illnesses, particularly in children.
C. Monoclonal antibody-purified Factor VIII-C concentrate is currently in use; minor bleeds require 10–20 U/kg as an initial dose, followed by one-half of that dose approximately every 12 hr; major bleeds require ~40 U/kg as the initial dose.
D. Recombinant Factor VIII-C is also available.
E. Concentrates of the vitamin K–dependent factors are a source of factor IX (Konyne, Proplex) for patients with factor IX deficiency. Monoclonal antibody purified Factor IX products are now commercially available.
F. Home care, with prompt infusion of product after the onset of a bleed, is essential to prevent serious joint damage in severe hemophiliacs.

VII. Monitoring
A. The level of the factor being replaced should be monitored serially; an aPTT alone is not adequate.
B. Improvement in clinically evident bleeding at the affected site(s) is also important.
C. Minor bleeds require Factor VIII-C or Factor IX levels in the ~30% range, while major bleeds require higher levels.
D. Rate of blood loss and T½ of the factor determine the frequency of infusion of the specific product.
E. Expected (calculated) versus actual factor levels achieved in-vivo are different for different products.
F. Duration of therapy depends on the cause of the bleed.

VIII. Prognosis
A. Rapid treatment of acute bleeding has improved survival.
B. Elimination of virally transmitted illnesses from blood products is the next goal.
C. About 20% of hemophiliacs develop inhibitors to Factor VIII-C; bleeding in these patients cannot be corrected by simple replacement with this factor.
D. Acquired immunodeficiency syndrome is currently a major cause of death in hemophiliacs.
E. Viral hepatitis occurs frequently.
F. Patients receiving concentrates of the vitamin K–dependent factors (Feiba, Konyne) can develop disseminated intravascular coagulation (DIC) due to the presence of activated coagulation factors.

Factor XI Deficiency

A. Occurs mainly in people of Jewish ancestry; variable bleeding is seen even in the same patient.

B. Autosomal recessive disorder.

C. Factor XI levels of 10–20% seen in heterozy-gotes.

D. Only available source of Factor XI is fresh frozen plasma.

Dysfibrinogenemia and Hypofibrinogenemia

Mainly laboratory curiosities; associated rarely with spontaneous clinical bleeding and even more rarely with thrombosis.

Factor XIII Deficiency

A. Autosomal recessive inheritance.

B. Excessive bleeding from the umbilicus at birth, lifelong bleeding disorder, recurrent spontaneous miscarriages, and intracranial bleeding may occur in homozygotes, with Factor XIII levels <1%.

C. Poor wound healing may also occur.

D. Only a urea solubility test (screening test) or a specific Factor XIII assay will detect the abnormality.

E. Routine tests such as the aPTT and PT are normal. Fresh frozen plasma or cryoprecipitate can be the source of Factor XIII.

Inherited Thrombotic Disorders

Antithrombin III (AT III) Deficiency

A. Physiologically very important serine protease inhibitor.

B. Deficiency, due either to an ~50% level of protein or to functional activity, is associated with a predilection for venous thromboembolic disease.

C. Incidence is ~1:2,000.

D. Heparin potentiates the ability of AT III to neutralize several serine proteases of the coagulation pathway.

E. Acquired deficiency occurs in liver disease, in DIC, and in some patients receiving estrogens.

Deficiency of Proteins C and S

A. Vitamin K–dependent proteins.

B. Thrombin bound to thrombomodulin on the endothelial cell surface activates protein C (APC).

C. APC rapidly degrades Factor V_a and Factor VIII_a and increases fibrinolysis.

D. Protein S is a cofactor for APC.

E. Approximately a 50% level of activity of protein C or a reduction in the level of free protein S is associated with a predilection for venous thromboembolic disease.

F. The frequency of heterozygous protein C deficiency is ~1:300; not all heterozygously deficient individuals have thrombotic symptoms.

G. Administration of warfarin sodium to heterozygous protein C- or protein S-deficient patients in the absence of concomitant adequate heparin may result in coumarin necrosis (hemorrhagic, painful, necrotic skin lesions which can progress to muscle necrosis).

H. A drop in protein C or S to homozygously deficient levels (<10%), triggers this process.

I. Lesions identical to those of purpura fulminans.

J. Immediate administration of IV heparin and discontinuation of warfarin sodium can abort the process.

Defective Fibrinolysis

A. Dysplasminogenemia resulting in impaired fibrinolysis and dysfibrinogenemias with an increased ability to form fibrin have been described. Very rare.

B. The condition predisposes to thrombotic disorders.

Arterial Thrombotic Disorders

A. Premature onset of ischemic heart disease, stroke, peripheral vascular disease, or a positive family history of such disorders should lead to an evaluation for the presence of known hyperlipidemic states. An increased frequency of a genetic inability to handle homocysteine has also been suggested as a cause.

Acquired Bleeding Disorders

Disseminated Intravascular Coagulation (DIC)

I. **Definition**

A. Clinical: Excessive generalized bleeding.

B. Histologic: The presence of fibrin deposits in the microcirculation, with special target organs affected in humans.

C. Laboratory: Excess generation of thrombin causes rapid disappearance of fibronogen, which leads to an altered fibrinogen level, an increase in thrombin–AT III complexes, fibrin monomers, and D-dimer-type fibrin degradation products.

II. Etiology

Activation of the coagulation pathway through contact factors (i.e., vessel wall damage—sepsis, Rocky Mountain spotted fever), release of tissue thromboplastin (tissue injury—abruptio placentae, dead fetus, brain injury, carcinomas), antigen–antibody interactions (purpura fulminans, mismatched blood transfusions), shock, stasis, and reticuloendothelial damage (Kassabach-Merritt syndrome) can all result in an accelerated "consumption" of coagulation factors.

III. Pathophysiology

A. Excess thrombin generation results in:
  1. Increased conversion of fibrinogen to fibrin.
  2. Thrombin bound to thrombomodulin on the endothelial cell surface activates protein C to activated protein C; the latter rapidly degrades Factors V_a and VIII_a and increases fibrinolysis by interfering with plasminogen activator inhibitor.
  3. Thrombin is the most potent physiologic platelet aggregating agent; it causes thrombocytopenia.
  4. Thrombin releases plasminogen activator and its inhibitor from the endothelial cell.
  5. Thrombin activates Factor XIII, resulting in crosslinking of fibrin polymers.
  6. Increased generation of plasmin, through Factor XII activation, through APC, and through plasminogen activator release from endothelium; plasmin degrades fibrin- and fibrinogen-producing degradation products.
  7. AT III levels drop due to binding with serine proteases and rapid clearance of complexes.
  8. Other effects of thrombin include chemotactic activity, initiation of cell division, and cleavage of complement components.
B. The liver plays a critical role in synthesizing coagulation factors and their inhibitors and clears activated coagulation factors, thus minimizing their effects.
C. Stasis and liver disease can have significant deleterious effects on a patient with DIC.

D. Balance between the rates of thrombin generation and consumption of factors versus the rate of production of factors determines the amount of reduction of coagulation factors.

IV. Diagnosis

A. Clinical manifestations vary widely.
B. Presence of an underlying disease state associated with DIC, a generalized bleeding disorder, classic skin lesions with a hemorrhagic-necrotic center and an erythematous periphery, or vital organ dysfunction (renal failure, adult respiratory distress syndrome, neurologic dysfunction) may be clues to the presence of a decompensated DIC.
C. DIC may be classified as compensated, overcompensated, or decompensated, depending on the fibrinogen level.
D. DIC may also be classified as acute or chronic, depending on the clinical circumstances.

V. Laboratory Findings

A. Laboratory tests are the key to diagnosis in this disorder.
B. In acute decompensated DIC, severe reductions in fibrinogen, Factor VIII-C, Factor V, increased fibrin monomers, fibrin degradation products, particularly D-dimers, and thrombocytopenia are found.
C. A low-grade or chronic DIC may present with an increased fibrinogen level and thrombocytopenia.
D. The effects on global tests such as the aPTT or PT depend on the amount of reduction of coagulation factors.
E. Coagulation changes in advanced liver disease and acute decompensated DIC look alike, except for normal or increased Factor VIII-C in the former.

VI. Differential Diagnosis

Excessive bleeding may be due to causes other than DIC, which may include:
A. Coagulopathy of liver disease.
B. Transfusion of large volumes of stored whole blood.
C. After open heart surgery.
D. Acquired inhibitors directed against specific coagulation factors.
E. Vitamin K deficiency or excessive oral use of anticoagulants.
F. Certain snake bites.

VII. Treatment

A. Treat the underlying cause; correct hypotension, acidosis, and sepsis.

B. DIC is usually self-correcting if precipitating factors are eliminated.

C. In chronic DIC, low-dose heparin is useful (Kassabach-Merritt syndrome, carcinomas); in purpura fulminans, heparin is essential.

VIII. Monitoring

Monitor the function of vital organs, along with the levels of fibrinogen and split products, to assess the response to therapy.

IX. Prognosis

Dependent on the course of the underlying disease.

Purpura Fulminans

A. "Purpuric lesions" occur in critically ill patients.

B. Lesions have a dark, firm, blackish center with a surrounding erythematous border; central necrosis may develop.

C. Acute decompensated DIC is common.

D. Biopsy shows widespread thrombosis of capillaries and venules, with a perivascular inflammatory infiltrate.

E. Urgent IV heparin is necessary to prevent the progression of lesions.

F. Skin lesions are similar to those of coumarin necrosis.

Vitamin K Deficiency

A. Vitamin K is essential to add γ-carboxy groups to the glutamic acid residues of the vitamin K–dependent factors; this cycle occurs in the liver.

B. Vitamin K–dependent proteins include Factors VII, IX, X, and II; proteins C, S, and Z, and osteocalcein.

C. The γ-carboxy site gives the proteins their coagulation function, chelates calcium, and attaches the coagulation factor to phospholipid membranes.

D. Food and gut bacteria are the usual sources of vitamin K in the diet.

E. Patients with obstructive jaundice, malabsorption syndromes; those who use antibiotics and intravenous feeding; those who ingest vitamin K antagonists; and newborns and malnourished people can all have vitamin K deficiency.

F. Prolonged PT with reduction in Factors II, VII, IX, and X, without any reduction in fibrinogen and Factors V, VIII-C, XI, and XII, is characteristic of a pure vitamin K deficiency.

G. Oral vitamin K is absorbed very rapidly. If malabsorption is a problem, or to correct severe prolongation of the PT due to oral anticoagulant excess, a slow IV infusion of vitamin K_1 should be given (e.g., 1 mg given over 5 min). Avoid large, rapid boluses.

H. In patients who have ingested large doses of warfarin sodium or following accidental ingestion of superwarfarins (rodenticides), it is essential to administer repeated, large doses of vitamin K_1 IV until the PT remains corrected.

Liver Disease

All coagulation factors are synthesized by the liver. Exceptions are factor VIII, tissue-type plasminogen activator (t-PA), its inhibitors (PAI-1,2), and urokinase-type plasminogen activator (u-PA).

I. Definition

A. Mild liver disease is characterized by some reduction of vitamin K–dependent factors; vitamin K is ineffective.

B. Moderately severe liver disease has, in addition, reductions in Factor V and fibrinogen.

C. Advanced liver disease has severe reduction in all factors with the exception of Factor VIII-C, thus differentiating it from an acute, decompensated DIC.

II. Pathophysiology

A. The γ-carboxy–vitamin K cycle in the liver is easily damaged.

B. Coagulopathy is due to:

1. Decreased synthesis of procoagulants (both vitamin K dependent and vitamin K independent).

2. Decreased clearance of activated coagulation factors predisposing to DIC.

3. Decreased levels of physiologic inhibitors.

4. Increased fibrinolysis due to reductions in α_2-antiplasmin and persistence of plasminogen activator released from the endothelium.

5. Platelet dysfunction due to alteration of platelet lipids and thrombocytopenia related to splenomegaly.

C. The liver removes activated coagulation factors.

D. Acute massive hepatic necrosis can be associated with a decrease in vitamin K production, as well as a DIC.

III. Treatment

A. Fresh frozen plasma to raise Factors II, V, and X into the ~30–40% range.

B. Fibrinogen, >50–80 mg%, is sufficient for normal hemostasis.

C. Platelets replaced as necessary.

D. Volume overload is a significant problem with fresh frozen plasma; plasma exchange addresses this problem.

IV. Monitoring

Serial coagulation tests for the adequacy of factor levels and decrease in bleeding.

V. Prognosis

Dependent on the cause of liver disease.

Extracorporeal Circulation

A. Exposure to a foreign surface can cause acute DIC.

B. Excess heparin can occur due either to inadequate neutralization with protamine sulfate or to heparin rebound.

C. Thrombocytopenia and platelet dysfunction can significantly prolong the bleeding time.

D. Uncommonly, excessive fibrinolysis may occur.

E. Most common cause of excessive bleeding after coronary bypass surgery is a surgical bleeder in the wound.

Prostatic Surgery

A. u-PA, synthesized in the genitourinary tract and released at the time of prostate surgery, may cause excessive local fibrinolysis, leading to hematuria.

B. Excessive postoperative bleeding can be well controlled by administration of ε-aminocaproic acid (EACA), given in a loading dose of 5 g followed by 1 g/hr.

Massive, Stored Blood Transfusion

A. Stored whole blood loses activity of Factors V and VIII-C, reaching levels of ~30% of normal in a few days.

B. Platelets undergo degranulation, loss of shape, and loss of metabolic activity within days.

C. Transfusion of large volumes of stored blood for massive bleeding can result in reductions of above.

D. In addition, shock and acidosis will precipitate a DIC.

Inhibitors to Coagulation Factors

I. Specific Antibodies

A. Immunoglobulins directed against a specific coagulation factor result in loss of activity of that factor, causing a severe bleeding disorder. The most common antibody is an IgG Factor VIII-C inhibitor.

B. About 20% of Factor VIII–deficient hemophiliacs receiving concentrate on a regular basis develop inhibitors.

C. Patients with autoimmune diseases or neoplasia; following drug reactions, surgery, or delivery, or without any apparent underlying disease may develop such inhibitors.

D. Excessive bleeding into skin, from the gastrointestinal tract, from venepuncture sites, or into vital organs including the abdomen can occur.

E. The condition is diagnosed by a prolonged aPTT, severe reduction to an undetectable level of one coagulation factor, and lack of correction of a prolonged aPTT in-vitro by the addition of normal plasma.

F. Bethesda units are a measure of the titer of antibody.

G. Treat only severe bleeding with:
1. Porcine Factor VIII.
2. Recombinant Factor VII_a.
3. Factor VIII inhibitor bypassing activity (FEIBA) in concentrates of vitamin K–dependent factors.
4. "Overwhelming" inhibitor by transfusing a large excess of Factor VIII-C.
5. Simultaneous administration of IV immunoglobulin and steroids.
6. Chronic therapy with immunosuppressives and chronic Factor VIII-C replacement to induce immune tolerance have also been used.

II. Monclonal Proteins

Can prolong the thrombin time by interfering with fibrin monomer polymerization, and can also inhibit platelet function.

III. Nonspecific Inhibitors

Anticardiolipin antibodies are not directed at specific coagulation factors but rather at phospholipids participating in coagulation.

A. Not associated with a bleeding disorder despite abnormal in vitro coagulation tests.

B. Large body of literature suggests an association with venous thrombosis, strokes, and recurrent miscarriages, but a cause-and-effect relationship has not been established.

C. A positive aPTT inhibitor test, an abnormal dilute Russel's viper venom test, a thromboplastin dilution test using human or rabbit brain thromboplastin, and correction of the prolonged aPTT with platelet extracts have all been proposed as coagulation tests to detect this type of inhibitor.

D. The phospholipids used to perform the aPTT determine whether the anticardiolipin antibody will be detected in coagulation tests.

E. The rapid plasma reagin test (RPR), IgG, and/or IgM anticardiolipin antibodies are other tests used to detect this problem.

F. Nonspecific inhibitors are seen in a variety of clinical conditions, including idiopathic thrombocytopenic purpura, systemic lupus erythematosus, and chronic inflammatory disorders, as well as in the absence of underlying diseases.

G. Clinical significance is unclear.

Acquired Arterial Thrombotic Disorders

A. Dietary factors, obesity, and hypertension are major risk factors.

B. Other diseases, such as diabetes mellitus and renal failure, can be associated with accelerated atherosclerosis.

Bibliography

Beutler E, Erslev AJ, Lichtman MA, et al. Hematology, ed 4. New York, McGraw-Hill, 1990.

Colman RW, Hirsh J, Marder VJ, et al. Hemostasis and Thrombosis. Basic Principles and Clinical Practice, ed 2. Philadelphia, Lippincott, 1987.

McKenna R. Acquired hemostatic disorders. In Schwartz G, Cayten CJ, Mangelson MA, et al (eds). Principles and Practice of Emergency Medicine, ed 3. Philadelphia, Lea and Febiger, 1991.

CHAPTER 74

Disorders of Primary Hemostasis

Rajalaxmi McKenna, M.D.

Platelet–Von Willebrand Factor–Endothelial Cell Disorders

The components of primary hemostasis are platelets, von Willebrand factor (vWF), and the vessel wall.

Inherited Bleeding Disorders

Von Willebrand's Disease (vWD)

I. Definition

A bleeding disorder due to abnormalities of von Willebrand factor.

II. Etiology

A. Quantitative or qualitative abnormalities of Factor VIII vWF.

B. Most common type is inherited as an autosomal dominant trait; homozygous, double heterozygous, and recessive forms also exist.

C. Patients with severe vWD have deletion of both alleles; others have heterozygous deletion or deletion of a large segment of the gene. Abnormalities at the 3' and 5' segments have also been reported. These result in major alterations of Factor VIII vWF.

D. Most patients do not have any identifiable genetic abnormalities.

III. Pathophysiology

An abnormal platelet–vessel wall interaction due to a reduced or altered Factor VIII vWF results in excessive mucosal–type bleeding.

IV. Diagnosis

A. Estimates of the frequency of the classical form are as high as 1:100.

B. Clinical symptoms and the laboratory phenotype vary.

C. People with blood group O have significantly lower levels of vWF antigen and ristocetin cofactor activity (R Co).

D. Mucocutaneous bleeding is characteristic: epistaxis, easy bruising, menorrhagia, gingival bleeding. Gastrointestinal bleeding in young patients is uncommon. Bleeding can occur following surgery.

E. Severe bleeding, including joint bleeding, is rare but can occur in the homozygous or recessive forms.

F. Older patients may have colonic angiodysplasia or associated hereditary hemorrhagic telangiectasia.

G. Symptoms appear in childhood and improve by the second or third decade of life.

H. Types of vWD and laboratory features

1. Routine studies should include a platelet count; activated partial thromboplastin time (aPTT); modified Ivy bleeding time; Factors VIII-C, VIII-vWF Ag, and VIII–R Co(in vitro measure of Factor VIII vWF "function"); a dose-response curve of ristocetin-induced platelet agglutination; and multimer analysis of Factor VIII-vWF antigen.

2. It is essential to study the patient serially several times.

3. Other components of hemostasis, including the prothrombin time (PT), Factor XIII, and platelet functions, should be tested at the first visit.

4. The patient should arrive for testing after being off all medications for 2 weeks prior to the studies.

5. *Type I vWD:* Most frequent type (70% of patients); autosomal dominant trait.
   a. Factors VIII-C, VIII-R Co activity, and VIII-vWF Ag are reduced to a similar extent.
   b. All multimeric forms of Factor VIII-vWF Ag are present but are reduced in amount in type IA, the most common variety.
   c. Bleeding time is inversely related to platelet R Co activity.
   d. Several variants of type I have been described.

6. *Type II vWD:* Characterized by absence of the largest, or the largest and intermediate-size multimers of Factor VIII-vWF Ag in plasma.
   a. There is reduced plasma Factor VIII-R Co activity but high to normal activity of Factors VIII-C and VIII-vWF Ag.
   b. Platelet vWF antigen shows similar abnormalities.
   c. Several subtypes have been described.
   d. Type II represents about 10–15% of patients with vWD.

7. *Type III vWD*
   a. Rare (0.5–5.3 per million).
   b. Low or undetectable level of Factors VIII-R Co and VIII-vWF Ag, with the level of Factor VIII-C varying from 3% to 10%.
   c. Platelet and plasma levels are similar.
   d. Consanguinity in parents is common.
   e. Antibodies to vWF may develop.

8. *Platelet type vWD (pseudo vWD)*
   a. This is a platelet defect in which the platelets have a high affinity for normal high molecular weight vWF.
   b. Plasma lacks the largest vWF multimers.
   c. Low concentrations of ristocetin and cryoprecipitate agglutinate the patient's platelets.
   d. 1-Deamino-8-D-arginine vasopressin (DDAVP) or cryoprecipitate causes thrombocytopenia in these patients.

9. *Acquired vWD*
   a. Hypothyroid patients can have significant reductions in Factor VIII–related activities and a prolonged bleeding time.
   b. Myeloproliferative disorders may be associated with a reduction in the largest vWF multimers and with a prolonged bleeding time.
   c. Patients with noncyanotic congenital cardiac defects may lose the largest Factor VIII-vWF Ag multimers and have a prolonged bleeding time.
   d. Circulating inhibitor (usually IgG) occurs in patients with B-cell disorders or without any underlying disease.
   e. Acquired vWD may be associated with angiodysplasia and Ehlers-Danlos syndrome; an endothelial defect resulting in both disorders has been postulated.

V. Differential Diagnosis

A. All other causes of a prolonged bleeding time should be excluded (i.e., platelet dysfunction, renal failure, thrombocytopenia).

B. Drug-induced prolongation of the bleeding time, particularly acetylsalicylic acid (ASA)–alcohol combination, must be excluded.

VI. Treatment

A. The goal is to improve the bleeding time and Factor VIII–related activities.

B. Cryoprecipitate and newer concentrates of Factor VIII (e.g., Humate P) have the necessary large vWF multimers to improve the bleeding time.

C. Factor VIII-C has a longer T½ in patients with vWD than in those with hemophilia A.

D. It is easier to correct the Factor VIII-C level than to obtain persistent correction of bleeding time.

E. Replacement is empiric, with the use of one bag of cryoprecipitate per 10 kg of body weight.

F. Repeat every 24 hr for 7–10 days after major surgery or severe bleeding.

G. DDAVP (Desmopressin) causes a sustained

increase in Factor VIII-C and vWF levels, particularly in type I vWF.

H. It enhances fibrinolysis by increasing tissue-type plasminogen activator (t-PA).

I. Arterial thrombi can develop; therefore, avoid using DDAVP in patients with known arterial thrombotic disease.

J. Give an IV dose of 0.3–0.4 μg/kg over 15 min. Protect DDAVP from light.

K. Repeated doses will result in a decreased response of Factor VIII–related activities. If factor levels post DDAVP are inadequate, cryoprecipitate should be used.

L. Recent studies in Europe confirm the utility of intranasal DDAVP.

M. Patients with type I vWD benefit from DDAVP.

N. The response of patients with type IIA vWD is variable; DDAVP is contraindicated in this type if thrombocytopenia develops after DDAVP.

O. Patients with platelet-type vWD require platelet transfusions.

P. ε-Aminocaproic acid can be used to minimize bleeding from mucous membranes and after dental extractions.

VII. Monitoring

Factor VIII-C and VIII vWF levels should be maintained in the desired range.

VIII. Prognosis

A. Severe vWD requiring frequent blood product transfusions places the patient at a risk of virally transmitted diseases.

B. As patients with vWD age, manifestations of gastrointestinal angiodysplasia may develop.

Bernard-Soulier Syndrome

A. Platelets are deficient in membrane glycoprotein Ib/V, resulting in an inability of platelets to adhere to endothelial cells in the presence of vW factor.

B. Inheritance is autosomal recessive, with frequent consanguinity.

C. Serious bleeding starts in childhood: epistaxis, ecchymoses, posttraumatic bleeding, menorrhagia. Death can occur due to bleeding.

D. Laboratory findings include a markedly prolonged bleeding time (>20 min), variable thrombocytopenia, large platelets on a peripheral smear, and failure to agglutinate with ristocetin while other in-vitro platelet aggregation is normal.

E. Therapy consists of repeated platelet transfusions as needed. Patients may develop antibodies to the missing membrane glycoprotein.

Glanzmann's Thrombasthenia

A. Platelets are abnormal or deficient in the membrane glycoprotein IIb/IIIa complex.

B. This glycoprotein complex interacts with vWF, fibronectin, and vitronectin outside the platelet and with actin within the platelet. It is also deficient in α-granule fibrinogen.

C. Deficiency of Pl^{A1}, Pl^{A2}, Bak^a (LeK^a), and Pen^a antigens on thrombasthenic platelets has been reported.

D. Inheritance is autosomal recessive, with frequent consanguinity.

E. Mucocutaneous bleeding starts in infancy.

F. Laboratory findings include a markedly prolonged bleeding time, absence of in-vitro platelet aggregation in response to all agonists, and absent or abnormal clot retraction.

G. Platelet count, morphology, aPTT, and PT are normal.

H. Chronic platelet transfusions are necessary, and may result in antibodies to the specific antigens they are missing.

Deficiency of Storage Pool or Deficient Secretion

A. α-Granule (Gray platelet syndrome) or α-granule (dense granule) deficiencies are associated with a milder bleeding disorder than the above.

B. Marrow fibrosis in α-granule deficiency may be due to secretion of platelet-derived growth factor into the marrow.

C. In α-granule deficiency, there is no adenosine diphosphate in the dense granule contributing to the disorder.

D. DDAVP may be tried as initial therapy prior to platelet transfusions.

Acquired Bleeding Disorders

Idiopathic Thrombocytopenic Purpura (ITP)

I. Definition

A. There is a reduced platelet count, with or without platelet dysfunction, due to autoantibodies directed against the platelets.

B. A compensated thrombocytolytic state may be associated with a normal platelet count.

II. Etiology

Platelet destruction due to an autoplatelet antibody, generally a 7S IgG.

III. Pathophysiology

A. Antibody-coated platelets are removed from the circulation by the spleen, resulting in a shortened life span of platelets.

B. Production of platelets by bone marrow is increased, consistent with the presence of increased colony-forming units and megakaryocytes in marrow.

C. Some autoantibodies may inhibit megakaryocyte colony formation, thereby decreasing production.

D. The spleen is a major site of autoantibody production, showing reactive germinal centers in the lymphatic nodules in the white pulp, an increase in plasma cells, and platelet destruction by macrophages.

IV. Diagnosis

A. Clinical features

1. Acute ITP (postinfectious) is a disease of childhood (2–9 years), with an acute onset of severe thrombocytopenia, generally preceded by a viral infection; it can also occur following immunization with live vaccines.

2. Chronic ITP is a disease of adults, with a female:male ratio of 3:1; a preceding viral syndrome is uncommon.

3. Bleeding manifestations are abrupt in onset in children and insidious in adults.

4. Symptoms include petechiae, ecchymoses, and hemorrhagic bullae in the mouth if the thrombocytopenia is acute in onset and severe.

5. Bleeding from the gums, gastrointestinal tract, and genitourinary tract can start suddenly (within a few hours) in children.

6. Menorrhagia and iron deficiency anemia occur in women.

7. Intracranial hemorrhage can occur, particularly when mucocutaneous bleeding manifestations are prominent.

8. Significant hepatosplenomegaly or prominent adenopathy should raise concerns about other underlying disorders.

9. "Shotty" adenopathy is common in children.

10. Associated diseases include systemic lu-

pus erythematosus, lymphoproliferative disorders, thyroid disease, other autoimmune disorders such as Crohn's disease, and myasthenia gravis.

B. Laboratory tests

1. Thrombocytopenia: severe in the acute form and variable in the chronic form.

2. Increased to normal levels of bone marrow megakaryocytes.

3. Normal or prolonged bleeding time, depending on the platelet count and the presence of platelet dysfunction.

4. Increased levels of platelet-associated IgG may be a nonspecific phenomenon.

5. Serum "autoantibody" tests detect platelet-directed antibodies as well as immune complexes.

6. Anticardiolipin antibodies (lupus anticoagulant) can be found.

7. Less frequently, specific antibodies directed against platelet membrane glycoproteins IIb and/or IIIa and Ib are found.

8. About 2% of patients with chronic ITP have systemic lupus erythematosus.

9. Coombs'-positive hemolytic anemia can occur with ITP in the Evans syndrome.

V. Differential Diagnosis

A. Other causes of thrombocytopenia must be excluded prior to making the diagnosis of ITP.

B. These causes include sepsis (bacterial, viral, fungal, etc.), human immuno-deficiency virus-1 (HIV-1), immune complexes such as those in chronic hepatitis or solid tumors; alloimmunization, drug-induced thrombocytopenia; posttransfusion purpura, disseminated intravascular coagulation (DIC), and decreased platelet production.

VI. Treatment

A. Acute ITP in children usually resolves spontaneously in 4–8 weeks.

B. Give IV IgG in a dose of 400 mg/kg daily for 5 days; a response is likely in younger patients. This therapy allows better survival of transfused platelets.

C. Prednisone (1–2 mg/kg/day) is the mainstay of therapy in adults. Its effectiveness is due to inhibition of phagocytosis in the spleen and reduction of antibody production, resulting in longer survival of platelets.

D. Decreased capillary fragility and improved bleeding time are other beneficial effects.

E. The length of prednisone therapy is dependent on the time and adequacy of the response and the duration of high-dose prednisone therapy.

F. Long-term, high-dose prednisone therapy is unacceptable due to its serious side effects.

G. Splenectomy is the second major therapeutic modality used when an adequate trial of steroids fails to restore a reasonable platelet count.

H. Platelet transfusions should be used for severe bleeding manifestations, even though these platelets are rapidly destroyed.

I. Danazol (400–800 mg/day), colchicine (1.2 mg/day), α-interferon (3×10^6 units/three times a week × 12 doses), vincristine (1–2 mg/week × 3 or 4 doses), and, infrequently, anti-Rh$_o$ (D) immunoglobulin (200–1,000 μg) have been unsed in refractory ITP.

J. Concern about second malignancies should restrict the use of immunosuppressives such as cyclosporin, cyclophosphamide, and azathioprine in patients with persistent, refractory thrombocytopenia with severe bleeding complications.

VII. Monitoring

Serial platelet counts, along with follow-up of clinical bleeding.

VIII. Prognosis

A. The majority of patients respond to steroids and splenectomy.

B. Refractory ITP is a cause of serious complications, including death.

Pregnancy with ITP

A. Transplacental passage of maternal IgG antiplatelet antibody can cause fetal death and recurrent miscarriages.

B. The platelet count in the fetus is unpredictable. However, thrombocytopenia is more likely to occur if the mother's platelet count is reduced at the time of labor.

C. More centers are now beginning to perform percutaneous umbilical cord blood samplings (PUBS) to obtain platelet counts on the fetus prior to delivery.

HIV-1-Associated Thrombocytopenia

A. Immune complexes, autoplatelet antibody, and the inhibitory effect of the virus on megakaryocytes have all been postulated as causes.

B. Thrombocytopenia can occur even at an early phase of HIV infection.

C. The bone marrow aspirate is usually hypercellular.

D. Steroids, IV immunoglobulin, splenectomy, α-interferon, anti-Rh° (D), and anti-c antibody have all been used.

E. Azathioprine (AZT) can improve the platelet counts.

Drug-Induced Immune Thrombocytopenia

A. Drug-induced antibodies bind to platelets by their Fab regions to platelet membrane glycoproteins GPIb/IX, GPIIb/IIIa, and GPV.

B. Immune complexes, autoantibodies, or hapten-dependent antibodies may attack platelets.

C. Frequently implicated drugs include quinidine, quinine, sulfonamides, gold, heparin, and procainamide.

D. A careful history is critical.

E. Thrombocytopenia is abrupt in onset and severe, occasionally associated with the development of chills and a warm sensation within minutes of ingesting the drug.

F. Petechiae, ecchymoses, hemorrhagic bullae in the oral mucosa, and hemorrhage from the gastrointestinal and genitourinary tracts can occur.

G. Discontinuation of the drug should result in improvement of the platelet count over several days.

H. Use available laboratory techniques to confirm the diagnosis.

I. Only if alternative drugs are not available should rechallenge be necessary; this test should be performed cautiously.

J. Heparin-induced thrombocytopenia may be associated with arterial thromboses.

PostTransfusion Purpura

A. High-titer, platelet-specific antibodies develop about 7–10 days after exposure to blood products.

B. Thrombocytopenia is severe, abrupt in onset, and associated with serious bleeding complications, including central nervous system (CNS) hemorrhage and death.

C. Pl^{A1} (Zw^a), Pl^{A2} (Zw^b), Bak^a, Bak^b, and Pen^a (Yuk^b) are platelet antigens which have been implicated.

D. These platelet antigens are generally noted to occur in multiparous women.

E. Plasma exchange is a very effective treatment. IV IgG may be helpful. Steroids are usually administered, but are not useful as a single modality of therapy.

Immune Complex Thrombocytopenia

A. This can be caused by bacterial (*Escherichia coli*, atypical mycobacteria), viral, or protozoal (malaria) infections or by tumors.

B. It responds poorly to steroids and splenectomy; best response obtained by adequate treatment of the underlying disease.

Acquired Thrombohemorrhagic Disorders

Thrombotic Thrombocytopenic Purpura (TTP) and Hemolyticuremic Syndrome (HUS)

I. Definition

A. Both TTP and HUS are characterized by thrombocytopenia, Coombs'-negative hemolytic anemia, microvascular thrombosis, and fever.

B. TTP affects adults, with prominent CNS involvement and variable renal failure.

C. HUS occurs in children, with prominent renal failure and "less frequent" CNS involvement.

II. Etiology

The precipitating factor appears to cause platelet and endothelial injury; HIV-1, toxemia of pregnancy, systemic lupus erythematosus, and chemotherapeutic agents may cause such injury. Certain verocytotoxin-producing strains of *E. coli* have been related to mass illnesses.

III. Pathophysiology

A. Appearance of platelet-agglutinating protein in the plasma of patients with TTP.

B. Increase in large Factor VIII-vWF multimers, absence of protective immunoglobulin, and prostacyclin-related abnormalities have all been postulated to cause the syndrome.

IV. Diagnosis

A. Clinically, an acute or, less commonly, a chronic relapsing syndrome may occur. Clinical findings depend on the organ(s) involved.

B. Hemostatic tests indicate predominant platelet consumption. The presence of schistocytes in peripheral blood is the sine qua non of this disorder.

C. Histologically, intracapillary and intra-arteriolar hyaline thrombi composed of platelets and fibrin are found. Gingival, rectal, and kidney biopsies have been done to establish a diagnosis.

V. Differential Diagnosis

Exclude Evans' syndrome, other causes of thrombocytopenia, anemia, and organ dysfunction.

VI. Treatment

A. TTP is treated with serial plasma exchanges coupled with prednisone; HUS is treated primarily with dialysis.

B. Platelet transfusions may cause platelet deterioration by increasing microvascular thrombosis; they should be used only for severe bleeding.

C. ASA is administered when the platelet count rises above $60,000/mm^3$.

VII. Monitoring

Serial platelet and reticulocyte counts, serum lactic dehydrogenase levels, and clinical manifestations guide the frequency and duration of plasma exchanges.

VIII. Prognosis

There is an ~80% survival rate with modern management.

Henoch-Schönlein Purpura

A. IgA-containing immune complexes are deposited in blood vessels, causing a leukoclastic vasculitis.

B. Young children are primarily affected, but the disease is seen even in elderly people.

C. A viral infection is followed by crops of a copper-colored, itchy rash, malaise, colicky abdominal pain (guaiac-positive stools, occasional intussusception), and polyarthralgias, followed in the third week by renal involvement (mainly hematuria; infrequently, hypertension and renal failure).

D. Torsion of the testes may develop; serious CNS involvement may occur.

E. Clinical manifestations are extremely variable.

F. The majority of patients do well, although both morbidity and mortality can occur.

G. Routine coagulation tests and platelet counts are normal.

H. Skin and kidney biopsies are diagnostic.

I. Steroids should be used for serious complications.

J. Treatment is mainly symptomatic.

K. The prognosis is excellent except for a minority of patients who develop renal dysfunction.

Approach to Patients with Bleeding Disorders

I. Problem

Excessive, spontaneous, posttraumatic or post-surgical bleeding.

II. Differential Diagnosis

Necessary to determine whether the problem is related to defects in the plasma coagulation mechanism or to defects in primary hemostasis.

III. Focus of the History and Physical Examination

A. Was the bleeding problem present since birth or did it develop later in life?

B. What is the duration of the problem, and are the symptoms still present?

C. Is there a consistent history of excessive bleeding in the past?

D. Did the excessive bleeding start recently?

E. Was it preceded by other illnesses or intake of drugs, including alcohol?

F. What is the pattern of organ involvement?

G. Is the type of bleeding consistent with a plasma coagulation-type defect or a mucosal-type bleed, or both?

H. The presence of petechiae and ecchymoses suggests a mucosal-type defect, whereas bleeding into the joints and muscles suggests a plasma coagulation defect.

I. The presence of large hemangiomas and prominent capillary angiomas around the lips or skin may be clues to the anatomic abnormalities.

J. Are other family members afflicted with the problem?

K. Is the pattern of excessive bleeding similar in other family members?

IV. Diagnostic Approach

A. Laboratory tests are the key to diagnosing the type of defect.

B. Simple tests include aPTT; PT; fibrinogen level; thrombin time; fibrin split products; Factors II, V, VII, and X; and euglobulin lysis time as an initial screen of the coagulation system.

C. Perform a urea solubility test if appropriate.

D. Tests for primary hemostasis include a platelet count, review of the peripheral blood smear for the appearance of platelets, bleeding time, and platelet function studies.

E. Based on the above screening tests, further workup should include mixing experiments with the patient's and normal plasma; assays of the early coagulation factors such as Factors VIII-C, IX, and XI; and other Factor VIII–related activities such as Factor VIII vWF Ag, VIII vWF activity (R Co), Factor VIII multimer analysis, and so on.

F. If a DIC-type process is suspected, attention should also be paid to the type and quantity of fibrin split products (e.g., D-dimers, thrombin–antithrombin III complexes).

Approach to Patients with Thrombotic Disorders

A. The approach to these disorders is similar to that used in patients with bleeding disorders.

B. The diagnosis, history, and focus of the physical exam will differ, depending on whether the disorder is a venous thrombotic problem or an arterial thromboembolic problem or, rarely, both.

C. A history of coumarin necrosis may suggest abnormalities in the protein C and protein S systems.

D. Oral contraceptives are known to be associated with reductions in antithrombin III.

E. The diagnostic approach in venous thrombotic disorders centers on obtaining samples, in a *steady state* for protein C activity, protein S (free and bound and activity assays), antithrombin III activity, and functional plasminogen assay as the initial steps.

F. It is necessary to keep in mind that acute disease affects the levels of these proteins, as do drugs like heparin and warfarin sodium.

G. In patients with arterial thrombotic disease, a detailed dietary history, fasting lipids including cholesterol, high-density lipoprotien, low-density lipoprotein, very-low-density lipoprotein, and lipoproteins form an initial simple screen. It is essential to exclude systemic diseases such as diabetes mellitus, renal failure, and hypothyroidism.

H. Free and bound homocysteine levels and loading tests to diagnose adults with an inherited inability to handle homocysteine constitute the next step.

Bibliography

Beutler E, Erslev AJ, Lichtman MA, et al. *Hematology*, ed 4. New York, McGraw-Hill, 1990.

Colman RW, Hirsh J, Marder VJ, et al. *Hemostasis and Thrombosis. Basic Principles and Clinical Practice*, ed 2. Philadelphia, Lippincott, 1987.

McKenna R. Acquired hemostatic disorders, in Schwartz G, Cayten CJ, Mangelson MA, et al (eds), *Principles and Practice of Emergency Medicine*, ed 3. Philadelphia, Lea and Febiger, 1991.

Transfusion Medicine

Richard J. Sassetti, M.D.

I. Introduction

Transfusion requires a patient-specific assessment of the indications and risks before it can be justified. Elective surgery should stimulate consideration of various forms of autologous transfusion, giving the patient sufficient information to consider the options, which will be discussed below.

A. Two possible goals for transfusion:
1. Therapeutic
2. Prophylactic

B. Prevention or reversal of the consequences of the deficiency requires achievement of an effective blood level for the specific component, not a return to normal levels. To avoid as much as possible the untoward consequences of blood transfusion:
1. Select the most effective form of the component available.
2. Determine the minimum effective dose.

C. Patient and donor processing: The steps taken to ensure minimum risks include the following serologic tests of the donor blood: rapid plasma reagin, hepatitis B surface antigen, the serum alanine transaminase (alanine aminotransferase, serum glutamic-onaloace-

tic transaminase), and antibodies to the hepatitis B core antigen, hepatitis C, human immunodeficiency virus-1, and human T-cell lymphotropic virus-I. Selected donors are tested for the anti-cytomegalovirus (CMV) antibody.

D. Patient screening
1. The ABO and Rh(D) type, direct antiglobulin or Coombs' test (DAT), and indirect antiglobulin or Coombs' test (IAT) are done. Immunosuppressed patients are tested for antibody to CMV to determine the necessity of administering CMV-negative blood products.
2. The final step to ensure safety in the case of red blood cell–containing transfusions is a crossmatch.

II. Blood Components

A. Whole blood: Whole blood is indicated when oxygen delivery and volume deficits coexist. Immunosuppression by transfusion is related to its leukocyte content and further diminishes the already limited value of whole blood transfusion.

B. Indications
1. Massive transfusion requiring more than one blood volume in 24 hr.

2. Autologous transfusion.
3. Transfusion from an intended related kidney donor.
C. Various packed red blood cell products differ in the amount of contamination by undesirable elements in whole blood.
   1. Packed red blood cells (contains all of the red blood cells and one-third of the plasma of whole blood).
   2. Washed packed red blood cells are free of plasma components and free of 95% of the contaminating leukocytes and platelets.
   3. Frozen washed packed red blood cells are free of plasma and free of 98% of contaminating leukocytes.
   4. Leukocyte-filtered packed red blood cells contain 35% of the plasma of whole blood but are less than 1% contaminated with leukocytes. The advantage of leukocyte-filtered products lies in the limitation of sensitization to human leukocyte antigen (HLA) antigens.
   5. In immunodeficient or immunosuppressed patients, it is important that the red blood cells be irradiated with at least 15 Gy to destory any viable lymphocytes capable of initiating a graft-versus-host reaction. It is also necessary to ensure that CMV antibody-negative immunosuppressed individuals receive only CMV antibody-negative products.
D. Indications
   1. Acute blood loss of more than 25% of the blood volume
   2. Preoperative patient with a hematocrit less than 24%. Documented pulmonary or cardiac problems may warrant transfusion at a higher hematocrit.
   3. Refractory anemias.
   4. Anemia in the presence of insufficient oxygen-carrying capacity, congestive heart failure, or coronary artery disease.
E. Alternatives to homologous transfusion of red blood cells
   1. Autologous donation
      a. Predeposit for elective surgery: The patient may be able to donate sufficient numbers of units of blood to cover anticipated needs during surgery. Freezing allows storage beyond the usual shelf life in the liquid state. Use of erythropoietin and/or oral iron may allow predeposit to be done in a shorter period of time.
      b. Intraoperative isovolemic hemodilution of 20–30% of blood volume, using the withdrawn blood as replacement during or after surgery.
      c. Surgically shed blood from areas free of bacterial contamination may be transfused after passage through a blood-salvaging apparatus.
      d. Blood shed postoperatively from the same areas can be used for transfusion.
F. Platelets
   1. The dose of platelets (4×10^{11}) necessary to achieve a satisfactory posttransfusion platelet increment in the recipient requires eight whole-blood donors. Special apheresis technology allows recovery of that number of platelets from a single donor, significantly reducing donor exposure, and expands the variety of platelet products available.
      a. Platelet packs: Made up of a pool of platelets harvested from four to eight random blood donations of compatible blood type to achieve the necessary number. Because red blood cell and plasma contamination is small, it is not necessary to match the blood type of the platelet pool to that of the recipient. One or two of these packs are used to achieve the appropriate number of platelets. Platelet packs should be restricted to patients whose need for platelets is limited.
      b. Single random donor platelets: Used to support patients whose need is expected to be protracted, such as those undergoing vigorous chemotherapy or bone marrow transplantation. Since these platelets are not HLA matched, there is a random probability that the patient will become refractory to them. If only one or a few donors are used over the period of thrombocytopenia, donor exposure is markedly reduced and unresponsiveness is delayed.
      c. "Crossmatch"-compatible, single-donor platelets: Selected for patients who have become refractory to some but not all HLA-unmatched donors.
      d. Cross-reactive, HLA-typed, single-donor platelets: Many HLA antigens cross-react and are slow to elicit specific antibodies. The use of these platelets forestalls the need to switch to HLA-

matched, single-donor platelets. These platelets should be reserved for patients who have become refractory to other platelet products.

   e. HLA-matched, single-donor platelets: These platelets have the highest probability of producing a significant post-transfusion increment in an otherwise refractory patient. Since matching is done for the major HLA loci only, these platelets will not prevent sensitization by antigens mismatched at the minor loci.

2. Indications
   a. Myelophthisic or chemotherapy-induced thrombocytopenia with a platelet count of less than 20×10^9/liter.
   b. Active bleeding with a platelet count less than 50×10^9/liter and/or an abnormal bleeding time.
   c. Abnormal platelet function, with a bleeding time greater than two times normal.
   d. Transfusion (more than one blood volume)-induced dilutional thrombocytopenia with a platelet count less than 75×10^9/liter.
   e. Disseminated intravascular coagulation with active bleeding or before an invasive procedure.
   f. Platelets count less than 75×10^9/liter at the time of an invasive procedure.

3. Contraindications
   a. Immune thrombocytopenia.
   b. Prophylactically following cardiac surgery, massive transfusion, or aplastic anemia.
   c. Thrombotic thrombocytopenic purpura (TTP) or related disorders.

4. Immunodeficient or immunosuppressed patients should receive only CMV antibody–negative and irradiated platelets.

G. Plasma
1. Plasma is available only as fresh frozen plasma. Because the content of coagulation factors is relatively dilute, it is difficult to achieve significant increases in deficient factors without producing hypervolemia.
   a. Indications
      (1) Multiple coagulation factor deficiency with a prothrombin time (PT) or an activated partial thromboplastin time (aPTT) greater than $1.5 \times$ normal.
      (2) Vitamin K deficiency or coumadin therapy with PT and aPTT greater than 1.5 times normal, which requires rapid reversal.
      (3) Significant single or multiple factor deficiency with bleeding or before an invasive procedure.
      (4) DIC with bleeding or PT and aPTT greater than 1.5 times normal.
      (5) TTP or related disorders.
      (6) Massive transfusion, with PT and aPTT greater than 1.5 times normal.
      (7) Antithrombin-III deficiency.
   b. Contraindications
      (1) Volume expansion.
      (2) Prophylactic use for massive transfusion or cardiac surgery.
   c. Fresh frozen plasma is free of cellular components and therefore does not carry the risks for which irradiation is indicated. However, it is argued, but not proven, that it may contain spilled leukocyte cytoplasmic contents and may have the potential to transmit CMV. The common practice is to not require CMV-negative plasma for immunosuppressed patients.

H. Granulocytes
1. There are no circumstances in which granulocyte transfusion in adults has been clearly shown to be efficacious. Because the yield:dose ratio from routine donations is so small, granulocytes are available only as apheresis products. There are approximately 1×10^{10} granulocytes in each product.
   a. Indications
      (1) Neutropenia to levels less than 0.5×10^9/liter.
      (2) Febrile course unresponsive to antibiotics for 24 to 48 hr.
      (3) Demonstrable bone marrow hypoplasia.
      (4) Reasonable chance of marrow recovery.
   b. Contraindication: prophylanis.

I. Cryoprecipitate
1. Cryoprecipitate is prepared from freshly drawn plasma and contains approximately 100 units of Factor VIII-C, 50 units of Factor VIII-vWF, 30 units of Factor XIII, and 250 mg of fibrinogen in about 20 ml of plasma. For these selected factors it repre-

sents a concentrate which allows for high dosage, with little or none of the hypervolemia risk of plasma.

   a. Indications
      (1) Factor VIII deficiency.
      (2) Von Willebrand's disease with active bleeding unresponsive to 1-deamino-(8-D-arginine)-vasopressin (DDAVP) or with an invasive procedure.
      (3) Hypo- or dysfibrinogenemia with bleeding or with an invasive procedure.
      (4) Factor XIII deficiency
      (5) DIC with active bleeding or with an invasive procedure.
      (6) Uremia-induced thrombocytopathy unresponsive to DDAVP or with an invasive procedure.

III. Risks of Transfusion
   A. Immune Effects
      1. The universal induction of a mild immunosuppressive effect not fully understood but attributed to the transfer of viable antigen recognition cells from the donor.
      2. The induction of graft-versus-host disease from engraftment of viable donor lymphocytes. These two effects can be eliminated by irradiation of donor blood with 15 to 25 Gy.
      3. The production of alloantibodies directed to donor cellular or plasma antigens. Alloimmunization is not an inevitable consequence but is dependent on the degree of antigenic difference between the donor and the recipient and on the responsiveness of the recipient. Alloimmunization is responsible for the febrile, allergic, and hemolytic transfusion reactions, as well as for platelet refractoriness, to be discussed below.
   B. Disease transmission
      1. Diseases with the potential for transmission by transfusion for which donors are not routinely tested are HIV-2, malaria, babesiosis, borreliosis (Lyme disease), toxoplasmosis, leukemia, American trypansomiasis, and Epstein-Barr (EB) virus. All these, with the exception of EB virus, are rare in the United States, but with increasing movement to and from endemic areas, these diseases may become a significant threat to transfusion recipients.
      2. A more important ongoing source of infection is the seronegative, asymptomatic, in-

fectious blood donor. None of the currently available serologic tests are 100% efficient. This must always be kept in mind when discussing transfusion alternatives with patients. The percentage estimated prevalence of seronegative infectious blood donors is as follows: hepatitis, 1:500, HIV; 1:100,100.

IV. Transfusion reactions
   A. A heterogeneous variety of deleterious responses which are grouped together because they are temporally and causally related to the transfusion.
   B. Alloimmune reaction
      1. Urticarial: The result of recipient allergy to usually unknown reagins passively transferred in the donor plasma. The symptoms consist of pruritus, urticaria, edema, and occasionally dyspnea. Treatment consists of:
         a. Termination of transfusion of the blood product, with maitenance of IV access.
         b. The administration of parenteral antihistamines (diphenhydramine, 50 mg IM).
         c. In more severe cases, administration of parenteral corticosteroids (dexamethasone, 4 to 20 mg IV) or
         d. 0.5 to 1 ml epinephrine 1:1,000 aqueous solution given slowly IV may be necessary.
         e. Prophylactic antihistamines are effective but problematic because, due to the idiosyncratic nature of the reaction, prevention may only rarely be necessary.
      2. Anaphylaxis may occur in a patient with severe IgA deficiency with preexisting anti-IgA antibodies. Onset may be so rapid and so severe as to require immediate major resuscitative intervention. Patients with proven anti-IgA antibodies should receive only IgA-free blood products, either washed red blood cells, platelets, and plasma or cryoprecipitate drawn from donors with documented severe IgA deficiency.
      3. Febrile reactions are due to preformed antileukocyte antibodies elicited by fetal white blood cells (WBCs) during pregnancy (usually in multiparous women) or by previous transfusion with products containing WBCs. The onset is sudden, with a temperature rise of 1°C or more within

minutes of the commencement of the transfusion, with accompanying chills and rigors. Temperature elevations of lesser magnitude or occurring much later are difficult to ascribe to the transfusion. Treatment consists of:

a. Interrupting the transfusion of the blood product, with maintenance of IV access.

b. Administration of appropriate antipyretics. Since fever may be the first evidence of a more serious reaction, such as a hemolytic or anaphylactic one, it is important to interrupt the transfusion while the likelihood of a major mismatch is assessed and the patient is observed for progression of signs and symptoms (see below). If there is no evidence suggesting the possibility of an acute hemolytic reaction, and transfusion may be restarted after the administration of antipyretics.

4. Hemolytic reactions result from immunization during pregnancy or prior transfusion. Isohemagglutinins are responsible for the most severe reactions and are the most frequent cause of fatal hemolytic transfusion reactions. Their obligatory presence mandates that the ABO blood grouping be respected whenever there is incompatibility. Compatibility around the ABO blood groups is as follows:

Blood Group	Antibodies Present	Compatible Cells
A	Anti-B	A, O
B	Anti-A	B, O
O	Anti-A, anti-B	O
AB	None	AB, A, B, O

a. Preformed antibody results in immediate, rapid intravascular and extravascular hemolysis. The activation of the complement pathway liberates anaphylatoxins and other vasoactive amines, producing hypotension. The immune complexes activate Hageman factor and bradykinin; the latter is a vasoactive substance which contributes to the hypotensive effects and the activation of the coagulation system, producing DIC.

These effects are dose dependent. Hypotension can be sufficient to produce some degree of renal failure, requiring dialysis, or severe enough to produce bilateral renal cortical necrosis. DIC can vary from a mild, transient, self-limited impairment of coagulation to a life-threatening hemorrhagic diathesis.

b. The signs and symptoms of acute hemolysis are variable and consist of flank pain, severe dyspnea (probably related to agglutinated red blood cells reaching the pulmonary arterioles), headache, a sense of impending doom, a sensation of burning over the course of the superficial vein into which the blood is flowing, and a generalized sense of warmth. Signs include fever, tachycardia, cardiac arrhythmias, hypotension, pallor, cyanosis, and diaphoresis. The plasma will be pink and in the laboratory will be shown to contain free hemoglobin. If the patient is not anuric the urine may contain hemoglobin. The DAT will be positive. Other laboratory data are as listed in Table 67-2. A comparison of pre- and posttransfusion blood samples will reveal most discrepancies, which are due to previous misidentification of the patient or the patient's blood sample on which testing was performed. Treatment consists of:

(1) Immediate interruption of the transfusion while maintaining IV access.

(2) Careful hydration and diuresis.

(3) Administration of low (renal)-dose vasopressors.

(4) Alkalinization of the urine.

Rarely, antibodies to blood group antigens other than ABO can produce acute hemolytic transfusion reactions in patients who have been pregnant or previously transfused when either the antibody concentration is below the threshold of the screening IAT or the antibody is missed during preparation of blood for transfusion. These reactions are seldom as severe as those due to ABO mismatch, but they should be treated similarly.

5. Delayed hemolytic transfusion reactions are the result of sensitization to allogeneic

antigens which may represent either a primary or an anamnestic response.

a. In a primary response, transfusion is the sensitizing exposure to the antigen. Ten to 14 days later, the production of antibody reaches a level sufficient to sensitize the red blood cells producing a weakly reactive DAT. The cells are cleared from the circulation and the DAT reverts to negative, while the IAT becomes positive. The reaction is self-limited and is often missed.

b. In a secondary response, within a few days of transfusion the patient may manifest some signs of hemolysis, such as a dropping hemoglobin level, mild elevation of the direct bilirubin level, and a positive DAT (again typically mixed field). The reaction is self-limited, the DAT reverting to negative with a normalization of other indicators of red blood cell destruction and the IAT converting to positive. Occasionally the antibody elicited (anti-Jk, Fy, Rh, or K) is capable of producing intravascular hemolysis which is self-limited; however, if the dose of antigen-positive red blood cells was large, interventions to minimize the effects of intravascular hemolysis may be necessary.

6. Platelet refractoriness follows transfusion of large quantities of platelet products containing large quantities of leukocytes. Most frequently, the antigens involved are HLA antigens.

a. Alloimmunization to HLA antigens occurs in about one-third of patients receiving large numbers of platelet transfusions. As a result, they fail to show a post-transfusion platelet increment and no clinical response to the transfusion.

b. Reducing the leukocyte contamination of the transfused product will reduce the frequency of sensitization. Selecting HLA-matched products will reduce it further. The most efficient use of the limited supply of HLA-specific platelet products is achieved by following the usage pattern outline earlier.

7. Noncardiogenic pulmonary edema (NCPE) or acute respiratory distress syndrome (ARDS) is occasionally seen with transfusion. Its pathogenesis appears to be due to cellular aggregates entering the pulmonary circulation. The inducing events include:

a. The transfusion of blood in which microaggregates have formed near the end of its shelf life.

b. The infusion of leukocyte-containing blood into an individual who has developed leukoagglutinins.

c. The infusion of plasma from an individual found to have high-titer leukoagglutinins or HLA antibodies.

8. Diagnosis and treatment requires termination of the transfusion and initiation of the steps listed in Section IV B.

Bibliography

Dutcher J. Platelet transfusion therapy, in Wernick P, Cannelos G, Kyel R, et al (eds), *Neoplastic Diseases of the Blood.* New York, Churchill Livingstone, 1991, p 881.

Holland P. The diagnosis and management of transfusion reactions and other adverse effects of transfusion, in Petz L., Swisher S (eds), *Clinical Practice of Transfusion Medicine*, ed 2. New York, Churchill Livingstone, 1989, p 713.

Kickler T. The challenge of platelet alloimmunization management and prevention. *Transfus Med Rev* 4(Suppl 1):8–18, 1990.

Pisciotto P. *Blood Transfusion Therapy: A Physician's Handbook*, ed 3. Arlington, Va., American Association of Blood Banks, 1989, p 1.

Apheresis

Bruce C. McLeod, M.D.

I. Definition

Apheresis refers to extracorporeal procedures that exchange or extract a blood component. There are two kinds of instruments.

A. Centrifugal: Separate by density as blood is flowing into the device.
   1. Intermittent flow: Must be stopped to empty red blood cells from the centrifugal element.
   2. Continuous flow: Separate all desired components without interruption of flow.

B. Membrane: Separate plasma (only) in a microporous element similar to a dialysis membrane.

II. Donor Apheresis

A. Plateletpheresis produces $3–6 \times 10^{11}$ single-donor platelets. Advantages over pooled platelets include:
   1. A lower infection risk.
   2. Fewer alloantigen exposures.
   3. A lower intrinsic leukocyte content.
   4. Matched donors are possible.

B. Leukopheresis produces $1–2 \times 10^{10}$ granulocytes. Although seldom used due to dosing limitations and a high likelihood of alloimmunization, these may be helpful in patients with:
   1. Severe neutropenia ($<200/\mu l$).
   2. Documented bacterial infection.
   3. Documented unresponsiveness to appropriate antibiotics.

C. Donor plasmapheresis (donation of 500 ml of plasma) supplies material for fractionation into albumin, gamma globulin, and clotting factors.

III. Therapeutic Apheresis

A. Plateletpheresis may be beneficial for patients with platelet counts $>1,000,000/\mu l$ and either thrombotic or hemorrhagic complications.

B. Leukopheresis may be indicated for:
   1. Hyperleukocytosis syndromes associated with acute or chronic leukemia. Emergent therapy is necessary if leukostasis is present or if the blast count is $>200,000/\mu l$. Consider prophylactic treatment for blast counts $>100,000/\mu l$.
   2. Immune diseases favorably influenced by removal of lymphocytes.
   3. Harvesting peripheral blood stem cells for cryopreservation and subsequent marrow reconstitution.

C. Red blood exchange may be indicated:
   1. To raise hemoglobin A levels to 50–70% of

normal in patients with hemoglobinopathies who suffer:

  a. Severe forms of infarctive crisis (e.g., stroke, acute chest syndrome).

  b. Frequent debilitating pain crises.

  c. Surgical problems requiring general anesthesia.

  d. Increased risk of maternal or fetal morbidity.

2. To remove infected red blood cells in heavily parasitized patients with malaria or babesiosis.

D. Therapeutic plasmapheresis (plasma exchange) is the most common apheresis treatment.

  1. The usual goal is removal of a harmful macromolecule, often an autoantibody. Efficiency deteriorates progressively, so that exchange of one plasma volume will deplete only 65% of intravascular stores. Most patients require multiple exchanges of 1–1.5 plasma volumes.

  2. Colloid must be supplied in the plasma replacement to prevent hypoproteinemia. Five percent albumin eliminates the risk of infection and is preferred for most patients, even though its use causes a transient coagulopathy. Donor plasma is recommended for thrombotic thrombocytopenic purpura (TTP); consider partial plasma replacement for other patients with preexisting bleeding tendencies.

3. Numerous disorders have been treated with plamapheresis. Its value is well established in the following types of conditions:

  a. Neurologic: myasthenia gravis, acute Guillian-Barré syndrome.

  b. Hematologic: TTP, post transfusion purpura (PTP), hyperviscosity.

  c. Renal: Goodpasture's syndrome, rapidly progressive glomerulonephritis.

  d. Rheumatologic: systemic lupus erythematosus, cryoglobulinemia.

Bibliography

Simon TL. Apheresis: principles and practice. In Rossi EC, Simon TL, Moss GS, eds. Principles of Transfusion Medicine, Williams and Wilkins, NY, 1991, pp. 521–526.

Price TH. Plateletpheresis and leukapheresis. In Rossi EC, Simon TL, Moss GS, eds. Principles of Transfusion Medicine, Williams and Wilkins, NY, 1991, pp. 527–536.

Nydegger UE, ed. Therapeutic Hemapheresis in the 1990s. Karger, Basel, 1990.

SECTION 9

Oncology

Chemotherapy of Malignant Diseases: Single and Multiple-Agent Chemotherapy—Mechanisms of Action and Toxicity

William Leslie, M.D.

ABVD (*A*driamycin, *B*leomycin, *V*inblastine, *D*acarbazine = DTIC)

I. **Classification**
   Combination chemotherapy.

II. **Indication**
   Treatment of advanced stages of Hodgkin's disease. This combination is non-cross-resistant with MOPP (nitrogen mustard, oncovin-vincristine, procarbazine, prednisone). It can be used as a salvage regimen in patients who relapse after MOPP chemotherapy or alternating with MOPP as an initial induction regimen.

III. **Dosages**
   A. Adriamycin: 25 mg/m^2 IV on days 1 and 15.
   A. Bleomycin: 10 U (units)/m^2 IV on days 1 and 15.
   C. Vinblastine: 6 mg/m^2 IV on days 1 and 15.
   D. Dacarbazine: 375 mg/m^2 IV on days 1 and 15.
   E. The cycle is repeated every 28 days.

IV. **Interactions and Complications**
   A. Acute toxicity: nausea and vomiting, hair loss, leukopenia, thrombocytopenia.
   B. Long-term toxicity: ABVD does not produce the high rate of male sterility seen with MOPP. The risk of acute nonlymphocytic leukemia is thought to be less than with MOPP. Adriamy-cin has cardiac toxicity in higher cumulative doses, and bleomycin has pulmonary toxicity. Patients who are receiving "mantle" radiation therapy to the chest need to be evaluated carefully to prevent synergistic toxicity.
   C. Response rates are at least as good as those with MOPP, and some studies suggest that they are slightly better.

Aminoglutethimide (Cytadren)

I. **Classification**
   Aromatase inhibitor.

II. **Mechanism of Action**
   Inhibits steroidogenesis. It inhibits the adrenal conversion of cholesterol to pregnenolone and the peripheral aromatization of androstenedione to estrone. Patients must be treated concurrently with hydrocortisone because of adrenal insufficiency resulting from aminoglutethimide.

III. **Indications**
   Used for estrogen receptor–positive metastatic breast cancer. Aminoglutethimide is usually given as third-line hormone therapy, but it is as effective as tamoxifen or megesterol acetate. It is

also active as a second- or third-line hormone therapy in metastatic prostate cancer.

IV. Dosages

Give 250 mg orally four times a day with hydrocortisone in divided doses. Initially, hydrocortisone is given in a dose of 20 mg orally four times per day, but it can later be tapered to 40 mg/day (20 mg twice a day) or even 30 mg/day (20 mg every morning, 10 mg every night) in divided doses. Lower doses of aminoglutethimide (e.g., 250 or 125 mg twice a day) also have been used recently.

V. Interactions and Complications

A. Central nervous system (CNS) toxicities include somnolence, depression, and ataxia. These effects are most common in the first 2–3 weeks and then may improve.

B. A pruritic rash may begin after 2 weeks, but is often temporary and can resolve despite continuation of the drug.

C. Idiosyncratic fevers and myelosuppression have been reported.

Bleomycin

I. Classification

Antibiotic.

II. Mechanism of Action

Inhibits DNA synthesis by causing scission of DNA strands.

III. Indications

Active in non-Hodgkin's lymphoma, Hodgkin's disease, testicular carcinoma, and squamous cell carcinoma of the head and neck. It can also be used to sclerose pleural effusions.

IV. Dosages

Give 10–15 units/m^2 IV, IM, or SC; it can be given weekly.

V. Interactions and Complications

A. Fever is frequent. Patients can be given acetaminophen prior to treatment.

B. There are reports of hypotension and anaphylaxis in patients with lymphoma. A small test dose is recommended.

C. Pulmonary interstitial fibrosis. This is dose related and clinically significant; pulmonary toxicity is seen in 10% of patients receiving a total dose of over 450 units. First signs are cough, dyspnea, and bibasilar pulmonary infiltrates on chest x-ray.

D. Dermatologic changes are seen, including erythema, hyperpigmentation, thickening

and desquamation of the skin on the palms and fingers.

E. Relatively nonmyelotoxic.

Chlorambucil (Leukeran)

I. Classification

Oral alkylating agent.

II. Mechanism of Action

Crosslinks DNA strands.

III. Indications

Used in chronic lymphocytic leukemia and indolent non-Hodgkin's lymphomas.

IV. Dosages

Usual dose is 0.1–0.2 mg/kg/day orally for 3–6 weeks or longer.

V. Interactions and Complications

Myelosuppression is slow in onset and reversible when the drug is discontinued.

CHOP (Cyclophosphamide, Adriamycin-*H*ydroxydaunorubicin, *O*ncovin-vincristine, *P*rednisone)

I. Classification

Combination chemotherapy.

II. Indication

Treatment of non-Hodgkin's lymphomas of high or intermediate grade type.

III. Dosages

A. Cyclophosphamide: 750 mg/m^2 IV on day 1.

B. Adriamycin: 50 mg/m^2 IV on day 1.

C. Vincristine: 1.4 mg/m^2 IV on day 1.

D. Prednisone: 100 mg orally every day for 5 days.

E. Given every 3 weeks for six to eight cycles.

IV. Interactions and Complications

A. Nausea and vomiting, hair loss, leukopenia, thrombocytopenia.

B. Complete responses occur in up to 58%, but up to half of these patients may relapse within 2 years.

C. About 30% of the patients remain in complete remission for more than 7 years.

CMF (Cyclophosphamide, *M*ethotrexate, 5-*F*luorouracil)

I. Classification

Combination chemotherapy.

II. Indication
Treatment of breast cancer. CMF is used both for metastatic disease and as adjuvant chemotherapy.

III. Dosages
A. Cyclophosphamide: 100 mg/m² orally on days 1–14.
B. Methotrexate: 40 mg/m² IV on days 1 and 8.
C. 5-Fluorouracil: 600 mg/m² IV days 1 and 8.
D. The cycle is repeated every 28 days. For patients receiving adjuvant therapy, six cycles are given.

IV. Interactions and Complications
A. Acute toxicity: mild nausea and vomiting, leukopenia, thrombocytopenia, mild alopecia, occasional mucositis and diarrhea.
B. Chronic toxicity: premenopausal women may have ovarian dysfunction ranging from reversible amenorrhea to sterility.

Cyclophosphamide (Cytoxan)

I. Classification
Alkylating agent.

II. Mechanism of Action
Inhibits DNA synthesis; the cell cycle phase is nonspecific.

III. Indications
Active in many malignancies, including breast cancer, non-Hodgkin's lymphoma, ovarian cancer, and sarcoma.

IV. Dosages (Examples)
A. Oral: 100 mg/m²/day for 14 days.
B. IV: 750 mg/m² every 3 weeks.

V. Interactions and Complications
A. Hematologic toxicity is usually dose-limiting.
B. Nausea, vomiting, and alopecia are common with IV administration.
C. Hemorrhagic cystitis: prevented by high fluid intake.
D. Syndrome of inappropriate antidiuretic hormone (SIADH) rare.

Dacarbazine (DTIC)

I. Classification
Synthetic compound.

II. Mechanism of Action
Inhibits RNA and protein synthesis. Also has an inhibitory effect on DNA synthesis.

III. Indications
Active in malignant melanoma, Hodgkin's disease, and sarcomas.

IV. Dosages (Example)
Give 250 mg/m² IV per day five times every month.

V. Interactions and Complications
A. Severe nausea and vomiting common.
B. Hematologic toxicity may be dose-limiting.
C. Flu-like syndrome with fever, myalgias, and malaise can be seen.

Etoposide (VP-16)

I. Classification
Plant alkaloid, semisynthetic derivative of podophyllotoxin.

II. Mechanism of Action
Interacts with DNA topoisomerase II, causing breaks in DNA.

III. Indications
Active in testicular cancer, lymphomas, lung cancer (small cell and non–small cell), and acute nonlymphocytic leukemia.

IV. Dosages (Examples)
A. IV: 50–100/m² IV daily for 3–5 days.
B. Oral: 50 mg/m² daily for up to 3 weeks.

V. Interactions and Complications
A. Hematologic toxicity is usually dose-limiting.
B. Alopecia is frequent.
C. Orthostatic hypotension may develop with rapid IV administration.
D. Severe neutropenia is sometimes seen with prolonged oral administration. The white blood cell count should be monitored closely.

Cisplatin (Cisplatinum)

I. Classification
Heavy metal compound.

II. Mechanism of Action
Acts like a bifunctional alkylating agent and crosslinks DNA.

III. Indications
Active in testicular cancer, ovarian cancer, bladder cancer, lung cancer (small cell and non–small cell), head and neck cancers, cervical cancer, and osteogenic sarcomas.

IV. Dosages
Give 60–120 mg/m² IV every 3 weeks; 20 mg/m² IV daily for 5 days every 3 weeks.

V. Interactions and Complications
A. Renal toxicity is dose-limiting. Serum creati-

nine should be measured prior to giving each dose. Patients should receive IV hydration before cisplatin administration.

B. Ototoxicity is seen but usually is subclinical, with loss of high-frequency hearing.

C. Peripheral neuropathy is seen at high doses.

D. Nausea and vomiting are frequent. This reaction may be prevented by giving high-dose metoclopramide or ondansetron.

E. Hematologic toxicity is usually moderate, but anemia can be seen.

5-Fluorouracil (5-FU)

I. Classification
Antimetabolite.

II. Mechanism of Action
Interferes with DNA synthesis by inhibiting thymidylate synthetase. Also interferes with RNA synthesis.

III. Indications

A. Active in adenocarcinomas of the colon, stomach, pancreas, breast, squamous cell carcinomas of the head and neck, esophagus, anus, and skin.

B. It may be given by continuous infusion to act as a radiation sensitizer.

C. Activity is enhanced by administration with leucovorin.

IV. Dosages (examples)

A. Weekly: 500–600 mg/m^2 IV.

B. Loading doses: 12–15 mg/kg IV daily for 5 days.

C. Continuous infusion: 1000 mg/m^2 over 24 hr daily for 5 days or more.

V. Interactions and Complications

A. Stomatitis and diarrhea are frequent and may be an indication to interrupt therapy. These reactions are seen more commonly with continuous infusion therapy or when 5-fluorouracil is given with leucovorin.

B. Leukopenia can be dose-limiting; this is more common with bolus administration.

C. Myocardial ischemia is seen occasionally with continuous infusion.

D. Hand-foot syndrome is seen with long-term, continuous infusion; paresthesias and hyperpigmentation on the palmar surface of the hands and feet.

E. Cerebellar ataxia seen rarely.

F. Can cause acute and chronic conjunctivitis.

Doxorubicin (Adriamycin)

I. Classification
Anthracycline antibiotic.

II. Mechanism of Action
Intercalates between DNA base pairs and inhibits DNA-dependent RNA synthesis.

III. Indications
Active in breast cancer, Hodgkin's disease, non-Hodgkin's lymphomas, sarcomas, bladder cancer, small cell lung cancer, thyroid cancer, hepatoma, prostate cancer, myeloma, and acute nonlymphocytic leukemia.

IV. Interactions and Complications

A. Cardiac toxicity: causes a cumulative dose-dependent cardiomyopathy. The risk of congestive heart failure increases markedly with cumulative doses greater than 550 mg/m^2. Doxorubicin may also cause acute cardiac changes such as sinus tachycardia, electrocardiographic changes, and arrhythmias.

B. Hematologic toxicity is a major dose-limiting toxicity.

C. Alopecia is common.

D. Extravasation during IV administration can cause severe local reactions; deep ulcerations can develop that are slow to heal.

E. Red urine due to renal excretion of the red-colored compound may be seen.

F. The dose should be reduced with hepatic dysfunction.

Melphalan (Alkeran)

I. Classification
Oral alkylating agents.

II. Mechanism of Action
Crosslinks DNA strands.

III. Indications
Active in multiple myeloma. Formerly used in adjuvant treatment of breast cancer and ovarian cancer.

IV. Doses
For multiple myeloma, give 0.25 mg/kg/day for 4–7 days every 4–6 weeks.

V. Interactions and Complications

A. Leukopenia and thrombocytopenia are dose-limiting.

B. Mild nausea and vomiting can be seen.

C. Chronic use may cause an increase in secondary acute nonlymphocytic leukemia.

Methotrexate

I. **Classification**
Antimetabolite.

II. **Mechanism of Action**
Inhibits dihydrofolate reductase, decreasing the availability of tetrahydrofolic acid, which is important in the synthesis of DNA and RNA.

III. **Indications**
A. Active in acute lymphocytic leukemia, non-Hodgkin's lymphomas, breast cancer, squamous cell carcinoma of the head and neck, sarcomas, bladder cancer, and choriocarcinoma; can be given intrathecally for carcinomatous meningitis.

B. High doses are given followed by leucovorin rescue to treat sarcomas and non-Hodgkin's lymphomas.

C. Low doses are given chronically to treat psoriasis.

IV. **Dosages (examples)**
A. Low dose: 2.5–5 mg orally daily.

B. Standard dose: 30 mg/m^2 orally daily for 14 days, 40–60 mg/m^2 IV q week.

C. High-dose leucovorin rescue is used with doses exceeding 100 mg. High doses may range from 200 mg/m^2 to 3 g/m^2 or higher.

D. The dose of leucovorin can be adjusted by measuring serum methotrexate levels.

E. Intrathecal: 12-mg dose given by lumbar puncture or Ommaya reservoir.

V. **Interactions and Complications**
A. Usual dose-limiting toxicities are mucositis and myelosuppression. Diarrhea is an indication to interrupt therapy. Hematologic toxicity is common.

B. If the patient has an effusion, methotrexate may be sequestered and slowly released, causing increased toxicity.

C. Methotrexate is excreted renally, and toxicity may be increased by renal dysfunction. Renal function must be carefully monitored in patients receiving high-dose methotrexate.

D. Chronic low-dose oral treatment, given for psoriasis or acute lymphoblastic leukemia, may cause hepatic fibrosis.

E. Acute pneumonitis is seen uncommonly, with fever, cough, and interstitial infiltrates.

F. Intrathecal administration can cause acute arachnoiditis, subacute neurotoxicity, or a chronic demyelinating syndrome.

Mithramycin (Plicamycin)

I. **Classification**
Antibiotic.

II. **Mechanism of Action**
Inhibits DNA-dependent RNA synthesis.

III. **Indications**
Used to treat refractory hypercalcemia of malignancy. Active in testicular cancer but generally no longer used for this disease.

IV. **Dosages**
For hypercalcemia, give 15–25 µg/kg IV every day for up to 3 days.

V. **Interactions and Complications**
A. Nausea and vomiting seen with higher doses. Fever, myalgias, and headache may occur.

B. Hemorrhagic diathesis can be seen with daily dosing; decreased platelet count, decrease of Factors II, V, VII, and X, and prolongation of the prothrombin time may occur.

C. Hepatic toxicity and renal toxicity are seen.

Mitomycin-C

I. **Classification**
Antibiotic.

II. **Mechanism of Action**
Inhibits DNA synthesis by intrastrand and interstrand crosslinking.

III. **Indications**
Active in gastric adenocarcinoma, pancreatic adenocarcinoma, colon carcinoma, and breast cancer.

IV. **Dosages**
Give 10–20 mg/m^2 IV for 6–8 weeks.

V. **Interactions and Complications**
A. Myelosuppression is the major dose-limiting toxicity. It is often delayed and cumulative.

B. Uncommon side effects include interstitial pneumonitis, nephrotoxicity, and cardiomyopathy.

C. Can cause a hemolytic-uremic syndrome with microangiopathic hemolytic anemia and renal failure.

MOPP (Nitrogen Mustard, Oncovin-vincristine, Procarbazine, Prednisone)

I. **Classification**
Combination chemotherapy.

II. Indication

Treatment of advanced stages of Hodgkin's disease.

III. Dosages

A. Nitrogen mustard: 6 mg/m^2 IV on days 1 and 8.

B. Vincristine: 1.4 mg/m^2 IV on days 1 and 8.

C. Procarbazine: 100 mg/m^2 orally on days 1–14.

D. Prednisone: 40 mg/m^2 orally on days 1–14.

E. A cycle of chemotherapy is given every 28 days for a minimum of six cycles.

IV. Interactions and Complications

A. Acute toxicities: nausea and vomiting, hair loss, leukopenia, thrombocytopenia, neurotoxicity.

B. Long-term toxicities: sterility in almost all men and in one-half of women. Increased risk of later development of acute nonlymphocytic leukemia.

C. Complete remissions are seen in 80% of patients. Fifty-five percent of all patients will remain free of disease for over 5 years and are considered cured.

PEB (Cisplatin, VP-16-*Etoposide, Bleomycin*)

I. Classification

Combination chemotherapy.

II. Indication

Treatment of testicular cancer.

III. Dosages

A. Cisplatin: 20 mg/m^2 IV on days 1–5.

B. VP-16: 100 mg/m^2 IV on days 1–5.

C. Bleomycin: 30 units IV on days 1, 8, and 15.

D. The cycle is repeated every 3 weeks for four cycles.

IV. Interactions and Complications

A. Acute toxicity: nausea and vomiting, hair loss, leukopenia, thrombocytopenia.

B. Long-term toxicity—mild decrease in creatinine clearance can be seen. Pulmonary toxicity due to bleomycin may develop. Chronic vascular toxicity is reported, including Raynaud's phenomenon.

C. Complete responses are seen in up to 97% of patients with minimal metastatic disease, 77% with moderate metastatic disease, and 48% with advanced metastatic disease.

Procarbazine

I. Classification

Hydrazine derivative with a structure similar to those of some monoamine oxidase inhibitors.

II. Mechanism of Action

Inhibits DNA, RNA, and protein synthesis.

III. Indications

Primarily used in Hodgkin's disease as part of the MOPP (nitrogen mustard, oncovin-vincristine, procarbazine, prednisone) regimen.

IV. Dosages

Give 100 mg/m^2 per day orally on days 1–14 each month.

V. Interactions and Complications

A. Decreased appetite and moderate nausea seen.

B. Drowsiness and depression may be related to inhibition of monoamine oxidase.

C. Patients should avoid foods that contain tyramine, such as wine, cheese, and yogurt. Other monoamine oxidase inhibitors should not be given concomitantly.

D. Interacts with alcohol, causing a disulfiram (Antabuse)-like reaction.

E. Can cause neurotoxicity with paresthesias of the extremities.

Tamoxifen (Nolvadex)

I. Classification

Nonsteroidal antiestrogen.

II. Mechanism of Action

Binds to estrogen receptors which are primarily located in the nucleus. This leads to altered protein synthesis and altered cell proliferation.

III. Indications

For breast cancer, tamoxifen is used to treat metastatic disease or as adjuvant therapy following surgery for stage II patients. Tamoxifen may also have some activity in malignant melanoma.

IV. Dosages

A. Give 10 mg orally twice a day.

B. No significant increase in response is seen with higher doses.

V. Interactions and Complications

A. The most common side effect is hot flashes. This is seen in 10–20% of postmenopausal women. Occasional nausea is seen in up to 100% of patients.

B. When therapy is initiated, a flare in disease activity can be seen with increased bone pain and, infrequently, hypercalcemia.

C. Uncommon side effects include vaginal irritation, vaginal bleeding, edema, headache, depression, thrombophlebitis, thrombocytopenia, and leukopenia.

D. Long-term use may cause a slight increase in endometrial cancer.

E. A significant decrease in total cholesterol and in low-density-lipoprotein cholesterol is seen after 18 months.

Vinblastine (Velban)

I. **Classification**
Plant alkaloid.
II. **Mechanism of Action**
Binds to tubulin and arrests cells in metaphase.
III. **Indications**
Active in non-Hodgkin's lymphoma, Hodgkin's disease, testicular cancer, breast cancer, choriocarcinoma, Kaposi's sarcoma, and bladder cancer.
IV. **Dosages**
Give 0.1–0.2 mg/kg IV.
V. **Interactions and Complications**
A. Leukopenia is often the dose-limiting toxicity.
B. Neurologic toxicity is less common than with vincristine but may cause constipation, ileus, or peripheral neuropathy.
C. Mucositis seen at higher doses.

Vincristine (Oncovin)

I. **Classification**
Plant alkaloid.

II. **Mechanism of Action**
Binds to tubulin and arrests cells in metaphase.
III. **Indications**
Active in acute lymphocytic leukemia, breast cancer, Hodgkin's disease, non-Hodgkin's lymphomas, sarcoma, Wilms' tumor, Kaposi's sarcoma and sometimes used in refractory immune thrombocytopenia (ITP).
IV. **Dosages**
A. Give 1.4 mg/m^2 IV.
B. The dose generally does not exceed 2 mg.
V. **Interactions and Complications**
A. Neurologic toxicity: sensory peripheral neuropathy is common; constipation due to parasympathetic neuropathy may be seen.
B. Alopecia is uncommon.
C. Leukopenia is unusual. Platelet counts may increase in ITP.
D. May stimulate antidiuretic hormone release, rarely causing the syndrome of inappropriate antidiuretic hormone.

Bibliography

Carter S, et al. *Chemotherapy of Cancer.* New York, Wiley, 1981.

DeVita V, Hellman S, Rosenberg S. *Cancer. Principles and Practice of Oncology,* ed 3. Philadelphia, Lippincott, 1989.

Gilman A, et al. *Goodman and Gilman's The Pharmacological Basis of Therapeutics,* ed 8. New York, Pergamon Press, 1990.

Wittes R. *Manual of Oncologic Therapeutics.* Philadelphia, Lippincott, 1989.

CHAPTER 77-A

Head and Neck Cancer

Samuel G. Taylor IV, M.D.

I. **Definition**

Head and neck cancer classically refers to carcinomas originating in the upper aerodigestive tract, comprising the oral cavity, oropharynx, nasopharynx, paranasal sinuses, and nasal cavity, and the major and minor salivary glands. The vast majority of these cancers arise from the epithelial lining of these regions; thus 95% or more are of squamous cell origin. While sarcomas, lymphomas, and melanomas may also occur in the head and neck areas, these cancers are considered separately as having a biological basis in common with cancers of similar histology in other sites that determines their management. Excluding cancers of the skin, approximately 42,000 new cases occur yearly, comprising about 5% of all cancers. There is a male predominance, with a male:female ratio of approximately 5:1.

II. **Etiology**

A. Mucous membrane exposure to the combined effects of alcohol and tobacco is the most common cause of these cancers in the United States. Tobacco smoking alone is not associated with an increased incidence of cancers in these sites, with the exception of the larynx. Snuff, chewing tobacco, and cigar and pipe smoking cause cancers in those sites that are directly exposed to the tobacco product.

B. On the Indian subcontinent, use of various betel nut and tobacco preparations intraorally, often in quid form that is left in the mouth for several days, has caused head and neck cancers to become the most common cancers in India and surrounding countries.

C. General factors
1. Poor dentition
2. Low intake of vitamin A–rich foods.

D. Specific factors
1. Nasopharyngeal carcinomas
   a. Keratinizing squamous cell carcinomas have the same risk factors as noted above but are less common than cancers in other sites due to reduced exposure by the nasopharynx to ingested carcinogens.
   b. Nonkeratinizing lymphoepitheliomas and undifferentiated carcinomas are associated with Epstein-Barr (EB) viral genome and with a high intake of smoked and salt-prepared foods, es-

pecially if begun in childhood, leading to a high incidence of such cancers in China, Southeast Asia, Africa, the Middle East, and in Eskimos.

2. Paranasal sinus and nasal cavity carcinomas are associated with woodworking and with nickel and cadmium exposure.

III. **Pathophysiology**

A. Upper aerodigestive tract cancers are >95% squamous cell carcinomas.

1. Well differentiated (grade I)

   a. More common in the lip, oral cavity, and glottic larynx.

   b. Better prognosis than grade III/IV

   c. Bleomycin responsive.

2. Moderately well differentiated (grade II)

   a. Predominates in the oropharynx and supraglottic larynx.

   b. Prognosis is more like that of well-differentiated tumors.

3. Poorly differentiated (grade III, no keratinization)

   a. Predominates in the nasopharynx and hypopharynx.

   b. Prognosis with surgery and/or radiation therapy less favorable than grade I/II tumors.

   c. More responsive to most chemotherapy regimens, but tends to recur more quickly with chemotherapy alone.

   d. Prognosis improved with combined chemotherapy and radiation regimens.

4. Undifferentiated (grade IV)

   a. Predominates in the nasopharynx, and occasionally in the oropharynx or hypopharynx.

   b. Usually there are bulky regional nodal metastases and an increased risk of hematogenous dissemination.

   c. Very responsive to chemotherapy.

5. Variants

   a. The spindle cell variant may be confused with the sarcomas, but its behavior and chemotherapy responsiveness are similar to those of poorly differentiated squamous cell carcinomas.

   b. Verrucous carcinoma is a variant of well-differentiated squamous cell carcinoma considered by some to respond poorly to or to dedifferentiate with radiation therapy. It may respond to surgery or to combined chemotherapy and radiation therapy.

c. Lymphoepithelioma is a poorly differentiated carcinoma with a lymphoid stroma. The carcinoma cells contain the EB viral genome. Stage for stage, these cancers are more treatable than keratinizing squamous cell cancers due to their high degree of radiation responsiveness.

B. Paranasal sinuses: Squamous cell carcinomas predominate, but adenocarcinomas and occasionally adenoid cystic carcinomas also occur.

C. Salivary glands

1. Squamous cell carcinomas are unusual. Adenoid cystic carcinomas, mucoepidermoid carcinomas, and adenocarcinomas are most frequent.

2. Adenoid cystic carcinomas are notable for their characteristic growth along nerve sheaths and fascial planes, their often slow growth that may evolve over 10–20 years, and the late development of pulmonary metastases.

IV. **Patterns of Spread**

A. Regional metastases are determined by the lymphoid drainage from the primary site. Lymphoid drainage favors the jugulodigastric nodes in virtually all cancers of the head and neck. Low neck nodes and supraclavicular lymphadenopathy are rarely the first forms of nodal involvement from upper aerodigestive primary sites.

1. Sites with <10% risk of regional nodal involvement

   a. Lip

   b. Sinuses

   c. Glottic larynx

2. Sites with early nodal involvement

   a. Nasopharynx

   b. Oropharynx

   c. Hypopharynx

B. Hematogenous dissemination of squamous carcinomas of the head and neck is unusual at the time of initial presentation and accounts for 15–30% of patients who fail primary therapy. Distant spread occurs first in lung or bone and is associated with patients who initially presented with multiple or large (>6 cm) neck nodes.

V. **Diagnosis**

Any adult presenting with a lump in the middle or upper neck, unilateral sore throat or ear pain, or unilateral nasal symptoms or persistent hoarseness should be considered suspect for a cancer of the upper aerodigestive tract. The presence of other risk factors places an increased obligation on the physician to exclude this possibility. It should be emphasized that because of associated medical problems arising from alcohol abuse and chronic tobacco exposure, most patients with head and neck cancers have visited a physician within the year prior to diagnosis.

A. Methods of diagnosi
   1. Biopsy or scraping of the suspicious areas; needle aspiration of neck nodes.
   2. Open biopsy of suspicious neck nodes is discouraged due to the contamination of fascial planes and reduced ability to perform a subsequent therapeutic neck dissection.
B. Evaluation of disease extent
   1. Staging of the primary tumor requires a meticulous examination under anesthesia, with mapping biopsies to determine the extent of the primary and exploration of the entire upper aerodigestive tract, the esophagus, and the lower airway to exclude the possibility of multiple primary cancers. Computed tomography (CT) and/or magnetic resonance imaging (MRI) scanning may be helpful to evaluate the local extent of disease, bone involvement, and neck disease.
   2. Because of the infrequency of hematogenous dissemination at presentation, unless N3 disease exists (any lymph node enlargement >6 cm), chest x-ray alone is considered adequate. A bone scan should also be considered if N3 disease is present. Because liver and brain involvement are rare unless lung or bone involvement is present and because liver scans may be associated with a high false-positive rate, liver scans are poor screening tests for metastases.
C. Multiple primary cancers occur in 20–30% of patients, either simultaneously (approximately 5% of cases) or metachronously (1 to 3% per year), depending on the length of follow-up and the patient's ability to alter the responsible carcinogen exposure.
D. Carcinoma in cervical nodes without an obvious primary site by indirect ear, nose, and throat (ENT) examination requires examination under anesthesia, biopsy of any suspicious area, and blind biopsies from the nasopharynx, oropharynx, and hypophar-

ynx to ascertain the site of origin. If these biopsies are negative, the cancer is determined to be one of unknown primary. Most such cancers are ultimately found to originate in the nasopharynx, oropharynx, or hypopharynx.

VI. **Staging**
Staging of head and neck cancers is remarkable in that the stage IV designation includes patients with advanced local or regional disease in addition to those with hematogenous dissemination. Thus, a proportion of patients with stage IV disease may yet be curable based on recognized prognostic variables of T stage, N stage, primary site location, and performance status.
A. Stage I: T $\leq$2 cm or involving one area; no suspicious lymphadenopathy.
B. Stage II: T 2–4 cm or involving two areas; no suspicious lymphadenopathy.
C. Stage III: Larger T, not involving adjacent structures and/or one lymph node $\leq$3 cm.
D. Stage IV: T involving adjacent bone, muscles, or regions and/or N >3 cm or multiple and/or hematogenous metastases.

VII. **Treatment**
Because head and neck cancers are predominantly regional problems, treatment depends primarily on methods giving local control with the least toxicity.
A. Surgery offers immediate treatment with no long-term sequelae, except for the results of the surgical defect. Its limitation is thus the initial morbidity of the procedure and the effects on swallowing, speech, and alteration in appearance. Early lateral oral cavity, oropharyngeal, and laryngeal lesions may be treated with modern surgical techniques with minimum toxicity.
B. Radiation therapy avoids surgical defects but requires 7–8 weeks of treatment and causes acute toxicities of mucositis, loss of taste and anorexia, and long-term xerostomia. It is best considered for all nasopharyngeal cancers, early hypopharyngeal and many laryngeal primaries, and more centrally located oral cavity and oropharyngeal primaries. More advanced stage III and stage IV cancers are traditionally treated with combined surgery and radiation therapy. Recent evidence suggests that these advanced lesions may be treated with combined radiation therapy and chemotherapy programs, avoiding surgery on the primary altogether in selected patients. Neutron ra-

diation has been especially effective in the management of bulky or inoperable salivary gland cancers.

C. Chemotherapy

1. Active, commonly used drugs include methotrexate, cisplatin, carboplatin, 5-fluorouracil (5-FU), bleomycin, mitomycin-C, hydroxyurea and taxol.

2. The most frequently used combination is cisplatin, 100 mg/m^2 on day 1, and 5-FU, 1000 mg/m^2 continuous infusion over 24 hr on days 1–5 (120 hr).

3. Multiple regimens of chemotherapy have been used prior to other regional treatment (induction chemotherapy). With two to three cycles of cisplatin-based combinations, response rates of 70–90% are achieved, with 20–60% of patients having complete responses. Several randomized trials, however, show that this treatment causes no survival improvement over regional treatment alone and increases the duration of treatment and its toxicity. Recent studies suggest that patients who have a good response to chemotherapy may avoid surgery and be treated definitively with radiation therapy alone.

4. Adjuvant chemotherapy after regional treatment has had a limited trial and is difficult to perform due to the stresses of regional treatment in this patient population.

5. Chemotherapy may be given during radiation therapy, and randomized studies have shown improved regional control with 5-FU, cisplatin, bleomycin, and mitomycin-C using this approach. With the failure of induction chemotherapy to cause any such benefit, combining chemotherapy with radiation simultaneously is becoming increasingly accepted for inoperable and difficult-to-manage cancers.

6. Chemotherapy as a single modality of treatment in recurrent or metastatic cancers is strictly palliative, without curative potential. Cisplatin, as a single agent, has been shown to improve survival over supportive care alone and may be especially effective in aneuploid cancers. The addition of other agents may offer a higher response rate but limited survival advantage. The median duration of the response to chemotherapy varies from 2 to 6 months, with median survival rarely being more than 8 months.

VIII. **Survival is dependent on: Prognosis**

A. Stage

I: 80–95% curative potential

II: 70–90% curative potential

III: 40–75% curative potential

IV: 0–50% curative potential

B. Site: Lip and glottic larynx > oral cavity, supraglottic larynx and oropharynx > nasopharynx and hypopharynx.

C. Performance status: Asymptomatic > symptoms but fully ambulatory > in bed less than 50% of the day > bedridden more than 50% of the day.

Bibliography

Heyne KE, Lippman SM, Hong WK. Chemoprevention in head and neck cancer. *Hematol. Oncol. Clin. North Am.,* 5:783–795, 1991.

Jacobs C. The internist in the management of head and neck cancer. *Am. Intern. Med.* 113:771–778, 1990.

Taylor SG IV. Head and Neck Cancer. Cancer Chemotherapy and Biological Response Modifiers Annual 13, H.M. Pinedo, D.L. Longo and B.A. Chabner, (eds). Elsevier Science Publishers B.V., 1992, pp. 440–454.

Chapter 77-B

Lung Cancer

Philip D. Bonomi, M.D.

I. Incidence
   A. Bronchogenic carcinoma has been the leading cause of death from cancer deaths in American men for decades.

   B. During the 1980s, lung cancer also became the leading cause of cancer-related death in American women.

   C. Approximately 161,000 new cases of lung cancer were diagnosed in 1992, and only 8% of these patients will be long-term survivors.

II. Etioloy
   A. Approximately 85% of the cases of lung cancer are related to cigarette smoking.

   B. A higher "dose" of cigarette smoking increases the risk of bronchogenic carcinoma.

     1. Cigarette dose is often expressed as the number of packs smoked daily multiplied by the number of years of smoking, that is, pack-years.

   C. Although cessation of cigarette smoking reduces the risk of developing lung cancer, it requires approximately 15 years after stopping for the risk to return to the level of a person who has never smoked.

   D. Timed-release transdermal nicotine patches have been relatively effective in overcoming cigarette addiction.

   E. Continued educational efforts by physicians and continued pressure from nonsmokers rights groups are needed to reduce the number of first-time smokers.

   F. Passive smoking, exposure to asbestos, and exposure to uranium dust also increase the risk of lung cancer.

III. Screening
An early detection program in which chest x-rays and sputum cytologic specimens were obtained every 4 months failed to produce a significant impact on mortality from lung cancer.

IV. Pathology
   A. There are four major histologic types of lung cancer:

     1. Squamous cell.

     2. Large cell.

     3. Adenocarcinoma.

     4. Small cell.

   B. The first three histologic types are generally

combined and referred to as *non–small cell lung cancer*.

C. It is essential for pathologists to distinguish non–small cell from small cell lung cancer because there is a marked difference in treatment for these groups of patients.

   1. Pulmonary resection is the primary treatment for early-stage, non–small cell lung cancer.

   2. In contrast, combination chemotherapy is the primary treatment for small cell lung cancer.

D. Small cell tumors are neuroendocrine carcinomas which contain neurosecretory granules and neural filaments. These subcellular elements are detected by electron microscopy.

   1. Neuroendocrine cells synthesize and may secrete polypeptide hormones such as antidiuretic hormone (ADH) and adrenocorticotropic hormone (ACTH).

V. Natural History

A. Symptoms from the primary tumor and regional lymph node metastases

   1. Cough, hemoptysis, and fever from post-obstructive pneumonia.

   2. Chest pain from pleural or chest wall invasion.

   3. Dyspnea from bronchial obstruction, pleural effusion, or a paralyzed diaphragm.

   4. Horner's syndrome and/or arm pain from a pancoast tumor (neoplasm involving the superior sulcus of the thoracic cavity).

   5. Hoarseness from recurrent laryngeal nerve palsy.

   6. Cardiac arrhythmia and tamponade from pericardial involvement.

   7. Dysphagia from esophageal obstruction.

B. Symptoms from sites of distant metastases

   1. Pain from bone metastases.

   2. Headache with or without neurologic deficits secondary to brain metastases.

   3. Back or radicular pain with or without neurologic deficits from spinal cord compression. Coughing or sneezing frequently dramatically increases pain and causes a characteristic band-like pain around the trunk when thoracic vertebral segments are involved.

   4. Right upper quadrant abdominal, right flank, or right shoulder pain is due to hepatic metastases.

C. Paraneoplastic syndromes

   1. Weight loss (>5% of usual weight) is the dominant feature of lung cancer. It occurs with or without anorexia.

   2. Hypercalcemia secondary to ectopic parathyroid hormone production occurs almost exclusively in squamous cell tumor.

   3. The syndrome of inappropriate antidiuretic hormone (SIADH) occurs in 5–10% of small cell lung cancer patients.

   4. Clinical evidence of hypercortisolism secondary to ectopic ACTH production occurs in 1–2% of small cell lung cancer patients.

   5. Clubbing occurs most commonly with adenocarcinoma of the lung and may be the first sign of the presence of potentially curable lung cancer. This phenomenon virtually never occurs in small cell lung cancer.

VI. Diagnosis

A. Histologic or cytologic confirmation of bronchogenic carcinoma can be established in approximately 85% of cases by bronchoscopy if the lesion is located centrally.

   1. The yield from bronchoscopy falls to about 40% for peripheral lesions.

   2. Transbronchial needle biopsy of subcarinal nodes during bronchoscopy (Wang needle biopsy) provides a histologic diagnosis and important staging information.

B. Computed tomography (CT) scan–directed needle biopsy may provide a histologic diagnosis for lesions not diagnosed by bronchoscopy.

   1. Peripheral masses surrounded by lung tissue (coin lesions) and with no evidence of metastases to nodal areas or to distant sites can be resected without establishing a tissue diagnosis preoperatively.

   2. CT-directed fine needle or core biopsies are particularly useful for lesions which are invading the chest wall, such as superior sulcus (pancoast) tumors.

   3. Needle biopsy of a lung lesion can establish a tissue diagnosis in patients with metastatic disease.

C. Mediastinoscopy is useful for detecting metastases to mediastinal lymph nodes and therefore provides important staging information.

   1. Mediastinoscopy may also provide a means to establish a tissue diagnosis if

bronchoscopy and needle biopsy have failed to do so.

   D. It is important to palpate the supraclavicular areas carefully because metastases to this site provide staging information which will prevent an unnecessary pulmonary resection.

      1. Biopsy of a supraclavicular node can also provide a relatively easy way to make a histologic diagnosis.

VII. Staging

   A. Staging of any neoplastic disease is essential to determine appropriate treatment for individual patients and for reporting the results of clinical trials.

   B. TNM staging definitions

      1. T definition refers to the size and invasiveness of the primary tumor.

      2. N tumor definition refers to metastases to regional lymph nodes.

      3. M definition refers to distant metastases.

   C. Type of staging

      1. Clinical diagnostic: all preoperative information including bronchoscopy, mediastinoscopy, scans, biopsies.

      2. Postsurgical pathologic: information from the surgical-pathologic report.

   D. Stage groups

      1. The specific details can be obtained from *Chest* 89 (Suppl):225S-233S, 1986, but the following are general descriptions:

         a. Stage 0: carcinoma in situ.

         b. Stages I and II: resectable for cure.

         c. Stage III: locally advanced disease; pulmonary resection is not curative except in highly selected cases.

         d. Stage IV: distant metastases.

   E. Generally the TNM staging system is applied to non–small cell lung cancer but not to small cell tumors.

      1. Instead patients who have small cell carcinomas are categorized as having limited or extensive disease.

      2. Limited disease is defined as tumor confined to one hemithorax.

         a. Malignant pleural effusions exclude a patient from the limited-disease category.

      3. Extensive disease consists of disease at all other sites, including metastases to the brain, bone liver, adrenals, and other distant sites.

VIII. Functional Evaluation

   A. Performance status

      1. Eastern Cooperative Oncology Group (ECOG) performance status: 0–1: ambulatory

      2. ECOG performance status 2–3: nonambulatory

      3. Poor performance status is associated with significantly worse survival.

   B. Weight loss

      1. None versus <5% versus ≥5%.

      2. Weight loss is associated with a poor prognosis.

   C. Cardiac status

      1. Myocardial infarct within 3 months is an absolute contraindication to surgery because the mortality rate is 20% when lung cancer surgery is performed in this group of patients.

   D. Pulmonary function

      1. In patients whose pulmonary function is compromised, the predicted postoperative forced expiratory volume (FEV) should be ≥1 liter/sec.

      2. A quantitative ventilation-perfusion lung scan may provide important information in patients with poor respiratory reserve. For example, if a patient with an FEV of 1.4 liters/sec requires a right pneumonectomy because of lung cancer and the quantitative lung scan shows that the right lung is receiving only 20% of the pulmonary perfusion, the predicted postoperative FEV will be (1.4 liters/sec)(80%) = 1.12 liters/sec. Therefore the patient is a candidate for resection.

   E. Age

      1. Elderly patients (>70 years) with acceptable cardiopulmonary function should not be denied potentially curative lung cancer surgery.

IX. Determining the Extent of Disease

   A. History

      1. Symptoms of distant disease warrant appropriate scans: CT brain scan with infusion or MRI brain scan in patients with compromised renal function, nuclide bone scan, CT scan of the liver, which is routinely included with the CT scan of the chest.

   B. Physical examination

      1. Signs of distant metastases warrant scans or x-rays. Particular attention should be given to the supraclavicular areas, which are frequent sites of nodal metastases and which may provide an easy method to establish a tissue diagnosis and will imme-

diately exclude the patient from pulmonary resection.

C. Laboratory tests
    1. Elevated levels of alkaline phosphatase and/or lactic dehydrogenase warrant bone and liver scans in patients being considered for surgery.

D. Radiographic studies
    1. CT scan of the chest is done routinely in patients with chest x-rays suggesting pulmonary neoplasm. These studies provide information about the local extent of disease and may suggest the best approach to establish a tissue diagnosis.
    2. Bone and brain scan are not done routinely unless there are signs, symptoms, or laboratory abnormalities suggesting metastases to these sites.

E. Bronchoscopy
    1. This not only provides tissue diagnosis in most lung cancer patients but may also provide important staging information such as invasion of the trachea or carina.

F. Mediastinoscopy
    1. This can be used to detect the presence of metastases in ipsilateral or contralateral mediastinal nodes. If metastases are found in these sites, these patients are excluded from surgical therapy.

X. Surgical Treatment of Non–Small Cell Lung Cancer

A. Pulmonary resection is the primary treatment.

B. Approximately 30% of all such patients are surgical candidates.
    1. These patients have clinical stage I and II and selected stage III disease.

C. Survival rates for patients whose disease has been completely resected are as follows:

Surgical Pathologic Stage	Five-Year Survival (%)
Stage I	60
Stage II	40
Stage III	28*

*This rate was obtained in a highly selected group of stage III patients.

D. Patients with metastases to ipsilateral mediastinal lymph nodes (N_2 disease) are not considered surgical candidates unless they are being treated on a clinical trial basis.

E. However, within N_2 disease there are different prognostic groups:

N_2 Group	Five-Year Survival (%)
Nodal metastasis evident on chest x-ray	5
Nodal metastasis detected by mediastinoscopy	10
Microscopic nodal metastases discovered only at the time of surgery	25–30

F. Stage III patients whose tumors invade the chest wall or mediastinal pleura without lymph node metastases (T_3N_0) are good surgical candidates.
    1. Five-year survival rates are 40–45% for this group.

G. Operative mortality
    1. Lobectomy: 3%.
    2. Pneumonectomy: 6%.

XI. Radiotherapy for Non–Small Cell Lung Cancer

Curative versus palliative radiation therapy:

A. Curative radiation therapy consists of a higher dose given over a longer period of time.

B. The objective of curative radiation therapy is to irradiate the primary tumor and metastases to regional lymph nodes.

C. Although many doses and schedules are used, one of the more commonly used schedules seen in 6000 cGy (rads) over 6 weeks.

D. The 5-year survival rate is approximately 5%, and the median survival is 9–12 months.

E. Palliative radiation therapy involves a lower dose of thoracic radiation given over a relatively short time. This treatment is used to reduce the following symptoms from the primary tumor and regional lymph node metastases:
    1. Dyspnea.
    2. Hemoptysis.
    3. Cough.
    4. Chest pain.
    5. Postobstructive pneumonia.

F. Radiation therapy is also effective for relieving symptoms from distant disease sites, including.

1. Brain metastases.
2. Spinal cord compression.
3. Osseous metastases.

XII. **Chemotherapy for Non–Small Cell Lung Cancer**

A. Combination chemotherapy produces partial remission in approximately 25% of stage IV non–small cell lung cancer patients
1. The median survival in stage IV patients is 4–5 months.
2. Randomized trials comparing supportive care to treatment with chemotherapy have shown conflicting results. In a trial which showed improved survival from chemotherapy, the median survival was increased by 2–4 months.
3. Many oncologists believe that stage IV patients should be treated only in clinical trials or with supportive care alone.

B. The remission rate with combination chemotherapy appears to be higher (50%) in stage III non–small cell lung cancer patients.
1. This group of patients who have locally advanced non–small cell lung cancer are usually treated with radiation therapy alone.
2. However, at least two randomized trials which compared radiation therapy alone to chemotherapy followed by radiation therapy have shown improved survival in patients treated with the combined therapy. The 2-year survival rates for chemotherapy-radiation therapy versus radiation therapy alone were 25% and 12%, respectively.
3. Two other randomized trials which compared radiation therapy alone with chemotherapy followed by radiation therapy failed to show a survival difference.
4. Additional information will become available from current randomized trials which are testing the concept of chemotherapy followed by radiation therapy.
   a. The use of chemotherapy followed by local therapy is often referred to as *neoadjuvant* treatment.
5. Randomized trials have also evaluated the use of radiation therapy and concurrent single-agent chemotherapy (cisplatin). In one of these studies, treatment with small daily doses of cisplatin was associated with improved survival compared to treatment with radiation therapy alone.

a. However, other randomized studies showed no survival difference for radiation therapy versus radiation and concurrent cisplatin therapy. Additional studies are needed to resolve this issue.
6. Two randomized trials have tested the use of postoperative adjuvant chemotherapy in patients with completely resected stage II–III non–small cell lung cancer. Both trials showed that chemotherapy produced a modest improvement in median survival, but there was no improvement in long-term survival. Therefore, the use of postoperative adjuvant chemotherapy should be limited to clinical trials.

XIII. **Treatment of Extensive Small Cell Lung Cancer**

A. Combination chemotherapy is the primary treatment for disseminated small cell lung cancer.
1. Initial response rates are approximately 60%, but drug-resistant cells emerge in virtually all patients.

B. Median survival duration for untreated patients is 2 months; for chemotherapy-treated patients it is 8–10 months.
1. There are virtually no long-term survivors.

C. Most commonly used regimens
1. Etoposide (VP-16)-cisplatin.
2. Cyclophosphamide-doxorubicin (Adriamycin)-vincristine.

D. None of the regimens have been shown to be clearly superior with respect to survival.

E. Similarly, the use of more than three drugs or of higher doses failed to produce clinically meaningful improved survival compared to standard regimens.

F. Recent studies suggest that treatment with single-agent chemotherapy (etoposide) may produce survival durations which are comparable to those observed with combination regimens.
1. Etoposide alone may be an appropriate way to treat patients with extensive disease, particularly elderly patients and those with poor performance status.

G. Radiation therapy is used to palliate symptoms from the primary tumor and/or from distant disease in patients who have chemotherapy-resistant tumors.

XIV. Limited Small Cell Lung Cancer

    A. The same combination chemotherapy regimens utilized for extensive disease are the primary treatment for limited small cell lung cancer.

    B. Treating intrathoracic disease with radiation results in approximately a twofold increase in the 2-year survival rate (from 12% to 25%).

    C. Increasing reports of trials including cisplatin-etoposide and concurrent thoracic radiation therapy are showing 2-year survival rates of 35–40%. This combined-modality regimen appears to be most effective for limited small cell lung cancer.

    D. There is a high incidence of brain metastases in small cell lung cancer patients.

        1. The incidence is particularly high in long-term survivors (≥2 years).

        2. Prophylactic radiation therapy reduces the recurrence of brain metastases but does not result in improved survival.

        3. There are reports of dementia and dystaxia following prophylactic cranial irradiation (PCI).

    E. Therefore, the use of PCI is controversial. Many oncologists recommend PCI in patients who are in complete remission.

    F. Rarely, small cell lung cancer patients present with early-stage disease (T_1N_0, T_2N_0). It is appropriate to resect these tumors and to give chemotherapy postoperatively.

    G. Superior vena cava syndrome occurs in 5–10% of small cell lung cancer patients.

        1. A cytologic or histologic diagnosis should be established.

        2. Then, if small cell lung cancer is found, chemotherapy with or without radiation therapy should be started.

Bibliography

Minna JD, Pass H, Glatstein E, et al. Cancer of the lung, in De Vita Vt Sr, Hellman S, Rosenberg SA (eds). *Cancer: Principle and Practice of Oncology*. Philadelphia, Lippincott, 1989, pp 591–705.

Ihde DC. Chemotherapy of lung cancer. *N Engl J Med* 327:1134–1141, 1992.

Mountain CF. A new international staging system for lung cancer. *Chest* 89 (Suppl): pp 225–233, 1986.

Chapter 77-C

Breast Cancer

Melody A. Cobleigh, M.D.

I. Definition

Breast cancer is a disease of the breast in which the epithelial cells lining the terminal ducts undergo malignant change. There will be 183,000 cases, with 46,000 deaths in the United States in 1993 alone. Breast cancer is the most common form of cancer affecting women and is second only to lung cancer as a cause of death from cancer.

II. Etiology

The cause of breast cancer is unknown. However, certain risk factors have been enumerated.

A. Major risk factors
1. Family history of breast cancer, especially in a first-degree relative with bilateral or premenopausal breast cancer.
2. Personal history of breast cancer.
3. Hereditary syndromes (LiFraumeni).

B. Minor risk factors
1. Early menarche (before age 12).
2. Late menopause (after age 55).
3. Late first pregnancy (after age 30).
4. Nulliparity.
5. Use of estrogen replacement therapy for prolonged periods (>5–10 years).
6. Consumption of a diet high in polyunsaturated fat.
7. Obesity.
8. High socioeconomic status.
9. Exposure to ionizing radiation, such as in survivors of atomic bomb blasts, patients treated with radiation for acne, and patients undergoing repeated chest fluoroscopy.
10. Use of oral contraceptives, especially before age 20.

III. Pathophysiology

A. Breast cancer begins in the terminal ducts. Atypical cells gradually undergo malignant change and fill the lumen. When these cells acquire the ability to spread through the basement membrane of the duct wall, the disease changes from one which is virtually 100% curable (intraductal carcinoma) to one that can spread throughout the body (invasive cancer).

B. Breast cancer cells spread simultaneously to locoregional (axillary) nodes and through the bloodstream. This predilection for spread by both routes makes axillary node dissection the most sensitive means of defining the likelihood of spread of cancer cells which originated in the breast to the rest of the body. For

Table 77C-1. Factors Affecting Breast Cancer Cell Growth

Stimulates
  Estrogen
  Transforming growth factor-α
  Insulin-like growth factor I
  Insulin-like growth factor II
  Her-2-neu ligand
  Epidermal growth factor
Inhibits
  Transforming growth factor-β
  Mammostatin

example, among node-positive patients, 75% will succumb after removal of the breast and no further treatment. Among node-negative patients, only 25% will succumb after removal of the breast and no further treatment.

C. In recent years, a number of growth factors have been discovered to have positive or negative effects on breast cancer cell growth. They are enumerated in Table 77C-1. Highly investigational treatments promise to harness the regulatory control of these molecules in order to induce remission in patients with breast cancer.

IV. **Diagnosis**
  A. Screening
    1. Mammography: Screening mammography significantly reduces the risk of death from breast cancer. Current screening recommendations of the American Cancer Society, endorsed by a number of medical societies, are shown in Table 77C-2.
    2. Breast self-examination: This should be conducted monthly from the time a patient begins menstruating. If the patient is still menstruating, the best time to perform it is during the week following the menstrual period.
    3. Examination by a physician: Breast examination should be a routine part of the annual physical examination by a physician.
  B. Biopsy: The only way to diagnose breast cancer definitively is through biopsy. There

Table 77C-2. Screening Guidelines for Early Detection of Breast Cancer

Baseline: Age 35
Biannually: Between ages 40 and 50
Annually: After age 50

are several ways of doing this, each with advantages and disadvantages (discussion is beyond the scope of this text):
    1. Fine needle aspiration.
    2. True-cut needles.
    3. Incisional.
    4. Excisional.
  C. Staging: The TNM staging system for breast cancer is shown in Tables 77C-3 and 77C-4. It is rooted in assessment of clinical and pathologic material. Patients with operable breast cancer should undergo a few diagnostic tests (Table 77C-5).

V. **Treatment**
Treatment is dependent upon the stage of the breast cancer and should be divided into treatment of the breast and treatment of the remainder of the body.
  A. Noninvasive breast cancer (carcinoma in situ);
    1. Treatment of the breast: Ductal carcinoma in situ (DCIS) and lobular carcinoma in situ (LCIS) are the two forms of noninvasive breast cancer. DCIS tends to be a unilateral process, whereas LCIS tends to be a marker of bilateral disease at some point in the patient's life. DCIS has two forms; the comedo variety, which is more aggressive and has a higher tendency to recur after lumpectomy, and the micropapillary/cribriform variety, which tends to remain localized and may be more amenable to cure by lumpectomy. There are no published prospective, randomized trials comparing breast preservation (lumpectomy) to mastectomy for carcinoma in situ. The National Surgical Adjuvant Breast Project (NSABP) conducted a study of over 600 women with ductal car-

Table 77C-3. Clinical Stage Grouping

	T Stage	N Stage	M Stage
Stage I	1a or 1b	0 or 1a	0
Stage II	0	1b	0
	1a or 1b	1b	0
	2a or 2b	0, 1a, or 1b	0
Stage IIIA	1a or 1b	2	0
	2a or 2b	2	0
	3a or 3b	0, 1, or 2	0
Stage IIIB	4	0, 1, or 2	0
	Any	3	0
Stage IV	Any	Any	1

Table 77C-4.   TNM Staging for Breast Cancer

TUMOR CHARACTERISTICS

TX   Primary Tumor cannot be assessed
T0   No evidence of primary tumor
         T_{is} Carcinoma in situ: intraductal carcinoma, lobular carcinoma in situ, or Paget's disease of the nipple with no tumor.
T1   Tumor ≤2 cm in greatest dimension
         a. No fixation to underlying pectoral facia or muscle.
         b. Fixation to underlying pectoral fascia or muscle.
T2   Tumor >2 cm but not >5 cm
T3   Tumor >5 cm
         a. No fixation to underlying pectoral facia or muscle.
         b. Fixation to underlying pectoral fascia or muscle.
T4   Tumor of any size, with direct extension to skin or chest wall (serratus anterior, ribs, intercostal muscles; does not include pectoralis).
         a. Fixation to chest wall.
         b. Edema (including peau d'orange), ulceration of the skin of the breast, or satellite skin nodules confined to the same breast.
         c. Both (a) and (b).
         d. Inflammatory carcinoma.

NODAL CHARACTERISTICS

NX   Regional lymph nodes cannot be assessed (i.e., previously removed).
N0   No palpable ipsilateral axillary nodes.
N1   Movable ipsilateral axillary nodes.
         a. Nodes not considered to contain cancer.
         b. Nodes considered to contain cancer.
N2   Ipsilateral axillary nodes containing growth and fixed to one another or to other structures.
N3   Metastasis to ipsilateral internal mammary nodes.

STAGING OF DISTANT METASTASIS IN BREAST CANCER

MX   Presence of distant metastasis cannot be assessed.
M0   No evidence of distant metastasis.
M1   Distant metastasis present, including skin involvement beyond the breast area or metastasis to ipsilateral supraclavicular nodes.

Table 77C-5.   Staging Evaluation for Patients with Breast Cancer

History, physical exam, chest X-ray, serum alkaline phosphatase, lactic dehydrogenase (LDH), serum glutamic-oxaloacetic transaminase (SGOT), serum glutamic pyruvic transaminase (SGPT).

If above tests are normal, proceed with surgery.

Bone scan: If there is bone pain or elevated alkaline phosphatase

Computed tomography of the liver: If there is hepatomegaly or elevated alkaline phosphatase, SGOT, SGPT, or LDH.

cinoma in situ. Women were randomly assigned to receive lumpectomy alone versus lumpectomy plus irradiation of the remaining breast tissue. While we await the publication of the results, it seems unreasonable to deny these patients breast preservation, which has proven to provide equal survival when compared with mastectomy in patients with more advanced stages of breast cancer. Axillary node dissection is not indicated in patients with carcinoma in situ when the lumpectomy specimen has been carefully evaluated and there are no areas of invasion or microinvasion. Carcinoma in situ can also be treated by mastectomy. The role of radiation therapy after lumpectomy for in situ cancers is unknown. However, nonrandomized trials suggest that irradiation of the remaining breast tissue decreases the likelihood of breast recurrence.

2. Treatment of the body: Adjuvant systemic treatment is not indicated for patients with carcinoma in situ.

B. Stages I, II, and IIIA

1. Treatment of the breast: Several prospective, randomized trials comparing mastectomy and axillary node dissection with less aggressive breast surgery (lumpectomy) and axillary node dissection, followed by breast irradiation, have concluded that survival is identical with either treatment. Some contraindications to breast preservation exist (Table 77C-6).

2. Adjuvant treatment: The National Institutes of Health (NIH) have held three consensus development conferences on this topic. The consensus statements are summarized in Table 77C-7. Consensus

Table 77C-6. Contraindications to Breast Preservation

Collagen vascular disease (contraindicates irradiation)

Poor cosmetic result (i.e., large tumor in a small breast)

Unreliable patient (will not complete irradiation; will not pursue follow-up mammographic screening)

Synchronous cancers in the same breast at sites remote from each other

Residual mammographic abnormalities after lumpectomy (i.e., widely scattered microcalcifications)

Table 77C-8. Prognostic Factors in Operable Breast Cancer

1. Number of involved nodes: The greater the number of nodes, the worse the prognosis.
2. Tumor size: The larger the tumor mass, the worse the prognosis.
3. S-phase: The higher the S-phase, the worse the prognosis.
4. Ploidy: Aneuploidy has a worse prognosis than diploidy.
5. Epidermal growth factor receptor: overexpression correlates with a worse prognosis.
6. Her-2-neu: Overexpression correlated with a worse prognosis.
7. Cathepsin D: High levels correlate with a worse prognosis.
8. Heat shock proteins HSP-27, HSP-70, and HSP-90: The presence of each correlates with a worse prognosis; the greater the number present, the worse the prognosis.
9. Nuclear grade: A poor grade correlates with shorter survival.

statements are by their very nature conservative. They echo advances which are proven beyond the shadow of a doubt. For this reason they cannot reflect cutting-edge research or even necessarily the opinions of specialists in the field (medical oncologists). This topic is best divided into adjuvant treatment of node-negative and node-positive patients.

a. Node-negative patients: Approximately 25–30% of these patients will relapse and die from breast cancer if no adjuvant treatment is administered. Some investigators have attempted to identify high-risk patients on the basis of prognostic factors (Table 77C-8). Thus far, these factors have not been proven to impact survival when used to select adjuvant chemotherapy for node-negative patients. What is sorely needed is a national data base large enough to incorporate all of these factors into a multivariate model so that meaningful studies can be designed to

test their validity in the adjuvant therapy setting.

(1) Adjuvant treatment: Ten randomized trials have evaluated the efficacy of adjuvant treatment. Adjuvant treatment significantly reduces the risk of recurrence by about one-third. Original publications of the largest trials did not show a significant difference in survival. However, updates of these trials at national meetings have now shown a survival advantage as well. Three of the largest studies will be reviewed briefly here.

Table 77C-7. Consensus Development Recommendations for Adjuvant Treatment of Early Breast Cancer

Year	Nodal status	Menopausal status	Receptor Status	Consensus
1980	Positive	Premenopausal	Positive	Chemotherapy
	Positive	Premenopausal	Negative	Chemotherapy
1985	Positive	Postmenopausal	Positive	Tamoxifen
1990	Negative*	Premenopausal	Positive	Adjuvant Rx
	Negative*	Premenopausal	Negative	Adjuvant Rx
	Negative*	Postmenopausal	Positive	Adjuvant Rx
	Negative*	Postmenopausal	Negative	Adjuvant Rx

*For tumors >1 cm.

(a) The NSABP B-13 trial compared 12 months of methotrexate, 5-fluorouracil, and leucovorin with no treatment in 679 women with receptor-negative, pre- or postmenopausal breast cancer. The risk of relapse was significantly lower in the group who received chemotherapy.

(b) In a companion protocol, NSABP B-14, the same group of investigators evaluated over 2,644 women with estrogen receptor–positive pre- or postmenopausal breast cancer. Tamoxifen given for 5 years was compared with placebo treatment. The risk of relapse was significantly lower in the group who received tamoxifen. Interestingly, the incidence of cancers in the opposite breast was significantly reduced by treatment with tamoxifen.

(c) The Intergroup randomly assigned 536 pre- and postmenopausal women to 6 months of (CMFP) versus no further therapy. These were women with estrogen receptor–negative tumors of any size or estrogen receptor–positive tumors larger than 3 cm. The risk of relapse was significantly lower in the group receiving chemotherapy. No information exists as to the effectiveness of combined chemohormonal treatment in node-negative patients, but studies are underway. No studies have compared tamoxifen therapy with chemotherapy.

(2) In its consensus development statement, the NIH stopped short of stating that adjuvant treatment of women with node-negative breast cancer was necessary. Instead it suggested that patients should be entered in clinical trials and, when this was not possible, they should be informed of the relative risks and benefits of adjuvant treatment.

b. Node-positive; chemotherapy: Approximately 75% of node-positive patients will relapse without adjuvant treatment. Sixteen trials have compared adjuvant chemotherapy with a no-treatment control group. An excellent review of this subject is available. Pooling the estimates of the effect of adjuvant chemotherapy compared with a no-treatment control group on disease-free survival (DFS) and survival, the following general statements can be made:

(1) Chemotherapy significantly prolongs DFS and survival.

(2) Combination chemotherapy is more effective than single-agent chemotherapy in prolonging DFS and survival.

(3) Chemotherapy has a greater impact on DFS in women under the age of 60, among whom competing causes of death are less common.

(4) Three to 6 months of chemotherapy appears to be as effective as longer durations of treatment.

c. Node-positive; hormonal therapy: Eight trials have compared oophorectomy or ovarian irradiation with no further treatment in premenopausal patients. None have shown a significant improvement in DFS or survival. Ten trials have compared tamoxifen with no further treatment. Most of these trials have been conducted in postmenopausal women. The following general statements can be made:

(1) Tamoxifen improves DFS in postmenopausal women.

(2) Tamoxifen is more effective in estrogen receptor–positive women.

(3) In general, tamoxifen does not significantly improve DFS or survival in premenopausal patients. However, there are few studies addressing this issue, and important clinical trials are underway.

(4) Tamoxifen significantly reduces the risk of new (contralateral) breast cancers.

(5) Longer treatments (5 years) are, in general, more effective than briefer 1- to 2-year) treatments. Current trials are evaluating 10-yr treatment with tamoxifen versus treatment for 5 years.

d. Node-positive; combined chemohormonal therapy: These studies are relatively recent. There are two types:

(1) Trials comparing adjuvant chemotherapy with a chemohormonal treatment: Six trials have been published in which the chemotherapy consisted of combinations of drugs and the hormone treatment was tamoxifen. The following general statement can be made: There is a trend toward improved relapse-free survival (RFS) among postmenopausal patients who received combined chemohormonal treatment.

(2) Trials comparing adjuvant hormone therapy with a chemohormonal treatment: Studies of this nature are the least mature. The NSABP has demonstrated improved RFS and survival among tamoxifen-responsive patients over age 50 who were treated with chemotherapy plus tamoxifen compared with tamoxifen alone.

The Ludwig group reported improved DFS among postmenopausal patients receiving combination chemotherapy, prednisone, and tamoxifen compared with prednisone and tamoxifen alone.

C. Stage IIIB: These patients are curable with combined-modality approaches that include induction chemotherapy followed by appropriate local treatment. This should include irradiation, with or without surgery, depending on the response of the breast cancer to induction chemotherapy.

D. Stage IV: These patients are categorically incurable. Experimental procedures using marrow-ablative doses of chemotherapy followed by autologous bone marrow rescue show promise but have not yet been shown to produce longer survival than standard treatment approaches. Outside the context of a clinical trial, the appropriate approach to such patients is palliative.

1. Endocrine manipulations may be used under appropriate circumstances (Table 77C-9). Premenopausal patients may undergo oophorectomy or tamoxifen therapy as a first-line hormone manipulation. Tamoxifen is generally regarded as the initial hormonal treatment of choice for postmenopausal patients. Patients who re-

Table 77C-9. Endocrine Treatment in Patients with Metastatic Breast Cancer

INDICATIONS
Receptor-positive tumor
Long disease-free interval (>1 year)
Metastasis predominantly to soft tissue or bone
CONTRAINDICATIONS
Rapidly progressive visceral disease
Lymphangitic lung metastasis
Liver metastasis with threat of liver failure
Bone marrow failure due to metastatic
Breast cancer
Short disease-free interval (<1 year)

spond to and then fail a first-line hormone manipulation will frequently respond to a second-, third-, fourth-, or even fifth-line treatment. Other hormone treatments include progestins (Megace), estrogens in superphysiologic dosages (diethylstilbestrol), and androgens (Halotestin).

2. Chemotherapy is reserved for a time when endocrine treatment has failed or is inappropriate. Combination chemotherapy is more effective in including remission than single agents (60% versus 15% in previously untreated patients). Treatment will depend in large measure on whether and what type of chemotherapy was administered in the adjuvant setting and on the disease-free interval.

3. Radiation therapy plays an extremely important part in the palliation of metastatic breast cancer (Table 77C-10).

4. Surgery is occasionally used in patients with metastatic breast cancer and can be exceedingly valuable in palliating problems that cannot be alleviated by systemic treatment or irradiation (Table 77C-11).

VI. Patient Monitoring
Patients are examined at regular intervals (Table

Table 77C-10. Indications for Radiation Therapy in the Palliation of Metastatic Breast Cancer

Painful bony lesions
Prophylactic treatment of bone lesions with impending fracture
Spinal cord compression
Brain metastasis
Chest wall recurrences

ment in survival rate (5-year survival is 35% vs. 20% for surgery alone).

  c. Postoperative radiotherapy

    (1) Reported results vary, depending on the extent of disease found at surgery.

    (2) Overall advantage is similar to that of preoperative radiotherapy.

  d. Palliative radiotherapy

    (1) Most patients are not eligible for curative treatment.

    (2) From 70% to 100% of patients with dysphagia are relieved of symptoms with minimal toxicity.

3. Chemotherapy

  a. Adjuvant chemotherapy (postoperatively)

    (1) No documented benefit in esophageal cancer.

  b. Neoadjuvant chemotherapy (preoperative)

    (1) Theoretical advantage is "downstaging" of the primary tumor, especially in borderline cases, and eradication of micrometastases to achieve local control and prevent distant spread.

  c. Single agents

    (1) Many active drugs are available.

    (2) Most active: cisplatin, 5-fluorouracil (5-FU) as infusion, mitomycin C, bleomycin, and methotrexate.

    (3) Response rate is 17–77%, with occasional complete responses.

  d. Combinations of drugs

    (1) Most active combination seems to be cisplatin and infusional 5-FU.

    (2) Overall response rates of 42–66% achieved, with 12–39% complete responses.

    (3) More effective than each drug individually.

    (4) Best role probably in the combined-modality or neoadjuvant setting.

4. Multimodality approach to esophageal cancer

  a. Chemoradiotherapy without surgery

    (1) In stage I and II disease, survival rates similar to those of surgery alone.

    (2) Two-year survival 22–40%; 5-year survival 18%.

    (3) An intergroup trial proved that chemoradiotherapy is better than radiotherapy alone.

      (a) Complete response, documented by endoscopy biopsy, achieved in 77% of patients vs. 30% ($p = .0011$)

    (4) Chemotherapy regimens include infusional 5-FU with or without cisplatin with or without mitomycin with or without bleomycin.

  b. Preoperative (neoadjuvant) chemoradiotherapy

    (1) Nonrandomized trials suggest superior results compared to histologic controls.

    (2) Randomized results needed to determine the optimal regimen.

    (3) Since current therapy is mostly ineffective because of distant disease, aggressive chemotherapy is likely to be part of any successful program.

V. Prognosis

  A. Overall prognosis is poor with less than 5% long term survivors.

  B. Select patients benefit from therapy with improvement in survivability as described under various treatment modalities above.

Bibliography

Klumpp TR, MacDonald JS. Esophageal Cancer. In: Ahlgren SD, MacDonald JS, eds. Gastrointestinal Oncology. Philadelphia, JB Lippincott, 1992, pp 69–147.

Roth JA, Lichtes AS. Cancer of the Esophagus. In: DeVita VT, Hellman S, Rosenberg SA, (eds). Cancer—Principles and Practices of Oncology. Philadelphia, JB Lippincott, 1993, pp 776–817.

Gastrointestinal Cancers

Edward H. Kaplan, M.D.

I. **Definition**

Cancers arising from the gastrointestinal tract which includes esophagus, stomach, small intestine, liver, pancreas, biliary tree, colon and rectum.

II. **Etiology and Epidemiology**

Gastrointestinal (GI) tract cancers account for the majority of adult solid tumors.

A. Widespread global health problem, with more than 2 million cases diagnosed yearly.
1. Over 1.5 million deaths per year.
a. Twice the death rate from lung cancer and over six times the death rate from breast cancer.

III. **Incidence**

A. In the United States more than 225,000 cases occur yearly.
1. The disease causes approximately 125,000 deaths per year.

IV. **Detection and Treatment**

A. Usually the disease is difficult to detect until the development of symptoms, usually at an advanced stage.
1. The anatomic location often creates vague symptoms.

2. Current screening techniques, although insufficient and relatively insensitive, are underutilized.

B. Surgery is the most common successful treatment for GI cancer patients.
1. In the past, the surgeon was the only clinician involved in the care of these patients.
2. Newer therapeutic approaches require a multimodality team, with surgery, radiation therapy, and/or chemotherapy being utilized to afford the best outcome.

C. Tumor markers
1. Occasionally useful in following the response to therapy or monitoring for relapses.
2. Not considered appropriate for screening of the general population.
a. Lack of sensitivity and specificity
3. Commonly available tumor markers in GI malignancies:
a. Carcinoembryonic antigen (CEA): Colorectal (especially advanced disease), gastric, and pancreatic.
b. (CA)19-9: Pancreatic, hepatobiliary, gastric, colorectal.

   c. α-Fetoprotein: hepatocellular.
4. Markers not yet routinely available
   a. CA-50 (pancreatic), DU-PAN-2 (pancreas, hepatocellular, biliary tract)
   b. (CSAp) (colon), (LSA) (nonspecific).

Bibliography

Ahlgren SD, MacDonald JS, eds. Gastrointestinal Oncology. Philadelphia, JB Lippincott, 1992.

Gastric Cancer

Edward H. Kaplan, M.D.

I. Definition

  A. Any malignancy arising from the stomach, which begins at the gastroesophageal junction and ends at the pylorus.

II. Etiology and Epidemiology

  A. Wide geographical variation.

  B. Appears to be closely related to the environment.

  C. Incidence of gastric cancer can decrease in high-risk populations who have immigrated and changed their dietary habits (especially Japanese-Americans).

  D. Dietary risk factors

    1. Low consumption of fresh fruits and vegetables.

    2. High intake of salts and nitrates.

    3. Decreased incidence span with a diet rich in grains.

    4. Alcohol *not* apparently related to risk of stomach cancer.

    5. Tobacco use has recently been conclusively linked to gastric cancer.

      a. There is a 2.5 to 5 times greater risk in smokers.

  E. Other risks

    1. People with blood type A (weakly linked).

    2. Gastric resection for peptic ulcer disease, especially the Billroth II procedure.

      a. Thought to be secondary to loss of increased gastric pH and intestinal metaplasia.

    3. Pernicious anemia

      a. Assumed to be secondary to atrophic gastritis and achlorhydria.

      b. Some studies suggest no increased risk.

    4. Ataxia telangiectasia

    5. Occupational hazards

      a. Coal mining.

      b. Nickel refining.

      c. Rubber and timber processing.

      d. May be associated with the standard of living rather than toxic exposures.

    6. *Helicobacter pylori* infection may be associated with gastric carcinogenesis.

III. Incidence

  A. Incidence of adenocarcinoma of the stomach has decreased by 60% between 1930's and 1970's but stable over the last 20 years.

B. Incidence equals approximately 10 per 100,000 whites in the United States and 90 per 100,000 in Japan.

IV. Pathology

A. Adenocarcinoma
1. Accounts for more than 90% of stomach cancers.
2. Most cancers formerly involve the distal stomach, but an apparent shift over the last 20–30 years has resulted in more proximal and gastroesophageal junction tumors.
3. Most clinically significant factor is ulcerating exophytic-type versus infiltrating, poorly differentiated, diffuse carcinoma (linitis plastica).

B. Leiomyosarcoma

C. Gastric lymphoma
1. Mostly of B-cell origin.

V. Patterns of Spread

A. Direct extension
1. Omentum
2. Surrounding organs

B. Nodal metastases

C. Hematogenous spread
1. Liver
2. Bone
3. Lung
4. Brain

D. Intraperitoneal metastases
1. Ovarian mass (Krukenberg tumor)
2. Blumer's rectal shelf
3. Disseminated intraperitoneally (clinically, Sister Mary Joseph's periumbilical nodes)

VI. Clinical Presentation and Diagnosis

A. Early disease associated with elusive, non-specific symptoms suggestive of gastritis or peptic ulcer disease.

B. Later disease associated with dysphagia, gastrointestinal bleeding, or related to distant metastases.

C. Upper endoscopy is indicated when dyspepsia persists after 2 weeks of medical treatment with an H_2 antagonist.

D. All gastric ulcers should be biopsied at least once.

E. Gastric cancer may ulcerate, but benign ulcers rarely become malignant.

VII. Staging

A. TNM staging is used.

B. Stage groupings
1. Stage I: limited to the mucosa or submucosa (5-year survival: 80%).

2. Stage II: into or through the scrosa, without invasion of adjacent tissue and without nodal involvement (5-year survival: 50%).
3. Stage III: lymph node involvement and/or involvement of immediately adjacent structures (5-year survival: 20%).
4. Stage IV: distant intra-abdominal nodes or distant metastases present (5-year survival: <5%).

VIII. Treatment

A. Surgery
1. Primary treatment modality.
2. Provides the best chance for cure and for palliation.
   a. Often resectability (and curability) can be determined only at surgical exploration.
   b. Preoperative evidence of lymphatic or adjacent visceral involvement does not always mean unresectability.
3. Extended lymph node dissection may improve survival without increasing morbidity and mortality.
4. Subtotal gastrectomy is as effective as total gastrectomy as long as all gross and microscopic disease is removed.
   a. Total gastrectomy has high morbidity and mortality rates.
      (1) Major cause of morbidity is an anastomotic leak.
      (2) Other postgastric problems
         (a) Dumping syndrome
         (b) Vitamin B_{12} deficiency
         (c) Malabsorption from blind syndrome
            i) Symptoms include epigastric fullness, hyperperistalsis, nausea and vomiting, and diarrhea.
            ii) Managed with small, frequent meals and a low-carbohydrate, high-fat diet.
   b. Preoperative evidence of lymphatic and adjacent visceral involvement does not always indicate unresectability.
   c. Complete surgical resection with margins free of macroscopic disease is possible in 30–50% of patients.
   d. Routine splenectomy is not indicated.

B. Radiation therapy
1. Cannot replace surgery as the primary treatment.
2. May control some inoperable or residual

macroscopic disease, but with very few (<6%) long-term survivors.

3. Adjuvant for microscopic residual disease
   a. Few controlled trials have been done, involving suboptimal radiotherapy.
   b. A few studies suggest that radiotherapy may reduce the local recurrence rate.
   c. Currently not routinely recommended except in the setting of an experimental protocol.

C. Chemotherapy
   1. Compared to other sites of the gastrointestinal tract, the stomach appears to be most responsive to chemotherapy.
   2. Numerous single agents exist, with response rates of up to 48%.
      a. Very few complete or long-lasting responses.
   3. Multiple-drug combination chemotherapy improves the chances of a response.
      a. FAM (5-fluorouracil [5-FU], Adriamycin, and mitomycin-C), traditionally considered to be standard, has approximately a 25% overall response rate but <5% complete responders.
      b. More recent programs—FAMTX (5-FU, Adriamycin, methotrexate), EAP (etoposide, Adriamycin, and cisplatin), and ELF (etoposide, leucovorin, and 5-FU)—have overall response rates of 43–72%, with 12–20% complete responders.

D. Multimodality approach

1. Several clinical trials have shown modest improvement in patients survival in certain subgroups (T_3 and T_4 tumors) given postoperative adjuvant chemotherapy.
2. Early studies suggest that preoperative (neoadjuvant) chemotherapy may "downstage" tumors, allowing a better chance of resection and cure in patients with locally advanced disease.
   a. Must be confirmed in phase III trials
3. Postoperative chemotherapy and radiation therapy currently being compared to surgery alone in a randomized nationwide intergroup stomach trial.

IX. **Prognosis**
   A. Depends on the extent of disease and treatment.
      1. All nodes negative: 73–81% 5-year survival.
      2. Perigastric nodes positive: 18% 5-year survival with simple dissection but 60% with extensive dissection.
      3. Regional nodes positive: 21% 5-year survival with extensive dissection.

Bibliography

Alexander HR, Kelsen DP, Tepper JE. Cancer of the Stomach. In: Devita VT, Hellman S, Rosenberg SA, (eds) Cancer - Principles and Practices of Oncology Philadelphia, JB Lippincott, 1993, pp 818–848.

Macdonald JS, Hill MC. Gastric Cancer. In: Ahlgren SD, MacDonald JS, eds. Gastrointestinal Oncology. Philadelphia, JB Lippincott, 1992, pp 149–193.

Chapter 77-G

Colorectal Carcinoma

Edward H. Kaplan, M.D.

I. Definition

  A. Colon Cancer

    1. Any malignancy arising in the large bowel.

      a. For cancer treatment purposes, disease may be classified by location: free intraperitoneal or retroperitoneal.

        (1) cecum, transverse colon and sigmoid are intraperitoneal structures.

  B. Rectal Cancer

    1. Rectum comprises area from upper valve of Houston to anal verge.

    2. Location of a tumor is defined as the distance between the lower margin and the anal verge.

II. Etiology and Epidemiology

  A. Wide international geographic variation.

    1. Highest incidence in most industrialized countries (except Japan).

    2. Lowest incidence in developing countries.

  B. Some environmental influence is probable.

    1. Increases in migrants from low-risk to high-risk countries.

    2. Varies among different ethic groups.

    3. Changes in dietary patterns may contribute to increased risk within 20–30 years.

    4. Environmental factors appear to impact on risk more rapidly than in other cancers.

      a. Probably determined by adult diet or dietary effect occurs more rapidly.

    5. Risk can also decline with migration.

      a. Scottish and British migrants to Australia have a decreased risk.

    6. Higher risk in urban than rural populations.

    7. Lower risk among Mormons and Seventh Day Adventists.

      a. Not totally explained by dietary habits.

  C. Genetic risks

    1. Intestinal polyposis syndrome

      a. Familial adenomatosis polyposis

        (1) Autosomal dominant trait: more than one-third not familial; new sporadic mutations.

        (2) Gene found on long arm of chromosome 5.

        (3) Accounts for 1% of all colorectal cancers.

        (4) Without colectomy, the risk of developing cancer is almost 100%.

      b. Peutz-Jeghers syndrome

(1) Multiple gastrointestinal hematomas.

(2) Lifetime risk of developing colorectal cancer is more than 2% (16× normal).

2. Nonpolyposis genetic syndrome

   a. Lynch syndromes I and II

      (1) I is colon specific; II is associated with cancers of the breast, endometrium and ovary.

      (2) Account for 6% of colon cancer.

      (3) Associated with predominantly right-sided colonic lesions.

      (4) Children of patients with this syndrome have a 50% risk of developing colon cancer.

   b. Family history (without a recognizable syndrome)

      (1) A two- to threefold increased risk in first-degree relatives of patients with colorectal cancer.

3. Inflammatory bowel disease

   a. Ulcerative colitis

      (1) Increased risk first observed in 1925.

      (2) Mean age of occurrence is 49 years (compared to 69 years in the general population).

      (3) Twenty-five percent of the patients developed cancer after 20 years of disease.

      (4) Frequently multifocal.

      (5) Usually occurs in sites of inflammatory disease and is preceded by dysphasia.

      (6) "Normal" mucosa may also develop malignancy.

      (7) Only true form of prevention is total colectomy.

   b. Crohn's disease

      (1) Risk not as striking as with ulcerative colitis.

         (a) A 7–20 times expected incidence compared to the general population.

         (b) May involve a genetic predisposition.

         (c) One-third of lesions found in grossly normal mucosa.

         (d) May occur anywhere in the small and large bowels.

D. Dietary risks

   1. Dietary fat

      a. Strong correlation between occurrence

of colorectal cancer and consumption of animal fat (*not* vegetable fat).

      b. Effect of cholesterol intake is ambiguous; no clear-cut relationship exists.

   2. Bile acids

      a. Fecal bile acids increased in patients with colonic adenomas and colon cancer.

   3. Dietary fiber

      a. Removal of insoluble fiber from food is associated with increased risk of colon cancer.

      b. Can bind carcinogens and tumor promotors.

III. **Incidence**

A. Over 150,000 new cases and 55,000 deaths expected in the United States (500,000 new cases worldwide) in 1994.

B. Accounts for 15% of newly diagnosed cancers in women and 14% in men.

IV. **Pathology of Colonic Polyps**

A. Nonneoplastic (one-third of polyps removed at colonoscopy).

   1. Hyperplastic polyps

   2. Mucosal tags

   3. Inflammatory polyps

B. Adenomas

   1. Benign neoplasms with malignant potential (two-thirds of polyps removed at colonoscopy).

   2. Patterns of growth

      a. Tubular, villous, or tubulovillous.

      b. All patients have at least mild dysplasia.

         (1) Five percent have severe dysplasia or carcinoma in situ.

         (2) Two and one-half percent have a component of invasive cancer.

      c. More likely to have severe dysplasia and villous > tubulovillous > tubular pattern.

V. **Diagnosis**

A. Screening for colorectal cancer

   1. Best chance of cure exists when no symptoms are present.

   2. Three true screening tests are available.

      a. Digital rectal exam

         (1) Simple and safe.

         (2) Detects less than 10% of colorectal cancers.

         (3) Apparently of decreasing importance with proximal migration of colorectal cancers.

      b. Fecal occult blood test

(1) Two separate samples required daily for 3 days.

(2) Ideally, a strict diet should be maintained.

(3) From 1% to 5% of asymptomatic patients have a positive test. Of these patients, 10% have cancer and 30% have adenomas.

    (a) The majority of cancers detected are in the early stage (Duke's A or B).

c. Sigmoidoscopy

(1) A 60-cm, flexible sigmoidoscope is preferred to a 25-cm, rigid one for screening.

(2) Reaches the rectum and part of the sigmoid colon.

(3) Fifty-eight cancers were detected in over 25,000 people screened; 81% were Duke's A or B, and 15-year survival was 90%.

(4) May be more useful in detecting polyps suggesting a need for full colonoscopy.

d. American Cancer Society recommendations

(1) Annual digital rectal after 40.

(2) Annual stool hemoccult test after age 50.

(3) Annual sigmoidoscopy for 2 years after age 50; then, if negative, every 3–5 years.

B. Presenting symptoms

1. Bright red blood per rectum.
2. Abdominal pain.
   a. Usually crampy and intermittent.
3. Change in bowel habits
   a. Constipation, diarrhea, change in caliber.
4. Iron deficiency anemia (from clinically silent bleeding).
5. Severe localized pain in rectal cancer.

C. Methods of diagnosis

1. Air contrast barium enema
   a. Radiologic procedure of choice in suspected colon carcinoma.
   b. Not to be utilized if perforation is suspected or following biopsy.
   c. May reveal early polypoid cancer (<2 cm).
2. Colonoscopy
   a. More sensitive (but more expensive) than barium enema.
   b. Allows biopsy for immediate diagnosis.

Table 77G-1. Staging of Colorectal Cancer

Duke's	AJCC/UICC*	TNM	5-year Survival (%)
A	I	$T_1N_0M_0$	95
B_1	I	$T_2N_0M_0$	85–90
B_2	II	$T_3N_0M_0$	60–80
B_3	II	$T_4N_0M_0$	30
C_1	III	$T_{1-2}N_{1-3}M_0$	50–60
C_2	III	$T_3N_{1-3}M_0$	40–50
C_3	III	$T_4N_{1-3}M_0$	20–30
D	IV	$T_xN_xM_1$	<5

*American Joint Committee on Cancer (AJCC) International Union Against Cancer (UICC)

c. Can investigate and identify other areas in the colon.

VI. **Staging and Prognosis** (Table 77G-1)

TNM criteria

T_1: Involves the submucosa

T_2: Invades the muscularis propria

T_3: Penetrates through the muscularis propria and may penetrate into the serosa or pericolic fat

T_4: Invades other organs or the free peritoneal cavity

N_0: No nodes

N_1: One to three pericolic or perirectal nodes

N_2: Four or more pericolic nodes

M_0: No distant metastases

M_1: Distant metastases

VII. **Primary Treatment**

A. Surgery

1. Mainstay of treatment.
2. Fifty percent of patients cured.
3. Rectal cancer
   a. Middle third: low anterior resection.
   b. Lower rectum (2–3 cm to anorectal ring): proctectomy with colorectal anastomosis.
   c. If fixed or adjacent to anal sphincter, abdominoperitoneal resection is required (colostomy necessary).
4. Poor prognostic factors
   a. Symptomatic patient
   b. Obstruction
   c. Perforation
   d. Advanced stage
   e. Total lymph nodes involvement (involvement of four or more nodes is worse than involvement of me to three)
   f. High histologic grade

g. Mucinous or scirrhous adenocarcinoma

h. Abnormal DNA ploidy

B. Radiation therapy

1. Mostly used in advanced and unresectable disease for palliative purposes.

2. In very early rectal cancer (possibly with local excision), may be sphincter sparing and as effective as traditional surgeries.

VIII. Adjuvant Therapy

A. Rectal cancer

1. Radiation therapy

a. Postoperative radiation therapy is included in most programs because of a local recurrence rate >50% overall.

b. By itself, has no impact on survival compared to surgery alone.

c. Preoperative versus postoperative radiation therapy

(1) Preoperative therapy is still considered experimental.

(2) Results of studies are ambiguous.

(3) Theoretically better because it may improve resectability by shrinking the primary tumor and may be easy to administer than postoperative therapy.

d. Not indicated for stage I disease because of the high surgical cure rate.

2. Chemotherapy

a. Historically, 5-fluorouracil (5-FU) plus semustine (MeCCNU) is the only effective program when given with radiation therapy.

b. MeCCNU is too toxic (acute nephrotoxicity and chronic leukemogenesis).

c. 5-FU with levamisole and/or with leukovorin is currently being investigated.

3. Combined-modality treatment

a. Only survival advantage shown involves local radiation therapy and 5-FU–based chemotherapy.

b. Current National Cancer Institutes (NCI) recommended adjuvant treatment for stage II or III rectal cancer: local radiation (45 Gy over 4–6 weeks) with 5-FU as radiosenitizer and 5-FU alone before and after the radiation.

c. Active investigations

(1) 5-FU *infusion* as radiosensitizer, with postoperative and/or preoperative radiation therapy.

(2) 5-FU before and after radiation therapy with levamisole and/or leucovorin.

B. Colon cancer

1. 5-FU plus levamisole

a. Considered the standard of care (NCI consensus).

b. A 39% reduction and recurrence and a 31% improved overall 5-year survival compared to that achieved with 5-FU alone (p < 0.005).

c. Therapy consists of a loading dose of 5-FU (daily for first week) followed by weekly intravenous 5-FU for a total of 1 year. Levamisole is taken orally for 3 days every 2 weeks for the year.

d. Other programs (i.e., 5-FU plus leucovorin plus or minus levamisole) undergoing clinical trials.

IX. Prognosis

Varies according to stage (see Table 77G-1).

Bibliography

Alabaster O, Gilinsky NH. Colorectal Cancer. In: Ahlgren SD, MacDonald JS, eds. Gastrointestinal Oncology. Philadelphia, JB Lippincott, 1992, pp 241–395.

Cohen AM, Minsky BD, Schilsky RL. Colon Cancer. In: Devita VT, Hellman S, Rosenberg SA, (eds) Cancer - Principles and Practices of Oncology, Philadelphia, JB Lippincott, 1993, pp 929–976.

Cohen AM, Minsky BD, Schilsky RL. Rectal cancer. In: Devita VT, Hellman S, Rosenberg SA, (eds) Cancer - Principles and Practices of Oncology, Philadelphia, JB Lippincott, 1993, pp 978–1004.

Krook JE, Moertel CG, Gunderson LL, et al. Effective Surgical Adjuvant Therapy for High-Risk Rectal Carcinoma. *New Engl J Med* 324:709–715, 1991.

Moertel CG, Fleming TR, Macdonald JS, et al. Levamisole and Fluorouracil for Adjuvant Therapy of Resected Colon Carcinoma. *New Engl J Med* 322:352–358, 1990.

Steele G. Combined-Modality Therapy for Rectal Carcinoma The Time Has Come. *New Engl J Med* 324:764–766, 1991.

Wolmark N, Rockette H, Fisher B, et al. Leucovorin-modulated 5-FU as Adjuvant Therapy for Primary Colon Cancer: NSABP C-03, Proceedings of the American Society of Clinical Oncology 12:192, 1993.

Chapter 77-H

Biliary Tract Cancer

Edward H. Kaplan, M.D.

I. **Definition**
  A. Biliary tract cancers include malignancies of the gallbladder intrahepatic and extrahepatic bile ducts, ampulla of Vater and the adjacent duodenal mucosa.

II. **Etiology and Epidemiology**
  A. Most common in 60- to 70-year-old persons.
  B. Gallbladder cancer more common in women (70%).
  C. Cholangiocarcinoma more common in men (60%).
  D. Increased risks seen
    1. Chronic inflammatory states
      a. Cholelithiasis
      b. Calcification ("porcelain" gallbladder)
      c. Chronic cholangitis
      d. Typhoid carriers
        (1) Sixfold increased risk
      e. Ulcerative colitis
    2. Familial polyposis
    3. Liver fluke infestation
    4. Biliary stasis
    5. Exposure to carcinogens: rubber and chemical workers, automotive workers, wood-finishing workers.

III. **Incidence**
  A. Approximately 8,000 cases occur yearly.
  B. Less than 4% of all gastrointestinal malignancies.
  C. Includes gallbladder cancer and cholangio-carcinoma.

IV. **Natural History**
  A. Usually present with signs and symptoms mimicking common benign diseases.
  B. Symptoms usually reflect local spread of disease with obstructive liver disease.
  C. Most tumors discovered at surgery; diagnosis is rarely made preoperatively.
  D. Patients with early disease may have a favorable prognosis.
    1. Overall median survival is 4–6 months.
    2. For very early-stage disease, 5-year survival is more than 90%.
      a. Accounts for 5–10% of cases.

V. **Treatment**
  A. Surgery
    1. Usually palliative.
    2. Curative for early disease found incidentally.
  B. Radiation therapy
    1. Usually palliative.

2. May prolong survival when used with surgery.
   a. Improved outcome may occur with intraoperative radiation therapy.
C. Chemotherapy
   1. No established role.
   2. Overall response rates 10 to 24%.
   3. 5FU, Adriamycin and Nitrosureas are most active drugs.

VI. Prognosis
A. Average median survival for patients with resected disease is 20 months
   1. Mean operative mortality 9%

B. Average median survival for unresectable patients is 9 months

Bibliography

Lotze MT, Flickinger JC, Cair BI. Hepatobiliary Neoplasms. In: Devita VT, Hellman S, Rosenberg SA, (eds) Cancer - Principles and Practices of Oncology. Philadelphia, JB Lippincott, 1993, pp 900–907.

Wanebo HJ, Ahlgren JD, Hill MC. Cancer of the Biliary Tract. In: Ahlgren SD, MacDonald JS, (eds). Gastrointestinal Oncology. Philadelphia, JB Lippincott, 1992, pp 399–416.

CHAPTER 77-I

Renal Cell Carcinoma

Jules E. Harris, M.D.

I. Definition

In the United States in 1993 27,000 cases of kidney cancer were diagnosed. Of these, some 85% were renal cell carcinoma. That year, 11,000 persons died of the disease. The incidence of renal cell carcinoma has gone up some 30% over the past 20 years. Renal cell carcinoma is the third most common genitourinary tumor. It makes up 3% of all cancers seen in the United States. The term *hypernephroma* is also used to describe renal cell carcinoma. This term was first applied in the late nineteenth century, when it was widely believed that renal cell carcinoma arose from adrenal rests within the kidney. It is now known that renal cell carcinoma is an adenocarcinoma which arises from the proximal convoluted tubule cells of the kidney. The term *renal cell carcinoma* is preferred in the description of this malignancy.

II. Etiology

A. The male:female ratio for occurrence of renal cell carcinoma is 2–3:1.

1. This tumor occurs predominantly in the sixth and seventh decades of life. About 100 such tumors have been described in children under the age of 14. In this group, the sex ratio is approximately reversed. Renal cell carcinoma has been described in a child as young as 4 months.

2. The male:female ratio for occurrence of this tumor in adult life has been attributed to the activation by male hormones of enzymes in the kidney which catalyze the production of mutagens from substances such as dimethylnitrosamine.

3. Renal cell carcinoma occurs more often in urban areas and among higher socioeconomic groups in the United States. It appears to be more common in individuals of German or Scandinavian background.

B. Smoking is perhaps the single most important etiologic consideration in the development of renal cell carcinoma.

1. Approximately one-third of all cases that occur in men and about one-quarter of all cases that occur in women can be directly attributed to smoking cigarettes. The risk of renal cell carcinoma increases with the time and amount smoked. Cigar smoking, pipe smoking, and tobacco chewing are also associated with an increased risk of renal cell carcinoma.

2. Renal cell carcinoma has been reported to

occur more often in workers exposed to cadmium (used in batteries) and in coke-plant workers.

C. High relative weight in both men and women has been reported as a risk factor for renal cell carcinoma.

1. Weight gain in middle life associated with a high intake of animal fat may be the risk factor involved.

2. Diet pill use has been linked to the development of renal cell carcinoma; the use of diuretics such as hydrochlorothiazide and furosemide may increase the risk of this malignancy. Acquired renal cystic disease, which occurs in about 35% of patients on long-term intermittent hemodialysis, is associated in 6% of cases with the development of renal cell carcinoma. In the majority of instances, the disease is localized.

3. There is an increased risk of renal cell carcinoma associated with phenacetin use.

4. A low intake of vitamin A may contribute to the development of renal cell carcinoma.

D. There is an increased incidence of renal cell carcinoma in persons affected by the von Hippel-Lindau syndrome.

1. This autosomal dominant disorder involves an inherited susceptibility to hemangioendotheliomas of the central nervous system, angiomas of the retina, angiomas of the spinal cord, angiomas or cysts of the skin, lung, pancreas, liver, epididymis, kidney, pheochromocytoma, and renal cell carcinoma.

2. Individuals who develop renal cell carcinoma with this syndrome tend to develop the disease earlier in life, generally during the third and fourth decades. Some 10–25% of the individuals with the syndrome will develop renal cell carcinoma. There is a greater tendency for the disease to be bilateral. In this disease, the sexes are equally affected by renal cell carcinoma.

3. The syndrome is associated with a deletion in the short arm of chromosome 3. A sporadic familial form of renal cell carcinoma is also associated with abnormalities of the short arm of chromosome 3. In these cases, there is a translocation of the short arm of chromosome 3 to chromosome 8. Sporadic renal cell carcinoma of the nonfamilial type may also be associated with other abnormalities in the short arm of chromosome 3. These may involve dele-

tions of chromosomal areas which direct suppressor gene function. Other chromosomes which may be also involved with abnormalities in the sporadic nonfamilial form of renal cell carcinoma are chromosomes 7, 11, 13, and 17.

III. **Pathology and Staging**

A. Pathologic considerations in this disease involve appreciation of the cytoplasmic appearance and patterns of tumor growth.

1. Four pathologic types of this tumor, based on cytoplasmic appearance, are recognized. These are, with the relative frequency in parentheses, clear cell (25%), granular cell (12%), mixed (50%), and spindle or sarcamoid (15%). Granular and sarcamoid variants of this tumor may have less favorable prognoses.

2. The pattern of tumor growth in renal cell carcinoma may be solid, cystic, trabecular, tubular, or papillary. The last tumor growth variant is relatively avascular and has an approximately 1.5 times better 5-year survival than do the others.

B. There is a TNM staging classification for renal cell carcinoma, but the more widely used staging method remains that of Robson.

1. By the Robson staging, stage I renal cell carcinoma is characterized by tumor confined within the renal capsule. Stage II involves tumor invasion of perinephric fat, with the tumor still confined to Gerota's fascia. Stage III disease is associated with tumor involvement of regional lymph nodes and/or the renal vein and inferior vena cava. Stage IV disease describes tumor involvement of the adjacent organs or distant metastases.

2. At the time of initial presentation, 45% of patients have either stage I or II disease, 20% stage III disease, and 30% stage IV disease. Survival is dependent upon the stage of the disease, with the 5-year survival for stage I disease being 70%, stage II disease 60%, stage III disease 35%, and stage IV disease 5%.

3. The right and left kidneys are equally affected in the sporadic form of the disease; the disease occurs bilaterally in its sporadic form in less than 2% of cases. For reasons not known, the survival of patients with renal cell carcinoma of the left kidney is 1.5 times better than that of patients with the cancer in the right kidney.

IV. Diagnosis

The diagnosis of renal cell carcinoma is frequently made serendipitously because of the many varied and unusual clinical presentations of the disease.

A. Renal cell carcinoma has classically been described as presenting clinically with the triad of hematuria, groin pain, and a renal mass. In actual practice, these findings occur together in only about 10–15% of patients on initial presentation.

   1. When the triad does occur together, it is associated in more than 40% of cases with metastatic disease. Some 30–40% of patients have none of the classic triad of signs and symptoms at any time during their clinical course.

   2. About 30% of patients present with only weakness, anemia, and weight loss. Renal cell carcinoma should be considered in the differential diagnosis of any prolonged, wasting disease.

   3. Hematuria is found in about 40% of patients on initial presentation. It occurs in another 35% of patients at some time during their clinical course. In 70% of cases the hematuria is microscopic. In about one-half of those who present with localized disease, however, there is gross hematuria. Proteinuria is found in 90% of patients.

B. Metastatic disease is found in about 30% of patients on initial diagnosis.

   1. In those patients who have metastatic disease, the lung is involved in 50%. Metastatic deposits in the lung tend to localize in the endobronchial area. Hemoptysis and the coughing up of a tumor plug may result.

   2. Bone may be involved in up to 30% of patients with metastatic disease. The metastatic lesions to bone are characteristically osteolytic and oval in shape. The location of bone metastases is similar to that found with other solid tumors, with the axial skeleton frequently involved. Hypercalcemia may complicate this feature of metastatic disease. Cord compression may result from vertebral column metastases and should be suspected with complaints of back pain, especially with a radial distribution.

   3. The liver is involved in 30% of instances, and the tumor may spread in 10% of cases to the adrenal, colon, and spleen. Tumor may spread to the brain in 25% of cases and to the thyroid as well in 25% of cases. Uncommon sites of metastases are found. Tumor may spread to the iris, epididymis, corpus cavernosum, the gallbladder, and bladder.

   4. The presence of regional lymph node metastases in the retroperitoneal space correlates frequently with the existence of lymph node metastases above the diaphragm. There may be spread to the supraclavicular nodes by way of the thoracic duct. Axillary and inguinal lymph nodes may be involved in the absence of regional nodal spread.

   5. Ten percent of patients who live for more than 10 years following apparently successful surgical resection of primary disease will develop metastatic disease at a late stage in their clinical course. Metastatic disease may develop 30 years or more after a primary resection. In 1–3% of cases where metastatic disease results, the metastatic deposit is a solitary focus of disease. Surgical resection of the solitary metastasis in the lung is associated with a 35% 5-year survival. Survival following the development of metastatic disease is dependent on the time from initial diagnosis, the patient's performance status, and the number of metastatic sites of disease.

C. Paraneoplastic conditions occur in 30% of patients with renal cell carcinoma at some time during their clinical course.

   1. A nonspecific anemia is found in 40% of patients due to a toxic marrow factor or decreased production of erythropoietin. Hypochromic, microcytic anemia has been reported due to sequestration of iron by the tumor. On the other hand, about 4% of patients at diagnosis have erythrocytosis and an elevated hematocrit. Eosinophilia, leukemoid reactions, and thrombocytosis have been reported with renal cell carcinoma.

   2. An intermittent, variable fever may occur in 17% of patients; in 2% of cases this may be the only presenting sign. Renal cell carcinoma should be included in the differential diagnosis of fever of unknown origin. The fever results from an endogenous pyrogen produced by the tumor. It resolves with resection of the primary tumor.

   3. A hepatopathy with reversible hepatic dysfunction is found in 10% of cases

(Stauffer's syndrome). Histopathologically, the liver shows a nonspecific, reactive hepatitis of varying severity. The most constant finding is of proliferating Kupffer cells forming clusters and nodules. Inflammatory cell infiltrates with fatty degenerative changes are also seen. This syndrome may be associated with hepatosplenomegaly.

4. Amyloidosis may occur in association with renal cell carcinoma in 3–5% of cases. It may produce a nephrotic syndrome or hepatosplenomegaly. It is unaffected by removal of the primary tumor. A neuromyopathy (peripheral myopathy, polyneuritis, or muscular dystrophy) may develop with a similar frequency. It may improve with resection of the primary disease.

5. Hypertension can develop during the clinical course of renal cell carcinoma. It results from renin release due to either renal artery obstruction or compression of renal parenchyma. Hypertension or high-output failure may result from arteriovenous fistulas in either the primary tumor or its metastases. Release by the tumor of excessive amounts of prostaglandins may give rise to hypotension in a previously hypertensive patient. An acute varicocele which does not collapse with recumbency and which results from obstruction of the left internal spermatic vein may be a presenting sign of renal cell carcinoma.

6. Gonadotropin production by this tumor may rarely result in feminization or masculinization. Prolactin production may be associated with galactorrhea.

7. Other paraneoplastic conditions seen rarely in renal cell carcinoma include recurrent thrombophlebitis, spontaneous subcapsular renal hemorrhages, and immune complex glomerulonephritis.

8. Spontaneous regression of metastatic disease has been reported in renal cell carcinoma, but this probably occurs in less than 1% of cases. In the majority of cases where this does occur—90% of cases or more—the metastatic disease has involved the lung. Metastatic lung disease may resolve following removal of the primary in the kidney. Occasional resolution of metastatic disease of the lung has followed radiation therapy to the primary. Spontaneous regression does not necessarily mean cure; in 50% or more of the cases where spontaneous regression has been observed, there will be recurrence of disease with death following in as long as 15 years. There is no justification for the removal of a primary in the hope that spontaneous regression of metastatic disease will result. Operative mortality for surgical removal of a primary in such a setting may be as high as 2–10%. However, wherever possible in situations where patients present with metastatic disease, an effort should be made to remove the primary. Reasons for removal of the primary in the presence of metastatic disease are to prevent hematuria, pain, and a local tumor mass effect at a later stage in the patient's clinical course. Removal of the primary may prevent the development of hypercalcemia. Removal of a primary, thus "debulking" disease may make the patient more responsive to therapy with a biological response modifier such as interferon or interleukin-2.

V. **Treatment**

Curative therapy for localized renal cell cancer involves surgery alone. There is no satisfactory or effective systemic therapy for metastatic disease with either hormone therapy or cytotoxic drugs. Radiation therapy is reserved for the palliative treatment of bone pain due to bone metastases or for the local treatment of pain or obstruction by infiltrating disease.

A. Renal cell cancer may have estrogen and progesterone receptors in 15–85% of cases.

   1. When it was found in the 1940s that renal cell tumors could be produced in male Syrian golden hamsters with prolonged administration of estrogen, it was suggested that hormone therapy might be effective in renal cell carcinoma.

   2. Studies done in the late 1960s and early 1970s reported a 10–15% response rate using progestational agents. Responses obtained, however, were probably subjective, and rigorous evaluation of the results claimed for hormone therapy show no more than 1–3% of patients responding. The use of progestational agents, however, may provide symptomatic, palliative support for renal cancer patients no longer responsive to other forms of therapy.

B. The use of cytotoxic drugs in advanced, disseminated renal cell carcinoma produces infrequent and incomplete responses which last for very short periods of time.

1. Vincaleukoblastine and the nitrosoureas give response rates of no more than 10–15%. These response rates are almost always partial, and it is unlikely that they affect overall patient survival. Combination chemotherapy has not shown any benefit over the use of single drugs.

C. Biological response modifiers which stimulate or augment antitumor immune responses have been used successfully to treat renal cell cancer. Here, too, however, response and survival benefits are limited.

1. Varying doses, routes of administration, and schedules of interferon therapy give 15–30% response rates. A dose-response effect has been demonstrated with this agent. Responses seen have rarely been complete. Good prolongation of disease-free intervals following the response to therapy has been seen mainly in patients with pulmonary metastases with good performance status and a long interval between resection of the primary disease and the development of metastatic disease. The use of interferon for the adjuvant therapy of surgically resected patients with a bad prognosis is currently being evaluated.

2. Interleukin-2, given alone or with lymphokine activated killer cells (LAK) cells, produces the same response rate as with interferon, but about 10% of those patients who respond have a complete response and some of these responses have been durable, in excess of several years. Such responses may be seen in patients who have widespread metastatic disease involving liver, lung, and intra-abdominal tissue.

VI. Prognosis

Prognosis in renal cell carcinoma may be more a function of the biological nature of the disease than of therapy. At the time of initial presentation regional lymph node involvement in Stage III disease carries a worse prognosis than renal vein involvement (15% vs. 35% 5 year survival). Renal cell carcinoma is a disease which can, even in metastatic form, "smoulder" for many years. Non-resectable disease, however, is associated with a less than 2% 5 year survival. The median survival for patients who develop metastatic disease is about 8 months.

Bibliography

Holland JM. National history and staging of renal cell carcinoma. *CA* 25:121–153, 1975.

Laski M, Virgrin D. Paraneoplastic syndromes in hypernephroma. *Sem Nephrol* 7:123–130, 1987.

Malek R, Omess P, Benson R, et al. Renal cell carcinoma in von Hippel-Lindau Syndrome. *Am J Med* 82:236–238, 1987.

Neidhart J, Anderson S, Harris J. Vinblastine fails to improve response of renal cancer to interferon. *J Clin Oncol* 9:832–837, 1991.

Weiss G, Margolis K, Aronson F. A randomized phase II trial of continuous infusion interleukin-2 or bolus injection interleukin-2 plus lymphokine-activated killer cells for advanced renal cell carcinoma. *J Clin Oncol* 10:275–282, 1992.

Prostate Cancer

Jules E. Harris, M.D.

I. Definition

In the United States in 1993 there were 165,000 newly diagnosed cases of prostate cancer. In that year 35,000 men died of the disease. If a man in the United States lives to the age of 85 years, he has a 1/7 chance of developing prostate cancer; it is the single most common malignancy to affect males in the United States. The age-adjusted death rate due to prostate cancer has not changed in more than 40 years. Ninety-five percent of prostate cancers are adenocarcinomas which arise from the acinar epithelium of the prostate; about 2–3% of prostate cancers are transitional cell tumors or intraductal adenocarcinoma.

II. Etiology

A. Prostate cancer is primarily a disease of middle-aged and elderly males.

   1. The mean age at which prostate cancer occurs is between 65 and 70 years. This cancer is rare among men younger than 40 years. The youngest reported case has been in a man aged 34 years.

   2. In no other malignancy does the incidence of disease increase with age as much as in prostate cancer.

B. In the United States, prostate cancer occurs more often among blacks than among whites.

   1. The overall incidence of prostate cancer is 69 per 1,000,000; the incidence rises to 488 per 100,000 in whites aged 70–75 years and to 852 per 100,000 in blacks aged 70–75 years. Over the past 20 years the incidence has been increasing in both whites and blacks, but at a more rapid rate in the latter group (55% compared to 20%).

C. This is a cancer in which prevalence exceeds incidence.

   1. Some 50% of males in the United States over the age of 70 years may have histopathologic evidence of prostate cancer in situ (latent carcinoma) without clinical evidence of disease. This incidence of in situ disease is similar to that found among Japanese men who live in Japan. However, Japanese men who live in Japan have about 1/10th the clinical incidence of prostate cancer that black and white men in the United States have. When Japanese men move to the United States, their incidence

of clinical prostate cancer begins to approximate that of blacks and whites within one or two generations. An environmental influence is suggested by these epidemiologic observations; a high dietary consumption of fat may be the factor involved.

D. No definitive hormonal basis for the development of this cancer has been established.

    1. Suggestive evidence that some form of hormonal imbalance may be involved in the pathogenesis of this disease comes from the following observations:

        a. The disease is uncommon in patients with cirrhosis of the liver where levels of estrogen are high.

        b. Eunuchs do not develop prostate cancer, and the malignancy is uncommon in patients who develop bilateral testicular atrophy following paraplegia.

    2. Familial aggregations of prostate cancer have been reported, with the incidence being up to three times more common in men whose fathers or brothers have the disease.

    3. The disease may be more common in men who have been sexually active with many female partners.

    4. Prostate cancer may be more common among workers in the rubber and cadmium industries.

III. Pathology and Staging

A. There is a TNM staging system for prostate cancer, but the commonly used and accepted method for staging remains one based on stages A–D.

    1. Stage A disease is found on initial presentation in no more than 5% of patients. It cannot be detected on clinical examination of the prostate. It is most commonly found incidentally in prostatectomy specimens obtained following surgery for the clinically benign disorder of benign prostatic hypertrophy (BPH). With three or fewer microscopic foci of well-differentiated tumor, the stage reported is A1; with more than three such microscopic foci or with a high-grade or poorly differentiated tumor, the stage assigned is A2. Some 10% of patients operated on for BPH will be found to have stage A prostate cancer; one-third of these will have A2 disease. Stage A2 disease may be associated with pathologic spread outside the prostate in up to 20–25%.

    2. Stage B disease is palpable disease which is limited on clinical examination to the prostatic capsule. A lesion measuring up to 1.5 cm and confined to one lobe is considered to be stage B1 disease. Stage B2 disease is a single lesion larger than 1.5 cm involving one lobe or a lesion which involves both lobes. At the time of presentation, 5–10% of patients will have stage B disease.

    3. Stage C disease shows clinical evidence of spread beyond the prostate capsule to involve seminal vesicles or the side wall of the pelvis. Some 45% of patients present clinically with stage C disease. However, about half of these patients will have pathologic stage D disease.

    4. Stage D prostate cancer represents metastatic disease. About 45% of these patients present with this stage of disease. It is further substaged as stage D1 disease, with only pelvic lymph node involvement, and stage D2 disease, with involvement of extraregional lymph nodes, bone, or viscera.

    5. The overall 5-year and 10-year survival for prostate cancer patients is 60% and 40%, respectively. The 5-year survival by stage is: A 75%, B 70%, C 40%, and D 20%. Approximately 10% of stage D patients will live for 10 years, but 10% die within a year.

B. Prostatic cancers are evaluated by degree of cellular differentiation on a Gleason scale of 1–10.

    1. The more undifferentiated tumors of higher Gleason grade are more likely to have pathologic evidence of lymph node involvement at any stage of disease.

IV. Diagnosis

A. Most patients with prostate cancer present initially with symptoms of lower urinary tract obstruction.

    1. Some 65% of patients with prostate cancer present with symptoms of decrease in the force of their urinary stream, frequency, dysuria, retention, or hematuria. Occasional patients present with rectal obstruction due to prostatic enlargement or with edema of the lower extremities as the result of iliac lymphatic or venous involvement by tumor. Perineural involvement by tumor may produce pain referred to the bladder, urethra, rectum, sacrum, perineum, or gluteal regions. The pain may mimic sciatic pain.

B. In addition to complaints which may be referable to the lower genitourinary tract, the majority of patients who present with disseminated prostate cancer will have symptoms of bone metastases.

1. Patients with metastatic prostate cancer have bone involvement in 75–85% of cases. They usually complain of poorly localized lower back pain or stiffness or have signs of pathologic fractures of the vertebral column or long bones. Metastases to bone are osteoblastic in 80% of cases, mixed osteoblastic/osteolytic in 16%, and purely osteolytic in 4%. X-rays may be negative in 50% of patients with bone metastases; a bone scan is a necessary part of the diagnostic workup.

2. Metastatic involvement of viscera, chiefly the lung, liver and adrenals, does occur. Visceral involvement is found in 40% of patients at autopsy.

3. Despite the fact that lung involvement is found at autopsy in 25–40% of prostate cancer patients, x-ray evidence of lung involvement is found in only 5–10% of patients ante mortem. Pulmonary metastases may be nodular in appearance or may involve lymphangitic spread, with associated hilar adenopathy and respiratory insufficiency.

C. Digital rectal examination remains the single most important procedure in the clinical diagnosis of prostate cancer.

1. The digital rectal examination is a necessary part of any complete physical examination but is an absolutely essential part of the physical evaluation of males over the age of 50 years. A palpable hard nodule in a male over the age of 50 years has about a 50% chance of being malignant. Lesions as small as 2–3 mm in diameter may be palpable. The differential diagnosis of a palpable nodule includes acute or chronic prostatic calculus and prostatic infarct or thrombosis.

2. Palpable abnormalities suspicious for prostatic cancer include differences in the firmness or size of the prostatic lobes.

3. Transrectal ultrasound may be used to help determine the nature of suspicious palpable rectal lesions. When used in conjunction with digital rectal examinations, rectal ultrasound may increase diagnostic specificity and sensitivity. Studies using this approach for the screening of appropriate aging populations are now underway in the United States.

D. The use of prostate-specific antigen (PSA) determinations has increased the ability of clinicians to diagnose and monitor the clinical course of prostate cancer.

1. PSA is a glycoprotein of 33,000–34,000 molecular weight; it is produced in the prostatic alveolar and ductal epithelial cells. It is a proteolytic enzyme responsible for the dissolution of seminal gel formed immediately after ejaculation.

2. PSA is found in normal benign and malignant prostate tissue. Its level in the blood may be increased in BPH, acute or chronic prostatitis, prostatic infarction; during clinical, surgical, or diagnostic manipulation of the prostate; and in prostate cancer. A normal nonvigorous rectal examination of the prostate should not produce false elevations in PSA. Narrow ranges of 0–2.5 ng/ml for the polyclonal antibody assay and 0–4.0 ng/ml for the monoclonal antibody assay have been established. The results of one assay cannot be readily translated into results for the other assay. The half-life of PSA is about 2–3.5 days. Elevations in PSA correlate with advanced prostatic cancer but do so with less reliability in early localized disease. PSA determinations alone cannot be used for the screening of prostate cancer. Care must be taken in the interpretation of results which are less than 10 ng/ml. In the absence of clinical evidence of prostate cancer, these may be associated with BPH. Levels of PSA in excess of 10 or 20 ng/ml may be suspicious for prostate cancer but must be interpreted in the light of clinical findings. The use of PSA determinations has largely replaced the measuring of serum levels of prostatic acid phosphatase in prostate cancer diagnosis and follow-up. The measurement of prostate acid phosphatase is a relatively unreliable and insensitive measure of prostatic cancer activity.

3. The use of digital rectal examination, ultrasonography, and PSA determinations in conjunction may increase the specificity and sensitivity of efforts to diagnose prostate cancer in appropriate populations. There is as yet insufficient evidence of clinical benefit to justify widespread

screening utilizing PSA determinations and transrectal ultrasonography together.

4. The monitoring of PSA levels is of value in evaluating the effectiveness and completeness of surgical prostatectomies and the effectiveness of radiotherapeutic approaches to localized prostatic cancer.

5. The definitive diagnosis of prostatic cancer is dependent on histopathologic examination of prostate biopsy material.

E. Lymphangiography and computed tomography (CT) scans of the abdomen have been used in the diagnostic workup of prostate cancer patients to detect pelvic and intra-abdominal lymph node involvement.

   1. Lymphangiography is not commonly used to detect lymph node involvement because of the high (30%) false-positive rate (due to fatty infiltration of nodes in older men) and the high (30%) false-negative rate. It is not accurate for the detection of obturator, hypogastric, and presacral nodes.

   2. CT scans may detect lymph node enlargement in about 60% of cases. It is frequently possible to confirm the presence of tumor in these cases by fine needle biopsy.

   3. In disease which appears to be clinically localized, a growing practice is to sample surgically for the presence of iliac lymph node metastases at the time of laparotomy or by laparoscopy before efforts are made to perform a radical prostatectomy or implant radioactive seeds in the prostate.

V. Treatment

A. The treatment for stage A or B prostate cancer is radical prostatectomy.

   1. Advances in surgical technique make possible the sparing of neurovascular structures during radical prostatectomy and the preservation of potency in many cases. Radical prostatectomy may be complicated by urinary incontinence and urinary strictures. Patients with prostate cancer are frequently elderly, with other systemic disease, contraindicating radical surgery. Carefully directed radiotherapy alone or in combination with the placement of radioactive seeds in the prostate during exploratory laparotomy to sample pelvic lymph nodes for metastases may produce cures or long-term control of localized disease.

B. Radiotherapy is the treatment of choice for patients with stage C disease.

   1. The 5- and 10-year survival rates for patients with stage C disease treated with radiotherapy are 35% and 30%, respectively. Radiotherapy is associated with impotence in a number of patients and with lower incidences of urethral structure, enteritis, proctitis, or cystitis.

C. The treatment of stage D disease involves either orchiectomy or hormone therapy.

   1. Some 80% of patients with stage D disease have some symptomatic relief frequently associated with objective decreases in measurable disease and PSA levels following bilateral orchiectomy. Responses are rarely complete. This remains for many the treatment of choice for stage D prostate cancer. In the past, similar results were obtained by treating patients with low doses of oral diethylstilbestrol.

   2. Diethylstilbestrol, which was formerly associated with thrombophlebitis, fluid retention, and sometimes aggravation of preexisting arteriosclerotic heart disease, has now largely been replaced by the use of Leutinizing hormone releasing hormone (LHRH) agonists such as leuprolide. These agents have the advantage of being given parenterally only every 4–5 weeks. They produce the same type of response and response duration as does orchiectomy. They may be more effective when given in combination with the testosterone antagonist flutamide. Flutamide will at least prevent the clinical flare in disease activity frequently observed on initiation of LHRH therapy.

   3. Long-term control of metastatic disease for up to a decade or more may be seen with orchiectomy or hormone manipulation. However, the average patient treated in this manner has no more than about 18 months' control of disease. Active, progressive disease usually develops within 2–3 years. Salvage therapy with progestational agents or other testosterone antagonists may provide some additional measure of control for a few months. However, the median time to death following initial failure of either orchiectomy or primary hormone management is 7 months. About 80% of all patients die in 18 months.

   4. Various cytotoxic drugs such as 5-fluorouracil and cyclophosphamide, given alone or in combination, have given partial re-

sponses in hormone-insensitive prostate cancer in 15–30% of cases. Such responses rarely last for more than a few months.

5. Suramin, a binding inhibitor of epidermal growth factor (EGF), has been used in clinical trials for metastatic prostate cancer. Some partial responses of limited duration have been reported. A defined role for this agent in prostate cancer will await additional clinical and basic research.

VI. Prognosis

The prognosis in prostate cancer is for the most part dependent on stage of disease. This has focused increasing attention on efforts to diagnose the disease at an early stage in populations at risk, i.e., men over the age of 55 years in whom 95% of prostate cancer will occur. Annual digital rectal examination and PSA determinations are rapidly becoming an integral part of normal physical examinations for all North American men over the age of 50 years. This may result in an increased diagnosis of prostate cancer at an earlier stage; studies are currently being conducted to see whether this is associated with increased survival. A large clinical trial is also being conducted by the NCI (U.S.) to determine whether the use of finasteride, a 5-alpha-reductase inhibitor, will delay or prevent the development of prostate cancer in men over the age of 55 years.

Bibliography

Cupp M, Oesterling J. PSA, digital rectal examination, and transrectal ultrasonography: Their roles in diagnosing early prostate cancer. *Mayo Clin Proc.* 68:297–306, 1993.

Johansson J, Adami H, Andersson S. High 10-year survival rate in patients with early untreated prostate cancer. *JAMA* 267:2191–2196, 1992.

Littrup P, Lee F, Mettlin C. Prostate cancer screening; Current trends and future implications. *Ca* 42:198–210, 1992.

Nakao M, Babaian R. Limitations of early prostate cancer detection. *Cancer Bulletin* 44:24–31, 1992.

Naslund M. New concepts in the diagnosis and treatment of prostate cancer. *Update Series Comprehensive Oncology* 1:1–9, 1993.

Gynecologic Cancer

Sarah T. Lincoln, M.D.

I. Introduction
Gynecologic malignancies are common, representing 12.5% of female cancers, 4.6% of all cancer deaths, and 1.1% of national mortality. They affect women and children of all ages.

Cancer of the Corpus Uterus

I. Etiology
  A. Related to estrogen stimulation.
    1. Unopposed postmenopausal replacement.
    2. High-fat diet.
    3. Obesity.
  B. Familial in 10–25% of cases
    1. Alone.
    2. With breast and/or ovarian cancer.
    3. With colon cancer.

II. Incidence
  A. Most common gynecologic tumor (50%).
  B. Common female cancer (8%).
  C. Sixth leading cause of cancer deaths among women.
  D. Has increased over the last 20 years.

III. Epidemiology
  A. Median age of occurrence: 60 years.

IV. Pathology
  A. Adenocarcinoma (90%)
    1. Pure
      a. Papillary serous variant behaves like ovarian carcinoma and has a particularly bad prognosis.
    2. Adenoacanthoma (benign squamous elements).
    3. Adenosquamous carcinoma (both elements malignant-appearing).
  B. Mesenchymal
    1. Pure
      a. Endometrial stromal cell sarcoma (ESS).
      b. Leiomyosarcoma.
    2. Mixed Mullerian tumors (MMT)
      a. Homologous form = carcinosarcoma: Both glandular and mesenchymal elements are normally found in the endometrium.
      b. Heterologous mesenchymal elements *not* normally found in the endometrium (i.e., bone, cartilage, central nervous system) in addition to malignant glands.

V. Diagnosis

A. Most common symptom is postmenopausal bleeding.
B. Evaluation
   1. Office-based transvaginal endometrial biopsy.
   2. Same-day surgery: fractional dilatation and curettage.

VI. **Staging**
A. FIGO
   1. Stage I: Confined to the corpus
      IA: No invasion
      IB: Invasion <1/2 of myometrium
      IC: Invasion >1/2 of myometrium, not serosa
   2. Stage II: Extension to cervix
      IIA: Endocervical gland involvement
      IIB: Cervical stromal invasion
   3. Stage III: Pelvic or nodal metastasis
      IIIA: Serosal or adnexal disease plus washings
      IIIB: Vaginal metastasis
      IIIC: Pelvic or para-aortic nodes
   4. Stage IV: Other metastasis
      IVA: Bladder or rectal mucosal invasion
      IVB: Distant metastasis, including intra-abdominal or inguinal.
B. CT scan or MRI can identify pelvic and nodal metastases, but direct inspection and biopsy at surgery is more accurate and required for documentation, making these modalities redundant.
C. Ultrasound can identify pelvic masses and may suggest invasion, but again, hysterectomy is more accurate.
D. Barium enema may be obtained because of the frequent association of a second primary in the colon, although the cost effectiveness of this procedure has been questioned.
E. CA-125 levels are usually elevated only in patients with advanced disease but may be useful as a marker in that subgroup.
F. Clinical prognostic factors include uterine sounding (worse outcome when >8 cm) or by endocervical curetting (worse outcome when positive).

VII. **Treatment**
A. Stage I to include:
   1. Total abdominal hysterectomy–bilateral salpingo-oophorectomy (TAH-BSO).
   2. Sampling lymphadenectomy.
   3. Washings.
   4. Adjuvant external radiation therapy
      a. Grade 3, any substage.

      b. Stage IC, any grade.
B. Stage II to include:
   1. Radical hysterectomy (including lymphadenectomy).
   2. Washings.
   3. Adjuvant external radiation therapy.
C. Stage III options:
   1. Post-operative external radiation therapy if extent of disease is not appreciated preoperatively.
   2. Preoperative external and internal radiation therapy, followed by TAH-BSO if extent of disease is detected on clinical preoperative evaluation.
D. Stage IVA: Similar to above.
E. Stage IVB options:
   1. Chemotherapy.
   2. Palliative radiation therapy.
   3. Palliative TAH-BSO.

VIII. **Prognosis**
Stage I: 90%
Stage II: 75%
Stage III: 50%
Stage IV: 10%

Cancer of the Cervix (Mark Karides, M.D.)

I. **Etiology**
A. Women at increased risk for development of cervical cancer include those with early initial sexual activity, multiple sexual partners, early pregnancy, multiparity, and a history of sexually transmitted disease.
B. Almost 50% of the cases of cervical cancer show evidence of human papilloma virus (HPV) infection. HPV types 16 and 18 are common in cervical intraepithelial neoplasia (CIN).

II. **Incidence**
A. Third most common female cancer.
B. There are 13,000 new cases of invasive cancer and 7,000 deaths each year.
C. Peak age incidence is 48–55. Carcinoma in situ has a peak age incidence of 25–40.
D. The only female genital cancer which can be prevented by screening techniques (Pap smear).

III. **Clinical Signs and Physical Findings**
A. Early invasive cervical carcinoma can produce a vaginal discharge or bleeding. Pelvic pain is a late symptom.
B. Tumor mass can impinge on lumbosacral nerve roots, causing low back or leg pain.

C. Involvement of the bladder and rectum can lead to urinary frequency, hesitancy, hematuria, tenesmus, and rectal bleeding.

IV. **Pathophysiology**

A. Exact mechanisms for the development of cervical cancer are not known, but it appears that viral infection plays an important role.

B. Cervical dysplasia and carcinoma in situ precede invasive cervical carcinoma. Squamous cell carcinoma usually arises from the squamocolumnar junction of the cervix. Squamous cell carcinoma accounts for 90% of cervical cancer, adenocarcinoma 5%, adenosquamous carcinomas 2–5%, and clear cell carcinoma 1–2%.

C. Cervical cancer spreads by direct extension into the paracervical tissue, vagina, or endometrium; metastases occur primarily by the lymphatics.

V. **Diagnosis**

A. Cervical dysplasia, carcinoma in situ, and invasive cervical cancer can be detected by a Pap smear.

B. The American Cancer Society recommends that asymptomatic women 20 years of age and older and those under 20 who are sexually active have a Pap smear for 2 consecutive years and then one every 3 years. Women considered to be at risk should have a yearly Pap smear.

C. Abnormal Pap smears should be evaluated by colposcopy, with subsequent biopsy. All visible cervical lesions should be biopsied.

D. Routine staging for patients with cervical carcinoma includes a pelvic exam, liver function tests, creatinine, chest roentgenograms, cystoscopy, flexible sigmoidoscopy, and intravenous pyelography. CT scan is helpful in evaluating retroperitoneal lymph nodes.

VI. **Staging**

A. Stage 0: Intraepithelial carcinoma

B. Stage I: Confined to the cervix
  IA: Preclinical
  IA1: Minimal stromal invasion
  IA2: Measurable invasion <5 mm deep and 7 mm across
  (Note: Society of Gynecologic Oncologist SGO criterion for microinvasion used in United States is <3 mm invasion.)
  IB: Lesions >5 × 7 mm, confined to cervix

C. Stage II: Beyond cervix but not to distal vagina or pelvic wall

IIA: Upper two-thirds of vagina, not parametria
IIB: Obvious parametrial involvement

D. Stage III: To pelvic wall or distal vagina or hydronephrosis
  IIIA: Distal third of vagina
  IIIB: To pelvic wall and hydronephrosis

E. Stage IV: Other metastasis
  IVA: Bladder or rectal mucosal invasion
  IVB: Distant metastasis

VII. **Treatment**

A. Stage 0, which consists of carcinoma in situ or intraepithelial carcinoma, is managed with TAH. Women who wish to have children can be managed with cervical conization and close follow-up.

B. Microinvasive (stage 1A1, 1A2) carcinoma is managed with TAH.

C. Stage 1B and 2A carcinoma of the cervix can be managed by either radical hysterectomy and pelvic lymphadenectomy or radiation therapy.

D. Stage IIB and III disease is treated either with radical hysterectomy and pelvic lymphadenectomy or with radiation therapy. More advanced tumors are managed solely with external radiation therapy.

E. Stage IV disease is treated with radiation therapy and surgery.

F. Chemotherapy: Used in patients with stage IIIB and IV disease who have recurrent disease after surgery and radiation therapy and in patients who present with para-aortic nodal disease. It has also been used along with radiation therapy as a radiation sensitizer. Cisplatin is the chemotherapeutic agent with the best activity in cervical cancer.

VIII. **Prognosis** (5-Year Survival)
Stage I: 90%
Stage II: 75%
Stage III: 50%
Stage IV: 10%

Cancer of the Ovary

I. **Etiology**

A. Higher incidences of ovarian cancer have been reported in industrialized nations.

B. There is an association between the development of ovarian cancer and disordered endocrine function.

C. An increased incidence is found with nulliparity and a lower mean number of pregnancies.

D. Oral contraceptives reduce the risk, and there is no association between ovarian cancer and synthetic estrogen use.

E. Familial associations do occur but are infrequent.

II. Incidence

A. Ovarian cancer is the leading cause of death from gynecologic malignancy in the United States, surpassing that of cervical and endometrical cancer combined. It is the fourth most common cause of cancer death in women.

B. Roughly 1 in 70 women will develop the disease in their lifetime, with a peak incidence between the ages of 55 and 60.

III. Pathophysiology

A. Epithelial tumors constitute more than 85% of ovarian malignancies, with less than 10% arising from stromal cells and less than 5% from germ cells.

B. Epithelial tumors arise from coelomic epithelium and spread by intraperitoneal dissemination, lymphatic spread or, rarely, hematogenous spread.

C. Extraovarian spread most often involves the peritoneum. Locally, however, it can involve the contralateral ovary, uterus, fallopian tubes, and regional lymph nodes.

D. Distant metastases can involve the liver, lung, pleura, kidney, bone, adrenal gland, bladder, spleen, and CNS, in that order.

IV. Diagnosis

A. Early ovarian cancer is often asymptomatic and symptoms, when present, are often vague and ignored.

B. Seventy-five percent of patients will have disease which has spread out of the pelvis at diagnosis. Signs and symptoms include abdominal discomfort, abdominal swelling, vaginal bleeding, and, to a lesser extent, gastrointestinal and urinary tract symptoms.

C. At the present time, there are no useful tumor markers or noninvasive tests accurate enough to be used as screening tools.

D. Patients suspected of having ovarian cancer should have a thorough history and physical exam, including breast and pelvic exams, as well as a Pap smear.

E. Complete blood count, chemistry profile, and Ca-125 should also be obtained.

F. Chest roentgenograms, pelvic ultrasound, and complete CT scans of the abdomen and pelvis aid in determining the extent of disease.

G. Patients with urinary symptoms should be evaluated with intravenous urograms and cystoscopy.

H. Patients with gastrointestinal symptoms should be further evaluated with barium enemas and proctoscopy.

I. Staging laparotomy is performed on all patients and establishes the stage of disease as well as allowing for tumor debulking.

V. Staging

A. Stage I: Growth limited to ovaries
   1. Stage IA: Growth limited to one ovary: no ascites present containing malignant cells. No tumor on the external surface; capsule intact
   2. Stage IB: Growth limited to both ovaries: no ascites present containing malignant cells. No tumor on the external surfaces; capsules intact
   3. Stage IC: Tumor classified as either state IA or IB but with tumor on the surface of one or both ovaries; or with ruptured capsule(s); or with ascites containing malignant cells present or with positive peritoneal washings

B. Stage II: Growth involving one or both ovaries, with pelvic extension
   1. Stage IIA: Extension and/or metastases to the uterus and/or tubes
   2. Stage IIB: Extension to other pelvic tissues
   3. Stage IIC: Tumor either stage IIA or IIB but with tumor on the surface of one or both ovaries; or with capsule(s) ruptured; or with ascites containing malignant cells present or with positive peritoneal washings

C. Stage III: Tumor involving one or both ovaries with peritoneal implants outside the pelvis and/or positive retroperitoneal or inguinal nodes. Superficial liver metastasis equals stage III. Tumor is limited to the true pelvis but with histologically proven malignant extension to small bowel or omentum
   1. Stage IIIA: Tumor grossly limited to the true pelvis with negative nodes but with histologically confirmed microscopic seeding of abdominal peritoneal surfaces
   2. Stage IIIB: Tumor of one or both ovaries with histologically confirmed implants of abdominal peritoneal surfaces none ex-

ceeding 2 cm in diameter; nodes are negative

3. Stage IIIC: Abdominal implants greater than 2 cm in diameter and/or positive retroperitoneal or inguinal nodes

D. Stage IV: Growth involving one or both ovaries, with distant metastases. If pleural effusion is present, there must be positive cytologic findings to allot a case to stage IV. Parenchymal liver metastasis equals stage IV.

VI. **Treatment**

A. Early ovarian cancer

1. Patients with stage IA or IB disease with well or moderately well differentiated histology are managed with surgery alone. Long-term survival in this group of patients is 85%.

2. For patients with stage IC–IIC disease, chromic phosphate given intraperitoneally and oral melphalan both produce 80% 5-year survival.

3. Patients with stage IB, II, and asymptomatic stage III disease have achieved 78% 5-year and 64% 10-year survival rates with whole-abdominal irradiation.

B. Advanced ovarian cancer

1. Three-fourth of women with ovarian cancer present with stage III or IV disease. Response to therapy of bulky disease is dependent on tumor debulking to less than 2 cm in diameter. This is followed by platinum-based chemotherapy.

2. In patients who obtain a clinical complete response (normal physical exam, normal Ca-125 level, and normal CT scan of the abdomen and pelvis), second-look laparotomy may be indicated.

3. A variety of second-line therapies exist, including retreatment with platinum-based regimens and Taxol.

C. Miscellaneous therapies

1. Intraperitoneal chemotherapy: Has theoretical appeal for patients with minimal residual or recurrent disease.

2. Taxol: This new chemotherapeutic agent is a derivative of the Pacific Northwest yew tree. It has recently been approved as a second-line agent in refractory ovarian cancer. In this setting, objective response rates of 30% have been reported. The use of Taxol as a first-line agent is under investigation.

VII. **Prognosis**

A. Stage I: 80%
B. Stage II: 60%
C. Stage III: 20%
D. Stage IV: 10%

Special Topics

I. **Primary peritoneal adenocarcinoma**

A. Absent or uninvolved ovaries.
B. Similar to ovarian cancer in:
1. Presentation.
2. Clinical course.
3. Response to chemotherapy.
C. Thus, is treated like ovarian cancer.

II. **Fallopian tube cancer**

A. Rare.
B. Early-stage disease presentation.
1. Similar to endometrial cancer.
2. Treated with postoperative pelvic radia6tion therapy.
C. Advanced-stage disease presentation:
1. Similar to ovarian cancer.
2. Treated with postoperative platinum-based chemotherapy.

III. **Tumors of low malignant potential**

A. Epithelial ovarian cancer.
B. Well-differentiated, grade 1 histology.
C. No evidence of stromal invasion.
D. However, disease may involve other structure (e.g., lymph nodes, omentum).
E. Indolent natural history.
F. Treatment is surgery.
G. Chemotherapy and radiation therapy are of questionable value.

IV. **Germ cell tumors**

A. Median age of development: 20 years.
B. Pathology
1. Dysgerminoma (analogous to seminoma in males).
2. Teratoma.
3. Embryonal cell.
4. Yolk sac tumor (endodermal sinus tumor).
C. Previously, surgical approach was similar to that for epithelial ovarian cancer, including:
1. Second- and third-look evaluations, but using:
2. Non-platinum-based chemotherapy for a prolonged course.
D. Recently, the treatment approach has been similar to that for testicular germ cell cancers.
1. Surgery for diagnosis only.

2. Short course of platinum-based chemo-
    therapy.
3. Clinical follow-up.

V. Gestational trophoblastic disease (GTD)

A. Rare (<1% of female gynecologic cancers)

B. Spectrum of neoplasia
   1. Benign hydatidiform molar pregnancy.
   2. Locally invasive molar pregnancy.
   3. Choriocarcinoma.

C. May occur following:
   1. Molar pregnancy (50%).
   2. Abortion.
   3. Ectopic pregnancy.
   4. Normal term pregnancy.

D. Quantitative serum beta-human chorionic
   gonadotropin (β-hCG) titer
   1. Sensitive.
   2. Specific.
   3. Directly correlates with disease volume.
   4. Should be within normal limits within
      8–16 weeks of completion of pregnancy
      (delivery, evacuation, etc.).
   5. Used to follow the response to treatment.

E. Staging
   1. FIGO staging
      Stage I: Confined to uterus
      Stage II: Pelvic metastasis
      Stage III: Pulmonary metastasis
      Stage IV: Other metastasis
   2. Hammond classification
      a. Nonmetastatic GTD: No evidence of
         disease outside uterus.
      b. Good prognosis for metastatic GTD
         (1) <4 months from antecedent preg-
             nancy.
         (2) hCG <40,000 mIU/ml serum.

(3) No liver or brain metastasis.
(4) No antecedent term pregnancy.
(5) No prior chemotherapy.

c. Poor prognosis metastatic GTD: The
   opposite of the above.

3. WHO scoring system Table 77K-1.

F. Diagnosis
   1. CT scans of the head, chest, abdomen,
      and pelvis provide information about the
      presence of metastatic disease.
   2. Chest x-ray also will document pertinent
      lung metastases, since patients with lung
      metastases found on CT but not on chest
      x-ray respond to chemotherapy just like
      patients without metastatic disease.
   3. MRI or ultrasound may help to identify
      coexisting pregnancy or myometrial in-
      vasion by trophoblast.
   4. Serum hCG level is mandatory; patients
      with placental trophoblastic tumors may
      have elevations of human placental lacto-
      gen (hPL) as well.

G. Treatment
   1. Molar pregnancy
      a. Moles, both partial and complete, are
         treated with suction evacuation. Pito-
         cin should be given once the cervix has
         been dilated.
      b. Patients with uteri >16 weeks in size
         should be monitored invasively to de-
         tect trophoblastic embolization and
         pulmonary edema.
   2. Malignant GTD
      a. Nonmetastatic and good-prognosis
         metastatic GTD can be treated with
         methotrexate (protocols vary).

Table 77K-1. World Health Organization (WHO) Scoring System

Factor	0	1	2	3
Age	≤39	>39		
Prior pregnancy	Mole	Ab, ectopic	Term	
Months from end of pregnancy to therapy	≤4	4–6	7–12	≥12
hCG at initial therapy (mIU/mL serum)	<1,000	1–10,000	10,000–100,000	>10,000
ABO blood group			B or AB	
Largest tumor (cm)	<3	3–5	>5	
No. of metastases		1–4	4–8	>8
Site of metastases		Kidney, spleen	GI, liver	Brain
Prior chemotherapy			Single drug	≥2 drugs

Risk score: Low risk = ≤4, intermediate = 5–7, high = 8.

b. Most patients who fail can be salvaged with single-agent actinomycin-D every 2 weeks.

c. Patients who fail salvage therapy are treated as high risk.

d. Patients should receive two cycles of treatment after negative titers.

3. High-risk metastatic GTD

a. Can be cured with intensive multi-agent chemotherapy. Regimens include methotrexate, actinomycin-D and chlorambucil MAC and etoposide, methotrexate, actinomycin-D, cyclophosphamide, vincristin EMA-CO.

b. Radiation therapy to the brain may improve the prognosis for patients with brain metastases. Patients should receive three cycles of treatment after negative titers.

Cancer of the Vulva

I. Etiology

A. May develop from dystrophic or in situ lesions.

B. May be found in conjunction with Human papilloma virus (HPV), but it is not clear that the virus plays the etiologic role it may play in cervical lesions.

II. Incidence

Comprises 3–5% of gynecologic cancers and 0.3% of all female cancers.

III. Epidemiology

A. Median age of occurrence: 60 years.

IV. Pathology

A. Squamous cell: 90%

B. Basal cell: 3%

C. Paget's carcinoma in situ (cis) of glandular or ductal origin which spreads to the epidermis.

D. Verrucous peculiar cis of squamous epithelium.

E. Melanoma

V. Diagnosis

A. Often insidious—ignored by both patients and physicians.

B. Common symptoms

1. Pruritus

2. Bleeding

3. Pain

4. Asymptomatic in 20% of cases

C. Punch biopsy or wide local excision of small lesions is most common method of diagnosis.

D. Acetic acid applied directly may aid in delineating the abnormal area and target it for biopsy.

VI. Staging

A. Lymphatic spread is common and is usually orderly, from superficial inguinal to deep inguinal to pelvic lymph nodes.

B. TNM staging system (carcinoma of the vulva is the only gynecologic cancer staged by this system)

1. Stage 0: Intraepithelial carcinoma (Tis)

2. Stage I: Tumor ≤2 cm, confined to vulva (T1N0M0)

3. Stage II: Tumor >2 cm, confined to vulva (T2N0M0)

4. Stage III: Any size tumor with spread to the urethra, vagina, or anus (T3N0M0) and/or unilateral inguinal nodes (T1-3N1M0)

5. Stage IV: Other metastases

   IVA: Tumor invading the upper urethra, bladder mucosa, rectal mucosa, or bone (T4N0-1M0) or bilateral inguinal nodes (T1-4N2M0)

   IVB: Distant metastasis (T1-4N0-2M1)

C. Computed tomography (CT) scan or lymphangiogram may identify occult pelvic metastases requiring radiation therapy.

D. Cystoscopy or proctoscopy may be useful when tumors extend into the urethra or anus.

VII. Treatment

A. Primarily surgical, although radiation therapy may play a role and can be effective in unresectable lesions.

B. Stage 0 (noninvasive) options:

1. Simple vulvectomy

2. Wide local excision

3. "Skinning" vulvectomy

4. Radical vulvectomy; advocated by some as protection against the possibility of microscopic and unsuspected invasion found on pathologic review.

C. Stages I and II: Modified radical vulvectomy with ipsilateral (lateral lesions) or bilateral (central lesions) superficial lymphadenectomy. Nodes should be frozen intraoperatively and deep nodes dissected if superficial ones are positive. Patients with positive nodes should receive inguinal and pelvic radiation therapy.

D. Stage III: Radical vulvectomy with complete lymphadenectomy. Adjuvant radiation therapy for patients with positive nodes. Experiments with neoadjuvant chemoradiation therapy before surgery are promising.

E. Stage IV: If isolated in the pelvis and not fixed to bone, perform exenteration or give radiation therapy. If distant metastases exist, perform local excision to palliate symptoms and give chemotherapy or local palliative radiation therapy.

F. Paget's disease
  1. May require extensive surgery due to the glandular component.
  2. May be difficult to eradicate.

G. Verrucous tumors
  1. Also may be locally invasive, recurrent, and difficult to control.
  2. Radiation therapy and chemotherapy have no impact.
  3. Some feel that radiation therapy may accelerate tumor growth.

VIII. Prognosis
Stage 0: 100%
Stage I: 90%
Stage II: 80%
Stage III: 70%
Stage IV: 30%

Cancer of the Vagina

I. Etiology
A. Squamous cell carcinoma
  1. May be found in conjunction with HPV, but it is not clear that the virus plays the etiologic role it plays in cervical cancer.
B. Clear cell adenocarcinoma
  1. Often result of in utero exposure to diethylstilbestrol taken by the mother during pregnancy.
  2. Greater risk with exposure earlier in pregnancy ie within first one-third to one-half of pregnancy.

II. Incidence
Comprises 2% of all gynecologic cancers.

III. Epidemiology
  1. Median age of occurrence: 60 years.
  2. Median age: 20 years.

IV. Pathology
A. Squamous cell: >90%.
B. Adeno <10%.
C. Vaginal intraepithelial neoplasia (VIN)
  1. Refers to epithelioid lesions only i.e. squamous cell

  2. Analogous to but much less common than cervical intraepithelial neoplasia (CIN).
D. Verrucous
  1. Similar to verrucous lesions of the vulva.
  2. Very hyperplastic but noninvasive.
  3. However, can cause significant, life threatening problems due to obstruction etc.
E. Melanoma
F. Sarcoma botryoides: generally found in childhood.

V. Diagnosis
A. Usually found by abnormal Pap smear.
B. Common symptoms
  1. Bleeding
  2. Discharge
  3. Pain
  4. Often asymptomatic.
C. Cervical primary must be ruled out with four-quadrant negative cervical biopsies.
D. Colposcopy as follow-up for abnormal Pap with ascetic acid and directed biopsies.

VI. Staging
A. Spread
  1. Direct extension.
  2. Extensive lymphatic network.
    a. Upper vagina-pelvic and para-aortic lymph nodes.
    b. Lower vagina-inguinal and femoral lymph nodes.
B. International Federation of Gynecology and Obstetrics (FIGO)
  1. Stage 0: Intraepithelial carcinoma
  2. Stage I: Vaginal wall only
  3. Stage II: Subvaginal tissue
  4. Stage III: Extension to pelvic wall
  5. Stage IV: Extension to bladder or rectum or distant disease
    a. IVA: Bladder or rectal mucosal invasion
    b. IVB: Distant metastasis

VII. Treatment
A. Radical surgery and radiotherapy both play a role.
B. Stage 0 options:
  1. Wide local excision.
  2. Partial vaginectomy.
  3. Laser/cryosurgery.
C. Stage I options:
  1. Internal and external radiation therapy
  2. Radical hysterectomy/vaginectomy with lymphadenectomy.
D. Stages II, III, and IV: Radiation therapy, both internal and external.

VIII. Prognosis

Stage 0: >95%

Stage I: 80%

Stage II: 50%

Stage III: 30%

Stage IV: 20%

CHAPTER 77-L

Sarcomas

John L. Showel, M.D.

I. **Definition**
Sarcomas are tumors derived from mesoderm (Table 77L-1)
Note: Lymphomas, leukemias, and genitourinary tumors are not included in this classification.

II. **Etiology**
Unknown, except where sarcomas have been induced by high doses of radiation during therapy.

III. **Pathophysiology**
  A. Primarily that of massive, space-occupying tumors which have the capacity to invade, cause tissue destruction, and metastasize.
  B. Some sarcomas have curious predilections, such as embryonal rhabdomyosarcomas presenting as proptosis or vaginal bleeding (botryoid tumors) or adult osteosarcomas in a focus of Paget's disease.
  C. Some lesions grow and recur locally, producing massive, painful, destructive tumors before they metastasize. Examples are liposarcomas, angiosarcomas, leiomyosarcomas, and hemangiopericytomas.
  D. Others metastasize early in their development, usually to the lungs and occasionally to other sites, including bones and liver.

Examples are osteogenic sarcoma, Ewing's sarcoma, malignant fibrous histiocytoma, and rhabdomyosarcoma.

IV. **Diagnosis**
  A. Clinical presentation as a painful mass, often in the extremities, abdomen, or limb girdles.
  B. Radiographs are sometimes characteristic, as with osteogenic sarcomas.
  C. An adequate incisional biopsy is important. Plans for excision cannot be made without a firm histologic diagnosis. Electron microscopy and special histochemical stains may be useful.
  D. The local extent of the tumor must be defined as accurately as possible. Useful radiographic measures include limb computed tomography (CT) scanning and magnetic resonance imaging (MRI). Angiography may be helpful.
  E. A chest CT is mandatory in tumors which have a tendency to metastasize early.

V. **Differential Diagnosis**
  A. Other tumors must be distinguished from sarcomas by histologic criteria.
  B. High index of suspicion is required for persistent limb or limb girdle pain in children

Table 77L-1. Classification of Sarcomas

Childhood	Adult
Embryonal rhabdomyosarcoma	Liposarcoma
Ewing's sarcoma	Malignant fibrous histiocytoma
Osteogenic sarcoma	Angiosarcoma
Giant cell tumor of bone	Hemangiopericytoma
Chondrosarcomas	Neurofibrosarcoma
Synovial sarcomas	Leiomyosarcoma

and adolescents; x-rays should be done early.

C. A benign or low-grade process must be carefully differentiated from a malignant tumor because the treatment and prognosis will differ dramatically.

VI. Treatment

A. Wide local excision; this should be done by an experienced cancer surgeon. Limb-sparing procedures should be done when feasible.

B. Chemotherapy (systemic, with or without local infusion) should be employed early—sometimes prior to surgery in tumors which metastasize early, such as osteogenic sarcoma or Ewing's sarcoma.

C. Radiation therapy may be a useful adjunct to surgery where excision is, of necessity, marginal.

D. Metastatic disease is occasionally curable with chemotherapy or limited surgery.

VII. Follow-up

A. Physical examination every 3 months for the first 2 years, then every 6 months thereafter.

B. Chest films every 3–6 months for the first 2 years, depending on the tumor type.

C. Routine blood counts and chemistries every 3–6 months or as indicated, depending on whether the patient is receiving chemotherapy.

D. Early detection of recurrence is important because an occasional patient can be cured by excision of local metastatic disease.

VIII. Prognosis

A. Small tumors are usually curable with expert surgery and chemotherapy where indicated.

B. Widespread metastatic disease is rarely curable.

C. Chemotherapy has made a major impact on childhood tumors. This is not the case in adult tumors.

Bibliography

Bearhrs OH, Henson DE, Huttes RBP, et al. *Manual for Staging of Cancer*, ed 3. Philadelphia, Lippincott, 1988.

Del Regato JA, Spjut HJ, Cox JD. Sarcoma, in *Ackerman and Del Regato's Cancer*, ed 6. St Louis, Mo, Mosby, 1985, pp 907–967.

Table 77L-2. Sarcoma Staging

Stage	Grade	Size	Nodes	Metastases
IA	I	<5 cm	0	0
IB	I	>5 cm	0	0
IIA	II	<5 cm	0	0
IIB	II	>5 cm	0	0
IIIA	III	<5 cm	0	0
IIIB	III	>5 cm	0	0
IVA	Any	Any	+	0
IVB	Any	Any	Any	+

Source: Adapted from DeJong (1967) (see Bibliography).

Neurologic Tumors

John L. Showel, M.D.

I. Definition

Tumors arising in or invading the brain, spinal cord, or eye. Tumors of the nervous system may be divided by location or tissue of origin (Table 77M-1).

A. Orbital tumors
1. Ocular tumors
   a. Retinoblastoma
   b. Melanoma
2. Optic nerve tumor
3. Lymphoma
4. Embryonal rhabdomyosarcoma

II. Etiology

Unknown

III. Clinical Features (Table 77M-2)

IV. Diagnosis

A. Computed tomography and magnetic resonance imaging almost always helpful and frequently diagnostic.

B. Tissue is highly desirable, but patient safety must be considered.

C. Cerebrospinal fluid required for diagnosis of meningeal involvement with leukemia, lymphoma, or carcinoma.

V. Differential Diagnosis

A. Vascular lesions and hemorrhages

B. Infections

C. Psychogenic disorders

D. Trauma

VI. Treatment

A. Depends on whether the lesion is primary or metastatic and on the patient's general condition.

B. Glucocorticoid therapy should be started immediately and tapered slowly.

C. Excision is the treatment of choice except for lymphoma and myeloma.

D. Radiation is the definitive treatment for lymphomas of the spine and myelomas and is a necessary adjunct in the treatment of most other tumors.

E. Solitary brain metastases may be excised in selected patients.

F. Definitive stabilization procedures should be included where possible in the surgical management of localized spine tumors, even if they are metastatic.

G. Chemotherapy is beneficial in grade III astrocytomas and brain lymphoma. Intrathecal chemotherapy is beneficial in most patients with leukemic or lymphomatous involvement of the leptomeninges and is

Table 77M-1. Classification of Neurologic Tumors by Location and Histology

	Brain	Intramedullary	Extramedullary	Extradural
Neuroectodermal	Astrocytoma Oligodendroglioma Ependymoma Pinealoma Ganglioneuroma Neuroblastoma Glioblastoma multiforme Medulloblastoma	Glioma Oligodendroglioma Ependymoma	Ganglioneuroma	
Meningeal	Benign Anaplastic Dural sarcomas Angiomatous		Benign Anaplastic Sarcoma Angiomatous	
Nerve sheath	Rare			

Lymphoma	Primary
	Spread from
	  outside CNS
			Primary intradural
			  lymphoma
				Spread from
				  outside CNS
				Primary extradural
				  lymphoma

Vascular	Hemangioblastoma Monstrocellular sarcoma	Hemangioblastoma	Vascular tumors	

Rare tumors and
  tumor-like
  conditions
	Xanthoma
	Primary melanotic
	Craniopharyngioma
			Lipomas
			Other sarcomas
				Chondroma
				Chondrosarcoma
				Osteogenic sarcoma
				Ewing's sarcoma
				Soft tissue sarcoma
				Myeloma

Metastatic tumors	Lung Breast Renal Germ cell Others	Rare (lung)		Prostate Breast Renal Lung Others

Table 77M-2. Clinical Features of Neurologic Tumors

Brain	Intramedullary Cord	Extramedullary Cord

Seizures (focal or generalized)
Increased intracranial pressure
  (headache, confusion, lethargy)
Focal signs and symptoms (e.g.,
  aphasia, ataxia)
Temporal lobe seizures
Personality changes
	Burning pain that is poorly
	  localized
	Spotty defects in sensation
	Saddle area symptoms not
	  marked
		Radicular pain
		Contralateral loss of pain and
		  temperature with ipsilateral
		  loss of proproception
		Saddle area symptoms more
		  marked than those at level of
		  lesion
		Pyramidal tract finding early and
		  marked
		Spinal subarachnoid block early
		  and marked

Source: Adapted from DeJong (1967) and Zulch (1986) (see Bibliography).

occasionally beneficial in meningeal carcinomatosis.

VII. Patient Monitoring

A. Postoperative monitoring should be frequent and careful, watching for early signs of hemorrhage or infection or increased pressure from fluid collections.

B. Mental and neurologic deterioration usually indicates tumor growth.

C. Dilantin toxicity indicated by lethargy and ataxia. Serum levels should be kept therapeutic to avoid seizures.

VIII. Prognosis

A. Glioblastoma multiforme has a poor prognosis, with survival rarely exceeding 1 year.

B. Other brain tumors, depending on their location, have variable courses. Low-grade lesions are sometimes cured.

C. The above statements apply to intramedullary cord tumors.

D. Early, adequate intervention in extradural tumors can preserve function for the remainder of the patient's course.

E. Patients who are paraplegic from metastatic disease are miserable and rarely live for more than a few weeks. This is especially tragic if the rest of the patient's disease is well controlled.

Bibliography

DeJong, RM. *Neurological Tumors*. New York, Holber Medical Division, Harper and Row, 1967.

Zulch KJ. *Brain Tumors*, ed 3. Berlin, Springer-Verlag, 1986.

CHAPTER **77-N**

Malignant Melanoma and Its Precursors

Janet M. Wolter, M.D.

I. Definition and Description

A. Malignant melanoma is a cancer of melanocytes, the cells in the skin that produce the protective pigment melanin. When transformed, these cells grow without control. Usually the pigment-producing ability is retained, and melanomas and even metastases from them are brown or black. A few lose the pigment-producing ability and are flesh-colored, or amelanotic, melanomas.

B. Precursor lesions are abnormal moles, or dysplastic nevi, that may occur sporadically or in families. They occasionally develop into melanomas and also serve as markers for individuals at higher than average risk of developing a melanoma.

C. There are five types of cutaneous melanoma.

1. Superficial spreading melanoma
   a. About 70% of patients.
   b. Often occurs in preexisting nevi.
   c. Usually larger than 1 cm.
   d. May start as a heavily pigmented area in an ordinary mole.
   e. Flat initially, then gradually becomes papular.

f. Borders may be notched.
g. Usually grows slowly initially, then more rapidly.

2. Nodular melanoma
   a. From 15% to 30% of patients.
   b. More aggressive tumor with a shorter growth period.
   c. Raised from inception.
   d. Pigmentation dark and uniform.
   e. Clearly defined border.
   f. Usually 1–2 cm in diameter (but may be smaller).

3. Lentigo maligna melanoma
   a. From 4% to 10% of patients.
   b. Slow growth pattern, with little propensity to metastasize.
   c. Generally large (more than 3 cm) and flat.
   d. Usually occurs over the age of 50.
   e. More common in women than in men.
   f. Average history is 10 years.

4. Acral lentiginous melanoma
   a. From 2% to 8% of white patients, 35–60% of blacks, Orientals, and Hispanics.
   b. Usually large, 3 cm or more in diameter.

c. Occurs on palms and soles or beneath nail beds.

d. Majority occur on soles of feet.

e. Occurs in older people.

f. Usually flat, resembling a stain on the sole or palm.

g. Borders are irregular.

h. More aggressive and more likely to metastasize than lentigo maligna melanomas.

5. Subungual melanoma

   a. Accounts for 2% of whites and for a larger percentage in pigmented people.

   b. Seen in older patients.

   c. More than 75% occur on thumbs and big toes.

   d. Black or brown discoloration in nail bed.

   e. Hard to differentiate from subungual hematoma.

   f. Often identified by nodal metastases.

D. Differential diagnosis

1. Seborrheic keratoses

   a. Waxy.

   b. Appear to be "stuck on."

   c. Edge can be lifted.

2. Junctional nevi

   a. Usually about 15 per person.

   b. Most smaller than 1 cm.

   c. Round with smooth edges.

   d. Evenly pigmented.

   e. Flat.

3. Compound nevi

   a. As above but palpable.

   b. May be slightly darker than junctional nevi.

4. Dermal nevi

   a. Dome-shaped (due to collection of deep melanocytes).

   b. Very little pigment.

   c. May be congenital.

5. Hemangiomas

   a. Should empty and then refill on pressure/release with a glass slide.

   b. May appear blue-black. If blood clotted, the emptying sign may be absent.

6. Blue nevus

   a. Small.

   b. Blue-black color.

   c. Slightly palpable.

   d. Unchanging through the years.

7. Pigmented basal cell cancer

   a. Common.

   b. Long, slow course.

   c. Raised from the beginning.

   d. Pearly appearance may be distinguished through the pigment.

8. Spitz nevus

   a. Children aged 5–10 (when melanoma is very rare).

   b. Surface smooth.

   c. Not deeply pigmented.

9. Dysplastic nevi

   a. Hardest to distinguish from melanoma.

   b. Often larger than 1 cm.

   c. Borders are irregular.

   d. Pigmentation may be irregular.

   e. Often a pinkish cast to pigmentation.

   f. Usually flat.

   g. Occur in sun-exposed areas but also outside of such areas.

     (1) Breasts

     (2) Abdomen and buttocks.

   h. Often multiple. Patients with dysplastic nevus syndrome (DNS) may have more than 100.

   i. Sporadic dysplastic nevi may become melanomas, and persons with DNS are more likely to develop melanomas.

   j. Persons with the characteristics of DNA should have at least one lesion biopsied for histologic confirmation, should be taught self-examination, and should be inspected by experts on a regular basis (at least once a year).

10. Because pictures are much better than words, the National Cancer Institute has available color photographs of these lesions in a free booklet called "What You Need to Know About Dysplastic Nevi." Order from 1-800-4-CANCER.

E. When there is any doubt, excisional biopsy should be performed by an individual trained to think of the consequences of incision orientation and possible subsequent wider excision. Skin biopsy specimens should be examined by trained dermatopathologists unless the diagnosis is obvious (seborrheic keratoses or basal cell carcinoma).

II. Etiology and Demographics

A. Sun exposure is the most important known risk. Highest incidence occurs in sunny areas such as:

1. Southern United States.
2. Australia.
3. Israel.
B. Acquired dysplastic moles increase the risk. These occur as follows:
   1. Sporadic: 5–10% of the population.
   2. Familial: rarer but also carries a higher risk.
C. Congenital moles (birth marks) carry increased risk. Should be removed if small and accessible.
D. Although seen from puberty on, incidence increases with age.
E. Seen more often in people with a family history of melanoma.
F. Highest incidence in fair-skinned, blue-eyed blonds or redheads who sunburn or freckle easily.
G. Incidence increased in people who spend a great deal of time in the sun, especially if they sustained severe sunburns in their teens or early twenties.

III. Incidence
A. Most rapidly increasing cancer.
B. While the U.S. population increased 11% from 1980 to 1989, the number of melanomas increased 94%.
C. Risk was 1:1,500 in 1935 but will be 1:90 by 2000 (Figure 77N-1).
D. Thought to be due to increased sun exposure:
   1. More leisure time.
   2. Less protective clothing.
E. Mortality rate down somewhat over the past 10 years, presumably due to increased early detection, leading to more cures.

IV. Pathology
A. Histologic features with prognostic significance
   1. Tumor thickness (Breslow measurement)
      a. Distance from upper level of epidermis to deepest part of tumor.
      b. Done with ocular micrometer on microscope.
      c. Sections must be carefully oriented vertically.
      d. Single most important indicator of the prognosis.
   2. Level of invasion (Clark) of malignant cells
      a. Level I: In epidermis.
      b. Level II: Into papillary dermis.
      c. Level III: To base of papillary dermis.
      d. Level IV: Into reticular dermis.
      e. Level V: Into subcutaneous fat.
      f. Not easy to determine when there has been regression or fibrosis.
      g. Does not apply to polypoid or mucosal melanomas.
      h. Good (but not the best) correlation with prognosis.
   3. Ulceration: very bad prognostic sign.
   4. Growth pattern
      a. Horizontal: may not have metastatic potential.
      b. Vertical: metastatic potential.
      c. Correlates with (1) and (2) above.
      d. Mitotic activity.
         (1) May be an independent prognostic factor.
         (2) Generally correlates with thickness of tumor.
      e. Regression: significance still uncertain.
      f. Lymphocytic reaction correlates with thickness (deeper lesions have fewer lymphocytes).
      g. Risk factors (Table 77N-1).
   5. Staging
      a. Original
         (1) Stage I: Localized primary melanoma.
         (2) Stage II: Metastases to regional nodes or metastases in transit.
         (3) Stage III: Disseminated disease.

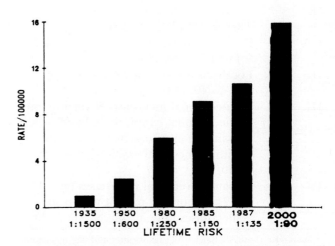

Figure 77N-1. Projected lifetime risk for developing malignant melanoma in the United States: past, present, and future. (From Rigel DS, Kopf AW, Friedman RJ. Incidence and mortality rates of malignant melanoma in the U.S. *The Melanoma Letter* 7(1):2–3, 1989.)

Table 77N-1. Melanoma: Major Factors Predicting Clinical Course

Factor	Unfavorable If:
Stage I (localized melanoma lesion)	
Thickness of tumor	>1.5 mm
Ulceration	Present
Gender	Male
Location	Trunk
Stage II (regional metastases)	
Number of lymph nodes with demonstrable metastases	More than one
Ulceration	Present
Gender	Male
Stage III (distant metastases)	Viscera
Number of sites	More than one

     b. American Joint Committee on Cancer (Table 77N-2)

V. Surgical Management

  A. Identification

    1. Excisional biopsy for lesions 1.5 cm or less (best done by the person who will do the definitive surgery, should that be necessary).

Table 77N-2. Melanoma Staging: American Joint Committee on Cancer

Stage	Criteria
IA	Localized melanoma ≤0.75 mm or level II+ (T1, N0, M0)
IB	Localized melanoma 0.76–1.5 mm or level III* (T2, N0, M0)
IIA	Localized melanoma 1.5–4 mm or level IV* (T3, N0, M0)
IIB	Localized melanoma >4 mm or level V* (T4, N0, M0)
III	Limited nodal metastases involving only one regional lymph node basin or less than five in-transit metastases but without nodal metastases (any T, N2, M0)
IV	Advanced regional metastases (any T, N2, M0) or any patient with distant metastases (any T, any N, M1 or M2)

Source: Ketcham AS, Balch CM. Classification and staging systems, in Balch CM, Milton GW (eds), *Cutaneous Melanoma: Clinical Management and Treatment Results Worldwide.* Philadelphia, Lippincott, 1992, p 59.

*When the thickness and level of invasion criteria do not coincide within a T classification, thickness should take precedence.

    2. Should include a narrow margin (2 mm) of normal skin (more is too much for a benign lesion and may be too little for a malignant one).

    3. Incision should be oriented with careful attention to possible necessity of more extensive surgery.

    4. Incision (preferably punch from the center) for lesions too large for excision or in an area where the extent of skin removed is critical (e.g., the face).

  B. Definitive treatment

    1. Complete excision is mandatory even if skin graft is necessary for closure.

    2. Surgical margins

      a. For anatomic sites where specific margins cannot be attained, widest practical margin must be accepted.

      b. Optimum margin width still not known.

        (1) Used to be very wide.

        (2) 1–3 cm margin has been shown to yield no increased incidence of recurrence.

        (3) Randomized trial of wide versus narrow margins (Sept., 1993) showed no survival difference in 1–4 mm. melanomas.

      c. Removal of deep margin (fascia) adds nothing to survival, but excision should be down to fascia.

    3. Elective regional node dissection

      a. Still controversial.

      b. Many trials performed.

      c. Recent randomized trial (dissection vs. no dissection) not yet published.

      d. Many surgeons do dissection only when it can conveniently be done in-continuity (one incision to remove both the melanoma and draining lymph nodes).

      e. May be beneficial in patients with lesions 1.5–4 mm deep.

        (1) Probably not justifiable in lesions less than 1.5 mm thick.

        (2) Not justifiable in lesions deeper than 4 mm because chance of systemic disease is very high.

      f. Elective lymph node dissection may be therapeutic but also may identify candidates for adjuvant treatment when an effective one becomes available.

      g. Morbidity can be considerable, especially in lower extremities.

4. Therapeutic regional node dissection is always indicated if there is no evidence of systemic disease and one or more lymph nodes can be demonstrated to contain melanoma. This can be done at the time of primary removal or at any later date when the node is detected.

VI. Adjuvant Treatment

A. None clearly beneficial.
1. Chemotherapy programs have not worked.
2. Biological response modifier programs still in early analysis.
    a. Interferon-α.
    b. Interferon-γ.
    c. Even if trials prove to be slightly positive, toxicity is troublesome.
3. Immunostimulants alone and in combination with chemotherapy do not work.
    a. Bacille Calmette-Guérin (BCG) and Methanol Extracted Residue of BCG (MER).
    b. BCG plus various chemicals.

B. Vaccines: Still under investigation.
1. Viral oncolysates.
2. Gangliosides.
3. Anti-idiotype monoclonal antibodies.

C. High-risk patients should be entered into clinical trials. No adjuvant treatment justifiable outside a trial.

VII. Treatment of Metastatic Disease

A. Evaluation
1. Gallium scan frequently helpful.
2. Chest x-ray, liver function tests, complete blood count, computed tomography scans.
3. Brain evaluation essential before embarking on major therapy.
    a. Brain metastases frequent.
    b. Unlike most other tumors, may go directly to brain without involving regional nodes or lungs.

B. Surgical treatment
1. Solitary metastases can be removed if necessary, even in the brain.
2. May be very useful for painful or potentially hemorrhagic sites such as the small bowel.
3. Regional perfusion and hyperthermia of an extremity with metastases in transit may be helpful.

C. Medical treatment
1. Chemotherapy
    a. Very low response rate to single drugs.

b. Dacarbazine (DTIC) produces the most frequent responses (±15%).
c. Bischloronitrosourea (BCNU) and other nitrosoureas are the next most active drugs.
d. In the past, combinations were not better (and were more toxic) than single drugs.
e. Newer effective drugs.
    (1) Cisplatin.
    (2) Carboplatin.
    (3) Taxol.
f. One promising new combination is DTIC, BCNU, cisplatin, and tamoxifen.
    (1) Has a 52% response rate.
    (2) Does not work when tamoxifen is left out.
    (3) High incidence of thromboembolic events needs to be addressed.
2. Biological therapy
    a. Interferon-α2: 16% response rate.
    b. Interleukin-2: 25% response rate.
    c. Interleukin-2 plus Lymphokine-Activated Killer (LAK) cells: 20% response rate.
    d. Interleukin-2 plus tumor-infiltrating lymphocytes: 42% response rate.
    e. All are very toxic.

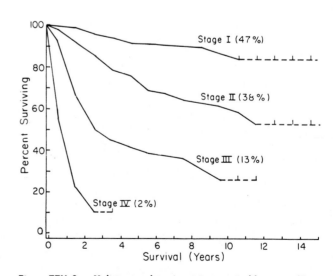

Figure 77N-2. Malignant melanoma: patient survival by stage. (From: Ketcham AS, Balch CM. Classification and staging systems, in Balch CM, Milton GW (eds), *Cutaneous Melanoma: Clinical Management and Treatment Results Worldwide.* Philadelphia, Lippincott, 1992, p 59.)

(1) Interferon: malaise, flu-like syndrome, liver toxicity.
(2) Interleukin-2: fluid-leak problems in lungs and fever. May require monitoring in the intensive care unit.
3. Vaccines and monoclonal antibodies under early study.

VIII. Prevention
A. With such a deadly disease, all health care professionals should learn to recognize precursor lesions and urge sun protection.
B. No such thing as a "healthy" tan.

IX. Prognosis
A. Depends on the depth and stage of the tumor.
B. Almost all early (thin) melanomas can be cured.
C. As depth and stage increase, the danger increases (Figure 77N-2).
D. Metastatic disease is a rapid killer.

Bibliography

Balch CM. The role of elective lymph node dissection in melanoma: Rationale, results, and controversies. *J Clin Oncol* 6:163–172, 1988.

Balch CM, Houghton A, Peters L. Cutaneous melanoma, in De Vita VT, Hellman S, Rosenberg SA (eds), *Cancer: Principles and Practice of Oncology*, ed. 3. Philadelphia, Lippincott, 1989, pp 1499–1542.

Balch CM, Urist MM, Karakousis CP, et al. Efficacy of 2-cm surgical margins for intermediate-thickness melanomas (1–4 mm). *Ann Surg* 218:262–267, 1993.

Greene MH, Clark WH Jr, Tucker MA, et al. Acquired precursors of cutaneous malignant melanoma. *N Engl J Med* 312:91–97, 1984.

Koh HK. Medical progress: Cutaneous melanoma. *N Engl J Med* 325:171–182, 1991.

National Institutes of Health Consensus Development Conference. NIH Consensus statement: Diagnosis and treatment of early melanoma. *NIH* 10(1):1–25, 1992.

Rigel DS, Kopf AW, Friedman RJ. The rate of malignant melanoma in the United States: Are we making an impact? *J Am Acad Oncol Dermatol* 17:1050–1053, 1987.

CHAPTER 78

Cancers of Unknown Primary Sites

Charles R. Thomas, Jr., M.D.

I. **Definition**

Cancers of unknown primary sites (CUPS) are biopsy-proven malignancies which lack clear cut histologic characteristics of a primary organ.

A. There is no evidence of a primary tumor site after a directed diagnostic evaluation.

B. From 0.5% to 7% of patients presenting with metastatic disease have CUPS. Up to two-thirds of these tumors are multifocal.

II. **Etiology**

By definition, no clear-cut etiologic determinants can be ascertained in CUPS.

III. **Pathology**

A. It is critical that enough tissue be obtained to undertake the appropriate pathologic assessment of the characteristics of the tumor in question. One-third of the specimen should be snap frozen for immunocytochemistry (ICC); one-third should be fixed in glutaraldehyde for electron microscopic analysis; and one-third should be fixed in formalin for light microscopic analysis.

B. Histologic examination can yield myriad tumor cell types, especially if a tissue section specimen is available; as opposed to a fine needle aspiration (FNA).

1. Adenocarcinoma
   a. Has a more glandular pattern of variation.
   b. Over one-third of adenocarcinomas are poorly differentiated.
2. Undifferentiated carcinoma.
3. Poorly differentiated carcinoma.
4. Squamous cell carcinoma.
5. Germ cell tumors.
6. Neuroendocrine tumors.
7. Less common types include sarcomas (partially characterized by spindle-cell morphology), melanoma, and non-Hodgkin's lymphoma.

C. Tumor markers can be helpful in determining the organ of origin, as well as in predicting the likelihood of response to selected therapeutic intervention strategies.

1. Carcinoembryonic antigen (CEA) is often elevated in epithelial cell tumors such as breast cancer, gastrointestinal tract tumors, liver metastases, and non–small cell lung cancer (NSCLC).
2. CA 19-9 may be elevated in patients with a clinical spectrum suggestive of pancreatic cancer.

3. CA 125 is elevated in ovarian cancer and in any other tumor that may invade the coelomic epithelium.

4. CA 15-3 may be elevated in breast cancer.

5. Alpha-fetoprotein (AFP) is classically elevated in hepatocellular carcinoma and germ cell neoplasms. It is also elevated, but to a lesser degree, in an assortment of benign liver diseases.

6. Neuron-specific enolase (NSE) is elevated in small cell lung cancer (SCLC), neuroendocrine tumors, and neuroblastoma.

7. Prostate-specific antigen (PSA) is elevated in prostate cancer but may also be elevated in benign prostatic disease, though to a lesser extent.

8. Beta-human choriogonadotrophin (B-HCG) is elevated in germ cell tumors.

D. Immunohistochemistry
1. The stains most often utilized are mucin, which is often positive for adenocarcinomas, and glycogen, which is often positive for renal cell carcinoma.

E. Immunocytochemistry (ICC)
1. ICC use has become widespread since the advent of unconjugated immunoenzyme techniques, such as the peroxidase-antiperoxidase Table 78-1 (PAP) and the avidin-biotin immunoperoxidase complex (ABC) methods.

2. Staining for tumor markers such as CEA, epithelial membrane antigen (EMA), leukocyte antigen (LCA), S-100, and estrogen/progesterone (ER/PR) status may prove useful.
   a. CEA may indicate that the tumor might behave like a gastrointestinal tract, lung, or breast primary.
   b. EMA is more representative of breast cancer.
   c. Keratin, via the AE1/AE3 monoclonal antibodies, can be expressed in squamous cell tumors from a variety of sites (i.e. NSCLC, anal, esophagus, cervix, and head and neck.
   d. LCA may be elevated in lymphomas.
   e. S-100 may be expressed in melanomas, as may Factor VIII–related antigen in angiosarcomas.

F. Electron microscopy.
G. Molecular diagnosis.

IV. **Diagnosis**
A directed evaluation should be undertaken. It should be based on the patient's age, sex, available

Table 78-1. Useful Immunoperoxidase Staining Patterns in the Differential Diagnosis of Poorly Differentiated Neoplasms

Tumor Type	Immunoperoxidase Staining Characteristics
Carcinoma	Epithelial stains (e.g., cytokeratin. EMA) (pos.)
	LCA, S-100, vimentin (neg.)
Melanoma	S-100, vimentin (pos.)
	NSE often (pos.)
	Epithelial stains (neg.)
Lymphoma	LCA (pos.)
	EMA occasionally (pos.)
	All other studies (neg.)
Sarcoma	
Mesenchymal	Vimentin (pos.)
Rhabdomyosarcoma	Desmin (pos.)
Angiosarcoma	Factor VIII antigen (pos.)
Neuroendocrine tumor	NSE, chromogranin (pos.)
	Epithelial stains (pos.)
Germ cell tumor	hCG and/or AFP (pos.)
	Epithelial stains (pos.)
Prostate cancer	PSA (pos.)
	Epithelial stains (pos.)

EMA, epithelial membrane antigen; LCA, leukocyte common antigen; NSE, neuron-specific enolase; hCG, human chorionic gonadotropin: AFP, α-fetoprotein; PSA, prostate-specific antigen.
Source: Hainsworth JD, Greco FA. Treatment of patients with cancer of unknown primary site, in *Important Advances in Oncology 1991.* Philadelphia, Lippincott, 1991, p 174. Used by permission.

histology (via light microscopy), and overall clinical presentation. More than half of all CUPS will have multiple sites of involvement. The most common sites of disease, in descending order, are liver > bone > lymph nodes (mostly in the cervical region) > pleural effusions = ascites > brain. It is imperative to try to readily identify curable neoplasms or those most likely to respond to chemotherapy or radiotherapy. Up to 30% of primaries will be identified antemortem, while 75% will be determined at autopsy. Most of the latter group will be infradiaphragmatic, usually occult pancreatic primaries.

A. History
1. Lung primaries often include a history of cough and other associated respiratory tract complaints.
2. Gastrointestinal tract primaries may present with evidence of bleeding, bowel obstruction, jaundice, or localized abdomi-

nal discomfort. A complaint of abdominal pain which distinctly radiates to the back should serve as a clue to a possible pancreatic cancer primary.

3. Skeletal pain, specifically involving the ribs, lumbar or thoracic spine, or hip area (including the proximal femur) is commonly seen in metastatic breast, prostate, and lung cancer. If the facial bones are involved, multiple myeloma may be present. Most important is to detect, readily diagnose, and treat an impending cord compression, a common finding with any of the aforementioned tumors.

4. B-symptoms, such as a 10% weight loss in the preceding 6 months, fever, or adenopathy, serve as indicators of primary hematologic malignancy, such as Hodgkin's disease or non-Hodgkin's lymphoma.

B. Clinical manifestations

1. Pleural effusions may be seen with a host of solid tumors, most commonly lung, breast, ovarian, and mesothelioma. A diagnostic thoracentesis, to determine if the pleural fluid is an exudate (supportive of a malignant process) or a transudate, is required. A separate specimen should be send for cytologic analysis.

2. Ascites is an indicator of hepatic compromise. It can either be malignant or benign. Metastatic lesions to the liver can result in significant ascites if a majority of the liver parenchyma is replaced with tumor *or* the hepatic veins are blocked (i.e., Budd-Chiari syndrome). Studding of the peritoneum with metastatic deposits of tumor may also result in ascites. Frequent bowel obstruction may accompany this scenario. Ovarian, hepatocellular, gastric, colon, pancreatic, and rectal primaries may all present with ascites. A diagnostic paracentesis is essential.

3. Adenopathy can be generalized (often with hematologic malignant primaries) or focal. Of the latter, isolated cervical adenopathy is most common. A workup, including a panendoscopy exam and FNA should be performed for cervical nodal presentations. A high or midcervical node may represent regional spread of an occult nasopharyngeal, tonsillar, tongue base, or hypopharyngeal primary tumor. Low cervical lesions are most commonly seen as a consequence of gastric (Virchow's node),

pancreatic, breast, or lung primaries. If FNA fails to yield an adequate tissue sample, cervical exploration with frozen section examination and excisional biopsy is required.

C. Diagnostic tests

1. General tests: Following a complete history and physical examination, a directed diagnostic workup should be undertaken. It should include some general laboratory tests, including a complete bloot count, serum electrolytes, serum liver function tests, a chest radiography (posteroanterior and lateral), and a computed tomography (CT) scan of the abdomen/pelvis.

   a. If respiratory complaints are part of the presenting clinical spectrum, then sputum cytologic examination should be done. A bronchoscopy should follow if there is an obvious mass on the chest radiograph or if the rest of the directed workup is normal and the respiratory complaints predominate.

   b. All females should receive bilateral breast mammograms, with a recent-generation machine and read by a dedicated radiologist. Pap smears should be performed on all female patients.

   c. Rectal exams should be performed on all patients, but all males also require a prostate exam. If it is enlarged in an asymmetric manner, a transrectal ultrasound scan should follow. FNA of any suspicious nodules is important.

   d. Obvious pleural fluid on a chest radiograph or ascites on an abdominal CT scan should undergo diagnostic sampling. It is important to perform a cytologic examination, stain for E/R status using the enzyme radioimmunocytochemistry assay, mucin, and CEA.

      (1) If a hepatic lesion is noted and is the only site of disease, AFP stains should be performed.

2. Specific tests: There are some situations in which more directed and selective tests should be undertaken.

   a. Cervical lymphadenopathy should make a primary head and neck cancer a high likelihood. A panendoscopy will help to make a definitive diagnosis. Squamous cell or adenocystic histology is strongly suggestive of a supraclavicular primary site of origin.

b. An enlarged supraclavicular lymph node may indicate a primary gastric cancer, especially if the FNA histology reveals an adenocarcinoma pattern. An upper gastrointestinal (UGI) barium swallow, with small bowel follow-through, should be performed if either there are symptoms of UGI discomfort or if the general diagnostic workup is unrevealing. If the UGI is normal, then further workup of the GI tract will probably be of no benefit.

   (1) If the FNA reveals a papillary adenocarcinomatous pattern, then thyroid gland imaging is warranted, since the type of treatment recommended would be different from that of a primary GI tract tumor.

c. An enlarged axillary lymph node warrants an FNA in all patients; females should also receive a high-quality mammogram (bilateral), if this has not previously been done. For females, if there is a lesion on the mammogram, it should be biopsied. The case should then be treated like any stage II breast carcinoma (mastectomy or lumpectomy plus axillary node dissection), as long as there are no other distant metastatic sites of disease. For males, a further directed workup may be indicated, depending on other observed associated symptom complexes.

d. Any patient with an abnormal chest radiograph should have a chest CT scan performed, with images extended through the liver and adrenals.

e. All patients with a guiac-positive stool should have this test repeated, while no longer ingesting animal meats in the diet. If this test is still positive, then a lower gastrointestinal (LGI) barium series should be obtained. If an abnormality is noted, then a colonoscopy of the large bowel should follow as soon as an adequate bowel preparation can be performed. If the LGI is normal, then a UGI with small bowel follow-through should be performed. Any abnormality in either the esophagus, stomach, or proximal duodenum, can be biopsied via an upper endoscopy. Obviously, a primary esophageal tumor presenting with a guiac-positive stool would most likely involve a more predominant associated complaint of dysphagia. Patients with no bowel-related symptoms or signs should not routinely undergo upper and lower barium studies.

f. Patients with elevated serum CEA and associated complaints of abdominal fullness (and/or right upper quadrant pain) should have the liver imaged with either ultrasound or CT. We advocate the latter. A dynamic bolus CT scan of the liver may reveal enhancement of lesions. If there are multiple lesions, an experienced liver surgeon should consider resection. If resection is considered and there is no evidence of distant metastatic spread outside of the liver, then either a CT portagram (via the portal vein) or a CT angiogram (via the hepatic artery) will delineate the anatomy more clearly. If the latter is performed, a baseline arteriogram of the celiac axis can be obtained to guide the surgical resection.

g. Patients with an abnormal prostate exam should undergo a transrectal ultrasound scan followed by a biopsy of suspicious lesions. Elevated PSA has been shown to be a fairly reliable indicator of prostate cancer. Very high levels of this serum marker usually indicate that the tumor has spread distantly (stage IVB), regardless of whether the rest of the diagnostic workup is normal or not (i.e., bone scintigraphy).

V. **Treatment**

A. After a directed search for the primary site has been undertaken, treatment should be based on the tumor type most likely to yield a response to therapy in the individual case. Regional (single-site) disease which is amenable to local therapy, such as surgical resection and/or radiotherapy, should be treated locally and observed for relapse. The obvious exception to this rule involves females who have adenocarcinomas within an axillary lymph node and who lack any GI clinical manifestations. Such cases should be managed as primary breast cancers. There is a 65% 10-year survival following surgery and radiotherapy in women presenting in this fashion.

B. Patients who appear to have germ cell cancers, neuroendocrine cancers, or poorly differentiated carcinomas, as well as those who progress following localized therapy, warrant a trial of platinum-based combination chemotherapy. Up to two-thirds of such patients will have an objective response, while one-fourth will obtain a complete response to such treatment. Overall, 15–20% of patients with poorly differentiated characteristics via light microscopy will have a long-term disease-free survival (>5 years). Patients with adenomatous features may benefit from an initial trial of infusional 5-fluorouracil-based therapy (see below). Women who present with CUPS, in the form of malignant ascites with poorly differentiated or undifferentiated adenocarcinomatous cytology, should receive platinum-based chemotherapy similar to an ovarian cancer protocol.

1. Published phase 2 trial combinations include cisplatin, etoposide, and bleomycin (BEP); cisplatin and 5-fluorouracil (PF); PF plus leucovorin (PFL); cisplatin and etoposide (PE); cyclophosphamide, doxorubicin, and cisplatin (CAP); and 5-fluorouracil, doxorubicin, and mitomycin-C (FAM). Platinum-based regimens have yielded the best responses. For patients with CUPS who progress on a platinum-based chemotherapy, a trial of continuous-infusion 5-FU (for 5 days or 4–6 weeks) is warranted in patients with good performance status.

C. The option of no treatment should be strongly considered in patients who have failed a platinum-based chemotherapeutic regimen and/or who have a declining performance status (unable to conduct the normal activities of daily living and spending more than 50% of their time in bed). In such cases, comfort should be the main goal of treatment. *Under no circumstances should patients with terminal and uncurable cancer receive hyperalimentation.*

VI. Prognosis

A. Most patients with CUPS will die of their disease. Most will present with multiple sites of disease. The overall period of median survival is around 9–10 months. From 15% to 20% of such patients will be long-term survivors.

B. Favorable subsets include the following:
   1. Patients with germ cell or neuroendocrine features, lymphomas, or isolated cervical nodal disease (especially squamous cell histology).
   2. Those with predominant midline tumors including nodal, mediastinal, or retroperitoneal disease.
   3. Those with good performance status.
      a. Able to perform activities of daily living with minimal or no assistance.
      b. Spend less than 50% of their time in bed.
      c. Those who obtained a good response if pretreated.
      d. Those <50 years of age.
      e. Female patients with a positive ER/PR status on the tissue specimen.

Bibliography

Bates SE. Clinical applications of serum tumor markers. *Ann Intern Med* 115:623–638, 1991.

Greco FA, Vaughn WK, Hainsworth JD. Advanced poorly differentiated carcinoma of unknown primary sites: Recognition of a treatable syndrome. *Ann Intern Med* 104:547–553, 1986.

Hainsworth JD, Greco FA. Poorly differentiated carcinoma and germ cell tumors. *Hemat Oncol Clin North Am* 5:1223–1231, 1991.

Hainsworth JD, Greco FA (eds.). Unknown Primary. *Seminar in Oncology* 20(3):205–291, 1993.

Hainsworth JD, Johnson DH, Greco FA. Poorly differentiated neuroendocrine carcinoma of unknown primary site: A newly recognized clinicopathologic entity. *Ann Intern Med* 109:364–371, 1988.

Hainsworth JD, Wright EP, Johnson DH, et al. Poorly differentiated carcinoma of unknown primary site: Clinical usefulness of immunoperoxidase staining. *J Clin Oncol* 9:1931–1938, 1991.

Mackay B, Ordonez NG. Tumors of unknown origin: The role of the pathologist. *Adv Oncol* 5:13–19, 1990.

Chapter 79

Paraneoplastic Syndromes

Kenning M. Anderson, M.D., Ph.D.

I. **Definition**
Paraneoplastic syndromes (PNPS) represent the metabolic changes in tissues initiated by but remote from a cancer or its metastases.

II. **Etiology**
There are several etiologies, depending on the inciting cancer. Genetic depression with synthesis of inappropriate RNA or protein products, including various growth factors and receptors, some of which may be defective; cell- or humoral-mediated immune phenomena; neuroendocrine mechanisms; "forbidden contact," with initiation of abnormal biologic responses; or other unknown reasons are the most common explanations.

III. **Pathophysiology**
   A. This varies with the type of cancer.
   B. The metabolic reaction of an affected tissue depends on its response to the inciting etiology.
   C. Consequently, the means of diagnosis employed varies according to the symptoms encountered.

IV. **Incidence**
   A. From 20% to 50% of cancer patients may exhibit such syndromes. According to one estimate, about one-third of patients with PNPS exhibit endocrine and metabolic sequelae, one-third connective tissue or dermatologic disease, one-sixth neurologic or psychiatric disorders, and the remainder hematologic, vascular, gastrointestinal, or overtly immunologic complications.

V. **Pathology**
   A. Syndromes due to ectopic hormone synthesis
      1. Definitive diagnosis of ectopic hormone production includes demonstration of synthesis by and increased concentration of a hormone in a cancer and its venous blood; the cells of origin not normally synthesizing clinically significant amounts of the product; remission of the endocrine syndrome after effective treatment of the underlying malignancy; and its return on recurrence of the cancer.
      2. This clinically demanding research is rarely performed.
   B. Hypercalcemia
      1. This is most often due to malignant disease. In addition to metastases, breast and lung cancers can cause resorption of bone by several mechanisms that depend on ectopic hormone synthesis.

2. Parathyroid hormone (PTH)-like activity is associated with squamous cell carcinomas, sarcomas and lymphomas.

3. Paracrine factors including prostaglandin E2 in breast cancer, 1,25-dihydroxyvitamin D in lymphomas, melanomas and small cell lung cancer, osteoclast-activating factor in multiple myeloma, and transforming growth factors α and β may be present.

4. Primary hyperparathyroidism must be excluded.

5. Ectopic PTH does not react with radioimmunoassays for *both* amino- and carboxy-terminal PTH.

6. Hypercalcemia can present as an oncologic emergency, to be discussed subsequently.

C. Ectopic adrenocorticotropic hormone (ACTH) syndrome

1. This is considered the second most frequent PNPS, especially in association with small cell lung cancer and with cancers of the thymus, pancreatic islet cells, and other endocrine organs; salivary glands; renal neoplasms; and neural crest tumors.

2. Hypokalemic alkalosis, glucose intolerance, and muscle weakness are usually much more prominent than physical findings of Cushing's syndrome.

3. Concentrations of ACTH in excess of 200 pg/ml, increased products of cortisol and 17-dehydroisoandrosterone, and inability to suppress their synthesis with exogenous dexamethasone characterize ectopic synthesis of ACTH.

D. Inappropriate secretion of antidiuretic hormone (ADH)

1. This condition, with hyponatremia, normal blood urea nitrogen, reduced serum osmolality, and increased urine sodium, in the absence of dehydration, oliguria, edema, or hypertension, is often associated with small cell lung cancers (Schwartz-Bartter syndrome).

2. The syndrome (SIADH), present biochemically in a high proportion of patients with small cell lung cancer, is clinically significant in only about 15% of patients.

3. The lethargy and somnolence remit with successful treatment of the malignancy when restriction of fluid intake, hypertonic saline, and intravenous furosemide are employed acutely, and with the use of demeclocycline or lithium carbonate in less urgent situations.

E. Ectopic gonadotropins

1. These include human chorionic gonadotropin and human chorionic somatomammotropin, both of which exhibit actions similar to those of leutinizing hormone (LH) and hormone activities similar to those of follide-stimulating hormone (FSH) and LH.

2. Ectopic synthesis is seen with gonadal and extragonadal germ cell malignancies, trophoblastic and lung cancers, and teratomas.

3. Increased β-chain of human chorionic gonadotropin (hCG) can be synthesized by pulmonary, gastrointestinal, and endocrine cancers.

4. Symptoms of precocious puberty, gynecomastia, hirsutism and amenorrhea depend on the age and sex of the patient.

F. Thyrotropin

1. Ectopic synthesis of thyroid-stimulating hormone (TSH) in patients with trophoblastic tumors (choriocarcinoma, hydatidiform mole, embryonal carcinoma of the testes) can be associated with biochemical elevations of T_4 and tachycardia, frequently without eye signs or tremor.

G. Pancreatic islet cell syndromes

1. These include the Zollinger-Ellison syndrome with a gastrin-secreting, non-B-cell pancreatic neoplasm, associated in up to one-third of patients with a multiple endocrine meoplasia I syndrome (MEN I, parathyroid, adrenal, or pituitary gland tumors).

2. Although the hyperglycemia syndrome due to excess secretion of glucagon by α-cell tumors is not really an example of ectopic hormone synthesis, such cancers are associated with diabetes, skin rashes, hemolytic anemia, and edema.

3. Non-β-cell cancers can give rise to the WDHA syndrome (watery diarrhea, hypokalemia, and metabolic acidosis) from the synthesis and release of vasoactive intestinal polypeptide (VIP). Gastric inhibitory peptide (GIP) is associated with reduced gastric secretion.

H. Carcinoid syndrome

1. This occurs in tumors of the enterochromaffin cells, which are distributed throughout the gastrointestinal tract.

2. Patients with carcinoids producing serotonin or kallikrein that drain into the liver have few associated symptoms, while those with carcinoids emptying into the general circulation experience symptoms including flushing, diarrhea, and bronchial constriction and can develop telangiectasias.

I. Ectopic calcitonin
1. Medullary carcinomas of the thyroid originating from thyroid C cells may secrete calcitonin without developing significant hypocalcemia, possibly due to compensatory synthesis of PTH.
2. About 10% of these patients exhibit other signs of the MEN IIa syndrome (medullary carcinoma of the thyroid, pheochromocytoma, parathyroid adenomas, or hyperplasia).
3. A variant (MEN IIb) is associated with a marfanoid habitus.
4. Paraendocrine synthesis of calcitonin has been observed in neural crest and small cell lung cancers, intestinal and bronchial carcinoids, and pheochromocytomas.
5. Calcitonin is employed as an indicator of residual or recurrent medullary carcinoma of the thyroid.

J. Erythrocytosis
1. Fifty percent of paraneoplastic erythrocytosis is due to renal neoplasms, although benign renal diseases can also be responsible.
2. The absence of pancytosis and splenomegaly, as well as a normal arterial oxygen saturation, exclude polycythemia vera and secondary erythrocytosis.

K. Somatotropin and the HPO syndrome
1. Some adenocarcinomas of the lung synthesize somatotropin (growth hormone).
2. The hypertrophic pulmonary osteoarthropathy syndrome (HPO), which includes clubbing of the distal phalanges and gynecomastia, has been associated with ectopic formation of hCG, but a neuroendocrine mechanism or ectopic somatotropin may contribute to the osteoarthropathy.
3. Involvement of the mediastinum by lung or nasopharyngeal neoplasms or by Hodgkin's disease has been associated with HPO.

L. Bombesin
1. This is a tetradecapeptide with unknown function in man associated with small cell lung cancer, without identified symptoms.

2. It may promote the autocrine growth of small cell lung cancer.

M. Cancer cell growth factors
1. Synthesis of multiple growth factors by cancer cells, including epidermal and other cell-derived factors, various cytokines, transforming, angiogenesis, and invasive factors capable of inducing autocrine, paracrine, or other responses is a subject of increasing importance for understanding cancer cell biology.

N. Connective tissue and dermatologic syndromes
1. About 20% of patients with a polymyositis-like myopathy have an underlying malignancy.
2. Dermatomyositis, or a rheumatoid arthritis-like or lupus erythematosus-like syndrome, can occur with different cancers.
3. Acanthosis nigricans should suggest secretion of an melanocyte-stimulating hormone (MSH)-like hormone by an intestinal malignancy, cutaneous flushing, carcinoid, migratory thrombophlebitis, an intra-abdominal malignancy such as carcinoma of the pancreas (Trousseau's syndrome), porphyria cutanea tarda, a hepatoma, pruritus due to lymphoma, or cold urticaria from cryoglobulinemia.
4. A variety of dermatoses including exfoliative, pemphigoid, psoriatic, erythematous, toxic, vesicular, or bullous lesions and Raynaud's phenomenon have been associated with various cancers.
5. Bowen's disease is characterized by scaly plaques occurring with different solid cancers, and generalized melanosis may develop in melanoma, lymphomas, and hepatomas.
6. Autoimmune responses to normal or cancer cells and neuroendocrine or paracrine/autocrine mechanisms may be responsible for some of the lesions mentioned in this section.
7. Kaposi's sarcoma occurring in patients with the acquired immunodeficiency syndrome seems to develop in response to a locally synthesized paracrine/endocrine factor.

O. Neurologic and psychiatric syndromes
1. Dementia, cerebellar degeneration, myelopathies, posterior root degeneration, and peripheral neuropathies have been associated with cancer.

2. Progressive multifocal leukoencephalopathy, seen in immunosuppressed individuals, may be due to polyoma virus infection.

3. Dementia and subacute cerebellar degeneration are more common than optic neuritis and limbic encephalitis.

4. Spinal cord syndromes resembling amyotrophic lateral sclerosis and sensorimotor neuropathies have been described.

5. Peripheral neuropathy, the most common neurologic PNS, may precede detection of a malignancy and may be primarily sensory or mixed.

6. Unlike the response of most PNPS, surgical removal of an underlying breast or other solid cancer usually does not lead to neurologic improvement.

7. Carcinomatous myasthenia (Eaton-Lambert syndrome) resembles myasthenia gravis, except that continued electrical stimulation increases neuromuscular transmission.

8. Generally, in patients with cancer, metastases, thrombosis, hemorrhage, or infection accounts for the neurologic symptoms.

P. Hematologic, gastrointestinal, renal, vascular, and miscellaneous syndromes

1. Erythrocytosis has been mentioned.

2. Normocytic normochromic anemia of chronic disease (ACD) is characterized by reduced red blood cell mass, serum iron, and saturation of transferrin; increased plasma volume; moderate hemolysis; and a normocytic marrow with normal ratios of erythroid to myeloid precursors.

3. The etiology of ACD can include "toxic" depression of erythropoiesis similar to that seen in many chronic diseases or due to chemotherapy, hemolysis, blood loss, malnutrition, and so on. Megaloblastic, hyperchromic anemias occur in carcinoma of the stomach (reduced vitamin B_{12}) or in folic acid deficiencies due to lymphoma invasion of the small bowel.

4. Leukemoid reactions with circulating myeloid precursors occur with hepatomas, with metastatic disease in bone, and with various solid cancers.

5. Erythrocyte agnegenesis is found in 2% of patients with thymoma.

6. Myelophthistic anemia results from replacement of bone marrow by cancer.

7. Disseminated intravascular coagulation and abnormal fibrinolysis are seen in lung, prostate, pancreas, liver, and other cancers.

8. Microangiopathic hemolytic anemia associated with mucin-secreting adenocarcinomas and autoimmune hemolytic anemias represent other immune-mediated hematologic responses to cancer which may overlap one another in mechanism and clinical findings.

9. Thrombocytopenia can be due to autoimmune mechanisms, among other factors.

10. The monoclonal gammopathies include relatively benign Waldenström's macroglobulinemia and the malignant multiple myeloma with urinary Bence Jones protein, hyperuricemia, hypercalcemia, and anemia.

11. Increased serum viscosity due to elevated concentrations of M or IgM protein can lead to thrombotic events, as in Waldenström's macroglobulinemia.

12. Nephrotic syndromes due to amyloidosis from carcinomas or lymphomas, renal tubular and Fanconi-like syndromes in hypergammaglobulinemic states, hypokalemia, hypercalcemia, or hyperuricemic nephropathies, as well as renal vein thrombosis due to intravascular coagulation, are some of the renal syndromes associated with different cancers.

13. Membranous glomerulopathy with proteinuria occurs in gastrointestinal malignancies. Secondary amyloidosis can complicate multiple myeloma, Waldenström's macroglobulinemia, and lymphomas.

Q. APUD tumors and the MEN syndromes

1. APUD cells (high *a*mine, amine *p*recursor *u*ptake, amino acid *d*ecarboxylation), derived from the primitive neural crest, also include sensory and sympathetic neuroganglia, melanocytes, and Schwann cells.

2. They are characterized by a high content of 5-hydroxytryptamine; amine precursors including 5-hydroxytryptophan, amino acid decarboxylases, and neurosecretory granules; and the release of polypeptide or amine hormones, including ACTH, calcitonin, gastrin, insulin, glucagon, MSH, and vasoactive peptides.

3. "Apudomas" are seen in the familial paraendocrine syndromes MEN I and MEN II.

4. Some of the hormones synthesized by these cells are appropriate for their cells of origin, but others such as somatotrophins are not, and these probably should be considered paraneoplastic.

VI. General Systemic Effects of Cancers

A. Fever, anorexia, and weight loss in cancer patients with increased energy expenditure, as reflected in an increased basal metabolic rate, diabetic-like glucose tolerance curves, and enhanced gluconeogenesis, are not well explained but appear due to activities of unidentified paracrine/endocrine factors.

B. Fever may be related to the production of interleukin-1, either from the cancer or from tumor-associated infiltrating inflammatory cells. Hypernephroma, metastatic liver cancer, and lymphomas are often responsible.

C. Lactic acidosis associated with leukemia or lymphoma, especially those that extensively infiltrate the liver, is characterized by an increase in lactate to 4–8 mmol/liter, probably due to increased release from the tumor.

D. Hypoglycemia due to retroperitoneal sarcomas, mesotheliomas, and other nonpancreatic cancers may result from excess utilization of glucose or ectopic release of an insulin-like material.

VII. Diagnosis and Treatment

A. The presenting symptoms of some patients can be due to paraneoplastic manifestations of an occult malignancy.

B. Diagnosis of paraneoplastic syndromes depends on excluding nonmalignant conditions and identifying a primary cancer and any metastases.

C. Procedures of general internal medicine are used to define nonmalignant causes of the patient's symptoms and/or to positively identify a cancer responsible for the paraneoplastic syndrome.

D. Successful treatment of an underlying malignancy generally results in remission of an associated paraneoplastic syndrome. Otherwise, treatment is symptomatic, including the therapies appropriate for acute oncologic emergencies.

E. While the diagnosis and treatment of paraneoplastic syndromes includes many aspects of general internal medicine, specialized information directed toward the identification and treatment of specific cancers may be required; for these the reader is referred to the Bibliography.

Bibliography

Bitran JD, Ultmann JE. The paraneoplastic syndromes, in Kelley WN (ed-in-chief), *Textbook of Internal Medicine*, vol. 1. Philadelphia, Lippincott, 1989, pp 1352–1357.

Bunn PA, Ridgway EC. Paraneoplastic syndromes, in DeVita VT, Hellman S, Rosenberg SA (eds), *Cancer. Principles and Practice of Oncology* ed 3. Philadelphia, Lippincott, 1989, pp 1896–1940.

Moossa AR, Schimpff SC, Robson MC (eds). *Comprehensive Textbook of Oncology*, ed 2. Baltimore, William & Wilkins, 1991, pp 1663–1683.

CHAPTER 80

Cancer Emergencies

Ritwick Panicker, M.D.
Charles R. Thomas, Jr., M.D.

Cancer emergencies are fairly common in medical practice. They may present as the first manifestation of cancer, as a result of therapy, or as a consequence of metastasis. All organ systems may be involved, either singly or multiply.

Metabolic Emergencies

Hypercalcemia

I. **Definition**

Elevated serum calcium level directly related to an underlying malignancy.

II. **Etiology**

A. Metastatic tumors: The most common are breast, lung (non–small cell), esophageal, and head and neck cancers.

B. Hematologic malignancies: The most common is myeloma; less common are Hodgkin's disease, non-Hodgkin's lymphoma, and leukemias.

C. Humoral hypercalcemia of malignancy (HHM): Though hypercalcemia in several of the above-mentioned cancers may result from the local production of humoral factors, HHM generally refers to hypercalcemia observed in the absence of metastatic disease.

III. **Pathophysiology**

A. Local and/or systemic production of various factors: osteoclast-activating factor in myeloma, prostaglandins, colony-stimulating factors, and tumor necrosis factors.

B. Parathyroid hormone-related protein (PTHrP) recently identified and gene cloned.

1. Partially similar to PTH in structure and function.

2. Increased levels result in hypercalcemia, hypophosphatemia, and increased nephrogenic cyclic cAMP.

3. Effects similar to those seen with elevated PTH.

C. Direct bone resorption and increased gastrointestinal absorption of calcium.

D. The above mechanisms, alone or in combination, cause pathologic fractures, bone pain, anorexia, constipation, neuromuscular symptoms, and other manifestations of hypercalcemia of malignancy.

IV. **Diagnosis**

Unlike the outpatient population, in which hyperparathyroidism is the most common cause of hypercalcemia, cancer is the most important cause in the hospitalized patient.

A. History
1. Anorexia, weight loss, polydipsia, polyuria, constipation, altered sensorium, lethargy, and weakness are common.
2. Clues to the presence of an underlying cancer include pathologic fractures, bone pain, abnormal masses, fever, night sweats, and cough with or without hemoptysis.

B. Physical findings
1. Due to hypercalcemia: Muscle weakness, hyporeflexia, psychosis, bradycardia, atrial or ventricular arrhythmias.
2. Due to underlying cancer: breast lumps, hepatosplenomegaly, pleural effusions and lung collapse, ascites, and lymphadenopathy.

C. Tests
1. Elevated serum calcium, corrected for albumin and elevated ionized calcium (normal range, 9–10.5 mg/dl).
2. Phosphate may be low or normal; paraprotein in myeloma (1–5% of myeloma patients may have nonsecretory myeloma and may fail to reveal paraprotein, though hypercalcemia may be present).
3. X-rays may reveal bony metastases, lytic lesions, generalized osteopenia, or specific evidence of malignancy (e.g., lung nodules, breast shadows).
4. Computed tomography (CT) scanning of the abdomen and thorax is commonly included in the workup to exclude lesions that may be missed by conventional radiographs.
5. Assays of PTH and PTHrP are available at most major centers and may help resolve the issue in cases that defy diagnosis; however, these tests should be performed only when the patient is clinically stable.

V. Differential Diagnosis

A. Primary hyperparathyroidism is the most important differential. An inappropriately high PTH level for a given serum calcium level strongly suggests the diagnosis. The presence of renal calculi, radiographic changes in industrial hand films, and the absence of systemic symptoms such as weight loss suggests this diagnosis.

B. Other considerations, which are rarer, include sarcoidosis, milk-alkali syndrome, and thiazide toxicity. These can usually be distinguished by a good history and physical exam.

VI. Treatment

A. Acute management includes vigorous hydration with normal saline, coupled with administration of IV furosemide (Lasix). This promotes rapid excretion of calcium by the kidneys. If renal function is compromised, as is often the case in myeloma patients, hydration and diuresis should still be attempted but done cautiously, with close monitoring of the patient's weight and fluid status.

B. Glucocorticoids are a useful adjunct, especially in patients with myeloma, lymphoma, and breast cancer. Give hydrocortisone, 200–400 mg IV every 6 hr, followed by oral prednisone, 20–40 mg/day.

C. Diphosphonates (e.g., etidronate), given IV or orally, have emerged as front-line agents for the treatment of hypercalcemia. They act by inhibiting osteoclast activity by binding to hydroxyapatite. IV etidronate, in doses of 2.5–7.5 mg/kg/day, will often normalize serum calcium levels in 48–72 hr. One can then continue maintenance therapy with oral etidronate.

D. Gallium nitrate has been shown to be highly effective in acute control of cancer-related hypercalcemia in controlled clinical trials (dose: 200 mg/m^2 by continuous infusion daily for 5 days).

E. Calcitonin, given as 4 IU/kg SC, has been used for several years in refractory cases. Gallium nitrate has been proven to be superior and is preferable.

F. Mithramycin and IV phosphates are rarely used in current practice but should be remembered as possible alternatives.

G. Hemodialysis with a low-calcium dialysate is still very useful in severe cases, especially if renal function is compromised.

H. Pamidronate (Aredia) is a new bisphosphonate that is given by continuous intravenous infusion over 24 hours in a dose of 60 to 90 mg. It is highly effective in treating hypercalcemia.

Tumor Lysis Syndrome, Urate Nephropathy, and Hyperphosphatemia

I. Clinical Picture

A. These conditions are most commonly seen in patients with hematologic malignancies, lymphoproliferative disorders, and bulky solid tumors, especially after chemotherapy.

B. Breakdown of cancer cells and the consequent release of intracellular ions results in hyperuricemia, hyperkalemia, hyperphosphatemia, hypocalcemia and elevated serum lactate dehydrogenase levels.

C. Clinical features include azotemia, renal failure, and neuromuscular weakness.

II. Treatment

A. Prophylaxis is crucial in patients at risk. This can be achieved with aggressive hydration, urine alkalinization, and allopurinol.

B. In established cases, expedient hemodialysis should be considered. This is often successful in reversing the electrolyte abnormalities and in clearing uric acid from the circulation.

Neuro-Oncologic Emergencies

Back Pain and Epidural Cord Compression

I. Definition

Involvement of the spine and spinal cord by primary or metastatic tumor, leading to bony destruction, cord and nerve root compression, and subsequent neurologic sequelae.

II. Etiology

Most common causes include cancers of the lung, breast, and prostate.

III. Pathophysiology

A. The tumor may involve the vertebral body and the surrounding bony structures.

B. It may compress the spinal cord as an extrinsic soft tissue epidural mass.

C. It may metastatize to the intramedullary region.

D. It may also result in vertebral subluxation, vertebral collapse, and local hemorrage.

E. Any or all of these conditions can result in back pain, spinal cord compression, sensorimotor weakness, paraplegia, and bladder and bowel signs.

F. The tumor can also invade the nerve roots, leading to radicular symptoms and signs.

IV. Diagnosis

Early diagnosis is vital to prevent serious neurologic dysfunction.

A. History and physical signs

1. The patient presents with back pain, progressive weakness, and a sensory deficit. Urinary and fecal incontinence or retention may be present.

2. The patient presents with back pain; the neurologic exam is normal. Useful clues to impending cord compression include radiation of pain to several dermatomes, worsening of pain when recumbent, and, most important, the presence of focal percussion tenderness on the spine.

3. The patient presents with radicular symptoms and signs only.

4. Cauda equina syndrome: Multiple root signs (L-1 to S-5); lower extremity weakness; bladder and bowel signs occur late.

5. Conus medullaris syndrome: Saddle numbness and early sphincter dysfunction.

B. Tests

1. Plain films of the spine are useful in detecting focal lesions. These may show vertebral collapse and/or fracture, erosion of vertebral appendages, and lytic lesions. It should be noted that plain films may be entirely normal.

2. CT scanning with a myelogram is useful in delineating the level and extent of obstruction to the spinal canal.

3. Magnetic resonance imaging (MRI) scanning, done with gadolinium diethylenetriamine pentaacetic acid (DPTA) enhancement, is best for detecting leptomeningeal spread of tumor.

4. Bone scans are useful, especially if the plain films are normal, and could be done prior to the MRI scan.

5. The myelogram is best for cauda and conus lesions.

V. Differential Diagnosis

A. Traumatic injury to the spine.

B. Osteoporosis and concomitant vertebral fractures.

C. Degenerative disc disease.

D. Spinal stenosis.

E. Primary neurologic disease (e.g., transverse myelitis).

VI. Treatment

A. Prompt institution of corticosteroids is mandatory. Dexamethasone 10 mg over 15 min, should be given as soon as possible before starting an imaging procedure, followed up by oral dexamethasone, 4 mg every 6 hr.

B. Definitive treatment is provided by radiation therapy or surgery. Radiotherapy should be given to the affected area if the patient has not had previous radiation therapy. Surgery is the preferred approach if the tumor is radioresistant, if a tissue diagnosis is required, or if previous radiation exposure precludes its use for cord compression. If vertebral collapse and destabilization are present, surgery is needed to stabilize the spine.

C. Once the acute phase is past, neurologic deterioration is halted, and the patient's condition is stable, decisions regarding further therapy (e.g., chemotherapy) can be made.

VII. Prognosis

A. ikelihood of improvement with radiation therapy or surgery depends on the level of function at the time of diagnosis and the tumor type.

1. Eighty percent of ambulatory patients with radiosensitive tumors will improve compared to less than 15% of patients with paraplegia.

2. For more radioresistant tumors, 70–80% of ambulatory patients will show improvement, whereas almost no patient with paraplegia will show improvement.

3. Patients with lymphoma, myeloma, and breast cancer have better outcomes than others.

B. The above statements emphasize the need for early detection and treatment of cord compression.

Altered Mental Status, Focal Deficits, and Acute Weakness

I. Pathology

Acute or subacute deterioration in mental status requires prompt evaluation. Multiple causes exist.

A. Chemotherapy-induced changes may range from transient confusion and florid hallucinations due to ifosfamide to diffuse encephalopathy secondary to 5-fluorouracil (5-FU), methotrexate, procarbazine, and cytosine arabinoside (Ara-C).

B. Cerebellar toxicity is a well-recognized complication of Ara-C therapy.

II. Manifestations

A. Concomitant metabolic derangements, such as hypercalcemia and hyponatremia, should be ruled out.

B. Patients with meningeal carcinomatosis may present with cranial nerve signs; meningitis in an immunocompromised patient can often occur without any focal signs.

C. Leptomeningeal disease usually occurs in the advanced stages of cancer.

D. Carcinoma of the breast and lung and melanoma are the most common solid tumors; leukemias and lymphomas are well known to involve the meninges, both at presentation and in their subsequent course.

E. Focal neurologic deficits raise the possibility of brain metastasis, though intracranial hemorrhage or thrombosis may present in a similar manner.

F. Cerebral herniation syndromes must be considered in any patient with rapid obtundation.

G. In addition to the conditions discussed above, acute muscle weakness can be caused by an acute ascending polyneuropathy (Guillain-Barré syndrome) and by the Eaton-Lambert syndrome seen in small cell lung cancer. These conditions are discussed elsewhere.

III. Diagnosis

A. Evaluation of patients with neuro-oncologic disorders includes a detailed history and physical exam to elicit subtle neurologic signs and an accurate assessment of mental status.

B. Laboratory tests should attempt to rule out any metabolic derangements, neutropenia, and thrombocytopenia.

C. Urgent imaging using either a CT or MRI scan of the head should be done as soon as the clinical situation has stabilized.

D. In deeply obtunded patients, the airway should be secured, an IV line established, and the blood pressure stabilized.

E. Signs of herniation, if present, should be treated with the administration of dexamethasone, 10 mg IV STAT, followed by mannitol, 0.5–1.0 mg/kg, and, if necessary, hyperventilation.

F. If brain imaging fails to reveal elevated intracranial pressure and the platelet count is satisfactory ($50,000/mm^3$ is an arbitrary cutoff often used), a lumbar puncture should be considered. This procedure is crucial to diagnose leptomeningeal disease and conditions such as the Guillain-Barré syndrome.

IV. Treatment

A. Definitive treatment includes surgical resection of metastases, especially if it will relieve herniation, and radiation therapy if feasible and if the tumor is at least partially radiosensitive.

B. Once leptomeningeal disease is confirmed, placement of an Ommaya reservoir and intraventricular therapy with methotrexate or Ara-C is recommended.

C. Patients with acute muscle weakness may require ventilatory support.

D. A realistic assessment of the patient's prognosis should be made once the acute crisis has been stablized and the etiology of the neurologic derangement ascertained.

Seizures

Seizures in a cancer patient may result from any of the causes discussed earlier. Status epilepticus, defined as repetitive seizures without resumption of consciousness, is a neurologic emergency. Recurrent, poorly controlled seizures also often require emergent treatment. Standard measures include securing the airway, establishing a good IV line, administration of IV 50% dextrose; diazepam, 2 mg/min (up to 20 mg IV) or ativan, 2–4 mg for immediate effect, followed by a loading dose of phenytoin, 17 mg/kg (no more than 50 mg/min). Maintenance therapy, preferably with one anticonvulsant, can be started once the patient is stable.

Cardiovascular Emergencies

Superior Vena Cava Syndrome

I. Definition
Constellation of symptoms resulting from partial or complete obstruction to the superior vena cava.
II. Etiology
   A. Most common etiology is bronchogenic carcinoma, followed by lymphoma.
   B. Other causes include thymomas, leukemias, teratomas, breast cancer, and ovarian cancer.
III. Pathophysiology
   A. Extrinsic compression of the superior vena cava is most common; tumor infiltration of SVC can also occur; true thrombosis of the superior vena cava is uncommon but possible.
   B. Impairment of venous drainage results in facial and upper extremity swelling, tracheal and brain edema, and development of collateral venous channels which may be visible on the chest wall.
IV. Diagnosis
   A. History
      1. Dyspnea, conjunctival redness, and eyelid puffiness are common.
      2. Stridor and dysphagia signify tracheal and esophageal obstruction.
      3. Symptoms of underlying cancer (e.g., hemoptysis, weight loss, fever, night sweats) must be sought.
   B. Physical signs
      1. Collaterals on chest wall, conjunctival and eyelid edema, and swollen facies and arms are common.
      2. Careful examination of lymph nodes is vital.
      3. Abnormal signs in the chest, such as a pleural effusion or lung collapse, may be present.

   C. Tests
      1. Chest x-ray and CT scanning of the chest have become integral to the workup of any patient with superior vena cava syndrome. These tests may demonstrate mediastinal widening, lymph node enlargement, and lung masses, and may also outline the degree of obstruction to the vasculature, trachea, and esophagus.
      2. The next step is to obtain tissue for diagnosis as expeditiously as possible. Biopsy of an enlarged lymph node, sputum cytology, bronchoscopy, and transthoracic needle aspiration are all useful, depending on the clinical situation.
      3. Mediastinoscopy or mediastinotomy with biopsy of lymph nodes (especially if a paratracheal mass is present) are widely accepted procedures in this situation.
         a. They are relatively well tolerated, with minimal morbidity and mortality, and clearly outweigh the risks of instituting emergent treatment without obtaining a proper histologic diagnosis.
         b. Only the patient with mental status changes and impending airway obstruction merits immediate therapeutic intervention.
V. Treatment
   A. It is best to await a diagnosis before instituting specific therapy, since in the overwhelming majority of cases the condition is not life-threatening.
   B. Initial measures include head elevation, supplemental oxygen, and gentle diuresis. Corticosteroids are helpful in reducing local vascular edema and should always be started.
   C. Specific treatment includes chemotherapy for small cell lung cancer and lymphomas, and radiotherapy as an adjunct or as the primary therapy for radiosensitive tumors. Radiotherapy is most helpful in life-threatening situations. Surgical bypass is reserved for patients with acute airway obstruction or altered mentation due to brain edema.

Malignant Pericardial Effusion and Cardiac Tamponade

I. Definition
II. Etiology
   A. Most common causes of malignant pericardial effusions include cancers of the lung and breast, lymphomas, and leukemias.

B. The rate of accumulation of fluid in the pericardial sac is more important than the total amount of fluid in determining the severity of symptoms and the need for emergent intervention.

C. Compromised diastolic filling leads to decreased stroke volume, low blood pressure, increased peripheral vascular resistance, and tachycardia.

III. Diagnosis

A. Symptoms: The patient develops dyspnea, chest pain, cough, and general weakness. Physical examination may reveal hypotension, tachycardia, thready pulse with pulsus paradoxus, hepatomegaly, increased jugular venous distension, distant heart sounds, and cyanosis. Edema and ascites are more common in chronic cases.

B. Chest x-rays may show pleural effusion, cardiomegaly with an irregular cardiac silhouette, a widened mediastinum, or a hilar mass. Electrocardiographic changes include tachycardia, nonspecific ST-T changes, low-voltage QRS complexes, atrial fibrillation, conduction abnormalities, and electric alternans.

C. An emergency echocardiogram is the single most useful test in these patients. It can assess the size of the effusion, wall motion and thickness, degree of diastolic filling compromise, and the presence of pericardial masses.

IV. Treatment

A. Treatment of choice is an emergency pericardiocentesis under echocardiographic control. This also serves as a diagnostic procedure; the fluid is sent for cytology and other appropriate tests.

B. In case of rapidly accumulating pericardial effusions, it is often essential to leave some form of long-term access for future drainage (e.g., a pigtail catheter). Subsequent management depends on the underlying diagnosis.

Gastrointestinal Emergencies

Gastrointestinal Bleeding

I. Etiology

A. Gastrointestinal bleeding is a common oncologic emergency. It is most commonly caused by hemorrhagic gastritis, peptic ulcer disease, the tumor itself, candida esophagitis, and thrombocytopenia.

B. Tumors that often bleed include lymphoma, leiomyoma, carcinoid, and metastatic melanoma.

II. Diagnosis

A. The patient may present with upper or lower gastrointestinal bleeding.

B. A history of previous cancer, recent chemotherapy, past surgery, dysphagia, alteration in bowel habits, weight loss, and diarrhea is important.

C. The physical exam should be thorough, with special emphasis on lymphadenopathy, hepatosplenomegaly, abdominal masses, and a rectal exam.

D. Endoscopy is the next step, especially if the etiology is unknown. Besides helping to establish a diagnosis, endoscopy can perform therapeutic interventions in the form of heater probe, laser treatment, or injection therapy.

III. Treatment

Treatment begins by establishing good intravascular access and fluid resuscitation, including blood and platelet transfusions. This is followed by endoscopic treatment, as described above, or by another therapy (e.g., chemotherapy for lymphomas).

Gastrointestinal Obstruction

I. Etiology

A. This can be acute or subacute.

B. Common causes are colorectal cancer, gastroesophageal neoplasms, metastatic cancer (especially ovarian), and metabolic derangements (e.g., hypokalemia and hypercalcemia).

II. Clinical Picture and Diagnosis

A. Clinically, the patient presents with abdominal pain, vomiting, constipation or obstipation, and abdominal distention.

B. Physical examination may reveal abdominal tenderness, absent or high-pitched bowel sounds, and masses in the pelvis or rectum.

C. Diagnostic tests include flat and upright plain x-rays of the abdomen, abdominopelvic CT scans, and upper and lower gastrointestinal endoscopy.

D. A gastrograffin enema may be useful in detecting large-bowel lesions.

III. Treatment

A. Treatment includes IV fluids, bowel rest, nasogastric suction, and broad-spectrum antibiotics if fever and leukocytosis are present.

B. Surgical decompression is often necessary,

and serves as both a diagnostic and a therapeutic tool.

Neutropenic Enterocolitis

I. **Definition**

Neutropenic enterocolitis, also known as *typhylitis*, *ileocecal syndrome*, and *necrotizing enteropathy*, is a life-threatening condition associated with acute leukemia and some solid tumors.

II. **Pathophysiology**

This includes leukemic infiltration of the bowel wall, direct toxic effects of chemotherapy, and bacterial invasion of the bowel wall.

III. **Clinical Picture and Diagnosis**
   A. The clinical picture consists of abdominal distention, watery diarrhea, fever, right-sided abdominal tenderness, neutropenia, and thrombocytopenia.
   B. Acute appendicitis is the most important differential diagnosis, others being pseudomembranous enterocolitis and diverticulitis.
   C. Plain films of the abdomen may show an ileus pattern with a distended cecum.
   D. CT scans typically show a thickened bowel containing air.
   E. Flexible sigmoidoscopy helps to rule out pseudomembranous enterocolitis.

IV. **Treatment**
   A. Medical management consists of bowel rest, nasogastric suction, broad-spectrum antibiotics, and total parenteral nutrition.
   B. If the patient shows no improvement in 2–3 days, surgical intervention should be considered.

Hematologic Emergencies

Thromboembolic Disorders

I. **Definition**

These include deep vein thrombosis, pulmonary embolism, and arterial thrombii.

II. **Etiology**

Commonly associated with cancer of the pancreas, stomach, colon, lung, breast, ovary, and prostate, as well as and unknown primary malignancies.

III. **Pathophysiology**

Increased levels of fibrinogen, Factors V, VII, IX, X, and XI; decreased levels of protein C and S.

IV. **Diagnosis**
   A. Deep vein thrombosis
      1. Symptoms of leg swelling, pain, and local warmth; patient may be asymptomatic.
      2. Physical exam is unreliable.
      3. Tests are usually necessary and include venography (the gold standard) and impedance plethysmography, which detects obstruction in proximal veins but is unable to distinguish between thrombotic and nonthrombotic occlusions.
      4. Doppler ultrasound is useful in documenting proximal lesions and can be done at the bedside.
   B. Pulmonary embolism
      1. Symptoms include acute onset of pleuritic chest pain, dyspnea, and scanty hemoptysis.
      2. Physical exam reveals tachypnea, tachycardia, and, less commonly, a pleural friction rub.
      3. Tests
         a. Arterial blood gas reveals a respiratory alkalosis with a widened A-a gradient.
         b. Electrocardiogram may only show tachycardia or features of right heart strain, P pulmonale, and right axis deviation.
         c. Chest x-rays are usually normal.
         d. Ventilation/perfusion scan should be performed; a normal perfusion scan alone rules out a pulmonary embolism.
         e. If the above tests are inconclusive, a pulmonary arteriogram will confirm the diagnosis and should be performed if the patient is hemodynamically stable.

V. **Treatment**
   A. Heparin is the initial treatment of choice in both cases. A bolus of 5,000 units should be given, followed by a maintenance infusion to keep the partial thromboplastin time at 1.5–2.5 times normal. Coumadin is begun 48–72 hr later and maintained for at least 3–6 months.
   B. Fibrinolytic therapy has a role in the treatment of deep vein thrombosis and pulmonary embolism and is discussed elsewhere.
   C. Patients in whom anticoagulation is contraindicated are candidates for balloon interruption of the intravenous catheter (e.g., placement of the Greenfield filter).

Disseminated Intravascular Coagulation (DIC)

I. **Definition**

DIC results from excessive activation of the coagulation and fibrinolytic pathways. These events may occur independently of each other.

II. **Etiology**
   A. Most common are prostate carcinoma, leukemia, especially acute nonlymphocytic leukemia of the M3 phenotype (also known as acute *promyelocytic leukemia*) and Burkitt's lymphoma.
   B. Less common are lung cancer and adenocarcinomas.

III. **Pathophysiology**
   A. Leukemic blasts contain urokinase and other proteolytic enzymes that activate fibrinolysis.
   B. Some leukemic cells also express procoagulant enzymes which initiate coagulation at the endothelial cell level.
   C. Circulating cancer cells may damage endothelial cells, promoting coagulation.

IV. **Diagnosis**
   A. Clinical features include widespread bleeding, purpura, microangiopathic hemolytic anemia, and arterial thrombosis in purpura fulminans.
   B. Laboratory tests
      1. These tests show prolongation of the prothrombin time, partial thromboplastin time, thrombin time, and, in most cases, thrombocytopenia.
      2. Decreased fibrinogen levels and elevated fibrin split products (FSP greater than 40 μg/ml) reflect fibrinolysis.
      3. The crosslinked D-dimer assay measures a subpopulation of FSP and is more specific.

V. **Treatment**
   A. Replacement of coagulation factors and fibrinogen with fresh frozen plasma and/or cryoprecipitate.
   B. Heparinization prior to initiation of chemotherapy in patients with acute promyelocytic leukemia.
   C. Most importantly, treatment of the underlying malignancy.

Hyperleucocytosis

I. **Definition**
   A white blood cell (WBC) count over 100,000/μl.

II. **Etiology and Clinical Manifestations**
   A. It occurs in chronic myelogenous leukemia (especially in blast crisis), acute myelogenous leukemia, acute lymphoblastic leukemia, and chronic lymphoid leukemia.
   B. Clinical manifestations represent organ system compromise secondary to the elevated WBC count and include respiratory insufficiency from capillary leak and central nervous system (CNS) dysfunction manifested by blurred vision, dizziness, vertigo, headache, and altered mental status.

III. **Treatment**
   A. When the patient is symptomatic, emergent treatment is necessary. This includes hydration, urine alkalinization, and allopurinol.
   B. Leukopheresis and prompt institution of appropriate chemotherapy should follow the initial measures. The need for leukopheresis is determined by the WBC count and the clinical symptoms and should be individualized for each patient.

Polycythemia

I. **Definition**
   A. Altered sensitivity to erythropoitin leading to an elevated red blood cell mass.
   B. May be primary (polycythemia rubra vera) or secondary to certain cancers, most importantly renal cell carcinoma and hepatoma.

II. **Clinical Manifestations**
   Clinical features include headache, weakness, dizziness, mild to severe CNS compromise with cerebral infarction or bleeding, Budd-Chiari syndrome, and splenomegaly.

III. **Treatment**
   A. Polycythemia, when severe (hematocrit greater than 60%) and symptomatic, merits emergent treatment.
   B. Apheresis, sequential phlebotomies, and hydroxyurea are the mainstays of treatment.

Thrombocytosis

I. **Definition**
   An abnormal elevation of the platelet count.

II. **Etiology**
   A. Increased platelet count may be associated with myeloproliferative disorders such as chronic myelogenous leukemia, essential thrombocytosis, polycythemia vera, and myeloid metaplasia.
   B. It is also observed in many cancers as a secondary phenomenon (e.g., in lung and liver cancer).
   C. Platelet plugs cause vascular occlusion and tissue ischemia, and platelet function defects

lead to a bleeding diathesis. The latter is more common and may manifest as purpura or as intracranial or gastrointestinal hemorrhage.

D. Thrombotic manifestations include cerebral thrombosis, transient ischemic attacks, myocardial infarction, and digit ischemia.

III. Treatment

A. Symptomatic patients may need emergent treatment, which includes platelet pheresis, hydroxyurea (30 mg/kg/day) or anagrelide, a new agent.

B. Chronic management is discussed elsewhere.

Thrombocytopenia

I. Definition

A decrease in the platelet count.

II. Etiology

A. This is most often secondary to chemotherapy, but it may be directly due to an underlying cancer, as seen in acute leukemias, and to bone marrow invasion by solid tumors (e.g., breast cancer).

B. Immune-mediated thrombocytopenia can occur in chronic lymphoid leukemia and lymphomas.

III. Treatment

A. Platelet counts below 20,000/μl require prophylactic platelet transfusions.

B. Patients with acute bleeding (e.g., gastrointestinal hemorrhage) often need more frequent platelet transfusions to keep their platelet counts around 50,000/μl.

C. Immune-mediated thrombocytopenia, diagnosed by the presence of increased numbers of megakaryocytes in the bone marrow, is treated with corticosteroids and immune globulin. The underlying cause is also treated.

Bibliography

Berger M. (editor). Oncologic Emergencies. Seminars in Oncology. 16:461–588, 1989.

DeVita V, Hellman S, Rosenberg S. Cancer: Principles and Practice of Oncology. Ed 3. J.B. Lippincott Co. 1989.

SECTION 10

Nephrology

CHAPTER 81

Approach to the Patient with Renal Disease

Edmund J. Lewis, M.D.

I. Identification of the Patient With Renal Disease
  A. History
    1. Nephrotoxins
      a. Antibiotics
        (1) Aminoglycosides
        (2) Sulfa agents
        (3) Penicillins and cephalosporins
        (4) Pentamidine
        (5) Amphotericin
      b. Radiocontrast agents
      c. Nonsteroidal anti-inflammatory agents
      d. Chemotherapeutic agents
        (1) Cis-Platinum
        (2) Methotrexate
        (3) Mitomycin-C
      e. Penicillamine
      f. Gold
    2. Family History
      a. Polycystic kidney disease
      b. Deafness
      c. Hematuria
      d. Hypertension
    3. HIV risk factors
    4. Intravenous drug abuse
    5. Systemic diseases
      a. Rheumatologic disease
      b. Diabetes
      c. Hypertension
    6. Infections
    7. Clinical signs and symptoms
      a. Edema
      b. HTN
      c. Hematuria
      d. Uremia
        (1) Nausea and vomiting
        (2) Lethargy
        (3) Pruritus
      e. Oliguria
      f. Nocturia
  B. Physical exam
    1. Blood pressure
    2. Edema
    3. Flank tenderness
    4. Rash
    5. Arthritis
    6. Pericardial rub
    7. Asterixis
    8. Mental Status
  C. Laboratory evaluation (See Chapter 82: Diagnostic Methods):
    1. Urinalysis
    2. BUN, creatinine, potassium, sodium, bicar-

bonate, anion gap, calcium, phosphorus, magnesium
3. Complete blood count
4. Autoimmune serology when indicated

II. Renal Syndromes
A. Fluid and electrolyte disorders
  1. Hypo/Hypernatremia: (See Chapter 83: Disorders of Salt and Water Metabolism)
  2. Hypo/Hyperkalemia: (See Chapter 83: Disorders of Salt and Water Metabolism)
B. Acid base disorders: (See Chapter 84: Disorders of Acid-Base Metabolism)
C. Hematuria
  1. Nephrolithiasis: (See Chapter 88: Nephrolithiasis)
  2. Urologic diseases
    a. Tumors
    b. Nephrolithiasis
    c. Papillary necrosis
    d. Infections
    e. Trauma
    f. Vascular malformations
  3. Glomerulonephritis
  4. Sickle cell disease and trait
  5. Renal vascular diseases
    a. Renal vein thrombosis
    b. Renal infarction
D. Proteinuria: (See Chapter 89: Glomerulonephritis and Nephrotic Syndrome)
  1. Tubular
    a. Interstitial disease
  2. Glomerular
    a. Nephrotic syndrome
    b. Nephritic syndrome
  3. Overflow
    a. Light chains
    b. Lysozymuria
  4. Orthostatic
E. Acute renal failure: (See Chapter 85: Acute Renal Failure)
  1. Pre-renal
  2. Parenchymal
  3. Post-renal
F. Chronic renal failure: (See Chapter 86: Chronic Renal Failure)
G. Nephrolithiasis: (See Chapter 88: Nephrolithiasis)
H. Hypertension
  1. Essential
  2. Renovascular
  3. Renal disease

Bibliography

Coe FL. Clinical and Laboratory Assessment of the Patient with Renal Disease. In: Brenner BM, Rector FC Jr. (eds). The Kidney. W.B. Saunders Co, Philadelphia 1986, pp. 703–734.

Epstein M, Perez GO. Pathophysiology of the edema-forming states. In: Narins RG (ed) Clinical Disorders of Fluid and Electrolyte Metabolism. McGraw-Hill Inc., New York 1994, pp. 523–544.

Fairley KF. Urinalysis. In: Schrier RW, Gottschalk CW, (eds). Diseases of the kidney. Little, Brown & Co., Boston. 1988, pp 359–392.

CHAPTER 82

Diagnostic Methods

Samuel Saltzberg, M.D.

I. Urinalysis
  A. Procedure
    1. External genitalia should be gently cleaned, foreskin retracted or labia separated, and midstream urine specimen collected.
    2. Urine should be examined within 30–60 min of voiding.
    3. Dipstick: Commercially available plastic strip with chemically impregnated paper squares which change color on exposure to urine. Measures or detects pH, leukocytes, hemoglobin, protein, glucose, ketones, and bile.
    4. Microscopy: Urine is centrifuged at 3,000 rpm for 3–5 min, supernatant is removed, and sediment is resuspended and examined under low and high power.
  B. Indications
    1. Routine screening.
    2. Hypertension: Rule out renal etiology or evidence of nephrosclerosis.
    3. Edema: Rule out nephrosis or nephritis.
    4. Flank pain: Rule out renal stones, pyelonephritis, acute glomerulonephritis, and renal infarction.
    5. Dysuria: Rule out urinary tract infection, urethritis, renal stones.
    6. Fever: Rule out urinary tract infection and glomerulonephritis.
    7. Renal insufficiency: See chapters 85 & 86.
    8. Systemic diseases: Rheumatologic/collagen vascular disease, diabetes mellitus, hemoptysis.
    9. Gross urinary abnormalities
      a. Macroscopic hematuria: See chapters 88 & 89.
      b. Foamy urine: Rule out proteinuria; see Section II, C and chapter 90.
  C. Potential Findings
    1. pH:
      a. Under normal conditions, will vary with the amount of acid/alkali in the diet.
      b. pH >5.5 in setting of metabolic acidosis is suggestive of distal renal tubular acidosis (type I RTA); see chapter 84.
      c. pH >7.0 in presence of pyuria is suggestive of infection with urease splitting organism.
    2. Specific gravity: Poor man's urine osmolarity.

a. Under normal conditions, will vary with free water requirements.

b. Will be disproportionately higher than urine osmolarity when high molecular weight molecules are present in urine (i.e., glucose, radiocontrast material).

c. Urine osmolarity is important diagnostically in conditions of abnormal water balance: hyponatremia, hypernatremia, polyuria. See chapter 83, Section I.

d. Urine osmolarity may be helpful in distinguishing between acute tubular necrosis (ATN) and prerenal azotemia; see chapter 85.

e. Isosthenuria: Fixed urine specific gravity of 1.010 (equal to plasma) suggests tubulointerstitial disease.

3. Glucose: Presence of glucosuria in the absence of hyperglycemia suggests proximal tubular cell abnormality.

4. Proteinuria

a. Can be measured with dipstick or sulfosalicylic acid test. Dipstick is most sensitive to albumin; sulfosalicylic acid test detects all proteins.

(1) False-positive dipstick: Urine pH >8, macroscopic hematuria, presence of phenazopyridine.

(2) False-negative dipstick: Light and heavy chain fragments of immunoglobulins: will be detected by sulfosalicylic acid test.

(3) False-positive sulfosalicylic acid test: Macroscopic hematuria, radiocontrast material, high levels of penicillin or cephalosporin, tolbutamide, tolmetin, sulfonamide.

b. Since the dipstick and the salfosalicylic acid test measure urinary protein concentration, the degree of positivity will vary with urine concentration. Therefore, the degree of proteinuria is best quantitated by a 24-hr urine collection. See Section II, C.

5. Hematuria

a. Dipstick will detect hematuria, hemoglobinuria, and myoglobinuria. Dipstick positive for heme, with no red blood cells (RBCs) seen on microscopic examination of urine, is suggestive of hemolysis or rhabdomyolysis, with resulting hemoglobinuria or myoglobinuria, respectively, or hemolysis of RBCs in urine with low specific gravity (<1.006).

b. Normal: Fewer than two RBCs per high-power field (HPF) on microscopic examination.

c. Origin may be glomerular or extraglomerular; see chapters 88 & 89.

d. Presence of RBC casts indicative of glomerular lesion.

6. Pyuria:

a. Normal: Fewer than four white blood cells (WBCs) per HPF on microscopic examination.

b. Contamination by periurethral or vaginal secretions is suggested by the presence of many squamous epithelial cells.

c. Infection: Pyelonephritis, cystitis, prostatitis, urethritis.

d. Tubulointerstitial disease: see chapter 85. Eosinophiluria (best detected by Hansel stain) is suggestive of but not diagnostic of drug-induced allergic interstitial nephritis.

e. Glomerulonephritis: Usually associated with hematuria and significant proteinuria.

f. Presence of WBC casts suggests glomerulonephritis, interstitial nephritis, or pyelonephritis.

7. Tubular epithelial cells

a. Nonspecific marker of tubular injury. May be increased in ATN, pyelonephritis, glomerulonephritis, or nephrotic syndrome.

b. In nephrotic syndrome, tubular cells may undergo fatty degeneration, forming oval fat bodies which reveal "Maltese crosses" under polarized light.

8. Lipid:

a. Lipiduria is typically present in nephrotic syndrome (chapter 90).

b. Free lipid can be confused with RBCs; however, lipid droplets are more refractile, exist in variable sizes, and are anisotropic under polarized light.

9. Casts: Cylindrical structures with an organic matrix (Tamm-Horsfall glycoprotein). Presence of cells within casts indicates intrarenal origin of the cells.

a. Hyaline casts

(1) Clear casts with optical density only slightly greater than that of urine.

(2) Normal finding; not indicative of renal pathology.

(3) Increased in acidic, concentrated urine and after diuretic use.

b. RBC casts: Indicative of glomerulonephritis.

c. WBC casts: Indicative of glomerulonephritis, interstitial nephritis, or pyelonephritis.

d. Epithelial cell casts: Seen in ATN, tubulointerstitial disease, and glomerulonephritis.

e. Fatty casts: Seen with moderate to heavy proteinuria.

f. Granular casts

(1) Felt to be formed from degeneration of cellular casts or aggregated serum proteins trapped within casts.

(2) Large numbers of muddy brown granular casts are commonly seen in ATN.

g. Waxy casts

(1) Casts with high optical density.

(2) Suggests markedly diminished nephron flow and therefore advanced renal disease.

h. Broad casts

(1) Formed within large or dilated tubules.

(2) Suggests advanced renal disease.

10. Crystals: presence does not necessarily imply abnormal condition.

a. Uric acid

(1) Pleomorphic.

(2) Seen in acid urine.

(3) May be present in large numbers in acute renal failure (ARF) of tumor lysis syndrome.

b. Calcium oxalate

(1) "Envelope" appearance.

(2) May be present in large numbers in ARF of ethylene glycol ingestion.

c. Calcium phosphate

(1) Wedge-shaped stellate appearance.

(2) Seen in alkaline urine.

d. Cystine

(1) Hexagonal.

(2) Pathologic; indicates cystinuria.

e. Triple phosphate (ammonium magnesium phosphate) crystals

(1) "Coffin-lid" appearance.

(2) Suggests infection with a urease-splitting organism.

11. Amorphous material: Urates in acid urine, phosphates in alkaline urine.

II. Functional Analysis

A. Creatinine clearance (CrCl)

Assuming that creatinine is completely filtered by the glomerulus and is not secreted (see Section II.A.4.b. below), reabsorbed, or metabolized by the renal tubule, creatinine clearance can give an estimate of the glomerular filtration rate.

1. Procedure

a. Patient voids at the start of the urine collection. This initial urine specimen is discarded.

b. For a specified time period (usually 24 hr), all voided urine is collected.

c. At the end of the collection period the patient voids, and this final urine is added to the collection.

d. Total urine volume and urine creatinine concentration are measured.

e. CrCl = [Urine creatinine concentration × urine volume]/[Plasma creatinine concentration × time]; units are adjusted so that final value is in milliliters per minute.

f. If the patient's plasma creatinine is not stable (i.e., patient has ARF), the time-averaged plasma creatinine concentration must be used in the denominator. If the rise in creatinine is linear, the mean of the plasma creatinines obtained at the start and finish of the collection will give an approximation.

g. Creatinine clearance in a patient in steady state can be approximated from the plasma creatinine without a urine collection by the following formula:
CrCl = [(140 − age) × (lean body weight) × (0.85 in women)]/[Plasma creatinine concentration × 72]

2. Indications

a. To determine presence and severity of renal insufficiency.

b. Serial measurements may be useful in following disease progression.

3. Potential findings

a. Normal creatinine clearance is 120 ± 25 ml/min in men, 95 ± 20 ml/min in women, with loss of 1 ml/min/year over age 40.

4. Limitations
  a. Inaccurate collection
    (1) Not all urine produced during the collection period is recovered.
    (2) Patient does not or cannot void completely at the beginning or end of the collection period.
    (3) Patient does not collect urine for the specified period of time.
    (4) Suspect incomplete collection if the amount of creatinine recovered in 24 hr is less than <20–25 mg/kg of lean body weight in men or <15–20 mg/kg of lean body weight in women.
  b. Creatinine is in fact secreted.
    (1) Creatinine clearance will tend to overestimate the glomerular filtration rate (GFR).
    (2) Relative amount of creatinine secreted to creatinine filtered increases with progressive renal failure.
    (3) Drugs that interfere with creatinine secretion (i.e., cimetidine, trimethoprim, probenecid, triamterene, spironolactone, amiloride) will decrease creatinine clearance while not affecting GFR.
  c. Compounds that interfere with plasma creatinine determination (i.e., noncreatinine chromagens, acetoacetate, cefoxitin, flucytosine) will make creatinine clearance determination uninterpretable.
  d. As renal disease progresses, some nephrons may hyperfiltrate to compensate for other nephron loss. Therefore, in early renal disease (<25–33% nephron loss), total renal creatinine clearance may remain stable despite disease progression.
B. Urine electrolytes
  1. Urine Na$^+$
    a. In normal subjects, urine Na$^+$ excretion will vary with Na$^+$ intake.
    b. Will be low (<20 mEq/liter) in conditions of decreased effective circulating volume, glomerular ischemia, and acute glomerulonephritis.
    c. Indications
      (1) Hyponatremia (see chapter 83)
        (a) Less than 20 mEq/liter in volume depleted or volume overloaded (congestive heart failure, cirrhosis, nephrosis) states.
        (b) More than 20 mEq/liter in syndrome of inappropriate antidiuretic hormone, salt-wasting nephropathy, osmotic diuresis, after diuretics use, and adrenal insufficiency.
      (2) Acute renal failure (ARF): ATN vs. prerenal azotemia (see chapter 85)
        (a) Less than 20 mEq/liter in prerenal conditions.
        (b) More than 40 mEq/liter in ATN.
        (c) Fractional excretion of Na$^+$ more accurate in distinguishing between these two conditions.
      (3) A 24-hr urine collection for absolute Na$^+$ excretion will
        (a) Determine compliance with Na$^+$ restricted diet.
        (b) Determine whether saline diuresis is responsible for polyuria.
  2. Urine Cl$^-$
    a. Generally correlates with urine Na$^+$ excretion.
    b. Metabolic alkalosis (see chapter 84)
      (1) The presence of bicarbonaturia will result in increased urinary Na$^+$ excretion even in the presence of effective volume depletion; therefore, urine Cl$^-$ is more useful.
      (2) Urine Cl$^-$ <10 mEq/liter suggests effective volume depletion (chloride-responsive metabolic alkalosis).
  3. Urine K$^+$:
    a. In normal subjects, urine K$^+$ excretion will vary with K$^+$ intake.
    b. Hypokalemia (see chapter 83).
      (1) K$^+$ excretion <30 mEq/24 hr suggests nonrenal K$^+$ wasting, poor K$^+$ intake, or prior diuretic use.
      (2) K$^+$ excretion >30 mEq/24 hr suggests renal K$^+$ wasting.
    c. Hyperkalemia: Not useful in the work-up of chronic hyperkalemia, as urinary K$^+$ secretion must be inadequate if patient has persistent hyperkalemia.

4. Urine anion gap
   a. $[Na^+] + [K^+] - [Cl^-]$
   b. Typically negative secondary to unmeasured cation ammonium, NH_4^+.
   c. Useful in metabolic acidosis to distinguish between nonrenal acidosis (i.e., diarrhea, urine anion gap markedly negative secondary to appropriate NH_4^+ production by the kidney) vs. inadequate renal acid excretion (i.e., type I and IV renal tubular acidosis [RTA] and renal insufficiency, anion gap positive secondary to inadequate NH_4^+ production).

C. Proteinuria
   1. Degree
      a. Normal: <150 mg/25 hr, mainly Tamm-Horsfall mucoprotein.
      b. Less than 3.5 g/24 hr: Suggests glomerular lesion (see chapter 90). From 150 mg to 3.5 g/24 hr
         (1) Can be tubular or glomerular in origin.
         (2) Predominance of low molecular weight proteins (lysozyme and β_2-microglobulin) as opposed to albumin suggests tubular origin.
      c. Microalbuminuria (albuminuria >30 mg/24 hr)
         (1) Strongly predictive of development of diabetic nephropathy in diabetics.
         (2) Will not be detected with routine urinalysis.
   2. Pattern
      a. Intermittent
         (1) Exercise
         (2) Fever
         (3) CHF
      b. Orthostatic
         (1) Normal amount of proteinuria during recumbency; significant proteinuria occurs only in upright position.
         (2) Typically found in younger patients (age <25 years).
         (3) Benign course; renal biopsy not indicated.
      c. Persistent
         (1) Secondary to glomerular lesion, tubulointerstitial disease, high right-sided pressure (i.e., constrictive pericarditis, CHF), renal artery stenosis, chronic obstruction, light or heavy chain immunoglobulin fragments, lysozymuria (acute leukemia).
         (2) Presence of >2 g/24 hr of proteinuria, active urine sediment (RBCs, WBCs, cellular and granular casts), hypertension (HTN), and/or renal insufficiency suggests more severe disease; and renal biopsy should be considered (see Section IV).

III. **Imaging Techniques**
   A. Plain film
      1. Detects renal or urinary tract calcifications.
      2. Renal nephrotomogram helpful in determining size and shape of kidneys.
   B. Intravenous urography
      1. Useful in evaluation of pelvicaliceal system and ureters: rule out renal stones (including radiolucent stones), papillary necrosis, ureteral obstruction, and medullary sponge kidney.
      2. Detects renal masses (cannot distinguish cystic from solid masses).
      3. Determines renal size and shape (i.e., scarring from renal infarction or chronic pyelonephritis).
      4. Risk of ATN, especially in patients with underlying renal insufficiency.
      5. Poor opacification in patients with moderate to severe renal insufficiency.
   C. Retrograde urography
      1. Allows evaluation of ureters and pelvicaliceal system without risk of IV radiocontrast.
      2. Best method of evaluating collecting system in patients with significant renal impairment.
   D. Ultrasound
      1. Noninvasive way of evaluating renal size and shape.
      2. Detects renal masses and distinguishes between simple cysts, complex cysts, and solid masses.
      3. Detects perinephric fluid collections (i.e., abscesses, hematomas).
      4. Detects both radiopaque and radiolucent renal stones (may not visualize small or ureteric calculi).
      5. Detects hydronephrosis and hydroureter (false negatives can be seen in patients with acute obstruction or retroperitoneal disease).

6. Procedure limited in obese patients.

E. Computed tomography (CT) scan
1. Excellent for evaluating renal masses, as well as retroperitoneal and perinephric processes.
2. Useful for preoperative staging of renal carcinomas.
3. Detects hydronephrosis and hydroureter, small renal cysts (rules out polycystic kidney disease), and renal stones.
4. Risk of ATN if radiocontrast is used, especially in patients with underlying renal insufficiency. Noncontrast study recommended only for evaluation of renal or perirenal calcification or hemorrhage or to rule out urine extravasation.

F. Magnetic resonance imaging
1. Provides anatomic detail of kidney for evaluation of masses and cysts.
2. Advantage over CT in ability to avoid nephrotoxic radiocontrast material.
3. Inferior to CT in detection of small masses and in identifying calcific or fatty structures.
4. Renal stones, because of lack of mobile protons, are detected by absence of signal.
5. May be useful in evaluating renal vasculature (i.e., renal artery aneurysms, arteriovenous malformations, renal vein thrombosis).

G. Angiography
1. Direct visualization of renal vascular system.
2. Best technique for evaluating large- and small-vessel stenoses, aneurysms, and malformations.
3. Renal venography can detect renal vein thrombosis or tumor invasion.
4. Used to evaluate renal vasculature prior to renal surgery.
5. Angioplasty of stenosis or embolization of aneurysm or arteriovenous fistula can be performed during the procedure.
6. Used to diagnose and stage renal carcinoma; largely supplanted by ultrasound and CT.
7. Risks include ARF from radiocontrast nephrotoxicity, renal artery dissection or occlusion, or atheroembolic disease.

H. Radionuclide studies
1. Agents:
a. Glomerular filtration
(1) ^{51}Cr EDTA; chromium ethylene diamine tetraacidic acid

(2) ^{99}Tc^m DTPA; technetium diethylene triamine pentaacetic acid
b. Effective renal plasma flow
(1) ^{131}IOIH: radioiodinated ortho-hippurate
(2) ^{99}Tc^m MAG3: technetium mercaptoacetyl triglycine
c. Tubular fixation
(1) ^{99}Tc^m DMSA: technetium dimercaptosuccinate
(2) ^{99}Tc^m aprotinin
2. Indications
a. Document renal perfusion: Rules out renal artery occlusion
b. Determine relative contribution of each kidney to total renal function.
c. Determine whether renal mass contains functional nephrons.
d. Diagnose obstructive uropathy.
e. Used with and without captopril to evaluate renovascular disease.

IV. **Renal Biopsy**
A. Procedure
1. Percutaneous biopsy
a. Establish normal platelet count, prothrombin time, partial thromboplastin time, and bleeding time.
b. Place patient in prone position.
c. Kidney typically localized by ultrasound, CT, or fluoroscopy.
d. Skin over biopsy site is prepped and local anesthetic administered.
e. Lower pole of kidney identified with "locating" needle.
f. Biopsy is performed using modified Vim-Silverman needle, Travenol Trucut disposable needle or automated biopsy gun.
g. Patient remains at bed rest for 24 hr, with frequent monitoring of blood pressure, pulse, and hematocrit.
2. Open biopsy
a. Performed in operating room under general anesthesia with direct visualization of the kidney.
b. Performed when there is a strong indication for renal biopsy in a patient for whom a percutaneous biopsy would be too risky (i.e., solitary or horseshoe kidney, bleeding abnormality, uncooperative patient).
B. Indications: Renal biopsies are performed to diagnose intrinsic renal disease that cannot be diagnosed by other means, to determine the

severity of disease, and to determine the response to therapy. There are no universally accepted indications, and the risk/benefit ratio must be determined on a case to case basis.

1. Proteinuria
   a. Less than 2 g/24 hr
      (1) In the absence of hematuria, HTN, renal insufficiency, or systemic disease, the prognosis is generally good, and unless there is a need for a specific diagnosis, many nephrologists would observe.
      (2) The presence of hematuria, HTN, and/or azotemia suggests more severe renal disease; a biopsy may be indicated if the specific diagnosis cannot otherwise be made.
   b. More than 2 g/24 hr
      (1) Suggests more severe disease.
      (2) In children with nephrotic syndrome, because of the high probability of the diagnosis of minimal change disease, most nephrologists would first treat empirically with corticosteroids as opposed to performing a renal biopsy.
      (3) In adults with nephrotic syndrome this is controversial, with some nephrologists first attempting an empiric trial of corticosteroids and others proceeding directly to renal biopsy.
2. Hematuria (see chapter 89)
   a. If hematuria of glomerular etiology is suspected, a renal biopsy should be considered.
   b. Asymptomatic patients with no or minimal proteinuria (<1 g/24 hr), no granular or cellular casts, no HTN, and normal renal function have a good prognosis, and many nephrologists will observe.
3. ARF
   a. ARF in hospitalized patients is commonly secondary to prerenal azotemia, ATN, drug-induced interstitial nephritis, or obstruction. Usually the diagnosis can be made clinically, and a renal biopsy is not necessary.
   b. ARF with an active urinary sediment (i.e., RBCs, WBCs) when the diagnosis is uncertain should strongly be considered for renal biopsy, as delay in diagnosis and treatment may result in permanent loss of renal function.
4. Chronic renal failure
   a. Renal biopsy in patients with chronic severe renal failure (especially with small kidneys on imaging) carries increased risk and is likely to reveal nondiagnostic scarring, and the disease process will likely not be amenable to treatment.
   b. In less advanced disease, biopsy should be considered if it will alter the therapeutic approach, if a specific diagnosis is necessary for prognostic reasons, or if it will assist in diagnosing a systemic disease.

C. Potential findings
   1. Light microscopy
      a. Glomeruli
         (1) Focal (only some glomeruli involved) vs. diffuse (all glomeruli involved).
         (2) Segmental (only a portion of the glomerulus involved) vs. global (whole glomerulus involved).
         (3) Cellular proliferation (extracapillary, endocapillary, mesangial) and necrosis.
         (4) Mesangial deposits or expansion.
         (5) Sclerosis.
         (6) Basement membrane abnormalities (thickness, splitting, defects): Evaluated with periodic acid–Schiff and silver stains.
      b. Tubules
         (1) Evidence of tubular necrosis and regeneration (ATN).
         (2) Evidence of tubular atrophy, dropout, and dilatation (chronic irreversible damage).
      c. Interstitium
         (1) Cellular infiltrates (acute interstitial nephritis).
         (2) Fibrosis (chronic irreversible damage).
      d. Vasculature
         (1) Arteriolar sclerosis (HTN).
         (2) Fibrinoid necrosis (malignant HTN, scleroderma).
         (3) Intravascular thrombi (fibrin: hemolytic-uremic syndrome, thrombotic thrombocytopenic purpura, malignant HTN, scleroderma; im-

mune complex: cryoglobulinemia).

    (4) Cholesterol emboli.

    (5) Inflammation (vascular rejection in transplant, vasculitis).

  2. Immunofluorescence

    a. Can detect immunoglobulins, complement, fibrin, albumin.

    b. Linear staining of basement membrane for IgG (anti–glomerular basement membrane disease, diabetes mellitus DM).

    c. Granular subepithelial deposits (membranous nephropathy, post-strepto-coccal glomerulonephritis).

    d. Granular subendothelial deposits (membranoproliferative glomerulo-nephritis, systemic lupus erythematosus, endocarditis, cryoglobulinemia).

    e. Mesangial (IgA, IgG, IgM, light chains, C_3).

  3. Electron microscopy

    a. Epithelial cells: Foot process fusion [(minimal change disease, focal segmental glomerulosclerosis (FSGS)].

    b. Immune complex deposits (mesangial, subepithelial, subendothelial).

    c. Basement membrane abnormalities

      (1) Thin basement membrane disease

      (2) Splitting in Alport's syndrome

      (3) Thickened in diabetic nephropathy

D. Limitations

  1. Insufficient tissue.

  2. Sampling error.

  3. Many different disease processes can have similar histologic appearances.

E. Contraindications

  1. Single functioning or horseshoe kidney.

  2. Bleeding disorder.

  3. Uncontrolled hypertension.

  4. Renal mass.

  5. Renal artery aneurysm.

  6. Sepsis.

  7. Renal abscess or pyelonephritis.

  8. Uncooperative patient.

F. Complications

  1. Bleeding

    a. Majority of patients have some peri-nephric or intrarenal bleeding, which is usually self-limited.

    b. One out of 10 patients will have gross hematuria (blood clots can cause obstruction).

    c. One out of 100 patients will require a blood transfusion.

    d. One out of 1,000 patients will require a nephrectomy.

  2. Arteriovenous fistula

    a. From 5% to 15% of biopsies

    b. Can cause hematuria, HTN, pain, and high-output heart failure.

  3. Puncture of other organ (liver, intestine)

Bibliography

Hricak H. Radiologic assessment of the kidney. In: *The Kidney* ed 4, Brenner BM, Rector FC (eds.). Saunders, Philadelphia, 1991, pp. 868–892.

Levey AS, Madaio MP, Perrone RD. Laboratory assessment of renal disease: clearance urinalysis and renal biopsy. In: *The Kidney* ed 4, Brenner BM, Rector FC (eds.). Saunders, Philadelphia, 1991, pp. 919–968.

Rose BD. Clinical assessment of renal function. In: *Pathophysiology of Renal Disease*, ed 2, Rose BD (ed.). McGraw-Hill Book Company, New York, 1987, pp. 1–37.

Skemesh O, Golbetz H, Kriss JP et al. Limitations of creatinine as a filtration marker in glomerulopathic patients. *Kidney Int* 28:830–836, 1985.

Disorders of Salt and Water Metabolism

Susan Hou, M.D.

Physiology of Salt and Water Excretion

I. Salt Excretion

A. Intravascular volume, as sensed by the kidney, is the major determinant of sodium excretion. The kidney filters approximately 24,000 mEq of sodium per day and reabsorbs approximately 99% of it. Small changes in the rate of reabsorption cause major changes in total body sodium.

B. From 50% to 80% of filtered sodium is reabsorbed in the proximal tubule by active transport, the amount depending on the renal blood flow.

C. The loop of Henle reabsorbs 25–40% of the filtered load of sodium. The thick ascending limb of the loop of Henle is impermeable to water, so sodium is absorbed, leaving water behind, a process that results in the formation of a dilute urine. The distal convoluted tubule reabsorbs approximately 10% of filtered sodium.

D. Sodium is added to the filtrate in the early segment proximal to the macula densa and reabsorbed distal to the macula densa.

E. The collecting tubule, responsible for reabsorption of 10% of filtered sodium aldoster-one, controls the rate of sodium reabsorption in this segment, increasing it in states of volume depletion and increasing it in states of volume overload.

II. Water Excretion

A. Abnormalities in serum sodium concentration result primarily from disordered excretion of water. As long as the kidney excretes the solute load produced by the body daily (approximately 800 mOsm/day), there is an obligate water loss determined by the concentrating ability of the kidney. If the kidney can produce a maximally concentrated urine of 1,600 mOsm/kg, 0.5 liter of urine must be excreted. Insensible loss is approximately 500–1,000 ml, depending on activity and body temperature. When water intake exceeds water loss through solute excretion and insensible loss, the kidney must excrete water by making a more dilute urine. Water is freely filtered at the glomerulus. It is reabsorbed passively following active sodium reabsorption in the proximal tubule. The descending limb of the loop of Henle is permeable to water, and water moves into the hypertonic medullary interstitium.

B. The ascending limb of the loop of Henle is impermeable to water. Here sodium and chloride are reabsorbed without water, leading to the formation of a dilute urine. Final determination of water excretion depends on the effect of antidiuretic hormone (ADH) on the collecting duct. In the absence of ADH, the collecting duct is impermeable to water and the dilute urine formed in the loop of Henle is excreted unchanged. When ADH is present, the collecting duct becomes permeable to water and water is moved into the hypertonic medullary interstitium. A concentrated urine is formed.

C. Factors leading to release of ADH
1. Increased osmolality.
2. Decreased effective circulating blood volume.
3. Decreased blood pressure.
4. Stress

Hypernatremia

I. Definition and Etiology

A. Hypernatremia with hypovolemia: Loss of water in excess of sodium. Hypernatremia occurs only when water is not available or the thirst mechanism is disordered.
1. Disordered thirst: In normal individuals, osmoreceptors in the anterolateral hypothalamus result in thirst when serum osmolality exceeds 295 mOsm. Severe hypovolemia may also result in thirst. The thirst mechanism can be disrupted by:
   a. Tumors impinging on the hypothalamus.
   b. Trauma.
   c. Granulomatous diseases.
   d. Vascular disease affecting the anterior communicating artery.
2. Extrarenal loss: Occurs when there is insensible loss or loss from sweat, which in the untrained individual contains about 70 mEq/liter of sodium; when water is not available for replacement; or, in the case of an ill patient, when the thirst mechanism is not normal.
3. Renal losses
   a. Central diabetes insipidus: This occurs with loss of 75% of the vasopressin secretory potential of the neurohyophysis. Many of the disorders that depress

the thirst mechanism can cause central diabetes insipidus.
   (1) Trauma and surgery.
   (2) Tumor: Primary brain tumor or lymphoma, leukemia.
   (3) Granulomatous diseases.
   (4) Infection: Tuberculosis, meningitis, encephalitis.
   (5) Vascular: Sheehan's syndrome, carotid aneurysm.
   (6) Gestational: Results from overproduction of vasopressinase, with failure of the pituitary to keep up with breakdown.
   b. Nephrogenic diabetes insipidus
   (1) Familial: X-linked recessive disorder.
   (2) Metabolic: Hypercalcemia, hypokalemia.
   (3) Drug-induced
      (a) Lithium: Polyuria occurs in 10% of patients treated with lithium. Interferes with the effect of ADH on the kidney at a point beyond cyclic AMP generation. Initially reversible but may become permanent.
      (b) Amphotericin.
      (c) Demeclocycline: in high doses. Used for treatment of the syndrome of inappropriate antidiuretic hormome (SIADH).
      (d) Obstructive uropathy.
      (e) Sickle cell disease or trait.
   c. Osmotic diuresis: Causes both salt and water losses, with disproportionately greater water losses. In the proximal tubule, where sodium is actively reabsorbed and water passively follows, the osmotically active substance remains in the tubular lumen and prevents water from being reabsorbed along its concentration gradient. Since the total amount of filtrate reaching the loop of Henle is increased, transit time is shortened in the loop as well as in the collecting duct, and the time for water reabsorption is decreased. The medullary gradient on which water reabsorption depends is washed out.
   (1) Metabolic: Hyperglycemia.
   (2) Drugs: Mannitol, radiographic contrast.
   (3) Postobstructive diuresis. Additive to

concentrating defect in obstructive uropathy

B. Hypernatremia with normal or expanded intravascular volume: Usually iatrogenic. Also requires disordered thirst or lack of access to water. Usually results from administration of normal saline without taking into account hypotonic losses.

II. Clinical consequences

A. Predominantly central nervous system (CNS) findings, including irritability, lethargy, ataxia, and seizures.

B. Acute hypernatremia with serum sodium greater than 160 mEq/liter carries a 50–75% mortality rate, and neurologic sequelae are common. However, the clinical picture is confusing since hypernatremia frequently develops in the setting of CNS abnormalities.

III. Differential Diagnosis

A. Distinction between renal and extrarenal losses: With extrarenal losses of both salt and water, urine sodium is <10 mEq/liter. With renal losses it is usually >20mEq/liter.

B. Central vs. nephrogenic diabetes insipidus: Measure changes in serum and urine osmolality and, when available, serum vasopressin levels, following a 4- to 6-hr dehydration test. Vasopressin is given at the end of the test, and changes in urine osmolality are observed. The patient with central diabetes insipidus should concentrate the urine following vasopressin intake, while the patient with nephrogenic diabetes insipidus will not respond.

IV. Treatment

A. Acute treatment: Water deficit can be calculated by using the following formula:

$$\frac{\text{Current serum sodium}}{\text{Ideal serum sodium}} \times \text{total body water} = \text{ideal TBW}$$

Ideal TBW − actual TBW = water deficit

1. In acute treatment of hypernatremia, water can be given in the form of D5W at a rate calculated to lower the serum sodium 10–15 mEq/day. Ongoing losses need to be included in the calculations.

B. Chronic treatment
1. Central diabetes insipidus can be treated with intranasal administration of the vasopressin analog desmopressin.
2. Nephrogenic diabetes insipidus: Often irreversible when secondary to drug use or,

as in the case of lithium, when there is no satisfactory alternative to the drug. Thiazide diuretics suppress sodium reabsorption in the diluting segment of the nephron, which results in mild volume contraction and increased reabsorption of sodium and water in the proximal tubule. Thiazides can bring about a modest decrease in polyuria.

V. Prognosis: Mortality in acute hypernatremia is 30–60%. Chronic hypernatremia is better tolerated and neurologic symptoms with a serum sodium as high as 160 mEq/L are generally reversible.

Hyponatremia

I. Definition and Etiology

A. Hyponatremia without hypoosmolality
1. Hyperglycemia: Glucose which cannot be transported into cells results in movement of water from the intracellular space, resulting in a drop in serum sodium by dilution.
2. Mannitol: Accumulates only in the presence of renal failure, but when it does, it results in hyponatremia by the same mechanism as glucose.
3. Hyperlipidemia: The water content of plasma is decreased, resulting in a decreased sodium concentration even while the sodium concentration in the water phase of plasma remains the same.
4. Paraproteinemia: Some mechanism as hyperlipidemia

B. Hyponatremia with hypovolemia: When any salt and water loss is replaced with water alone, when a critical volume loss is reached, hyponatremia occurs through three mechanisms:
1. Avid sodium reabsorption in the proximal tubule results in decreased delivery of filtrate to the diluting segment of the nephron.
2. The collecting duct is not completely impermeable to water, and when transit time is slowed by a decrease in filtrate, water may be reabsorbed.
3. When a critical degree of volume contraction occurs, ADH is released in response to volume in spite of low serum osmolality.

C. Hyponatremia with hypervolemia: Renal plasma flow is reduced in edema-forming states, and water is retained. There is decreased effective circulating volume, and the kidney responds to decreased renal perfusion with increased proximal sodium reabsorption and decreased delivery of filtrate to the diluting segment of the nephron. In the case of renal failure there may be no water excretion, and serum sodium is simply a function of salt and water intake and extrarenal losses.

1. Congestive heart failure.
2. Cirrhosis of the liver.
3. Acute and chronic renal failure.

D. Hyponatremia with euvolemia
  1. SIADH
    a. Tumors, particularly bronchogenic carcinoma, may secrete ADH without any relationship to plasma osmolality. This has been described with other tumors, including gastric, pancreatic, duodenal, bladder, and prostate.
    b. Pulmonary diseases.
    c. Neurologic diseases.
    d. Psychiatric diseases.
    e. Reset osmostat: Some individuals retain the ability to completely suppress ADH secretion, but do so at a lower serum osmolality than normal people.
  2. Endocrine causes
    a. Adrenal glucocorticoid insufficiency: Causes water retention through hemodynamically mediated release of ADH and possibly by changes in renal hemodynamics.
    b. Hypothyroidism: Decreased delivery of filtrate to the diluting segment of the nephron and persistent ADH release result in a water-excreting defect in hypothyroidism. It rarely leads to clinically important hyponatremia.
  3. Drugs
    a. Thiazide diuretics can lead to hyponatremia by unknown mechanisms. The patient may be either hypovolemic or euvolemic. In a small minority of patients, hyponatremia develops rapidly and may lead to death or permanent brain damage.
    b. Chlorpropamide causes hyponatremia in 4% of patients by increasing renal tubular sensitivity to ADH.
    c. Carbamazepine: Mechanism unclear
    d. ? Phenothiazines, tricyclic antidepressants, monoamine oxidase inhibitors. It is not clear whether the drug or the underlying disease is responsible.
    e. Cytoxan: May enhance tubular sensitivity to ADH. Water intoxication may be a problem because patients receiving high-dose cytoxan are vigorously hydrated.
    f. Vincristine.
    g. Clofibrate: Increases ADH release.
    h. Narcotics.
  4. Postoperative hyponatremia: ADH release is increased in the postoperative period. It is not clear whether this is the result of pain, emesis, or narcotic administration. Hyponatremia is not uncommon in postoperative patients given hypotonic fluids. It is usually mild, but a small subset of healthy women undergoing routine operations develops severe hyponatremia, resulting in severe brain damage and death.
  5. Psychogenic polydipsia.

II. Clinical Consequences

A. Hyponatremia may be associated with nausea, anorexia, lethargy, confusion, seizures, irreversible brain damage, and death. The severity of the symptoms depends on the rate of fall of the serum sodium.
B. Some investigators believe that a drop from 140 to 125 mEq/liter within 24 hr may be associated with permanent brain damage.
C. People who experience a slow drop in serum sodium are frequently asymptomatic even at very low levels of serum sodium.

III. Differential Diagnosis

A. Volume status may be evident on physical exam.
B. Urine sodium: In congestive heart failure, cirrhosis, or volume contraction, urine sodium is generally <20 mEq/liter and Fractional excretion of sodium (Fe_{Na}) will be <1%. The use of diuretics raises the urine sodium in these conditions. In renal failure, urine sodium is generally >20 mEq/liter and Fe_{Na} is >1%. SIADH is usually associated with mild volume expansion not apparent on physical exam. Accordingly, urine sodium is >20 mEq/liter and Fe_{Na} is >1%. If an individual with SIADH become volume contracted, urine sodium will drop. Urine sodium is elevated in adrenal insufficiency.
C. SIADH is accompanied by other subtle signs of volume expansion. The creatinine is <1 mg/dl, and blood urea nitrogen (BUN) is <10 mg/dl if underlying renal function is normal. Uric acid is depressed.
D. Adrenal insufficiency is usually associated with elevated serum potassium and slightly

elevated BUN and creatinine due to mineral-ocorticoid deficiency. The diagnosis can be made by the Cortrosyn stimulation test.

E. Urine osmolality is inappropriately high in all types of hyponatremia except psychogenic polydipsia, where water intake exceeds the ability of the normal kidney to excrete it.

F. Measurement of thyroxine and thyroid-stimulating hormone can be used to exclude hypothyroidism.

G. Drug use should be apparent from the patient's history but in surreptitious diuretic use, serum and urine measurements of diuretics may be necessary.

H. Measurements of serum ADH levels are becoming increasingly available for use in the diagnosis of SIADH.

IV. Treatment

A. Hyponatremia with hypovolemia: Normal saline will correct volume depletion and reverse the processes that result in water retention. Adequate filtrate will be delivered to the diluting segment of the nephron, and ADH release in response to volume stimuli will be turned off.

B. Correction of hyponatremia in edema-forming states includes water restriction, discontinuation of diuretics if they are being used, and, if possible, treatment of the underlying condition.

C. Treatment of euvolemic hyponatremia

1. In drug-induced hyponatremia, the drug is discontinued.
2. Adrenal insufficiency and hypothyroidism are treated with specific hormonal replacement.
3. All euvolemic forms of hyponatremia respond to water restriction.
4. Water restriction may be difficult in forms of SIADH which are not reversible. Drugs which cause nephrogenic diabetes insipidus can be used chronically. Lithium has been used, but it does not impair urinary concentration in all patients and is complicated by neurologic and gastrointestinal side effects even at therapeutic doses. Demeclocycline predictably causes increased water losses in doses of 1,200 mg daily.
5. Vasopressin antagonists are being developed to treat SIADH.

D. The controversy surrounding the treatment of hyponatremia centers on the treatment of severe, symptomatic hyponatremia. Severe, acute hyponatremia can be associated with irreversible brain damage. However, rapid correction of hyponatremia has been associated with central pontine myelinolysis manifested by pseudobulbar palsy, quadriparesis, swallowing difficulties, and inability to speak. Symptoms may develop after transient improvement. Some investigators have argued that the development of this syndrome is either the result of hyponatremia itself or of correction to hypernatremic levels or hypoxia associated with the underlying disease. We offer the following guidelines for correction of hyponatremia:

1. Asymptomatic hyponatremia can be treated with water restriction alone, including the elimination of hypotonic intravenous fluids.
2. Care should be taken not to raise the serum sodium acutely above 120 mEq/liter when hyponatremia is chronic or 130 mEq/liter when acute.
3. Acute hyponatremia can be corrected at a rate of 2 mEq/liter/hr.
4. Chronic hyponatremia should not be corrected at a rate faster than 0.5 mEq/liter/hr.
5. Hypertonic saline (3%) should be given in 100-ml infusions, with careful monitoring of the serum sodium when hyponatremia is severe ($\leq$115 mEq/L) and the patient has neurologic symptoms. Lasix can be given and urinary sodium losses replaced in the form of 3% saline. The patient with SIADH is usually volume expanded, and whatever sodium is given will be excreted in the urine until the patient becomes euvolemic.

V. Prognosis

The mortality of chronic hyponatremia has been estimated to be anywhere from 10–30% although death is frequently the result of underlying disease rather than hyponatremia per se. Complete recovery is the rule if the serum sodium does not drop below 125 mEq/L in acute hyponatremia, as long as the underlying disease is reversible. There is a high incidence of death or permanent brain damage in healthy young women who become hyponatremic postoperatively, with 27% mortality and 60% chronic vegetative state in one series. Death secondary to central pontine myelinolysis has been seen with rapid correction or over correction of hyponatremia.

Bibliography

Arieff AI: Hyponatremia, convulsions, respiratory arrest, and permanent brain damage after elective surgery in healthy women. *N Engl J Med* 314:1529–1535, 1986.

Cluitmans FHM, Meinders AE: Management of severe hyponatremia: rapid or slow correction? *Am J Med* 88:161–166, 1990.

Hantman D, Rossier B, Zohlman R, et al: Rapid correction of hyponatremia in the syndrome of inappropriate secretion of antidiuretic hormone. *Ann Intern Med* 78:870–875, 1973.

Simard M, Gumbiner B, Lee A, et al: Lithium carbonate intoxication. *Arch Intern Med* 149:36–46, 1989.

Sterns RH, Riggs JE, Schochet SS: Osmotic demyelination syndrome following correction of hyponatremia. *N Engl J Med* 314:1535–1542, 1986.

Chapter 83-B

Disorders of Potassium Homeostasis

Susan Hou, M.D.

Potassium Distribution

Potassium is the major intracellular cation. Of the approximately 3,000 mEq of potassium in the body, only about 65 mEq is in the extracellular fluid. The intracellular potassium concentration is maintained by sodium potassium ATPase, which actively transports potassium into cells to offset potassium leakage out of cells along a concentration gradient. Serum potassium is maintained within a narrow range, and even small changes in serum potassium may compromise vital cell functions. The ability of humans to tolerate a wide range of dietary potassium intake depends of the ability to transport potassium into cells and the ability of the kidney to excrete potassium. Fluctuations in serum potassium do not always reflect changes in total body potassium.

Potassium Excretion

I. Renal Handling

Normally, the kidney accounts for 90% of potassium excretion. Potassium is freely filtered by the glomerulus. Most of the filtered load is reabsorbed in the proximal tubule. Potassium enters the tubular lumen in the descending limb of the loop of Henle and leaves in the thin ascending limb. Regulation ofpotassium secretion depends on the distal nephron, including the distal convoluted tubule and the collecting duct. Usually 5–15% of the filtered load is excreted, but excretion may be much higher.

II. Factors Affecting Potassium Secretion by the Distal Nephron
A. Flow rate of filtrate.
B. Tubular sodium concentration.
C. Aldosterone.
D. Transepithelial potential difference.
E. The distal nephron decreases potassium secretion and may reabsorb potassium in the face of potassium deficiency.

III. Potassium Secretion
Potassium is secreted by the colon. Secretion is increased in renal failure and decreased in potassium depletion.

Hyperkalemia

I. Definition: Serum potassium ≥5.0 mEq/L
II. Etiology

A. Increased dietary intake of potassium rarely causes hyperkalemia in the absence of an excretory defect or difficulty with transport into cells. Rapid administration of potassium salts can lead to hyperkalemia even in individuals with no excretory defect.

B. Increased endogenous load through cell lysis: Crush injuries, tumor lysis.

C. Decreased excretion
   1. Renal failure: Hyperkalemia commonly occurs in acute renal failure, particularly oliguric. In chronic renal failure, renal and colonic adaptations make it possible to excrete a normal potassium load until the glomerular filtration rate (GFR) is reduced to 10 ml/min.
   2. Hyporeninemic hypoaldosteronism (type IV renal tubular acidosis): GFR >20 ml/min. Hyperchloremic metabolic acidosis. Low renin. Low aldosterone. More frequent in diabetics.
   3. Primary hypoaldosteronism.
   4. Addison's disease.
   5. Tubular K excreting defects not secondary to decreased aldosterone: Seen in lupus and sickle cell disease.
   6. Miscellaneous unusual causes: genetically determined enzyme defects, pseudohypoaldosteronism.
   7. Drugs: Potassium-sparing diuretics, angiotensin-converting enzyme inhibitors, nonsteroidal anti-inflammatory agents, cyclosporine, heparin.

D. Altered distribution between extracellular and intracellular potassium.
   1. Insulin deficiency.
   2. Acidosis.
   3. Beta-adrenergic blockade.
   4. Exercise.
   5. Other drugs: Succinyl choline, arginine hydrochloride

III. **Clinical Consequences**
A. Cardiac: Ventricular fibrillation or cardiac arrest.
   1. Electrocardiographic (ECG) changes start with peaked T waves, followed by flattening of the P wave, prolongation, widening of the QRS complex, and, finally, a sine wave immediately before arrest.
B. Neuromuscular: Ascending paralysis similar to that of Guillain-Barré syndrome.

IV. **Treatment of Acute Hyperkalemia**
A. Calcium does not change the serum potassium but protects the heart from the effects of hyperkalemia. Used when ECG changes other than peaked T waves are present. Give calcium gluconate, 10 ml of a 10% solution; effective for 15–20 min.

B. Glucose and insulin: Insulin promotes the transport of potassium into cells, thereby lowering serum potassium. Glucose is given to prevent the induction of hypoglycemia by the insulin. An initial dose of 10 units of regular insulin can be given with 50 ml of a 50% dextrose solution. The initial bolus can be followed by an infusion of D10W with 50 units of insulin. Onset of action: 15–30 min.

C. Sodium bicarbonate: Shifts potassium into cells. Given in 50-mEq ampules every 15 min unless circulatory overload or hypernatremia develops. Onset of action: 15–30 min. Most effective if acidosis is present.

D. Kayexalate (sodium polystyrene sulfonate): Given orally in hyperosmotic solution or as a retention enema. It is a cation exchange resin which removes 1 mEq of potassium per gram when given orally and 0.5 mEq/g when given as an enema. Dose 50 grams. Onset of action: 60–120 min. May be associated with bowel perforation or ulceration if used in the immediate postoperative period.

E. Dialysis: Hemodialysis is preferred over peritoneal dialysis for severe hyperkalemia.

V. **Treatment of Chronic Hyperkalemia**
A. Restrict dietary potassium to 50 mEq/day. Avoid salt substitutes.
B. Diuretics.
C. Mineralocorticoids. May be complicated by volume overload.
D. Correction of acidosis.
E. Chronic use of exchange resins. Usually poorly tolerated.
F. Dialysis.

Hypokalemia

I. **Definition:** Serum potassium less than 3.5 mEq/L
II. **Etiology**
A. Inadequate intake: Prolonged potassium-poor diet or anorexia nervosa.
B. Extrarenal losses: After 5 days, renal potassium excretion is reduced to 20 mEq/day or a fractional excretion of 6%.
   1. Gastrointestinal: Potassium loss from diarrhea is one of the most common causes of hypokalemia. Laxative abuse and villous

adenoma of the colon are other causes of gastrointestinal loss.

2. Perspiration: Sweat contains 9 mEq/liter of potassium. Massive losses may occur during exercise in a hot environment. Renal adaptation does not occur in this form of hypokalemia.

C. Renal potassium losses

1. Diuretic therapy: The most common cause of renal potassium loss. Increased delivery of filtrate and sodium to the distal tubule results in increased potassium secretion. Chloride depletion is also associated with increased potassium secretion. The drop in serum potassium is 0.3–0.6 mEq/liter, but 10% of patients drop below 3.0 mEq/liter.

2. Other diuretic states, including postobstructive diuresis, recovery from acute tubular necrosis (ATN), osmotic diuresis. In diabetic ketoacidosis, a second mechanism of potassium loss occurs in association with ketoanions.

3. Magnesium depletion: Mechanism of renal wasting is unknown.

4. Excess mineralocorticoid: primary hyperaldosteronism. Presents with hypertension and hypokalemia, frequently with an exaggerated drop in potassium from diuretics. Other causes of increased mineralocorticoid activity include adrenal genital syndromes. licorace ingestion, and Liddle's syndrome.

5. Ectopic adrenocorticotropic hormone (ACTH) production causes hypokalemia through glucocorticoid-mediated potassium wasting.

6. Bartter's syndrome: Primary disorder of chloride reabsorption and potassium secretion. Potassium depletion leads to prostaglandin production, which, in turn, leads to other features of the syndrome, including low blood pressure, resistance to the pressor effects of angiotensin, and hyperplasia of the juxtaglomerular apparatus. Chloride wasting leads to metabolic alkalosis. It usually presents in childhood. In adults, diuretic abuse should be considered.

7. Renal tubular acidosis (RTA)

a. In distal RTA potassium secretion is increased in response to a decreased ability to secrete hydrogen ions and due to secondary hyperaldosteronism resulting from volume contraction.

b. Hypokalemia occurs in type 2 RTA primarily when treatment results in an increase in serum bicarbonate and filtered bicarbonate, with increased delivery of sodium bicarbonate to the distal tubule after the proximal tubule fails to reabsorb it.

8. Drugs

a. Penicillins: Penicillin salt represents a nonreasborbable anion which must be accompanied by a cation.

b. Cisplatinum: Secondary to tubular magnesium wasting.

c. Streptozotocin: Fanconi's syndrome with multiple proximal tubular abnormalities.

d. Aminoglycosides: Altered distal tubular permeability to potassium.

e. Amphotericin B.

D. Hypokalemia due to shifts from extracellular to intracellular space.

1. Alkalosis: Potassium shifts are less marked than in metabolic acidosis.

2. Drugs

a. Insulin.

b. β-Agonists, including inhaled β-agonists given for astham.

c. Glucose through endogenous insulin release.

3. Rapid incorporation into cells, particularly following treatment of megaloblastic anemia.

4. Hypokalemic periodic paralysis: Either an autosomal dominant disorder or acquired in association with thyrotoxicosis in Orientals.

III. **Clinical Consequences**

A. Neuromuscular: Weakness, cramps, tetany, rhabdomyolysis.

B. Cardiac: Digitalis toxicity, ventricular irritability, ECG changes including flattened T waves, U waves, and ST-segment depression.

C. Gastrointestinal: Ileus, constipation.

D. Endocrine: Carbohydrate intolerance.

E. Renal: Nephrogenic diabetes insipidus.

IV. **Treatment**

A. Estimation of potassium deficit: The estimate is always approximate because most potassium is intracellular. Each 1 mEq/liter drop in serum potassium represents a deficit of about 350 mEq. Below 2 mEq/liter, the deficit is usually more than 1000 mEq/liter and the correlation with serum potassium is poor.

B. Rate of replacement: Intravenous potassium should not be given at a rate greater 10 mEq/hr without ECG monitoring. A dose of 30 mEq/hr can be given with ECG monitoring in an intensive care unit for life-threatening emergencies. If there are no ongoing losses, oral potassium replacement can be accomplished with 40–100 mEq/day in divided dose.

C. Route of replacement: Intravenous potassium should be used only if the patient cannot take oral potassium or if life-threatening complications of hypokalemia are present. Intravenous potassium should not be used based solely on the serum potassium. When intravenous potassium is used, the patient should be monitored for sudden overshoot with the development of hyperkalemia.

D. Coexisting hypomagnesemia should be corrected.

E. Chloride deficiency should be corrected by administering potassium chloride.

F. Administration of glucose and correction of acidosis will aggravate hypokalemia.

G. Potassium replacement in individuals treated with diuretics: Potassium should be prescribed only after hypokalemia has been demonstrated. Patients with a serum potassium less than 3 mEq/liter should be treated with replacement or potassium-sparing diuretics. Those who are taking digitalis, who are at risk for arrhythmias, and who have type 2 diabetes should be given potassium supplements to keep the serum potassium above 3.5 mEq/liter. Potassium-sparing diuretics should not be used in individuals with renal insufficiency.

Bibliography

Ponce SP, Drug-induced hyperkalemia. *Medicine* 64:357,

Reeves WB, Andreoli TE. Tubular sodium transplant, in Schrier RW, Gottschalk CW (eds), *Disease of the Kidney*. Boston, Little, Brown, 1988, pp

Robertson GL, Berl T. Pathophysiology of water metabolism, in Brenner, Rector (eds), *The Kidney*. Philadelphia, Saunders, 1991, pp

Tannen RL. Disorders of potassium balance, in Brenner, Rector (eds), *The Kidney*. Philadelphia, Saunders, Philadelphia, 1991, pp.

CHAPTER 84

Disorders of Acid-Base Metabolism

Janis Orlowski, M.D.

Introduction

The normal serum concentration of hydrogen ions is 35–45 nEq/liter, or, as more commonly denoted, a serum pH of 7.35–7.45. pH is defined as the negative log concentration of hydrogen ions (pH = $\log_{10}$ $1/[H^+]$). The hydrogen ion concentration in healthy individuals, seldom deviates from a pH value of 7.40 by more than a few nanoequivalents per liter. Proper cellular function appears to be extremely sensitive to hydrogen ion concentration. The homeostatic mechanisms which maintain this careful balance are the buffering systems and renal acid excretion.

I. Buffers

A. A buffer is a pair of substances that can denote or accept hydrogen ions in a manner that moderates the serum concentration of hydrogen ions. For example, $Na_2HPO_4 + HCl \approx NaH_2PO_4 + NaCl$. In this example, phosphate acts to remove hydrogen ions from the body fluids.

B. There are many buffers in serum, including red blood cells, proteins, and, most important for the acute changes in serum concentration of hydrogen ions, the bicarbonate–carbonic acid buffering system.

C. As defined by the Henderson-Hasselbach equation, the serum concentration of hydrogen ions is buffered by bicarbonate ions to produce carbonic acid. Carbonic acid is in equilibrium with the concentration of carbon dioxide and water. Therefore:

$$H^+ + HCO_3^- \approx H_2CO_3 \approx CO_2 + H_2O$$

D. Bicarbonate will be depleted to buffer the serum against elevation in the hydrogen ion concentration. Hydrogen ions will eventually be excreted by the kidney and the buffer bicarbonate generated to restore the normal serum concentrations of these substances.

II. Renal Acid Excretion

A. Reabsorption of bicarbonate: Filtered bicarbonate is reclaimed in the proximal tubule epithelium. Carbonic acid within the proximal tubule epithelium is metabolized to bicarbonate, which is reabsorbed into the tubular blood, and hydrogen ion, which is actively excreted into the lumen of the tubule. Through the presence of the enzyme carbonic anhydrase, which is present in the luminal brush border of the proximal tubule epithelium, carbonic acid is formed from the secreted hydrogen ion and the filtered bicarbonate ion. Carbonic acid will then dehydrate to water and carbon dioxide. The end result is the generation of a bicarbonate ion with the excretion of a hydrogen ion.

B. Excretion of titratable acid: Phosphates and, to a lesser extent, sulfates and creatinine will buffer hydrogen ion excreted into the lumen of the tubule. Phosphates are weak salts freely filtered by the glomerulus. Hydrogen ions are actively secreted into the tubule lumen and bind with the phosphates to produce a salt, which is then excreted.

C. Excretion of ammonium: Ammonium excretion will vary based on the acid load to the kidney. This is the major adaptive mechanism and begins with the deamination of glutamine to ammonia (NH_3) in the renal tubule. NH_3 will freely diffuse across the cell to the lumen of the tubule, where it combines with hydrogen ions to produce NH_4^+. The trapped hydrogen ion cannot back-diffuse into the tubular cell and is therefore excreted as an ammonium salt.

Metabolic Acidosis

I. **Definition**

Acidosis is defined as an elevation in the normal serum concentration of hydrogen ions. Therefore, acidosis is a condition with a serum pH less than 7.35. *Metabolic acidosis* is the result of an underlying physiologic disturbance which is *initiated* either by the loss of bicarbonate or by the addition of hydrogen ions to the serum, leading to the elevation of hydrogen ions.

II. **Pathophysiology**

One can approach the differential diagnosis of a metabolic acidosis by looking at those conditions in which hydrogen ions are added to the serum, those in which hydrogen ions are not excreted, and, finally, those in which there is a primary loss of bicarbonate.

A. Hydrogen ion addition to the serum
   1. Intrinsic generation of acid
      a. Lactic acidosis: This form of metabolic acidosis is the most common form for the hospitalized patient. Lactic acid is produced during anaerobic metabolism or mitochondrial dysfunction from pyruvic acid. Excessive lactic acid pro-

duction can be found in the following clinical situations:

(1) Increased oxygen demands: Excessive motor activity such as seizure or severe exercise can increase the metabolic demands of muscles, resulting in increases in the anaerobic end products of metabolism.

(2) Reduced oxygen delivery: Reduced tissue perfusion will result in reduced oxygen delivery and, therefore, an increase in anaerobic metabolism. Conditions resulting in reduced oxygen delivery include:
   (a) Hypotension.
   (b) Cardiac arrest.
   (c) Congestive heart failure.
   (d) Low cardiac output.

(3) Reduced arterial oxygen content
   (a) Asphyxia.
   (b) Anemia.
   (c) Carbon monoxide poisoning.
   (d) Hypoxemia.

(4) Toxins
   (a) Cyanide: This drug blocks oxidative metabolism, resulting in an increase in anaerobic metabolism.
   (b) Ethanol: Lactate production may be normal, but hepatic dysfunction can interfere with hepatic conversion to bicarbonate.
   (c) Fructose infusions: Causes depletion of cellular stores of energy, specifically adenosine triphosphate.
   (d) Phenformin: This drug, as well as other biguanides, has been shown to have a direct effect on the induction of lactic acidosis.

(5) Miscellaneous causes of lactic acidosis
   (a) D-Lactic acidosis: Bacterial overgrowth of the gut in patients with a blind loop or jejunoileal bypass has rarely been found to metabolize glucose to *d*-lactic acid, which is then absorbed into the body, resulting in a systemic acidosis.
   (b) Malignancy-associated lactic acidosis: An increase in serum lactic acid has occasionally been associated with malignancies. The etiology of the increased lactate production is not known, but it is corrected with primary treatment of the malignancy.

b. Diabetic ketoacidosis: During states of relative or absolute insulin depletion, the body is unable to utilize glucose for metabolism and so begins to utilize free fatty acids, which leads to the production of the ketones: acetoacetic acid and 3-hydroxybutyric acid.

c. Alcoholic ketoacidosis: May be associated with starvation and binge drinking. An increase in fatty acid metabolism producing acetoacetic acid and 3-hydroxybutyric acid occurs because of unknown mechanisms of lipolysis.

d. Starvation ketosis: Similar to the acidosis in diabetic ketoacidosis, the ketones acetoacetic acid and 3-hydroxybutyric acid are produced from the metabolism of free fatty acids. In this circumstance, the cause is the breakdown of adipose tissue and not the lack of insulin.

e. Infantile organic acidoses: congenital errors of metabolism.

2. Extrinsic toxins leading to acid production

a. Methyl alcohol intoxication: Liver metabolism to formaldehyde and then to formic acid leads to severe metabolic acidosis and blindness.

b. Ethylene glycol intoxication: Metabolized to oxalic acid.

c. Paraldehyde intoxication: Toxic metabolite not clearly differentiated.

d. Salicylate intoxication.

e. Hydrochloric acid administration.

f. Ammonium chloride administration.

g. Cationic amino acid administration.

B. Hydrogen ions not excreted

1. Renal tubular acidosis.

2. Renal insufficiency.

3. Adrenal insufficiency.

C. Loss of bicarbonate

1. Definition: The intestinal juices distal to the pylorus are bicarbonate-rich solutions. Hence, diarrhea, drainage of pancreatic juice, or duodenal drainage can lead to massive loss of bicarbonate from the body.

2. Differential diagnosis

a. Diarrhea

b. Pancreatic drainage

c. Biliary drainage

d. Urinary diversion

e. Renal carbonic anhydrase inhibition

f. Bicarbonate-wasting renal diseases

g. Dilutional acidosis: The potential change in the ratio of carbonic acid to bicarbonate that occurs if there is a sudden increase in the amount of water in the extracellular fluid.

III. Diagnosis

A. Unmeasured anions (the "anion gap"): It is convenient to determine the cause of metabolic acidosis by determining the plasma concentration of anions that are not ordinarily measured by routine blood chemistry determination. This is carried out by simply adding the serum HCO_3 and the serum Cl (measured anions) and subtracting this from the serum concentration of Na^+ (measured cation). In the normal physiologic situation, the value obtained is usually less than 12.

B. Acidosis may occur with or without an increase in the unmeasured anions.

Acidosis with No Increased Anion Gap

Diarrhea	Bicarbonate loss
Ureterosigmoidostomy	Bicarbonate loss by colon
Ammonium chloride ingestion	NH_4 $NH_3 + H^+$
Renal tubular acidosis Decreased H^+ secretion	Renal bicarbonate loss or
Pyelonephritis (some cases)	Decreased H^+ secretion

C. In contrast, causes of metabolic acidosis associated with an increased concentration of unmeasured anions include those in which there is either endogenous or exogenous addition of acid to the cellular fluids.

Acidosis with an Increased Anion Gap

Renal insufficiency	Decreased H^+ secretion by kidney and retention of phosphate and sulfate
Diabetic ketoacidosis	Acetoacetic, β-hydroxybutyric acids
Lactic acidosis	Lactic acid
Paraldehyde (deteriorated)	Acetic acid
Methyl alcohol intoxication	Formic acid
Ethylene glycol intoxication	Formic acid
Salicylate intoxication	Lactic acid

IV. Compensated Metabolic Acidosis

    A. When the extracellular fluid concentration of bicarbonate decreases, resulting in acidemia, the central respiratory center is stimulated and the rate of respiration increases. This results in the removal of CO_2 by the lungs at an increased rate. The reduction of pCO_2 thus restores the H^+ concentration toward normal.

    B. This respiratory compensation, while tending to restore the H^+ concentration toward normal, never really restores the H^+ concentration to precisely normal.

Metabolic Alkalosis

I. Definition

Metabolic alkalosis is a disorder of acid-base metabolism in which there is an increase in the serum concentration of bicarbonate with no concomitant change in the pCO_2, causing an increase in the extracellular fluid pH. Metabolic alkalosis may be induced by:

    A. Administration of alkali.

        Retention of bicarbonate

        1. Organic anions.

        2. Administration of alkali.

        3. Milk-alkali syndrome.

    B. Chloride depletion due to loss of gastric secretions.

        1. Vomiting: Initiation of the alkalosis is due to loss of hydrogen ions from the stomach

        2. Nasogastric tube suctioning: Initiation of the alkalosis is due to loss of hydrogen ions from the stomach

        3. Villous adenoma.

        4. Chloride diarrhea.

    C. Chloride depletion due to the effects upon the kidney.

        1. Diuretics.

        2. Nonreabsorbable anions.

        3. Hypercalcemia.

    D. Chloride and potassium depletion due to excessive steroids.

II. Respiratory Compensation for Metabolic Alkalosis

In contrast to the ability of the respiratory system to compensate in situations of metabolic acidosis, it is a curious phenomenon that respiratory compensation in metabolic alkalosis is an irregular and unpredictable event. In theory, an increase in the blood pH should be associated with a decreased respiratory drive and an increase in the pCO_2. This would tend to normalize the ratio of bicarbonate to carbonic acid and normalize the pH.

Respiratory Acidosis

I. Definition

Respiratory acidosis is an abnormality in acid-base balance due to failure of the lungs to eliminate the normal amount of carbon dioxide. This leads to an increase in the pCO_2 and, therefore, an increase in the plasma carbonic acid level.

II. Etiology

    A. Depression of the central nervous system (CNS) respiratory center: CNS disease and certain drugs.

    B. Intrinsic lung or airway disease, causing decreased ventilation or decreased diffusion.

    C. Diseases of the chest wall, causing loss of the normal bellows action of the thorax.

III. Compensation for Respiratory Acidosis

Elevation of the plasma pCO_2 causes metabolic compensation, which is mediated by the kidney. The renal response to increased pCO_2 is increased excretion of acid as titratable acid and ammonium. The net increase in the total amount of hydrogen ions secreted by the renal tubule results in increased bicarbonate reabsorption. In this way, the kidney compensates for the respiratory acidosis by increasing the serum bicarbonate and restoring the ratio of bicarbonate to carbonic acid to the normal 20:1 value. Renal response to an elevated pCO_2 takes approximately 6–12 hr to begin and is not complete for several days.

Respiratory Alkalosis

I. Definition

Respiratory alkalosis is a decrease in the plasma content of carbon dioxide, causing an increase in the pH. It is due to hyperventilation, which results in increased excretion of carbon dioxide by the lungs.

II. Etiology

    A. Primary stimulation of the CNS respiratory center (emotion, certain drugs).

    B. Reflex stimulation of peripheral chemoreceptors, causing increased respiratory center activity.

    C. Reflex stimulation of the respiratory center due to intrathoracic stretch receptors (localized pulmonary disease).

D. The hallmark of all of the above causes of respiratory alkalosis is increased alveolar ventilation.

III. Compensation for Respiratory Alkalosis

A. The kidney is involved in the metabolic compensation for respiratory alkalosis. Increased excretion of bicarbonate occurs in association with sodium and potassium. Perhaps the most accurate observations regarding this reaction have been made on individuals who reside for prolonged periods at high altitudes. Such persons consistently have normal blood pH values, as the serum bicarbonate value has been decreased due to renal excretion and a normal ratio of bicarbonate to carbonic acid (20:1) has been reestablished.

Primary Acid-Base Disturbances

Disorder	Primary Event	Effect on H^+	Compensation
Metabolic acidosis	↓HCO_3	↑	↓ pCO_2
Metabolic alkalosis	↑HCO_3	↓	↑ pCO_2
Respiratory acidosis	↑pCO_2	↑	↑ HCO_3
Respiratory alkalosis	↓pCO_2	↓	↓ HCO_3

B. Common equations used to evaluate acid-base disorders and their compensatory mechanisms, above, include the following:

Metabolic acidosis: $\Delta PCO_2 \sim 1.2\ \Delta HCO_3$

Metabolic alkalosis: $\Delta PCO_2 \sim 0.7\ \Delta HCO_3$

Respiratory acidosis

　　Acute: $\Delta H^+ \sim 0.75\ \Delta pCO_2$

　　Chronic: $\Delta H^+ \sim 0.30\ \Delta pCO_2$

Respiratory alkalosis

　　Acute: $\Delta H^+ \sim 0.75\ \Delta pCO_2$

　　Chronic $\Delta HCO_3 \sim 0.5\ \Delta pCO_2$

C. Approach to an acid-base problem

1. The history and physical exam should alert the physician to the type of problem.
2. Determine the pH. Is this an acidosis or an alkalosis?
3. Determine if the abnormality is primarily metabolic or respiratory.
4. If a metabolic acidosis exists, determine the anion gap.
5. Determine if there is adequate or inadequate compensation.
6. Clues to a mixed acid-base disorder:
   a. HCO_3 <15: Metabolic acidosis.
   b. HCO_3 >45: Metabolic alkalosis.
   c. Blood gas normal but anion gap abnormal.
   d. Compensation is different than predicted.

Bibliography

Burton Rose. In: Clinical Pathophysiology of Acid-Base and Electrolyte Disorders, ed 3., McGraw Hill, New York, 1989.

Cohen JJ, Kassirer P. (eds) In: Acid-Base, Little, Brown & Co., Boston, 1982.

CHAPTER 85

Acute Renal Failure (ARF)

Roger Rodby, M.D.

I. **Definition**

An acute reduction of the glomerular filtration rate (GFR) expressed clinically as the retention of nitrogenous waste products in the blood, often accompanied by a decrease in the urine volume. There are three major pathophysiologic categories.

A. Prerenal ARF: A decrease in GFR secondary to inadequate blood flow to functionally and structurally intact kidneys.

B. Parenchymal ARF: A decrease in GFR secondary to renal parenchymal disease.

C. Postrenal ARF: A decrease in GFR secondary to obstruction to the outflow of urine.

II. **Prerenal ARF**

A. Etiology: Any reduction in renal blood flow may impair GFR and result in prerenal ARF.

1. Impaired cardiac output from intravascular volume depletion.

2. Impaired cardiac output from primary cardiac disease.

3. Normal or elevated cardiac output, but with blood being shunted away from the kidney.

4. Primary renal vasoconstriction.

B. Pathophysiology: Although renal blood flow is impaired in prerenal ARF, the microcirculation of the glomerulus is specially adapted to minimize the resultant decrease in GFR. Afferent arteriolar vasodilatation and efferent arteriolar vasoconstriction increases both the intraglomerular pressure and the filtration fraction (GFR/renal plasma flow) in an attempt to maintain the GFR. When this mechanism is not sufficient to prevent a significant reduction in GFR, ARF results.

C. Differential diagnosis

1. Intravascular volume depletion: Impaired renal blood flow secondary to reduced cardiac output as a result of intravascular volume depletion.

a. Exogenous losses

(1) Hemorrhage.

(2) Gastrointestinal losses: vomiting/nasogastric suction, diarrhea.

(3) Urinary losses: osmotic diuresis (glycosuria), diuretics.

b. Endogenous losses: Third space sequestration

(1) Movement of fluid from the intravascular compartment to the extravascular compartment (e.g.,

bowel catastrophe or muscle trauma).

    (2) Portal hypertension with ascites.

    (3) Nephrotic syndrome with hypoalbuminemia and edema.

    (4) Venous or lymphatic obstruction with edema.

2. Cardiac disease: Impaired renal blood flow secondary to decreased cardiac output as a result of primary cardiac disease.

    a. Cardiomyopathy.

    b. Valvular disease.

    c. Constrictive pericarditis.

    d. Pericardial tamponade.

3. Peripheral vasodilatation: Impaired renal blood flow secondary to shunting of blood away from the kidney, usually in the setting of a normal to high cardiac output and low systemic vascular resistance.

    a. Sepsis.

    b. Cirrhosis.

4. Primary renal vasoconstriction: Systemic hemodynamics may be normal, but vasoconstriction at the level of the kidney impairs renal blood flow and GFR.

    a. Hepatorenal syndrome (HRS): Severe liver disease accompanied by intense renal vasoconstriction and ARF.

        (1) May be mediated by an unidentified humoral factor circulating as a result of liver disease.

        (2) Diagnosis of HRS depends on the exclusion of intravascular volume depletion.

    b. Nonsteroidal anti-inflammatory agents (NSAIAs): By blocking prostaglandin-mediated afferent arteriolar vasodilatation, they can markedly decrease renal blood flow and GFR in the patient with an already impaired renal blood flow from any process (see Section II, B).

    c. Cyclosporine: Renal vasoconstriction may be a result of cyclosporine-mediated endothelin release.

    d. Hypercalcemia: Pathophysiology unclear.

D. Diagnosis

1. Historical data: A history of excessive fluid losses, hemorrhage, cardiac disease, liver disease, severe infection, and the usage of NSAIAs should be sought.

2. Physical findings

    a. Intravascular volume depletion with orthostatic hypotension and flat neck veins.

    b. Marked fluid overload, as seen with cardiac or liver disease.

    c. The presence of edema may accompany both intravascular volume expansion (cardiac disease) and depletion (third spacing).

    d. Unfortunately, renal blood flow can only be predicted with certain findings on the physical exam.

3. Diagnostic tests

    a. Central venous pressure monitoring or pulmonary artery catheterization for measurement of pulmonary artery wedge pressure may be necessary to define the patient's intravascular and hemodynamic status.

    b. Chemistries: The blood urea nitrogen (BUN)/creatinine ratio may be elevated (>20), but this finding is not highly sensitive or specific, since diet and the protein catabolic rate independently affect this ratio.

    c. Urine

        (1) Urinalysis: Specific gravity may be ≥ 1.020.

        (2) Urine chemistries reflect sodium and water reabsorption: $U_{Na} < 20$ mEq/liter, $U/P_{Creat} > 40$, $U_{Osm} > 500$ mOsm/liter, and fractional excretion of sodium (FE_{Na}) of $<1\%$:

$$FE_{Na}\,(\%) = ([U_{Na} \times P_{Creat}]/[U_{Creat} \times P_{Na}]) \times 100$$

(Table 85-1).

Table 85-1. Urine Chemistries ARF

	U_{Na}	U_{Osm}	U/P_{Creat}	FE_{Na}
Prerenal ARF	<20 mEq/liter	>500 mOsm/liter	>40	<1%
Nondiagnostic	20–40 mEq/liter	350–500 mOsm/liter	20–40	
Acute tubular necrosis	>40 mEq/liter	<350 mOsm/liter	<20	>1%

Note: The most useful urinary index is the FE_{Na} where there is little to no overlap between the values that differentiate prerenal from nonprerenal causes of ARF. $FE_{Na}\,(\%) = ([U_{Na} \times P_{Creat}]/[U_{Creat} \times P_{Na}]) \times 100$.

E. Treatment

Treatment focuses on the restoration of renal blood flow.

1. Reversal of abnormal hemodynamics should be attempted to increase cardiac output and renal blood flow. This may require placement of a pulmonary artery catheter for pressure monitoring, as well as cardiac output measurements.

2. NSAIAs should be discontinued.

3. Infection should be treated.

4. Liver transplantation is the only proven treatment for the hepatorenal syndrome.

5. If GFR cannot be restored, one may have to initiate a number of intake restrictions. Dialysis may be necessary (see Section V).

F. Prognosis: If renal blood flow is restored, there should be complete recovery from renal failure.

III. Parenchymal ARF

A. Etiology: Any process that affects the nephron's ability to create and process ultrafiltrate. This may be a result of damage to blood vessels, glomeruli, or tubules.

B. Pathophysiology: Processes include ischemia with or without infarction, barotrauma, and immunologic or toxic insults.

C. Differential diagnosis

1. Macrovascular disease: Diseases affecting the renal artery or vein requires involvement of *both* kidneys to cause renal failure unless the patient has only one functional kidney (congenital absence or prior infarction or removal).

   a. Renal infarction: May be accompanied by flank pain and hematuria but can be silent. Anuria common. Lactate dehydrogenase (LDH) should markedly increase (isoenzyme 1)

      (1) Arterial thrombosis: Usually associated with atherosclerotic disease. May be embolic. Diagnosis made by arteriogram. Surgical or thrombolytic intervention should be performed within 24 hr of event. Prognosis poor.

      (2) Aortic dissection.

      (3) Embolic: Usually in the setting of cardiac arrthymia, cardiomyopathy, or endocarditis.

   b. Renal vein thrombosis

      (1) Presentation: May present with flank pain and hematuria but can be silent. Kidney is swollen and may be palpable. Can embolize to lungs.

      (2) Pathophysiology: Seen in hypercoaguable or hemoconcentrated state: dehydration, pregnancy, oral contraceptive use, nephrotic syndrome, sickle cell disease; also seen with venous compression.

      (3) Diagnosis: Renal venogram, magnetic resonance imaging (MRI), computed tomography (CT) or occasionally ultrasound.

      (4) Therapy: Anticoagulation with or without thrombolytics.

      (5) Prognosis: Venous collaterals usually prevent infarction; renal prognosis good.

2. Microvascular disease: Arterioles and/or glomeruli. Diagnosis made by constellation of symptoms, serologic tests, and renal biopsy

   a. Vasculitic syndromes: Patient usually has signs of systemic disease. Urine usually quite active with protein, RBCs and RBC casts. Erythrocyte sedimentation rate (ESR) elevated. Complement levels are usually normal. May be elevation of antineutrophil cytoplasmic antibody (ANCA). Pathology demonstrates fibrinoid necrosis of blood vessel wall and/or segmental necrosis of glomerular tuft. Crescents may be present. Immune complexes rare.

      (1) Polyarteritis nodosa (PAN)

         (a) ANCA may be elevated, usually in perinuclear pattern (P-ANCA). Often associated with chronic hepatitis B surface antigenemia.

         (b) Therapy: Cyclophosphamide and steroids.

      (2) Wegener's granulomatosis

         (a) Usually accompanied by upper respiratory tract symptoms. Pulmonary hemorrhage can be life-threatening.

         (b) ANCA usually elevated: cytoplasmic pattern (C-ANCA).

         (c) Therapy: Cyclophosphamide and steroids.

      (3) Henoch-Schönlein Purpura (HSP):

         (a) Usually a self-limiting pediatric disease but can be seen in adults.

         (b) Purpuric rash on buttocks and lower legs. Often accompanied by abdominal pain and blood in stool (gastrointestinal vasculitis).

    (c) Immunoglobulin A (IgA) seen on immunofluorescence.

    (d) Therapy: May require cyclophosphamide and steroids.

(4) Allergic granulomatosis (Churg-Strauss vasculitis)

    (a) Similar to PAN clinically but with a history of asthma and eosinophilia.

    (b) Therapy: Cyclophosphamide and steroids.

(5) Mixed essential cryoglobulinemia

    (a) Purpuric rash on extremities, arthritis, Raynaud's phenomenon.

    (b) Often associated with chronic hepatitis B surface antigenemia or in infection with hepatitis C. Third component of complement (C3) depressed.

    (c) Glomerular lesion may include capillary loop occlusion by precipitated cryoglobulin.

    (d) Therapy: Cyclophosphamide, steroids, and plasmapheresis.

(6) Rheumatoid vasculitis

    (a) Seen occasionally in patients with severe rheumatoid arthritis.

    (b) Therapy: Cyclophosphamide and steroids.

b. Glomerulonephritic syndromes: Severe inflammation in some forms of glomerulonephritis produces ARF. Symptoms depend on an associated systemic disease. The urinalysis has protein, RBCs, and RBC casts. Gross hematuria may be present. The FE_{Na} may be <1%. The pattern of glomerular inflammation depends upon the diagnosis. When ARF is present, crescents are common.

(1) Poststreptococcal glomerulonephritis (PSGN)

    (a) Clinically apparent with fluid retention, gross hematuria 6–20 days following strep infection.

    (b) Immune complex mediated, with consumption of C3. The antistreptolysin O titer (ASO) should be elevated.

    (c) Large subepithelial immune complex, electron-dense deposits ("humps") seen on electron micrographs.

    (d) Usually self-limiting. Antibiotics given only to prevent spread of infection to close contacts.

(2) Subacute bacterial endocarditis

    (a) ARF not common but, when present, is usually associated with crescents.

    (b) C3 often depressed.

    (c) Immune complex GN with pathology very similar to that of PSGN.

    (d) Usually self-limiting with antibiotic therapy.

(3) Shunt nephritis

    (a) ARF rare.

    (b) Immune complex disease associated with chronic infection of ventriculoatrial shunt, often with chronic bacteremia.

    (c) C3 often depressed.

    (d) Self-limiting with resolution of infection (may require shunt removal).

(4) Visceral abscess–associated glomerulonephritis

    (a) When glomerulonephritis is present, ARF is common.

    (b) C3 may be normal.

    (c) May be a paucity of immune complexes similar to a vasculitis.

    (d) Recovery not always seen despite eradication of infection.

(5) Other Postinfectious glomerulonephritides (nonpoststreptococcal)

    (a) Pathogenesis similar to that of PSGN but rarely cause ARF.

    (b) Organisms include a number of bacterial, viral, fungal, protozoal, helminthic, and spirochetal agents.

(6) IgA Nephropathy

    (a) Gross hematuria 1–2 days following an upper respiratory tract infection. ARF rare but can occur when associated with crescents.

    (b) Usually self-limiting.

(7) Systemic lupus erythematosus (SLE)

    (a) Severe glomerular inflammation may cause ARF, usually associated with depression of C3, as well as elevation of the anti-double-stranded DNA titer, but this is not universal.

(8) Therapy: Steroids with or without cytotoxic agents.

(9) Prognosis: Good if treated early and aggressively.

(10) Anti-glomerular basement membrane antibody (anti-GBM)–mediated glomerulonephritis

    (a) May present with (Goodpasture's syndrome) or without pulmonary hemorrhage which can be life-threatening.

    (b) Diagnosis: Made by demonstration of circulating anti-GBM antibody and renal biopsy with linear (smooth) immunofluorescence of capillary loops.

    (c) Therapy: Plasmapheresis, steroids, and cyclophosphamide. Plasmapheresis particularly helpful for pulmonary hemorrhage.

    (d) Prognosis: Renal prognosis poor if patient is oliguric.

(11) Idiopathic, rapidly progressive glomerulonephritis

    (a) A nonimmune complex–mediated crescentic GN frequently associated with antineutrophil cytoplasmic antibodies (ANCA), similar to a vasculitis, but without symptoms of a systemic disease.

    (b) Diagnosis: By renal biopsy and exclusion of systemic disease.

    (c) Therapy: Steroids, cyclophosphamide with or without plasmapheresis.

c. Cortical necrosis: Formation of intravascular thrombi usually secondary to a microangiopathic syndrome causing ARF through patchy infarction of the renal cortex. Anuria is common. Endothelial damage with microangiopathy, schistocytes, and thrombocytopenia is common to all of these diseases. Urine may show protein and RBCs. Although recovery is common, significant renal failure may persist.

(1) Hemolytic-uremic syndrome (HUS)

    (a) More common in children. Often preceded by an *Escherichia coli* infection. Also seen with cy-

closporine and mitomycin C use. Also seen postpartum and after bone marrow transplantation.

    (b) Therapy: Antiplatelet agents and plasma exchange have possible benefits. Steroids do not appear to be helpful.

(2) Thrombotic thrombocytopenic purpura (TTP)

    (a) Similar to HUS but has more systemic symptoms. ARF less common in TTP than in HUS.

    (b) Therapy: Steroids, plasma infusions, or plasma exchange with or without antiplatelet therapy.

(3) Preeclampsia

    (a) May progress to a microangiopathic process with ARF.

    (b) Therapy: Induction of delivery.

(4) Disseminated intravascular coagulation (DIC)

    (a) Endotoxemia.

    (b) Amniotic fluid embolism.

    (c) Retained dead fetus.

d. Malignant hypertension

(1) Presentation: Usually a history of hypertension. May be seen in essential or secondary hypertension. Other acute end-organ damage (e.g., encephalopathy, retinopathy) usually present.

(2) Laboratory tests: Microangiopathy with schistocytes can be seen. Urine shows protein and RBCs.

(3) Pathophysiology and pathology: Vascular and glomerular damage resembling that of vasculitis (fibrinoid necrosis). Pathogenesis is not immunologic but is hemodynamic (direct barotrauma).

(4) Therapy: Reduction of blood pressure.

(5) Prognosis: Recovery common but may take months

e. Scleroderma

(1) Presentation: Patients may develop a phase of malignant hypertension and ARF (scleroderma renal crisis).

(2) Laboratory tests: Serologic tests consistent with scleroderma; schistocytes may be seen. Urine shows protein and RBCs.

(3) Pathophysiology: Appears to be related to ischemia and vasospasm;

possibly mediated by renin-angiotensin system.

    (4) Pathology: Histologically, may appear indistinguishable from malignant hypertension.

    (5) Therapy: Antihypertensives, especially angiotensin-converting enzyme inhibitors (ACEi).

    (6) Prognosis: Recovery common since advent of ACEi.

f. Atheroembolic disease

    (1) Presentation: Can be spontaneous but usually preceded by arterial angiographic procedure in patient with diffuse atherosclerotic disease. Can involve multiple organs both clinically and pathologically. Often confused with vasculitis. Emboli may be seen on retinal exam. Usually nonoliguric.

    (2) Laboratory tests: Eosinophilia is common. Hypocomplementemia has been reported. Urine is benign.

    (3) Pathology: Cholesterol clefts in arcuate and intralobular arteries.

    (4) Pathophysiology: Vessels appear only sparsely involved, and cause of ARF is unclear. Perhaps immunologic, as suggested by eosinophilia.

    (5) Diagnosis: Renal biopsy.

    (6) Therapy: none

    (7) Prognosis: Poor; related to renal failure and diffuse atherosclerotic disease.

3. Acute interstitial nephritis: ARF secondary to interstitial inflammation usually related to a pharmacologic agent. Originally described with methicillin and was accompanied by generalized hypersensitivity, fever, rash, and eosinophilia, but may occur without systemic symptoms.

a. Presentation: Nonoliguric ARF 1–2 weeks after initiation of drug. Other symptoms may occur (see above).

b. Laboratory tests: May see eosinophilia and eosinophiluria. Urine shows pyuria, mild proteinuria, and possibly WBC and epithelial cell casts.

c. Pathology: Interstitial edema with infiltration of lymphocytes, monocytes, plasma cells, and eosinophils.

d. Pathophysiology: Unclear but delayed hypersensitivity reaction to drug with lymphocyte sensitization and release of lymphokines. The direct cause of the decrease in GFR may be similar to acute tubular necrosis (see Section III,C,5).

e. Causative agents

    (1) Common: Penicillins, sulfonamides, rifampin, phenindione.

    (2) Less common: Allopurinol, diphenylhydantoin, cimetidine.

f. Diagnosis: Usually clinical but may require renal biopsy.

g. Therapy: Withdrawal of offending agent. Steroids may be of benefit in severe cases.

h. Prognosis: Recovery is usual.

4. Intrarenal tubular obstruction: ARF secondary to tubular obstruction from precipitation of one of a number of endogenous or exogenous substances. Crystallization occurs as a result of high filtered load, concentration of the urine, and low pKs making them relatively insoluble in the acidic environment of urine. Alkalinization of the urine, when possible, is often protective and/or therapeutic. Pathophysiology of ARF related to both obstruction and mechanisms similar to those of acute tubular necrosis (see Section III,C,5).

a. Uric acid (acute uric acid nephropathy)

    (1) Usually a result of excessive purine production from cellular breakdown after either chemotherapy for lympho/myeloproliferative diseases (tumor lysis syndrome) or rhabdomyolysis.

    (2) Laboratory tests: Urate usually >20 mg/dl. Urine urate/creatinine ratio >1.0.

    (3) Therapy: Allopurinol, hydration, alkalinization of the urine, initiated as early as possible or prior to event (if possible). Hemodialysis to lower urate level may be necessary in the oliguric patient.

b. Oxalate

    (1) Produced as a result of metabolism of:

        (a) Ethylene glycol (EG).

        (b) Methoxyflurane anesthesia.

    (2) Therapy: (EG) Intravenous ethanol, hydration, and usually hemodialysis for the severe metabolic acidosis

c. Sulfadiazine, sulfapyridine

    (1) Relatively insoluble sulfonamides:

Usage increasing, as often drug of choice for parasitic infections in acquired immunodeficiency syndrome (AIDS).

(2) Therapy: Hydration, urine alkalinization.

d. Acyclovir

(1) May precipitate in renal tubules.

(2) Therapy: Molecule has two pKs, one <5.0, one >7.0; optimal urine pH unknown.

e. Methotrexate

(1) May precipitate in renal tubules.

(2) Therapy: Has several pKs, all <6.0, and although not proven, urine alkalinization may be helpful.

5. Acute tubular necrosis (ATN): The most common cause of parenchymal ARF, usually initiated by a clearly defined event that damages the renal tubules; either ischemia (postischemic ATN) or exposure to a nephrotoxin (nephrotoxic ATN). Both are characterized by a similar pathologic description, clinical course, and pathophysiologic explanation for the decrease in GFR.

a. Etiology and differential diagnosis

(1) Ischemic ATN: Hemodynamic events that decrease renal perfusion for which autoregulatory mechanisms cannot prevent ischemia and subsequent tubular cell damage.

(2) Nephrotoxic ATN: Toxins directly toxic to tubular cells.

(a) Heavy metals.

(b) Halogenated hydrocarbons.

(c) Pigments: Myoglobin (rhabdomyolysis) and hemoglobin (acute hemolytic reaction) and other unknown products of cellular breakdown. Early in course, may be associated with FE_{Na} <1%. Coprecipitation with Tamm-Horsfall protein results in cast formation and tubular obstruction and may contribute to nephrotoxic process.

(d) Light chains/multiple myeloma (MM): Coprecipitation with Tamm-Horsfall protein results in cast formation and tubular obstruction and may contribute to nephrotoxic process. Hypercalcemia (see Section II,C,4,d), hyperuricemia (see Section

III,C,4,a), and amyloidosis may all be present in MM and may independently cause ARF. Increased risk of ARF from radiocontrast in present of light chainuria.

(e) Aminoglycosides.

(f) Radiocontrast: Early oliguric phase but usually nonoliguric. Hydration prior to administration may decrease risk of ARF. Nonionic dyes do not appear to be protective. Risk factors include diabetes, multiple myeloma, and any prerenal state. Early in course, may be associated with FE_{Na} <1%.

(g) Other pharmacologic agents: Antibiotics, diuretics.

b. Presentation: Characterized by an abrupt and severe reduction in GFR, often with oliguria.

c. Laboratory test: Urine

(1) Evidence of tubular damage with coarse granular casts and possibly tubular cell casts but otherwise benign.

(2) Isosthenuria: Specific gravity 1.010.

(3) Urine chemistries reflect defect in sodium and water reabsorption (Table 85-1). Most useful of these indices is the FE_{Na}, which is ≥1%.

d. Pathophysiology: Proposed mechanisms of decreased GFR are many. Most likely multifactorial, but vasomotor theory seems to predominate.

(1) Obstruction theory: Intratubular obstruction from swollen, necrotic tubular cells.

(2) Backleak theory: Filtration occurs, but filtrate leaks back into interstitium as a result of tubular damage. Appears to play a minor role.

(3) Vasomotor theory: Cortical blood flow has been shown to decrease markedly in ATN. In addition, there is afferent arteriolar constriction and efferent arteriolar dilatation, both of which contribute to a decreased filtration fraction (the opposite of prerenal states; see Section II,B). This decrease in renal blood flow in conjunction with a decreased filtration fraction is felt

to be the major factor responsible for the severe reduction in GFR.

    e. Pathology: Wide range of findings, including rare signs of tubular cell damage with regeneration (occasional mitotic figure) to severe tubular cell destruction with cell sloughing.

    f. Clinical course: Profound reduction in GFR may persist despite the normalization of systemic hemodynamics or removal of nephrotoxin. Recovery seen in days to weeks (rarely >8 weeks). Complete recovery is the rule unless cortical necrosis is involved (see Section III,C,2,c).

    g. Therapy: Normalization of hemodynamics and removal of nephrotoxins. Initiate a number of intake restrictions. Dialysis may be necessary (see Section V).

IV. Postrenal ARF

A. Etiology: Any disease that causes obstruction to the outflow of urine. This may occur as a result of either intrinsic obstruction or extrinsic compression at any level of the urogenital tract. Obstruction must be bilateral or must occur at the level of the urethra to cause ARF unless the patient has only one functional kidney (congenital absence, prior infarction or removal).

B. Pathophysiology: Obstruction to urine flow increases intratubular pressure and prevents glomerular ultrafiltration. This is followed by renal vasoconstriction; a decrease in renal blood flow appears to be involved as well.

C. Presentation
1. Anuria is highly suggestive of obstruction, but incomplete obstruction can be seen with any range of urine outputs.
2. A hyperchloremic, hyperkalemic acidosis (type IV RTA) may be seen.
3. Patients are frequently asymptomatic.
4. May see FE_{Na} <1% in first hours of obstruction.

D. Differential diagnosis
1. Urethral obstruction.
2. Bladder outlet obstruction.
    a. Prostatic hypertrophy/cancer.
    b. Bladder cancer.
3. Bilateral ureteral obstruction
    a. Nephrolithiasis.
    b. Cancer (intrinsic or extrinsic).
    c. Blood clots.
    d. Renal papillae.

    e. Surgical ligation.
    f. Retroperitoneal fibrosis.

E. Diagnosis
1. Dilatation of the urogenital tract occurs almost immediately upon obstruction.
2. Ultrasonography is quick, easy, and highly sensitive except when ureters are encased (preventing dilatation). This is termed *nondilated obstruction*.
    a. Tumor involving the retroperitoneum.
    b. Retroperitoneal fibrosis.
    c. Requires a high index of suspicion since usual screening test (ultrasound) is normal.
    d. May require cystoscopy with retrograde urography to diagnose.

F. Treatment
1. Relief of obstruction usually requires urologic procedure. If unsuccessful, may require percutaneous nephrostomy placement.
2. May see postobstructive diuresis.
    a. Excretion of retained solute (sodium, urea etc.).
    b. May have transient urine-concentrating defect as a result of damage to collecting duct.

G. Prognosis: With obstruction <2 weeks, complete recovery may be seen. Obstruction >2 weeks is usually associated with residual renal damage. Recovery may continue for several weeks if obstruction has been prolonged.

V. Approach to the Patient with ARF

A. Differential diagnostic clues
1. Anuria (<100 ml/24 hr)
    a. Obstruction (see Section IV,D).
    b. Total renal arterial or venous occlusion (see Section III,C,1).
    c. Cortical necrosis (see Section III,C,2,c).
    d. ATN: Unusual to be anuric but may occur
2. Urinalysis
    a. Hematuria and proteinuria: Glomerulonephritic and vasculitic disorders (see Section III,C,2,a,b).
    b. Pyuria, WBC casts: Acute interstitial nephritis (see Section III,C,3).
    c. Hematuria by dipstick but without RBCs on microscopic examination: Myoglobinuria or hemoglobinuria.
    d. Proteinuria negative by dipstick but positive by sulfosalicylic acid: Light chainuria.

3. ARF associated with FE_{Na} <1%. (see Section II,D,3,c).
   a. Prerenal ARF of any cause.
   b. Early radiocontrast-induced ARF.
   c. Early obstruction.
   d. Early pigment-induced ARF: myoglobinuria and hemoglobinuria.
   e. Hepatorenal syndrome.
   f. Acute glomerulonephritis.
4. ARF associated with eosinophilia.
   a. Atheroembolic disease (see Section III,C,2,f).
   b. Acute interstitial nephritis (see Section III,C,3).
   c. Allergic granulomatosis (see Section III,C,2,a).
5. ARF associated with hypocomplementemia
   a. Poststreptococcal glomerulonephritis (see Section III,C,2,b).
   b. SLE (see Section III,C,2,b).
   c. Mixed essential cryoglobulinemia (see Section III,C,2,a).
   d. Subacute bacterial endocarditis (see Section III,C,2,b).
   e. Shunt nephritis (see Section III,C,2,b).
   f. Hepatorenal syndrome: A severe defect in hepatic synthetic function can result in hypocomplementemia.
6. ARF associated with peripheral schistocytosis.
   a. HUS (see Section III,C,2,c).
   b. TTP (see Section III,C,2,c).
   c. Preeclampsia (see Section III,C,2,c).
   d. DIC (see Section III,C,2,c).
   e. Malignant hypertension (see Section III,C,2,d).
   f. Scleroderma renal crisis (see Section III,C,2,e).
   g. Any vasculitis: Less common.
7. ARF associated with hemoptysis or pulmonary hemorrhage (pulmonary-renal syndromes).
   a. Commonly associated
      (1) Anti-GBM disease (Goodpasture's syndrome).
      (2) Wegener's granulomatosis.
   b. Less commonly associated
      (1) Polyarteritis nodosa and other vasculitides.
      (2) SLE.
      (3) Subacute bacterial endocarditis.
      (4) Mixed essential cryoglobulinemia.
   c. Other

      (1) Renal vein thrombosis with pulmonary embolus.
8. ARF associated with rash
   a. Purpura: Henoch-Schönlein purpura, mixed essential cryoglobulinemia, SLE, subacute bacterial endocarditis, polyarteritis nodosa, Wegener's granulomatosis, HUS, TTP.
   b. Atheroembolic disease: May grossly appear to be vasculitic.
   c. Urticaria or erythema multiforme: Allergic interstitial nephritis.
B. Treatment of ARF: If ARF is not readily reversible, a number of interventions should be initiated.
   1. Fluid management (including sodium intake): Depends entirely on the volume status of the patient.
   2. Potassium restriction: <2 g/day.
   3. Protein restriction: Controversy exists. Protein restriction will delay uremia but should not be done at the expense of precipitating a severe negative nitrogen balance (unless dialysis is not available). Intake should not exceed 1 g/kg/day. There is no evidence that larger amounts will make the patient less catabolic, and they may only increase the need for dialysis.
   4. Caloric requirements: By supplying adequate calories, endogenous protein breakdown is minimized. This can be achieved by administering a minimum of 100 g of carbohydrate (500 ml of 20% glucose).
   5. Drug dosing: Adjustments in drug dose and dosage interval may be necessary, depending on the route of excretion. Loading doses are not usually altered.
   6. Dialysis: May be necessary, depending on volume, electrolyte, and acid-base status, as well as the development of uremic symptoms.

Bibliography

Bidani A, Churchill PC. Acute renal failure. *Disease-a-Month* 35:59–132, 1989.

Brenner BM, Lazarus JM (eds). *Acute Renal Failure*, ed 2. Churchill Livingstone, New York, 1988.

Miller TR, Anderson RJ, Linas SL, et al. Urinary diagnostic indices in acute renal failure: A prospective study. *Ann Intern Med* 89:47–50, 1978.

Schrier RW. Acute renal failure. *Kidney Int* 15:205–216, 1979.

CHAPTER 86

Chronic Renal Failure

Stephen Korbet, M.D.

I. **Definition**
   A. Chronic renal failure: Progressive, irreversible loss of renal function.
   B. Azotemia: Describes the retention of nitrogenous waste products from protein metabolism (such as urea) in patients with advanced chronic renal failure and is usually applied when the blood urea nitrogen (BUN) level reaches or exceeds 80 mg/dl.
   C. Uremia: Symptomatic azotemia results when renal function is extremely compromised (glomerular filtration rate ≤10 ml/min). In this setting the BUN is usually, but not always, >100 mg/dl and the serum creatinine ≥10 mg/dl. The patient is symptomatic, with complaints of headache, vomiting, and mental status changes. If the patient is toxic enough, uremia can lead to convulsions and coma. When uremia is present, the patient has reached end-stage renal disease (ESRD) and requires replacement therapy such as dialysis or transplantation in order to sustain life.

II. **Etiology**
   A. The primary causes of ESRD are diabetes mellitus, hypertension, and glomerulonephritis (Table 86-1).
   B. Early in the course of chronic renal failure, a renal biopsy may be performed and will lead to an accurate diagnosis. Without a biopsy, however, there are clinical and laboratory features which may help distinguish these entities.
      1. Glomerulonephritis: Hypertension is common, proteinuria is ≥3.5 g/dl, the urinary sediment is usually active with microscopic hematuria and red cell casts, urine volume is usually decreased, and the kidneys are small by ultrasound, with increased echogenicity (exceptions to this pattern occur in diabetes mellitus and amyloidosis, where the kidneys may be normal in size).
      2. Interstitial nephritis: Hypertension is uncommon, proteinuria is ≤1.5 g/dl, and urinary sediment is bland. However, pyuria and white blood cell casts may be present, urine volume is increased, and the kidneys are small and echogenic by ultrasound and may be irregular due to cortical scarring.

Table 86-1. Primary Causes of ESRD

Diabetes mellitus	33%
Hypertension	29%
Glomerulonephritis	15%
Cystic kidney disease	4%
Interstitial nephritis	3%
Other/unknown	12%

Table 86-2. Incidence of ESRD by Age

Age	Percentage
0–19	2
20–44	21
45–64	35
65–74	26
≥75	16

3. Nephrosclerosis: The patient is hypertensive, proteinuria may vary between 0.5 and 1.0 g/day, the urinary sediment is bland, the urine volume is decreased, and, by ultrasound, the kidneys are small and echogenic. On fundoscopic exam the patient should have evidence of hypertensive retinopathy.

C. It is important to distinguish acute renal failure from chronic renal failure, as the former is generally reversible.

1. Unlike patients with chronic renal failure, those with acute renal failure will have had previously normal serum creatinine values.

2. In acute renal failure, the kidneys will be normal in size and echogenicity, as determined by ultrasonography, and they will not have the metabolic stigmata of chronic renal failure such as anemia and osteodystrophy.

D. Patients with chronic renal failure may have superimposed acute renal failure. This should be considered in any patient with chronic renal failure who has a precipitous, unexpected decline in renal function.

III. **Incidence**

A. Over 190,000 patients in the United States have ESRD.

1. The number of patients developing ESRD increases at a rate of approximately 10% per year.

B. Males account for 55% and females 45% of the patients with ESRD.

C. The majority of patients affected are in the older age groups (Table 86-2), and 50% of patients presenting with ESRD are ≥61.

D. Even though 69% of patients presenting with ESRD are white and 28% are black, the incidence is four times greater in the black population than the white population.

IV. **Pathophysiology**

A. Progression to ESRD

1. Once chronic renal failure has developed (i.e., serum creatinine ≥1.5 g/dl), progression to ESRD is not uncommon, especially if there is no specific treatment for the primary renal process (i.e., diabetes mellitus, focal segmental glomerulosclerosis).

2. The decline in renal function, as followed by 1/serum creatinine, usually proceeds in a linear fashion.

a. Factors that may cause a precipitous decline in the loss of renal function

(1) Uncontrolled hypertension.

(2) Nephrotoxic drugs (i.e., nonsteroidal anti-inflammatory agents).

(3) Acute on chronic renal failure.

b. Factors which may improve or stabilize the loss of renal function

(1) Good blood pressure control.

(2) Low-protein diet.

(3) Achieving a remission from the underlying glomerular process, either spontaneously or due to therapy.

3. Potential causes for the progressive loss in renal function

a. Glomerular damage due to hyperfiltration.

b. Glomerular damage due to hemodynamic forces.

c. Secondary hyperparathyroidism.

4. As renal failure progresses, serum creatinine will double with every 50% reduction in glomerular filtration rate (GFR) (i.e., when the GFR declines from 100 to 50 ml/min, the serum creatinine increases from 1 to 2 mg%; a further reduction of 50% to a GFR of 25 ml/min results in an increase in serum creatinine to 4 mg%; and so forth).

B. Fluid and electrolytes

1. As total GFR decreases, single-nephron GFR increases in the remaining functional nephrons in order to maintain homeostasis.

2. It is only after >90% of the total nephron

mass is lost that the adaptive mechanisms of the kidney fail and ESRD results.

   a. This usually occurs at a GFR of ⩽10 ml/min or a serum creatinine of ⩾10 mg/dl.

3. Sodium

   a. The fractional excretion of sodium increases as the GFR decreases in order to maintain sodium balance.

   b. The kidney is able to conserve sodium as well as increase its excretion to a limited degree. However, the rate at which these adaptations occur is much slower than normal and may take up to 3–5 days.

     (1) Acute sodium restriction could lead to dehydration.

     (2) Acute increase in sodium intake could lead to volume overload and congestive heart failure.

4. Potassium

   a. The fractional excretion of potassium increases and may exceed 100% as the GFR declines.

   b. Aldosterone levels increase with decreasing GFR in order to increase renal and fecal excretion of potassium.

5. Acid-base homeostasis is maintained by increasing ammonia production, which facilitates hydrogen ion loss (see Chapter 84).

6. Water handling

   a. Fractional excretion of water increases with declining GFR.

   b. The ability to maximally concentrate as well as dilute the urine becomes progressively compromised.

     (1) The urine osmolality is usually similar to that of the serum (isosthenuric).

     (2) The ability to adjust to an acute water load or deprivation is compromised.

7. The fractional excretion of calcium, magnesium, and phosphorus increases as GFR declines.

C. Uremic toxins

1. GFR declines as products of protein metabolism begin to accumulate (urea, ammonia, guanidine, and guanidinosuccinic acid).

2. Other uremic toxins which are dependent upon glomerular filtration accumulate as well.

   a. Middle modules: Unknown substances which have molecular weights between 500 and 5,000.

   b. Parathyroid hormones.

   c. Beta$_2$-microglobulin: A low molecular weight protein (12,600) which is present on cell surfaces and depends upon glomerular filtration for excretion.

3. BUN is one of many potential uremic toxins that provides an easily measured marker for the treatment of uremia, as many of the symptoms of uremia seem to correlate with the BUN level.

D. ESRD (GFR ⩽10 ml/min) results in the ultimate failure of the above adaptive mechanisms to maintain homeostasis. Dialysis is required in order to prevent or treat the following:

1. Congestive heart failure due to sodium and water retention.

2. Hyperkalemia.

3. Acidosis.

4. Extrarenal manifestations of uremia (see below).

V. Extrarenal Manifestations of Uremia

A. Hematologic

1. Anemia: affects >90% of patients with chronic renal failure.

   a. Normocytic and normochromic, with an inappropriately low reticulocyte count.

   b. Etiology

     (1) Erythropoietin deficiency.

     (2) Decreased red blood cell survival.

     (3) A depressed response to erythropoietin due to uremic toxins.

   c. Symptoms: Easy fatigability, loss of energy, decreased exercise tolerance, and shortness of breath.

   d. Treatment

     (1) Transfusions

       (a) Only temporarily corrects anemia.

       (b) Risk of viral infection (i.e., human immunodeficiency virus, hepatitis C).

       (c) Iron overload (hemochromatosis) may occur with frequent transfusions.

     (2) Anabolic steroids

       (a) Effective in only 50% of the patients treated.

       (b) Takes ⩾6 months before an

effect on the hematocrit is seen.

(c) Work by stimulating erythropoietin production from the native kidneys.

(d) Potential adverse effects

   i) Hepatotoxicity, peliosis hepatitis, and hepatocellular carcinoma.

   ii) May cause virilization in women.

(3) Recombinant human erythropoietin (EPO)

(a) Physiologically and immunologically identical to human erythropoietin.

(b) Intravenous or subcutaneous administration.

   i) EPO appears to be more effective when given subcutaneously and therefore requires only one-half to one-third of the dose given intravenously in order to maintain a similar hematocrit.

(c) Therapeutic goal: Hematocrit between 30 and 36%.

(d) Failure to respond to EPO may be a result of iron deficiency, aluminum intoxication, or an acute or chronic inflammatory process such as infection, febrile illness, minor surgery, or a malignancy.

(e) Monitoring therapy

   i) Hematocrit: Checked weekly and then every other week once the patient is on a stable dose and the hematocrit is stable.

   ii) Ferritin level: Maintained at a level >100 ng/ml.

   iii) Iron saturation: Maintain a level >20%.

(f) Complications

   i) Hypertension may develop or is exacerbated in 35–40% of the patients.

   ii) Hyperkalemia, hyperphosphatemia, and increasing BUN may occur in a small percentage of patients due to dietary indiscretion and decrease in the efficiency of dialysis resulting from the increased hematocrit.

   iii) Seizures may rarely occur, usually due to malignant hypertension. A history of seizure is a relative contraindication to the use of EPO.

   iv) Iron deficiency: Patients should be started on iron supplementation when EPO therapy is initiated.

2. Coagulation disorders: prolonged bleeding times due to platelet dysfunction may be related to a decrease in platelet factor 3, platelet serotonin and thromboxane A_2. In addition, defects in platelet factor VIII/vonWillebrand factor has been described.

  a. Treatment

    (1) Dialysis.

    (2) Cryoprecipitate.

    (3) Estrogens.

    (4) Deamino-8-D-arginine vasopressin (DDAVP).

3. Immunologic abnormalities

  a. Decreased lymphocyte counts.

    (1) Decrease in delayed hypersensitivity.

    (2) Increased potential for viral and fungal infections.

  b. Decreased chemotaxis of neutrophils

    (1) Increased bacterial infections.

  c. Decreased opsonization.

B. Renal osteodystrophy (Figure 86-1)

1. Secondary hyperparathyroidism (osteitis fibrosa cystica): High-turnover bone disease associated with an elevated parathyroid hormone level, an increased alkaline phosphatase level, and radiographically by subperiosteal reabsorption, most noted in the phalanges and distal third of the clavicles.

2. Osteomalacia: Low-turnover bone disease generally associated with aluminum intoxication and decreased vitamin D levels. Parathyroid hormone levels are low or normal, alkaline phosphatase levels are normal, and serum calcium levels may be normal or elevated.

3. Metastatic calcification: Occurs when the calcium phosphate product level is ≥70.

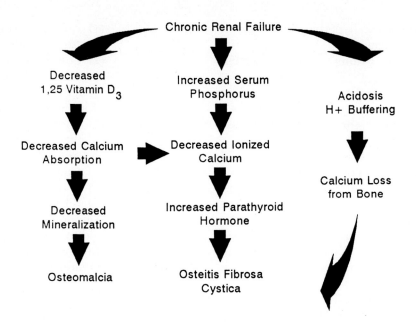

Figure 86-1. The development of renal osteodystrophy in chronic renal failure.

a. Vascular calcifications may occur, leading to insufficiency and ischemic ulcerations of the skin and gastrointestinal tract.

b. Periarticular calcification leading to arthritis.

c. Visceral calcifications leading to restrictive lung disease, cardiac conduction abnormalities and arrhythmias, and calcifications in skeletal muscle.

4. Treatment

  a. Normalization of serum phosphorus levels

    (1) Dietary restriction of phosphate intake.

    (2) Phosphate binders: Calcium carbonate, calcium acetate, and albumin hydroxide preparations.

      (a) Caution in using aluminum-containing phosphate binders should be observed, as prolonged use may be associated with aluminum intoxication.

        i) Aluminum intoxication is associated with microcytic anemia, low-turnover bone disease, and neurologic symptoms consisting of myoclonus and seizures.

    (3) Dialysis: Phosphate removal.

  b. Normalize ionized calcium levels.

    (1) Calcium supplementation: Calcium carbonate and calcium acetate.

    (2) 1-25 Dihydroxy vitamin D_3 supplementation: Enhances gastrointestinal absorption of calcium and bone mineralization.

  c. Aluminum removal: For patients with aluminum intoxication and low-turnover bone disease.

    (1) Discontinue aluminum-containing binders.

    (2) Chelation therapy with deferoxamine mesylate.

  d. Subtotal parathyroidectomy: Reserve for patients with uncontrolled high-turnover bone disease or severe hypercalcemia. Aluminum-induced osteomalacia should be ruled out prior to surgery, as aluminum deposition may be enhanced after parathyroidectomy.

C. Cardiovascular abnormalities

  1. Hypertension: Commonly a result of intravascular volumes and sodium excess managed with:

    a. Dietary restriction of sodium and fluid.

    b. Dialysis: Sodium and volume removal.

    c. Antihypertensive drugs (see Chapter 87).

2. Left ventricular hypertrophy: Found in 30–85% of patients.
   a. Secondary to long-standing hypertension.
   b. Diastolic dysfunction may be seen (due to poor ventricular compliance).
3. Atherosclerotic coronary artery disease can be seen in 25% of patients.
   a. May be a result of hypertension and abnormalities of lipid metabolism.
   b. Myocardial infarction is the most common cause of death in ESRD patients.
4. Pericarditis: The pericardial fluid is usually hemorrhagic in nature and may lead to tamponade (especially if the patient is volume expanded).
   a. Requires aggressive dialysis (i.e., four to seven times weekly).
   b. Pericardiocentesis is required if effusions are large and/or the patient is hemodynamically unstable.
   c. A pericardial "window" or pericardectomy may be required if the effusion recurs.
   d. Uremic pericarditis may rarely become constrictive.

D. Neurologic manifestations
1. Mental status changes: Irritability, difficulty concentrating, and insomnia.
   a. Progression to stupor and coma may occur if uremia goes untreated.
   b. Convulsions may occur and may be the result of electrolyte abnormalities (acidosis, hyponatremia, hypocalcemia), as well as an elevated BUN.
   c. Electroencephalographic (EEG) changes are observed and consist of generalized slowing.
   d. Contusion and subdural hematoma should be evaluated, for uremic patients are predisposed to these complications.
2. Peripheral neuropathy: Present in up to 65% of patients.
   a. "Restless leg syndrome: Patients have an uncomfortable sensation (prickling) in their lower extremities and gain relief with movement.
      (1) The sensations are worse in the distal extremity.
      (2) More prominent in the evenings.
          (a) May lead to sleep disturbances.
   b. Sensory neuropathy: Symmetric

(1) Painful, burning paresthesias in a "stocking glove" distribution.
(2) Loss of sensation to pain, light touch, vibration, and pressure (in legs more than arms).
   c. Motor neuropathy: Symmetric.
      (1) Lower extremities affected more than upper ones and distal extremities more than proximal ones.
      (2) May lead to wasting and weakness.
      (3) Bilateral foot drop may be seen.
   d. Autonomic neuropathy may occur and may lead to impotence and postural hypotension.
   e. Treatment
      (1) Dialysis: Will stabilize or improve most neurologic manifestations of uremia. Improvement in mental status changes, peripheral neuropathy symptoms, EEG and nerve conduction studies are observed.
      (2) Renal transplantation: More consistent improvement is noted. Improvement is noted progressively over 6–12 months.

E. Metabolic disturbances
1. Glucose intolerance: Occurs in up to 70% of patients and usually increases postprandially.
   a. Peripheral resistance to insulin.
   b. Increased gluconeogenesis and hepatic release of glucose.
2. Hyperlipidemia: Type IV
   a. Reduced lipoprotein lipase activity.
   b. Decreased levels of high-density lipoproteins (HDL).
      (1) May lead to acceleration of atherosclerosis.
3. Gonadal dysfunction
   a. Resistance to follicle-stimulating hormone/luteinizing hormone (FSH/LH).
      (1) Menstrual irregularity.
      (2) Infertility
   b. Decreased testosterone levels.
      (1) Reduced sperm counts.
      (2) Infertility.

VI. Dietary Management of ESRD
A. Goal: To prevent malnutrition, which can occur in up to 40% of dialysis patients, and to reduce the potential for uremic symptoms by appropriate dietary restrictions.

B. Calories: 36–38 kcal/kg/day are generally required.
   1. In peritoneal dialysis patients, glucose absorption adds to the caloric intake (approximately 71 kcal with 2 liters of 1.5% dextrose and up to 214 kcal with 4.25% dextrose).
C. Protein requirements
   1. Hemodialysis patients require 0.8–1.2 g/kg/day.
   2. Peritoneal dialysis patients require an increase in protein intake compared to hemodialysis patients (1.2–1.5 g/kg/day) due to peritoneal losses of protein into the dialysate (as much as 10–20 g/day)
D. Potassium restriction: 1 mEq/kg/day is recommended (50–70 mEq/day)
   1. Avoid high-potassium-containing foods (bananas, oranges, grapefruits, tomatoes).
E. Sodium restriction: 1–3 g/day of sodium is recommended (1 g of sodium = 43 mEq of sodium) or 2–6 g/day of sodium chloride (NaCl) (1 g of NaCl = 17 mEq of sodium).
F. Phosphorus restriction: 0.8–1.2 g/day is recommended.
   1. Avoid high-phosphorus-containing foods (eggs, cream, cheese, milk).
   2. Phosphate binders are generally required for adequate phosphorus control (calcium acetate, calcium carbonate, aluminum hydroxide preparations).
G. Fluid management: Must be individualized and should be adjusted for residual urine output, as well as fluid removed during dialysis.
   1. Hemodialysis patients should be restricted to 1,000–1,500 ml/day.
   2. Peritoneal dialysis patients may be allowed larger fluid intake due to increased fluid removal with hypertonic dialysate solutions.
      a. Two liters of 1.5% dextrose will generate 200 ml of ultrafiltrate per exchange.
      b. Two liters of 4.25% dextrose will generate 400–600 ml of ultrafiltrate per exchange.
H. Vitamin and mineral requirements
   1. Deficiency of water-soluble vitamins may occur due to poor intake and dialytic losses. Supplementation should include folic acid, pyridoxine, and vitamin C.
   2. Iron supplementation is required. Iron deficiency may occur due to blood loss in hemodialysis, as well as gastrointestinal bleeding from uremic gastritis or from increased utilization with EPO.
   3. Magnesium restriction is required due to decreased excretion. Avoid magnesium-containing antiacids.

VII. **Hemodialysis**
A. Patient population: 80% of patients on chronic dialysis are on hemodialysis.
   1. In-center hemodialysis: Patients are dialyzed at a dialysis facility.
      a. This represents approximately 80% of patients on chronic hemodialysis.
      b. The patient must go to a dialysis facility for each dialysis procedure.
   2. Home hemodialysis
      a. Represents 20% of patients on chronic hemodialysis.
      b. Allows patients to dialyze in the comfort of their own homes and to be involved with the dialysis procedure.
      c. However, requires the patient to be extremely motivated to do the dialysis procedure. The patient must have a partner to assist in the dialysis procedure and must have enough space in the home to perform the procedure as well as store the supplies required.
B. Technical aspects and requirements
   1. Basic principles
      a. Diffusion: The movement of solutes across a semipermeable membrane from a high- to a low-concentration gradient (the movement of urea, which is in high concentration in the blood, across the synthetic dialysis membrane and into the dialysate, which is urea free).
      b. Hemofiltration: The movement of water and solute (ultrafiltrate) through a semipermeable membrane as a result of hydrostatic pressure differences (increased hydrostatic pressure in the blood compartment in comparison to the dialysate compartment causes the formation of ultrafiltrate and hence allows the removal of solute and water from the body).
   2. Vascular access (Figure 86-2): This is essential in performing extracorporeal dialysis. The access allows blood to be removed and returned to the body at flow rates of 200–400 ml/min.

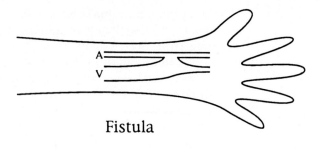

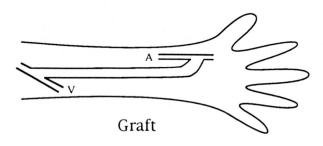

Figure 86-2. Vascular access in forearm
A = artery, V = vein.

a. Arteriovenous fistula (AVF): Created by the surgical anastomosis of an artery and a vein.
   (1) Most commonly used are the radial artery and cephalic vein.
   (2) Should be created in the nondominant arm.
   (3) Requires 4–6 weeks for appropriate maturization to occur (arterialization of the venous side—thickening of the venous wall to allow the insertion of dialysis needles).
b. Arteriovenous grafts: The formation of a vascular access with the use of foreign materials.
   (1) These are used when the patient's own vessels are felt to be inadequate, usually due to severe atherosclerotic changes.
   (2) Materials such as a bovine heterograft or a polytetrafluoroethylene graft (PTFE, Gortex) are utilized to form an anastomosis between an artery and a vein.
3. Dialysis machine: A highly technical piece of equipment which has essentially two primary purposes.
   a. Pump blood at a flow rate of 200–400 ml/min through the dialyzer.

   (1) Numerous gauges allow the monitoring of pressure within the system as the blood is being pumped to be sure that the circuit is functioning appropriately.
   (2) An error detection device monitors for air leaks to prevent an air embolus.
   b. Mix and pump dialysate through the dialyzer at a rate of 500 ml/min.
   (1) A conductivity meter on the machine ensures that water and dialysate concentrate are mixed in the appropriate proportions to give the exact electrolyte composition desired in the dialysis solution.
4. Dialyzer (artificial kidney)
   a. Semipermeable membranes composed of various symmetric materials (cuprophane and cellulose acetate are the ones most commonly used).
   b. Hollow-filter dialyzers (thousands of small-diameter capillaries through which blood flows) and parallel-plate dialyzers (membrane sheets arranged in parallel, forming compartments through which blood flows) are the most commonly used dialyzers.
   (1) Blood and dialysate solute are pumped through the dialyzers in a countercurrent fashion and are separated by the synthetic membranes.
   (2) In order to prevent clotting within the dialyzers, the patient is carefully anticoagulated with heparin during the dialysis procedure.
5. Dialysate: A water-electrolyte solution which allows the removal, by diffusion, from the blood of excess solutes and uremic toxins which have accumulated and the replacement, by diffusion, from dialysate to the blood of needed electrolytes and minerals such as base (in the form of acetate or bicarbonate) and calcium.
   a. The standard dialysate solution has the following electrolyte characteristics; sodium 140 mEq/liter, potassium 2 mEq/liter, chloride 102 mEq/liter, acetate 35 mEq/liter or bicarbonate 35 mEq/liter and calcium 2.5–3.5 mEq/liter.

b. It is imperative that a purified water supply be used in order to prepare the dialysate solution. This requires that the water be softened (to remove minerals), deionized (to remove electrolytes), and treated with reverse osmosis to further remove electrolytes and aluminum. Finally, the water must be passed through an ultrafilter prior to being used in order to remove bacteria and endotoxins.

6. Dialysis prescription: Patients are dialyzed for 3–4 hr three times weekly. Patients generally require 2,000–3,000 ml of fluid to be removed during each dialysis session in order to remain uvolemic.

C. Adequacy of dialysis: For effective dialysis (which has implications for morbidity and mortality), various parameters are measured and used to adjust the dialysis prescription accordingly.

1. Urea reduction ratio (URR)

a. $\text{URR} = \dfrac{\text{Predialysis BUN} - \text{postdialysis BUN}}{\text{Predialysis BUN}} \times 100$

b. URR should be $\geq 60\%$.

2. Urea kinetic modeling (Kt/V urea).

a. Kt/V is a dimensionless ratio in which K is equal to the dialyzer clearance of urea, t is the time on dialysis, and V is the volume distribution of urea (this is equal to the volume of the distribution of water).

b. $Kt/V < 0.8$ is associated with high morbidity and mortality; Kt/V of 1–1.4 constitutes adequate dialysis.

c. In order to provide adequate dialysis, as defined by the above parameters, a change in dialysis prescription may be required and may consist of increasing the blood flow rate, using a larger, more efficient dialyzer, and/or increasing the dialysis time. It is imperative, however, that the vascular access function appropriately. Any malfunction in the access (thrombosis) which alters blood access can contribute to inadequate dialysis and should be corrected.

D. Complications
1. Access related
a. Vascular "steal" syndrome: Ischemia of the hand distal to the vascular access as a result of blood being shunted through the vascular access. This is usually seen in patients with compromised circulation (diabetes, atherosclerosis).

(1) Symptoms: The extremity may be cool, cyanotic, and painful. Occasionally ulcers may develop on the hand or fingers.

(2) Surgical revision or ligation is required.

b. Infection: Most commonly occurs in patients with grafts (up to 20%).

(1) Gram-positive organisms (*Staphlococcus epidermidis* and *Staph. aureus*) are most common.

(2) Removal of the graft may be required to eradicate complicated infections.

c. Thrombosis: Often the result of venous outflow stenosis. Requires declotting and dilatation of the stenotic area by angioplasty or surgical revision.

2. Dialysis-associated hypotension: The cause is multifactorial.

a. Overaggressive hemofiltration leading to excessive volume removal.

b. Acetate dialysate: May cause vasodilatation as well as myocardial dysfunction in patients with underlying cardiac disease.

c. Autonomic neuropathy.

d. Antihypertensive medications: Patients should hold or reduce antihypertensive medication prior to dialysis.

3. Dialysis disequilibrium syndrome: Headache, nausea, vomiting, muscle twitching, and lethargy which may occur during or shortly after dialysis. In extreme forms, seizures and coma may occur.

a. Most commonly seen in a severely uremic patient who is too aggressively dialyzed. The urea concentration and osmolality within the brain do not drop as rapidly as within the serum. This leads to osmotic shifts, causing cerebral edema.

b. Preventive measures for patients who may be predisposed to this syndrome consist of short dialysis times and low blood flow rates in order to reduce the

BUN concentration more slowly during dialysis.

4. Dialysis dementia: A progressive disorder which begins with abnormalities of speech consisting of stuttering and stammering, personality changes, myoclonus, seizures, and progressive dementia leading to death.

   a. Generally occurs in patients who have been on dialysis for several years.

   b. Felt to be a result of aluminum intoxication from aluminum-containing phosphate binders and from water sources used in dialysis which are not treated well and can be high in aluminum content.

   c. Treatment consists of discontinuing aluminum-containing phosphate binders, better water treatment, and chelation therapy with deferoxamine mesolate.

5. Dialysis-induced amyloidosis

   a. Occurs in patients who have been on dialysis for $\geq$5–10 years.

   b. Causes arthropathy involving primarily large joints (shoulders, hips). On x-ray, deposits within bone appear as lytic lesions.

   c. A common cause of carpel tunnel syndrome in chronic hemodialysis patients.

   d. The amyloid deposits are felt to be comprised β_2-microglobulin, a low molecular weight (12,500) protein that is renally excreted and poorly cleared by dialysis. As a result, β_2-microglobulin levels are quite high in the serum of patients with chronic renal failure.

   e. Carpel tunnel syndrome, when severe, can be corrected surgically. Unfortunately, there is no specific therapy for dialysis-induced amyloidosis. It is thought that peritoneal dialysis may clear β_2-microglobulin better than hemodialysis and that levels may be lower in patients dialyzed with more biocompatible membranes.

VIII. Peritoneal Dialysis

A. Patient population: 15–20% of patients on chronic dialysis are on peritoneal dialysis.

1. Peritoneal dialysis is performed by the patient, allowing the patient to have an active role in his or her care. This gives the patient a feeling of independence. The dialysis procedure is performed at home but can also be easily performed in the workplace if a clean area can be provided. Since little equipment is required, patients have far more freedom and are able to vacation with a minimum of preplanning.

2. Peritoneal dialysis may be indicated in the following situations:

   a. Patients with cardiovascular instability: Since fluid is removed gradually on a daily basis, hypotension is less likely to occur.

   b. Patients with contraindications to systemic heparinization (angiodysplasia).

   c. Patients who fail hemodialysis because of vascular access problems.

   d. Patients who live a considerable distance from a dialysis facility.

3. Potential contraindications

   a. Loss of peritoneal surface area, which may result from intra-abdominal catastrophic events or multiple surgeries.

   b. The presence of ostomies (i.e., colostomies, ileostomies, nephrostomies).

   c. Recent abdominal surgery.

   d. Pleuroperitoneal communication.

   e. Abdominal hernias.

4. Chronic peritoneal dialysis is also contraindicated in patients with physical handicaps such as blindness or crippling arthritis, as well as those with mental handicaps unless a partner who can perform the procedure is willing and available.

B. Technical aspects and requirements

1. Basic principles

   a. Diffusion.

   b. Osmosis: The passage of solvent (water) through a semipermeable membrane from a low to a high osmotic concentration gradient.

2. Access to the intra-abdominal cavity is required. A Tenckoff catheter must be surgically placed to allow access. This has two Dacron cuffs which are placed in the subcutaneous tissue and rectus muscle. These provide stability to the catheter and a barrier to the external environment.

3. Dialysate used in peritoneal dialysis is a sterile fluid which has a specific electrolyte composition and uses lactate as the

source for base. Glucose is used to create the osmotic gradient required in peritoneal dialysis. Dialysate with 1.5% dextrose has an osmolality of 340 and removes 200 ml of ultrafiltrate after a 3- to 4-hr dwell. Dialysate with a 4.25% dextrose concentration has an osmolality of 500 and removes up to 900 ml of ultrafiltrate after a 4- to 6-hr dwell.

4. Dialysis prescriptions
   a. Continuous ambulatory peritoneal dialysis (CAPD): 2 liters of dialysate are instilled into the peritoneal cavity and allowed to dwell for 4–6 hr. Three such exchanges are usually performed during the day, using 1.5% dextrose. The fourth exchange, performed at night, usually has an 8-hr dwell time in order to allow the patient ample time to sleep; 4.25% dextrose is utilized to maintain ultrafiltration.
   b. Continuous cyclic peritoneal dialysis (CCPD): An automated cycler is used which performs four to six 2-liter exchanges during an 8- to 10-hr period overnight. A final 2-liter exchange is then performed at the end of the cycling period and is carried by the patient throughout the day until the next cycling period begins the next night. This option is preferred by patients who wish to be free of dialysis procedures during the day. It is also useful in patients who require a partner to assist in their dialysis.

C. Adequacy: Prescribed parameters have been established which define adequate dialysis in peritoneal dialysis patients. Achieving these parameters is associated with decreased morbidity and mortality.
   1. Total creatinine clearance equals residual renal creatinine clearance (liters/week) plus peritoneal creatinine clearance (liters/week) and should be ≥40–50 liters/week. In the average patient, this is achieved with the standard peritoneal dialysis prescription as described above.
   2. Peritoneal equilibration test (PET): This is designed to assess peritoneal function and allows individualization of peritoneal dialysis therapy. The procedure is as follows:
      a. Two liters of 2.5% dialysis solution are instilled in the patient and allowed to dwell for 4 hr.

   b. After this, a serum sample (P) and an aliquot of dialysate (D) are sent for determination of the creatinine concentration.
   c. Patients with average peritoneal transport properties: a D/P ratio of 0.5–0.8 can be adequately dialyzed with either standard CAPD or CCPD. Patients with high peritoneal transport properties (D/P > 0.81) or patients with low peritoneal transport properties (D/P < 0.5) may require adjustments in the PD prescription to ensure adequate dialysis. This can be done by adjusting the frequency and duration of exchanges performed.

D. Complications.
   1. Peritonitis: The most common complication encountered by patients on peritoneal dialysis. Approximately 60% of patients will have one episode of peritonitis within the first year.
      a. Diagnosis is made when the patient has cloudy fluid usually associated with abdominal pain and the peritoneal dialysis cell count is ≥100 white blood cells/mm^3, of which ≥50% are neutrophils.
      b. From 60% to 75% of peritonitis episodes are caused by gram-positive organisms, most commonly *Staph. epidermidis* and *Staph. aureus*. Twenty percent are caused by gram-negative organisms.
      c. Peritonitis is easily treated with appropriate antibiotic coverage given either intravenously or intraperitoneally.
      d. More complicated episodes of peritonitis (e.g., relapsing peritonitis) may be a result of catheter exit site or tunnel infection and may require catheter removal.
   2. Catheter failure: A poorly functioning catheter (difficulty instilling or draining the dialysate) may occur in obese patients or those with a large omentum, which may lead to catheter obstruction or malposition. In addition, fibrin may deposit on or within the catheter and prevent good flow. Finally, dialysate fluid may migrate through the tunnel and leak out of the exit site in catheters, especially early on when they have not healed in. This may result in catheter loss.

3. Hydrothorax may develop in patients on peritoneal dialysis. This is thought to be a result of fluid migrating through lymphatics in the diaphragm into the pleural space. Tapping of the pleural fluid can be diagnostic, as it will show an extremely elevated glucose concentration. The hydrothorax will resolve after peritoneal dialysis is discontinued. After a prolonged period of discontinuation, the communication may seal off spontaneously and peritoneal dialysis can be resumed.

4. Early in peritoneal dialysis, patients may complain of referred pain to the shoulder due to diaphragmatic irritation and may complain of abdominal pain which is thought to result from the hypertonic and ascitic PD fluid. Both of these problems usually improve after the patient has been on dialysis for several weeks to a month.

IX. Renal Transplantation

A. Renal transplantation is the definitive cure for uremia. Opportunities for transplantation come primarily from donors who are declared legally dead (cadaveric). When a parent or sibling is healthy, willing, and immunologically compatible, he or she may donate a kidney as a living related donor.

B. Demographics: Unfortunately, there are more recipients than donors. Presently, 20,000 potential recipients are awaiting transplantation. Approximately 10,000 transplants are performed yearly. Of these, 80% are a result of cadaveric donation and 20% are a result of living related donors.

C. Recipient selection
1. Otherwise healthy ESRD patients are considered potential candidates for renal transplantation.
   a. Potential recipients are evaluated by their nephrologist and a transplant surgeon to be sure that they are physically and mentally capable of undergoing renal transplantation.
   b. Potential living related donors are evaluated by a qualified internist or nephrologist to be sure that they are healthy, free of renal disease, and mentally able to proceed with the nephrectomy required for the donation process.
   (1) Risks

(a) Those associated with general anesthesia and surgery.
(b) Hypertension may develop in 20% of patients.
(c) Renal function, as determined by serum creatinine, and 24-hr urine protein excretion remain stable in the majority of patients.

D. Contraindications to renal transplantation
1. ABO incompatibility.
2. Active infection.
3. Malignancy.
   a. Patients who are considered cured of their malignancy after ⩾2 years may be reconsidered as potential candidates.
4. Active peptic ulcer disease.
   a. Patients may be reconsidered after this has resolved.
5. Significant and irreversible cardiac or pulmonary disease.
6. Malnourished or debilitated patients.
7. Underlying urologic problems leading to an unsuitable bladder or urethra.
8. Elderly patients (⩾60 years of age).
   a. This is an arbitrary cutoff which is made on the assumption that anesthesia, surgery, and immunosuppressive therapy will be poorly tolerated. Thus, the acceptable age of a patient must be individualized.

E. Technical aspects
1. Living related transplants: These are usually performed simultaneously by two surgical teams so that the harvesting of the donor kidney and the transplantation into the recipient can occur as rapidly as possible. As a result, postoperative function of the transplant is usually excellent.
2. Cadaveric renal transplant: The cadaveric organ generally comes from an outside institution. It is harvested and preserved in an iced saline solution called *Euro-Collins' solution* for preservation and transportation. Ideally, transplantation should occur within 24–36 hr after harvesting has occurred to reduced ischemic time and the potential for postoperative acute tubulonecrosis, which is common.

F. Pharmacotherapy
1. Steroids: Inhibit the activation of macrophages.

a. Used in maintenance immunosuppression, as well as for acute rejection.

b. Side effects include hypertension, cushingoid features, diabetes mellitus, aseptic necrosis, peptic ulcer disease, and psychosis.

2. Azathioprine: Inhibits proliferation of activated T cells.

a. Complications consist of granulocytopenia, megaloblastic erythropoiesis, liver disease, interstitial pneumonitis, and an increased prevalence of malignancy.

b. Allopurinol prolongs the half-life of azathioprine, requiring a reduction in the dose when the two drugs are used concurrently.

3. Cyclosporine: Inhibits the activation of helper T cells, as well as the release of several lymphokines.

a. Complications consist of hypertension, acute and chronic renal disease, thrombosis, tremor, gingival hyperplasia, and hirsutism, as well as malignancy and infection.

b. Drugs that increase cyclosporine levels: ketoconazole, cimetidine, diltiazem, and erythromycin. Therefore, close monitoring and adjustment of cyclosporine levels are required when these medications are used.

c. Drugs that decrease cyclosporine levels: phenytoin, phenobarbital, and ethanol.

4. Antilymphocyte globulin (ALG): This is usually used to treat acute rejection.

a. This may lead to a marked reduction in lymphocyte counts, predisposing to infection.

5. Monoclonal antibodies (e.g., OKT3): These interfere with the immunologic function of T lymphocytes and are used to treat acute rejection.

a. Complications of consist of fever, noncardiogenic pulmonary edema, and aseptic meningitis.

G. Complications

1. Renal

a. Arterial thrombosis or stenosis at the area of anastomosis may occur, leading to acute postoperative dysfunction of the transplant.

b. Lymphatic fluid may collect, causing a lymphocele, which can occasionally lead to ureteral obstruction by external pressure.

c. A urine leak may develop due to poor anastomosis of the ureter to the bladder, leading to transplant failure.

d. Posttransplant ATN may occur in up to 50% of cadaveric transplant recipients.

e. Acute as well as chronic rejection may occur, leading to transplant failure.

f. Recurrence of the underlying disease may occur in the transplanted kidney and lead to failure. This may occur in patients who have primary glomerulopathies such as FSGS and rarely in patients with systemic diseases such as diabetes mellitus.

g. De novo glomerular disease: Membranous glomerulopathy and transplant glomerulonephropathy may occur independent of the underlying renal disease in the transplanted kidney and may lead to transplant failure. This usually occurs >6 months posttransplant.

2. Extrarenal

a. Hypertension.

b. Infection, including:

(1) Viral: Cytomegalovirus, herpes simplex virus, and varicella-zoster virus.

(2) Opportunistic: *Pneumocystis carinii*.

(3) Central nervous system infections due to *Listeria*, *Cryptococcus*, and *Aspergillus*.

c. Malignancy may occur from 6 months to 2 years after transplantation.

(1) Squamous and basal cell skin cancers are common; therefore, sunscreen should be worn.

(2) Lymphomas are common, are usually extranodal, and generally involve the central nervous system.

Bibliography

Alfrey DL, Chan L. Chronic renal failure: Manifestations and pathogenesis, in Schiner RW (ed), *Renal and Electrolyte Disorders*, ed 4. Boston, Little, Brown, 1992, pp 539–579.

Glassock RJ (ed). *Current Therapy in Nephrology and Hypertension*, ed 3. St. Louis, MO, Mosby Year Book, 1992.

Tisher CC, Wilcox CS (eds). *Nephrology for the House Officer*. Baltimore, Williams and Wilkins, 1992.

United States Renal Data System 1991 Annual Data Report: Excerpts. *Am J Kidney Dis* 18(Suppl):1–127, 1992.

CHAPTER 87

Hypertension

Janis Orlowski, M.D.

Renal (Secondary) Hypertension

Renovascular Hypertension

I. **Definition**

Renovascular hypertension is defined as an anatomic abnormality in the renal artery or its branches leading to the development of excess blood pressure. Not all abnormalities of renal artery anatomy lead to hypertension, so further studies must be used to define the lesion as a true cause of hypertension in an individual patient.

II. **Goldblatt Hypertension Model**

A. Renovascular hypertension was first studied when Goldblatt and his associates clipped the renal artery of a dog in a study initially designed to investigate the renal contribution to hypertension (Figure 87-1). They found that there was an immediate rise in systemic blood pressure after clipping the right renal artery. This elevation in blood pressure is ameliorated by a right nephrectomy. Hypertension is again found when the single left renal artery is clipped. This has given rise to two classic models of renal mediated hypertension.

1. The first model is the two-kidney–one-clip model, which most closely approximates renovascular hypertension.
2. The second model is the one-kidney–one-clip model, which parallels hypertension associated with a decrease in renal mass. A cascade of events leads to the stimulation of the renin angiotensin system.

B. From 1940 to the early 1950s, patient's with hypertension, a unilateral small kidney, and/or a demonstrable lesion in their renal artery underwent nephrectomies, leading to only a 20–25% cure rate for their hypertension. This poor cure rate can be attributed to two separate factors:

1. Not all renal artery lesions lead to the development of hypertension.
2. Long-standing renovascular hypertension may lead to systemic arteriolar abnormalities which are not reversible.

III. **Incidence**

A. The true incidence of renovascular hypertension in the unselected hypertensive population is approximately 2%, with some studies showing the incidence increasing to as much as 6% if factors such as rapidly rising blood

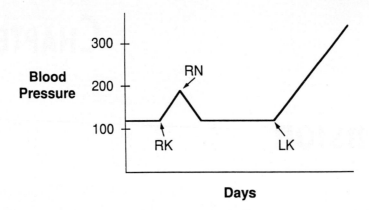

Figure 87-1. The Goldblatt hypertension experimental model demonstrates that there is a rise in blood pressure when the right renal artery is clipped (RK) (two-kidney–one-clip model of hypertension). This rise in blood pressure is ameliorated when the right kidney is removed (RN). After recovery from the right nephrectomy, systemic blood pressure again rises when the left renal artery is clipped (LK) (one-kidney–one-clip model of hypertension).

pressure, difficult-to-treat blood pressure, and/or abdominal bruit are used to select the population. Blacks, as a rule, have been found to have a much lower incidence of renovascular hypertension, as demonstrated by a study by Keith evaluating the cause of malignant hypertension. This study demonstrated renovascular hypertension as the etiology in 32% of whites but in only 4% of blacks who were referred to a tertiary center for evaluation of hypertension. This concept of a racial difference in the incidence of renovascular hypertension has recently come under scrutiny.

B. Svetkey et al. have reported that in 167 patients referred for evaluation of hypertension with one or more clinical findings of renovascular hypertension (i.e., persistently elevated or difficult-to-control blood pressure, age above 50 at onset, worsening of blood pressure, or an abdominal bruit), they found a 24% incidence of renal artery stenosis (39/167). Twenty-seven percent of the white patients and 19% of the blacks had renovascular stenosis, and 14% of the entire group had renovascular hypertension as defined by an improvement in their blood pressure after successful angioplasty or renal artery bypass surgery (23/167). This information suggests that previously held concepts about the rare occurrence of renovascular hypertension in the black population have to be reinvestigated based on the clinical presentation.

IV. Renovascular Lesions

The renovascular lesions seen can be categorized into two main types, followed by a series of more uncommon presentations.

A. Atherosclerotic disease as the cause of renovascular hypertension is seen in 65% of all patients with renovascular hypertension. This disease is seen most commonly in patients older than 50 years of age. The lesion affects the left kidney more commonly than the right, with bilateral disease seen in about a third of the patients. The lesion commonly affects the ostia and the first third of the renal artery. The disease is found most commonly in men with a history of smoking. Hyperlipidemic states are also a contributing risk factor.

B. Fibromuscular dysplasia is seen in approximately 30–35% of all patients with renovascular hypertension. These patients typically are women between the age of 20 and 50. The Mayo and Cleveland clinics have developed a morphologic classification of this type of lesion (Figure 87-2). Intimal fibroplasia has an incidence of 1%. Histologically, it is a proliferation of the endothelial cell. Medial fibroplasia occurs in 95% of the cases in this disease. The normal smooth muscle of the renal artery is replaced with thick collagenous bands. Finally, the rare adventitial and periarterial fibroplasias occur in less than 1% of cases.

C. Other uncommon forms of renovascular anatomic abnormalities leading to renovascular hypertension include:
   1. Extrinsic compression from tumors, masses, or inflammation.
   2. Intrinsic compression from tumors, aneurysms, emboli, or thrombi.

D. An important note is that Takayasu's arteritis (a giant cell vasculitis of the major arterial

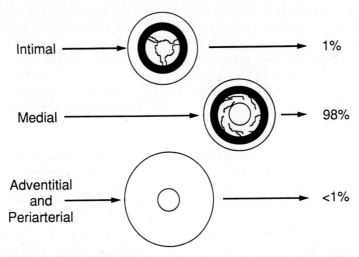

Figure 87-2. Pictorial representation of the Mayo Clinic classification of fibromuscular dysplasia. One percent of cases are attributed to intimal hyperplasia. The majority of cases (98%) are found pathologically to have hypertrophy of the smooth muscle of the renal artery or medial hyperplasia. Rarely, fibromuscular dysplasia is attributed to adventitial hyperplasia.

vessels) is the most common cause of renovascular hypertension in the Oriental population.

V. Clinical Characteristics

A. The typical clinical presentation of renovascular hypertension, as determined by the National Cooperative Study on Renovascular Hypertension, is that of a 35-year-old female with hypertension of short duration and no end-organ damage or a patient older than 50 with newly diagnosed hypertension or increased blood pressure (which is more difficult to control in patients with hypertension) and evidence of end-organ damage. The study also found that patients with renovascular hypertension are more often of ideal body weight in comparison to patients with essential hypertension, have a shorter duration of hypertension, more frequent onset of hypertension before age 50, less family history of hypertension, more severe retinopathy, more abdominal and flank bruits, higher blood urea nitrogen levels, and lower potassium levels compared to age-, gender-, race-, and diastolic pressure-controlled pairs with essential hypertension.

B. Renovascular hypertension has been documented in 10% of the renal transplant population, usually occurring 6 months after transplant.

1. Numerous causes, including stenosis at the renal artery anastomosis, progressive atherosclerotic disease, kinking of the renal artery leading to turbulent flow, and emboli, have been implicated in this process.

2. The clinical triad of elevated diastolic hypertension, progressive renal insufficiency, and a vascular bruit over the renal allograft should lead to further studies to evaluate the transplant patient for renovascular hypertension.

VI. Confirmatory Studies

A. Confirmatory studies are characterized by low specificity or sensitivity.

B. The rapid-sequence intravenous pyelogram (IVP) is 70–75% sensitive, with a false-positive rate of 10–15%.

C. Radionuclide studies are 75–85% sensitive but have a higher false-positive rate than the IVP.

D. Newer reports of angiotensin-converting enzyme inhibitor use prior to radionuclide studies show an increase in sensitivity to almost 90% but include the risk of sudden hypotension and acute renal failure.

E. The diagnostic gold standard, the angiogram, will correlate with surgical success only if the lesion is more than 50% stenosed or if there are multiple lesions, with the greatest lesion being approximately 50%. A nondiagnostic angiogram should be followed up with renal vein renin sampling to see if there is a 50% increase in renin in the "clipped" kidney compared to the inferior vena cava or the contralateral renal vein.

F. Surgery has a favorable blood pressure response in 80% of cases with fibromuscular dysplasia and in approximately 60% of cases caused by atherosclerotic disease. Reported surgical complications are approximately 3%.

G. Angioplasty has an 85–90% cure rate with fibromuscular dysplasia and a 75% success rate with nonoccluded, nonstial arteriosclerotic lesions.

VII. **Pathophysiology of Renal Hypertension**

A. Studies of laboratory animals using the original model of the two-kidney–one-clip model first developed by Goldblatt in 1934 have given us insight into the development and maintenance of renovascular hypertension (Figure 87-3).

B. Phase I (acute phase): This phase is marked by renal artery stenosis, usually greater than 70%, leading to renal ischemia. This decrease in renal perfusion results in a marked increase in renin excretion because of the decrease in arteriolar transluminal pressure in the juxtaglomerular apparatus, an increase in the stimulation of the renal sympathetic nerves, and other hormonal effects. Increased renin leads to the increase in angiotensin II production with marked concomitant systemic hypertension because of the effect of angiotensin II on peripheral vascular resistance. The rise in blood pressure has been attributed solely to the increase in the renin-angiotensin system, as evidenced by multiple studies which have attempted to inhibit this system (Figure 87-4).

C. Angiotensin-converting enzyme inhibitors have been clearly shown to block the hypertension caused by renovascular lesions accounting for the entire increase in blood pressure. Christlieb and colleagues studied the role of angiotensin by causing active immunization to angiotensin II, which also showed that hypertension did not develop. In 1985, Wood et al. demonstrated that a specific inhibitor of renin (CGP-29287) caused a normalization of blood pressure in marmosets with renovascular hypertension.

D. As reviewed more thoroughly elsewhere, the rise in blood pressure is solely related to the increase in the renin-angiotensin system, but the absolute rise is attenuated by many factors.

1. First, it has been shown that atrial natriuretic factor antagonizes the effects of angiotensin II.

2. In renovascular hypertension atrial natriuretic factor levels are found to be elevated.

3. Prostaglandins also attenuate the rise in blood by acting locally to counterbalance the effects of hypertension from angiotensin II.

4. Inhibition of prostaglandins in the presence of angiotensin II causes unchecked angiotensin II to increase afferent and efferent resistance, further worsening renal function in this model.

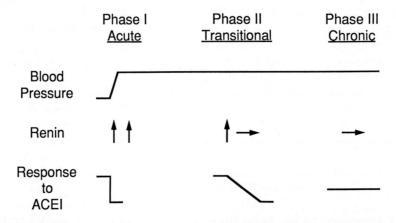

Figure 87-3. Pathophysiology of renal hypertension in the two-kidney–one-clip model of renovascular hypertension can be separated into several phases, as demonstrated by the renin level and the hypertensive response to angiotensin converting enzyme inhibitors (ACEI). Phase I reveals an immediate rise in blood pressure, with an elevated renin level secondary to the acute renal ischemia. ACEI usually provides an immediate fall in blood pressure. Phase II involves lowering of the renin level because of the increased blood flow to the clipped kidney as a result of the higher systemic pressures. ACEI is variable. Finally, phase III, the chronic phase, results in persistent hypertension due to arteriolar damage to the peripheral vessels. Renin levels are variable, as is the response to ACEI.

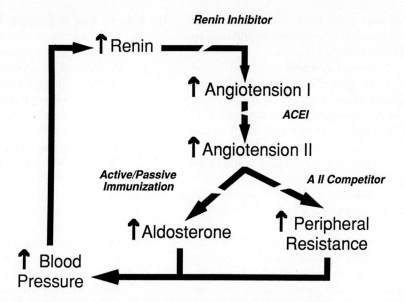

Figure 87-4. This diagram displays the renin-angiotensin system which leads to hypertension. Several investigators have demonstrated the roles of each level of the system by specifically inhibiting subsegments resulting in normalization of blood pressure. Wood et al. used a specific renin inhibitor to study the effects of renin. Christlieb et al. studied the immunization against angiotensin. Angiotensin-converting enzyme inhibitors are known to block the conversion of angiotensin I to angiotensin II, resulting in lower blood pressure.

5. The renal medulla is thought to be a source of a nonprostanoid vasodilator which again counterbalances the effects of angiotensin II.

6. Heptinstall et al. showed that ablation of the renal medullary interstitial cell caused a worsening of the hypertension.

7. Finally, it has been shown that the denervation of the kidney has an attenuating effect on blood pressure.

E. In phase I, the volume is usually normal to low as the contralateral kidney begins to excrete salt and water in response to the pressure effect. Angiotensin-converting enzyme inhibitors cause a sudden marked decrease in systemic pressure if administered at this stage. Removal of the clip to the kidney would cause an immediate return of the blood pressure to normal. This is not exactly the sequence seen in human cases of renovascular hypertension unless the renal artery occlusion occurs acutely, such as with emboli, thrombi, or dissection.

F. Phase II (transitional phase): This phase is marked by a decrease in renin-angiotensin because there is an increase in renal artery perfusion to the ischemic kidney as a result of the increase in systemic pressure and the volume expansion, which was mediated by increased aldosterone levels. However, the levels of renin are still abnormally high; hence, angiotensin-converting enzyme II inhibition can still provoke a moderate decrease in blood pressure. This effect can be enhanced by the use of diuretics. The contralateral kidney still excretes salt and water, but there is a shift in the pressure-natriuresis curve thought to be secondary to locally mediated effects of angiotensin II, as well as the increased level of aldosterone on the unclipped kidney.

G. Phase III (chronic phase): In this phase, if the renal artery is unclipped, systemic hypertension continues because of the arteriolar damage done to peripheral vessels and/or nephrosclerosis to the original unclipped kidney which withstood severe systemic hypertension.

Hypertension Associated with Renal Parenchymal Disease

I. Etiology

A. The etiology of the hypertension in renal disease is associated with:

1. The decreased ability of the kidney to excrete a sodium and water load.

2. The inability to respond to physiologic reactions which may cause an increase in the

intravascular volume or pressure, which, under normal circumstances, would lead to sodium and water excretion.

B. Renal parenchymal diseases can also cause ischemia at the juxtaglomerular apparatus, resulting in a physiologically inappropriate increase in renin-angiotensin system activity, resulting in retention of salt and water in the nonoliguric patient with renal insufficiency.

1. The increased volume initially leads to an increase in cardiac output.

2. This then leads to a persistent increase in peripheral resistance which results in elevated blood pressure.

C. Unlike the well-defined causes of hypertension, a disturbed sodium/water balance or an overactive renin-angiotensin system, the sympathetic nervous system does not appear to play a role in hypertension secondary to renal parenchymal disease. Not only are there normal levels of catecholamines, but there also appears to be a decreased responsiveness to catecholamines in patients with renal insufficiency prior to starting dialysis.

D. Whether other known causes of hypertension, such as abnormal vasoactive pressure depressant levels, lead to the hypertension seen with renal parenchymal disease needs to be further investigated.

II. Incidence

A. Hypertension in patients with renal parenchymal disease is very common. More than 80% of patients with end-stage renal disease are also hypertensive.

B. Hypertension is much more commonly found in patients with a glomerular cause for their renal insufficiency as opposed to those with a tubulointerstitial etiology.

C. Hypertension is commonly found in cases of nephritis with acute glomerular inflammation such as poststreptococcal glomerulonephritis or vasculitis.

D. Hypertension is also seen commonly in the nephrotic syndrome secondary to focal segmental glomerulosclerosis and much less frequently in minimal-change glomerulonephritis.

E. As mentioned, tubulointerstitial causes of renal disease uncommonly cause hypertension, but hypertension is reported with reflux nephropathy.

F. The incidence of hypertension increases with the increased loss of renal function.

The Kidney's Role in Essential Hypertension

A. Some of the accumulated medical literature suggests that essential hypertension can be thought of as a primary renal defect. Rettig and his colleagues have shown that transplantation of kidneys from spontaneously hypertensive rats or from rats with hypertension induced in the classic two-kidney–one-clip model (phase III, chronic hypertension) causes hypertension in normotensive animals. Kidneys transplanted from the setting of renovascular hypertension into a normotensive animal results in the continued expression of hypertension.

B. On the other hand, renal transplantation from a normotensive rate into the spontaneously hypertensive animal results in a continually normal blood pressure.

C. In humans, Guidi et al. have reported that a positive family history in a cadaver renal transplant donor is a factor in the amount of antihypertensive therapy necessary for blood pressure control after transplant, controlling for level of renal function, number of rejections, and amount of immunosuppressants used.

Pathophysiology of Essential Hypertension

Researchers believe that the sine qua non of primary hypertension is persistently elevated vascular resistance leading to hypertrophy and increased contractility of vessels. Fowler et al. have suggested that the initial cause of vascular contractility may be secondary to mildly increased levels of angiotensin II and that subsequent damage to the arteries may lead to a host of complicated, generalized changes. It is known that patients with hypertension have a lower blood volume. However, London et al. demonstrated that early, mildly hypertensive patients have elevated total body volume relative to controls, suggesting that there is a disturbance in the pressure-volume control in the kidney in early hypertension.

Guyton and fellow researchers demonstrated a rise in the pressure-volume control in the kidney in early hypertension. They found that with an increase in cardiac output or volume, the body will respond with autoregulation in this tissue; that is, because the increase in blood flow or volume is not needed, the tissue will cause an increase in peripheral vessel constriction to regulate this change in hemodynamics. The increase in peripheral vascular resistance leads to a decrease in cardiac output or a further regulation of volume. In a normal kidney, an increase in arterial pressure raises the excretion of salt and water. However, in primary hypertension this pressure-sodium curve is reset, resulting initially in a constriction of efferent arterioles, leading to an increase in filtration fraction, which favors sodium and water reabsorption. This increase in filtration fraction eventually leads to an increase in blood volume and a higher systemic pressure, eventually equilibrating at a new higher set point for sodium excretion.

Bibliography

Christlieb AR, Biber TUL, Hickler RB. Studies on the role of angiotensin in experimental renovascular hypertension: An immunologic approach. *J Clin Invest* 48:1506–1518, 1969.

Fowler W-L Jr, Johnson JA, Kurz KD, et al. Renin-angiotensin mechanisms in oral contraceptive hypertension in conscious rats. *Am J Physiol* 248(5pt2):H695–699, 1985.

Goldblatt H. Studies on experimental hypertension: III. The production of persistent hypertension in monkeys (Macaque) by renal ischemia. *J Exp Med* 65:671–675, 1937.

Goldblatt H, Lynch J, Hanzal RF, et al. Studies on experimental hypertension: I. The production of persistent elevation of systolic blood pressure by means of renal ischemia. *J Exp Med* 59:347–378, 1937.

Guidi E, Bianchi G, Rivolta EZ, et al. Hypertension in man with a kidney transplant: role of familial versus other factors. *Nephron* 41:14–21, 1985.

Guyton AC, Coleman TG, Cowley AV Jr, et al. Arterial pressure regulation overriding dominance of the kidneys in long-term regulation and in hypertension. *Am J Med* 52(5):584–594, 1972.

Heptinstall RH, Salyer DC, Salyer WR. Experimental hypertension: The effects of chemical ablation of the renal papilla on the blood pressure of rats with and without silver-clip hypertension. *Am J Pathol* 78:297–307, 1975.

Keith TA. Renovascular hypertension in black patients. *Hypertension* 4(3):438–443, 1982.

Lombard JH, Eskinder H, Kauser K, et al. Enhanced norepinephrine sensitivity in renal arteries at elevated transmurfal pressure. *Am J Physiol* 259(1pt2):H29–33, 1990.

London GM, Safor ME, Weiss YA, et al. Volume-dependent parameter in essential hypertension. *Kidney Int* 11:204–208, 1977.

Martinez-Maldanado M. Clinical conference: Pathophysiology of renovascular hypertension. *Hypertension* :707–719, 1991.

Morrison EG, McCormack EG. Pathological classification of renal arterial disease in renovascular hypertension. *Mayo Clin Proc* 46:161–168, 1971.

Rettig R, Folberth CG, Stauss H, et al. Hypertension in rats induced by renal grafts from renovascular hypertension donors. *Hypertension* 4:429–435, 1990.

Simon N, Franklin SS, Bleifer KH, et al. Cooperative study of renovascular hypertension. *JAMA* 220:1209–1218, 1972.

Svetky LP, Kadir S, Dunnick NR, et al. Similar prevalence of renovascular hypertension in selected blacks and whites. *Hypertension* 17:678–683, 1991.

Wood JM, Gulati N, Forgiarini P, et al. Effects of a specific and long-acting renin inhibitor in the marmoset. *Hypertension* 7:797–803, 1985.

CHAPTER 88

Nephrolithiasis

Samuel Saltzberg, M.D.

I. **Definition**
Concretions consisting of crystalline components in an organic matrix occurring in the urinary collecting system.

II. **Etiology**
Stones are usually composed of the following crystalline components:
A. Calcium stones: 75–85% of stones.
  1. Calcium oxalate: ~70% of stones.
  2. Calcium phosphate: ~10% of stones.
    a. Hydroxyapatite: $(Ca)_5(PO_4)_3OH$, most common.
    b. Brushite: $CaHPO_4 \cdot 2H_2O$.
    c. Witlockite (calcium orthophosphate).
    d. Octocalcium phosphate.
    e. Carbonate apatite: Commonly present in struvite stones.
B. Uric acid: 5–8% of stones
C. Magnesium ammonium phosphate (struvite): 5–15% of stones. Associated with infection with a urease-splitting organism. May also contain a component of carbonate apatite. Commonly forms staghorn calculi.
D. Cystine: 1–3% of stones.
E. Xanthine.
F. Triamterene.

G. 2,8-Dihydroxyadenine.
H. Silica.

III. **Pathophysiology**
Stones are formed by nucleation and subsequent crystal growth of crystalline components in a supersaturated urine. The process is promoted by either increased urinary concentration of crystalline components, decreased concentration of inhibitors, or environmental conditions that promote crystallization. Multiple disorders may be present in the same patient.
A. Calcium stones
  1. Hypercalciuria: Urinary calcium >300 mg/day (men), >250 mg/day (women). Present in 40–60% of stone formers.
    a. Secondary causes
      (1) Hyperparathyroidism
      (2) Hyperthyroidism
      (3) Cushing's syndrome
      (4) Granulomatous diseases (sarcoidosis, tuberculosis, silicosis, disseminated candidiasis, leprosy)
      (5) Immobilization
      (6) Vitamin D intoxication
      (7) Rapidly progressive bone disease

(8) Paget's disease
(9) Hypomagnesemia
(10) Renal tubular acidosis
b. Idiopathic
(1) Absorptive hypercalciuria: Primary increase in intestinal calcium absorption.
(2) Renal hypercalciuria: Impaired renal tubular reabsorption of calcium.
(3) Primary enhancement of 1,25-$(OH)_2$-vitamin D production
(4) Renal phosphate leak: Impaired renal tubular reabsorption of phosphate stimulates synthesis of 1,25-$(OH)_2$-vitamin D.
2. Hyperoxaluria: >45 mg/day
a. Hereditary: Rare autosomal recessive enzyme defect leads to oxalate overproduction.
(1) Type I: Deficiency of α-keto-β-OH-glutarate:glyoxalate.
(2) Type II: Increased conversion of hydroxypyruvate to L-glyceric acid.
b. Enteric: Small bowel disease and fat malabsorption.
(1) Unabsorbed fatty acids complex free calcium, leaving less calcium available to complex dietary oxalate, resulting in more free oxalate available for absorption.
(2) Unabsorbed bile salts and fatty acids increase intestinal permeability to oxalate.
c. Excess dietary oxalate: Chocolate, beets, rhubarb, green leafy vegetables, tea, nuts.
d. Hypervitaminosis C: Ascorbic acid (vitamin C) is metabolized to oxalate.
e. Ethylene glycol intoxication.
f. Methoxyflurane anesthesia.
3. Hyperuricosuria: >800 mg/day (men), >750 mg/day (women), 20% of calcium oxalate stone formers. Monosodium urate or uric acid crystals form a nidus for heterogeneous nucleation of calcium oxalate.
a. Excessive intake of purine: From meat, poultry and fish.
b. Primary urate overproduction.
4. Hypocitraturia: <320 mg/day, 15–30% of stone formers. Urinary citrate complexes calcium and reduces ionic calcium

concentration. Citrate also directly inhibits crystallization of calcium oxalate and calcium phosphate.
a. Metabolic acidosis: Enhances tubular reabsorption of citrate and impairs peritubular uptake and synthesis of citrate.
(1) Distal renal tubular acidosis
(2) Chronic diarrhea
(3) Thiazide-induced hypokalemia (intracellular acidosis)
(4) High sodium intake
(5) Excessive intake of animal proteins
b. Idiopathic
5. Hypomagnesiuria: <24 mg/day, 5–10% of stone formers. Urinary magnesium complexes with oxalate. In addition, magnesium depletion can cause hypercalciuria.
a. Malabsorption of magnesium
b. Inadequate magnesium intake
6. Reduced levels of other inhibitors
a. Inorganic pyrophosphate
b. Acid mucopolysaccharides
c. Glycopeptides: Nephrocalcin
7. Alkaline urine: Promotes calcium phosphate crystallization.
8. Low urine volume: high urinary concentration of crystalloid components.
9. Specific syndromes
a. Distal renal tubular acidosis
(1) Hypocitraturia from systemic acidosis and hypokalemia.
(2) Hypercalciuria and hyperphosphaturia from enhanced bone resorption of systemic acidosis.
(3) Alkaline pH of urine.
b. Chronic diarrhea
(1) Hypocitraturia from systemic acidosis and hypokalemia.
(2) Hyperoxaluria.
(3) Low urine volume.
B. Uric acid stones
1. Hyperuricosuria
a. Excessive intake of purine
b. Urate overproduction
(1) Lesch Nyhan syndrome: hypoxanthine-guanine phosphoribosyltransferase deficiency
(2) Malignant tumors
(3) Myeloproliferative disorders
(4) Idiopathic
2. Acidic urine: Shifts equilibrium from urate to less water-soluble uric acid.

3. Low urine volume: Increased concentration of uric acid.

C. Magnesium ammonium phosphate (struvite) stones: Associated with chronic urinary tract infections with urease-splitting organisms (*Proteus, Pseudomonas, Klebsiella*).

1. Magnesium ammonium phosphate crystal formation
   a. Production of large amounts of ammonia (NH_3) from urea.
   b. Formation of ammonium (NH_4^+) and alkalinization of urine ($NH_3 + H^+ \rightleftharpoons NH_4^+$).
   c. Alkalinization increases amount of trivalent phosphate.
   d. Ammonium, trivalent phosphate, and magnesium complex to form stone.
2. Carbonate apatite crystal formation
   a. H_2CO_3 dissociates to CO_3^{2-} (carbonate) in alkaline urine.
   b. Calcium complexes with carbonate to form carbonate apatite.
3. Other metabolic abnormalities: Metabolic abnormalities listed in Section III,A may be present and may predispose to calcium stone formation. These calcium stones may then contribute to chronic infection.

D. Cystine stones: Autosomal recessive trait (prevalence, 1 in 7,000) resulting in defective proximal tubular reabsorption of cystine and other dibasic amino acids. Stone forms secondary to low solubility of cystine in urine.

E. Xanthine stones: Overproduction of xanthine in patients with high purine metabolism treated with allopurinol.

F. Triamterene: Urinary triamterene precipitates in some patients taking this diuretic.

G. 2,8-Dihydroxyadenine: 2,8-dihydroxyadeninuria.

H. Silica: Urinary silica in patients taking trisilicate as an antacid.

IV. **Diagnosis**
A. History
   1. Symptoms
      a. Asymptomatic.
      b. Flank pain radiating to testicle or vulva.
      c. Hematuria.
      d. Frequency, urgency, and/or dysuria.
   2. Past medical history
      a. Gout.
      b. Chronic urinary tract infections.
      c. Chronic diarrhea.
   3. Family history of stones

B. Clinical signs
   1. Patient in severe pain. Typically has difficulty remaining in one position.
   2. Costovertebral angle tenderness.
   3. Signs of infection (e.g., fever).
C. Diagnostic tests
   1. Acute stone passage
      a. Urinalysis: Hematuria, evidence of urinary tract infection (pyuria, bacteria), cystine crystals, pH.
      b. Complete blood count: elevated white blood cell count with infection.
      c. Electrolytes: Hypokalemia, hypercalcemia, metabolic acidosis.
      d. Uric acid.
      e. Creatinine: Elevated only with unilateral obstruction in patient with one functioning kidney or in bilateral obstruction.
      f. KUBs: Calcium, struvite, and cystine stones are radiopaque. Uric acid, xanthine, and 2,8-dihydroxyadenine stones are radiolucent.
      g. Intravenous pyelogram: Anatomy of urinary tract, presence of radiolucent stones, and location of stones.
      h. Renal ultrasound: Presence of stones, evidence of hydronephrosis.
   2. Chronic stone disease
      a. Analysis of stone.
      b. Serum electrolytes, including calcium and phosphate.
      c. Parathyroid hormone level if calcium is elevated.
      d. Serum uric acid.
      e. Urinalysis: pH, cystine crystals.
      f. Three separate 24-hr urine collections for calcium, oxalate, uric acid, citrate, and volume.
      g. Qualitative test for urinary cystine.
      h. Dietary history.

V. **Differential Diagnosis**
A. Hematuria: Glomerular diseases, sickle cell disease and trait, tumor, vascular malformation, renal cysts, renal infarction, cystitis, prostatitis.
B. Flank pain: Musculoskeletal pain, pneumonia, pulmonary embolism, cholecystitis, pancreatitis, splenic infarct, pyelonephritis, acute glomerulonephritis, renal cysts, renal infarction.

VI. **Treatment**
A. Management of acute stone disease
   1. Conservative management: Fluids and

analgesia: most stones <5 mm pass spontaneously.

2. Stone removal: Indicated in presence of infection, severe obstruction, intractable pain, serious bleeding, and stones >10 mm.
   a. Retrograde passage of flexible basket.
   b. Pyelolithotomy and ureterolithitomy.
   c. Lithotripsy: Extracorporeal, percutaneous, or endoscopic. Not for staghorn calculi. Complications: perinephric hematoma, renin-mediated hypertension.

B. Long-term management: Most physicians treat aggressively only patients with recurrent stone disease. Maintenance of urine output >2,000 ml/day probably indicated in all patients who have had a stone.
   1. Calcium stones
      a. Hypercalciuria
         (1) Treatment of underlying disease in secondary causes.
         (2) Thiazide diuretic: Increases distal calcium reabsorption through a direct effect and increases proximal reabsorption by inducing mild volume depletion.
         (3) Amiloride: Increases calcium reabsorption when given with thiazide. Prevents thiazide-induced hypokalemia. Extreme caution needed if used with potassium citrate.
         (4) Sodium restriction: High sodium excretion increases calcium excretion.
         (5) Absorptive hypercalciuria
            (a) Reduce calcium intake: Caution—in patients with renal calcium wasting this may result in negative calcium balance.
            (b) Sodium cellulose phosphate: Binds calcium in gut. Caution: May result in negative calcium balance, magnesium depletion, and second hyperoxaluria.
            (c) Orthophosphate: Inhibits $1,25\text{-(OH)}_2$-vitamin D synthesis, binds intestinal calcium, and decreases saturation of calcium oxalate by increasing urinary pyrophosphate. Cau-

tion: May increase susceptibility to calcium phosphate stones.

   b. Hyperoxaluria
      (1) Pyridoxin: May be effective in some patients with hereditary oxalosis.
      (2) Workup and treatment, if possible, of any underlying malabsorption state.
      (3) Oxalate-restricted diet.
      (4) Fat-restricted diet.
      (5) Magnesium supplementation: Magnesium binds oxalate in intestine. Also corrects any hypomagnesiuria.
      (6) Calcium supplementation: Binds oxalate in intestine. Caution: Increased calcium absorption and resulting increase in urinary calcium excretion may counterbalance any beneficial effect from decrease in oxaluria.
      (7) Cholestyramine: Binds oxalate and bile salts in intestine. May not cause sustained reduction.
      (8) Oxabsorb®: An organic marine hydrocolloid reported to bind oxalate in intestine.
   c. Hyperuricosuria
      (1) Purine-restricted diet.
      (2) Allopurinol.
   d. Hypocitraturia
      (1) Potassium citrate: Corrects any underlying metabolic acidosis and increases urinary citrate excretion. Note: Sodium citrate may not be as effective, as it may increase calcium excretion by increasing sodium excretion.
      (2) Decrease intake of animal proteins.
   e. Hypomagnesiuria: Magnesium supplementation.
   f. Distal renal tubular acidosis: potassium citrate: Corrects metabolic acidosis, hypocitraturia, and hypokalemia.
   g. Chronic diarrhea
      (1) Potassium citrate: Corrects metabolic acidosis and hypocitraturia.
      (2) Treatment of hyperoxaluria (see Section VI,B,1,b).
      (3) Adequate fluid intake.

2. Uric acid stones
   a. Purine-restricted diet.
   b. Alkalinization of urine: Shifts equilibrium to more water-soluble urate.
   c. Allopurinol.
3. Magnesium ammonium phosphate stones
   a. Treatment of any correctable urologic abnormality.
   b. Workup and treatment of any metabolic disturbance described in Section III,A.
   c. Usually requires surgical stone removal followed by control of chronic infection.
   d. Acetohydroxamine: A urease inhibitor. Side effects include hemolytic anemia, thrombophlebitis, and nonspecific neurologic symptoms.
   e. Hemiacidrin: Acid citrate solution that may dissolve struvite. Requires irrigation of intact, unobstructed renal pelvis.
4. Cystine stones
   a. Hydration: May require an intake of more than 4 liters/day.
   b. Attempt to alkalinize urine to pH 7.0–7.5 with potassium citrate or sodium bicarbonate.
   c. Drug therapy: Thiopronin, penicil-lamine, captopril. These agents have sulfhydryl groups that react with cystine to form mixed disulfides, which are more soluble.

VII. **Patient Monitoring**
Careful follow-up to monitor recurrence of stones and to confirm compliance with dietary recommendations and drug therapy. Yearly KUBs examinations to monitor for new stones, stone passage, and stone growth in patients with radiopaque stones. Repeat metabolic studies to determine effect of therapy.

VIII. **Prognosis**
With selective therapy, individual stone formation may be reduced by over 90%. Treatment is generally less effective in patients with hyperoxaluria (especially hereditary), struvite stones, and cystine stones.

Bibliography

Coe FL, Favus MJ. Nephrolithiasis, in Brenner BM and Rector FC (eds), *The Kidney*, ed 4. Philadelphia, Saunders, 1991, pp 1728–1767.

Coe FL, Parks JH. Pathophysiology of kidney stones and strategies for treatment. *Hosp Pract* 23:195–168, 1988.

Pak CYC. Etiology and treatment of urolithiasis. *Am J Kidney Dis* 18:624–637, 1991.

Pak CYC. Citrate and renal calculi: New insights and future directions. *Am J Kidney Dis*, 17:420–425, 1991.

CHAPTER 89

Glomerulonephritis and Nephrotic Syndrome

Stephen Korbet, M.D.

Normal Glomerular Architecture

I. Glomerular Capillary Wall
 A. Epithelial cell.
 B. Glomerular basement membrane.
 C. Fenestrated endothelium.
  1. Glomerular permeability characteristics.
   a. Size selective: Molecules with molecular weights above 50,000 generally cannot permeate the glomerular capillary wall.
   b. Charge selective: The glomerular basement membrane and the epithelial cell layer are negatively charged. This is thought to be a result of the high sialic acid and heparin sulfate proteoglycan contents, which are negatively charged.

II. Mesangium

Proteinuria

I. Definition
 A. Normal: Usually the low molecular weight proteins and the small amount of albumin that are filtered are reabsorbed by the proximal tubule.

However, approximately 150 mg of protein can be excreted in the urine in a 24-hr period of time. Approximately one-third of the protein excreted normally is albumin, the remainder being Tamm-Horsfall glycoprotein, excreted by the distal nephron.
 B. Overflow proteinuria: The glomerulus and tubule function normally, and proteinuria is a result of excess production of freely filtered, low molecular weight protein such as Bench Jones protein or lysozyme.
 C. Tubular proteinuria: The glomerulus functions normally; however, the tubules are damaged and unable to reabsorb the normally filtered proteins (e.g., in acute or chronic tubulointerstitial diseases). Proteinuria generally does not exceed 1–2 g/day.
 D. Glomerular proteinuria: The glomerulopathy results in loss of large molecular weight proteins such as immunoglobulins and albumin. This results in protein excretion usually exceeding 3.5 g/day.

Nephrotic Syndrome
 I. Definition (See Table 89-1)

Table 89-1. Idiopathic Nephrotic Syndrome

Disease	Adults	Children
Minimal change disease	15%	75%
Focal segmental glomerulosclerosis and hyalinosis	15%	10%
Membranous nephropathy	50%	<5%
Membranoproliferative glomerulonephritis	15%	10%
Other	5%	<5%

A. Proteinuria greater than or equal to 3.5 g/24 hr.
B. Hypoalbuminemia.
C. Edema.
D. Hypercholesterolemia.
E. Lipiduria.

Minimal Change Disease

I. **Etiology**
  A. T-cell mediated disorder
II. **Clinical Presentation** (See Table 89-2)
  A. Idiopathic
  B. Secondary causes
    1. Hodgkin's disease.
    2. Drugs
      a. Nonsteroidal anti-inflammatory agents (usually associated with acute interstitial nephritis).
      b. Lithium carbonate.
III. **Histology**
  A. Light microscopy: Normal-appearing glomeruli.
  B. Immunofluorescence: Negative.
  C. Electron microscopy: Epithelial foot process fusion.
IV. **Clinical Course**
  A. Rarely leads to end-stage renal disease.
  B. Primary complications are those associated with the nephrotic syndrome (edema, pleural/pericardial effusions and ascites, hypercoaguability secondary to loss of antithrombin III, and infections as a result of loss of immunoglobulins and complement).

V.
  Therapy
  Extremely responsive to prednisone therapy, with complete remissions achieved in less than 12 weeks.

Focal Segmental Glomerulosclerosis and Hyalinosis (FSGS)

I. **Etiology**
  A. Idiopathic
  B. Secondary causes
    1. Human immunodeficiency virus (HIV) nephropathy.
    2. Heroin nephropathy.
    3. Reflux nephropathy.
II. **Clinical Presentation** (See Table 89-2)
III. **Histology**
  A. Light microscopy: Some glomeruli appear normal; however, characteristically, other glomeruli have segmental areas of scarring with hyalinosis. The segmental scars may at first be apparent only at the corticomedullary junction.
  B. Immunofluorescence: Generally negative, but granular deposits of IgM and complement may be seen in the mesangium.
  C. Electron microscopy: Epithelial foot process fusion and segmental scarring may be seen as well.
IV. **Clinical Course**
  A. In 10–20% of cases, disease may spontaneously remit.

Table 89-2. Presenting Characteristics

Disease	Hypertension	SCr ≥1.3 mg/dl	Microscopic Hematuria	Depressed Complement	Steroid Responsive
Minimal change disease	no	no	no	no	**yes**
FSGS	**yes**	**yes**	**yes**	no	no
Membranous GN	no	no	no	no	no
MPGN	**yes**	**yes**	**yes**	**yes**	no

B. The majority of patients (60%) progress to end-stage renal disease in 5 years.

V. Therapy

Prednisone: poorly responsive to steroid therapy.

Membranous Glomerulopathy (MGN)

I. Etiology
   A. Idiopathic
   B. Secondary causes
      1. Systemic disease: Systemic lupus erythematosus (SLE), rheumatoid arthritis.
      2. Drug induced: Penicillamine and gold (especially in patients with Human Lymphocyte Antigen (HLA Dr3), captopril.
      3. Infections: Secondary syphilis, chronic hepatitis B, malaria, schistosomiasis.
      4. Neoplasia: Carcinoma of the lung, colon, stomach, breast, etc.
   C. In situ immune complex formation.

II. Clinical Presentation (See Table 89-2)

An extremely uncommon lesion in children. Therefore, one should suspect an early presentation of lupus MGN when a child presents with this lesion.

III. Histology
   A. Light microscopy: Diffuse thickening of the capillary walls. By the silver stain (Jones stain), which stains primarily the mesangium and the glomerular basement membrane, characteristic spikes are seen.
   B. Immunofluorescence: IgG and complement are seen in a characteristic granular pattern around the capillary walls. The mesangial areas should be devoid of immunofluorescent material. If the mesangium is positive by immunofluorescence for immunoglobulins, consider SLE. If immunoglobulins IgM and IgA are also present, consider SLE. In idiopathic MGN, the mesangium is generally negative for immunoglobulin deposits.
   C. Electron microscopy: Demonstrates subepithelial electron-dense deposits encircling the glomerular capillary wall. Again, the mesangium is devoid of electron-dense deposits in idiopathic membranous GN.

IV. Clinical Course
   A. From 50% to 60% of patients progress to end-stage renal disease over 10–15 years.
   B. From 10% to 20% of patients spontaneously remit over the course of 5 years.
   C. The remaining 20% of patients have persistent proteinuria with varying degrees of renal insufficiency.

V. Therapy
   A. Prednisone.
   B. Prednisone plus chlorambucil.
   C. Prednisone plus cyclophosphamide.
   D. The above therapies have all been tried, and there is great debate over their effectiveness. However, some controlled studies report impressive results for therapies (b) and (c) with respect to sustained complete remissions.

Membranoproliferative Glomerulonephritis (MPGN)

I. Etiology
   A. Idiopathic
   B. Secondary causes
      1. Infections: Shunt nephritis, chronic viral infections such as hepatitis B.
      2. Systemic diseases: SLE, mixed connective tissue disease.
      3. Miscellaneous: sickle cell disease.

II. Clinical presentation (See Table 89-2)

III. Histology
   A. Light microscopy: Demonstrates glomerular capillary wall thickening with mesangial proliferation. By the silver stain (Jones stain) the characteristic tram tracking is identified, which represents the basement being split by the interposition of the mesothelial cell cytoplasm into the glomerular basement membrane.
   B. Immunofluorescence
      1. In type I MPGN, granular deposits of IgG may be seen in the capillary walls and mesangium, as well as complement.
      2. In type II MPGN, IgM may be present but immunoglobulins may be entirely absent; however complement is invariably present in the mesangium and capillary walls.
   C. Electron microscopy
      1. In type I MPGN, subendothelial electron-dense deposits are often noted, with marked peripheral capillary interposition of mesangial cells.
      2. In type II MPGN, electron-dense deposits are seen splitting the glomerular basement membrane, hence the name *dense deposit disease*.

IV. Clinical Course
   A. Type II MPGN may be associated with partial lipodystrophy.
   B. Type II MPGN (and, less often, type I MPGN) may be associated with extremely depressed C3 levels as a result of the presence

of C3 nephritic factor (an IgG autoantibody which stabilizes the C3 convertase and allows persistent utilization of C3).
C. Spontaneous remissions are uncommon.
D. From 40% to 50% of patients progress to end-stage renal disease over 5–10 years.

V. Therapy
A. Prednisone.
B. Persantine and aspirin.
C. Treatment with either of the above agents has generally not been very successful.

Glomerulonephritis

Defining features
A. Hypertension.
B. Active urinary sediment: Microscopic hematuria/red blood cell casts.
C. Renal insufficiency.
D. Proteinuria: Usually 2–3 g/24 hr.
E. Edema, anemia, and hypoalbuminemia as a result of decreased glomerular filtration rate and sodium and fluid retention.

Poststreptococcal Glomerulonephritis

I. Etiology
A. Group A: β-hemolytic streptococci resulting from either throat or skin infection with a nephrogenic strain.
B. A latent period of 1–2 weeks before presentation, allowing antibody production in excess of antigen production to form soluble immune complexes similar to those of serum sickness.

II. Presentation:
The classic features of glomerulonephritis previously described.

III. Serologic Findings
A. Elevation in antibody titers to streptococcal enzymes (antistreptolysin O, DNAse B, and hyaluronidase).
B. A decrease in C3 levels.

IV. Histology
A. Light microscopy: Diffuse proliferative and exudative glomerulonephritis.
B. Immunofluorescence: granular deposits of IgG and C3 are noted around the capillary walls.
C. Electron microscopy: Distinct electron-dense deposits are seen in the subepithelial region of the capillary wall and are classically referred to as "humps."

V. Clinical Course
Over 90% of patients have a spontaneous remission over the course of several weeks. Approximately 5% of patients may go on to develop a rapidly progressive glomerulonephritis. This is more common in adults than in children.
A. C3 levels return to normal within 8–16 weeks as do antibody titers.
B. Urinary sediment may be active for several months after clinical resolution.

VI. Therapy
A. Antibiotics do not prevent glomerulonephritis and do not alter the course once glomerulonephritis has become evident.
B. Palliative therapy is the primary goal until renal function returns to normal (diuretics, salt and water restriction).

IGA Nephropathy (Berger's disease)

I. Definition
A. IgA nephropathy is a primary glomerulopathy without systemic symptoms.
B. Henoch-Schönlein purpura is associated with a renal biopsy picture similar to that of IgA nephropathy.
C. The clinical spectrum is felt to be a systemic form of the disease associated with abdominal pain, purpuric lesions, and arthralgias.

II. Pathogenesis
Increase in circulating IgA immune complexes secondary to overproduction and/or decreased removal by the reticuloendothelial system.

III. Clinical Presentation
A. Common in young adults (80% of patients are between the ages of 16 and 35 years).
B. Upper respiratory tract infections may precede the disease by a few days.
C. Recurring episodes of gross hematuria.
D. Proteinuria usually less than 1 g/24 hr.
E. Renal function usually normal.

IV. Serologic Findings
A. Serum IgA levels elevated in 50% of cases.
B. Polymeric IgA primarily.
C. Complement levels are usually normal.

V. Histology
A. Light microscopy: Mesangial expansion and increased mesangial cellularity (may take on a segmental flavor). However, almost any renal lesion can be seen. Rarely, crescentic glomerulonephritis has been described.
B. Immunofluorescence: The lesion is defined by IgA as the sole or primary immunoglobulin localized in the mesangium.

C. Electron microscopy: Electron-dense deposits noted in the mesangium.

VI. Clinical Course

Generally benign. Only 20–30% of patients develop progressive renal insufficiency over the course of 20 years or more.

VII. Therapy

Supportive. Prednisone and cytotoxic agents have not been proven to be of any significant benefit.

Crescentic Glomerulonephritis

I. Definition

A pathologic term defining 50% or more of the glomeruli involved with cellular crescents.

Rapidly Progressive Glomerular Nephritis (RPGN)

I. Definition

The clinical term used to describe acute deterioration in renal function over 2–6 weeks secondary to glomerulonephritis. Since crescentic glomerulonephritis is generally seen with the clinical picture of RPGN, the terms are often used synonymously.

Immunopathologic Classification of Crescentic/Necrotizing Glomerulonephritis

I. Anti-GBM Nephritis (linear immune deposits): 20%.

A. Goodpasture's syndrome (if pulmonary hemorrhage is present).

B. Nephritis without pulmonary hemorrhage.

1. Circulating antibodies to the GBM are present. Antibody titers do not correlate with the severity of disease, but with reduction in disease activity the titers decline. Antibody titers can be measured directly and quantitatively or by an indirect assay.

2. Pulmonary hemorrhage: Usually associated with a previous history of smoking or viral pulmonary infections.

3. Clinical course: Untreated over 90% of patients progressed to end-stage renal disease. Pulmonary hemorrhage, if present, can lead to a fulminate respiratory death.

4. Therapy

a. Prednisone, cytoxan, and plasmapheresis.

b. Renal outcome is dependent upon the initial severity of disease involvement.

Patients with more than 50% crescents, or a serum creatinine level above 5 mg/dL and/or anuria have a poor prognosis.

II. Immune-Complex Nephritis (granular immune deposits): 40%

A. Systemic diseases: SLE, Henoch-Schönlein purpura, mixed essential cryoglobulinemia.

B. Postinfectious glomerulonephritis: Poststreptococcal GN.

1. Therapy: High-dose steroids, with or without cytoxan.

III. Pauci Immune Nephritis (no immune derposits): 40%

A. Idiopathic RPGN.

B. Systemic vasculitis.

1. Wegener's granulomatosis.

2. Polyarteritis nodosa.

a. Antineurophilic cytoplasmic antibodies (ANCA): Associated with Wegener's granulomatosis (cytoplasmic) and polyarteritis nodosa (perinuclear).

b. ANCA titer: Correlates with disease activity and declines as the patient goes into remission.

c. Therapy

(1) Pulse steroids.

(2) Steroids plus cyclophosphamide.

IV. Pulmonary-Renal Syndromes

A. Goodpasture's syndrome

B. Wegeners's granulomatosis

C. Churg-Strauss syndrome (allergic granulomatosis)

D. SLE

Bibliography

Korbet SM, Schwartz MM, Lewis EJ: Minimal change disease of adulthood. *Am J Nephrol* 8:291–297, 1988.

Korbet SM, Schwartz MM, Lewis EJ: The prognosis of focal segmental glomerular sclerosis of adulthood. *Medicine* 65:304–311, 1986.

Salant DJ: Immunopathogenesis of crescentic glomerulonephritis and lung purpura. Kidney Int 32:408–425, 1987.

Schena FP, Cameron JS: Treatment of proteinuric idiopathic glomerulonephritides in adults: A retrospective survey. Am J Med 85:315–326, 1988.

Schwartz MM, Korbet SM: Crescentic glomerulonephritis, in *Progress in Genitourinary Pathology*, Damjanov I, editor, Field and Wood Medical Publishers, Inc., 1989; pp 163–195.

Schriwer RW (Ed): Renal and Electrolyte Disorders, 3rd edition. Boston, Little, Brown, 1986.

Warren GU, Korbet SM, Schwartz MM, Lewis EJ: Minimal change glomerulopathy associated with nonsteroidal anti-inflammatory drugs. *Am J Kidney Dis* 13:127–130, 1989.

CHAPTER 90

Renal Disorders Associated with Systemic Diseases

Stephen M. Korbet, M.D.

Non-inflammatory Renal Disorders

Diabetic Nephropathy

I. **Incidence**
    This may occur in up to 50% of the patients having diabetes of 10–20 years' duration. It accounts for 25–40% of all patients on chronic dialysis.

II. **Pathology**
    The kidneys may be normal or larger than normal even in patients with end-stage renal disease.
    A. Diffuse glomerulosclerosis: This is characterized by expansion of the mesangium and glomerular basement membrane thickening. It is common in diabetics and is the major cause of proteinuria and renal failure but is not diagnostic of diabetes mellitus.
    B. Nodular glomerulosclerosis: Characterized by a cellular nodular expansion of the mesangium and classically referred to as the *Kimmelstiel-Wilson lesion*. This is seen in up to 50% of biopsy specimens. It is diagnostic of diabetes mellitus.
    C. Papillary necrosis: May lead to flank pain and hematuria resembling nephrolithiasis.

D. Neurogenic bladder: May lead to obstructive uropathy, incontinence, and/or recurrent pyelonephritis.

III. **Pathogenesis of Diabetic Glomerulosclerosis**
    A. May be a result of insulin deficiency, hyperglycemia, or glucose intolerance, all of which may lead to increased glycosylation of proteins.
    B. May be due to some genetic factor independent of hyperglycemia and insulin deficiency.

IV. **Clinical Features**
    Patients generally do not develop diabetic nephropathy until after 10–20 years of diabetes. Diabetic retinopathy is usually present at the time nephropathy becomes apparent. The urinary sediment in diabetic nephropathy is unremarkable for red blood cells or red blood cell casts. If a diabetic patient has an atypical presentation for diabetic nephropathy, other primary glomerulopathies should be considered and a renal biopsy entertained. In general, patients with a classic presentation for diabetes mellitus do not require a renal biopsy, as this generally adds nothing to the overall care.
    A. Increased glomerular filtration rate (GFR): Early in the course of diabetes, patients have a

super normal GFR. The mechanism for this is unknown but is thought to be multifactorial (i.e., due to elevated growth hormone levels, increased filtration pressure, and possibly increased permeability of the glomerular basement membrane).

B. Increased microalbuminuria may precede clinical evidence of proteinuria and is felt to be predictive of the eventual development of diabetic nephropathy. Clinical evidence of proteinuria is the hallmark of diabetic nephropathy and is generally associated with hypertension. Up to 70% of patients will ultimately develop the nephrotic syndrome (24-hr urine protein >3 g). This is usually associated with renal insufficiency as well.

C. Renal failure: Once proteinuria is evident, the majority of patients progress to end-stage renal disease over 3–5 years. Hypertension is common in diabetics with renal insufficiency. Hypertension may exacerbate the progression to end-stage renal disease; therefore, good blood pressure control is mandatory. Due to the potential precipitation of renal failure, intravenous contrast media should be avoided in patients with diabetic nephropathy and renal insufficiency.

V. **Treatment**

A. Careful control of hyperglycemia.

B. Control of hypertension.

C. Angiotensin-converting enzyme inhibitors: There is preliminary evidence that these may have a renal protective effect related to treatment of glomerular hypertension over and above the effects on systemic hypertension.

D. Diuretics: Along with salt and water restriction, may be beneficial not only in controlling blood pressure but also in treating the symptoms of the nephrotic syndrome.

E. Insulin requirements: These may decrease with progressive renal failure, as there is diminished renal inactivation of insulin.

F. Maintenance dialysis: This is recommended when the serum creatinine reaches 8 mg/dl because of the increased morbidity and mortality of diabetics compared to nondiabetics, which may be exacerbated by uremia.

G. Transplantation: Diabetics who are felt to be candidates for transplantation should undergo this surgery, as it is felt that their course with the renal transplant is substantially better than that of chronic dialysis. Diabetic nephropathy can recur in the transplanted kidney; this has been reported within 5 years after transplantation. However, this rarely leads to end-stage renal disease in the transplant.

Amyloidosis

I. **Definition**

A systemic infiltrative disease characterized by an eosinophilic extracellular protein that generally has a fibrillar ultrastructural appearance and a highly organized, β-pleated sheet pattern by x-ray diffraction. Amyloid is histochemically defined by the green birefringence noted on polarization microscopy after staining of the tissue with Congo red. Amyloidosis can also be classified by its biochemical composition (Table 90-1).

II. **Pathology**

As previously noted, the diagnosis is made by the characteristic staining properties of Congo red.

A. Renal amyloidosis: The glomerulus is primarily affected and may demonstrate marked expansion of the mesangium, with an occasional nodular appearance and pronounced thickening of the capillary wall due to infiltration of amyloid into the glomerular basement membrane. Ultrastructurally, nonbranching fibrils 10 nm in diameter can be seen in the mesangium, as well as in the glomerular basement membrane.

Table 90-1. Classification of Amyloidosis

New Classification	Common Name	Protein Composition
AL	Primary amyloid Myeloma-associated amyloid	Light chains
AA	Secondary amyloid, familial Mediterranean fever	Amyloid A protein
AF	Familial amyloid	Transthyretin (prealbumin)
SSA	Senile cardiac amyloid	Transthyretin (prealbumin)
$A\beta_2 M$	Dialysis amyloid	β_2-Microglobulin
AE	Medullary thyroid cancer	Calcitonin

B. Renal involvement also consists of interstitial, peritubular, and vascular deposits.

C. Infiltration of amyloid is commonly found in the liver, heart, skin, and gastrointestinal tract, as well as in peripheral nerves.

III. Clinical Features

A. Renal amyloidosis: Generally presents with proteinuria evolving to the nephrotic syndrome (75% of patients) and leads to renal insufficiency. Microscopic hematuria is occasionally seen. Although patients with amyloidosis generally have hypotension, hypertension can be found in 20–50% of patients, especially with advanced renal failure. The kidneys may be normal or enlarged even in patients with advanced renal insufficiency. Once proteinuria develops, the majority of patients progress to end-stage renal disease. The mean survival of patients with renal amyloidosis is approximately 20–30 months.

B. Extrarenal amyloidosis: Liver failure leading to cirrhosis and portal hypertension may occur; cardiac manifestations include congestive heart failure, cardiomegaly, and arrhythmias; gastrointestinal features include malabsorption, and neurologic involvement may result in peripheral as well as autonomic neuropathy (postural hypertension). The overall prognosis of patients with amyloidosis is strongly dependent upon the cardiac status. Those with congestive heart failure have a 1-year survival of only 30%.

IV. Treatment of Renal Amyloidosis

A. Other than familial Mediterranean fever, which is responsive to colchicine, there is no specific therapy for the other forms of amyloidosis.

B. Symptomatic therapy may be given for the nephrotic syndrome and chronic renal failure, but ultimately chronic dialysis is required.

C. Renal transplantation: Previously, patients with systemic amyloidosis were felt to be poor candidates for renal transplantation. Recent information indicates that patients with primary or secondary amyloidosis may have favorable outcomes after renal transplantation and therefore should be considered as candidates.

Gammopathies

I. Multiple Myeloma

There are several ways in which multiple myeloma affects renal function and structure (Table 90-2). The evaluation and diagnosis of multiple myeloma is described in Chapter 72D.

A. Bence Jones (light chain) proteinuria: Light chains are low molecular weight proteins which are easily filtered by the glomerulus. When these are made in large quantities, such as in multiple myeloma, overflow proteinuria may occur. This is not a result of glomerular or tubular dysfunction but a reflection of the fact that Bence Jones proteins (molecular weight 22,000) are freely filtered. This can lead to massive levels of proteinuria (greater than 10 g/day). It can be differentiated from the nephrotic syndrome by the fact that patients are not hypoalbuminemic. These proteins may be toxic to the kidney and can cause renal failure.

B. Myeloma kidney: Precipitation of proteinaceous casts within the renal tubules leading to intrarenal obstruction and associated with a giant cell reaction around the tubules. This commonly leads to renal failure. The casts have been shown to demonstrate IgG and kappa or lambda light chains. Treatment of the underlying multiple myeloma, as well as acute dialysis and occasionally plasmapheresis, may have therapeutic benefit for the acute renal failure by decreasing the production and serum concentration of the nephrotoxic paraprotein.

C. Nephrotic syndrome: May be a result of renal amyloidosis or light chain deposition disease (LCDD). Clinically, these two entities are indistinguishable. They may be differentiated only by renal biopsy. There is therapeutic importance in making a distinction, as patients with LCDD may have stabilization or improvement in their renal function with treatment of the multiple myeloma, whereas those with amyloidosis usually show no improvement in renal status with treatment.

Table 90-2. Renal Involvement in Multiple Myeloma

Glomerular lesions
  Amyloidosis
  Light chain deposition disease (LCDD)
Tubulointerstitial lesions
Myeloma kidney
Uric acid nephropathy
Hypercalcemic nephropathy
Pyelonephritis

D. Pyelonephritis.

E. Acute uric acid nephropathy: Hyperuricemia occurs as a result of purine release after treatment of multiple myeloma. This can lead to extremely high levels of uric acid, which results in precipitation within the kidney and leads to acute renal failure. This may be prevented by the use of allopurinol prior to therapy, as well as by adequate hydration of patients. Acute dialysis may be required in an attempt to reduce extremely high levels of uric acid and prevent acute renal failure.

F. Hypercalcemic nephropathy: Hypercalcemia secondary to multiple myeloma may lead to salt wasting and polyuria, which can result in volume depletion and may exacerbate underlying renal insufficiency.

G. Renal tubular dysfunction: Light chains have been shown to be toxic to renal tubular function and may result in Fanconi syndrome, distal tubular acidoss, and nephrogenic diabetes insipidus.

II. **Light Chain Deposition Disease (LCDD)**
Approximately 70% of patient with LCDD have multiple myeloma. In the remaining patients, myeloma is not present.

A. Essentially all patients with LCDD have evidence of free light chains in either the serum, the urine, or both when evaluated by immunoelectrophoresis.

B. This systemic disorder has been associated with deposits not only in the kidney but also involving the heart, liver, and nervous system. Similar to amyloidosis, it can lead to renal, cardiac, and liver failure, as well as peripheral neuropathies.

C. Renal pathology: The lesion associated with LCDD is a nodular glomerulosclerosis which resembles diabetic nephropathy. The diagnosis of LCDD, however, is made on immunofluorescence where a monoclonal light chain (either kappa or lambda) is deposited along the tubular basement membranes, as well as the glomerular basement membrane and mesangium. Ultrastructurally, fibrils may be seen in the expanded mesangium or glomerular basement membrane.

D. Clinically, the patient presents with massive light chain proteinuria but will also have evidence of the nephrotic syndrome with hypoalbuminemia. Progression to renal failure is common.

E. Treatment: Alkylating agents and prednisone may arrest or improve the renal disease in patients with LCDD. Therapy is most beneficial in patients whose serum creatinine is <5 mg/dl.

Immunotactoid (Fibrillary) Glomerulopathy (ITG)

I. **Definition**
Primary glomerulopathy with highly organized electron dense deposits in the form of microtubules/microfibrils. Diagnosis is made by excluding other diseases with similar ultrastructural appearance such as amyloidosis, cryoglobulinemia, light chain depositor disease, lupus nephritis and para proteinemias.

II. **Pathology**
This lesion is characterized histologically by highly organized ultrastructural deposits which appear to be composed of immunoglobulin and complement and are negative for amyloid when examined by Congo red stain. The deposits almost always involve the mesangium and usually the capillary walls. The tactoid/fibrils may range in diameter from 10 to 50 nm. They are relatively homogeneous in diameter and in most cases are around 20 nm. All current reports find IgG and complement in the glomeruli, with IgM and IgA present in approximately one-half of the cases. ITG does not appear to be a multisystemic disease process. Unlike amyloidosis and LCDD, involvement of other major organs is not found. ITG therefore represents a primary glomerulopathy.

III. **Pathogenesis**
Recent studies utilizing immunoelectron microscopy confirm the immunoglobulin composition of the tactoids/fibrils. It is not known, however, if the tactoids/fibrils represent organized immune complexes or monoclonal immunoglobulins.

IV. **Laboratory Evaluation**
Serologically, patients should be carefully screened for evidence of cryoglobulinemia, amyloidosis, systemic lupus erythematosus, or a paraproteinemia, disorders associated with glomerular deposits which also have a highly organized tactoidal or fibrillar characteristic.

V. **Clinical Features**
Patients with immunotactoid glomerulopathy present with proteinuria which is in the nephrotic range in over 60% of cases. Males are affected slightly more often than females (61% vs. 39%). Hypertension is a presenting feature in 66% of patients, and hematuria is reported in 78% of cases. Renal insufficiency is frequently a presenting feature in 47% of patients. Over an average course of follow-up of 4 years, 45% of patients

Table 90-3. Lupus Nephritis: Pathologic Features

Lesion	Mesangial	Focal Proliferative	Diffuse Proliferative	Membranous
Incidence	10%	20%	40–60%	10%
Light microscopy	Mild mesangial proliferation	Focal segmental proliferation ± necrosis	Diffuse endo-capillary pro-liferation with necrosis	Mesangial expansion with diffuse thickening of capillary walls
Immuno-fluorescence	Diffuse mesangial deposits of Ig* and complement	Diffuse mesangial and some capillary wall deposits of Ig and complement	Diffuse mesangial and capillary wall deposits of Ig and complement	Heavy staining for Ig and complement along capillary walls and mesangium
Electron microscopy	Mesangial deposits only	Mesangial, with some sub-endothelial and subepithelial deposits	Large, diffuse, mesangial, sub-endothelia, and subepithelial deposits	Mesangial and diffuse sub-epithelial deposits

*Ig = immunoglobulins (primarily IgG but also IgM and IgA)

reported to date have progressed to end-stage renal disease.

VI. Treatment

The experience in treating this disorder using prednisone and/or immunosuppression is quite limited and has not been impressive. Four patients have successfully undergone renal transplantation, but proteinuria recurred in two of them at 21 and 60 months, respectively, and was associated with the recurrence of immunotactoid glomerulopathy in the renal allograft.

Inflammatory Renal Disorders

Lupus nephritis

I. Definition

Auto-immune disease. Defined by specific criteria outlined by the American College of Rheumatology.

II. Incidence

The frequency of renal disease in patients with systemic lupus erythematosus (SLE) is approximately 60%. Lupus nephritis can be one of the most severe complications in patients with SLE, leading to end-stage renal disease.

III. Pathologic Classification and Features (see Table 90-3)

IV. Clinical Features at Presentation (see Table 90-4)

V. Treatment and Course

A. Mesangial lupus nephritis: This lesion has an extremely good prognosis and rarely if ever progresses to end-stage renal disease. As a result, treatment is usually dictated by the extrarenal manifestations and usually consists of low-dose glucocorticoid therapy. The 5-year renal survival is 100%.

B. Focal proliferative glomerulonephritis: With the use of moderate-dose glucocorticoid therapy, a reduction or complete remission in

Table 90-4. Lupus Nephritis: Clinical Features at Presentation

Lesion	Mesangial	Focal Proliferative	Diffuse Proliferative	Membranous
Hypertension	—	±	+	—
Renal insufficiency	—	±	+	—
Proteinuria	1+	2–3+	3+	4+
Active urinary sediment	±	+	+	—
Hypocomplementemia	—	+	+	±

+ = present.
— = not present.
± = occasionally present.

proteinuria occurs in over 50% of patients. Renal function usually stabilizes, and the 5-year renal survival is excellent at 90%.

C. Diffuse proliferative glomerulonephritis: Due to the severe nature of this lesion, high-dose glucocorticoid therapy is initiated cytotoxic agents such as cyclophosphamide are often utilized as well. Remission can be induced in approximately one-half of those patients with mild renal insufficiency at presentation (serum creatinine ≤ 2 mg/dl). The 5-year renal survival is 50%.

D. Membranous lupus nephritis: Remission of the nephrotic syndrome or a significant reduction in proteinuria can be achieved in approximately 30% of patients with the use of high-dose prednisone for 2 months. Due to the slowly progressive loss of renal function in those patients who remain nephrotic, the 5-year renal survival is 90%.

E. Response to therapy in patients with lupus nephritis is evaluated based on improvement in serologic parameters (normalization of serum complement levels and reduction in antinuclear antibody levels), urinary sediment (there should be no microscopic hematuria or red blood cell casts), proteinuria (the proteinuria may or may not completely resolve), and stabilization or improvement in serum creatinine levels.

F. It should be noted that patients with milder degrees of lupus nephritis may progress to more severe forms of lupus nephritis which may require a second renal biopsy for documentation, as this will change the patient's prognosis and require a reevaluation of the therapy to be utilized.

Polyarteritis Nodosa (PAN)

I. **Definition**
Two major types of PAN are described: (1) Classic PAN involves large arteries, and (2) microscopic PAN involves smaller arteries and is occasionally termed *hypersensitivity angiitis*.

II. **Clinical Features**
A. Renal involvement with classic PAN may consist of renal artery aneurysms, thrombosis, and renal infarctions, with hypertension, hematuria, and flank pain being the presenting features.

B. In microscopic PAN, focal segmental necro-

tizing glomerulonephritis is the predominant feature. Patients present with proteinuria, microscopic hematuria, and renal insufficiency. Middle-aged men appear to be more frequently affected than women and usually present with fatigue, low-grade fever, muscle aches, and weight loss. Purpuric skin lesions are occasionally found involving the lower extremities.

III. **Renal Pathology**
A focal and segmental, necrotizing, and proliferative glomerulonephritis, with or without necrotizing lesions of small arteries, is seen. This is a pauci immune form of glomerulonephritis; therefore, the immunofluorescence is generally unremarkable or negative, except that fibrin may be found in the segmental areas of inflammation. No unusual or characteristic features are noted by electron microscopy.

IV. **Laboratory Findings**
The erythrocyte sedimentation rate is elevated, antineutrophilic cytoplasmic antibodies (ANCA) are elevated, and characteristically the cytoplasmic-ANCA (antibody to proteinase 3) is elevated in patients with PAN. The ANCA level is useful in following disease activity and the response to therapy. Hepatitis B surface antigen may be positive in some patients. Cryoglobulin levels, rheumatoid factor, and serum immunoglobulin levels may be elevated in some patients. Complement levels may occasionally be low but are usually normal.

V. **Therapy**
Pulse intravenous glucocorticoid therapy given daily three to five times over the course of a week, followed by daily high-dose prednisone. In addition, cyclophosphamide is utilized for up to 6 months or more, depending upon the response and the course of the disease. Following renal function and urinary sediment are helpful as indicators of the response to treatment. However, following the sedimentation rate and ANCA is generally the method of disease activity and response to therapy serologically.

Wegener's Granulomatosis

I. **Definition**
A multisystemic disease classically involving the upper airway, ear, nose, lung, and kidney. Histologically it is characterized by a necrotizing granulomatous vasculitis. The kidney may be involved

in up to 50% of cases. Death may result from renal failure, sepsis, and/or pulmonary hemorrhage.

II. Renal Pathology

A focal and segmental necrotizing, proliferative glomerulonephritis is seen. The glomerular pathology is similar to that described in PAN. This also represents a pauci immune form of glomerulonephritis.

III. Laboratory Features

Elevated erythrocyte sedimentation rate and an elevated ANCA (more specifically, a peripheral ANCA which represents antibodies to myeloperoxidase). Patients generally have renal insufficiency, with an active urinary sediment (microscopic hematuria and red blood cell casts) and proteinuria which is rarely in the nephrotic range. X-rays of the lungs may demonstrate segmental pulmonic infiltrates with consolidation and cavitation.

IV. Therapy

High-dose glucocorticoids in combination with cyclophosphamide are utilized. The response to therapy can be followed in a fashion similar to that described for PAN, with evidence of remission based on a reduction in the erythrocyte sedimentation rate and ANCA levels, as well as improvement or stabilization in parameters of renal function. With the use of immunosuppressive treatment, survival at 1 year has risen to ≥80%.

Mixed "Essential" Cryoglobulinemia

I. Definition

Cryoglobulins are proteins which precipitate upon cooling and become soluble upon warming (Table 90-5).

II. Renal Pathology

Diffuse proliferative glomerulonephritis is seen. Immunofluorescence demonstrates granular deposits of immunoglobulin and complement involving the capillary wall and mesangium. Electron microscopy is most remarkable for large subendothelial or intracapillary deposits which, on close observation, have an organized ultrastructural appearance which is unusually fibrillary or tubular in nature.

III. Clinical Features

All patients present with recurrent palpable purpura, usually involving the lower extremities. Seventy percent have polyarthralgias, and renal disease is present in up to 55% of patients. Most patients with renal disease present with significant proteinuria (23% having the nephrotic syndrome). Hypertension and renal insufficiency are seen in 45% of patients.

IV. Laboratory Features

Classically, patients with mixed essential cryoglobulinemia have type II or III cryoglobulins (Table 90-5). Hypocomplementemia is frequently seen as well. Hepatitis B surface antigen, antibody, or both may be found in the serum or cryoglobulin in up to 60% of patients.

V. Treatment and Clinical Course

Steroids and cyclophosphamide are generally initiated to stop the production of the abnormal immunoglobulin, and plasmapheresis (usually 12 treatments are given over 4 weeks) is instituted to increase removal of the cryoglobulin from the serum. In most patient the renal disease is slowly progressive, leading to renal failure over a period of months to years.

Table 90-5. Classification of Cryoglobulins

Type	Immunoglobulin Class	Serum Level (mg/ml)	Associated Disease
Type I, Monoclonal	IgM > IgG	>1 (80% of cases)	Multiple myeloma, Waldenström's macroglobulinemia
Type II, mixed monoclonal-polyclonal (with rheumatoid factor)	IgM-IgG ≫ IgG-IgG	>1 (80% of cases)	Mutiple myeloma, autoimmune disease, mixed essential cryoglobulins
Type III, mixed polyclonal	IgM-IgG ≫ IgM-IgG-IgA	<1 (80% of cases)	Autoimmune disease, mixed essential cryoglubulins

Bibliography

Korbet SM, Lewis EJ: Cryoimmunoglobulinemia. In: Glassock RS, (ed). Current Therapy in Nephrology and Hypertension-2, BC Decker, Inc., Philadelphia, Pa., 1987, pp 142–144.

Korbet SM, Lewis EJ: Glomerulonephritis and the nephrotic syndrome. In: Gonick HC, (ed). Current Nephrology Volume 9, Year Book Medical Publishers, Chicago, Il., 1986, pp 209–247.

Korbet SM, Schwartz MM, Lewis EJ: Immunotactoid glomerulopathy. (review) *Am J Kidney Dis* 17:247–257, 1991.

SECTION 11

Rheumatology

Chapter 91

Approach to the Patient with Rheumatic Disease

Calvin R. Brown, M.D.

I. **General Approach to Patient with Rheumatic Disease**
   A. Rheumatic diseases are variable in expression and involve multiple organ systems. Their pathogenesis is often unknown.
   B. Categories of rheumatic diseases.
      1. Synovitis: Inflammation of the synovial membrane in the joint, with resultant damage to surrounding structures. Management is based on reduction of inflammation. Prototypic disease is rheumatoid arthritis.
      2. Enthesopathy: Inflammation where ligaments attach to bone, the enthesis. There is a predilection for involvement of the spine. Management is also based on reduction of inflammation. Prototypic disease is ankylosing spondylitis.
      3. Cartilage degeneration: Mechanical, genetic, and biochemical factors lead to failure of integrity of cartilage. Management is based on reduction of pain, mechanical relief, or joint replacement. Prototypic disease is osteoarthritis.
      4. Crystal-induced synovitis: Formation of microcrystals of inorganic material induce inflammation in joint fluid and synovium. Management is based on reduction of body levels of the precipitating substance and/or reduction of inflammation. Prototypic disease is gout.
      5. Septic arthritis: Infection occurs within closed joint space. Treatment is based on drainage and specific antibiotics.
      6. Systemic autoimmune diseases: Characterized by reaction of the immune system to multiple self tissues such as vessel walls, muscle, glomerulus, and so on. Managed by immunosuppression. There is no one prototypic disease; systemic lupus erythematosus, myositis, and vasculitis are examples.
      7. Generalized conditions: Heterogeneous group of conditions characterized by pain, often diffuse, without objective detectable abnormalities. The pathophysiology is poorly understood. There may be neurologic or psychologic manifestations similar to those of other "functional" diseases. Treatment is aimed at provided symptomatic relief; progressive degeneration does not occur. *Fibromyalgia* and *myofascial pain syndrome* are used to describe variants of these conditions.

II. **Approach to the Patient with Arthritis**
   A. History
      1. Determine that the joint itself is involved.

Table 91-1. Differential Diagnosis of Monoarthritis

Inflammatory
Gout
Calcium pyrophosphate deposition disease (pseudogout)
Septic arthritis
Calcium hydroxyapatite deposition disease

Noninflammatory
Osteoarthritis
Mechanical derangement of joint
Traumatic arthritis
Neuropathic arthropathy (Charcot's arthropathy)
Avascular necrosis of bone
Arthritis with bleeding disorders
Osteochondritis dissecans
Loose joint body
Pigmented villonodular synovitis
Juxta-articular bone tumors
Osteochondromatosis

Table 91-2. Differential Diagnosis of Polyarthritis

Inflammatory
Rheumatoid arthritis
Psoriatic arthritis
Reiter's syndrome
Ankylosing spondylitis
Connective tissue diseases (lupus, scleroderma, myositis)
Polymyalgia rheumatica
Rheumatic fever
Gout, pseudogout (usually monoarticular)

Noninflammatory
Generalized osteoarthritis

Pain occurs in the joint area itself and may also be referred to surrounding structures.
2. Determine the number of joint areas affected.
   a. One joint = monoarticular arthritis.
   b. More than four joints = polyarticular arthritis.
   c. Two to four joints = oligoarticular arthritis, often considered as or evolving into polyarticular arthritis.
3. Determine the sequence of involvement.
   a. Additive: Starts with involvement of one or few joints; over time, the number of joints continuously involved increases. Polyarthritis frequently begins in this fashion.
   b. Migratory: Involvement shifts from joint to joint; only one or a few joints are involved at one time. Usually evolves into monoarticular disease.
4. Determine the acuity of the condition.
   a. Acute: Onset rapid (over hours to days); becomes dramatic or catastrophic if not resolved in less than 6 weeks.
   b. Chronic: Onset is insidious; patient may not be able to recall when symptoms began. May progress for many weeks before medical help is sought.
5. Determine if symptoms of inflammation are present.
   a. Stiffness that worsens with rest or inactivity.
   b. Fever and fatigue are frequent systemic signs of inflammation.

   c. Swelling can be misleading since it is seen in both inflammatory and noninflammatory conditions; see Section II, B.
B. Physical exam
   1. Presence of any constitutional symptoms (fever, weight loss, weakness) indicates that inflammation is present.
   2. Range of motion of joint: limitation of motion confirms joint involvement; occurs in most types of advanced arthritidies.
   3. Presence or absence of inflammation: Warmth and soft tissue swelling indicate inflammatory arthritis. Fluid within joint space (effusion) and tenderness are nonspecific.
III. **Differential Diagnosis**
   Based on the history and physical exam.
   A. Determine the category of arthritis based on the following classification (Tables 91-1 and 91-2).
      1. Monoarthritis versus polyarthritis.
      2. Acute versus chronic arthritis.
      3. Inflammatory versus noninflammatory arthritis.
   B. Additional diagnostic methods are useful to define the diagnosis further within these categories.

Bibliography

Gall EP. Evaluation of the Patient. History and Physical Exam. In: Primer of the Rheumatic Diseases ed 10. Schumacher HR Jr, (ed) Arthritis Foundation. Atlanta, 1993, pp 60–64.

Michette CJ, Hunder GG. Examination of the Joints. In: Textbook of Rheumatology ed 4. Kelley WN, Harris ED Jr., Ruddy S (eds.) W.B. Saunders, Philadelphia, 1993, pp 351–367.

Diagnostic Methods

Evan M. Barton, M.D.
John R. Charter, M.D.

Radiology of the Rheumatic Diseases

I. Introduction

Standard radiography and other imaging techniques are a necessary adjunct to the history and physical examination of the patient with rheumatic complaints. Standard x-ray films have long been the first resource in this regard and can be used both to assist in making and to confirm a diagnosis. More important, they may often be used serially to document changes in bone or joint structures as the disease progress. Hence the initial radiologic examination of a patient suspected of having a rheumatologic disease will differ from that of a patient with an established diagnosis.

A. In the first instance, a survey of selected areas which have a high likelihood of producing positive (or negative) findings should be undertaken.

B. In the second instance, areas known to be affected by the disease process should be examined to support the clinical impression of stable or advancing disease.

C. In addition to standard radiography, this section will include brief discussions of computed tomography, magnetic resonance imaging (MRI), ultrasound, and arthrography.

D. Radioisotopic assessment of joints is a highly sensitive but less specific method of examination. Its greatest strength is in discovering areas which are somewhat remote from the site of clinical concern. It will be discussed in Chapter 92C.

II. Standard Radiography

When a patient is initially being evaluated for a suspected rheumatic disease, the following radiographic studies should be considered.

A. Both hands/wrists: Posterior-anterior, oblique (Norgaard, "ball-catching") and lateral views: The hand and wrist can be considered a single unit and placed on one film. Such studies are of particular value in assessing rheumatoid arthritis.

B. Cervical spine: The examination should include the anterior-posterior view; the "open mouth" view of C_1 and C_2; both oblique views; and two lateral views, one in neutral position and one in flexion. Particular attention is paid to the area of the odontoid process; to the alignment of the vertebrae; to disc spaces; and to encroachment by bony elements into the intravertebral foramina.

C. Pelvis: A single anterior-posterior view provides valuable information on hip joints as well as sacroiliac joints.

D. Lumbar spine: This is an important first examination in patients with low back pain, particularly if one suspects a spondylarthropathy or diffuse idiopathic skeletal hyperostosis. It is of less value in patients suspected of having rheumatoid arthritis.

E. Feet: If there is moderatre to severe clinical involvement here, an examination is in order. At times, characteristic erosive disease may be found in the absence of severe symptoms. If metatarsophalangeal or interphalangeal (toe) joints are involved, the area in question should be placed in the center of the film for better definition.

F. Other joints: Early involvement of knees, elbows, shoulders, and ankles may show minimal changes that are difficult to detect radiographically. However, if clinically important, a good film at this stage provides a baseline with which further progression may be compared. Views of the thoracic spine are important in young patients to delineate scoliosis, developmental processes, or effects of childhood diseases such as juvenile rheumatoid arthritis.

III. **Computed Tomography**

This is a very helpful examination when early sacroiliac disease is suspected and conventional films are equivocal or negative. It may provide crucial information in spinal cases when there is disc or bony encroachment on the neural structures. Loose bone fragments in the hip joint, subluxation of the shoulder joint, arthritis of the sternoclavicular joints, and resolution of complicated overlying structures in the upper cervical region and base of the skull are all circumstance conditions in which computed tomography may be helpful.

IV. **Magnetic Resonance Imaging**

This examination method relies heavily on differences in tissue contrast. Because the clinician can manipulate that contrast with different pulse sequences, a very powerful imaging tool is now available. This technique has replaced arthrography as the examination of choice for knee problems. It can display a heretofore only suspected phenomenon: intraosseous trauma or the "bone bruise." This concept allows a better un-

derstanding of the causes of pain around a joint or in an extremity after trauma when all other tests are negative.

Examination of the hip with MRI is very sensitive in the detection of osteonecrosis and nondisplaced hip fractures. Pigmented villonodular synovitis can have a very specific pattern. Fluid collections around joints (synovial cysts), in tendon sheaths, or in the soft tissues of extremities are easily detected with MRI.

Examinations of the shoulder with MRI are also very sensitive in detecting soft tissue abnormalities, especially in the rotator cuff. A problem here is that, in some instances, it is both "too sensitive" and "nonspecific." Techniques used to examine the wrist are evolving. However, better resolution will be required to detect some of the intracarpal ligaments on a regular basis. The ankle and foot examinations likewise are in evolution. As with the larger joints, fluid collection, tendon ruptures and tendon sheath disease can be easily detected. Smaller details will, however, require better resolution.

Finally, clinical investigation is progressing in the area of synovitis detection. The relative contributions of synovial proliferation and fluid accumulation to swollen, painful joints can be determined with MRI. An intravenous injection of gadolinium is required. It remains to be seen if information of this sort, obtained early in the course of rheumatoid disease, for example, would be helpful in planning early treatment, particularly when aggressive treatment may be beneficial.

V. **Ultrasound**

This examination is particularly helpful in detecting such fluid collections as a Baker's Cyst, an organizing hematoma, or an abscess. It is especially helpful as a guide for the percutaneous aspiration of these "masses." Ultrasound was used extensively to evaluate the rotator cuff at the shoulder. The examination proved to be very operator dependant and its popularity is waning.

VI. **Arthrography**

This examination is virtually no longer used for examination of the knee. However, it remains a very good technique for examining the shoulder for rotator cuff tears, largely because of its high specificity. It continues to be an excellent tool for examining the wrist, especially in ulnar sided pain. Some authors advocate a "triple compartment" examination while others maintain a "single compartment"—the radiocarpal joint—examination is adequate.

VII. Suggested Radiologic Procedures

A list of suggested radiologic procedures follows. It contains the usual sources of diagnostic information in known or suspected musculoskeletal diseases. Clinicians will do well to consider the diagnostic radiologist as a consultant in the case at hand and provide pertinent clinical information along with the request for any study.

A. Rheumatoid arthritis: Hands and wrists, cervical spine with lateral view in flexion (especially preoperatively if patient will be under general anesthesia); knees, anterior-posterior and lateral views, plus weight-bearing (standing) views; ultrasound for popliteal cysts.

B. Osteoarthritis: Hands, noting especially distal and proximal interphalangeal joints; hips, knees, anterior-posterior lateral and "sunrise" views, plus weight-bearing (standing) view. Spine: Anterior-posterior lateral and oblique views.

C. Avascular necrosis: Hips, knees, shoulders; standard radiography followed by MRI as clinically indicated.

D. Spondylarthropathies (Reiter's inflammatory bowel-related conditions): Standard views of affected peripheral joints, including heels, sacroiliac joints, and lumbar spine.

E. Ankylosing spondylitis: Sacroiliac joints, entire spine; peripheral joints if affected.

F. Crystal deposition diseases (gout, chondrocalcinosis, etc.): Knees, wrist, pelvis, and feet, including toes, midfoot, and hind foot.

G. Infectious arthritis: Serial films of affected joints at intervals timed to assess progressive destruction; rule out osteomyelitis in adjoining bone.

H. Tumors: Standard radiography of the lesion; MRI for soft tissue detail; scintigraphy for distant metastatic bone lesions from any source and for myeloma.

I. Neuropathic joints (Charcot joints, diabetes): Standard radiography of the affected part.

Bibliography

Firooznia H, Cornelia G, Mahvash R, et al: MRI and CT of the Musculoskeletal System. Mosby–Yearbook, 1992.

Weissman BN (Ed) Imaging of Rheumatic Diseases. In: Rheumatic Disease Clinics of North America. 17:3, 1991.

Serology

Denise Verges, M.D.

Acute Phase Reactants

I. Definition

A group of plasma proteins which are altered in response to tissue damage—inflammatory, infections, malignant, toxic, or chemical. Erythrocyte sedimentation rate (ESR) and C-reactive protein are most commonly measured.

  A. Erythrocyte sedimentation rate

    1. A nonspecific laboratory test which measures the distance in millimeters that erythrocytes fall in 1 hr.

    2. It is dependent on the aggregation of red blood cells and the formation of rouleaux.

    3. Increases in asymmetric proteins such as fibrinogens or immunoglobulins lead to rouleaux formation and an elevated ESR.

    4. The Westergren method is most commonly used.

    5. Normal value in males is less than 16; in females, less than 25.

    6. Increased levels are found in:

      a. Malignancy

      b. Infection

      c. Collagen vascular disease (very high in polymyalgia rheumatica or temporal arthritis)

      d. Waldenström's macroglobulinemia

      e. Pregnancy

      f. Advancing age

      g. Oral contraceptive users

      h. Anemia

      i. Heparinized blood

    7. Decreased levels are found in:

      a. Polycythemia

      b. Sickle cell anemia

      c. Hereditary spherocytosis

      d. Anisocytosis and poikilocytosis

      e. Hemoglobinopathy

      f. Pyruvate kinase deficiency

      g. Hypofibrinogenemia

    8. Clinical uses

      a. May be used judiciously to follow the course of disease and the response to therapy.

      b. Has no diagnostic specificity.

      c. Should not be used as a screening or diagnostic test.

    9. Disadvantages

      a. Difficult to correct for variability in size,

shape, and concentration of erythrocytes.

   b. Indirect reflection of acute phase reactants.

   c. No well-defined normal range.

B. C-reactive protein

  1. An acute phase protein of pentameric structure, named for its ability to precipitate with pneumococcal cell wall c-polysaccharides in the presence of calcium.

  2. Synthesized by hepatocytes; rises within a few hours of an acute inflammatory stimulus and peaks at 2–3 days.

  3. Present in trace amounts in all subjects.

  4. A level of 1–10 mg/dl is considered moderately elevated; greater than 10 mg/dl is considered markedly elevated.

  5. Has clinical applications similar to those of the ESR; the major difference is the more rapid elevation in response to inflammation.

  6. Rises in pregnancy and with oral contraceptive use.

  7. Detected by radial diffusion and electroimmunodiffusion, laser nephelometry, and enzyme immunoassays.

C. Complement: A system of plasma and membrane proteins which function as part of the immune system by mediating a variety of inflammatory effects.

  1. Methods of measurement

   a. Immunoassays for individual complement proteins: C_3 is most plentiful. C_4 is most sensitive to minor degrees of activation.

   b. CH50 measures the ability of complement in test serum to lyse 50% of a standard suspension of sheep red blood cells coated with rabbit antibody.

  2. Hypocomplement states arise from:

   a. Complement deficiency states

    (1) Early classical pathway deficiency associated with a systemic lupus erythematosus (SLE)-like syndrome and an increased susceptibility to infection; C_2 deficiency is most common.

    (2) C1q inhibitor deficiency-hereditary angioedema.

    (3) C3b inactivator deficiency-recurrent pyogenic infections.

    (4) Terminal component deficiencies: recurrent neisserial infections.

   b. Immune complex deposition: SLE

    (1) Rheumatoid arthritis

    (2) Systemic vasculitis

    (3) Essential mixed

    (4) Cryoglobulinemia

   c. Chronic antigenemia resulting from infection (e.g. subacute bacterial endocarditis, gram-negative sepsis).

   d. Glomerulonephritis

   e. Hepatic failure

   f. Malnutrition

  3. Low complement levels are associated with increased activity of SLE, specifically renal disease. They may be used in conjunction with the clinical picture to guide therapy.

  4. Elevated complement levels are found in rheumatoid arthritis (except when associated with vasculitis) or gout.

Rheumatoid Factor

I. Definition

A. Rheumatoid factors are autoantibodies which are specific for antigenic determinants on the F fragment of IGG molecules.

B. IgM, IgA, IgG, and IgE rheumatoid factors exist, but only IgM rheumatoid factor is measured by the standard serologic tests.

C. Since IgM rheumatoid factors are multivalent, they agglutinate antigen-coated particles efficiently.

II. Methods of Detection

A. Latex agglutination: Latex coated with human IgG is combined with serum. Agglutination occurs if IgM rheumatoid factor is present in the serum. The titer is expressed as the highest dilution yielding detectable agglutination.

B. Rose-Waaler reaction: An agglutination reaction using sheep red blood cells coated with human or rabbit IgG. It is more specific for rheumatoid arthritis but is rarely used because it is time-consuming.

C. Radioimmunoassay and enzyme-linked immunosorbent assay (ELISA): Able to detect all classes of rheumatoid factor. More sensitive than agglutination at higher titers of dilution.

III. Incidence

A. Occurs in a variety of acute and chronic inflammatory states; many conditions are associated with hypergammaglobulinemia or immune complex formation.

B. Present in 1–5% of the normal population.

C. Titers increase with advancing age.

D. Patients with rheumatoid arthritis tend to have higher titers than patients without rheumatic diseases. Up to 25% of patients with rheumatoid arthritis may be seronegative.

IV. Diseases Associated with Rheumatoid Factor

A. Rheumatic diseases: Rheumatoid arthritis, SLE, Sjorgren's scleroderma, polymyositis.

B. Infectious disease
1. Acute: Mononucleosis, hepatitis, influenza, other viral infections, parasitic infections.
2. Chronic: Subacute bacterial endocarditis, tuberculosis, leprosy, syphilis, brucellosis.

C. Noninfectious diseases
1. Neoplasms
2. Diffuse interstitial pulmonary fibrosis
3. Chronic liver disease
4. Cryoglobulinemia
5. Sarcoidosis
6. Waldenström's macroglobulinemia

Antinuclear Antibodies (ANA)

I. Definition

A group of autoantibodies directed against nuclear and cytoplasmic cellular antigens, which are present in the sera of many patients with rheumatic diseases.

II. Detection

A. Indirect immunofluorescence: In this most reliable screening test for ANA, test serum is applied to a slide containing frozen mouse liver sections or a human tissue culture line, then incubated and washed. Immunoglobulins in the serum with antinuclear specificity attach to the nuclei of the cellular substrate. Fluorescein-labeled rabbit anti-human IgG is applied. The bound anti-human IgG is then visualized by immunofluorescent microscopy.

B. Radioimmunoassay or ELISA: These allow more specific identification of autoantibodies.

C. Immunodiffusion and counterimmunoelectrophoresis: Insensitive; now used less frequently.

III. Patterns of ANA

These are less useful than identification of specific autoantibodies but are still of some value.

A. Homogeneous: All connective tissue diseases, drug-induced lupus.

B. Speckled: SLE, rheumatoid arthritis, scleroderma, Sjögren's disease.

C. Peripheral: SLE; correlates with anti-double-stranded DNA.

D. Nucleolar: Scleroderma, Sjögren's disease.

E. Centromere: CREST syndrome.

IV. Specific Autoantibodies

A. Anti-DNA: Detected by radioimmunoassay immunofluorescence on crithidia luciliae or ELISA
1. Anti-double-stranded DNA: Highly specific for SLE; present in 60% of SLE patients; fluctuates with disease activity.
2. Anti-single-stranded DNA: Less specific; also present in hepatitis, mononucleosis, rheumatoid arthritis, and drug-induced lupus; found in 92% of patients with SLE.

B. Antibodies to RNA protein antigens
1. Anti-Smith: Found in 35% of SLE patients; highly specific. Has been associated with isolated central nervous system disease in lupus erythematosus.
2. Anti-RNP: Present in all patients with mixed connective tissue disease; occurs less frequently in SLE, discoid lupus, and scleroderma. Lupus patients have a low frequency of renal disease.
3. Anti-RO (SSA): Associated with Sjögren's disease (70–95%), congenital heart block, and neonatal lupus dermatitis (100%). Less frequently associated with SLE and subacute cutaneous lupus erythematosus. Lupus patients with SSA have a high frequency of nephritis.
4. Anti-LA (SSB): Nearly all patients have anti-RO antibodies as well. Associated with diseases similar to anti-RO. Preset in up to 5% of the general population.
5. Anticentromere antibodies: Detected by immunofluorescence on tissue culture lines. Present in 50–90% of CREST patients; highly specific for CREST.
6. Anti-SCL 70: Highly specific for scleroderma; occurs in up to 25% of patients.
7. Anti-J01: Present in 30% of patients with polymyositis and in 10% of those with dermatomyositis.
8. Anti-Rana: Associated with the Epstein-Barr virus. Present in 90–95% of rheumatoid arthritis patients.

C. Antihistone antibodies: Detected by immunofluorescence. Reconstitution present in 30% of SLE patients and in nearly 100% of patients with drug-induced lupus.

D. Antiphospholipid antibodies
1. Anticardiolipin antibody and the lupus anticoagulant are two antiphospholipid antibodies found in up to 40% of patients

with SLE and in 2% of the general population.

2. They prolong phospholipid-dependent coagulation steps by competing with coagulation factors for binding to phospholipid.

3. Despite a prolonged activated partial thromboplastin time, they are associated with arterial and venous thrombosis.

4. Other complications include fetal loss, thrombocytopenia, livedo reticularis, hemolytic anemia, stroke, and vascular heart disease.

5. Primary antiphospholipid antibody syndrome occurs in patients without collagen vascular disease. Complications are similar to those of patients with associated collagen vascular disease.

6. Patients who have had a thromboembolic event should receive prolonged anticoagulation with coumadin and/or antiplatelet therapy.

Bibliography

Bedell SE, Bush BT. Erythrocyte sedimentation rate from folklore to facts. *Am J Med* 78:1001–1009, 1985.

Harley JB, Gather KK. Autoantibodies. *Rheum Dis Clin North Am* 14:43–53, 1988.

Sammaritano LR, Gharavi AE, Lockshin MD. Anti-phospholipid antibody syndrome: Immunologic and clinical aspects. *Semin Arthritis Rheum* 20:81–96, 1990.

Radioisotope Assessment of Joints

Paul Glickman, M.D.

Types of Isotopes Useful in Joint Imaging

I. **Technetium-99m Pertechnetate**
   This is mainly protein bound and localizes in inflamed joints because of increased vascularity and effusions.
   A. Uptake by normal joints should not exceed uptake by adjacent tissue.
   B. Nonspecific but correlates well with clinical examinations.
   C. Not suited to axial joint imaging.
   D. More sensitive than clinical examinations.
   E. When normal, helps to confirm the clinical diagnosis of fibromyalgia.
   F. May provide evidence of clinically obscure joint disease (e.g., steroid-treated early rheumatoid arthritis or polymyalgia rheumatica).

II. **Technetium-99m Phosphate**
   This is absorbed directly by bone. Two isotopes, technetium-99m pyrophosphate and technetium-99m methylene diphosphonate, are used.
   A. Primarily used to detect metastatic disease and osteomyelitis.
   B. Used to evaluate deep joints such as those of the axial skeleton. May demonstrate facet and costovertebral joints.

C. Normal joints show increased uptake compared to background, making diagnosing of peripheral joint arthritis difficult.
   D. May be useful in detecting sacroilitis, particularly when used with quantifying techniques.
   E. May detect osteonecrosis of the femoral head before radiologic changes occur. A cold central area surrounded by an area of increased uptake increases the specificity of the diagnosis.
   F. Useful in detecting osteonecrosis of other joints such as the knee and shoulder.
   G. May be useful in detecting osteomyelitis, osteoid osteoma, stress fractures, and primary bone tumors.
   H. Of little value in diagnosing advanced degenerative spinal disc or facet disease.
   I. Useful in demonstrating loosening of hip or knee prostheses, particularly when combined with gallium-67 or indium white blood cell imaging.

III. **Gallium-67**
   This attaches to neutrophilic leukocytes.
   A. May detect infection.
   B. However, may also concentrate in any inflammatory process, including tumors.

Table 92C-1. Indications for Bone and Joint Scans

Indication	Procedure	Radiopharmaceutical
Peripheral joint synovitis	Joint scintigraphy	Technetium-99m pertechnetate
Osteomyelitis Septic arthritis Disc-space infection Complications of arthroplasty	Joint scintigraphy followed by gallium or leukocyte scintigraphy	Technetium-99m diphosphonate Gallium-67 citrate Indium-111 leukocytes
Osteonecrosis Axial skeletal disease Sacroiliitis Stress fractures Primary bone tumors Osteoid osteoma	Bone scintigraphy	Technetium-99 m diphosphonate

IV. **Indium-Labeled Leukocytes**
   These may be useful in detecting early infection.
V. **Radionucleotide Arthrography**
   A. Technetium-99 sulfur colloid injected intra-articularly may demonstrate loosening of hip prostheses. Particularly useful when combined with contrast arthrography.

Bibliography

Gottschalk A. Hoffler PB, Potchen EJ. In: Diagnostic Nuclear Medicine, Williams and Wilkins publ., Baltimore 1988, pp 1046–1075.

Schumacher RH, (ed) In: Primer on the Rheumatic Disease. Ed 10. pp 74–80 The Arthritis Foundation 1993.

Chapter 92-D

Arthrocentesis and Synovial Fluid Examination

Calvin R. Brown, M.D.

I. **Purpose**

Provides useful information about processes occurring within joint spaces.

II. **Indications**

A. Helps differentiate inflammatory from non-inflammatory arthritis.

B. Useful in establishing a diagnosis when more than one form of arthritis is present.

C. Provides supporting evidence for a diagnosis when other information suggests the diagnosis.

D. May be therapeutic when draining tense effusions or products of inflammation, as well as in septic and crystalline arthritis.

E. Essential in making a correct diagnosis in inflammatory monoarthritis. Urgently indicated to rule out or establish the diagnosis of septic arthritis.

III. **Technique**

A. Frequently underperformed because of lack of appreciation of the information yielded and perceived lack of skill in performing this test.

B. Test may be performed at the bedside or in an ambulatory setting. Operator wears gloves to prevent contact with fluid. Skin cleansed with

iodine solution and kept sterile to prevent introduction of organisms into the joint. Skin infiltrated with Xylocaine or a topical anesthetic. Avoid instillation of anesthetic into deep structures or into the joint itself to avoid interfering with the results of the analysis.

C. If fluid is to be aspirated, a 20-gauge or larger needle is needed. If fluid is to be injected, a 25-gauge needle may be used. Size of syringe should correspond to estimated volume of the effusion to be drained. One milliliter of fluid is adequate to perform appropriate tests.

D. Complications

1. Infection of a previously sterile joint occurs <1 in 10,000 aspirations.

2. Local bleeding is usually minor.

3. Direct injury to cartilage by the needle is rare; avoided by avoiding movement of the needle within the joint space.

E. Approach to specific joints

1. Shoulder entered anteriorly just lateral to the coracoid process.

2. Elbow entered laterally between the olecranon process and lateral epicondyle.

3. Wrist aspirated from the dorsal surface at the radiocarpal joint.

4. Knee entered from the medial or lateral aspect at the midpoint of the groove between the patella and femur.
5. Ankle entered anteriorly, medial or lateral to the extensor hallicus tendon, avoiding the dorsalis pedis artery.
6. Interphalangeal joints approached from the dorsolateral direction.
7. Hip requires a fluoroscopic direction to enter.

F. If a joint is to be injected, the single-needle technique is preferred, with removal of the aspirating syringe while the needle is in the joint space and insertion of the injecting syringe into the needle for subsequent injection.

IV. Synovial Fluid Analysis

A. Appearance
1. Clear fluid is normal or noninflammatory.
2. Cloudy fluid indicates varying degrees of inflammation.
3. Bloody fluid indicates coagulopathy or trauma to a joint structure or bone; look for fracture or internal derangement of the joint.

B. Laboratory studies
1. Leukocyte count
   a. Less than 2000/mm^3; noninflammatory.
   b. From 2000/mm^3 to 50,000/mm^3; inflammatory.
   c. From 50,000/mm^3 to more than 100,000/mm^3: frequently septic; with early sepsis or in immunocompromised patients, may be as low as 20,000/mm^3.
   d. Noninflammatory fluid: less than 50% neutrophils; inflammatory fluid: 50–95% neutrophils; septic fluid: often more than 95% neutrophils.

2. Culture
   a. If fluid looks turbid or the differential diagnosis includes sepsis, obtain culture and Gram stain.
   b. Consider acid-fast and fungal cultures in immunocompromised patients and cloudy chronic arthritis.

3. Crystal analysis using polarized microscopy by an experienced observer within a few hours of obtaining a sample for crystals.
   a. Uric acid crystals are needle-shaped and strongly positively birefringent.
   b. Calcium pyrophosphate crystals are rhomboid-shaped and weakly positively birefringent.
   c. Other crystals include "maltese cross"–shaped lipid crystals and submicroscopic calcium hydroxyapatite crystals.

4. Glucose, viscosity, mucin clot, protein, and immunologic tests are of little value.

Bibliography

Fries JF. General approach to the patient with rheumatic disease, in Kelly WN, Harris E, Ruddy S, et al (eds), *Textbook of Rheumatology*, ed 2. Philadelphia, Saunders, 1985, p 361.

Gatter RA. *A Practical Handbook of Synovial Fluid Analysis*. Philadelphia, Lea and Febiger, 1984.

Polley HF, Hunder GG. *Rheumatologic Interviewing and Physical Examination of the Joints*. ed 2. Philadelphia, Saunders, 1978, pp 1–25.

CHAPTER 93

Classification of Rheumatic Diseases

Lynn Meisles, M.D.

I. **Diffuse Connective Tissue Diseases**
   A. Rheumatoid arthritis
   B. Juvenile rheumatoid arthritis
      1. Systemic onset (Still's disease)
      2. Polyarticular onset
      3. Pauciarticular onset
   C. Systemic lupus erythematosus
   D. Systemic sclerosis
   E. Polymyositis/dermatomyositis
   F. Necrotizing vasculitis and other vasculopathies
      1. Polyarteritis nodosa
      2. Hypersensitivity vasculitis
      3. Wagener's granulomatosis
      4. Giant cell arteritis
         a. Temporal arteritis
         b. Takayasu's arteritis
      5. Kawasaki disease
      6. Behcet's disease
      7. Cryoglobulinemia
      8. Juvenile dermatomyositis
   G. Sjögren's syndrome
   H. Overlap syndrome
II. **Seronegative Spondyloarthropathies**
   A. Ankylosing spondylitis
   B. Reiter's syndrome

   C. Psoriatic arthritis
   D. Arthritis associated with chronic inflammatory bowel disease
III. **Degenerative Joint Diseases**
   A. Primary
   B. Secondary
IV. **Infectious Agents Causing Arthritis, Bursitis, and Tenosynovitis**
   A. Direct
      1. Bacterial
         a. Gram-positive cocci (e.g., *Staphylococcus*)
         b. Gram-negative cocci (e.g., *Gonococcus*)
         c. Gram-negative rods
         d. Mycobacteria
         e. Spirochetes (e.g., Lyme disease)
         f. Others, including leprosy and mycoplasma
      2. Viral
      3. Fungal
      4. Parasitic
   B. Indirect (reactive)
      1. Bacterial
         a. Acute rheumatic fever
         b. Postdysenteric (e.g., *Shigella*, *Yersinia*)
         c. Intestinal bypass

2. Viral (hepatitis B)
V. Metabolic and Endocrine Diseases
  A. Crystal-induced conditions
    1. Monosodium urate (gout)
    2. Calcium pyrophosphate dihydrate (pseudogout)
    3. Apatite
    4. Oxalate
  B. Biochemical abnormalities
    1. Amyloidosis
    2. Hyperlipoproteinemias
    3. Hemoglobinopathies
    4. Hemochromatosis
    5. Ochronosis
    6. Others
  C. Endocrine diseases
    1. Diabetes mellitus
    2. Acromegaly
    3. Hyperparathyroidism
  D. Immunodeficiency diseases
    1. Primary
    2. Acquired immunodeficiency syndrome

VI. Neoplasms
  A. Primary (e.g., synoviosarcoma)
  B. Metastatic
  C. Multiple myeloma
  D. Leukemia and lymphoma
  E. Villonodular synovitis
  F. Osteochondromatosis

VII. Neuropathic Disorders
  A. Charcot joints
  B. Compression neuropathies
    1. Peripheral entrapment (e.g., carpal tunnel syndrome)
    2. Radiculopathy
    3. Spinal stenosis

  C. Reflex sympathetic dystrophy
VIII. Bone, Periosteal, and Cartilage Disorders
  A. Osteoporosis
    1. Generalized
    2. Localized
  B. Osteomalacia
  C. Hypertrophic osteoarthropathy
  D. Diffuse idiopathic skeletal hyperostosis
  E. Paget's disease
  F. Osteonecrosis
  G. Osteochondritis
  H. Costochondritis
  I. Osteomyelitis

IX. Nonarticular Rheumatism
  A. Myofascial pain syndrome
    1. Generalized (e.g., fibromyalgia)
    2. Regional
  B. Low back pain
  C. Tendinitis or bursitis
  D. Ganglion cysts
  E. Fasciitis
  F. Chronic ligament and muscle strains
  G. Vasomotor disorders (e.g., Raynaud's phenomenon)

X. Miscellaneous Disorders Associated with Arthritis
  A. Trauma
  B. Pancreatic disease
  C. Sarcoidosis
  D. Palindromic rheumatism

Bibliography

Kelley WN, Harris ED, Ruddy S, et al. Textbook of Rheumatology. Philadelphia, W.B. Saunders, 1993.

CHAPTER 94

Rheumatoid Arthritis

Lynn Meisles, M.D.

I. **Definition**
Rheumatoid arthritis (RA) is a chronic systemic disease most commonly presenting as a symmetrical arthritis. Joint inflammation may be remitting but, if continuous, can result in joint destruction, deformity, and disability.
  A. It is the most common inflammatory arthropathy, occurring in 1.5% of the adult population.
  B. Eighty percent of patients have a positive test for rheumatoid factor.
  C. Women are affected two to three times more often than men.
  D. Peak age of onset is between 35 and 45, but individuals of any age can be affected.
  E. Seventy percent of patients with RA are human leukocyte antigen (HLA)-DR4 positive.

II. **Etiology**
The etiology of RA remains unknown. Most likely many different stimuli in the immunogenetically susceptible host can trigger the disease.
  A. Infectious agents have been implicated.
    1. Polyarthritis occurs during many bacterial, viral, and spirochetal infections of humans and animals.
    2. Measles virus and parvovirus have been cultured from the joints of several patients with a seronegative arthritis.
    3. There are increased serum antibody titers to Epstein-Barr virus in patients with RA.
  B. The presence of rheumatoid factor (RF) has been questioned.

    1. RF contributes to synovitis through activation of complement and formation of immune complexes that are phagocytosed by polymorphonuclear neutrophils in synovial fluid.
    2. Immunogenetics researchers are studying to what degree the RF response in humans is associated with the genes that predispose to the disease.
  C. Metabolic, endocrine, and nutritional factors, as well as geographic, occupational, and psychosocial variables, have been investigated without revealing a clear link to the etiology.

III. **Pathophysiology**
Immunologic processes are responsible for the inflammation and tissue destruction that occur in RA.
  A. Immune complexes form in the joint, which activate and fix complement and attract neutrophils.
  B. Neutrophils ingest the immune complexes, triggering the release of hydrolytic enzymes, oxygen radicals, prostaglandins, and other mediators of inflammation.
  C. T lymphocytes with both helper/inducer (CD4) and cytotoxic/suppressor (CD8) phenotypes are abundantly present and activated in synovial tissue; macrophages are also common.
  D. These mononuclear cells are stimulated to release soluble products that cause inflam-

mation, synoviocyte proliferation, increased vessel permeability, and production of collagenase by synovial cells.

E. Synovium proliferates, hypertrophies, and forms granulation tissue (pannus).

1. Tendon sheaths and bursal linings show similar inflammatory changes.
2. Tendons may form nodules or adhesions or may rupture.
3. Bursitis may also develop.

F. Pannus erodes cartilage and bone.

G. Extra-articular manifestations may represent deposition of systemic immune complexes.

IV. Diagnosis

The diagnosis of RA is based primarily on clinical grounds. No laboratory finding, including RF, is specific for RA.

A. Historical data: Onset of symptoms is typically insidious, occurring over a period of weeks or months.

1. Systemic features include malaise, fatigue, and weight loss. Diffuse musculoskeletal pain may be the first nonspecific complaint.
2. Subsequently, specific joints exhibit pain, tenderness, swelling, and redness in a symmetric distribution.
3. Duration of morning stiffness is an accepted criterion of disease severity.
4. In a minority of patients (10%), the onset of RA is acute; symptoms occur over a period of days or may even be manifested overnight.

B. Clinical signs and physical findings include articular and extra-articular manifestations.

1. Joints: RA is typically a symmetrical polyarthritis mainly affecting the small joints of the hands (metacarpophalangeals [MCPs] and proximal interphalangeals [PIPs], with sparing of the distal interphalangeals [DIPs]), wrists, knees, feet, ankles, shoulders, and elbows.

a. Hands: Initial features are pain and swelling of MCP and PIP joints, leading to a spindle-shaped appearance of the fingers. Soft tissue laxity leads to ulnar deviation. In advanced cases, swan neck deformities develop through hyperextension of PIP joints with flexion of DIP joints. Boutonniere deformities occur by flexion deformity of PIP joints and extension of DIP joints.

b. Wrists: RA almost always causes palpable, boggy wrist synovium. Later, volar subluxation of the hand can occur. Synovial proliferation on the volar aspect may produce carpal tunnel syndrome by compressing the median nerve.

c. Elbows: Loss of full extension is common.

d. Shoulders: Glenohumeral, acromioclavicular, and thoracoscapular joints may be involved. Subacromial bursitis and rotator cuff lesions also commonly occur.

e. Neck: Neck pain and stiffness are common. Progressive erosion may lead to atlantoaxial subluxation, resulting in spinal cord compression and neurologic signs.

f. Hips: RA manifested as abnormal gait and limitation of joint motion. Groin discomfort is a frequent complaint.

g. Knees: Synovial hypertrophy and effusions are common. Effusions can be detected by balloting the patella or by a positive bulge sign. Baker's cysts may form and occasionally dissect or rupture, mimicking acute thrombophlebitis. Quadriceps atrophy, joint instability, and valgus or varus deformities can all occur.

h. Feet and ankles: Changes are similar to those described in the hands. MTP synovitis may be apparent by MTP "squeezing." Later, subluxation may occur, causing pain with ambulation.

i. Others: Almost any synovial joints may become involved, including temporomandibular joints, sternoclavicular and manubriosternal joints, and cricoarytenoids.

2. Extra-articular manifestations: Systemic symptoms including low-grade fever and minor lymphadenopathy often occur. As the disease progresses, muscle atrophy and weakness are common. Almost all organ systems may be involved.

a. Skin: Subcutaneous nodules develop in 20% of patients, associated with seropositive disease that is progressive and destructive. Occur over periarticular structures and areas subject to pressure.

b. Cardiac: Most frequent symptomatic lesion is acute pericarditis unrelated to the duration of arthritis. Pericardial effusions, constrictive pericarditis, and tamponade also occur. Lesions similar to rheumatoid nodules may involve the myocardium and valves, possibly leading to valvular insufficiency and conduction abnormalities.

c. Pulmonary: Pleuritis and pleural effusion may occur; effusion is typically exudative. Nodules, either subpleural or intraparenchymal, are also seen; nodules occur in association with a pneumoconiosis called *Caplan's syndrome*. Interstitial fibrosis with pneumonitis, and necrotizing bronchiolitis associated with gold and penicillamine use, may also occur.

d. Neurologic: Entrapment neuropathies (most often involving the median nerve), peripheral neuropathy, mononeuritis multiplex (in vasculitis), and cervical cord compression may all occur.

e. Ophthalmologic: Sjögren's syndrome (SS) may develop, causing eye dryness with possible corneal and conjunctival lesions. Scleritis, episcleritis, and scleromalacia may also occur.

f. Vasculitis: Small and medium-sized vessels affected; may lead to digital infarcts, gangrene, mononeuritis multiplex, and leg ulcers. Associated with manifestations of systemic disease and depression of serum complement.

g. Hematologic: Anemia, thrombocytopenia, and lymphadenopathy may occur. Felty's syndrome (neutropenia and splenomegaly) also seen in patients with active arthritis.

C. Diagnostic tests: Laboratory data and x-rays help confirm the clinical diagnosis.

1. Laboratory tests
   a. Raised erythrocyte sedimentation rate: Correlates with the size and number of affected joints and the activity of disease. May be greater than 100 mm/hr.
   b. Raised C-reactive protein.
   c. Anemia is common; normochromic, normocytic anemia of chronic disease or hypochromic microcytic iron deficiency anemia (possibly due to gastrointestinal [GI] bleeding).
   d. Thrombocytosis is common in active disease.

e. RF is positive in 80%. Positives occur in 30% of related diseases such as systemic lupus erythematosus (SLE), diabetes mellitus, SS, and periarteritis nodosa. RF may also be positive in various infectious and noninfectious diseases.

f. Antinuclear antibody is positive in 20%.

g. Synovial fluid is inflammatory, with 2,000–50,000 cells/mm^3.

2. X-rays are helpful for diagnosis, prognosis, and disease monitoring.
   a. X-ray changes include soft tissue swelling, periarticular osteoporosis, marginal erosions, and deformities.
   b. Cervical spine films required for neck symptoms and prior to intubation. Flexion and extension views are helpful in diagnosing subluxation of the atlantoaxial joint.
   c. Chest x-ray helpful for cardiac and respiratory complications of RA.

3. Biopsy may be helpful in difficult cases.
   a. Biopsy of a nodule shows central fibrinoid necrosis surrounded by a palisading cellular area.
   b. Synovial biopsy shows lymphocytes, plasma cells, and occasional giant cells infiltrating enlarged villi. These findings are not diagnostic.

V. **Differential Diagnosis**
Many of the inflammatory arthropathies may mimic RA, especially in its early stages.

A. Rheumatic diseases
   1. Osteoarthritis
      a. Erosive osteoarthritis characterized by inflammatory changes in PIP joints; most commonly occurs in middle-aged women.
      b. Osteoarthritis (OA) and RA approach each other clinically and pathologically as disease progresses.
   2. SLE
   3. Systemic sclerosis
   4. Gout and calcium pyrophosphate crystal deposition
   5. Psoriatic arthritis
   6. Sarcoidosis

B. Nonrheumatic diseases
   1. Lyme disease
   2. Whipple's disease
   3. Amyloidosis
   4. Malignancies

VI. **Treatment**
Management of RA is directed at reducing or suppressing inflammation, preserving joint

function, and providing pain relief. No curative therapy is available.

A. Nonsteroidal anti-inflammatory drugs (NSAIDs) should be started on every newly diagnosed patient with RA unless contraindicated; most effective analgesic and anti-inflammatory agents for first-line treatment. GI distress is the major side effect; it may make NSAIDs intolerable for some patients. Many preparations are available, and patients respond to different agents in individual ways.

B. Corticosteroids are used for relief of symptoms, but they are not curative and do not prevent progressive joint destruction.

1. Intra-articular corticosteroid injections are indicated for acute or subacute inflammatory synovitis; should not be repeated more than three or four times a year. Infection must be ruled out before injection when only one or two joints flare.

2. Low-dose oral steroids (5–10 mg/day) used when NSAIDs fail and while waiting for a slow-acting treatment to become effective.

3. Parenteral steroids used for surgical coverage and in severe, life-threatening complications such as systemic vasculitis.

C. Slow-acting drugs are considered second-line agents.

1. Indications

a. Severe synovitis that does not respond to NSAIDs alone.

b. Development of erosions on x-ray (especially of the hands or feet).

c. Presence of extra-articular manifestations, including nodules.

2. Individual drug preferences vary among physicians.

a. Hydroxychloroquine or sulfasalazine have the least toxicity and are common first choices.

b. Gold can be administered by injectable or oral routes. Auranofin has less toxicity than injectable forms but less efficacy as well. Onset of action is 3–6 months.

c. D-Penicillamine is as beneficial as injectable gold but has varied and unpredictable toxicity; should probably be used after a trial of gold has failed or when gold is contraindicated.

d. Methotrexate (low-dose, weekly pulse) is effective and has a reasonable

toxicity risk. Onset of action is relatively early, often within 3–4 weeks.

e. Azathioprine is also effective but has a longer onset of action.

f. Cyclophosphamide, chlorambucil, and experimental therapies are reserved for severe, resistant diseases and those with life-threatening complications.

g. Combination therapies may prove more effective; the goal is to maximally suppress immune responses.

D. Physical and occupational therapy promote muscle building and joint protection. Also provides help in ADLs.

E. Orthopedic surgery can be preventive or reparative.

VII. **Patient Monitoring**

Patients with RA need to be closely observed and treatment adjusted as needed. Monitoring includes:

A. Symptomatic deterioration, including worsening pain and increased morning stiffness.

B. Serial x-rays of involved joints to look for erosive disease.

C. Evidence of joint or ligament instability.

D. Evidence of extra-articular manifestations.

VIII. **Prognosis**

About 10% of RA patients proceed to develop severe disability. Features indicating a poor prognosis:

A. High-titer RF at first presentation or within 1 year of onset of RA.

B. Early appearance of erosions (within 1 year of onset of symptoms).

C. Extra-articular manifestations.

D. Presence of HLA-DR 4.

Bibliography

Fleming A, Benn RT, Corbett M, et al. Early rheumatoid disease II. Pattern of joint involvement. *Ann Rheum Dis* 35:361, 1976.

Fleming A, Crown JM, Corbett M. Early rheumatoid disease I. Onset. *Ann Rheum Dis* 35:357, 1976.

Jacoby RK, Jayson MIV, Cosh JA. Onset, early stages and prognosis of rheumatoid arthritis: A clinical study of 100 patients with 11 year follow-up. *Br Med J* 2:96, 1973.

McKenna F. Clinical and laboratory assessment of outcome in rheumatoid arthritis. *Br J Rheum* 27(Suppl. 1):12, 1988.

Wilkens RF. Rheumatoid arthritis: Clinical considerations in diagnosis and management. *Am J Med* 83(4B):31, 1987.

CHAPTER 95

Sjögren's Syndrome

John P. Huff, M.D., Ph.D.

I. Definition

Sjögren's syndrome (SS) is an autoimmune disorder characterized by decreased exocrine function. The lacrimal and salivary glands are affected, leading to the sicca complex of keratoconjunctivitis and xerostomia. Presentations are of three general types:

A. Primary SS, consisting of the sicca complex only.

B. Secondary SS, consisting of the sicca complex with an accompanying connective tissue disease such as rheumatoid arthritis (RA), systemic lupus erythematosus (SLE), and systemic sclerosis.

C. Lymphoproliferative SS, consisting of the sicca complex and lymphoproliferation of either a benign or malignant nature.

II. Etiology

As with other autoimmune diseases, multiple factors are probably involved in the etiology of this syndrome, including immunologic, genetic, hormonal, and environmental ones.

A. Up to 90% of patients have positive rheumatoid factor (RF) and up to 80% of patients have positive antinuclear antibody (ANA) (SS-A and SS-B are most common). Organ-specific antibodies are also frequently found against the thyroid, parietal cells, and so on. Lymphopenia, hyperglobulinemia, and T-cell and natural killer cell abnormalities may be present.

B. Human leukocyte antigen (HLA)-B8 and -DR3 are associated with primary SS, while HLA-DR4 is associated with secondary SS.

C. More than 90% of patients are women.

D. Viruses have been implicated with an antibody to Epstein-Barr virus–related nuclear antigen (RANA) frequently present in secondary SS with RA.

III. Pathophysiology

The sicca complex occurs due to a progressive lymphocytic infiltration and destruction of the exocrine glands. Biopsy of the minor salivary gland of the lower lip shows multiple lymphocytic aggregates infiltrating and destroying the acinar tissue. This leads to progressive gland dysfunction and the associated dryness. Similar changes in other exocrine glands can cause respiratory, gastrointestinal, hepatic, pancreatic, renal, auditory, and genital dysfuncion.

IV. Diagnosis

Diagnosis depends on two of three criteria being met: (1) definite keratoconjunctivitis sicca, (2) an associated extraglandular lymphoproliferative or connective tissue disorder, and (3) a salivary gland biopsy with a characteristic lymphocytic infiltrate. Certain conditions that can give false-positive results should be excluded.

A. Keratoconjunctivitis sicca can be verified by measuring tear flow or by loss of integrity of the corneal epithelial surface. Patients with keratoconjunctivitis and xerostomia only are said to have sicca syndrome.

   1. Schirmer's test directly measures tear flow. A filter paper strip folded 5 mm from the end is placed in the middle of the lower lid, with the 5-mm end in the trough. The filter paper is allowed to wick up the tears for 5 min. Wetting of less than 15 mm in young individuals and 10 mm in older ones is abnormal.

   2. Corneal epithelial integrity can be determined by instilling fluorescein or rose bengal stain. Collection of stain in the palpebral aperture is a positive test.

   3. Xerostomia can be diagnosed by the history and by an examination showing decreased salivation, by inability to swallow a cracker dry, and by no increased salivation in the presence of candy.

B. Associated connective tissue disorders, in order of frequency, are RA, SLE, systemic sclerosis, polyarteritis nodosa, and polymyositis.

C. Salivary gland biopsies should show an average of two lymphocytic foci/4 mm². Each focus should contain more than 50 lymphocytes.

D. Additional findings may include enlarged parotid glands (may be unilateral), thyroiditis, central nervous system dysfunction, vasculitis (periarteritis nodosa), increased drug allergies (especially to penicillin and possibly gold), and others.

E. Exclusion criteria include sarcoidosis, preexisting lymphomas, graft-versus-host disease, and viral infections including Epstein-Barr virus, mumps, human immunodeficiency virus, and others.

V. Differential Diagnosis

Other diseases, aging, and drugs can mimic the symptoms of SS.

A. Diseases include sarcoidosis, graft-versus-host disease, acquired immunodeficiency syndrome, and parotid tumors including lymphoma, adenoma, and carcinoma. Other causes include metabolic disorders and infections (e.g., alcoholism, malnutrition, pancreatitis, diabetes, tuberculosis, and actinomycosis).

B. The incidence of senile sicca syndrome is 3% (females more than males) in patients over 80 years of age.

C. Parasympathetic drugs, diuretics, antihypertensives, antidepressants, can also mimic the symptoms of SS.

VI. Treatment

Management is aimed at treating the symptoms and the underlying autoimmune process.

A. Symptomatic and localized therapy is aimed at limiting damage to organ systems.

   1. Ocular treatment can include artificial tears during the day and an ointment at night. Room humidifiers, wraparound glasses, and goggles worn during the day and/or night can be helpful. Closure of the puncta can help prevent drainage from the conjunctiva. Ophthalmologic exams should be done at 6-month intervals.

   2. Oral treatment can include water and artificial saliva to facilitate swallowing. Sugarless candy and a pilocarpine mouthwash can also stimulate saliva. Yeast infections occur frequently and can be treated with an oral antifungal lozenge. Bacterial infections of the salivary gland, though uncommon, can occur. Dental caries and gum disease are very common. Good dental care and frequent checkups are important.

   3. Generalized exocrine gland involvement can lead to hoarseness, bronchitis, and decreased vaginal secretions resulting in dyspareunia, constipation, loss of pancreatic secretions, hypo- or achlorhydria, and dermal dryness. Saturated solution of potassium iodide can be used as a mucolytic for respiratory and mucosal symptoms. Propionic acid gels can be used for vaginal dryness. A room humidifier can help decrease the drying of membranes.

B. Treatment of underlying autoimmune disease processes may result in significant improvement. Hydroxychloroquine has recently been shown to result in significant improvement in multiple laboratory parameters in primary disease and may be of benefit. Corticosteroid and immunosuppressive therapy in general should be reserved for severe functional disabilities or life-threatening complications.

VII. **Patient Monitoring**
- A. Therapeutic efficacy in the treatment of any underlying autoimmune disease should be monitored and altered to maximize beneficial effects. Vasculitis, cryoglobulinemia, and glomerulonephritis can develop.
- B. Ocular and oral examinations should be done on a regular basis. Lesions can develop at an accelerated rate and can result in significant morbidity.
- C. Hashimoto's thyroiditis develops in about 5% of patients.
- D. Salivary gland swelling for a prolonged period, or of a particularly hard or nodular nature, should be viewed as suspicious for neoplasia. Biopsy should be considered.

VIII. **Prognosis**
- A. Localized disease can and often does progress, resulting in significant dysfunction.
- B. There is a 44-fold increase in the incidence of non-Hodgkin's lymphoma.

Bibliography

Alexander EL, Malinow K, Lejewski JE, et al. Primary Sjogren's syndrome with central nervous system disease mimicking multiple sclerosis. *Ann Intern Med* 104:323–330, 1986.

Bloch K, Buchanan W, Wohl M, et al. Sjogren's syndrome: A clinical pathological, and serological study of 62 cases. *Medicine (Balt)* 44:187–231, 1965.

Fox RI, Chan E, Benton L, et al. Treatment of primary Sjogren's syndrome with hydroxychloroquine. *Am J Med* 85(Suppl 4A):62–67, 1988.

Talal N. Sjogren's syndrome, in Rose N, Mackey I (eds), *The Autoimmune Diseases*. New York, Academic Press, 1985, pp 145–159.

CHAPTER 96

Systemic Lupus Erythematosus

John P. Huff, M.D., Ph.D.

I. **Definition**
Systemic lupus erythematosus (SLE) is a chronic inflammatory disease which can involve almost every organ system in the body. It is the prototypical autoimmune disease characterized by multiple immunologic abnormalities, most consistent of which is the presence of antinuclear antibodies (ANA).

II. **Etiology**
The precise etiology of SLE is unknown but is most likely due to a combination of hormonal, genetic, and environmental factors. The reported incidence rate varies from 4 to 250/100,000 population. Most studies report rates in the 10 to 50/100,000 range.
A. Incidence is higher in females and peaks during the childbearing years.
   1. Sex is a factor, with a female:male ratio of approximately 8:1.
   2. Sex ratio is lower in children (2 to 5:1) and older persons (2:1), in whom hormones may be less of a factor, and highest in the childbearing years (20 to 30:1).
   3. Higher incidence in men with Klinefelter's disease.

4. Abnormalities in estrogen metabolism noted in both sexes with SLE.
   a. Estrogen may play role in occurrence of SLE.
   b. Androgens may ameliorate the disease.
B. Genetic factors, including race and familial occurrence, are risk factors for developing SLE.
   1. Occurrence in American blacks is four times that in whites.
   2. Americans of Hispanic and Asian heritage are at higher risk than whites.
   3. Familial aggregation occurs.
      a. About 10% of patients have an affected first-degree relative.
      b. Rate in monozygotic twins is four times that in dizygotic twins.
      c. Other autoimmune diseases also more common in first-degree relatives.
   4. Multiple human leukocyte antigen (HLA) associations have been reported.
      a. A1, B8, DR2, DR3, DRw52, DQw1, and DQw2 are associated risk factors.
      b. Null gene for complement factor 4

(C4), C4AQO, increases the risk, especially in association with DR2.

C. Environmental factors have been implicated.

  1. Drugs and chemicals can cause a lupus-like syndrome.
     a. Procainamide, hydralazine, isoniazid, chlorpromazine, phenytoin, and others.
     b. Exogenous estrogen in the form of oral contraceptives.
     c. L-Canavanine in alfalfa sprouts.
  2. Infectious agents such as retroviruses are under investigation.
  3. Injuries to skin from injuries and ultraviolet (UV) and thermal burns can precipitate an attack.

III. Pathophysiology

SLE is a chronic inflammatory disease that appears to be caused by a disturbance in immunoregulation, resulting in pathologic changes.

A. Pathogenesis is most likely due to a combination of genetic, environmental, hormonal, and immunoregulatory factors.

  1. Polyclonal B-cell activation results in development of antinuclear antibodies.
     a. Ninety-nine percent of patients have positive ANA.
     b. Anti-double-stranded (native) DNA antibodies are seen in about 50% of patients.
        (1) Highly specific for SLE.
        (2) Associated with renal involvement.
  2. Suppressor T-cell dysfunction and decreased numbers of T cells have been reported.
  3. Environmental stresses, UV and thermal burns, and physical injuries have been implicated in disease development and exacerbation.

B. Pathology is characterized by general and organ-specific findings.

  1. General findings
     a. Hemotoxylin bodies, which are aggregates of nuclear material similar to that found in lupus erythematosus (LE) cells, are found in almost all organ systems.
     b. Onion skin lesions, concentric layers of fibrosis around penicillary arterioles, are found in the spleen.
     c. Libman-Sacks verrucous endocarditis consists of rare lesions characteristic of SLE. Lesions occur most frequently at the mitral valve. Mitral stenosis and dysfunction of the chordae tendini and papillary muscles can occur.

  2. Skin involvement is second only to arthritis as a clinical manifestation in SLE.
     a. About 60% of patients develop a distinct erythematous malar rash (butterfly), which may also develop on the sun exposed V-neck and periungal areas.
     b. Follicular plugging and atrophy of dermal appendages similar to discoid lupus can occur.
     c. Histologic changes include edema, vacuolization, and perivascular cellular infiltrates at the dermal-epidermal junction in involved skin.
     d. Characteristic deposits that stain with fluorescent-labeled anti-IgG occur at the dermal-epidermal junction in both involved and uninvolved skin.

  3. Biopsies show that clinical and subclinical involvement of the kidney can occur. This occurs in most if not all SLE patients even if there is a normal urinary sediment.
     a. In mild disease, only some of the glomeruli and focal areas of the glomerulus are affected. Pathology consists of mesangial cell proliferation, with thickening of the mesangium or segmental (focal) proliferation of the capillary cells of the glomerular tufts.
        (1) Immunofluorescence shows immunoglobulins and C3 in the mesangium.
        (2) Subendothelial and subepithelial deposits can be seen in the focal proliferative form.
        (3) Changes may be clinically silent.
     b. In diffuse proliferative glomerulonephritis, a majority of glomeruli and most of each glomerulus are involved.
        (1) Cellular proliferation may fill in Bowman's space, forming cellular crescents. Thickening of Bowman's capsule can result in fibrous crescents.
        (2) Immunofluorescent and electron microscopic studies show subendothelial and subepithelial deposits of complement and immuno-

globulin in the glomeruli. This gives a characteristic "wire loop" appearance to the immunofluorescent history.

(3) The basement membrane may be affected, resulting in a "lumpy-bumpy" appearance.

c. In membranous lupus nephritis the basement membrane is usually uniformly thickened.

(1) There is usually little mesangial cell proliferation and thickening, in contrast to the diffuse proliferative form.

(2) The membranoproliferative form resembles the diffuse proliferative form in its clinical course.

d. Pathologic changes outside the glomeruli can occur or may be the only renal involvement.

(1) Tubular, interstitial, and vasculitic infiltrates may be present.

(2) The presence of interstitial infiltrates may worsen the prognosis.

IV. Diagnosis

The 1982 American College of Rheumatology revised criteria requires that 4 out of 11 criteria be met, in the absence of other explanations, for a diagnosis of SLE to be made (Table 96-1).

A. Criteria are used for classification and comparison of groups of patients and are not absolutely necessary for individual patient diagnosis.

1. Patients meeting four or more criteria are classified as having definite SLE.

2. Patients meeting fewer than four criteria are classified as having possible SLE.

B. Subacute cutaneous lupus erythematosus (SCLE) is a milder, limited form of disease in which the skin is the main disease target.

1. Lesions resemble discoid lupus but are usually nonscarring.

2. Strong association with HLA-DR3 and autoantibodies to Ro(SS-A).

C. Other related limited or atypical forms can be seen.

1. ANA-negative lupus is rare.

a. Many patients eventually convert.

(1) Many are or become Ro(SS-A) and/or La(SS-B) positive.

(2) SLE can have a low-titer rheumatoid factor and be mistaken for early rheumatoid arthritis.

b. High incidence of photosensitive and cutaneous involvement (SCLE) and arthritis.

c. Low incidence of renal and central nervous system (CNS) involvement.

2. Neonatal lupus is a rare complication resulting in rash, hemolytic anemia, thrombocytopenia, heart block, and/or fetal wastage.

a. Strongly correlated with presence of maternal Ro/SS-A antibodies.

b. In general, these infants do not develop SLE later in life.

3. Antiphospholipid antibody syndrome is associated with recurrent thrombotic events, abortions, and thrombocytopenia.

a. Patients often have ANA-negative, atypical, or incomplete lupus-like syndromes.

b. Presence of antibody can be determined by an assay for antiphospholipid antibodies, a false-positive Venereal Disease Research Laboratory (VDRL), or a prolonged prothrombin time (confirmed by the lupus anticoagulant test).

c. IgG and IgM isotype antibodies have been associated with arterial and venous thrombotic events, respectively.

d. Patients have a higher incidence of CNS disease and end-organ damage due to thrombotic disease.

4. Drug-induced lupus can be brought on by numerous medications, including procainamide (most frequent cause), hydralazine, sulfonamides, penicillins, hydantoins, chlorpromazine, isoniazid, alpha methyldopa, quinidine, propylthiouracil, and methimazole.

a. Clinical features include gradual onset of arthralgias, myalgias, polyarthritis, fever, pleuritic pain, and migraines.

b. Renal, CNS, cutaneous vasculitis, and severe hematologic abnormalities are unusual.

c. Positive LE prep with a positive ANA due to antihistone antibodies are found in over 90% of patients. Lupus anticoagulant and biological false-positive VDRL have been found. Immune complexes, hypocomplementemia, and anti-double-stranded DNA (dsDNA) antibodies are unusual.

Table 96-1. 1982 Revised Criteria for Classification of Systemic Lupus Erythematosus

Condition	Description
Malar rash	Fixed erythema, flat or raised over the mallar eminences, tending to spare the nasolabial fold.
Discoid rash	Erythematous, raised patches with adherent keratotic scaling and follicular plugging; atrophic scarring may occur in older lesions.
Photosensitivity	Skin rash as a result of an unusual reaction to sunlight, by patient history or physician observation.
Oral ulcers	Oral or nasopharyngeal ulceration, usually painless, observed by a physician.
Arthritis	Nonerosive arthritis involving two or more peripheral joints, characterized by tenderness, swelling, or effusion.
Serositis	Pleuritis-proven history of pleuritic pain or rub heard by a physician or evidence of pleural effusion or Pericarditis documented by electrocardiography, rub, or evidence of pericardial effusion.
Renal disorder	Persistent proteinuria (>0.5 g/day) or greater than 3+ if quantitation not performed or Cellular casts—may be red cell, hemoglobin, granular, tubular, or mixed.
Neurologic disorder	Seizures in the absence of offending drugs or known metabolic derangements (e.g., uremia, ketoacidosis, or electrolyte imbalance) or Psychosis in the absence of offending drugs or known metabolic derangements (e.g., uremia, ketoacidosis, or electrolyte imbalance).
Hematologic disorder	Hemolytic anemia with reticulocytosis or Leukopenia (<4,000/mm) on two or more occasions or Lymphopenia (<1,500/mm) on two or more occasions or Thrombocytopenia (<100,000/mm) in the absence of offending drugs.
Immunologic disorder	Positive LE cell preparation or Anti-DNA: antibody to native DNA in abnormal titer or Anti-Sm: presence of antibody to Sm antigen or False-positive serologic test for syphilis known to be positive for at least 6 months and confirmed by *Treponema pallidum* immobilization or fluorescent treponemal antibody absorption test.
Antinuclear antibody	An abnormal titer of ANA by immunofluorescence or an equivalent assay at any point and in the absence of drugs known to be associated with a drug-induced lupus syndrome.

d. Symptoms usually resolve with withdrawal of the offending drug. A short course of nonsteroidal anti-inflammatory drugs (NSAIDs) and/or corticosteroids may be necessary in some cases.

e. Syndrome is associated genetically with slow acetylators of drugs, HLA-DR4, and C4a and C4b null alleles.

V. **Differential Diagnosis**

The differential diagnosis includes other chronic inflammatory and autoimmune diseases, infections, medications, and neoplasms which can cause systemic symptoms and manifestations.

A. Chronic inflammatory and autoimmune diseases.

1. Rheumatoid arthritis (RA) and juvenile rheumatoid arthritis (JRA) are systemic diseases which can present with an intermittent course. Patients can be rheumatoid factor negative and have low-titer ANA (up to 1:160 Hep-2).

2. Mixed connective tissue disease and systemic sclerosis can overlap in presentation with SLE, with symmetric polyarthritis and a positive ANA.

3. Additional autoimmune diseases include polymyositis, dermatomyositis, Still's disease, vasculitis, cryoglobulinemia, Behcet's syndrome, familial Mediterranean fever, and sarcoidosis.

4. Other diseases include leukemia, lymphoma, idiopathic thrombocytopenia purpura, leprosy, urticaria, syphilis, and multiple sclerosis.

B. Chronic and acute infections can mimic systemic inflammatory diseases such as SLE. Subacute bacterial endocarditis, gonococcal and meningococcal septicemia, serum sickness, rheumatic fever, hepatitis, secondary syphilis, leprosy, and parvovirus B19 infection can all resemble the onset of SLE.

VI. Treatment

Treatment can be divided into three categories: nonmedicinal, medicinal, and experimental or unproven therapies.

A. Nonmedicinal therapies consist of patient education and physical therapy.

1. All patients and their families need to be educated about their disease. They need to know that SLE is a chronic inflammatory disease that will be with them for life. It waxes and wanes and can affect almost any organ in the body. However, with proper monitoring, treatment, and changes in lifestyle to avoid certain stresses, they can, in general, live a relatively normal life.

   a. Patients should avoid prolonged exposure to sunlight.

   b. Patients should get regular exercise. Participation in strenuous physical activities should be avoided by those with severe disease.

2. Physical therapy should be used in appropriate patients to maintain function and provide rehabilitation.

3. Some patients may benefit from psychological counseling.

B. Medications range from relatively benign NSAIDs to powerful disease-modifying immunomodulatory agents. Choice of medications depends on the severity of symptoms and on major organ involvement.

1. NSAIDs such as aspirin, ibuprofen, and indomethacin are the mainstay of treatment for systemic symptoms without major organ involvement. Indications for use include fatigue, fever, rash, arthralgias, arthritis, pleurisy, and pericarditis. They should be continued even when more powerful drugs are added for control of major organ involvement.

2. Antimalarials are used mainly for rashes of both the systemic (including mild cutaneous vasculitis) and discoid type and can also be beneficial for treatment of arthritis. Chloroquine can be started at 500 mg/day and tapered to 125 to 250 mg/day or every other day after a few weeks. Alternatively, hydroxychloroquine can be used at 200 to 400 mg/day after a few weeks at higher doses.

3. Glucocorticoids can be used in patients with severe systemic symptoms and/or major organ involvement.

   a. Moderate doses (0.5 mg/kg/day) will often result in a response of pericarditis or pleurisy that does not respond o an NSAID (preferably indomethacin) and antimalarials.

   b. Higher doses (1 to 2 mg/kg/day) should be reserved for more severe diseases, including renal, CNS, pulmonary, vasculitis, and severe thrombocytopenia and hemolytic anemia.

   c. Patients should, in general, be started on daily therapy and tapered off or placed on alternate-day therapy after the disease is under control.

   d. There are no hard rules for tapering of glucocorticoids, and every patient is different. Tapering down to levels of 1.0 mg/kg/day should be fairly rapid (over a 1-week period) to avoid toxicity when possible. Tapering down to 0.5 mg/kg/day can be done over 1 month. Complete tapering or tapering to alternate-day therapy may take many months. Flares occur frequently with tapering and often require reinstitution of higher doses for control. Some patients may require chronic low to moderate daily or preferably alternate-day glucocorticoid therapy.

C. Cytotoxic immunosuppressive agents used in SLE include the antimetabolites, methotrexate and azathioprine, and the alkylating agents, cyclophosphamide and chlorambucil. Controlled studies have shown that these drugs are not as effective in general as glucocorticoids in controlling symptomatic, multisystem disease, but they can and should be used as powerful steroid-sparing adjuncts in appropriate patients.

1. Methotrexate (MTX) has been shown to work well in another autoimmune disease, RA. A pilot study of MTX in SLE showed benefit in a majority of patients on the low dose of 7.5 mg/week. Doses of up to 15 mg/week have been used in RA with relative safety. MTX is an attractive drug, due to its steroid-sparing effect and relatively low toxicity, and should be considered as an alternative therapeutic option. Patients need to be monitored for myelosuppression and hepatitis.

2. Azathioprine appears to be less effective than cyclophosphamide in treating SLE but overall is considered safer. It can affect both antibody production and cell-mediated immunity, and it may be especially effective for patients with resistant discoid lupus or for those with glomerulonephritis and minimal scarring on renal biopsy. Doses range from 0.8 to 4.0 mg/kg/day. Patients need to be monitored for myelosuppression and hepatitis. An increased incidence of lymphomas has been reported with long-term use.

3. Chlorambucil at high doses suppresses all bone marrow cell lines, while at doses of 1.0 to 2.0 mg/kg/day it has a greater effect on lymphopoiesis and granulopoiesis. Toxicities include infections, gastrointestinal distress, hepatotoxicities, dermatitis, infertility, leukopenia, thrombocytopenia, and, rarely, irreversible bone marrow suppression. A late complication of increasing concern is leukemia. Chlorambucil should be considered only after other treatment options have failed.

4. Cyclophosphamide is superior in efficacy to azathioprine and at least equal to chlorambucil, with lower toxicity than chlorambucil. It suppresses both cell-mediated and humoral immunity through its effects on both B and T cells. Intravenous bolus therapy every 3 to 4 weeks at doses of 0.5 to 1.0 g/m^2 has been shown to have less toxicity than daily oral therapy at doses of 0.7 to 3 mg/kg/day. The aim of oral therapy is to maintain the granulocyte count at around 1,500/mm^3 or the total white blood cell count at 3,500 to 4,000. Counts may go lower with bolus therapy. Monitoring should be fairly frequent, especially if other drug changes are made. The drug is given in the morning with good hydration to avoid hemorrhagic cystitis. Other toxicities include shingles, other infections, bladder fibrosis, carcinoma, lymphopenia, granulocytopenia, cardiac dysfunction, pulmonary fibrosis, infertility, and inappropriate antidiuretic hormone secretion.

D. Experimental and future therapies

1. Total lymphoid irradiation has a profound, long-lasting immunosuppressive effect. Helper lymphocytes bearing the Leu 3 (T4) marker appear to be most severely affected, resulting in depressed cellular and humoral immunity. Improvement in renal function has been noted after treatment. Patients are at increased risk of infection.

2. Plasmapheresis reduces the amount of circulating inflammatory mediators such as immune complexes and antibodies, which appears to have a beneficial effect on cellular immunity as well. Exchanges of 40 ml/kg with 5% colloidal solution are done several times a week for 2 to 4 weeks. Effects appear to be transient. Immunosuppressive drugs can be given to suppress a rebound from the therapy. Long-term benefit from plasmapheresis in SLE is still questionable.

3. Intravenous immunoglobulin therapy has been shown to result in improvement in a limited number of patients with various collagen vascular diseases, including SLE.

4. Cyclosporin therapy is promising; however, no clinical trials have been reported to date.

E. Treatment of atypical lupus and specific syndromes

1. ANA-negative lupus patients have a high incidence of photosensitive cutaneous involvement (SCLE), arthritis, and Raynaud's syndrome and a lower incidence of renal and CNS involvement. Many patients develop or have autoantibodies to Ro(SS-A) and La(SS-B) and/or a positive latex fixation test. They have prolonged survival compared to ANA-positive patients. Treatment is with NSAIDs and glucocorticoids when needed, as outlined above.

2. End-stage renal disease in SLE patients can be successfully treated with both hemodialysis and peritoneal dialysis, as well as transplantation. SLE patients with acute exacerbations of renal disease can occasionally recover significant function and should therefore be treated aggressively. Patients may also experience a decrease in extrarenal disease activity during dialysis. Overall survival rates of SLE patients on dialysis and posttransplantation are similar to those of patients with end-stage renal failure from other causes.

3. Antiphospholipid antibody syndrome is associated with recurrent abortions and thrombocytopenia. Increased thrombotic episodes including strokes, deep venous thrombosis, and pulmonary embolism, other CNS disease including transient ischemic attacks, atypical migraines, and chorea also occur. Women who have had recurrent abortions and who become pregnant can be treated during pregnancy with high-dose prednisone and aspirin. Recurrent thrombotic events are treated by long-term anticoagulation.

4. Thrombocytopenia may be treated with many different therapies, depending on the severity of the disease and the response to therapy. Therapies include moderate- to high-dose corticosteroids, vinca alkyloids, vincristine and vinblastine, danazol, and high-dose intravenous gamma globulin. Splenectomy should be considered after less aggressive therapy has failed.

5. Significant hemolytic anemia is unusual in SLE, with most anemia being due to chronic disease. When anemia is severe and is due to hemolysis, initial therapy is high-dose steroids. Other therapies include immunosuppressive drugs and/or splenectomy.

6. Pregnancy and the neonatal lupus syndrome in general are treated with corticosteroids. Maternal flares are treated with prednisone, and disease in the fetus is treated with dexa- or betamethasone, which readily crosses the placenta. Mothers may be at increased risk for flares during pregnancy and in the immediate postpartum period. Recurrent abortions have been treated with prednisone and aspirin, as noted above in treating the antiphospholipid antibody syndrome; however, there is no consensus on the optimal treatment at present.

7. Drug-induced lupus can be caused by a variety of drugs (see Section IV,C,4). Treatment usually consists of withdrawing the offending drug. A short course of NSAIDs and/or corticosteroids may be necessary in strongly symptomatic cases.

VII. **Patient Monitoring**

Patients need frequent, regular monitoring to assess disease activity and change therapy. Prompt assessment of any abnormal signs or symptoms is mandatory.

A. Patients need to be educated to participate in monitoring their disease.

B. Regular visits to the doctor should occur at 3- to 6-month intervals.

1. Patients should receive a full general physical examination.

2. Assessment for physical signs and symptoms consistent with active disease, as outlined in Table 96-1, should be done. Subtle signs of disease activity such as fatigue, fever, and weight loss should also be assessed.

3. A laboratory evaluation to look for subclinical disease activity, done during regular visits, should include a complete blood count, chemistry panel, ANA titer, anti-dsDNA titer, complement, and urinanalysis.

C. SLE patients have an increased susceptibility to infections due to derangements in the autoimmune system.

1. Signs of infection should be dealt with immediately, as infection is a leading cause of death in SLE patients.

2. Flares in disease activity may be caused by infections; a documented flare therefore does not rule out the presence of infection. C-reactive protein may be helpful in evaluating infection as (unlike in RA) high levels tend to correlate with the presence of infection.

3. Patients should receive a yearly influenza vaccination and a pneumococcal vaccination. Prophylactic antibiotics have been advocated.by some physicians when patients undergo dental, genitourinary, or other invasive surgeries.

VIII. Prognosis

SLE patients as a group have a greater degree of morbidity and mortality than the general population. Clinical and laboratory factors that can identify a subset of patients at risk for a poor outcome have been identified.

A. Data from the Lupus Survival Study Group on survival in 1,103 SLE patients treated at university centers between 1965 and 1978 show an increased mortality rate.
   1. Survival rates were 96% at 1 year, 93% at 2 years, 86% at 5 years, and 76% at 10 years.
   2. Life expectancy curves level off with time.
   3. Longer survival is correlated with milder disease.
   4. Severe, life-threatening disease activity can occur even late in the disease.

B. Clinical and laboratory factors associated with outcome
   1. Clinical factors associated with a poor outcome include CNS involvement other than seizures during early febrile disease, renal involvement (especially with nephrotic syndrome), major and nonmajor organ involvement, nonresponsiveness to glucocorticoids, flares during tapering of steroids while still at high doses, and patient age of 15 to 30 years.
   2. Laboratory factors associated with a poor outcome include biopsy-proven signifi-

cant involvement of any major organ system, elevated urine protein, elevated serum creatinine, prolonged severe anemia, extremely low complement components, and antibodies to dsDNA and leukocytes. A rim or diffuse ANA pattern has a somewhat poorer prognosis than a speckled pattern.

C. Other factors that affect the prognosis are the expertise of the institution caring for SLE patients and the source of funding for care (socioeconomic).

Bibliography

Ballow M, Parke A. The uses of intravenous immune globulin in collagen vascular disorders. *J Allergy Clin Immunol* 84(4):608–612, 1989.

Euler HH, Gutschmidt HJ, Sachumecking M, et al. Induction of remission in severe SLE after plasma exchange synchronized with subsequent pulse cyclophosphamide. *Prog Clin Biol Res* 337:319–320, 1990.

Ginzler EN, Schorn K. Outcome and prognosis in systemic lupus erythematosus. *Rheum Dis Clin North Am* 14(1):67–78, 1988.

Kelley WN, Harris ED, Ruddy S, et al. *Textbook of Rheumatology*, ed 3. Philadelphia, Saunders, 1989, pp 1077–1146.

Nossent HC, Swaak TJ, Berden JH. Systemic lupus erythematosus: Analysis of disease activity in 55 patients with end-stage renal failure treated with hemodialysis or continuous ambulatory peritoneal dialysis. Dutch Working Party on SLE. *Am J Med* 89(2):169–174, 1990.

Rothenberg RJ, Graziano FM, Grandone JT, et al. The use of methotrexate in steroid-resistant systemic lupus erythematosus. *Arthritis Rheum* 31(5):612–615, 1988.

Rothfield N. Efficacy of antimalarials in systemic lupus erythematosus. *Am J Med* 85(4A):53–56, 1988.

Steinberg AD, Steinberg SC. Long-term preservation of renal function in patients with lupus nephritis receiving treatment that includes cyclophosphamide versus those Arthritis treated with prednisone alone. *Arthritis Rheum* 34(8):945–950, 1991.

Tan EM, Cohen AS, Fries JF, et al. The 1982 revised criteria for the classification of systemic lupus erythematosus. *Arthritis Rheum* 25:1271–1277, 1982.

CHAPTER 97

Scleroderma and Variants

Charlotte A. Harris, M.D.

Scleroderma

I. Definition

A. Systemic sclerosis is a generalized disorder of connective tissue characterized by proliferative and obstructive changes in the microvasculature that lead to intense fibrosis. The skin, blood vessels, synovium, skeletal muscle, gastrointestinal tract, lungs, heart, and kidneys can all be involved. The term *scleroderma* can also be used to describe localized areas of hidebound skin.

B. Classification

1. Diffuse disease
   a. Patients with diffuse disease have more rapidly progressive, widespread skin thickening.
   b. It affects the distal and proximal extremities, as well as the trunk.
   c. The classification criteria define skin involvement proximal to metacarpophalangeal or metatarsophalangeal joints as characteristic of diffuse scleroderma.
   d. Patients with diffuse disease have a higher incidence of visceral disease.

2. Limited disease
   a. Formerly known as *CREST* (calcinosis, Raynaud's syndrome, esophageal dysmotility, sclerodactyly, and telangiectasia).
   b. These patients have skin involvement limited to the distal extremities, fingers, and face.

II. Epidemiology

A. Age of onset is typically 30–60 years. Incidence increases with age.

B. Women outnumber men by a 3–4:1 ratio.

C. Very rare in childhood.

D. Unusual to have two cases of scleroderma in first-degree relatives, but other connective tissue illnesses may occur in family members.

III. Pathophysiology

A. Fibrosis

1. Fibrosis is due to the overproduction of collagen by fibroblasts present in the skin or viscera.
   a. Collagen overproduction is demonstrated by measuring the weight and hydroxyproline contents of skin biopsy specimens.

2. Dysregulation of dermal fibroblasts is also seen when these cells are maintained in tissue culture. Glycosaminoglycan is overproduced in this setting.

3. The process triggering collagen overproduction is the key to understanding the mechanism of this disease.

B. Vascular damage

1. Histology shows that there is vascular damage of medium-sized and small arteries in many organ systems in scleroderma. This has led to the idea that injury to the vascular endothelium is an important factor in causing scleroderma.

2. A serum endothelial cell cytotoxic factor has been described, but it has not been consistently reproducible. Endothelial cell injury leads to platelet aggregation, myointimal cell proliferation, reduction in vessel diameter, and distensibility.

3. In capillaries, which do not have myointimal cells, devascularization can occur. Capillaries can become dilated, and interstitial fibroblasts can be induced to produce collagen by platelet factors that move into the interstitium through damaged capillaries.

C. Immune abnormalities

1. Serologic factors

a. As noted in Section IV,B, multiple serologic abnormalities exist in scleroderma.

b. There is little correlation between the presence or titer of these antibodies and the clinical severity or prognosis.

2. Lymphocytes

a. Early in disease, lymphocytes and plasma cells accumulate in synovium, skin, the gastrointestinal tract, and lung.

b. In the dermis, most of the lymphocytes are T cells.

c. In peripheral blood, the number of T cells is diminished.

IV. **Diagnosis**

A. Raynaud's phenomenon

1. Vasospasm is induced by cold exposure or emotion.

2. This leads to well-demarcated blanching followed by cyanosis. It may be followed by erythema once the vasospasm subsides.

3. Raynaud's phenomenon is generally bilateral and can affect the toes, the ears, and the tip of the nose. There may be infarction of tissue, causing pitting scars or gangrene.

4. Raynaud's phenomenon is present in 95% of cases and can precede other manifestations of scleroderma by many years. It is the initial manifestation in 75% of cases.

B. Skin

1. At the onset of symptoms, patients experience diffuse swelling of the hands and occasionally of the feet. After a period of weeks to months, the puffiness of the fingers is replaced by thickened, firm skin.

2. Skin thickening of more proximal areas such as the forearms, face, and trunk is nearly always diagnostic of scleroderma.

3. Skin shows loss of normal folds and areas of hypo- or hyperpigmentation and develops a shiny appearance.

4. In diffuse disease, skin changes may progress rapidly to involve the upper arms, face, and trunk. Distal thickening is generally more severe than proximal thickening.

5. Patients with limited scleroderma usually have abnormal skin only over the fingers and face. About 5% of scleroderma patients do not have skin disease. This condition has been called *systemic sclerosis sine scleroderma*.

6. Skin biopsy during the phase of induration reveals a marked increase in densely packed collagen fibers in the reticular dermis. Arterioles demonstrate subintimal hyperplasia and hyalinization. T-cell infiltrates are present deep in the dermis.

7. With the passage of time, the skin thickening can resolve. This process usually begins proximally. The skin then becomes atrophic. Thinning of the skin may result in ulcers over contracted joints.

8. Telangiectasias may occur in both the limited and diffuse forms of the disease. They are generally more numerous in patients with limited disease. The most common locations are the fingers, face, lips, and tongue.

9. Calcinosis occurs more frequently in limited scleroderma. Areas of trauma tend to develop calcinosis; these include the fingers, forearms, elbows, and knees.

C. Musculoskeletal system
   1. Muscle is frequently affected in scleroderma.
      a. Inflammatory myositis can be part of scleroderma, with elevated muscle enzymes, an abnormal electromyogram (EMG), and infiltration of mononuclear cells on biopsy. This is identical to the myositis seen in systemic lupus erythematosus, polymyositis, and dermatomyositis.
      b. There is a more chronic type of myopathy seen in scleroderma that is generally not seen in other types of connective tissue illness.
         (1) Onset of weakness is gradual and mild, muscle enzymes are minimally elevated, and EMGs are normal.
         (2) Biopsy shows noninflammatory replacement of muscle cells by fibrosis.
         (3) Glucocorticosteroid therapy is not indicated for this indolent form of myopathy.
   2. Joints and tendons
      a. About 10% of patients with scleroderma present with a symmetrical polyarthritis. It is seronegative and nonerosive. Usually the synovitis subsides as the skin involvement of scleroderma develops. Synovial biopsy shows mononuclear inflammatory cells and, later, fibrosis.
      b. Carpal tunnel syndrome and leathery tendon rubs are manifestations of tenosynovial disease.
         (1) The leathery tendon rubs occur over the extensor and flexor tendons of the fingers, distal forearms, knees, and ankles.
         (2) The tendon rubs are present only in the diffuse form of the disease and are an indicator of more aggressive disease.
         (3) Findings on x-rays are usually restricted to diffuse osteopenia. Distal resorption of phalanges can occur.
D. Gastrointestinal tract: Most patients with scleroderma develop gastrointestinal disease. It is similar in patients with diffuse and limited disease.
   1. Esophagus

      a. Most common site of gastrointestinal disease. Ninety percent of patients with scleroderma have diminished propulsive force of the smooth muscular lining of the lower two-thirds of the esophagus.
      b. About 50% of these patients have clinical symptoms of dysphagia. The best tests for this condition are manometry and cine-esophography. The findings are quite specific for scleroderma and can be diagnostically helpful early in the disease.
      c. Incompetence of the lower esophageal sphincter develops, resulting in gastric reflux. There is a high incidence of peptic esophagitis that can be complicated by stricture or rupture.
      d. Long-standing disease can result in esophageal dilatation.
      e. Disease of the esophagus is caused by replacement of the muscularis with fibrous tissue and by collagen deposition in the lamina propria and submucosa. The myenteric plexi do not appear abnormal histologically. The mucosa of the distal esophagus shows metaplastic changes. This can predispose to adenocarcinoma of the esophagus.
   2. Duodenum
      a. This site can also have fibrosis of musculature, resulting in hypomotility and malabsorption.
      b. This causes symptoms of postprandial bloating and abdominal pain.
   3. Small intestine
      a. The small intestinal muscularis can also be replaced by fibrosis, but this is less common than the more proximal fibrosis, affecting about 20% of patients with diffuse scleroderma.
      b. Malabsorption is due to poor mixing of intestinal contents and overgrowth of bacteria that interfere with fat absorption. Patients present with weight loss, episodes of abdominal distention, pseudo-obstruction, and diarrhea. X-rays reveal small bowel dilatation, and 72-hr fecal fat excretion is increased.
      c. Pneumatosis intestinales is an x-ray finding of diffuse scleroderma. Atrophy of the muscularis allows entry of

air into the wall of the intestine. This condition is generally asymptomatic.

4. Colon: Smooth muscle of the large intestine can also become fibrotic. This results in the formation of sacculations of the intestinal wall. These wide-mouthed diverticula appear on the antimesenteric border of the transverse and descending colons. They are quite specific for scleroderma but are a late finding and thus are not helpful diagnostically.

E. Pulmonary system
1. Pleurisy or pleural effusion can be manifestations of pulmonary scleroderma. These findings are quite rare.
2. Pulmonary hypertension is more frequently seen in limited scleroderma but may also be present in diffuse scleroderma. Pulmonary hypertension may or may not be accompanied by interstitial fibrosis. It can be diagnosed by auscultation, echocardiography, roentgenography, or right heart catheterization. Patients with pulmonary hypertension have subintimal hyperplasia microscopically. The prognosis is very poor even with vasodilator therapy.
3. Diffuse pulmonary fibrosis is present in most patients with scleroderma, and is distributed evenly in both the limited and diffuse forms. Chest x-rays reveal bibasilar linear or nodular scarring, and pulmonary function tests demonstrate depressed vital capacity initially. This is followed by findings of restrictive lung disease. Because activity is limited, many patients do not develop dyspnea until fibrosis becomes severe. Patients with Scl-70 antibodies have a higher incidence of pulmonary fibrosis.

F. Cardiac disease occurs almost exclusively in patients with diffuse scleroderma.
1. Only about 10% have clinical symptoms, but testing using an echocardiogram or thallium exercise testing shows left ventricular dysfunction in a high proportion of patients. Patients with symptoms present with congestive heart failure and ventricular or atrial arrythymias. Pathologic exam reveals patchy myocardial fibrosis.
2. Pericarditis can occur but is not common. Myocarditis also occurs infrequently. It is usually accompanied by inflammatory myopathy of skeletal muscle.

G. Renal system
1. Renal crisis in scleroderma affects only about 10% of patients with diffuse scleroderma. Its onset can be abrupt, presenting with malignant hypertension, hyperreninemia, and hypertensive encephalopathy. It generally occurs early in the disease in a patient with rapidly progressive skin involvement. Patients usually develop rapidly progressive renal insufficiency if not treated. Rarely, blood pressure remains normal; in this case, microangiopathic hemolytic anemia is a feature of the disease. More subtle markers of renal disease, such as proteinuria and hypertension, are present in one-third to one-half of patients.
2. Pathologic findings are localized to arcuate and interlobular arteries and arterioles, where angiography demonstrates constriction accompanied by a marked decrease in cortical blood flow. Internal hyperplasia and fibrinoid necrosis are seen. Inflammatory infiltrates are lacking.

H. Diagnostic tests
1. Routine tests
   a. Anemia
      (1) Iron deficiency may be secondary to gastrointestinal blood loss.
      (2) Patients may develop anemia secondary to renal failure.
      (3) Very rarely, patients can develop hemolytic anemia that is immunologically mediated.
   b. The erythrocyte sedimentation rate is usually normal or mildly elevated.
2. Immunologically related tests
   a. Mild hypergammaglobulinemia due to elevated IgG may occur in over one-third of patients.
   b. From 25% to 30% of patients will have positive rheumatoid factor, usually in low titer.
   c. Nearly all patients have positive antinuclear antibodies (ANA).
      (1) Anticentromere antibodies are quite sensitive and very specific (over 50%) for the limited form of scleroderma. They occur in less than 5% of patients with diffuse scleroderma.
      (2) Anti-Scl-70 is present in about 30% of patients with diffuse scle-

roderma, although it has high specificity. It is directed against the nuclear enzyme topoisomerase, which acts to modify the conformation of DNA.

    d. Anti-PM-Scl is seen in patients who have an overlap between limited scleroderma and polymyositis.

    e. Hypocomplementemia and the presence of anti-DNA are unusual in either form of scleroderma.

V. Differential Diagnosis

When arthritis is a presenting feature of systemic sclerosis and the ANA is positive, scleroderma can be confused with systemic lupus erythematosus. Within a few months, other features of systemic lupus develop or skin tightening of scleroderma occurs and the two diseases can be distinguished. More often the patient will present with Raynaud's phenomenon and arthralgias. It can be difficult to distinguish between early scleroderma and idiopathic Raynaud's phenomenon. Serologic and nailfold capillary exams may be helpful.

VI. Treatment

A. No form of therapy has been shown to be effective in adequately controlled trials.

B. Glucocorticosteroids are useful in the management of myositis and acute pericarditis.

C. Penicillamine has been studied in uncontrolled retrospective studies. The results suggest that penicillamine, when given over prolonged periods, is accompanied by a decrease in skin thickness, a lower rate of new visceral organ involvement, and longer survival.

D. The most effective therapy is the use of inhibitors of the renin-angiotensin system in patients with renal scleroderma. These drugs significantly reduce the morbidity and mortality of scleroderma.

Variants

I. Eosinophilic Fasciitis

A. First described in the mid-1970s.

B. Affects males twice as often as females; age of onset is 30–60 years.

C. Onset frequently follows an episode of heavy exertion.

D. Patients rapidly develop tender swelling of the arms and legs that spares the face,

hands, and feet. Skin becomes indurated and thickened.

E. Raynaud's phenomenon is absent.

F. There is no visceral disease.

G. Laboratory studies reveal negative ANA, eosinophilia, and hypergammaglobulinemia.

H. Biopsy specimens from the epidermis down to the skeletal muscle demonstrate widespread inflammation and intense deposition of collagen in the deep fascia, the subcutis, and, less prominently, in the dermis.

I. Glucocorticoid therapy is helpful initially but may be difficult to taper. About half of these patients develop chronic fibrosis of the skin.

J. Major differences from scleroderma
1. Absence of Raynaud's phenomenon.
2. Nailfold capillaries are normal, whereas 90% of scleroderma patients have abnormalities.
3. Some eosinophilic fasciitis patients develop aplastic anemia.

II. Environmentally Induced Syndromes

A. Toxic oil syndrome
1. In May 1981, an acute illness appeared in Spain, consisting of noncardiogenic pulmonary edema, myalgia, rash, and eosinophilia. Over the next few months, patients developed skin thickening, polyneuropathies, and sicca syndrome. Pathologic exam revealed endothelial injury with an inflammatory infiltrate in the perivascular area. Chronic cases demonstrated fibrosis and atrophy.
2. This syndrome was linked epidemiologically to the use of adulterated toxic rapeseed oil in cooking. It is felt that this oil was a source of oxygen radicals which damaged the endothelium.
3. As in scleroderma, glucocorticoid therapy was helpful in the acute inflammatory phase but not in the chronic phase of the syndrome.

B. Eosinophilia myalgia syndrome
1. In November 1989, a syndrome of eosinophilia myalgia was identified and felt to be related to ingestion of L-tryptophan. L-Tryptophan was withdrawn from the market in the United States.
    a. Case definition
        (1) Eosinophil cell count greater than 1,000/mm^3.
        (2) Generalized myalgia of severity sufficient to affect a patient's abil-

ity to pursue his or her usual daily activities.

  (3) Absence of any infection or neoplasia that could account for factors (1) or (2).

2. The etiology of this syndrome was attributed to a contaminant in one manufacturer's lots of L-tryptophan. This syndrome sometimes overlapped with eosinophilic fasciitis. Visceral involvement also occurred, including pulmonary disease and polyneuropathies.

3. Treatment recommendations were to withdraw L-tryptophan. In mild cases, this may be sufficient; in more severe cases, courses of moderate to high doses of glucocorticoids have been given, depending on disease severity.

III. Localized Scleroderma

A varied group of disorders manifested by linear patches of scleroderma. There are no serologic or visceral signs of disease. This syndrome most frequently appears in young females.

A. Morphea

1. Starts with one or more erythematous patches of skin.

2. Later becomes sclerotic and ivory-colored.

3. Lesions are surrounded by erythematous borders when active and may increase to severe centimeters in diameter.

4. When they become widespread, the condition is called *generalized morphea*.

5. Later, hard skin may soften.

6. Biopsy reveals new collagen deposition in the dermis. This may be accompanied by heavy infiltrates of lymphocytes, plasma cells, and histiocytes.

B. Linear scleroderma

1. These lesions appear as long streaks or bands of thickened skin.

2. Most commonly they present on extremities, but they can occur on the trunk or face.

3. When they are present on the frontoparietal scalp, the condition has been called *en coup de sabre*. It is associated with atrophy of underlying tissue and can result in disfiguring facial asymmetry.

4. If linear scleroderma crosses a joint, it can cause joint contracture.

C. There can be overlap between morphea and linear scleroderma. These conditions may be associated with a peripheral eosinophilia, ANA—especially single-stranded DNA—and a positive rheumatoid factor. No beneficial therapy is known for these disorders.

Bibliography

Jimenez SA, Sigal SH. A 15 year prospective study of rapidly progressive systemic sclerosis with D-penicillamine. *J. Rheumat.* 18:1496–1502, 1991.

Kelley WN, Harris ED Jr, Ruddy S, et al. *Textbook of Rheumatology*, ed 4. Philadelphia, Saunders, 1993, pp 1113–1156.

LeRoy EC, Medsger TA Jr. The specter of scleroderma-related syndromes, in Schumacher HR (ed), *Primer on the Rheumatic Diseases*, ed. 9. Richmond, Va., William Byrd Press, 1988, p 117.

McCarty D. *Arthritis and Allied Conditions: A Textbook of Rheumatology*, ed 11. Philadelphia, Lea & Febiger, 1989, pp 1118–1165.

Seibold JR. Scleroderma, in Kelley WN, Harris ED Jr, Ruddy S, et al (eds), *Textbook of Rheumatology*, ed 3. Philadelphia, Saunders, 1989, p 1215.

Steen VD, Costantino VP, Shapiro AP. Crises in Systemic Sclerosis: Relation to angiotensin converting enzyme (ACE) inhibitors *AIM* 113:352–357, 1990.

Tiffanelli DL. Systemic scleroderma. *Med Clin North Am* 73(5):1167–1180, 1989.

Chapter 98

Polymyositis/Dermatomyositis

Thomas J. Schnitzer, M.D.

I. **Definition**

Polymyositis (PM) encompasses a group of inflammatory diseases of muscle. When the skin is also involved, this is called *dermatomyositis* (*DM*). Most cases are idiopathic, while others are associated with malignancy, other connective tissue disorders, and, rarely, infection. Childhood PM/DM has features distinct from those of adult-onset disease.

II. **Etiology**

PM/DM is believed to have an immunologic basis. The factor(s) precipitating the disease are unknown. Preceding viral infections, particularly with enteroviruses (e.g., coxsackievirus), have been implicated as a possible trigger of the immune response, especially in childhood disease.

III. **Pathophysiology**

The weakness seen in PM/DM is due to muscle destruction.

A. T cells are the predominant effector cell seen in inflammatory infiltrates in affected muscle.

B. Skeletal muscle is the primary target. Regenerating and atrophic fibers are seen.

C. Vasculitis is seen only in childhood PM/DM or in association with other connective tissue diseases.

IV. **Diagnosis**

A. There is a history of progressive muscle weakness.

1. Usual onset occurs over 3–6 months, occasionally acute and then often associated with myoglobinuria.

2. Difficulty is noted in climbing stairs, getting out of chairs or bathtub, lifting heavy objects overhead, or combing hair.

3. Gait may become clumsy, with a tendency to be unsteady and fall.

B. Major physical finding is objective weakness on formal strength testing.

1. Proximal muscles specifically are weak.

2. Distal muscles are rarely affected.

3. There is symmetrical distribution and diffuse involvement, unlike the pattern in specific myopathies.

4. Neck and paraspinal muscles are commonly involved.

C. Laboratory data confirm the diagnosis.

1. Creatinine phosphokinase (CPK) elevated in 95% of cases, and the level reflects disease activity.

2. Electromyography (EMG) should be done in the clinically involved (weak) muscle group.
   a. Insertional activity with fibrillation potentials and positive sharp waves at rest.
   b. Motor unit potentials show decreased amplitude and an increased proportion of polyphasic potentials.
   c. Increased irritability.
3. Biopsy should be done of clinically involved muscle but not at the site of prior EMG.
   a. Inflammatory infiltrate of predominantly T lymphocytes and monocytes is seen.
   b. Degenerating and regenerating muscle fibers; fiber size variation is present.
   c. Electron microscopy (EM) should be done to differentiate inclusion body myositis.

V. Differential Diagnosis
A. Neuromuscular diseases—numerous types.
B. Myopathies.
C. Endocrine myopathies: thyroid, pituitary, parathyroid.
D. Metabolic myopathies: uremia, hepatic failure, K^+ levels.
E. Toxic myopathies: alcohol, drugs.
F. Carcinoma-related myopathies.
G. Polymyalgia rheumatica.
H. Other connective tissue diseases.
I. Infections.
J. Inclusion body myositis.

VI. Treatment
A. Initial therapy consists of high-dose steroids (1 mg/kg) for 3–6 months as a minimum.
B. Add immunosuppressive/cytotoxic agents if no improvement occurs on prednisone alone.
C. Prednisone should be tapered *gradually* to 20 mg/day, which should be maintained for at least 1 year, then tapered even more slowly over another 1–2 years.
D. Non-steroidal anti-inflammatory drugs are of little or no benefit.

VII. Patient Monitoring
A. Clinical measure of strength is the most important parameter to follow.
B. CPK level reflects extent of muscle destruction and should be evaluated regularly; erythrocyte sedimentation rate is less helpful.

VIII. Prognosis
A. Patients with malignancy-associated disease have the poorest prognosis.
B. Overall survival is approximately 95% at 1 year, 85% at 2 years, and 80% at 5 years, though some series report significantly lower survival figures.
C. Complete remission is uncommon and occurs only after several years of therapy.

Bibliography

Bohan A, Peter JB, Bowman RL, et al. A computer-assisted analysis of 153 patients with polymyositis and dermatomyositis. *Medicine* 56:255, 1977.

DeVere R, Bradley WG. Polymyositis: Its presentations, morbidity and mortality. *Brain* 98:637, 1975.

Hochberg MC, Feldman D, Stevens MD. Adult onset polymyositis/dermatomyositis: An analysis of clinical and laboratory features and survival in 76 patients with a review of the literature. *Semin Arthritis Rheum* 15:168, 1986.

CHAPTER 99

Vasculitis

Lawrence Layfer, M.D.

Vasculitis consists of inflammation of blood vessels, encompassing a wide spectrum of illnesses, with symptoms and severity dependent on the type, size and location of affected vessels. Inflammation is often, but not always, due to an antigen–antibody reaction, with the inciting antigen varying in each illness. Classification systems are imperfect, often based on a combination of blood vessel size, pathology, and/or clinical features.

Small Vessel/Hypersensitivity Vasculitis

Leukocytoclastic Vasculitis

I. **Definition**
   Small vessel vasculitis caused by immune complex deposition, usually in response to some external antigen, with predominantly skin manifestations. Serum sickness reaction is the prototype of this category of vasculitis.
II. **Pathology and Pathophysiology**
   A. Inflammation of small skin vessels, usually postcapillary venules, by polymorph infiltration, causing destruction of vessel walls with extravasation of red blood cells (RBCs), lead-

ing to typical red, raised, purpural lesions. Destruction of polys leads to "nuclear dust," defining the term *leukocytocytoclastic* vasculitis.
   B. Caused by antibody–antigen reaction with complement, depositing in vessel walls, attracting polymorphs and inflammatory mediators. Multiple antigens may precipitate a reaction, including drugs (penicillin, sulfa, others), infections (streptococcus, hepatitis, subacute bacterial endocarditis [SBE]), or inflammatory illnesses (systemic lupus erythematosus [SLE], rheumatoid arthritis [RA], Sjögren's syndrome). Other illnesses with immune complexes (carcinoma, cryoglobulinemia), and other inflammatory illnesses (chronic active hepatitis, primary biliary cirrhosis, inflammatory bowel diseases) may cause similar lesions.
III. **Clinical Description**
   A. Skin manifestations: Skin lesions are usually found on the lower extremity, often in crops in the same stage of development. Involvement of buttocks and mucous membranes occurs. Palpable purpura, macular/papular lesions, and erythema multiforme are the most common types of lesions. Healing often

occurs with hyperpigmentation. Vesicle formation or ulceration of lesions occasionally occurs. Pain and edema are often noted in association with lesions.

B. Other organ involvement: Disease may occur in sites other than the skin and needs to be looked for: arthritis or arthralgias; gastrointestinal (GI) symptoms, often manifest as abdominal pain or melena; peripheral neuropathy; renal involvement from glomerulonephritis, often with hematuria; and, more rarely, other organs. Constitutional symptoms such as fever, malaise, or lassitude may occur.

IV. Diagnosis

Diagnosis is based on the typical clinical presentation and on biopsy of the skin lesion. An attempt should be made to categorize the type of vasculitis by antigen or by clinical circumstances, as noted in Section II.

V. Treatment

The offending antigen should be removed where possible. Often such illnesses are self-limited. Drug treatment depends on whether the illness is self-limited or persistent, systemic or local, life-threatening or only annoying. Mild, limited illness may be treated with nonsteroidal anti-inflammatory drugs (NSAIDs) or acetylsalicylic acid (ASA). Colchicine, dapsone, or hydroxychoroquine may be used for more resistant illness, as may short courses of prednisone. Long-term prednisone or cytotoxic/immunosuppressive medication should be reserved for life-threatening illness.

Other Hypersensitivity/Small Vessel Vasculitides

I. Henoch-Schönlein Syndrome

A. Triad of purpura, glomerulonephritis with hematuria, and abdominal pain with melena, most commonly seen in children. Arthralgias may occur. Springtime seems to be the favored season. Precipitating event is unknown, perhaps viral.

B. Skin lesions, often purpuric, are located on the lower extremities or on the buttock and arms. Lesions may ulcerate. Arthralgia or arthritis, usually affecting the knees and ankles, or GI lesions causing pain, bleeding, intussusception, protein loss, or perforation, are common. Diffuse edema may occur. Glomerulonephritis occurs with segmental necrotizing lesions associated with hematuria, casts, and proteinuria.

C. IgA and complement are usually found in blood vessels. Illness is often self-limited. Prednisone treatment may be helpful. Some chronic renal lesions may occur. Adults often have a more severe course than children.

II. Mixed Cryoglobulinemia

A. Cyroglobulins represent immune complexes which precipitate in the cold. Damage occurs through deposition of complexes in vessel walls, with subsequent complement fixation and vessel wall damage. The size of the vessel involved determines the symptoms: postcapillary venule involvement resembles hypersensitivity vasculitis, whereas muscular artery involvement resembles polyarteritis nodosa. Disease severity may vary from recurrent benign lower extremity petechiae to life-threatening organ system infarction or chronic glomerulonephritis. Treatment depends on the severity of the illness.

B. Cryoglobulins contain antigens of IgG, IgA, or IgM molecules, with other IgG or IgM molecules serving as antibodies to the antigen-immunoglobulin. Such anti-antibody antibodies have rheumatoid factor activity. Monoclonal-producing illnesses like myeloma often create cryoglobulins, as do infectious illnesses like hepatitis B or SBE, and autoimmune illnesses like SLE.

III. Hypocomplementemic Vasculitis

Urticaria associated with hypocomplementemia, often in episodes, with biopsy specimens showing necrotizing vasculitis. Lesions occur most commonly on the face, trunk, or upper extremity. They last for 24–48 hr and fade centrally. Purpura and vesicles may be seen. Fever, joint pain, arthritis or abdominal symptoms, and renal disease may occur.

IV. Overlap with Autoimmune Illnesses

RA, SLE, Sjögren's syndrome, mixed connective tissue disease (MCTD), or other similar illnesses may be associated with either hypersensitivity vasculitis or polyarteritis-type lesions. Diagnosis is made by the presence of other features of the underlying autoimmune illness with appropriate autoantibodies.

V. Panniculitis

Inflammation in venules (septal) or arterioles (lobar) of subcutaneous fat leads to skin lesions with or without systemic signs. Two classes of illness occur, depending on the type of vessel involved.

A. Septal (venule) involvement: Venule inflammation causes a syndrome of erythema nodosum, consisting of subcutaneous red, tender nodules, occasionally fluctuant. The size is usually 0.5 to 2.5 cm over the pretibial area; rarely, nodules occur in the upper extremity. Causes include idiopathic, infections (streptococcus, tuberculosis, fungi, other), drugs (sulfa, BCP), or diseases like Crohn's disease, Bechet's disease, or sarcoid (usually the Lofgren's syndrome variant, consisting of bilateral hilar adenopathy, ankle synovitis, and erythema nodosum). Biopsy may not be needed when the clinical picture is typical. Treatment is with NSAIDs and removal of the offending agent. Rarely, more severe or persistant illness is treated by corticosteroids or other drugs like hydroxychloroquine.

B. Arterial (lobar) involvement: Lobar involvement is often more disseminated in its location, located on both upper and lower extremities as well as the trunk, and often with larger lesions. Look for underlying illness like pancreatitis or pancreatic cancer. SLE may be associated with such lesions (lupus profundus). An idiopathic type (Weber-Christian syndrome) may occur. Erythema induration consists of a more granulomatous type vasculitis, usually confined to skin.

Vasculitides of Small and Medium-Sized Muscular Arteries

Polyarteritis Nodosa

I. Definition

Illness or inflammatory destruction of muscular arteries leading to dysfunction and/or destruction of multiple organs, including most commonly the gut, kidney, and nerve. The illness is frequently associated with severe constitutional symptoms, especially fever, and may exist by itself or be part of an underlying infectious or inflammatory illness.

II. Pathology and Pathogenesis

A. Inflammatory vasculitis of medium-sized and small muscular arteries is caused by immune complex deposition in the artery wall, with subsequent complement attachment and activation of immune mechanisms of destruction. This is best seen in hepatitis B, where immune complexes containing viral antigen and antiviral antibody, as well as complement, can be seen in serum as well as blood vessel walls, associated with blood vessel destruction.

B. Lesions are seen in all stages: active, scarred, and healed. Organ damage is caused by ob-

struction of the vessel, with ischemia/infarction to the underlying organ or aneurysm formation with subsequent rupture of the vessel.

C. The underlying antigen of the illness should be sought. Polyarteritis may be part of many systemic autoimmune illnesses, may overlap with small vessel vasculitis, or may exist as an illness on its own. Illnesses that should be sought include hepatitis B and C, cryoglobulinemia, autoimmune illness (SLE, RA, Sjögren's syndrome), or carcinoma (hairy cell leukemia). Idiopathic disease is the most common cause.

III. Clinical Presentation

A. Systemic symptoms: weight loss, fever, malaise, and fatigue.

B. Organ system involvement
   1. Renal: 80% glomerulonephritis from focal segmental necrosis, intrarenal arterial narrowing with hypertension, and/or infarction.
   2. Neurological
      a. Peripheral nerve: 50% mononeuritis multiplex with wrist or foot drop, stocking/glove neuropathy.
      b. Central nervous system: 25% CVA, seizure, confusion, myelopathy.
   3. Gastrointestinal: 30% organ infarct—bowel, liver, spleen, or occasionally gallbladder and appendix. Cramps and melena may be seen.
   4. Skin: 50% purpura, nodules, infarcts with ulcers, livido reticularis.
   5. Heart: 30% myocardial infarction, pericarditis, congestive heart failure.
   6. Joints: 50% arthralgia, arthritis.

IV. Diagnosis

A. Diagnosis is made by a consistent clinical picture associated with evidence of abnormal vessels. Such proof is available in two ways: by biopsy of available tissue (muscle, renal, sural nerve, testes), showing typical inflammatory changes (see above), or by angiography (celiac, mesenteric, renal, cerebral), showing the typical beading pattern of alternating aneurysm and scarring. Anti-neutrophilic cytoplasmic antibodies (ANCA) may be positive.

B. Necessary to rule out conditions that mimic the syndrome: atrial myxoma, cholesterol emboli, SLE.

V. Treatment

Treatment is aimed at improving the poor prognosis documented in the literature. High-doses of prednisone at levels of 40–60 mg/day are appropriate and have been shown to increase 5-year survival from 10% in untreated patients to 50–60%. Higher daily doses or pulse steroids may be appropriate in life-threatening situations. Cytotoxic drugs like cytoxan should be considered if failure to achieve an adequate response or failure to taper steroids to acceptable doses occurs. Monitoring for side effects of steroids, as listed in Chapter 117, must be done.

Other Vasculitides of Small and Medium-Sized Muscular Arteries

I. **Churg-Strauss Disease**
Systemic vasculitis similar to polyarteritis associated with allergic rhinitis, asthma, and pulmonary infiltrates that may be migratory. Peripheral eosinophilia and elevated IgE titers are seen, as are extravascular granulomas and eosinphilic infiltrates. Differential diagnosis includes sarcoid, Wegener's granulomatosis, eosinophilic pneumonias, and bronchopulmonary aspergillosis. Other aspects of clinical illness, evaluation, and therapy are similar to those of periarteritis nodosa.

II. **Kawasaki Disease**
Also called the *mucocutaneous lymph node syndrome*. Characteristics are an acute febrile illness, usually occurring in children 5 years of age and under, with mucous membrane redness, conjunctivitis, erythema, and vesicle formation of skin on the trunk and extremities, associated with adenopathy. Pancarditis may occur. Coronary vasculitis is seen with aneurysm formation in up to 60% of patients by angiography. Lesions smaller than 8 mm usually heal spontaneously, with resolution of illness in 4–6 weeks. Larger lesions may persist. Therapy with ASA or gamma globulin may be useful. Steroids are thought to increase aneurysm formation.

III. **Cogan's Syndrome**
Triad of audiovestibular signs, ophthalmic nonsyphilitic interstitial keratitis, and arthralgia. Ten percent of patients have vasculitis of the skin, nervous system, viscera, or kidney. Aortitis with aortic valve insufficiency may occur, as may systemic symtoms. Males and females are equally affected. The average age at presentation is 25 years. Treatment with steroids or cytotoxic agents may be needed.

IV. **Buerger's Disease**
This disease, also called *thromboangiitis obliterans*, is an inflammatory illness of small and medium-sized arteries and veins leading to arterial obstructive signs of claudication, ulceration, gangrene, pulselessness, and Raynaud's syndrome in distal extremities. [Superficial venous thrombophlebitis occurs.] Most patients are males with a strong smoking history. The history, as well as angiography or Doppler exam, is usually diagnostic. The best treatment consists of cessation of smoking, although vasodilatory drugs or sympathectomy may help.

V. **Isolated CNS Vasculitis**
Diffuse CNS vasculitis of parenchymal and leptomeningeal arteries is seen on angiogram or biopsy. It is most common in men of middle age, presenting with headache, confusion, obtundation, and focal signs or seizures. Fever and hypertension may occur. In elderly women, Sjögren's syndrome may be present. Abnormalities of the electroencephalogram (EEG) and cerebrospinal fluid (CSF) are noted. Treatment with high-dose prednisone, with or without cytotoxic agents, is appropriate.

VI. **Postzoster Vasculitis**
Ipsilateral granulomatous angiitis of CNS arteries of the middle cerebral branches 1–2 weeks following an episode of herpes zoster opthalmicus. Contralateral hemiplegia or cranial nerve abnormalities result. Elevated erythrocyte sedimentation rate (ESR) rate with focal abnormalities on EEG and CSF pleocytosis and elevated protein occur. Angiography reveals typical irregularity and beading. No systemic disease is seen. Vasculitis is thought to be secondary to direct viral invasion of vessel walls, with a subsequent granulomatous reaction.

Granulomatous (Wegener's) Vasculitis

I. **Definition**
Systemic granulomatous vasculitis involving the facial sinuses, upper and lower airways, and renal glomeruli.

II. **Pathology and Pathophysiology**
The hallmark of Wegener's vasculitis is necrotizing granulomatous lesions of the upper and lower respiratory tracts. Focal necrotizing vasculitis of small arteries and veins in multiple organs is also noted. Focal necrotizing glomerulonephritis is commonly noted on renal biopsy. Diffuse prolif-

erative lesions with crescent formation, as well as interstitial nephritis and renal vasculitis, may be seen.

III. Clinical Presentation

A. General
1. Occurs from 8 to 80 years of age.
2. Mean age of presentation is 45 years. Male patients outnumber females.

B. Upper airway: Sinusitis, rhinitis, nasal mucosal ulceration, serous otitis from eustachian tube involvement with hearing loss. Bony destruction may occur, with saddle nose deformity. Secondary bacterial sinusitis is common. Inflammation of the trachea or bronchi occurs, with resultant stenosis in 55%.

C. Lower airway: 90% have lung involvement, with pulmonary infiltrates which often cavitate. Cough, dyspnea, and hemoptysis may occur. Pleural effusions may be seen.

D. Renal: 85% have focal glomerulonephritis, often with crescent formation. Granulomas not seen. Urine may show protein, red blood cells, or casts.

E. Other conditions: Joint pain and mild inflammation in 50%. Eye inflammation in 50% with iritis and uveitis. CNS involvement in 20%; peripheral neuropathies may occur. Skin lesions in 50% include purpura and nodular ulcers.

F. Laboratory tests: Anemia, leukocytosis, ESR elevation, and normal complement levels with occasional immune complexes may be seen. Antinuclear antibodies (ANA) are negative but rheumatoid factor (RF) is often present. Antineutrophilic cytoplasmic antibodies (ANCA) are seen in 90%, with elevations during active illness and decreased levels with remission.

IV. Diagnosis

The diagnosis should be suspected in patients with systemic illness and sinusitis, upper airway ulcerations, cavitary or noncavitary lung infiltrates, and renal sediment abnormalities. Confirmation is made by biopsy and by the presence of typical antibodies (ANCA). Consider other granulomatous illnesses (sarcoid, lymphoma, Churg-Strauss syndrome, and lethal midline granuloma).

V. Treatment

High-dose prednisone (60 mg/day) must be supplemented with cytoxan therapy, 2–3 mg/kg/day, as prednisone alone has failed to significantly impact mortality of 90% 2-year survival, while cytoxan has made survival the rule. Trimethoprim-sulfamethonasole has been used for milder disease, and azathioprine or other alkylating agents have been used in cytoxan failures or complications. ANCA may prove to be an effective means of documenting remission or predicting exacerbation.

Vasculitis of Large Arteries

Takayasu's Arteritis

I. Definition

Large vessel granulomatous vasculitis involving the aortic arch and its branches, usually at their origins, leading to ischemic symptoms and signs, most commonly in the extremities.

II. Pathology and Pathophysiology

A. Lymphocytes, plasma cells, and, more rarely, polymorphs or giant cells may be noted. Early on, most disease is found in the adventitia, but panarteritis may develop. Later, thrombosis or fibrosis with scar formation and narrowing may occur. Aneurysms or dissections may result.

B. The etiology remains unknown. Racial and certain human leukocyte antigen associations suggest that genetics plays some role.

III. Clinical Presentation

A. Patients are usually female and often Oriental, although males and Caucasions may develop the illness.

B. Symptoms reflect large vessel involvement (iliac, femoral, subclavian, or brachial), with pulselessness, claudication, ischemia, and Raynaud's phenomenon in the extremities. Bruits are a common physical finding. Carotid involvement leads to cardiovascular accident–type symptoms. Renal artery involvement leads to hypertension. Aortitis may lead to aortic valve incompetence or aortic dissection. Mesenteric, coronary, pulmonary, or other large arteries may become involved.

C. Systemic symptoms such as fever, weight loss, myalgia, arthralgia, and nondeforming arthritis may also occur.

D. Elevated ESR and nonspecific inflammatory indicators, as well as anemia, are common. Because biopsies of large vessels are difficult to obtain, arch angiography is used to visualize narrowings of arch vessels.

IV. Diagnosis

Recognition of clinical symptoms, as well as laboratory and angiographic confirmation, leads to the diagnosis. One or a few lesions noted on the angiogram may be confused with atherosclerosis (especially in the presence of hypertension) or other vascular abnormalities.

V. Treatment

Prednisone, in doses of 40–60 mg/day, will suppress inflammation and results in a 5-year survival rate of 90% or more. After the inflammatory phase, replacement of stenotic arterial segments may be needed to restore blood flow. The ESR is an accurate predictor of activity or remission.

Giant Cell Arteritis (see Chapter 117)

Bibliography

Conn DL (ed). *Rheumatic Disease Clinics of North America*, Vol 16, No 2: *Vasculitis*. Philadelphia, Saunders, 1990, pp 251–497.

Conn DL. Vasculitis and related disorders, in Kelly WN, Harris ED, Ruddy S, et al (eds), *Textbook of Rheumatology*, ed 3. Philadelphia, Saunders, 1989, p 1167.

CHAPTER 100

Relapsing Polychondritis

Joel A. Block, M.D.

I. **Definition**
   A. Relapsing polychondritis (RP) is a progressive systemic disease consisting of relatively quiescent periods which are punctuated by episodes of inflammatory involvement of cartilage-containing structures, frequently accompanied by involvement of the sense organs and the cardiovascular system.
   B. The absence of a known etiologic agent or mechanism renders the definition of the disease imprecise.

II. **Etiology and Pathophysiology**
   A. The etiology of RP is obscure. No pathogenic source which would explain the constellation of symptoms and signs has been identified.
   B. Evidence suggests that RP is an autoimmune disease, either triggered by an abnormal response to cartilage-related antigens or due to cross-reactivity of unrelated antigens with epitopes present on cartilage.
      1. Pathologically, involved sites demonstrate a lymphocytic and plasma cell infiltration in addition to depletion of cartilage matrix components. The ultimate result is chondrocyte death and fibrosis.
      2. Antibodies against cartilage and cartilage components (e.g., type II collagen) have been described in the sera of affected patients, although no currently identifiable antibody is either specific or sensitive for RP.
      3. Circulating immune complexes, as well as immune complex deposition at involved sites, are typically identified and likely play a role in the pathophysiology of the disease.
      4. Autosensitization to cartilage components has been described.

III. **Diagnosis**
   As with many systemic inflammatory diseases, there are no specific signs or tests which are pathognomonic for RP, and the diagnosis is usually made on clinical grounds.
   A. Clinical features
      1. Epidemiology: Predominantly Caucasian; no apparent familial tendency; affects males as commonly as females; affects persons of all ages, but more than half of all reported cases had onset between the ages of 40 and 60 years.

2. Presenting symptoms: Typically, the patient experiences sudden onset of pain, tenderness, and erythematous swelling of cartilaginous structures, most commonly one or both pinnae. If untreated, early flares generally last several days to several weeks prior to subsiding spontaneously.

3. Organ involvement during the disease course
   a. Ears
      (1) Pinnae: Recurrent and chronic inflammatory episodes result in loss of cartilage and drooping of ears; involved in approximately 90% of cases during the course of disease.
      (2) Internal ears: Both *conductive* hearing losses from collapse of the external auditory canal and middle ear inflammation and *neurosensory* losses due to vasculitis of auditory and vestibular nerves occur.
   b. Arthropathy: Joint involvement, including both transient arthralgias and inflammatory arthritis, is the second most common manifestation of symptomatic disease.
      (1) Classically, there is an asymmetric, episodic, nondeforming arthritis which responds to nonsteroidal anti-inflammatory drugs (NSAIDs).
      (2) Occasionally, spondylitis, tenosynovitis, and costochondritis are associated.
      (3) Noninflammatory effusions may be seen.
   c. Nose: Nasal chondritis is seen in the majority of cases during the course of disease. Recurrent inflammation results in a saddle-nose deformity.
   d. Laryngotracheal/bronchial involvement: Occurs in approximately half of patients during the course of their disease and tends to be a poor prognostic sign.
      (1) Symptoms: Hoarseness, nonproductive cough, dyspnea, aphonia.
      (2) Signs: Tenderness over thyroid cartilage and anterior trachea, stridor.
      (3) Loss of tracheal structure requires a tracheostomy. If the lesion is intrathoracic, a tracheostomy will be ineffective.

   e. Ocular involvement: Approximately half of affected patients will have eye involvement during their disease course. This may include uveitis, conjunctivitis, scleritis/episcleritis, and sicca syndrome.
   f. Cardiovascular system: Frequent complications include aortic valve insufficiency due to dilation of the aortic ring or destruction of the valve cusps, aneurysms of large arteries, pericarditis, myocarditis, and inflammatory endocarditis.
   g. Cutaneous: There are no specific dermal findings. However, associations include leukocytoclastic vasculitis, livedo reticularis, and erythema nodosum.

B. Laboratory evaluation: There are no laboratory tests which are diagnostic for RP. Rather, the laboratory evaluation is typically consistent with a nonspecific systemic inflammatory process.
   1. Blood tests
      a. The erythrocyte sedimentation rate is usually abnormal; the degree of elevation is roughly in proportion to disease activity.
      b. Anemia of chronic disease is typical.
      c. Leukocytosis is mild to moderate, including occasional eosinophilia.
      d. Rheumatoid factor and antinuclear antibody (ANA) may be positive.
      e. Circulating immune complexes (e.g., C1q and Raji cells) are often present.
      f. Complement is usually normal.
      g. Anti–type II collagen and anti-cartilage antibodies are unpredictable and nonspecific.
   2. Urine: There are reports of elevated urinary glycosaminoglycan levels in patients with active RP.
   3. Radiographic evaluation: Cartilage is radiolucent. Therefore, routine radiographic exams are most useful in diagnosing complications of the disease (e.g., pneumonia and atelectasis).
      a. Computed tomography is helpful in demonstrating tracheobronchial collapse and destruction.
      b. Gallium scintigraphy may demonstrate bronchial inflammation.
      c. Magnetic resonance imaging has not been extensively studied in RP but has

proven useful in imaging cartilaginous structures.

4. Pathology: Biopsy of involved sites is usually not necessary for diagnosis. When performed, patchy inflammatory infiltrates are seen; granulation tissue with fibrosis replacing cartilage occurs in destructive disease.

C. Coexistent diseases: As with all autoimmune diseases, there is occasional association and overlap with other inflammatory diseases.

1. Rheumatologic diseases: RP has been reported in association with rheumatoid arthritis, lupus erythematosus, seronegative spondylarthropathies, scleroderma, and the vasculitides.

2. Thyroid disease, including Graves' disease, Hashimoto's thyroiditis, and myxedema, has been reported in association with RP.

3. Rarely, RP has been seen in association with inflammatory bowel disease, myeloproliferative diseases, and primary biliary cirrhosis.

4. MAGIC syndrome: An overlap of RP and Behçet's disease has been termed the "*Mouth And Genital Ulcers with Inflamed Cartilage*" syndrome.

D. Proposed diagnostic criteria: McAdam et al. have proposed the following as diagnostic criteria for RP. For definite RP, three or more of the clinical features must be present.

1. Bilateral auricular chondritis
2. Nonerosive, seronegative inflammatory polyarthritis
3. Nasal chondritis
4. Ocular inflammation
5. Respiratory tract chondritis
6. Auditory and/or vestibular dysfunction

IV. Differential Diagnosis

A. Infectious: Inflammation of the auricular or nasal cartilage needs to be distinguished from pyogenic cellulitis; in populations at risk, leprosy and syphilis need to be excluded.

B. Inflammatory: Wegener's granulomatosis commonly affects the nasal and paranasal regions, and polyarteritis variants may mimic some of the features of RP. The arthropathy may be confused with rheumatoid arthritis early in the disease course. The ocular involvement may be confused with the seronegative spondylarthropathies, Behçet's disease, and sarcoidosis.

C. Traumatic: Auricular trauma, cold-induced injury, and hematomas may mimic early RP.

V. Treatment

A. Medications

1. NSAIDs, including aspirin, effectively suppress the inflammatory response and are the mainstay of therapy in mild or early disease.

2. Steroids (e.g., prednisone at a dose of 0.5–1.0 mg/kg) are effective in controlling more severe exacerbations and may diminish the frequency of flares, although they probably do not alter the natural history of the disease. Tapering needs to be individualized, but it should be as expeditious as possible consistent with preventing a flare. Most patients will require continuous low-dose prednisone.

3. Dapsone has been used commonly in an attempt to control the inflammatory component of RP. Although data to support its efficacy are scanty, anecdotal reports suggest that it may be helpful.

4. Cyclophosphamide, azathioprine, cyclosporin A, and methotrexate have all been tried in refractory cases, with mixed results.

B. Supportive measures

1. Tracheostomy needs to be considered early in the course of tracheobronchial involvement.

2. Valve replacement is needed for severe valvular involvement; aneurysm repair should be done when indicated.

3. Surgical reconstruction after nasal involvement is felt to exacerbate rather than palliate the disease and is not generally recommended.

VI. Prognosis

A. Both the course and the severity of RP are variable. Thus, for an individual patient, the prognosis remains obscure. Michet et al. reported a median survival of 11 years from the time of diagnosis.

B. The classical course consists of episodic flares which resolve over time; however, chronic low-grade disease, as well as acute fulminant disease, are frequently seen.

C. Complications

1. Major complications include infection, airway collapse, dissecting aneurysm, and congestive heart failure.

2. Cosmetic problems include saddle nose and floppy ears.

Bibliography

Arkin CR, Masi AT. Relapsing polychondritis: Review of current status and case report. *Semin Arthritis Rheum* 5:41–61, 1975.

Herman JH. Polychondritis, in Kelley WN, Harris ED, Ruddy S et al (eds), *Textbook of Rheumatology*, ed 4. Philadelphia, Saunders, 1993, pp 1400–1411.

Hoang-Xuan T, Foster CS, Rice BA. Scleritis in relapsing polychondritis. Response to therapy. *Ophthalmologica* 97:892–898, 1990.

McAdam LP, O'Hanlan MA, Bluestone R, et al. Relapsing polychondritis: Prospective study of 23 patients and a review of the literature. *Medicine* 55:193–215, 1976.

Michet CJ, McKenna CH, Luthra HS, et al. Relapsing polychondritis. Survival and predictive role of early disease manifestations. *Ann Intern Med* 104:74–78, 1986.

Orme RL, Nordlund JJ, Barich L, et al. The MAGIC syndrome (mouth and genital ulcers with inflamed cartilage). *Arch Dermatol* 126:940–944, 1990.

Chapter 101

Ankylosing Spondylitis

Robert Katz, M.D.

I. **Definition**
   A. Ankylosing spondylitis is an inflammatory disease of the spine. It begins in the sacroiliac joints and may or may not progress upward to the lumbar spine and other areas of the spine.
   B. Enthesopathy: An enthesis is the area where ligament or tendon attaches to bone. This is a common area of inflammation and, later, bony proliferation in patients with ankylosing spondylitis.
   C. Spondylitis occurs in ankylosing spondylitis and also may occur in association with psoriasis, Reiter's syndrome, and inflammatory bone disease.

II. **Etiology**
   A. Genetic factors: Approximately 90% of U.S. Caucasians with ankylosing spondylitis test positive for the human leukocyte antigen (HLA)-B27 gene compared to an 8% prevalence of this gene in the general population. The gene expresses itself as an HLA-B27 antigen detectable on the surfaces of all nucleated cells in the body.
   B. Environmental factors: There is probably a still unidentified environmental factor which can trigger the onset of ankylosing spondylitis in susceptible individuals. Some have suggested *Klebsiella* as a possible etiologic agent, but convincing evidence is lacking. Certain amino acid sequences are similar in *Klebsiella* and the HLA-B27 antigen.

III. **Pathophysiology**
   A. Peripheral arthritis: ankylosing spondylitis is associated with an asymmetrical inflammatory arthritis of peripheral joints, particularly those in the lower extremities. Inflammation can occasionally lead to loss of cartilage and joint damage and also to bony proliferative changes, reducing range of motion.
   B. Enthesopathy in spondylitis: Initially, inflammatory changes can occur at the enthesis and also over the anterior portion of the annulus fibrosus of the intervertebral disks. Later, bony proliferative change may occur, bony spurs over the enthesis and in the spine, and bony syndesmophytes bridging vertebral bodies. When severe, these syndesmophytes may produce an inflexible "bamboo" spine.
   C. Interaction between genetic and environmental factors: It is possible that the HLA-

B27 antigen acts as a site of fixation for an organism or that HLA-B27 is closely linked to an immune response gene that is responsible for causing an abnormal immune response resulting in spine and joint inflammation. Finally, it is possible that an organism may have many antigenic similarities with the HLA-B27 gene, and this may allow it to enter the body and cause tissue damage without being well detected by the immune system; alternatively, antibodies against the organism may cross-react against the HLA-B27 antigen on tissues cells in the body.

IV. **Clinical Diagnosis**
  A. Tends to occur in young males (age of onset below 40 years), although some studies have shown a closer male:female ratio, suggesting that spondylitis may be underdiagnosed in females.
  B. Onset is gradual.
  C. Morning stiffness and stiffness after sitting for a long time, such as when getting out of a car, occurs. The stiffness decreases with exercise.
  D. Stiffness is generally in the area of the buttocks and low back. It may radiate into one or both thighs.
  E. Inflammatory synovitis of peripheral joints, especially lower extremity ones, occurs.
  F. Pain develops in the plantar or Achilles heel.
  G. Iritis develops.
  H. Costovertebral involvement occurs, causing chest pain with deep breathing.
  I. Rarely, aortitis and aortic insufficiency develop.
  J. Cardiac conduction disturbances are found.
  K. Upper lobe pulmonary fibrosis appears.
  L. Physical findings
    1. A relatively normal back exam if only the sacroiliac joints are involved. In this case, the lumbosacral spine may move quite well.
    2. Decreased extension and flexion of the lumbosacral spine. The finger-to-floor distance can be measured when the patient bends over.
    3. Abnormal Schober test: A mark is made over the lower spine at about the level of the so-called dimples of Venus, and another mark is made 10 cm above the first one. Normally, the distance between these two marks increases to 15 cm or more when a person bends over; an in-

crease of less than 10 cm is abnormal. However, the test is not specific for ankylosing spondylitis.
    4. Diminished chest expansion: Chest expansion is normally more than 2 in. between total exhalation and total inhalation. Expansion of less than 1 in. is abnormal.
    5. With cervical involvement, there is restriction of lateral rotation and extension of the neck. The distance between the occiput and the wall can be measured when the patient is standing with the back and heels to the wall. Normally, the neck can easily extend backward to touch the wall.
    6. Inflammatory arthritis: Joints typically involved in ankylosing spondylitis are lower extremity joints such as the knee and ankle, and also joints adjacent to the spine—the shoulders and hips. Decreased range of motion of the shoulders and hips is common in patients with chronic spondylitis.

V. **Radiographic Abnormalities**
  A. Sacroiliac joints
    1. Periarticular sclerosis.
    2. Irregularity of the joint margins.
    3. Erosions.
    4. Narrowing and finally fusion of the sacroiliac joints.
  B. Radiographs of the lumbosacral spine, thoracic spine, and cervical spine may show syndesmophytes, the vertical bony bridges that start in the annulus fibrosus and extend from one vertebra to another. These are different from osteophytes, which start off horizontally and are parrot beak shaped and broad-based.
  C. Bony proliferative changes in peripheral sites of tendon attachment, the heel, pelvis.
  D. Changes in peripheral joints: Joint space narrowing and sometimes bony proliferative changes. In advanced cases, hip ankylosis and severe shoulder involvement can occur.

VI. **Laboratory Findings**
  A. HLA-B27 positive.
  B. Elevated sedimentation rate.
  C. Mild anemia of chronic disease.
  D. Over 2,000 white blood cells per cubic millimeter in peripheral joint effusions.

VII. **Differential Diagnoses**
  A. Lumbar radiculopathy with pain in the back extending down into the leg.

B. Osteoarthritis of the spine.

C. Spinal stenosis.

D. Fibromyalgia with pain in the location of the back and spine.

E. Diffuse idiopathic skeletal hyperostosis (DISH): In this condition there are bony bridges extending up and down the spine, but they start off horizontally and move vertically, and the sacroiliac joints are normal.

VIII. **Treatment**

A. Nonsteroidal anti-inflammatory drugs such as indomethacin and diclofenac are helpful.

B. Sulfasalazine has been shown in some studies to be effective when combined with nonsteroidal anti-inflammatory drugs.

C. Some practitioners recommend the use of a neck collar when patients ride in a car if they have cervical involvement. This is done to avoid spinal fractures from sudden whiplash injuries.

D. Patients should avoid using many pillows under the head; they may aggravate a cervical flexion deformity.

E. Exercises that emphasize spine extension, resisting the tendency of the disease to produce spine curvature and loss of height.

IX. **Prognosis**

Many patients with ankylosing spondylitis have mild involvement, but the spondylitis may ascend up the spine to involve the lumbosacral, thoracic, and cervical spines. Spinal fractures can occur.

Bibliography

Ferrza BF, Tugwell P, Goldsmith CN, et al. Meta-analysis of sulfasalazine in ankylosing spondylitis. *J Rheumatol* 17:1482–1486, 1990.

Gaston JSH. How does HLA-B27 confer susceptibility to inflammatory arthritis? *Clin Exp Immunol* 82:1–2, 1990.

Khan, Mohammed A, Van der Linden, Sjet M. Ankylosing Spondylitis and Other Spondyloarthropathies: *Rheumatic Disease Clinics of North America*. Volume 16, part 3, 1990, p 551–579.

Tsuchiya N, Husby GH, Williams RC. Studies of humoral and cell-mediated immunity to peptides shared by HLA-B27.

CHAPTER 102

Reiter's Syndrome and Enteropathic Arthritis

Robert Katz, M.D.

I. Definitions

Reiter's syndrome: A collection of symptoms first described by Dr. Hans Reiter in 1916.

A. Reiter's triad
1. Inflammatory arthritis
2. Urethritis
3. Conjunctivitis

B. Enthesopathy: Inflammatory changes and proliferative bone growth may occur at the junction between tendon and bone and between ligament and bone. These areas are called *entheses*.

C. Reactive arthritis: Inflammatory arthritis occurring generally 1–3 weeks after an episode of urethritis or gastroenteritis. The arthritis is not infectious but probably occurs as an immunologic reaction, primarily in genetically susceptible individuals.

D. Enteropathic arthritis: Arthritis associated with inflammatory bowel disease, that is, ulcerative colitis or Crohn's disease.

II. Etiology

A. Genetic factors: Approximately two-thirds of patients who develop Reiter's syndrome or reactive arthritis are born with the human leukocyte antigen (HLA)-B27 gene com-

pared to an 8% prevalence of the same gene in the U.S. population.

B. Environmental factors: Some of the organisms known to precipitate Reiter's syndrome or reactive arthritis in susceptible individuals include *Shigella*, *Salmonella*, *Chlamydia*, *Yersinia*, *Mycoplasma*, and *Campylobacter*. Frequently, the arthritis, eye disease, and mucocutaneous changes follow an episode of urethritis or gastroenteritis.

C. Enteropathic arthritis: Is most often associated with the activity of inflammatory bowel disease. In this illness, it is also possible that bacteria or bacterial antigens from the gut enter the circulation and stimulate an immunologic reaction that leads to joint inflammation.

D. Interplay of genetic and environmental factors: Presumably, certain organisms gain access to the circulation from the genitourinary or gastrointestinal tract. In individuals who are genetically susceptible, primarily those who have the HLA-B27 gene or other gene cross-reactive with HLA-B27 (B7, B22, B42), the organism induces arthritis by one of several possible mechanisms.

1. Molecular mimicry: Part of the antigenic structure of the organism may be similar to that of the HLA-B27 gene. Therefore, the body does not recognize the organism as a foreign invader and allows it to cause tissue damage. It is possible that antibodies made to the organism cross-react with the HLA-B27 antigen.

2. The organism may attach itself directly to the HLA antigen, which rests on the surface of most cells in the body. The antigen may then act as a receptor for the organism.

3. The HLA-B27 gene may be closely related to certain immune response genes that are responsible for directing an abnormal immunologic reaction leading to joint inflammation.

E. The organisms responsible for provoking Reiter's syndrome cannot be cultured from the joint, and the illness is not due to persistent infection.

F. Enteropathic arthritis may occur when bacteria or bacterial antigens gain access to the circulation and stimulate an immunologic response. Tissue damage may occur through:

1. Circulating immune complexes.

2. Antibodies to microorganisms that cross-react with joint tissue.

3. Production of antiepithelial cell (anticolon) antibodies which cause tissue damage.

4. Cytotoxic cells directed at antigens on intestinal epithelial cells.

III. Diagnosis

A. Reiter's syndrome: The diagnosis of Reiter's syndrome depends on the clinical collection of symptoms and sometimes a positive HLA-B27 antigen test.

1. Arthritis
   a. Inflammatory—warmth, swelling.
   b. Oligoarticular—one to five joints.
   c. Asymmetric.
   d. Preference for lower extremity joints, particularly the knee and ankle.
   e. The inflammation is often extremely intense and begins rather abruptly.
   f. Dactylitis—diffuse swelling of a toe or finger, producing a "sausage digit."
   g. Sacroilitis and spondylitis—sometimes more asymmetric and with more skipped areas than ankylosing spondylitis
   h. Enthesopathy—inflammation at the

site where ligaments attach to bone (plantar fascitis, patella tendon, Achilles tendon).

2. Eye findings
   a. Conjunctivitis.
   b. Iritis.

3. Mucocutaneous lesions
   a. Keratoderma blennorrhagica—a scaly rash on the palms and soles.
   b. Circinate balanitis—a rash on the glans penis.
   c. Onycholysis and subungual hyperkeratosis—but no nail pitting, as in psoriasis.
   d. Stomatitis, often painless.

4. Aortitis—which can lead to aortic insufficiency.

5. Cardiac conduction disturbance (increased PR interval, heart block).

6. Cervicitis.

B. Enteropathic arthritis
   1. Inflammatory—with warm, swollen joints.
   2. Oligoarticular (five or fewer joints), usually lower extremity joints (knees, ankles, hips).
   3. Asymmetric.
   4. Peripheral arthritis generally correlates with active inflammatory bowel disease. Episodic, sometimes recurrent.
   5. Sacroilitis and spondylitis.
   6. Not directly related to HLA-B27.
   7. Erythema nodosum.
   8. Pyodema gangrenosum.
   9. Iritis.

IV. Differential Diagnosis

A. Psoriatic arthritis.

B. Gonococcal arthritis, skin pustule, one joint often predominant.

C. Bechet's disease.

D. Septic arthritis.

E. Gout, pseudogout, and calcium pyrophosphate crystal disease.

F. Acquired immunodeficiency syndrome (AIDS)—Reiter's syndrome has been seen in some patients with this disease.

G. Ankylosing spondylitis.

H. Rheumatoid arthritis.

I. Rheumatic fever.

J. Noninfectious arthritis associated with infections such as meningococcemia.

V. Laboratory Findings

A. Synovial fluid
   1. More than 2,000 white blood cells per cubic millimeter in synovial fluid.

B. Poor viscosity, poor mucin clot (these findings are also suggestive of inflammatory synovitis).

C. HLA-B27 is positive in two-thirds of patients with Reiter's syndrome. It is controversial whether or not the test supports the diagnosis and whether it should be ordered. The diagnosis of Reiter's syndrome and reactive arthritis needs to be made primarily on clinical grounds, but some clinicians still find the HLA-B27 test quite helpful. HLA-B27 does not help with the diagnosis of enteropathic arthritis.

D. Other laboratory findings
1. The erythrocyte sedimentation rate may be increased.
2. Mild anemia of chronic disease may occur.
3. Occasionally the white blood cell count is increased.
4. Negative rheumatoid factor and antinuclear antibody (ANA).
5. Some patients will have sterile pyuria in Reiter's syndrome.

VI. X-Ray Findings
A. X-rays are often normal in Reiter's syndrome and enteropathic arthritis.
B. Abnormalities on x-rays include typical findings of inflammatory arthritis such as:
1. Periarticular osteoporosis.
2. Joint space narrowing from cartilage loss.
3. Bony erosions.
4. Hypertrophic bone changes.
   a. Proliferative bony changes at the enthesis, such as the heel, pelvis, and metatarsals.
   b. Sclerosis and irregularity of the sacroiliac joints.
   c. Bony bridging between vertebral levels. The bony bridges (syndesmophytes) in Reiter's disease are asymmetrical and spotty with skip areas.

VII. Course and Prognosis
A. Reiter's syndrome: The arthritis of Reiter's syndrome is often quite intense and lasts for

about a year in many cases. However, there are three courses:
1. An acute episode lasting for 6–18 months.
2. Intermittent attacks over many years.
3. Chronic smoldering arthritis that does not remit spontaneously.

B. Enteropathic arthritis: Most episodes parallel activity of the bowel disease and are not as intense as those of Reiter's syndrome and subside within 6 months. However, if sacroiliitis or spondylitis develops, the course may be chronic and may not parallel the bowel disease.

VIII. Treatment
A. Nonsteroidal anti-inflammatory drugs: Indomethacin or diclofenac are often the drugs of first choice, but other nonsteroidal anti-inflammatory drugs can be used.
B. Systemic steroids, although they are less effective than in rheumatoid arthritis.
C. Corticosteroid injection of inflamed joints with long-lasting, insoluble preparations.
D. In chronic cases, sulfasalazine, methotrexate, or azathioprine may be added to anti-inflammatory drug therapy.
E. Iritis responds to topical or, when necessary, systemic steroids.
F. Control of the inflammatory bowel disease often is associated with control of the inflammatory joint symptoms.

Bibliography
Hammer RE, Maika SD, Richardson JA, et al. Spontaneous inflammatory disease in transgenic rats expressing HLA-B27 and human B2m; an animal model of HLA-B27-associated human disorders. *Cell* 63:1099–1112, 1990.

Keat A. Reiter's syndrome and reactive arthritis in perspective. *N Engl J Med* 309:1606–1615, 1983.

Seronegative Spondyloarthropathies. Current Opinion in Rheumatology. Volume 3. Number 4. 1991.

Simenon G, Van Gossum A, Adler M, et al. Macroscopic and microscopic gut lesions in seronegative spondyloarthropathies. *J Rheumatol* 17:1491–1494, 1990.

CHAPTER 103

Behçet's Syndrome

Calvin R. Brown, M.D.

I. **Definition**
   Originally described as a triad of recurrent oral and genital ulcers with uveitis. Now recognized as a multisystem disease involving the eyes, skin, joints, and gastrointestinal and neurologic systems. Most prevalent in Japan and the Mediterranean countries.

II. **Diagnostic Criteria**
   A. Major criteria
      1. Recurrent oral or apthous ulcers
      2. Skin lesions
      3. Ocular lesions
      4. Iridocyclitis
      5. Retinal uveitis
      6. Genital ulcers
   B. Minor criteria
      1. Arthritis
      2. Gastrointestinal lesions
      3. Epididymitis
      4. Vasculitis
      5. Central nervous system lesions
      6. Pulmonary lesions
      7. Glomerulonephritis
   C. Criteria needed for diagnosis
      1. Complete: Four major criteria.
      2. Incomplete: Three major or two major and two minor criteria.
      3. Suspected: One or more major or minor criteria.

III. **Clinical Features**
   A. Oral ulcers, painful with purulent exudate, usually the first symptom. Similar ulcers appear on the scrotum or vulva but occur less commonly.
   B. Various skin lesions, pustules, and skin hypersensitivity.
   C. Recurrent anterior and posterior ocular uveitis.
   D. Mildly inflammatory oligoarticular arthritis.
   E. Gastrointestinal ulcers, erosions, and bleeding.
   F. Small vessel vasculitis and thrombosis.
   G. Acute focal central nervous system lesions and cerebrovascular accidents.
   H. Glomerulonephritis.

IV. **Pathogenesis**
   A. Pathogenesis unknown. Polyclonal hypergammaglobulinemia and presence of antibodies to multiple tissues found; elevated acute phase reactants indicates that the immune system plays a role.

B. Human leukocyte antigen (HLA)-B5 and -B51 found frequently in Japanese and Mediterranean patients, but not in Europeans or Americans.

V. Treatment

A. Colchicine, 0.6 mg two to four times per day, is useful for mild disease.

B. Corticosteroids are advocated for more severe cases; high doses (60 mg prednisone equivalent) is needed for severe disease or central nervous system involvement.

C. Chlorambucil and cyclosporin are effective for devastating ocular involvement but are potentially toxic.

VI. Prognosis

Life expectancy in affected morbidities can include blindness and the effects of CNS disease.

Bibliography

Lakhanpal S, Tani K, Lie JT, et al. Pathologic features of Behçet's syndrome. *Hum Pathol* 16:790–795, 1985.

Shimizu T, Erlich GE, Inaba G. Behçet's disease. *Semin Arthritis Rheum* 8:223–260, 1979.

Yazici H, Pazarli H, Barnes C, et al. A controlled trial of azathioprine in Behçet's syndrome. *N Engl J Med* 322:281–285, 1990.

CHAPTER 104

Psoriatic Arthritis

Joel A. Block, M.D.

I. **Definition**
   A. The diagnosis of psoriatic arthritis applies when a patient has psoriasis *and* an inflammatory arthritis in the absence of rheumatoid factor (a seronegative arthropathy).
      1. The coincident presence of rheumatoid factor–positive symmetric arthritis and psoriasis is not classed as psoriatic arthritis, but rather as rheumatoid arthritis with psoriasis.
      2. Although the clinical manifestations of both the arthritis and the skin disease in psoriasis may be protean, psoriatic arthritis has a distinct epidemiology and clinical course and is therefore properly considered a syndrome.
   B. Psoriatic arthritis is classified as one of the seronegative spondyloarthropathies.

II. **Etiology**
   As with many rheumatologic conditions, the etiology and pathophysiology of psoriatic arthritis are poorly understood. However, several associations have been described.
   A. Familial predisposition
      1. First-degree family members of affected individuals have a prevalence of psoriasis of greater than 20% and a prevalence of psoriatic arthritis of greater than 5%.
      2. The risk of developing psoriatic arthritis may be increased 40-fold among family members of patients.
   B. HLA associations
      1. Human leukocyte antigen (HLA)-B27 is present in the majority of psoriatics with spondylitis; it is less strongly associated with arthritis restricted to the nonaxial skeleton.
      2. Less successful attempts have been made to correlate HLA antigens with the other clinical presentations of the arthritis. Controversy exists regarding the significance of associations with HLA-B17, -DR4, and -DR7.
   C. Environmental effects on susceptible patients
      1. Bacterial antigens may trigger arthritis in a manner similar to the reactive arthritides. There have been reports of antibodies against streptococcal and staphylococcal antigens which are elevated in psoriatic arthritis relative to patients who have psoriasis without arthritis.
      2. Unconfirmed reports suggest that local

trauma may precipitate arthritis and synovitis in psoriatics.

III. Pathology and Pathophysiology

A. Synovial involvement

1. The synovitis of the peripheral arthritis is pathologically similar to the synovitis of rheumatoid arthritis and includes synovial edema and thickening, lymphocytic infiltrates, hypertrophic villi, and articular destruction.

2. Psoriatic arthritis has a greater tendency than rheumatoid arthritis toward ankylosis and joint fusion.

3. Immune deposition in involved joints tends not to include rheumatoid factor.

B. Immune system activation

1. The majority of psoriatic arthritics have elevated serum levels of IgG, IgA, and detectable circulating immune complexes.

   a. Approximately twice as many psoriatics with arthritis have elevated Raji cell immune complexes compared to psoriatics without arthritis.

   b. There is no apparent correlation between the serum levels of IgG, IgA, or immune complexes and the severity or activity of disease.

2. Although the total level of T lymphocytes is normal, there are reports of a functional reduction in helper cell activity; this is likely due to the psoriasis rather than to the arthritic component.

IV. Differential Diagnosis

A. Seronegative spondyloarthropathies: The distinction of psoriatic arthritis from ankylosing spondylitis depends on the presence of dermal psoriasis. Reiter's syndrome with keratoderma blennorrhagicum can mimic pustular psoriasis and needs to be distinguished by other manifestations. In addition, Reiter's syndrome has a greater propensity to involve the lower extremities; psoriatic arthritis tends to involve the upper extremities more severely than the lower extremities.

B. Inflammatory osteoarthritis involves the distal interphalangeal joints in a manner similar to the distal interphalangeal variant of psoriatic arthritis; however, osteoarthritis occurs in the context of osteophytes rather than osteolysis and ankylosis.

C. Gout and polyarticular gout need to be distinguished by analysis of synovial fluid for uric acid crystals, especially if the serum uric acid is elevated.

V. Diagnosis

A. History

1. The most common age at onset of disease is the mid-thirties to the mid-forties.

2. The male:female ratio is approximately 1:1.

3. Typically, psoriatic skin involvement precedes articular involvement by several months to a few years; occasionally, arthritis may present prior to detectable skin disease, but definitive diagnosis must await the onset of skin or nail involvement.

B. Clinical signs and physical findings

1. Articular disease: The pattern of joint findings is heterogeneous, and presenting patterns frequently evolve into different patterns during the disease course. Almost all patients have some peripheral articular involvement, and almost half develop spondylitis.

   a. Mono- and asymmetric pauciarticular involvement is the most common presenting form.

      (1) The distal and proximal interphalangeal joints of the hands or feet, as well as the wrists, elbows, ankles, or knees, can be involved. Typically, the small joints of individual digits are inflamed, giving rise to the "sausage digit" appearance; the upper extremities are somewhat more commonly involved than the lower extremities.

      (2) Inflammatory arthritis of the distal interphalangeal joints occurs in 5–10% of patients and represents the classical appearance of psoriatic arthritis.

      (3) With severe disease progression, osteolysis and phalangeal bone resorption occur, giving rise to *arthritis mutilans*; this is often restricted to individual digits and is called *telescoping*. Telescoping is associated with severe psoriatic skin disease, earlier age, and systemic symptoms.

   b. Symmetric polyarthritis occurs in approximately one-quarter of patients and is similar to seronegative rheumatoid arthritis, although the distal interphalangeal joints may be involved.

   c. Spondylitis and sacroiliitis are frequently present in association with all forms of peripheral arthritis but occur uncommonly in the absence of peripheral arthritis (less than 10% of patients).

    (1) Sacroiliitis is present in more than 20% of patients and is commonly asymmetric.

    (2) Spondylitis, which occurs in more than 40% of patients, can involve any portion of the spine and frequently involves the cervical spine. Syndesmophytes are common, but evolution to the "bamboo spine" of ankylosing spondylitis is rare.

  d. Enthesitis, or inflammation at the sites of tendon insertion, is common.

2. Cutaneous disease must be demonstrated to definitively diagnose psoriatic arthritis.

  a. Nail involvement is present in most patients with psoriatic arthritis and may be the only skin manifestation.

    (1) It typically includes nail pitting, thickening, and separation.

    (2) Nail pitting frequently overlies involved distal interphalangeal joints.

  b. Skin involvement needs to be sought in the scalp, extensor surfaces, and perianal and periumbilical areas.

3. Other involved areas

  a. Ophthalmologic inflammation, including conjunctivitis, iritis, and episcleritis, occurs in approximately one-third of patients.

  b. Aortic insufficiency and pulmonary interstitial fibrosis have been described as infrequent associations.

C. Diagnostic tests: There are no specific or sensitive laboratory procedures which diagnose psoriatic arthritis.

1. Blood work: There may be mild elevation of the erythrocyte sedimentation rate, and anemia of chronic inflammation may be present. Serum uric acid is elevated in approximately 20% of patients. Rheumatoid factor is negative and serum immunoglobulin levels are usually normal, although there may be nonspecific elevations. Circulating immune complexes are often detectable.

2. Synovial fluid: A typical mild to moderately inflammatory effusion, with neutrophil predominance, is expected.

3. Radiographic evaluation

  a. Peripheral joint appearance includes erosions, phalangeal resorption, joint fusion, and the "pencil-in-cup" deformity.

  b. Axial skeleton involvement includes asymmetric and symmetric sacroiliac erosions and fusion, asymmetric and isolated syndesmophytes, and occasionally cervical subluxation.

D. The diagnosis of psoriatic arthritis depends on documenting the presence of psoriasis in the presence of an inflammatory seronegative arthritis.

VI. Treatment

A. Supportive measures

1. Instruction in joint protection.

2. Daily range-of-motion exercises to maintain joint mobility.

B. Medication

1. Nonsteroidal anti-inflammatory agents (NSAIDs) are the mainstay of therapy for pain and mild to moderate inflammatory disease. Some rheumatologists consider indomethacin more effective than other NSAIDs in the treatment of psoriatic arthritis.

2. Steroid injections: Intra-articular glucocorticoid injections are effective in controlling mono- or oligoarticular synovitis and when a few joints are particularly severely involved in polyarticular disease. Care should be taken to avoid injecting through psoriatic skin lesions in light of the risk of infection.

3. Gold: Parenteral gold is probably as effective in suppressing psoriatic arthritis as it is for rheumatoid arthritis and is considered to be somewhat better tolerated by psoriatics. Recent studies suggest that oral gold is less effective than parenteral gold.

4. Methotrexate has been used effectively for the treatment of cutaneous psoriasis for almost 40 years, and is well tolerated and considered effective in the treatment of psoriatic arthritis.

5. Photochemotherapy

  a. PUVA: The combination of oral psoralens with exposure to ultraviolet A has long been considered effective treatment for psoriasis. Patients with peripheral arthropathy have shown a concomitant improvement with PUVA therapy, possibly related to their skin improvement; spondylitics, however, do not appear to respond as well.

    b. Photopheresis: Extracorporeal irradiation of lymphocytes with ultraviolet A after sensitization with psoralens has shown some efficacy in the treatment of psoriatic arthritis but probably is ineffective for treating skin lesions.

  6. Other agents which have been tried and may be somewhat effective include antimalarials, cyclosporine A, retinoids, oral vitamin D, and azathioprine.

C. Surgery

  1. Psoriatics are at increased risk for postoperative wound and implant infections, probably because of the colonization of skin plaques.

  2. Joint replacement is effective, although the results of hand surgery tend to be less satisfactory than for rheumatoids.

VII. Prognosis

A. For the majority of patients, the disease course tends to consist of relatively quiescent periods punctuated by acute flares of inflammatory arthritis.

  1. Patients with pauciarticular disease tend to have less disability and less progression to arthritis mutilans.

  2. Patients with severely mutilating arthropathy also tend to have severe skin involvement.

B. Mortality is not increased from the arthritis itself, although various risks from treatment exist, including myelosuppression, osteoporosis, and sepsis.

Bibliography

Gladman DD, Anhorn KAB, Schachter RK, et al. HLA antigens in psoriatic arthritis. *J Rheumatol* 13:586–592, 1986.

Kammer GM, Soter NA, Gibson DJ, et al. Psoriatic arthritis: A clinical, immunologic and HLA study of 100 patients. *Semin Arthritis Rheum* 9:75–97, 1979.

Lambert JR, and Wright V. Psoriatic spondylitis: A clinical and radiological description of the spine in psoriatic arthritis. *Q J Med* 46:411–425, 1977.

McHugh NJ, Laurent MR, Treadwell BLJ, et al. Psoriatic arthritis: Clinical subgroups and histocompatibility antigens. *Ann Rheum Dis* 46:184–188, 1987.

Michet CJ. Psoriatic arthritis, in Kelley WN, Harris ED, Ruddy S, et al (eds), *Textbook of Rheumatology*, ed 4. Philadelphia, Saunders, 1993, pp 974–984.

Moll JMH, Wright V. Familial occurrence of psoriatic arthritis. *Ann Rheum Dis* 32:181–197, 1973.

Palit J, Hill J, Capell HA, et al. A multicentre double-blind comparison of auranofin, intramuscular gold thiomalate and placebo in patients with psoriatic arthritis. *Br J Rheumatol* 29:280–283, 1990.

Stern SH, Insall JN, Windsor RE, et al. Total knee arthroplasty in patients with psoriasis. *Clin Orthop Rel Res* 248:108–110, 1989.

Wilfert H, Hönigsmann H, Steiner G, et al. Treatment of psoriatic arthritis by extracorporeal photochemotherapy. *Br J Dermatol* 122:225–232, 1990.

CHAPTER **105**

Acute Rheumatic Fever

Judith E. Frank, M.D.

I. **Definition**

Acute rheumatic fever (ARF) is an inflammatory disease that occurs as a delayed sequel to an antecedent group A streptococcal pharyngitis infection. It primarily involves the heart, joints, central nervous system, and skin.

II. **Etiology**

ARF is the result of a preceding group A β-hemolytic streptococcal pharyngeal infection. Other sites of strep infection (i.e., skin, wound, or pneumonia) do not result in ARF.

III. **Pathogenesis**

Although the etiology of ARF has been established, the pathogenesis of the disease remains in question.

IV. **Diagnosis**

There is no clinical feature or laboratory test that is diagnostic of ARF. Therefore criteria were developed by Jones in 1944 (modified in 1965) to help establish the correct diagnosis. Two major criteria or one major and two minor criteria indicate a high probability of ARF if supported by evidence of a preceding streptococcal infection (i.e., recent scarlet fever, positive throat culture for group A streptococcus,

increased antistreptolysin O or other strep antibody titers).

A. Major manifestations

1. Arthritis

   a. The most common presenting symptom and possibly the only manifestation in adults.

   b. Involves the large joints: Knees, ankles, elbows and wrist.

   c. Migratory polyarthritis with an average of seven joints involved over a 2- to 6-week period.

   d. Fever.

   e. Lag period of approximately 18 days after the strep pharyngitis (range, 1–5 weeks).

2. Carditis: Common in children but rare in adults (15%).

   a. New or changing heart murmur with mitral regurgitation as the most common murmur.

   b. Cardiomegaly.

   c. Congestive heart failure.

   d. Pericarditis.

3. Sydenham's chorea: Neurologic disorder

characterized by involuntary, purpose-less, rapid movements which disappear with sleep.

    a. Rarely, if ever, occurs in adults.

    b. Occurs after other symptoms have subsided.

4. Erythema marginatum: An evanescent, pink, macular rash which begins on the trunk.

    a. Rare in adults.

5. Subcutaneous nodules: Pea-sized, pain-less, firm nodules that usually occur over extensor surfacs and bony prominences.

    a. Rarely, if ever, occur in adults.

    b. Nodules last for periods ranging from days to weeks.

B. Minor manifestations

1. Fever occurs in almost all attacks and can last for 1 month.

2. Arthralgias.

3. Previous rheumatic fever.

4. Elevated erythrocyte sedimentation rate (ESR) or C-reactive protein (CRP).

5. Prolonged PR interval on electrocardio-gram.

C. Laboratory findings

1. Throat Cultures: Usually negative by the time ARF occurs.

2. Antibodies to streptococcal extracellular products: peak 4–5 weeks after strepto-coccal pharyngitis.

    a. Antibodies to ASO: Most available.

    b. Anti-DNase B: Remains elevated longest.

    c. Others: Antihyaluronidase and anti-streptokinase.

3. Acute phase reactants: ESR or CRP.

4. Anemia: Normochronic normocytic.

5. Echocardiogram: With Doppler tech-nique can now diagnose carditis.

V. Differential Diagnosis

The arthritis in ARF is similar to other causes of polyarticular arthritis in adults.

A. Reactive arthritis

B. Gonococcal arthritis

C. Rheumatoid arthritis

D. Systemic lupus erythematosus

E. Subacute bacteria endocarditis

F. Viral infections (rubella and hepatitis)

VI. Treatment

A. Complete course of penicillin to eradicate the group A strep pharyngitis.

1. A 10-day course of oral penicillin (PCN).

2. Single-injection benzathine PCN: 1.2 million units IM.

B. Anti-inflammatory drugs

1. Nonsteroidal anti-inflammatory drugs (NSAIDs) or salicylates.

2. Corticosteroids.

VII. Prognosis

Neither salicylates, NSAIDs, nor glucocorti-coids shorten the course of ARF.

A. In 80%, subsides in 6 weeks.

B. In 5%, persists for more than 6 months.

C. Prognosis is worse if carditis is present.

VIII. Prevention

A. Primary prophylaxis: Proper therapy of streptococcal pharyngitis prevents initial at-tacks.

B. Secondary prophylactic: ARF does not re-cur when streptococcal disease is prevented. Since infections may be asymptomatic, all patients with a history of ARF need prophy-lactic therapy. The length of this treatment is still controversial, but 5 years is presently recommended.

1. Most effective: monthly IM benzathine PCN, 1.2 million U.

2. Oral PCN V, 250 mg twice a day, or sulfadiazine, 500 mg twice a day, or erythromycin, 250 mg twice a day.

Bibliography

Bisno Al, Shulman St, Dajani AS. The rise and fall (and rise ?) of rheumatic fever. *JAMA* 259(5):728–729, 1988.

Markowitz M. The decline of rheumatic fever. Role of medical intervention. *J Pediatr* 105:545, 1985.

Schumacher HR Jr. *Primer on the Rheumatic Diseases*, ed 9 Arthritis Foundation, Atlanta, 1988, pp 156–159.

Stollerman GH. Rheumatic fever, in Kelly WN, Harris ED, Ruddy S, et al (eds), *Textbook of Rheumatology*, ed 3. Philadelphia, Saunders, 1989, p 1312.

Wallace MT, Garst PD, Papdinos TJ, et al. The return of acute rheumatic fever in young adults. *JAMA* 262(18):2557–2561, 1989.

CHAPTER 106

Adult Onset Still's Disease

Judith E. Frank, M.D.

I. **Definition**

Adult-onset Still's Disease (AOSD) is a form of seronegative polyarthritis similar to systemic juvenile rheumatoid arthritis (JRA) in children. This disease usually affects young adults between the ages of 20 and 35. Both sexes are equally affected.

II. **Etiology**

The etiology of AOSD is still unknown.

III. **Clinical Signs and Physical Findings**

A. Fever (96%): High spiking with chills ("quotidian fever").

B. Rash (86%): Erythematous, nonpruritic, salmon-colored, maculopapular rash predominantly over the trunk, most apparent when patients are febrile.

C. Pharyngitis (49%).

D. Polyarthritis (94%): Predominantly involves the wrist, metacarpophalangeals, (MCPs), proximal and knees.

E. Lymphadenopathy (52%).

F. Splenomegaly (42%) or hepatomegaly (27%).

G. Pleuropulmonary disease (33%).

H. Pericarditis (36%) or carditis (3%).

IV. **Diagnostic Tests**

There are no specific laboratory tests for AOSD, but nonspecific abnormalities are common.

A. Elevated erythrocyte sedimentation rate: Often over 100 mm/hr.

B. Leukocytosis.

C. Anemia.

D. Negative tests for RF, antinuclear antibody, and antistreptolysin O.

E. Abnormal liver function tests.

F. X-ray findings.

1. Ankylosis of PIP, DIP and carpometacarpal (CMC) joints.

2. Cervical apophyseal joint involvement.

V. **Differential Diagnosis**

Infection (subacute bacterial endocarditis, rubella, meningococcal, gonococcus, hepatitis, syphilis) and reactive arthritis (Reiter's syndrome or acute rheumatic fever) must be ruled out.

A. Proposed criteria

1. High-probability or definite AOSD: 6 weeks of high, spiking fever, arthritis, evanescent rash, and neutrophilia.

2. Probable AOSD: Fever, arthritis, rash, or

neutrophilia plus any minor manifestation (serositis, pharyngitis, hepatosplenomegaly, lymphadenopathy).

VI. **Prognosis and Treatment**
The prognosis is generally good, although the majority of patients will require corticosteroids.
A. High-dose salicylates or a nonsteroidal anti-inflammatory drug for mild disease.
B. Corticosteroids for systemic disease at a dose of 1–2 mg/kg/day.
C. Persistent articular disease can be treated with gold, antimalarial agents, penicillamine, azathioprine, or methotrexate.

Bibliography

Cush JJ, Medsger TA Jr, Christy WC, et al. Adult-onset Still's disease: Clinical course and outcome. *Arthritis Rheum* 30:186–194, 1987.

Onta A, Yamaguchi M, Kaneokah, et al. Adult Still's disease: Review of 228 cases from the literature. *J Rheumatol* 14:1139–1146, 1987.

Reginato AJ, Schumacher HR, Baker DJ, et al. Adult onset Still's disease: Experience with 23 patients and literature review with emphasis on organ failure. *Semin Arthritis Rheum* 17:39–57, 1987.

Schumacher HR Jr. *Primer on the Rheumatic Diseases,* ed 9. Arthritis Foundation, Atlanta, 1988, pp 170–171.

CHAPTER 107

Osteoarthritis

Jovan M. Popovich, M.D.

I. Definition

Osteoarthritis is a degenerative disease of the cartilage of joints. It is of diverse etiology and obscure pathogenesis.

II. Etiology

A. Generalized or localized idiopathic osteoarthritis; the underlying cause is unknown.

B. Secondary osteoarthritis associated with underlying local or systemic factors.

1. Developmental disorders
   a. Slipped capital femoral epiphysis
   b. Multiple epiphyseal dysplasia
   c. Congenital dislocation of the hips
   d. Legg-Calve-Perthes disease

2. Heritable metabolic disorders
   a. Hemochromatosis
   b. Wilson's disease
   c. Alkaptonuria

3. Physical factors
   a. Meniscectomy
   b. Trauma (acute, chronic, occupational, sports, fractures through the joint)
   c. Joint laxity
   d. Avascular necrosis

4. Endocrine disorders
   a. Hypothyroidism
   b. Acromegalic arthropathy
   c. Hyperparathyroidism
   d. Diabetes mellitus
   e. Obesity

5. Inflammatory joint disease with residual joint damage
   a. Rheumatoid arthritis
   b. Gout
   c. Septic and tuberculous arthritis
   d. Psoriatic arthritis
   e. Hemophilic arthropathy

6. Calcium deposition disease
   a. Calcium pyrophosphate deposition disease
   b. Apatite arthropathy

7. Neuropathic arthropathy

8. Miscellaneous
   a. Frostbite
   b. Hemoglobinopathies

III. Pathogenesis

In the pathogenesis of osteoarthritis, multiple biochemical, mechanical, immunological, and inflammatory factors play a role.

A. Unknown primary insult leads to changes in the chondrocyte microenvironment, leading to activation of chondrocyte and altering the balance between synthesis and degradation, causing cartilage loss.

B. Subchondral bone osteoblasts increase the rate of synthesis; bone stiffness is increased; subchondral microfractures develop.

C. Peripheral synovial cells become metaplastic; attempts at repair produce osteophytes.

D. Formation of pseudocysts occurs in trabecular bone. Volume and density of all articular and periarticular structures are increased.

IV. **Diagnosis**

Diagnosis of osteoarthritis is made on the basis of the history, physical examination, and x-ray studies.

A. History
 1. Pain after joint use early in the course of the disease, pain at rest and at night late in the course of the disease.
 2. Stiffness of short duration (usually less than 30 min), localized to involved joints, on awakening in the morning or after inactivity.

B. Clinical signs and physical findings
 1. Bony enlargement of the joints
 2. Crepitus
 3. Localized tenderness
 4. Limitation of motion and pain on motion.
 5. Small effusion and transient inflammatory episodes.

C. Diagnostic tests
 1. No specific laboratory abnormalities. Laboratory tests are useful only to exclude other rheumatic diseases or a metabolic cause. Synovial fluid shows minimal abnormalities; it is clear and viscous, with a leukocyte count less than 2,000/mm^3.
 2. Roentgenographic findings of osteoarthritis
   a. Diarthrodial joints
     (1) Normal x-ray does not rule out early degenerative changes as a cause of symptoms.
     (2) Asymmetric joint space narrowing is an early finding. Presence of pain correlates poorly with the radiologic appearance of the joint.
     (3) Osteophyte formation.
     (4) Subchondral bony sclerosis.
     (5) Subchondral bone cysts.
     (6) Erosive osteoarthritis: subchondral erosions and gull wing appearance in distal interphalangeal (DIP) and proximal interphalangeal (PIP) joints.

   b. Spine
     (1) Disc space narrowing.
     (2) Anterior and lateral spinous osteophytes: spondylosis.
     (3) Facet joint and associated posterior bony structural changes.
     (4) Spondylolisthesis.
     (5) Ligamentous calcification: Diffuse idiopathic skeletal hyperostosis (DISH).

V. **Clinical Subsets of Osteoarthritis**

A. Idiopathic generalized osteoarthritis
 1. Three or more joint groups involved.
 2. Family history positive.
 3. Occurs in middle-aged women, often rapid and inflammatory.
 4. Radiologic changes exceed clinical findings.

B. Localized forms of osteoarthritis
 a. Osteoarthritis of the hip
   (1) More common in men than in women.
   (2) Superolateral, commonly unilateral, involvement has a worse prognosis.
   (3) Medial involvement, with a better prognosis, is associated with polyarticular joint involvement.

 b. Osteoarthritis of the knee
   (1) More common in obese women with varus deformity.
   (2) Follows trauma or meniscal operation in men.
   (3) Chondromalacia patellae, seen most often in young adults, characterized by softening and erosion of patellar articular cartilage and by pain around the patella that is aggravated with activity such as walking up and down the stairs.

 c. Osteoarthritis of the spine
   (1) Apophyseal
   (2) Intervertebral disk
   (3) Spondylotic
   (4) Diffuse idiopathic skeletal hyperostosis
     (a) Flowing ossification of anterolateral aspects of four or more continuous thoracic vertebrae without loss of disc height.

 d. Osteoarthritis of the hands
   (1) DIP, PIP, and carpometacarpal (CMC) involvement is frequent.
   (2) Occurs predominantly in middle-aged women.

(3) May have a episodic course with an abrupt inflammatory onset.

(4) Familial aggregation is frequent.

e. Erosive osteoarthritis

(1) Distribution similar to that of nodal osteoarthritis of the hands.

(2) Postmenopausal women most often affected.

(3) Familial aggregation frequent.

(4) Recurrent episodes of inflammation lead to joint deformity and occasionally ankylosis.

VI. Differential Diagnosis

Atypical presentation leads to diagnostic difficulties.

A. Inflammatory osteoarthritis of the hands may suggest the diagnosis of seronegative rheumatoid arthritis, psoriatic arthritis, or Reiter's syndrome.

B. Osteoarthritis of the hip can be confused with aseptic necrosis or pigmented villonodular synovitis.

C. Osteoarthritis of the knee should be differentiated from internal joint derangement, osteochondritis, chronic infection, and anserine bursitis.

VII. Treatment of Osteoarthritis

Treatment is symptomatic and for the most part empiric.

A. Drugs

1. Analgesic agents such as acetaminophen or propoxyphene hydrochloride on an as-needed or continuous basis.

2. Nonsteroidal anti-inflammatory agents

a. Considerable variation among patients in terms of tolerance and benefit.

b. If one drug fails to reduce symptoms, it is always worthwhile to evaluate another.

c. Each drug should be used regularly for a period of 2–3 weeks; not only the initial response but also the consequences of cessation of therapy should be assessed.

3. Muscle relaxants.

4. Intra-articular steroid injections are useful in management of acute flares. They should be used infrequently and cautiously. The usual dose in large joint is 40 mg of methylprednisolone or its equivalent. An acute, self-limited synovitis may follow corticosteroid injection in 1–10% of cases.

B. Physical therapy: Rehabilitative treatment in osteoarthritis is aimed at controlling regional pain, reducing impairment of function, and providing joint protection. Different techniques have been used.

1. Local rest during periods of inflammation.

2. Treatment with various modalities

a. Heat and cold modalities (ultrasound, diathermy, hot and cold packs).

b. Transcutaneous nerve stimulation.

3. Mobilization techniques: Traction.

a. Lumbar traction not markedly successful.

4. Range-of-motion exercises.

5. Muscle-strengthening exercises (isometric, isotonic, isokinetic).

6. Aerobic exercises.

7. Orthotics.

8. Assistive devices and adaptive aids.

C. Surgery: Surgery is considered for relieving severe pain or for correction of deformity causing severe disability, stabilization of joints, redistribution of joint forces, decompression of neural impingement, or removal of the loose body from the joint. Surgical procedures include arthroplasty, osteotomy, fusion, and partial or total joint replacement. Arthroscopic techniques can be used early for irrigation, debridement, removal of loose bodies, and smoothening of irregular joint surfaces.

Bibliography

Bland JH. Diagnosis and treatment of osteoarthritis. *Curr Opinion Rheumatol* 1:315–324, 1989.

Brandt KD, Mankin HJ: Osteoarthritis. In Kelly W. Textbook of Rheumatology, ed 4. 1993, pp 1355–1399.

Mankin HJ, Brandt KD, Shulman LE. Workshop on etiopathogenesis of osteoarthritis. Proceedings and recommendation. *J Rheumatol* 13(6):1130–1160, 1986.

McCarthy DJ, Koopman WJ: Section on osteoarthritis in Arthritis and Allied Conditions, ed. 12. 1992, pp 1699–1769.

CHAPTER 108

Infectious Arthritis

Judith E. Frank, M.D.

I. Definition

Although infectious agents such as viruses, fungi, and mycobacteria may cause arthritis, bacterial arthritis is the most destructive form and therefore requires immediate recognition and treatment. Bacterial arthritis is usually divided into two types: those caused specifically by *Neisseria gonorrhoeae* and those caused by all other bacteria. Organisms may enter the joint from the bloodstream or from an adjacent osteomyelitis, or they may be introduced directly through a needle, penetrating wound, or during surgery.

Nongonococcal Bacterial Arthritis

II. Etiology

A. Gram-positive: Most common cause of nongonococcal bacterial arthritis.
   1. *Staphylococcus aureus:* The most common and most destructive organism; it may be methicillin resistant. It is seen in 80% of joint infections in patients with forms of chronic arthritis such as rheumatoid arthritis (RA).
   2. *Staph. epidermidis:* An important cause of prosthetic joint infections.
   3. Streptococci: Both the group-A and non-group-A types can cause arthritis. Pneumococcal arthritis is seen in alcoholics and other immunocompromised hosts. It rarely causes joint damage.

B. Gram negative: Seen in immunocompromised host such as neonates, the elderly, intravenous drug users, cancer patients, and those with underlying chronic diseases.
   1. *Escherichia coli:* Most common in the elderly.
   2. *Haemophilus influenzae:* Most common cause of bacterial arthritis in children.
   3. *Pseudomonas aeruginosa:* Intravenous drug users.
   4. *Pasteurella multocida:* Animal bite.
   5. *Salmonella:* Underlying sickle cell disease or systemic lupus erythematosus (SLE).

C. Anaerobic: Most infections occur postoperatively and are polymicrobial
   1. *Bacteroides fragilis:* RA patients.
   2. *Fusobacterium, Corynebacterium:* Other.

D. Polymicrobial: Reported in 2–10% of nongonococcal arthritis.

E. *Brucella:* Needs special media for growth. Disease is transmitted to humans by infected animals.
   1. *B. abortus:* United States.
   2. *B. melitensis:* South and Central America.

III. **Pathophysiology**
   A. Hematogenous: The synovial lining is extremely vascular, so organisms in the blood may be trapped in the synovial space. There the bacteria multiply and cause an inflammatory response, with release of proteolytic enzymes which cause destruction.
   B. Puncture wound: Rarely from joint aspiration (1/500–1/5,000).
   C. Skin infection.
   D. Osteomyelitis.
   E. Predisposing factors: Bacterial arthritis is most common in the very young, the elderly, and those with chronic illnesses.
      1. RA: 75% of cases caused by *Staph. aureus.*
      2. Crystal disease: Gout and calcium pyrophosphate deposition disease CPPD.
      3. Osteoarthritis.
      4. Chronic systemic diseases: Cancer, liver disease, diabetes mellitus, and collagen vascular diseases.
      5. Intravenous drug use: Usually due to *Staph. aureus* or *P. aeruginosa.* Has a predilection for sacroiliac, sternoclavicular, and intervertebral joints.
      6. Prosthetic joints.

IV. **Diagnosis**
   A. History and physical findings
      1. Elicit a history of predisposing risk factors.
      2. Monarticular arthritis (80–90%)
         a. Abrupt onset of pain, swelling, and heat in a joint with limited range of motion.
         b. Knee: Most common site.
         c. Fever.
      3. Polyarticular: Usually seen in those with underlying chronic diseases such as RA, with *Staph. aureus* being the most common organism.
   B. Diagnostic tests
      1. Joint aspiration: The most important diagnostic procedure.
         a. Gram stain: Positive in 75% of *Staph. aureus* infections but in less than 50% of negative infections.
         b. Culture and sensitivity: Plate immediately or inoculate in blood culture bottles.
         c. Leukocyte count: Usually greater than 50,000, wbc/ml with more than 80% polymorphonuclear leukocytes.
         d. Glucose: Less than 50% of fasting simultaneous blood sugar.
      2. Blood tests
         a. Blood cultures: Most important blood test, with 50% positive. May be positive when synovial fluid culture is negative.
         b. Leukocytosis: Nonspecific.
         c. Elevated erythrocyte sedimentation rate: nonspecific.
      3. Radiologic evaluation
         a. Plain films: Obtain at baseline film and follow for progression. Also necessary to rule out osteomyelitis.
            (1) Immediate: Joint effusion.
            (2) One week: Periarticular osteoporosis.
            (3) Two weeks or more: Joint space narrowing with erosions.
         b. Bone scintigraphy: Detects bone changes earlier than x-ray but is nonspecific. Useful for axial joints such as sacroiliac and vertebral joints.
         c. Computed tomography: may be used to guide joint aspirations (sacroiliac or sternoclavicular).

V. **Differential Diagnosis**
   Includes crystal disease, other infectious agents, and acute presentation of systemic rheumatic diseases such as SLE, RA, or Reiter's syndrome.

VI. **Treatment**
   A. Antibiotics: Patients should receive at least 2 weeks of intravenous therapy followed by 1–2 weeks of oral therapy. Treatment must be started immediately after joint aspiration, with adjustment in antibiotics once the results of the Gram stain and culture are known.
      1. Positive Gram stain:
         a. Gram-positive cocci: Nafcillin or vancomycin.
         b. Gram-negative cocci: Penicillin (PCN) or cephalosporin.
         c. Gram-negative bacilli: Aminoglycosides and a β-lactam antibiotic or third-generation cephalosporin.
      2. Negative Gram stain:
         a. Healthy young adult: PCN or cephalosporin.
         b. Elderly or compromised host: Need to cover for methicillin-resistant *Staph. aureus* and gram-negative bacilli.

B. Joint drainage: At this time, there are no clear guidelines for using repeated closed needle aspiration or surgical drainage (arthroscopic versus open drainage) to remove the fluid from an infected joint.
  1. Large-bore needle aspiration: Must be repeated at regular intervals if fluid reaccumulates.
  2. Surgery: Usually the initial procedure in these situations.
    a. Hip infections in children.
    b. Difficult or impossible to drain adequately with a needle.
    c. Coexisting osteomyelitis.
C. Rehabilitation
  1. Passive and non-weight-bearing.
  2. Active.

VII. Prognosis
Nongonococcal bacterial arthritis is a serious illness and without adequate treatment has a 5–10% mortality rate.
A. *Staph. aureus* and gram-negative bacilli: Worst outcomes, with only 50% complete recovery.
B. *Strep. pneumoniae:* Complete recovery in more than 80%.
C. Anaerobic and polymicrobial infections: Poor outcomes.

Disseminated Gonococcal Infection

I. Definition
Disseminated gonococcal infection (DGI) generally occurs in young, healthy females and is now the most common cause of bacterial arthritis in the United States.

II. Etiology
Neisseria gonorrhoeae.

III. Pathophysiology
Various host–bacteria interactions are important in both local and disseminated gonorrhea infections.
A. Bacterial virulence factors: Pili, outer membrane proteins, and cell wall lipopolysaccharides.
B. Complement deficiencies: Increased risk of *Neisseria* infections with terminal complement deficiencies of C_5–C_9.
C. Local factors: Endometrial pH and the increased prevalence of DGI early in the menstrual cycle and in pregnancy.
D. DGI strains: Nearly all sensitive to penicillin.

IV. Diagnosis
A. History and physical findings
  1. Time from sexual contact to DGI ranges from 1 day to 2 months, and most patients have no symptoms of local infection.
  2. Migratory or additive polyarthralgias.
  3. Physical exam.
    a. Tenosynovitis: Most often over the dorsum of the hand, wrist, ankle, or knee.
    b. Synovitis: Purulent in 25–50%, usually involving multiple large joints.
    c. Dermatitis: Small maculopapular or vesicular lesions usually found over the extremities. They are usually asymptomatic and require careful inspection to be detected.
    d. Fever.
B. Diagnostic tests
  1. Synovial fluid: In contrast to bacterial arthritis, synovial fluid cultures are positive in less than 25%.
  2. Blood cultures: Rarely positive.
  3. Genitourinary, rectal, and pharyngeal cultures: Positive in approximately 75% of patients; therefore, should be done in all patients suspected of having DGI.

V. Differential Diagnosis
Includes hepatitis, subacute bacterial endocarditis, viral arthritis, acute rheumatic fever, Lyme disease, and Reiter's syndrome.

VI. Treatment
The treatment is generally very effective; therefore, this therapeutic response can be used for diagnostic purposes. Patients usually become afebrile within 24–48 hr of antibiotic therapy, with dramatic improvement of joint and skin disease in 1–3 days.
A. Antibiotics
  1. PCN: Until recently, all DGI strains were sensitive to PCN, but reports of PCN-resistant organisms have been reported. Give 10 million U of PCN G intravenous until improvement is noted and oral PCN or ampicillin for 7–10 days.
  2. Ceftriaxone: Recommended for PCN-resistant organisms.
B. Joint drainage: Large, purulent joints should be drained, but generally DGI is not a destructive process; therefore, drainage is not essential for complete recovery.

VII. Prognosis
Most patients have rapid and complete recovery

from DGI. Recurrent infection is rare except in cases of terminal complement deficiencies.

Other Causes of Infectious Arthritis

I. **Viruses**
   A. Hepatitis B.
   B. Rubella.
   C. Parvovirus.
   D. Others: Alphaviruses, paramyxoviruses, enteroviruses, adenovirus.
II. **Mycobacteria**
   A. M. tuberculosis
   B. Atypical mycobacteria
III. **Fungi**
IV. **Lyme disease:** *Borrelia burgdorferi*

Bibliography

Goldenberg DL. Bacterial arthritis, in Kelly WN, Harris ED, Ruddy S, et al (eds), *Textbook of Rheumatology,* ed 3. Philadelphia, Saunders, 1989, p 1567.

Goldenberg DL, Reed JI. Bacterial arthritis. *N Engl J Med* 312:441–446, 1982.

O'Brien JP, Goldenberg DL, Rice PA. Disseminated gonococcal infection: A prospective 49 patients and a review of pathophysiology and immune mechanisms. *Medicine* 62:395–406, 1983.

Rompalo AM, Hook EW 3d, Roberts PL, et al. The acute arthritis-dermatitis syndrome. The changing importance of *Neisseria gonorrhea* and *Neisseria meningititis. Arch Intern Med* 147(2):281–283, 1987.

Rosenthal J, Bole GG, Robinson WD. Acute mongonococcal infectious arthritis. *Arthritis Rheum* 23:889–897, 1980.

Schumacher HR Jr. *Primer on the Rheumatic Diseases,* ed 9. Atlanta, 1988, pp 181–188.

CHAPTER 109

Sarcoid Arthropathy

Margaret Michalska, M.D.

I. Definition

Sarcoid arthropathy (SA) occurs in 5–37% of patients with sarcoidosis. Two distinct clinical patterns are recognized in adults. The acute form is associated with bilateral hilar adenopathy (Löfgren's syndrome) and erythema nodosum. The chronic form accompanies multiorgan sarcoidosis.

II. Etiology

The etiology remains unknown. An unusual reaction to *Mycobacterium tuberculosis* has been postulated, but the organism has not been identified in sarcoid lesions.

III. Pathophysiology

Noncaseating granulomas are the hallmark of sarcoidosis. Large numbers of T lymphocytes enriched with T4 cells are present in these lesions.

IV. Diagnosis

The presence of hilar adenopathy, skin lesions, uveitis, impaired delayed hypersensitivity, elevated serum angiotensin-converting enzyme levels, hypercalcemia, and hypercalciuria support the diagnosis of sarcoidosis. Tissue biopsy showing typical granulomas establishes the diagnosis.

A. Löfgren's syndrome
   1. Physical findings: Acute onset of articular and periarticular swelling, usually accompanied by hilar adenopathy, fever, and erythema nodosum. Ankles and knees are most frequently affected. Pain and impairment are much less than expected in the presence of dramatic inflammation.
   2. Investigations: X-rays show soft tissue swelling. Chest x-ray reveals bilateral hilar adenopathy. The erythrocyte sedimentation rate is elevated. The latex test for rheumatoid factor is positive in 15–40% of cases. Hyperuricemia is detectable in 25% of cases.
   3. Treatment: Joint manifestations subside over 2 weeks to 4 months. Nonsteroidal anti-inflammatory drugs (NSAIDs) and colchicine are used to shorten attacks.
   4. The prognosis is excellent.

B. Chronic sarcoid arthritis
   1. Physical findings: Episodes of recurrent, protracted oligoarthritis or monarthritis with polysynovitis. Severe arthritis is most common in patients with multisystem granulomatous disease. Tenosynovitis can be seen.
   2. Investigations: Noncaseating granulomas

found on synovial biopsy confirm the diagnosis. X-ray shows osteolytic lesions and a lacy trabecular pattern.

3. Treatment: NASIDs and colchicine are used. Chloroquine has been shown to improve the cutaneous manifestations of sarcoidosis. Corticosteroids are used particularly in severe ocular disease, pulmonary parenchymal disease, and central nervous sytem involvement.

4. The prognosis is good. Even with severe systemic disease arthritis is usually mild but cases of recurrent and protracted synovitis also occur. Joint destruction however is infrequent.

Bibliography

Gumpel JM, Johns CJ, Shulman LE. The joint disease of sarcoidosis. *Ann Rheum Dis* 26:194–205, 1967.

James DG, Neville E, Carstairs LS. Bone and joint sarcoidosis. *Semin Arthritis Rheum* 6(1):53–81, 1976.

Sokoloff L, Bumin JJ. Clinical and pathological studies of joint involvement in sarcoidosis. *N Engl J Med* 260:842–847, 1959.

Thomas PD, Hunninghake GW. Current concepts of the pathogenesis of sarcoidosis. *Am Rev Respir Dis* 135(3):747–760, 1986.

CHAPTER 110

Reflex Sympathetic Dystrophy Syndrome

John P. Huff, M.D., Ph.D.

I. **Definition**

Reflex sympathetic dystrophy syndrome (RSDS) is one of a family of related somatic pain conditions attributable to overactivity of the peripheral sympathetic nervous system involving somatic structures.

II. **Etiology**

The etiology of RSDS is unclear.

A. Over 50% of cases are associated with antecedent major or minor trauma.

B. Twenty-five percent of cases are idiopathic.

C. Hemiplegia, myocardial infarction and ischemia, peripheral nerve injury, and exposure to drugs such as barbiturates and isoniazid have also been related to the development of RSDS.

III. **Pathophysiology**

A central and peripheral nervous system role has been suggested in the initiation and propagation of RSDS. Peripheral sympathetic nervous system overactivity and reactivity occurs by an unknown mechanism. Men and women of all ages are affected equally.

IV. **Diagnosis**

Presence of a combination of signs and symptoms is necessary for diagnosis.

A. A severe burning pain, usually in a distal extremity.

B. Tenderness often associated with allodynia (pain with touch) and hyperpathia (overreaction to repetitive stimulation).

C. Swelling: pitting or nonpitting.

D. Dystrophic skin changes consisting of a shiny complexion, loss of wrinkling, atrophy, and hypertrichosis.

E. Vasomotor changes in the affected area with sweating, temperature, and color changes.

1. Warm and flushed in early disease.

2. Cool, dusky, and pallid in late disease.

F. Radiologic changes.

1. A nonspecific, patchy osteopenia.

2. A unique three-phase bone scan showing unequal blood flow in the first phase, asymmetric pooling of the radionucleotide in soft tissues in the second phase, and increased (less commonly, de-

creased) periarticular radionucleotide uptake in the delayed or third phase.

G. Alleviation of symptoms after sympathetic nerve block.

V. Differential Diagnosis

Localized pain from many causes can be confused with RSDS.

A. Trauma.
B. Overuse injuries.
C. Regional osteoporosis.
D. Myofascial pain syndrome.
E. Arthritis: Degenerative and inflammatory.
F. Infection: Cellulitis or septic arthritis.
G. Fractures.
H. Tendinitis and bursitis.
I. Peripheral vascular disease.
J. Regional lymphatic or venous obstruction.
K. Psychogenic.

VI. Treatment

Early recognition and treatment are important.

A. Early disease
   1. Physical therapy for mobilization and range of motion.
   2. Analgesics as needed.
   3. Nonsteroidal anti-inflammatory drugs.
B. Nonresponsive or late disease
   1. Trial of prednisone, 15 mg four times per day, tapered over 2–3 weeks.
   2. Sympathetic nerve block if steroids fail.
   3. Range-of-motion exercise.
C. Transcutaneous electrical nerve stimulators (TENS) can offer some relief.
D. Surgical sympathectomy in cases partially responsive to sympathetic nerve block.
E. Regional intravenous guanethidine and bretylium have been effective experimentally.

VII. Patient Monitoring

Patients need frequent monitoring.

A. Prolonged disease is more difficult to treat.
B. Can progress to permanent disability.

C. Relapses can occur.
D. Mild exacerbations can occur after steroids are discontinued. These usually last for only a few weeks.

VIII. Prognosis

The prognosis in general is dependent on the length of time the disease is present.

A. Early disease responds to conservative therapy.
B. Mild disease and disease with a positive bone scan usually responds to corticosteroid therapy.
C. Late and severe disease usually responds best to repeated sympathetic nerve block.
D. Surgical sympathectomy can elicit a good response in cases that have partially responded to sympathetic nerve block.
E. Nonresponse is unusual, but can occur and usually leads to marked physical and psychological disability.

Bibliography

Dietz FR, Mathews KD, Montgomery WJ. Reflex sympathetic dystrophy in children. *Clin Orthop* 258:225–231, 1990.

Garrett RA. Chronic pain syndromes, in Kelley WN (ed), *Textbook of Rheumatology*, ed 3. Philadelphia, Saunders, 1989, p 1893.

Kozin F, McCarty DJ, Sims J, et al. The reflex sympathetic dystrophy syndrome. I. Clinical and histologic studies: Evidence for bilaterality, response to corticosteroids, and articular involvement. *Am J Med* 60:321–331, 1976.

Loh L, Nathan PW, Schott GD, et al. Effects of regional guanethidine infusion in certain painful states. *J Neurol Neurosurg Psychiatry* 43:446–451, 1980.

Werner R, Davidoff G, Jackson MD, et al. Factors affecting the sensitivity and specificity of the three-phase technetium bone scan in the diagnosis of reflex sympathetic dystrophy syndrome in the upper extremity. *J Hand Surg (AM)* 14:520–523, 1989.

CHAPTER 111

Familial Mediterranean Fever

Margaret Michalska, M.D.

I. **Definition**
Familial Mediterranean fever (FMF) is an autosomal recessive disorder occurring primarily in persons from the Mediterranean area. It is characterized by recurrent attacks of fever, abdominal pain, and chest pain, as well as asymmetric oligoarthritis. Amyloidosis can develop.

II. **Etiology**
The etiology of FMF is unknown.

III. **Pathophysiology**
Acute nonspecific peritoneal inflammation has been found, with predominance of polymorphonuclear leukocytes (PMNs) in the exudate. Pleural and joint inflammation is also nonspecific.

IV. **Diagnosis**
  A. History: Attacks first occur between ages 5 and 15. The family history reveals a close relative with similar symptoms or a consanguineous marriage.
  B. Clinical signs
    1. Fever without shaking chills, usually lasting for a few hours.
    2. Abdominal crises resembling acute peritonitis lasting for 12–24 hr.
    3. Acute chest pain involving one hemithorax, occasionally accompanied by pleural effusion or pericarditis.
    4. Intermittent asymmetric arthritis involving, in order of decreasing frequency, the knees, ankles, hips, shoulders, feet, toes, elbows, wrists, and hands.
  C. Diagnostic tests
    1. Laboratory findings are nonspecific. Elevated erythrocyte sedimentation rate and fibrinogen levels are seen. Both rise at the outset of attacks.
    2. Leukocytosis is common; leukopenia can occur in the presence of splenomegaly.
    3. Proteinuria and nephrotic syndrome are seen in the presence of amyloidosis.
    4. Joint fluid contains PMNs early and lymphocytes late during an acute attack.
    5. Radiologic examination frequently shows osteoporosis with pseudocyst formation. With chronicity, degenerative changes develop. Widening and sclerosis of sacroiliac joints has been described.

V. **Differential Diagnosis**
  A. Acute febrile illness, acute appendicitis, and pancreatis; porphyria; cholecystitis.

B. Inherited forms of hyperlipidemia.

C. Acute arthritis: Septic, crystalline, and rheumatic disease.

VI. Treatment

A. Acute attacks respond to nonsteroidal anti-inflammatory drugs.

B. Prophylaxis with colchicine, 0.6 mg two or three times per day, greatly reduces the frequency of attacks, as well as the incidence of amyloidosis.

VII. Prognosis

The prognosis is good, and patients remain free of symptoms between attacks. Amyloidosis, when it occurs, is associated with splenomegaly and nephrotic syndrome, frequently leading to death.

Bibliography

Goldstein RC, Schwabe AD. Prophylactic colchicine therapy in familial Mediterranean fever: A controlled double blind study. *Ann Intern Med* 81:792–794, 1974.

Heller H, Gafni J, Michaeli D, et al: The arthritis of familiar Mediterranean fever. *Arthritis Rheum* 9:1–17, 1966.

Heller H, Sohar E, Sherf L. Familial Mediterranean fever. *Arch Intern Med* 102:50–71, 1958.

Matzner Y, Ayesh SK, Hochner-Celniker D, et al. Proposed mechanism of the inflammatory attacks in familial Mediterranean fever. *Arch Intern Med* 150(6):1289–1291, 1990.

CHAPTER 112

Crystal Diseases

Denise Verges, M.D.

Crystal diseases are a group of arthropathies characterized by crystal deposition in and around joints, leading to variable clinical, radiographic, and pathologic abnormalities.

Gout

I. Definition

A heterogeneous group of genetic and acquired diseases resulting from tissue deposition of monosodium urate crystals.

II. Etiology

Hyperuricemia, in combination with various etiologic influences (hereditary, pathologic, pharmacologic, and dietary), leads to the clinical syndrome. Hyperuricemia results from overproduction (10%) or underexcretion (90%).

A. Hyperuricemia

   1. Excessive production of uric acid (10%)

      a. Idiopathic.

      b. Inherited enzyme defects: hypoxanthine guanine phosphoribosyl transferase deficiency, phosphoribosylpyrophosphate synthetase superactivity, glucose-6-phosphatase deficiency.

      c. Increased cell turnover: Myeloproliferative and lymphoproliferative disorders, hemolytic anemia, psoriasis, obesity.

      d. Increased purine nucleotide catabolism—tissue hypoxia; glycogeneses types III, V, and VII; drug-induced ethanol, fructose, and cytotoxic agents.

      e. Increased purine ingestion: Purine-rich diets, pancreatic extract.

B. Impaired renal uric acid excretion: (90%)

   1. Idiopathic.

   2. Renal disease: Chronic renal failure, lead nephropathy, polycystic kidney disease, hypertension.

   3. Abnormal metabolic states: Starvation, dehydration, salt restriction, lactic acidemia, ketonemia, glycogenesis type I, diabetic ketoacidosis, eclampsia, Bartter's syndrome.

   4. Endocrinopathies: Hyperparathyroidism, hypothyroidism, nephrogenic diabetes insipidus.

   5. Drug-induced: Diuretics; low-dose salicylates, ethanol, ethambutol, pyrazinamide; levodopa; methoxyflurane; laxative abuse.

6. Other: Sarcoidosis, beryllium disease, Down's syndrome.

III. Pathophysiology

A. The inciting event is the deposition of monosodium urate crystals from supersaturated extracellular fluid in the connective tissue of joints.

1. Subsequently, crystals are discharged into the joint cavity from local trauma or metabolic change.
2. Immunoglobulin coats crystals, enhancing phagocytosis and leading to superoxide generation by neutrophils.
3. Neutrophils are used by the crystals, releasing lysosomal enzymes and more crystals.
4. Acute synovitis and articular damage result.
5. Urate crystals also stimulate monocytes to release pyrogens, leading to fever.

B. Other factors thought to be involved
1. Fibrinogen, complement, albumin, acid phosphatase
2. β-Glucuronidase
3. Crystal structure
4. pH
5. Temperature
6. Cation concentrations
7. Mechanical stimuli

C. The complete role of crystals in the pathogenesis of gout is not understood, as they can be found in asymptomatic joints.

IV. Epidemiology

A. Prevalence is 2–2.6/1,000.
B. Males predominate, with a 15:1 ratio; peak age of onset is the fifth decade.
C. After menopause, the incidence in female patients reaches that of men.
D. Associations
1. Obesity
2. Ethanol abuse
3. Diabetes mellitus
4. Hyperlipidemia
5. Hypertension
6. Atherosclerosis
7. Calcium oxalate urolithiasis

V. Diagnosis

A. History: Emphasize:
1. Age at onset of symptoms.
2. History of kidney stones or previous arthritis.
3. Symptoms of underlying disease, such as anorexia, weight loss, or fatigue.
4. Current medications (especially diuretics or low-dose aspirin) or a recent change in medication.
5. Family history of gout or arthritis.
6. Dietary intake and alcohol use.
7. Recent acute illness.

B. Clinical signs and physical findings
1. Asymptomatic hyperuricemia
   a. Serum urate value exceeds the limit of solubility of monosodium urate in serum.
   b. Upper limit of normal is 7.0 mg/dl in males and 6.0 mg/dl in females.
   c. Occurs in 5% of normal persons in adulthood.
   d. Present for 20–30 years before the first attack of gout.
2. Acute gouty arthritis
   a. The most common early manifestation of gout.
   b. Onset in patients under 30 should lead to a search for an enzymatic defect or another underlying cause.
   c. Initial attack is monarticular in 90% of cases; the most frequently involved joint is the first metatarsophalangeal (50–70%), followed by insteps, ankles, heels, knees, wrists, fingers, and elbows.
   d. Six percent of patients develop polyarticular gout; a past history of gout is usually present.
   e. Onset begins abruptly, frequently at night; fever may be present.
   f. Affected joints are warm, red, and extremely tender.
   g. Desquamation of the skin may occur with resolution of inflammation.
   h. Untreated gout has a variable course; early mild attacks may last for hours; severe attacks can last for weeks.
   i. Can be triggered by trauma, alcohol, drugs, surgical stress, or acute medical illness.
3. Intercritical gout
   a. The asymptomatic period between attacks.
   b. A second episode may not occur or many years may pass between attacks.
   c. Subsequent episodes are increasingly frequent, more severe, of longer duration, and more likely to be polyarticular.
4. Chronic tophaceous gout
   a. A tophus is a chronic foreign body

granuloma surrounding a core of monosodium urate crystals.

   b. Its presence correlates with the degree of hyperuricemia and the duration of disease.

   c. Fifty percent of inadequately treated patients develop tophi.

   d. The average duration of gout prior to the development of tophi is 11.6 years.

   e. Tophi occur most often in the synovium, subchondral bone, tendons and bursae, over bony prominences, and on the pinna; they may involve any joint, the heart valves, or vocal cords.

   f. Tophaceous gout is usually painless, but it can cause stiffness and aching of joints; joint destruction and deformities may result.

   g. White chalky material may extrude from the tophi; rarely, suppuration occurs.

  5. Renal disease

   a. Nephrolithiasis

    (1) From 10% to 25% of patients with gout develop kidney stones, both uric acid and calcium.

    (2) The incidence is twice as high in patients with secondary gout as it is in those with primary gout.

    (3) Stone formation increases with the serum urate concentration and with urinary uric acid excretion.

   b. Acute uric acid nephropathy

    (1) The precipitation of uric acid crystals in collecting ducts and ureters can lead to acute renal failure.

    (2) It occurs most commonly after aggressive chemotherapy for leukemia or lymphoma—the acute tumor lysis syndrome.

   c. Urate nephropathy

    (1) Deposition of urate crystals occurs in the medullary interstitium, papillae, and pyramids.

    (2) One-third of gouty patients have albuminuria and isosthenuria.

    (3) Impaired renal function in these patients cannot be attributed to hyperuricemia alone; hypertension and atherosclerotic disease appear to be involved.

C. Tests

  1. Laboratory tests

   a. Intra- or extracellular monosodium urate crystals are present; rod- or needle-shaped crystals are negatively birefringent (bright yellow) and parallel to the axis of slow vibration.

   b. Synovial fluid is cloudy; the leukocyte count ranges from 2,000 to 100,000 mm^3, mainly neutrophils; coexistent infection must be ruled out.

   c. Serum uric acid level may be normal, especially with aspirin use or initiation of a uricosuric agent.

   d. Mandatory laboratory work includes a complete blood count and platelet count, urinalysis, serum uric acid, blood urea nitrogen, creatinine, triglycerides, albumin, serum glutamic-oxaloacetic transaminase, calcium, phosphate, 24-hr urinary uric acid excretion, and creatinine clearance.

  2. Radiographs

   a. They play a minor role in the initial attack of gout; only soft tissue swelling is present.

   b. Tophi lead to an asymmetric polyarthropathy with eccentric soft tissue swelling.

   c. Sharply defined gouty erosions, with sclerotic margins and an overhanging edge, are characteristic.

   d. Secondary osteoarthritic changes occur late.

VI. Differential Diagnosis

  A. Septic arthritis

  B. Pseudogout

  C. Cellulitis

  D. Thrombophlebitis

  E. Rheumatoid arthritis

VII. Treatment

  A. Asymptomatic hyperuricemia: Only marked uric acid overexcretors should be treated to protect against nephrolithiasis. In all other cases, no therapy is recommended.

  B. Acute gout

   1. May be treated with colchicine, nonsteroidal drugs, or steroids.

   2. Drugs affecting the serum urate concentration should not be changed (started or stopped).

   3. Colchicine

    a. Inhibits production of a chemotactic factor, which limits the amount of inflammation.

    b. The half-life is about 30 hr.

    c. It is excreted by hepatic, renal, and intestinal routes.

d. For the initial attack, the recommended dosage is 0.5 or 0.6 mg orally every 1–2 hr until:
   (1) Objective reduction of joint inflammation occurs.
   (2) Gastrointestinal (GI) toxicity develops.
   (3) The maximum oral dosage (8–10 mg in 24 hr) has been given.
e. The oral dosage must be adjusted in the presence of renal or hepatic dysfunction.
f. Colchicine may be given intravenously, but only to patients with normal renal and hepatic function. A single dose is 2 mg; the cumulative dose in 24 hr should not exceed 4 mg.
g. Toxicity of colchicine
   (1) G.I: Nausea, vomiting, abdominal cramping, diarrhea (mainly with oral use).
   (2) Bone marrow suppression.
   (3) Renal, hepatic, and central nervous system (CNS) dysfunction.
   (4) Myopathy and neuropathy.
   (5) Disseminated intravascular coagulation.
   (6) Local chemical thrombophlebitis or tissue necrosis from extravasation (intravenous use only).
4. Nonsteroidal anti-inflammatory drugs
   a. Have largely replaced colchicine because of the lower incidence of GI side effects.
   b. Effective even after therapy has been delayed for several days.
   c. Inhibit inflammation by interfering with prostaglandin synthesis.
   d. The response to nonsteroidals is not specific for gout.
   e. The most commonly used agent is indomethacin, but all others have been proven efficacious.
   f. The main reason to pick one drug over another is the difference in toxicity.
   g. Full dosages of anti-inflammatories should be given and tapered after there is clinical improvement.
   h. Side effects
      (1) GI: Ulceration and bleeding of the esophagus, stomach, and duodenum; epigastric pain, dyspepsia, and nausea.
      (2) Renal: Papillary necrosis, neph-

rotic syndrome, acute renal failure, interstitial nephritis.
      (3) CNS: Drowsiness, headache, vertigo, confusion.
      (4) Rarely, abnormalities of liver function and bone marrow depression.
   i. Caution should be exercised in patients with renal dysfunction or a history of peptic ulcer disease.
5. Corticosteroids
   a. Indicated when colchicine and nonsteroidal agents have failed, are poorly tolerated, or are contraindicated.
   b. Can use adrenocorticotropic hormone, 20 U intravenously or 40–80 U intramuscularly every 6–12 hr for 1–3 days.
   c. Prednisone, at dosages of 15–30 mg/day, may resolve the attack.
   d. Intra-articular corticosteroid injections may help if only a few joints are involved.
   e. Rebound flares are common with discontinuation of therapy; simultaneous use of colchicine (0.6 mg twice per day) or nonsteroidal agents is recommended.
C. Prophylaxis of acute gout
   1. The prophylactic benefit of colchicine in preventing recurrent acute attacks has been demonstrated.
   2. Renal and hepatic function must be normal to use colchicine on a chronic basis.
   3. Since the frequency of acute gouty attacks may increase with the initiation of antihyperuricemic therapy, some recommend simultaneous colchicine prophylaxis for the first 6–12 months of treatment.
D. Treatment of hyperuricemia
   1. Indications for normalizing serum uric acid levels in gout
      a. Presence of tophi.
      b. Major uric acid overproducers (urinary excretion >1100 mg of uric acid in 24 hr) because of the increased risk of tophaceous deposition and stone formation.
      c. Frequent gouty attacks unresponsive to prophylactic colchicine or nonsteroidal agents.
      d. Recurrent uric acid renal calculi.
      e. Recurrent calcium oxalate renal calculi when associated with hyperuricosuria.
   2. Uricosuric drugs

a. Interfere with the tubular reabsorption of filtered urate. Include:
   (1) Probenecid
   (2) Sulfinpyrazone
   (3) High-dose salicylates
   (4) Radiocontrast agents
   (5) Glyceryl quaiacolate
   (6) Several nonsteroidal agents
b. The two agents used in the United States, probenecid and sulfinpyrazone, are equally effective.
   (1) Probenecid
      (a) Begin with the lowest effective dose and titrate to normal uric acid levels; 50% of patients require 1 g/day.
      (b) Increase fluid intake at the initiation of therapy to avoid uric acid deposition in the kidney.
      (c) There is a reduced response to probenecid or sulfinpyrazone in patients with renal insufficiency.
      (d) Acetylsalicylate blocks the effects of both agents.
      (e) Interferes with the renal excretrion of many medications, including penicillin, ampicillin, indomethacin, acetazolamide, and dapsone.
      (f) Side effects
         i) Gastric intolerance—8%
         ii) Hypersensitivity and rash 5%
         iii) New uric acid stone: Prevent by forcing fluids or alkalinizing urine.
         iv) Increased frequency of new attacks at initiation of therapy: Prevent with simultaneous use of colchicine.
   (2) Sulfinpyrazone
      (a) An analog of a phenylbutazone metabolite which has no anti-inflammatory effects.
      (b) Initiate use of the drug in low doses and titrate to normalize the serum urate level; average maintenance dose is 300–400 mg/day.
      (c) Side effects: Gastric intolerance (5%), rash and hypersensitivity (rare), and bone marrow suppression (rare).

E. Allopurinol
   1. It inhibits xanthine oxidase, which converts hypoxanthine to xanthine and xanthine to uric acid.
   2. Its chief metabolite, oxypurinol, is also a xanthine oxidase inhibitor and has a half-life of 20 hr.
   3. The dosage should be started at 100 mg and titrated until normouricemia is maintained.
   4. Patients with renal insufficiency should receive a reduced dosage.
   5. Allopurinol may increase the toxicity of the chemotherapeutic agents 6-mercaptopurine and azathioprine because they are inhibited by xanthine oxidase.
   6. Side effects: 5% of patients discontinue therapy because of side effects.
      a. Pruritic maculopapular rash.
      b. Hypersensitivity syndrome: An immunologic reaction to the drug. It is more common in patients with renal insufficiency. Mortality rate is 27%. Symptoms include:
         (1) Fever
         (2) Eosinophilia
         (3) Leukocytosis
         (4) Worsening renal function
         (5) Hepatocellular injury
         (6) Vasculitis
      c. Bone marrow suppression
      d. Kidney stones
      e. GI intolerance
   7. Uricosuric drugs versus allopurinol
      a. Frequency of toxicity with probenecid, sulfinpyrazone, and allopurinol is similar, but the severity is greatest with allopurinol.
      b. A uricosuric drug should be the drug of choice in all patients except those who are major overexcretors, or who have renal insufficiency or a history of kidney stones.
      c. Allopurinol is preferred for the prevention of acute tumor lysis syndrome.

Calcium Pyrophosphate Deposition Disease (CPDD)

I. Definition
A form of crystalline arthropathy characterized by a wide spectrum of clinical patterns.
II. Etiology

A. Hereditary: Autosomal dominant, with variable penetrance.
B. Sporadic
  1. Most common form encountered.
  2. No evidence of familial predisposition or underlying disorder associated with CPDD.
  3. Aging and previous joint trauma or surgery are predisposing factors.
C. Metabolic
  1. Strong associations
    a. Hyperparathyroidism
    b. Hemochromatosis
    c. Hypomagnesemia
    d. Hypophosphatasia
    e. Wilson's disease
    f. Gout
  2. Likely associations
    a. Hypothyroidism
    b. Ochronosis
    c. Amyloidosis
    d. Hypocalciuric hypercalcemia

III. Pathophysiology
A. Calcium pyrophosphate deposition probably results from various antecedent metabolic aberrations. Hypotheses include:
  1. The accumulation of pyrophosphate; through an enzyme system involving increased nucleoside triphosphate (NTP) pyrophosphohydrolase levels and diminished pyrophosphatase levels.
  2. Biochemical or structural changes in the cartilage matrix.
B. Preformed deposits of crystals in cartilage are shed into the joint cavity.
  1. Factors which enhance calcium pyrophosphate solubility—such as a fall in ionized calcium, which occurs after trauma—may trigger the crystal shedding.
  2. Mechanisms of inflammation induced by calcium pyrophosphate crystals are similar to those by monosodium urate crystals.

IV. Diagnosis
A. History: Emphasize:
  1. Age at onset.
  2. Family history.
  3. Location of symptoms.
  4. Previous joint trauma or surgery.
  5. Presence of other medical conditions.
  6. Antecedent illness or surgery.
B. Clinical presentation
  1. Asymptomatic
    a. The most common form of CPDD; present in 44% of persons over age 84.
    b. The incidental finding of chondrocalcinosis in radiographs of asymptomatic joints.
  2. Acute synovitis (pseudogout)
    a. Acute onset of severe pain, stiffness, and swelling in a joint.
    b. Overlying erythema and florid synovitis are present.
    c. Fever, malaise, and confusion may be seen.
    d. Most commonly involved joint is the knee (50%), followed by the wrist, shoulder, and ankle.
    e. It is usually spontaneous but can follow trauma, intercurrent illness, or surgery.
    f. It is most often self-limited, resolving in 1–3 weeks.
    g. Patients are usually asymptomatic between episodes.
    h. Ten percent of cases are polyarticular.
  3. Chronic pyrophosphate arthropathy (pseudo-osteoarthritis)
    a. A chronic low-grade synovitis in numerous joints, with evidence of joint degeneration.
    b. Pattern of involvement is similar to that of pseudogout.
    c. Chronic pain, stiffness, and limited range of motion occur.
    d. It may be associated with acute attacks of pseudogout.
    e. On exam, bony swelling, crepitus, joint line tenderness, and decreased range of motion are present.
    f. Distinguished from osteoarthritis by the location of the affected joints, degree of inflammation, and greater severity.
    g. Other forms include pseudoneuropathic joints and a severely destructive arthropathy of the knees, shoulders, and hips.
    h. Pseudo-rheumatoid arthritis demonstrates subacute or chronic symmetric arthritis of large joints.
    i. Atypical presentations simulate ankylosing spondylitis or polymyalgia rheumatica.
C. Tests
  1. Synovial fluid: Rhomboid or linear crystals, weakly positive or nonbirefringent, intra- and extracellular.
  2. Screening for associated metabolic condi-

tions should include serum calcium, phosphorus, alkaline phosphatase, iron, total iron-binding capacity, magnesium, and thyroid function tests.

3. Radiographs
   a. Chondrocalcinosis: Linear and punctate calcifications of fibrocartilage and articular cartilage.
   b. The most commonly involved fibrocartilages are the knee menisci, the triangular fibrocartilage of the wrist, and the symphysis pubis.
   c. CPDD may deposit in tendons or bursae.
   d. Pyrophosphate arthropathy can resemble osteoarthritis, but the distribution over joints and marked hypertrophy help to distinguish them.

V. Differential Diagnosis
   A. Pseudogout
      1. Septic arthritis
      2. Gout
      3. Rheumatoid arthritis
   B. Pyrophosphate arthropathy
      1. Osteoarthritis
      2. Neurotrophic joints

VI. Treatment
   A. Asymptomatic chondrocalcinosis: No therapy indicated.
   B. Pseudogout
      1. Aspiration of joint fluid.
      2. Nonsteroidal agents or intra-articular corticosteroids in resistant cases.
      3. Intravenous colchicine is effective, but rarely needed.
   C. Pyrophosphate arthropathy: therapy similar to that of osteoarthritis.
      1. Salicylates
      2. Nonsteroidal drugs
      3. Analgesics
      4. Physical therapy

Basic Calcium Phosphate Crystal Deposition Disease

I. Definition
A group of diseases associated with the deposition of basic calcium phosphate crystals (hydroxyapatite, octacalcium phosphate) in and around joints.

II. Etiology
   A. Idiopathic
   B. Secondary to local tissue damage
   C. Familial
   D. Associated with scleroderma, dermatomyositis, or systemic lupus erythematosus
   E. Metabolic
      1. Hypercalcemia
      2. Hyperphosphatemia
      3. Vitamin D intoxication
      4. Renal failure
      5. Hemodialysis
      6. Diabetes mellitus
      7. Associated with other forms of crystal deposition

III. Pathophysiology
Calcification is prevented in normal connective tissue by certain inhibitors (in vitro this has been demonstrated with inorganic pyrophosphate, proteoglycan aggregates, and noncollagenous proteins). Basic calcium phosphate deposition can occur if:
   A. Soluble concentrate is raised secondary to a metabolic disorder.
   B. Aging or tissue damage disrupts normal inhibition.
   C. Nucleating agents are present in the tissue.
   D. A cell-driven mechanism is present.

IV. Clinical Picture
   A. Asymptomatic (the majority of cases)
   B. Calcific periarthritis
      1. Can be unifocal, multifocal, or familial.
      2. The shoulder is the most frequently involved joint.
      3. Consider a metabolic cause if numerous joints are involved or if deposits are very large.
      4. The acute attack
         a. Usually occurs in persons under 40.
         b. Incidence in equal in males and females.
         c. Onset is abrupt; may follow trauma.
         d. Severe pain and local tenderness can occur.
         e. Symptoms resolve in a few days.
         f. Accounts for 7% of painful shoulders.
   C. Calcific tendinitis and bursitis
      1. There is inflammation of the tendon sheath or bursa associated with calcium deposition.
      2. There is abrupt onset of severe pain.
      3. This condition can mimic gout.
   D. Intra-articular basic calcium phosphate arthropathies
      1. Acute gout-like attacks.
      2. Erosive polyarticular disease.
      3. Mixed crystal deposition disease.
      4. Osteoarthritis: basic calcium phosphate

(BCP) crystals are found in 30–60% of patients; this may be an epiphenomenon.
E. Milwaukee shoulder syndrome
1. A rapidly destructive shoulder arthropathy found predominantly in elderly women.
2. The knee is involved in one-half of the cases (often asymptomatic).
3. There is painful reduced range of motion and large, cool effusions.
4. Predisposing factors: Joint trauma, CPPD deposition, recurrent dislocations, neurologic abnormalities, and dialysis.
5. Radiographs shows joint space narrowing, osteophytes, soft tissue calcifications, and subchondral cysts.
6. Laboratory tests
   a. Noninflammatory synovial fluid.
   b. Light microscopy of synovial fluid, with alizarin's stain.
   c. Electron microscopy of selected samples.
   d. Labeled pyrophosphates to detect apatite.
F. Secondary BCP arthropathies and periarthropathies
1. Associated conditions include:
   a. Chronic renal failure
   b. Calcinosis in collagen vascular diseases (scleroderma)
   c. Severe neurologic injury
   d. Postcorticosteroid injection
V. **Therapy**
A. Calcific periarthritis, tendinitis, or intra-articular arthropathies
1. Nonsteroidal drugs
2. Colchicine
3. Aspiration
4. Surgery for large calcific deposits
B. Milwaukee shoulder syndrome: Nonsteroidal drugs, analgesics, aspiration, surgery.
C. Calcinosis: warfarin, probenecid.

Bibliography

Becker MA. Clinical aspects of monosodium urate monohydrate crystal deposition disease. *Rheum Dis Clin North Am* 14:377–396, 1988.

Doherty M, Dieppe P. Clinical aspects of calcium pyrophosphate dihydrate crystal deposition. *Rheum Dis Clin North Am* 14:395–413, 1988.

Halverson PB, McCarty DJ. Clinical aspects of basic calcium phosphate crystal deposition. *Rheum Dis Clin North Am* 14:427–439, 1988.

Rubenstein J, Pritzker KP. Crystal associated arthropathies. *Am J Radiol* 1585–695, 1989.

Wallace SL, Singer JZ. Therapy in gout. *Rheum Dis Clin North Am* 14:441–457, 1988.

CHAPTER 113

Fibromyalgia Syndrome

Robert Katz, M.D.

I. Definition
  A. Fibromyalgia (fibrositis) is a clinical syndrome of diffuse musculoskeletal pain and points of musce tenderness.
  B. Myofascial pain syndrome is a more limited and regional distribution of pain.

II. Etiology
  The etiology of fibromyalgia is unknown. There is evidence of several possible causes.
  A. Affective spectrum disorder: Poor sleep and low energy. Some studies have shown an increased prevalence of depression in fibromyalgia patients and their relatives compared with controls. Furthermore, fibromyalgia may respond to low doses of antidepressants. It is possible that fibromyalgia is due, or aggravated by, an imbalance of neurotransmitters in the brain and spinal cord. Other illnesses that may be part of an "affective spectrum" include migraine, irritable bowel syndrome, dysmenorrhea, and chronic fatigue syndrome.
  B. Muscle disease: Perhaps fibromyalgia is a type of muscle disease related to ischemia of muscle or to abnormal muscle metabolism. Studies of muscle histology have not shown inflammation or significant abnormalities. Some histochemical studies have revealed a decrease in high-energy phosphates, and some investigators have concluded that energy metabolism in muscle may be abnormal in fibromyalgia.
  C. Stress: Although there is no direct evidence, some have theorized that fibromyalgia may be a stress-related disorder.
  D. Psychological disturbance: Investigators have found evidence of a somatizing tendency in some fibromyalgia patients. Abnormal psychological studies have been documented in fibromyalgia patients, and these are not explained by the intensity of pain.
  E. Sleep disturbance: There is abnormal deep (stage 4) sleep in fibromyalgia; this could be the cause of fatigue and possibly of the diffuse muscle aching. Sleep electroencephalograms have shown alpha waves (awake pattern) superimposed on delta waves (deep sleep pattern). This alpha-delta syndrome suggests that the patient never really enjoys deep, uninterrupted sleep.

III. Diagnosis
  Diagnostic criteria accepted by the American

College of Rheumatology have been developed. The primary criteria are widespread pain and many tender points in muscle.

A. Widespread pain: Pain is not well localized to the joints. The location of pain is generally above and below the waist, on both the left and right sides of the body, and affects the spine and peripheral areas.

B. Tender points: The presence of multiple tender points is characteristic. Typically, of 18 suggested sites, 11 or more points are tender. Tender point sites are the occiput, lower cervical spine, midpoint of the upper trapezius muscles, chest wall over the second rib, upper thoracic spine, elbows, gluteal muscles, medial knees, and lateral hips (greater trochanters).

C. Control points: Generally the thumbnail, forehead, and dorsal midfoot are not very tender in fibromyalgia patients.

D. Fibromyalgia may occur in association with systemic conditions such as rheumatoid arthritis or systemic lupus erythematosus, but it has no known connection to these disorders.

E. Other common features
1. Low energy.
2. Nonrestorative sleep, often with many awakenings.
3. Headaches.
4. Irritable bowel syndrome.
5. Pain at other locations, such as the pelvis and face.
6. Paresthesias; electromyographic (EMG) studies are normal.
7. Subjective joint swelling but no true swelling on physical examination.
8. Morning stiffness.
9. Hypersensitivity to weather conditions.

F. Laboratory studies: Typically, all laboratory studies are normal, including the complete blood count, sedimentation rate, and autoimmune studies. Not uncommonly, rheumatologists evaluate patients with positive antinuclear antibody (ANA) or other autoimmune tests who have chronic, diffuse muscle pain. These patients often have fibromyalgia; in these cases, there is no known association between the abnormal autoimmune tests and the fibromyalgia. X-rays and bone scans are also normal in fibromyalgia.

IV. **Differential Diagnosis**

A. Polymyalgia rheumatica: In elderly people the symptoms of polymyalgia rheumatica are proximal—the neck and shoulders, back, and upper thighs—not distal, and the sedimentation rate is high.

B. Systemic lupus erythematosus: Young women with a positive ANA and low energy may actually have fibromyalgia, the positive ANA being of unclear significance.

C. Polymyositis: Presents with weakness, a high creatinine phosphokinase level, but rarely pain.

D. Rheumatoid arthritis: Definite persistent joint swelling occurs.

E. Carpal tunnel syndrome: Paresthesias are common in fibromyalgia, but the EMG and nerve conduction studies are normal.

F. Cervical and lumbar radiculopathies: EMG and nerve conduction studies are normal in fibromyalgia.

G. Chronic fatigue syndrome: There is a great deal of overlap between the symptoms of chronic fatigue syndrome and fibromyalgia. Fibromyalgia is primarily a pain syndrome.

V. **Prevalence and Gender Association**

A. Some studies estimate that 3–6 million people or more in the United States have fibromyalgia.

B. Approximately 90% of these patients are women.

C. Age distribution: The peak incidence and prevalence are in the 20- to 50-year age group, but many patients first develop their symptoms in adolescence. Fibromyalgia is also not uncommon in the geriatric age group.

VI. **Patient Education: Booklets from The Fibromyalgia Network (Bakersfield, Ca) and the Arthritis Foundation.**

VII. **Treatment**

A. Amitriptyline: A low dosage, 10–50 mg at night, may be helpful in improving sleep and some of the other symptoms of fibromyalgia.

B. Cyclobenzaprine—especially at night; sedating.

C. Alprazolam and other benzodiazepines. Some patients respond but habituation may occur.

D. Tricyclic antidepressants: Some practitioners are more successful by treating with full antidepressant dosages of tricyclic antidepressant medication (i.e., 150–250 mg desipramine, etc.) Selective Serotonin reuptake inhibitors may also work. Fluoxetine may improve fatigue. Others sometimes help.

E. Soft tissue injections of lidocaine or lidocaine and a corticosteroid: These may be helpful if the pain is particularly intense over a confined region. This is certainly well known with chest wall pain, but it may work for other areas.

F. Nonsteroidal anti-inflammatory drugs: These may be somewhat helpful, but many patients tolerate them poorly.

G. Analgesics: Nonnarcotic analgesics may provide transient pain relief.

H. Hot bath or other forms of heat.

I. Aerobic exercise: Studies have shown that a regular program of low-impact aerobic exercises may improve well-being and function in patients with fibromyalgia.

J. Massage.

K. Biofeedback.

L. Stress reduction and informal psychotherapy by the physician may help patients to live with fibromyalgia.

M. Job modifications.

N. Those patients who mention an active lifestyle including regular active exercise tend to do better.

VIII. Prognosis and Course

Onset is usually gradual, although in some patients symptoms follow trauma such as automobile accidents or infections.

Bibliography

Goldenberg DL, Felson DT, and Dinerman H. A randomized, controlled trial of amitriptyline and naproxen in the treatment of patients with fibromyalgia. *Arthritis Rheum* 29:1371–1377, 1986.

Goldenberg, Don L. Fibromyalgia Syndrome, an Emerging but Controversial Condition: *JAMA* 257:2782–2787, 2802–2803, 1987.

The American College of Rheumatology 1990 Criteria for the Classification of Fibromyalgia: Arthritis Foundation, *Arthritis and Rheumatism*, Vol 33, No 2, 1990.

Wolfe, Frederick. Rheumatic Disease Clinics of North America: Fibromyalgia: *The Clinical Syndrome:* Vol 15, No 1, 1989.

CHAPTER 114

Hypertrophic Osteoarthropathy

Jan Clarke, M.D.

I. **Definition**

Hypertrophic Osteoarthropathy (HO) is a syndrome characterized by digital clubbing, long bone periostitis, and arthritis. It may be primary (hereditary with onset in childhood), associated with Graves' disease (thyroid acropachy), or secondary.

II. **Etiology and Pathogenesis**

Secondary HO is seen in association with malignancies (primary, especially bronchogenic, and metastatic tumors to lung), chronic infections (e.g., subacute bacterial endocarditis and bronchiectasis), chronic liver disease, inflammatory bowel disease, and infected aortic or axillary grafts. The pathogenesis is not clear; there is limited support for neurogenic and humoral theories.

III. **Diagnosis**

Diagnosis is established based on characteristic physical and radiographic findings.

A. History

1. In the case of isolated clubbing, there may be no symptoms, or only minor reports of burning or warmth of the fingertips.
2. Joint pain and swelling may be the presenting complaint in HO.
3. Severe, aching bone pain may be prominent in patients with lung cancer.

B. Clinical signs and physical findings of clubbing are characteristic but will not distinguish primary from secondary HO. The changes develop over months to years and may not be recognized by the patient. In HO, joint involvement may be seen.

1. Softening of the nail bed with a rocking sensation when the proximal nail is palpated.
2. Periungual erythema and warmth.
3. Increased sweating of the hands and feet; oily face and scalp, with coarsening of facial features (more prominent in primary HO).
4. Increase in the angle between the fingernail and nail base to more than 180 degrees (normal is 160 degrees).
5. Ratio of the circumference at the nail base to the circumference at the distal interphalangeal joint is greater than 1.
6. Edema at the wrists or ankles.
7. Joint effusions, with or without the appearance of inflammatory signs.

C. Diagnostic testing: The diagnosis of HO is

established with plain radiographs and radionuclide imaging; serum studies are not useful.
1. X-ray findings
   a. Periostitis is seen as periosteal new
      bone along the shafts of long bones
      (typically sparing the epiphyses), com-
      monly the tibiae, fibulae, radii, and
      ulnae.
   b. Nonspecific soft tissue swelling and
      clubbed digits; focal tuftal hypertrophy
      or resorption may be seen.
2. Radionuclide findings (frequently precede x-ray changes and correlate well with
   clinical manifestations)
   a. Diffuse, symmetric uptake along shafts
      of long bones, giving a "double stripe"
      appearance.
   b. Increased periarticular uptake in the
      presence of synovitis.

IV. **Differential Diagnosis**
Secondary HO is distinguished from primary
HO and thyroid acropachy by later onset and the
absence of a family history, and by absence of
pretibial myxedema and thyroid dysfunction,
respectively.

V. **Treatment**
A. For isolated clubbing, no treatment is required.

B. Painful bone and joint symptoms may respond drammatically to removal of the primary lung lesion—resection or other treatment of the tumor, treatment of the abscess,
   bronchiectasis, or pneumonia.
C. Intrathoracic vagotomy may provide significant pain relief.
D. Nonsteroidal anti-inflammatory agents, steroids, and chemical vagotomy have provided
   symptomatic relief.

VI. **Patient Monitoring**
Patients can be monitored by following their
symptoms; follow-up bone scan may be useful to
monitor for recurrent tumor.

VII. **Prognosis**
Prognosis for secondary HO is related to the
course of the underlying condition.

Bibliography

Resnick D, Niwayama G. Enostosis, hyperostosis and periostitis, in Resnick D, Niwayama G: *Diagnosis of Bone and Joint
Disorders*, ed 2. Philadelphia, Saunders, 1988, p 4073.

Schumacher HR. Articular manifestations of hypertrophic pulmonary osteoarthropathy in bronchogenic carcinoma: A clinical and pathologic study. *Arthritis Rheum*
19:629–636, 1976.

Chapter 115

Diffuse Idiopathic Skeletal Hyperostosis

Jan Clarke, M.D.

I. **Definition**
Diffuse idiopathic skeletal hyperostosis (DISH), known by many other names as well, is a common condition of unknown etiology affecting older adults (predominantly men). It is characterized by anterolateral spinal calcification or ossification and by spinal and extraspinal osteophytes.

II. **Diagnosis**
Diagnosis is established by plain radiography. The middle and lower thoracic regions are more involved than the cervical and lumbar spines.

III. **Clinical Findings**
Clinical findings are nonspecific and are typically quite mild despite extensive radiographic changes.
A. Radiographic criteria for diagnosis
  1. Flowing calcification and ossification along the anterolateral aspect of at least four contiguous vertebrae.
  2. Preservation of disc height.
  3. Absence of intra-articular bony ankylosis of the sacroiliac and apophyseal joints.
B. Other radiographic features considered to be characteristic of DISH.
  1. Proliferation or "whiskering" in the pelvis at sites of ligamentous and tendon attachment.

  2. Spurs at the posterior and inferior calcaneous, dorsal talus, certain tarsal bones, base of the fifth metatarsal, anterior patella, and olecranon.
C. The history is nonspecific and may include complaints of back stiffness and/or pain. With cervical involvement, dysphagia may be reported. Some patients have recurring heel and elbow pain consistent with tendinitis.
D. Clinical signs and physical findings are largely limited to moderate to severe limitation of range of motion of the spine. There may be tenderness over the entheses of the calcaneous or the olecranon during an episode of tendinitis; spurs may be palpable in those regions.

IV. **Differential Diagnosis**
Differential diagnosis includes other conditions associated with hyperostosis—degenerative disc disease, spondylosis deformans, ankylosing spondylitis (AS) and the other inflammatory spondyloarthropathies, acromegaly, hyperparathyroidism, fluorosis, ochronosis, neurarthropathy, trauma, and sternal hyperostosis.
A. Degenerative disc disease and spondylosis deformans show prominent disc space

changes—narrowing, vacuum phenomenon, and adjacent sclerosis—that are not features of DISH.

B. AS and other inflammatory spondyloarthropathies affect younger adults and are associated with prominent clinical features that can distinguish them from DISH. Radiographically, the bulky, flowing ossification and "whiskering" of DISH are distinct from the thin syndesmophytes and erosions at entheses seen in AS and related disorders.

V. Treatment
Treatment is symptomatic.

VI. Prognosis
The prognosis is quite good; DISH is not associated with progressive disability.

Bibliography

Resnick D, Niwayama G. Diffuse idiopathic skeletal hyperostosis (DISH): Ankylosing hyperostosis of Forestier and Rotes-Querol, in Resnick D, Niwayama G: *Diagnosis of Bone and Joint Disorders,* ed 2. Philadelphia, Saunders, 1988, p 1562.

CHAPTER 116

Drugs Used in Rheumatology

Delfin Santos, M.D.

Nonsteroidal Anti-inflammatory Drugs (NSAIDs)

I. Classification

A. Phenyl propionic acid derivatives
   1. Fluribiprofen (Ansaid)
   2. Ketoprofen (Orudis)
   3. Fenoprofen (Nalfon)
   4. Naproxen (Naprosyn)
   5. Naproxen sodium (Anaprox)
   6. Ibuprofen (Motrin, Advil, Medeprin, Rufen, Nuprin)

B. Indoleacetic acid derivatives
   1. Indomethacin (Indocin)
   2. Sulindac (Clinoril)

C. Pyrrole acetic acid derivatives
   1. Tolectin (Tolmetin)

D. Pyrrolo-pyrrole
   1. Ketorolac (Toradol)

E. Phenyl acetic acid derivatives
   1. Diclofenac (Voltaren)

F. Pyrazolones
   1. Phenylbutazone (Butazolidin)

G. Fenamates
   1. Mefenamic acid (Ponstel)
   2. Meclofenamate (Meclomen)

H. Naphthylalkanone
   1. Nabumetone

I. Oxicams
   1. Piroxicam (Feldene)

J. Pyrano carboxylic acid derivative
   1. Etodolac (Lodine)

K. Salicylates
   1. Aspirin
   2. Diflunisal (Dolobid)
   3. Magnesium choline salicylate (Trilisate)
   4. Salicyl salicylate (Disalcid, Mono-gesic, Salflex, Salsalate, Salsitab)

II. Mechanism of Action

A. NSAIDs inhibit prostaglandin and other forms of end product biosynthesis by inhibition of cyclooxygenase in the arachidonic acid pathway.

B. Inhibition of lipoxygenase enzymes by certain NSAIDs (e.g., diclofenac and indomethacin).

III. Indications

A. For relief of mild to moderate episodes of acute pain and inflammation.

B. Alone or in combination with second-line agents in chronic inflammatory or chronic painful conditions.

Table 116-1. Nonsteroidal Antiinflammatory Drugs

Drug	How Supplied (mg)	Dosing	Half Life (hours)	Maximum Dose (24 hours)
Fluribiprofen	100	bid, tid	3–4	200 mg
Ketoprofen	50, 75, *200	*qd, tid, qid	2–3	300 mg
Fenoprofen	200, 800, 800	tid, qid	2–3	2400 mg
Naproxen	250, 375, 500, *550	bid, tid	2–4	1500 mg
Ibuprofen	200, 400, 600, 800	tid, qid	2–3	3200 mg
Indomethacin	25, 50, 75 SR	bid, tid, qid	4–12	200 mg
Sulindac	150, 200	bid	8–10	400 mg
Tolectin	200, 400	tid, qid	1–2	1600 mg
Diclofenac	50, 75	bid, tid, qid	1–2	200 mg
Phenylbutazone	100	tid, qid	40–80	800 mg
Mefenamic acid	250	qid	2–4	1000 mg
Meclofenamate	50, 100	tid, qid	2–3	400 mg
Piroxicam	20	qd	30–80	20 mg
Diflunisal	250, 500	bid, tid	8–12	1500 mg
Etodolac	200, 300, 400	bid, tid	4–7	1200 mg
Nabumetone	500, 750	qd	3–4	200 mg
Oxaprozin	600	qd	20–25	1200 mg
Ketorolac	**10 ***30 mg/ml, 60 mg/ml	bid, tid, qid	4–6	150 mg

*Oruvail; **Oral, ***Parenteral.

IV. Dosages

A. There are many different strengths and dosages in the NSAID group (see Table 116-1).

V. Drug Interactions

A. Pharmacokinetic properties

1. Large doses of NSAIDs reduce the plasma prothrombin concentration and may enhance the effects of oral anticoagulants.

2. Salicylates may displace coumarin anticoagulants from plasma protein-binding sites and increase plasma levels of the anticoagulant.

3. Higher incidence of gastric bleeding when NSAIDs are used with thrombolytic or anticoagulant agents.

4. Decreased glomerular filtration rate when NSAIDs are given concomitantly with certain antihypertensive agents.

5. Decreased secretion of other organic acids.

   a. May elevate methotrexate to critical levels.

   b. May elevate digoxin levels.

6. Decreased natruretic effects of furosemide and thiazide diuretics.

7. Inhibit hepatic metabolism of other drugs.

   a. Especially common with phenylbutazone when used with oral hypoglycemic agents or phenytoin.

VI. Complications

A. Gastrointestinal

1. Gastritis and gastric ulceration, leading to occult or gross gastrointestinal bleeding and perforation.

2. Constipation, nausea, vomiting, or diarrhea.

3. Elevation of transaminases see, especially in patients with systemic lupus erythematosus (SLE) or juvenile rheumatoid arthritis.

   a. Liver function studies should be monitored at 3-month intervals in patients on chronic NSAID therapy.

B. Renal

1. Acute interstitial nephritis

2. Renal papillary necrosis

3. Nephrotic syndrome

4. Hyperkalemia

5. Hematuria, proteinuria

6. Acute renal shutdown with increasing azotemia secondary to inhibition of renal prostaglandins in patients with preexisting prerenal disease.

   a. Hypertension

   b. Congestive heart failure

   c. Cirrhosis

C. Neurologic

1. Aseptic meningitis

Table 116-2.   Intra-articular Corticosteroid Preparations: Recommended Doses for Rheumatoid Knee Synovitis and Duration of Action

Generic Name	Proprietary Name	Dose (mg)	Mean Duration of Response (days)
Hydrocortisone acetate		37.5–100.0	6, 40
Dexamethasone acetate	Decadron-LA	5	8
Prednisolone acetate	Meticortelone	30	8
Triamcinolone diacetate	Aristocort Forte	20–30	8
Methylprednisolone acetate	Depo-Medrol	30–40	
Betamethasone acetate and phosphate	Celestone Soluspan	0.6–5.0	9
Hydrocortisone tertiary butylacetate (TBA)		25.0–37.5	12, 30
Prednisolone TBA	Hydeltra-TBA	20–40	15
Triamcinolone acetonide	Kenalog-40	10–30	14
Triamcinolone hexacetonide	Aristospan	10–40	21, 59, 90

Source: Gray RB, Gottlieb NL (1983), with permission.

a. More likely to occur in patients with SLE or related connective tissue diseases.
b. Reported with only a few NSAIDs such as ibuprofen, sulindac, and tolmetin.
2. Headache, dizziness, vertigo, psychiatric disturbances
  a. Most frequently reported with indomethacin.
D. Hematologic
  1. Inhibition of platelet aggregation
    a. Increased bleeding time
  2. Agranulocytosis
    a. More common with phenylbutazone.
E. Endocrine
  1. Delayed parturition.
  2. Breast tenderness and enlargement.
F. Special senses
  1. Tinnitus.
VII. Contraindications
A. Known allergies to specific NSAIDs.
B. Allergies to aspirin or NSAIDs manifested by anaphylaxis, asthma, or hypotension.
  1. More common in patients with nasal polyps, rhinitis, and asthma.
C. During pregnancy unless absolutely necessary.
  1. Effect on fetal cardiovascular system.
    a. Early closure of ductus arteriosus during third trimester of pregnancy.

Corticosteroids

I. Definition
A. Synthetic analogues of cortisol.

II. Mechanism of Action
A. Maintenance of vascular responsiveness to circulating vasoconstrictive factors.
B. Prevents increase in cell wall permeability.
C. Prevents sticking and diapedesis of leukocytes through cell walls.
D. Inhibits cyclooxygenase, thus blocking prostaglandin synthesis.
E. Impedes cellular immunity.
F. Stabilizes lysosomal membranes and prevents release of lysosomal enzymes when given as an intra-articular injection.
G. Decreases levels of serum immunoglobulins and complement.

III. Indications
A. When potent anti-inflammatory action is essential to avoid serious complications, such as can occur with pericarditis, vasculitis, and scleritis.
B. As an intra-articular or soft tissue injection when local anti-inflammatory action is needed.
  1. Tendinitis, bursitis
  2. Carpal tunnel syndrome
  3. Fibromyalgia tender points
  4. Ganglion cysts
C. Steroids are used in rheumatoid arthritis, systemic lupus erythematosus (SLE), and other collagen vascular diseases when adequate anti-inflammatory effect has not been obtained with other agents.

IV. Dosages
A. Oral
  1. See Table 116-2.
  2. See Table 116-3.

V. Interactions

Table 116-3. Relative Potencies of Oral Steroids

Steroid	"Equivalent" Dose (mg)	Mineralocorticoid Activity	Serum Half-life (hr)
Short-acting			
Cortisone	25.0	++	8–12
Hydrocortisone	20.0	++	8–12
Intermediate-acting			
Prednisone	5.0	+	12–36
Prednisolone	5.0	+	12–36
Methylprednisolone	4.0	0	12–36
Triamcinolone	4.0	0	12–36
Long-acting			
Dexamethasone	0.75	0	36–54
Betamethasone	0.6	0	36–54

Table 116-4. Relative Potencies of Parenteral Steroids

Steroid	Equivalent Dose (Mg)	Range of Usual Mg/mL Dosage (mg)*
Injectable corticosteroids:		
Hydrocortisone tebutate (Hydrocortone-TBA)	50	25–100
Prednisolone tebutate (Hydeltra-TBA)	20	5–40
Betamethasone acetate and betamethasone sodium phosphate (Celestone Soluspan)	6†	1.5–6
Methylprednisolone acetate (Depo-Medrol‡)	20	4–40
Triamcinolone acetonide (Kenalog 40)	40	5–40
Triamcinolone (Aristocort Forte)	40	5–40
Triamcinolone hexacetonide (Aristospan)	20	5–40

*Amount will vary depending on the size of the joint to be injected.
†Available as 3 mg acetate and 3 mg phosphate.
‡Supplied in 20 mg/mL, 40 mg/mL, and 70 mg/mL preparations.

A. Increased requirements for insulin and oral hypoglycemic agents in diabetics.
B. Decreased corticosteroid blood levels when given with:
   1. Phenytoin
   2. Phenobarbital
   3. Rifampin
   4. Ephedrine
C. Decreased corticosteroid metabolic clearance when given with oral contraceptives.
D. Inhibition of response to coumarin.
E. Hypokalemia when given concomitantly with:
   1. Amphotericin B
   2. Potassium-depleting diuretics
F. Decrease the serum salicylate level by increasing its metabolism and clearance.

G. Decreases effectiveness of isoniazid by increasing its metabolism and clearance.
VI. **Complications**
A. Endocrine
   1. Cushing's syndrome, adrenal suppression, diabetes
   2. Growth suppression in children
   3. Menstrual irregularities
B. Fluid and electrolytes
   1. Fluid and sodium retention, leading to edema and hypertension
   2. Hypokalemia
C. Skin
   1. Atrophy at site of local injection
   2. Impaired wound healing
   3. Capillary fragility
   4. Acne

D. Musculoskeletal
 1. Myopathy
 2. Loss of muscle mass
 3. Osteoporosis
 4. Avascular necrosis
 5. Pathologic fractures
E. Gastrointestinal
 1. Peptic ulcer
 2. Pancreatitis
 3. Gastroduodenitis
F. Neurologic
 1. Convulsions
 2. Mental and mood changes
 3. Vertigo
 4. Headache
G. Intra-articular
 1. Steroid flare
 2. Tendon rupture
 3. Intra-articular calcifications

VII. Contraindications
A. Bacteremia or other serious infection
B. Intra-articular steroid injection just prior to joint replacement
C. Intra-articular injection through infected skin

Gold compounds

I. Classification
A. Parenteral
 1. Oil-based aurothioglucose (solganal)
 2. Water-based gold sodium thiomalate (myochrysine)
B. Oral
 1. Auranofin (ridaura)

II. Mechanism of Action
A. Not well understood; some proposed mechanisms:
 1. Inhibition of the activity of lysosomal and other cellular and extracellular enzymes.
 2. Inhibition of mononuclear phagocyte function.
 3. Possible immunosuppressant effects.

III. Indications
A. Progressive and severe rheumatoid arthritis after NSAIDs, physical therapy, and other first-line treatments have failed.

IV. Dosages
A. Solganal
 1. First dose, 10 mg; second and third doses, 25 mg; fourth and subsequent doses, 50 mg.
B. Myochrysine

 1. First dose, 10 mg; second and third doses, 25 mg; fourth and subsequent doses, 25 to 50 mg.
C. Ridaura
 1. Initially 6 mg per day, may increase to 9 mg per day if response inadequate after 6 months.

V. Interactions
Auranofin has been reported to increase phenytoin levels when used concomitantly.

VI. Complications
A. Bone marrow toxicity
 1. Thrombocytopenia
 2. Granulocytopenia
 3. Aplastic anemia
 4. Eosinophilia
B. Renal
 1. Proteinuria: Mild or nephrotic range
 2. Hematuria
 3. Acute or chronic renal failure
C. Skin
 1. Rash
 2. Stomatitis, pruritus, alopecia, and photosensitivity
D. Pulmonary
 1. Gold bronchitis
 2. Cough, shortness of breath
 3. Interstitial pneumonitis and fibrosis
E. Nitritoid
 1. Flushing, fainting, dizziness, and sweating.
  a. Most commonly reported with gold sodium thiomalate. If this occurs with sodium thiomalate, may switch to aurothioglucose.
F. Eye
 1. Iritis, corneal ulcers
G. Neurologic
 1. Encephalitis
 2. Peripheral neuritis
H. Gastrointestinal
 1. Diarrhea, nausea, vomiting
 2. Lower abdominal pain

VII. Contraindications
A. Uncontrolled diabetes
B. Hepatic dysfunction or a history of infectious hepatitis
C. Marked hypertension
D. Blood dyscrasias
E. Renal disease
F. SLE
G. Severe debilitation
H. Previous complications with gold therapy
 1. Necrotizing enterocolitis

2. Pulmonary fibrosis
3. Exfoliative dermatitis
4. Bone marrow toxicity

Penicillamine (depen, cuprimine)

I. Definition
A. Penicillamine, 3-mercapto-D-valine, is a chelating agent used as a disease modifying antirheumatic drug.

II. Mechanism of Action
A. Inhibits release of lysosomal enzymes and oxygen radicals, thus acting as an anti-inflammatory agent.
B. May decrease the cell-mediated immune response by selective inhibition of T-lymphocyte function.
C. Dissociates IgM rheumatoid factor in vitro and in vivo.

III. Indications
A. As a second-line agent in rheumatoid arthritis (RA) and juvenile rheumatoid arthritis (JRA).
B. RA associated with extra-articular manifestations such as Felty's syndrome or vasculitis.
C. Used in progressive systemic sclerosis.

IV. Dosages
A. Start low, 125–250 mg/day, with slow increments until a clinical response is obtained.
B. Increments should be made at 8- to 10-week intervals.
C. Give alone 1.5–2 hr before meals.
D. Maximum dose: 1,000–1,500 mg/day.
E. May be 2–3 months before a response is noted.
F. Blood count and liver function should be monitored.

V. Interactions
A. Should not be used with other drugs that have potential bone marrow toxicity.
B. May reduce digoxin levels.

VI. Complications
A. Skin
1. Early rash
2. Late rash
B. Gastrointestinal
1. Hypogensia, anorexia, nausea
2. Mouth ulcers
3. Pancreatitis
4. Hepatic dysfunction
C. Hematologic
1. Bone marrow depression: Thrombocytopenia, agranulocytosis, aplastic anemia

D. Renal
1. Proteinuria: Mild or nephrotic range
E. Immunologic
1. Polymyositis
2. Goodpasture's syndrome
3. SLE
4. Pemphigus
5. Myasthenia gravis
6. Sjögren's syndrome
F. Drug fever usually requires discontinuation of drug.

VII. Contraindications
A. Pregnancy
B. Penicillamine-related bone toxicity
C. Renal insufficiency

Sulfasalazine (azulfidine)

I. Definition
Compound of sulfapyridine and 5-aminosalicylic acid.

II. Mechanism of Action
A. Inhibits folate absorption and metabolism.
B. Inhibits prostaglandin synthesis and degradation.
C. Reduces leukotriene production by inhibiting the lipoxygenase pathway of arachidonic acid metabolism.

III. Indications
A. As a second-line treatment for RA and JRA.
B. Psoriatic arthritis, Reiters syndrome, ankylosing spondylitis and other undifferentiated spondyloarthropathies.

IV. Dosages
A. Give 500 mg four times per day, enteric coated; increase to 1 g three times per day if tolerated after 3–6 months and if clinical benefit has not been obtained.

V. Interactions
A. Sulfonamides may displace or be displaced by other highly protein-bound drugs.
B. Decreased blood level of sulfasalazine when given with ferrous sulfate.
C. Inhibition of folic acid absorption.
D. Decreased digoxin bioavailability.

VI. Complications
A. Blood dyscrasias
1. Macrocytic anemia, aplastic anemia, thrombocytopenia
B. Gastrointestinal
1. Stomatitis, hepatitis, pancreatitis
2. Diarrhea
3. Abdominal pain

C. Hypersensitivity
1. Stevens-Johnson syndrome
2. Skin eruptions, photosensitivity
3. Urticaria, serum sickness
4. Anaphylactoid reactions
D. Renal
1. Hematuria, proteinuria, nephrotic syndrome
2. Renal insufficiency
E. CNS
1. Headache, depression, convulsions, tinnitus, vertigo
2. Transverse myelitis
F. Reproductive
1. Reversible oligospermia
VII. **Contraindications**
A. Patients with allergies to salicylates or sulfasalazine.
B. Patients with porphyria may experience an acute attack.

Antimalarials

I. **Classification**
A. Chloroquine (Aralen)
B. Hydroxychloroquine (Plaquenil)
II. **Mechanism of Action**
A. Alters lysosomal and other cellular membrane functions, thus stabilizing lysosomes so that they malfunction.
1. Inhibition of chemotaxis.
2. Inhibition of lymphocyte and macrophage responses.
B. Interferes with DNA and RNA function, thus depressing protein synthesis.
C. Interferes with antigen–antibody reactions.
III. **Indications**
A. As a second-line agent in RA.
B. Used for discoid lupus and SLE.
IV. **Dosages**
A. Chloroquine: 250–500 mg/day.
B. Hydroxychloroquine: 200–400 mg/day.
V. **Interactions**
A. Absorption may be decreased when used with kaolin or magnesium trilisate.
VI. **Complications**
A. Gastrointestinal
1. Bloating, flatus
2. Irritable bowel syndrome
B. Muscular
1. Depressed muscle contractibility and possible unmasking of myopathies.

C. Grayish-blue pigmentation of skin, nail bed, and palate with prolonged therapy.
D. Retinal pigmentation
1. Requires regular ophthalmologic examinations.
E. CNS
1. Headache
2. Psychotic episodes
3. Convulsions
VII. **Contraindications**
A. Retinal or visual field changes
B. History of retinitis pigmentosa
C. Allergy to antimalarials
D. Pregnancy
E. Myasthenia gravis

Methotrexate (Rheumatrex)

I. **Definition**
A. Folic acid antagonist
II. **Mechanism of Action**
A. Potent inhibitor of dihydrofolate reductase.
1. Limits thymidylate synthesis.
B. Suppresses primary and anamnestic antibody responses.
C. It has been postulated that lymphocytes are killed or suppressed, resulting in a delayed response.
III. **Indications**
A. Second-line agent in resistant cases of RA
B. Psoriatic arthritis
C. Reiter's syndrome
D. Polymyositis
E. Temporal arteritis
IV. **Dosages**
A. Usual starting dose is 7.5 mg/week, either as a single oral dose or as 2.5 mg every 12 hr for a total weekly dose of 7.5 mg.
B. May be given IM.
C. Doses range from 7.5 to 40 mg/week; rarely, 25 mg or more is used.
V. **Interactions**
A. Concomitant use of NSAIDs and methotrexate may raise methotrexate to toxic levels.
1. Also displaced by sulfonamides, salicylates, tetracycline, and chloramphenicol.
B. Probenecid in combination with methotrexate has been reported to increase the toxicity of methotrexate through inhibition of renal tubular secretion.
VI. **Complications**
A. Bone marrow suppression

1. Anemia, leukopenia, thrombocytopenia and bleeding.
  B. Hepatoxicity
    1. Liver atrophy, necrosis, cirrhosis, and periportal fibrosis.
      a. Requires monitoring of transaminase levels
      b. Some authors advocate liver biopsy when the cumulative dose reaches 2–3 g.
  C. Gastrointestinal
    1. Nausea, vomiting, diarrhea
    2. Oral mucositis
  D. Predisposition to opportunistic infections.
  E. Abortions, teratogenesis, defective oogenesis and spermatogenesis, and oligospermia.
  F. Methotrexate pneumonitis.
  G. Peripheral eosinophilia at higher doses.
VII. Contraindications
  A. Pregnancy
  B. Human immunodeficiency virus (HIV)-infected individuals
    1. Reported to exacerbate illness
  C. Impaired renal function.
  D. In conjunction with heavy alcohol consumption.

Azathioprine (Imuran)

I. Definition
  A. Antimetabolite
  B. Imidazolyl derivative of 6-mercaptopurine.
II. Mechanism of Action
  A. Cell-cycle-specific antimetabolite.
  B. Decreases antibody response and delayed hypersensitivity reaction.
  C. Diminishes B-lymphocyte responsiveness.
  D. Purine antagonist which suppresses adenine and guanine.
III. Indications
  A. Severe erosive RA not responsive to first-line agents.
  B. As a steroid-sparing agent in patients dependent on high doses of steroids.
  C. Patients with SLE.
IV. Dosages
  A. Initial dose should be 1.0 mg/kg (50–100 mg) as a single dose or twice daily schedule.
  B. Dose may be increased at four week intervals by 0.5 mg/kg/day.
  C. Total daily dose should not exceed 2–5 mg/kg/day.
V. Interactions
  A. Allopurinol increases pharmacologic effects of azathioprine and requires that one-fourth to one-fifth of the usual dose of azathropine

be given when the two drugs are used concomitantly.
VI. Complications
  A. Hematologic
    1. Leukopenia, thrombocytopenia macrocytic anemia, selective erythrocyte aplasia.
  B. Gastrointestinal
    1. Nausea, vomiting
    2. Hepatoxicity
      a. Elevated alkaline phosphatase
      b. Elevated bilirubin
  C. Skin rashes, alopecia, fever.
  D. Increased incidence of secondary malignancy.
VII. Contraindications
  A. Hypersensitivity to azathroporine
  B. Pregnancy

Cyclophosphamide (Cytoxan)

I. Definition
Alkylating agent of the nitrogen mustard group.
II. Mechanism of Action
  A. Depletes both suppressor T and B lymphocytes.
    1. Suppresses humoral and cell-mediated immunity.
  B. Causes defects in lymphocyte function.
    1. Decreases antibody production.
III. Indications
  A. Severe erosive RA resistant to less toxic medications.
  B. SLE with active lupus nephritis or CNS lupus resistant to steroids.
  C. Steroid-resistant vasculitides.
IV. Dosages
  A. Initial dose: 1.5–2.0 mg/kg/day.
    1. Approximately 75–150 mg oral dose.
  B. May be increased to 3 mg/kg/day if no response occurs in first 6–8 weeks.
  C. May be given as 750–1,000 mg/m^2 as an IV bolus. Appropriate dose determined when leukocyte count drops to approximately 2,500 cells/mm^3 on day 7 or day 14 after treatment.
  D. Clinical response seen after 4–6 weeks.
  E. If an adequate response is achieved, the dose should be decreased by 25 mg/month to the lowest effective maintenance dose.
V. Interactions
  A. Use of allopurinol or thiazide diuretics may enhance bone marrow toxicity of cyclophosphamide.
  B. Chronic high doses of phenobarbital may increase the rate of metabolism and the leukopenic effect of cyclophosphamide.

C. May inhibit succinylcholine metabolism and result in prolonged apnea after anesthesia.

VI. Complications
A. Bone marrow suppression
   1. Leukopenia, thrombocytopenia.
B. Predisposes to secondary neoplasms.
C. Acute hemorrhagic cystitis in up to 12% of patients.
D. Gonadal suppression.
E. Renal
   1. Syndrome of inappropriate antidiuretic hormone
F. Interstitial pulmonary fibrosis.
G. Alopecia.
H. Infertility
   1. Depressed sperm motility
   2. Amenorrhea

VII. Contraindications
A. Pregnancy.
B. Bone marrow–suppressed patients.
C. Patients who have had an adverse reaction to cyclophosphamide in the past.

Chlorambucil (Leukeran)

I. Definition
A. Alkylating agent of the nitrogen mustard group.

II. Mechanism of Action
A. Suppresses all myeloid elements, thus suppressing immune function.
B. Interacts with cellular DNA to produce cytotoxic cross-linkage.
C. Less potent than cyclophosphamide.

III. Indications
A. Severe RA refractory to less toxic medications.

IV. Dosages
A. Oral dose between 0.5 and 0.2 mg/kg/day.

V. Interactions
A. May increase serum and urine uric acid levels.

VI. Complications
A. Hematologic
   1. Anemia, leukopenia, coma, thrombocytopenia, pancytopenia
B. Skin
   1. Alopecia, rashes
C. Amenorrhea
D. Susceptibility to infections
   1. Herpes zoster in up to 12% of patients
   2. Mycotic infections
   3. Bacterial infections

VII. Contraindications
A. Patients with known hypersensitivity.
B. Patients who have shown prior resistance to treatment with this drug.

Cyclosporin.

I. Definition
A. Cyclic polypeptide immunosuppressant agent.

II. Mechanism of Action
A. Noncytotoxic immunomodulatory agent.
B. Primarily inhibits the activation of T-helper-inducer lymphocytes by blocking interleukin-2 production.
C. Inhibits gamma-interferon and interleukin-3 production.

III. Indications
A. Under investigation as a second-line agent in RA.

IV. Dosages
A. 1–10 mg/kg/day

V. Interactions
A. Use with other nephrotoxic agents may increase renal toxicity.
B. Ketoconazole and amphotericin B have increased concentrations of cyclosporin.

VI. Complications
A. Nephrotoxicity
B. Neurotoxicity
   1. Hyperesthesia
   2. Tingling
   3. Nervousness
   4. Tinnitus, tremor
C. Hypertension
D. Gum hyperplasia
E. Bone marrow suppression
F. Gastrointestinal
   1. Nausea, vomiting, diarrhea
G. Susceptibility to infections
H. Hepatoxicity

VII. Contraindications
A. Hypersensitivity to cyclosporin or polyoxyethylated castor oil
B. Pregnancy

Colchicine

I. Definition
A. An alkaloid obtained from various species of *Colchicum*.

II. Mechanism of Action
  A. Inhibits leukocyte migration to inflamed area.
  B. Decreases lactic acid production, thus decreasing deposition of uric acid.
  C. Interferes with kinin formation.
  D. Diminishes phagocytosis.
  E. Inhibits release of histamine granules from mast cells.

III. Indications
  A. Acute gouty arthritis.
  B. Calcium pyrophosphate deposition disease (pseudogout).
  C. Familial Mediterranean fever.
  D. Prophylaxis against recurrent attacks of gout.
  E. Primary and secondary amyloidosis.

IV. Dosages
  A. Give 1–2 mg IV initially, then 0.5 mg every 6 hr for acute attacks.
    1. IV colchicine is falling into disuse because of toxicity.
  B. Oral dose: 0.5–0.6 mg every hr until one of three things happens:
    1. Therapeutic goals are met.
    2. Gastrointestinal side effects develop.
    3. Completion of maximum dose: 5–6 mg total dose in 24 hr.
  C. Dose should not be repeated for at least 1 week when maximum doses are given.
  D. Give 0.3–0.6 mg twice per day as prophylaxis.
  E. Dose adjustment required in renal and hepatic disease.

V. Drug Interactions
  A. No reported drug interactions.

VI. Complications
  A. Hematologic
    1. Bone marrow suppression
    2. Disseminated intravascular coagulation
  B. Renal shutdown
  C. CNS dysfunction
  D. Myopathy, neuropathy
    1. More common in patients with renal or hepatic disease.
  E. Hepatocellular failure
  F. Gastrointestinal
    1. Diarrhea, hyperperistalsis, nausea and vomiting.
  G. Skin
    1. Local chemial phlebitis if extravasates to skin.

VII. Contraindications
  A. Significant liver or kidney disease
  B. Neutropenia
  C. Pregnancy

  D. Recent IV course of colchicine
  E. IV colchicine after long-term oral regimen.
  F. Hematologic malignancy requiring chemotherapy

Allopurinol

I. Definition
  A. Inhibits xanthine oxidase which is the enzyme responsible for the conversion of hypoxanthine to xanthine and xanthine to uric acid.

II. Mechanism of Action
  A. Inhibits xanthine oxidase.
  B. Blocks the conversion of 6-thiouric acid.

III. Indications
  A. Treatment of primary hyperuricemia associated with gout.
  B. Hyperuricemia secondary to polycythemia vera and myeloid metaplasia.

IV. Dosages
  A. Initial daily dose of 100 mg, then increase to 300 mg/day in a single dose.
  B. Dose should be adjusted in patients with renal failure.
  C. Peak onset: 2–6 hr.
  D. Half-life: 2–3 hr.

V. Drug Interactions
  A. Purine analog chemotherapeutic agents are inactivated by xanthine oxidase. Increased toxicity can be seen if these drugs are used with allopurinol without a dose adjustment.
    1. Azathroprine
    2. Hypoxanthine arabinoside
    3. 6-Mercaptopurine
  B. Increases toxicity of cyclophosphamide.
  C. Prolongs half-life of probenecid by 50%.
  D. Inhibits hepatic microsomal drug-metabolizing enzymes that metabolize oral anticoagulants.
  E. Increased incidence of skin rash when given with ampicillin.
  F. Toxic effects enhanced when given with thiazide diuretics.

VI. Complications
  A. May precipitate acute gouty attack.
  B. Predispose to xanthine renal stones.
  C. Allopurinol hypersensitivity syndrome.
    1. Immunologic reaction to allopurinol characterized by fever, eosinophilia, leukocytosis, coma, renal failure, and hepatocellular injury.
  D. Headache, drowsiness, vertigo
  E. Nausea, vomiting, diarrhea

F. Peripheral neuritis

G. Bone marros suppression

H. Skin rash

1. Erythema multiforme

2. Toxic epidermal necrolysis

3. Erythematous maculopapular rash

I. Chronic renal disease and oral diuretics seem to predispose to complications.

VII. Contraindications

A. Patients with known allergy

B. Patients taking azathroprine unless dose is adjusted adequately.

Probenecid (Benemid)

I. Definition

A. Uricosuric and renal tubular transport blocking agent.

II. Mechanism of Action

A. Uricosuric agent that increases the quantity of urate filtered at the glomerulus.

B. Inhibits reabsorption of urate in the proximal tubules.

C. Potent inhibitor of certain glycerine conjugates.

III. Indications

A. Treatment of hyperuricemia in patients with gout who are underexcreters of uric acid.

IV. Dosages

A. Give 250 mg/day for 1 week, then 500 mg twice per day.

B. Children: 10–25 mg/kg daily dose.

V. Interactions

A. Prolongs plasma concentration of penicillin.

B. Influences pharmacokinetics of many drugs.

C. Acetylsalicylate blocks uricosuric effect of probenecid.

D. Subtherapeutic doses of heparin may have profound anticoagulant effect in patients taking probenecid.

E. May increase therapeutic doses of methotrexate to toxic levels.

VI. Complications

A. Acute gouty attack

B. Nephrolithiasis

C. Gastrointestinal irritation

VII. Contraindications

A. Blood dyscrasias

B. Uric acid kidney stones

C. History of hypersensitivity reaction to probenecid

D. Acute gout

E. Patients with creatinine clearance less than 80 will have no response to probenecid.

Sulfinpyrazone (Anturane)

I. Definition

A. Uricosuric agent, a derivative of phenylbutazone

II. Mechanism of Action

A. Uricosuric agent that inhibits tubular reabsorption of uric acid by competitive inhibition.

III. Indications

A. Treatment of patients with hyperuricemia and gout who are underexcretors of uric acid.

IV. Dosages

A. Give 100–200 mg/day for chronic gout (usual starting dose).

B. May be increased gradually until adequate lowering of uric acid is achieved—usually 100–400 mg/day in two to four doses.

C. Preferably given with meals.

D. Patient may require up to 800 mg/day.

E. Required high fluid intake and urine alkalinization.

V. Drug Interactions

A. When given with probenecid, an additional uricosuric effect is obtained because probenecid blocks tubular secretion of sulfinpyrazone.

1. Prolongs uricosuric effect.

B. Salicylate ingestion can block uricosuric effect of drug.

C. Same effect as probenecid on renal elimination of certain drugs.

VI. Complications

A. Gastrointestinal symptoms same as those of probenecid.

B. Uric acid stones.

C. Bone marrow toxicity.

D. Hypersensitivity reactions with rash and fever.

VII. Contraindications

A. Active peptic ulcer disease.

B. Known hypersensitivity to phenylbutazone or other pyrazoles.

C. Blood dyscrasias.

Bibliography

Brater CD. Drug–drug and drug–disease interactions with nonsteroidal anti-inflammatory drugs. *Am J Med* 80(Suppl 1A):62–77, 1986.

Brogden RN. Nonsteroidal anti-inflammatory analgesics other than salicylates. *Drugs* 32(Suppl 4):27–45, 1986.

Clissoid SP. Aspirin and related derivatives of salicylic acid. *Drugs* 32(Suppl 4):8–26, 1986.

Gray RG, Gottlieb NL. Intra-articular corticosteroids: An updated assessment. *Clin Orthop* 177:235–263, 1983.

Pugh MC, Pugh CB. Current concepts in clinical therapeutics: Disease-modifying drugs for rheumatoid arthritis. *Clin Pharm* 6:475–488, 1987.

Chapter 117

Polymyalgia Rheumatica and Giant Cell Arteritis

Lawrence Layfer, M.D.

Polymyalgia Rheumatica (PMR)

I. Definition

Clinical syndrome characterized by proximal muscle aching and stiffness of the hip, shoulder girdle, and neck in the elderly.

II. Etiology

Remains unknown. Reports in twins and families, as well as in human leukocyte antigen (HLA) associations, have suggested a genetic predisposition. Isolated cases are the rule, however. Aging may be a factor, but the mechanism remains unclear.

III. Pathophysiology

Remains unknown. Pathologic exam has revealed mild lymphocytic infiltrates in involved synovium, correlating with uptake noted in joints on technetium bone scan, suggesting that muscle symptoms are due to joint disease. No myositis or vasculitis has been found. Immune complexes have been noted in the serum of some patients, but their role in the causation of illness remains speculative.

IV. Diagnosis

  A. History

    1. Character: Pain, aching and stiffness, ex-acerbated in the morning, often described as having "shoveled snow the day before."

    2. Location: Proximal hip and shoulder girdle, occasionally neck or more peripheral joints.

    3. Onset: Sudden and bilateral, rarely insidious or unilateral.

    4. Associated symptoms: Weight loss, malaise, fatigue, low-grade fever, depression. Carpal tunnel syndrome or mild inflammatory synovitis of the knees and hands may be seen.

  B. Physical exam: Muscles may be tender to palpation but are not weak, although they may appear weak if pain is severe. Joints may have mild inflammation, as noted above. Temporal arteries must be examined in all patients.

  C. Diagnostic tests

    1. Erythrocyte sedimentation rate (ESR): Often elevated, occasionally normal. Other acute-phase reactants may be elevated but are not routinely checked.

    2. Anemia: Normochromic anemias are common. Platelets may be elevated.

3. Autoantibodies: Rheumatoid factor and antinuclear antibody (ANA) are usually absent. Immune complexes may be noted. HLA-DR4/CW3 has been slightly associated.

4. Other factors: Muscle enzymes, like creatinine phosphokinase and aldolase, are negative, as are muscle biopsies and electromyograms. Liver enzymes may be increased in 30%, especially alkaline phosphatase, reflecting mild hepatitis. Synovial fluid, when present, is generally noninflammatory. X-rays are unremarkable, but technetium bone scans may demonstrate uptake around large joints.

V. **Differential Diagnosis**
Based on typical clinical presentation and elevated ESR in the correct age group. Appropriate exclusions are polymyositis, hypothyroidism, chronic infection, tumor, depression, fibromyalgia, rheumatoid or inflammatory arthritis, and vasculitis.

VI. **Treatment**
A. Acetylsalicylic acid and nonsteroidal anti-inflammatory drugs: Up to 20% of patients may respond to these drugs, most only partially. Caution is needed because of gastrointestinal ulceration and renal insufficiency in this age group.

B. Corticosteroids
1. Doses of 15 mg/day of prednisone are quickly effective in most patients. Rarely, higher doses may be necessary. If no response occurs, another illness or giant cell arteritis (GCA) should be considered.
2. Steroid precautions should be taken. Watch blood pressure and glucose in early stages of therapy. Assess purified protein derivative status in all patients before use. Consider in this age group whether osteoporosis precautions or therapy are indicated.

VII. **Patient Monitoring**
Taper prednisone 1 mg every 2–4 weeks, following the ESR and clinical symptoms.

VIII. **Prognosis**
The prognosis is generally excellent, with little morbidity. Most patients can be taken off medications within 1–2 years. The main complications are untreated/silent GCA and the side effects of medication.

IX. **Relationship to Giant Cell Arteritis**
A. Fifty percent of patients with GCA have PMR. Up to 15% of patients with PMR have silent GCA by blind temporal artery biopsy. There is no clear evidence that vasculitis is the cause of the muscle pain or synovitis in PMR, however, leaving the relationship between the two illnesses purely a clinical, not a pathophysiologic, association.

B. PMR patients without symptoms of GCA need not undergo temporal artery biopsy routinely. However, failure to respond to low-dose corticosteroid therapy, presistent ESR elevation, GCA symptoms, or abnormal temporal arteries on exam should prompt such biopsy (see next section).

Giant Cell Arteritis (GCA)

I. **Definition**
Inflammatory giant cell vasculitis primarily affecting the extracranial head and neck vessels of the aortic arch branches, predominantly seen in the elderly and presenting more commonly with headache and sudden visual changes.

II. **Etiology**
Remains unknown. The considerations discussed in relation to PMR also apply to GCA.

III. **Pathophysiology**
A. Biopsy reveals large vessel involvement with multinucleated giant cells with lymphocytes, histiocytes, and occasional polymorphs centered about the internal elastic lamina with necrosis and thrombosis. The involvement of blood vessels of the extracranial circulation is directly responsible for the symptoms.

B. The cause of the inflammation remains unknown. A granulomatous reaction in the artery suggests cell-mediated immunity, perhaps to local arterial antigens such as elastic tissue. Immune complexes and complement deposition have also been noted. No firm conclusions can currently be drawn.

IV. **Diagnosis**
A. Clinical presentation
1. Onset: Headache (32%), PMR (40%), fever (15%), and visual change (7%) are the most common presenting complaints.
2. Arterial symptoms: Symptoms due to inflammation of blood vessels with resultant pain, ischemia, or infarction of structures fed by involved arteries.
a. Headache (68%): Unilateral or bilateral, throbbing or constant; scalp tender over the artery; the artery may

swell and have a bruit over it; the pulse may be decreased.

b. Visual symptoms (30%): Amaurosis fugax, transient or permanent, due to involvement of the retinal or ophthalmic artery. Diplopia, ptosis, or extraocular movement change may occur. Ophthalmoscopic exam may reveal pallor or edema of a disc. Optic atrophy, hemorrhage, or "cotton wool" exudates may be seen.

c. Tongue claudication: (6%): Symptoms of pain precipitated by use; infarction of the tongue may occur.

d. Jaw claudication: (45%): Occurs with chewing or talking.

e. Systemic vessels (7%): Disease may cause aneurysm or dissection of the aorta. Renal artery disease may lead to hypertension or renal failure. Raynaud's phenomenon is seen in 3% due to vessel involvement in extremities. Arch angiogram may be helpful.

3. Systemic symptoms: PMR is seen in 40% and fever in 40%, with 15% presenting as fever of unknown origin. Weight loss (50%) is common. CNS symptoms such as cardiovascular accident, mononeuritis or peripheral neuropathy may occur. Sore throat with cough is seen in 9%.

B. Diagnostic tests

1. Same as for PMR except for biopsy. Remember, the ESR may be normal in a small number of patients.

2. Biopsy of the superficial temporal artery is the gold standard for diagnosis. See section III for a discussion of pathology. Involvement is often patchy, with skip lesions, and disease may often be seen unilaterally. Therefore, to rule out GCA confidently in patients suspected of having the illness, a unilateral biopsy of 4–6 cm should be followed with a similar biopsy of the other artery. Treatment with steroids may alter biopsy appearance. Biopsy should be done early (within days). However, therapy should not be withheld in symptomatic patients. Occasionally, diagnosis is made in the presence of normal biopsy when clinical symptoms and signs are typical.

3. Angiograms of the temporal artery have not proved useful for routine use. Aortic arch angiograms may be useful in patients who present with suspected large vessel symptoms.

V. **Differential Diagnosis**

Based on clinical symptoms/signs with an elevated ESR. Biopsy and angiogram help to confirm the diagnosis. Appropriate differential diagnoses include isolated CNS vasculitis, Takayasu's arteritis, and other causes of headaches or sudden monocular blindness (transient ischemic attacks, cardiovascular accident, multiple sclerosis) or jaw pain.

VI. **Treatment**

A. Acute treatment: Patients with sudden visual loss and elevated ESR should be considered for immediate steroid therapy, 60–100 mg/day, and biopsy undertaken along with other evaluations within 48–72 hr.

B. Treatment for confirmed diagnosis: Prednisone, 40–60 mg/day, should be started immediately. For some patients, higher-dose or intravenous therapy may be appropriate early on. The ESR should be watched for a response, as should clinical signs.

VII. **Patient Monitoring**

Tapering should be 10% of the dose every 2–4 weeks, with reevaluation of the ESR and signs with each change. Flares should be treated with increased prednisone. Cytotoxics may occasionally be needed for patients who fail to respond or become too steroid toxic. Steroid precautions mentioned in the discussion of PMR should be followed.

VIII. **Prognosis**

A. Steroid therapy is usually effective in aborting damage from ischemia. Damaged eyes, however, may not recover once vision has been lost.

B. Illness may last for months to years, and patients need to be followed as their medication is tapered. Several patients have had flares in systemic arch vessels during tapering.

Bibliography

Ginsberg WW. Polymyalgia rheumatica, in Conn DL (ed), *Rheumatic Disease Clinics of North America*, Vol 16, part 2. Philadelphia, Saunders, 1990, p 325.

Hunder GG. Giant cell arteritis and polymyalgia rheumatica, in Kelly WN, Harris ED, Ruddy S, et al (eds), *Textbook of Rheumatology*, ed 3. Philadelphia, Saunders, 1989, p 1200.

Hunder GG. Giant cell (temporal) arteritis, in Conn DL (ed), *Rheumatic Disease Clinics of North America*, Vol 16, part 2. Philadelphia, Saunders, 1990, p 399.

SECTION 12

Endocrinology

CHAPTER 118

The Pituitary and Hypothalamus

C.R. Kannan, M.D.

Introduction

The pituitary gland is a small gland measuring 1.2–1.5 cm in its greatest diameter from side to side, with an anteroposterior diameter approximating 1 cm and a thickness of 0.5 cm. Couched in the bony sella turcica, the pituitary gland is connected to the hypothalamus by the pituitary stalk. The hypothalamus lies ventral to the thalamus, forming the floor and lower lateral walls of the third ventricle. The median eminence, an important area from which the pituitary stalk originates, is located at the base of the hypothalamus. Together, the hypothalamus and pituitary form a unit that functions as an integrated axis governing the function of the adrenal, the thyroid gland, the gonads, the breast tissue, and the growing end of the cartilage.

The hypothalamic-pituitary unit is clinically important for several reasons:

1. The pituitary gland can become the seat of tumor formation. Although benign, these tumors can wreak havoc by causing supra- and parasellar compression syndromes that can lead to blindness and death.

2. Functional abnormalities of the pituitary gland result in impressive clinical syndromes. Six major hormones are secreted by the anterior pituitary gland: growth hormone, (GH) prolactin, adrenocorticotropic hormone (ACTH), thyroid-stimulating hormone (TSH), luteinizing hormone (LH), and follicle-stimulating hormone (FSH). Perturbations of function can lead to hyperfunctional or hypofunctional syndromes (Table 118-1).

3. The pituitary gland can be involved by systemic processes such as metastatic disease, granulomatous disease, tuberculosis, collagen vascular diseases, and infectious processes.

This chapter will focus briefly on some of the important clinical syndromes that involve the pituitary gland and the hypothalamus.

Acromegaly

I. Definition
Acromegaly is a multisystemic disease resulting from sustained secretion of GH. The term *gigantism* is used when the disease starts before fusion of the cartilage. Acromegaly shortens the life span and causes considerable morbidity.

II. Etiology
A. The most common cause of acromegaly is a GH-secreting pituitary tumor called *soma-*

Table 118-1. Clinical Syndromes That Result from Pituitary Dysfunction

Hormone	Syndrome	Clinical Presentation	Common Etiologies
		Hyperfunctional	
GH	Acromegaly or gigantism	Increased growth, cardiovascular disease, change in appearance	GH-secreting pituitary tumor
Prolactin	Hyperprolactinemic syndromes	Galactorrhea, amenorrhea, impotence, osteopenia	Pituitary tumors, suprasellar disease, lactotrope hyperplasia
ACTH	Cushing's disease	Hypertension, diabetes, changing facial appearance, osteopenia, myopathy	Pituitary tumor
LH/FSH	Precocious puberty	Puberty that begins early	Idiopathic
TSH	Hyperthyroidism	TSH-induced thyrotoxicosis	Tumors, hyperplasia
		Hypofunctional	
GH	GH-deficient dwarfism	Growth retardation	Congenital, tumorous
Prolactin	Postpartum hypoprolactinemia	Inability to breast-feed	Sheehan's snydrome
ACTH	Secondary hypoadrenalism	Adrenal insufficiency	Tumors, vascular disease, isolated ACTH deficiency
LH/FSH	Kallmann's syndrome secondary hypogonadism	Puberty that never occurs; postpubertal gonadal failure	Gonadotropin-releasing hormone deficiency, tumors, Sheehan's syndrome, hemochromatosis
TSH	Secondary hypothyroidism	Thyroid failure	Tumors, isolated TSH deficiency
All hormones	Panhypopituitarism	Hypoadrenalism, hypothyroidism, hypogonadism	Sheehan's syndrome, tumor, apoplexy

totropinoma. These tumors can be small (*microadenoma* if less than 1 cm), medium-sized (*macroadenoma* if larger than 1 cm but confined to the sella), or invasive (with extension superiorly or laterally).

B. Less commonly, acromegaly can be caused by GH secretion from an ectopic source such as the lung.

C. Very rarely, GH secretion can be a result of ectopic secretion of GH-releasing hormone by other tumors. These are usually located in the pancreas or bronchus.

III. **Pathophysiology**

Regardless of the etiology, chronic hypersecretion of GH results in a spectrum of changes that involve virtually every organ system.

A. Metabolic changes: GH is an anabolic, lipolytic, mitogenic, and counterinsulin hormone. Thus, nitrogen retention, increased free fatty acids, increased growth of several tissues, and some degree of glucose intolerance are integral accompaniments of hypersomatotropism.

B. Visceral, acral, and cartilaginous overgrowth result from the growth-promoting actions of the hormone. These sets of actions are mediated by a peptide called *insulin-like growth factor I (IGF-I)*. This peptide is generated by the liver (and to a lesser extent by other tissues) in response to GH and mediates several but not all actions of GH at the tissue level. The growth-promoting actions of IGF-I, when sustained, result in increased size of the hands, jaw, heart, salivary glands, skin, peripheral nerves, thyroid gland, and viscera. Increased growth—initially with increased function—eventually results in exhaustion of organ function and decompensation.

IV. Clinical Features

Chronic hypersomatotrophism is one of the few endocrinopathies that permits instant recognition. The following constellation of clinical features may be present in varying degrees and in variable combinations.

A. Acral enlargement. The classic history of changing shoe size, glove size, and ring size may be obtained in two-thirds of patients.

B. Thickening and oiliness of skin, increased sweating, and coarsening of facial features are constant and yet so insidious that patients may not even notice these changes. An old photograph—taken 5–10 years earlier—may be invaluable in documenting progressive changes.

C. Headache and parasellar syndromes, most notably compression of the optic chiasm with bitemporal hemianopsia, are encountered with enlargement of the GH-producing tumor.

D. Cardiovascular complications represent an important cause of death in acromegaly. Acromegalic cardiomyopathy is a distinct entity characterized by severe biventricular failure, often progressive and refractory to medical therapy. In addition, hypertension, cardiac arrhythmias, and coronary heart disease are present in 20–25% of patients.

E. Peripheral neuropathy of the entrapment variety and chronic degenerative joint disease contribute to limitation of mobility in acromegalic patients.

F. Overt diabetes requiring insulin may be encountered in as many as 20% of patients with acromegaly.

V. Diagnosis

A. The presence of acromegaly can be confirmed by demonstrating abnormal GH dynamics as well as elevated levels of IGF-I (somatomedin-C) in the circulation. The two crucial tests to demonstrate abnormal GH dynamics are (1) failure of GH to suppress completely after a 100-g glucose load and (2) a paradoxical GH response to an intravenous bolus of thyrotropin-releasing hormone (TRH). Measurement of IGF-I in the plasma has become the most sensitive test to document acromegaly. IGF-I levels are elevated in all patients with active acromegaly and often correlate with the severity of illness.

B. After confirmation of acromegaly, pituitary imaging with computed tomography (CT), or preferably magnetic resonance imaging (MRI), is indicated to demonstrate the presence of a tumor and to define its extent. In addition, complete testing of pituitary reserve to document a deficiency of other pituitary hormones is mandatory.

C. Perimetry is needed to document field cuts.

VI. Treatment

A. The ideal treatment for acromegaly aims at removal of GH excess while preserving normal pituitary function. The chances for such a cure are best when acromegaly is caused by a microadenoma, which can be removed by transsphenoidal microadenomectomy without compromising the function of the normal pituitary. When the tumor is large, cure of acromegaly can seldom be achieved with anything less than total removal of the tumor, along with the entire pituitary. In such cases, hypopituitarism is an equitable trade-off for the cure of hypersomatotropism.

B. Medical: The use of bromocriptine has found acceptance as an adjunctive treatment for acromegaly. The drug reduces GH levels in 75% of patients with acromegaly but seldom normalizes the levels. The clinical and symptomatic improvement achieved in some patients can be impressive. Shrinkage of the tumor occurs in varying degrees, but this may require rather large doses, with attendant side effects of the drugs such as nausea, postural hypotension, leg cramps, and digital vasospasm. Somatostatin analogs (e.g., Sandostatin) have also been shown to decrease tumor size and reduce GH levels in acromegalics, but additional studies are needed to determine their role as sole agents for the treatment of acromegaly.

VII. Prognosis

A. Acromegaly is a devastating disease due to its effects on the cardiovascular system. In addition, several complications can punctuate the natural history of acromegaly. These include the following:

1. The development of apoplexy, a catastrophic bleed into the tumor, which can result in death.

2. Progressive encroachment on the normal pituitary tissue, resulting in hypopituitarism.

3. Blindness from compression of the optic chiasm and optic tracts.

4. A tendency to develop a variety of benign

and malignant neoplasms, most notably polyps of the colon, and adenocarcinoma of the colon, breast, and bronchus.

B. The heightened proclivity for tumor formation in acromegaly may be related to the mitogenic properties of GH, IGF-I, or both. Thus, it is evident that, unless treated effectively, acromegaly carries an extremely unfavorable prognosis.

Hyperprolactinemic Syndromes

I. Definition

Elevation of the prolactin level in the absence of pregnancy is defined as inappropriate hyperprolactinemia. A basal level greater than 20 ng/ml in females or greater than 15 ng/ml in males indicates perturbation in the control of prolactin secretion and may be associated with:

A. Oligomenorrhea or amenorrhea in females.

B. Impotence and erectile dysfunction in males.

C. Galactorrhea in either sex.

D. Patients with hypopituitarism or pituitary tumors.

E. Patients with clinical evidence of suprasellar disease (e.g., diabetes insipidus or visual field cuts).

F. Unexplained premature osteopenia.

II. Etiology

Prolactin secretion is controlled by tonic negative inhibition from the hypothalamus, which is mediated by dopamine (the *prolactin inhibitory factor*). Conditions that lead to depletion of hypothalamic dopamine from the tuberoinfundibular neurons or interruption of dopamine transport to the lactotropes will result in "lactotrope escape" and consequent hyperprolactinemia. The most common cause of hyperprolactinemia are:

A. Drug induced: Phenothiazines, tricyclic antidepressants, butyrephenones, metoclopramide, reserpine, α-methyldopa, estrogens, cimetidine, and opioids.

B. Hypothalamic disease: Suprasellar tumors (craniopharyngioma, germ cell tumors), granulomatous disease (sarcoid), and metastatic disease (especially from breast cancer).

C. Stalk disease: "Autosection" by a nonsecretory pituitary tumor extending superiorly and interrupting dopamine transport (*pseudoprolactinoma*).

D. Idiopathic hyperprolactinomia (nontumorous lactotrope hyperplasia).

E. Prolactinomas
   1. Microprolactinomas (less than 1 cm).
   2. Macroprolactinomas (more than 1 cm).
   3. Invasive macroprolactinomas (more than 1 cm with para- or suprasellar extension).

F. Decreased clearance, as in chronic renal failure and primary hypothyroidism.

G. Chest wall disease, as with herpes zoster infection, burns, or postthoracotomy.

H. Miscellaneous endocrinopathies: Thyroid disorders (both hypo- and hyperthyroidism), empty sella syndrome, Addison's disease, and polycystic ovaries.

III. Clinical Features

A. Menstrual and ovulatory dysfunction: The classic presentations of hyperprolactinemia, especially when caused by prolactinoma, are amenorrhea, oligomenorrhea, and infertility or some combination thereof; 25–30% of women with secondary oligomenorrhea or amenorrhea may have an underlying prolactin problem; infertility in females may be caused or complicated by an underlying prolactin problem in 10–18% of patients. Even when menses are regular, hyperprolactinemia can cause a shortened luteal phase and can contribute to subfertility. In general, the severity of symptoms correlates with the magnitude and duration of hyperprolactinemia.

B. Galactorrhea may be present in 40–80% of patients with sustained hyperprolactinemia.

C. Headaches, visual field cuts, and symptoms of hypopituitarism may develop when hyperprolactinemia is secondary to an invasive macroprolactinoma. Such *giant prolactinomas* are unusual in females but are the rule in males with prolactin-secreting tumors.

IV. Diagnostic Studies

A. Basal prolactin level, preferably done in the morning, with the patient resting and supine, is the initial test. The pulsatile nature of prolactin secretion may occasionally result in missing mild hyperprolactinemia.

B. The second step after documenting hyperprolactinemia is to exclude a drug use history (prescribed as well as recreational), primary hypothyroidism, chronic renal failure, and pregnancy. Thus, thyroid function tests (TFT), blood urea nitrogen, creatinine, and β-human chorionic gonadotropin, are necessary.

C. In the absence of the above, CT or MRI of the sella and suprasellar regions are necessary to exclude organic lesions in those areas. Most patients with microprolactinoma have basal prolactin levels in excess of 100 ng/ml. Basal prolactin levels show an excellent correlation with the size of prolactinoma.

D. If the CT or MRI study reveals the presence of a macroadenoma, the reserve of the other pituitary hormones should be tested.

V. Treatment

The therapeutic arena for prolactinomas is dominated by dopamine agonist therapy, represented by bromocriptine. This drug has found wide acceptance in the treatment of idiopathic hyperprolactinemia, microprolactinoma, and macroprolactinoma and even in selected cases of invasive macroprolactinomas. The clinical factors that direct treatment include objectives of the patient, presence of tumor in the pituitary, size of the tumor, degree of prolactin elevation, presence of suprasellar involvement, compliance and cost factors, and availability of neurosurgical expertise.

A. Medical: Bromocriptine has become the treatment of choice for the hyperprolactinemic syndromes for the following reasons:
   1. Bromocriptine lowers and normalizes the prolactin level in more than 90% of patients with hyperprolactinemia, regardless of the etiology.
   2. Within 2–6 months of instituting therapy, there is resumption of menstruation, ovulation, and adequacy of the luteal phase in 60–80% of patients with microprolactinomas.
   3. Shrinkage of tumor occurs with impressive frequency.
   4. Side effects can be minimized if treatment is phased in gently and gradually.

B. Surgical: The advantages of transsphenoidal microadenomectomy include successful restoration of menses and fertility, low morbidity, and a low incidence of hypopituitarism. However, the incidence of recurrent hyperprolactinemia ranges between 17% and 48%. The enthusiasm for transsphenoidal microadenomectomy as a method for treating microprolactinoma has fallen considerably since dopamine agonist drugs have found wide application. Surgery is still an option in patients who cannot take bromocriptine, or in the few who fail to respond to it, and in patients with invasive tumors that cause parasellar compression syndromes.

Hypopituitarism

I. Definition

Hypopituitarism occurs as a result of deficient secretion of one, more than one, or all tropic hormones secreted by the pituitary gland. Undiagnosed, this condition carries with it a high degree of morbidity and mortality.

II. Etiology

Pituitary failure can result from numerous causes.

A. Tumors: Tumors of the sella, suprasellar, and parasellar regions represent the most common cause of hypopituitarism. The frequency of subtle abnormalities in pituitary reserve exceeds the incidence of clinically overt hypopituitarism, which is a delayed expression of the disease.

B. Vascular conditions: Sheehan's syndrome and pituitary apoplexy represent the two common vascular etiologies of hypopituitarism.

C. Hypophysitis: Autoimmune destruction of the pituitary (*lymphocytic hypophysitis*) is rare, tends to occur in women, and is characterized by its temporal relation to pregnancy. The condition presents as a space-occupying lesion in the sella and can mimic the presentation of a pituitary tumor.

D. Miscellaneous: Metastatic disease (breast, lung, colon), metabolic disorders (hemochromatosis), and granulomatous disease (sarcoid, Hand-Schuller-Christians disease) represent rare etiologies.

III. Clinical Features

A. Constitutional symptoms such as weight loss, easy fatigability, anorexia, and weakness are often present.

B. Hypoadrenalism, caused by ACTH deficiency, can be the presenting symptom, often leading to acute adrenal crisis triggered by stress. The clinical clues to the presence of ACTH deficiency include low blood pressure, postural hypotension (although less severe than in primary adrenal insufficiency), loss of axillary hair (especially in females), and generalized hypopigmentation.

C. TSH deficiency leading to secondary hypothyroidism.

D. Gonadotropin deficiency, which is often an early marker of the disease. Decreased libido with erectile dysfunction in males, and oligomenorrhea, amenorrhea, and infertility in females, should raise the suspicion of hypopituitarism. Atrophy of breasts or testes may be evident in long-standing cases.

E. Prolactin deficiency becomes relevant only for the nursing mother in the postpartum period. The classic history of inability to lactate after delivery is pathognomonic for Sheehan's syndrome.

Table 118-2.   Pituitary Reserve Testing

Tropic Hormone	Basal Tests	Dynamic Tests
ACTH	Low cortisol with low ACTH	Cortisol response to ACTH
		Cortisol response to hypoglycemia
		Metyrapone test
		Corticotropin-releasing hormone test
TSH	Low T_4 index with low TSH	TRH-stimulation test
LH, FSH	Low LH, FSH with low sex steroid level	Luteinizing hormone-releasing hormone stimulation test
Prolactin	Low prolactin level	TRH stimulation test
GH	Low IGF-I level	GH response to levodopa, Clonidine, insulin, or growth hormone-releasing hormone

F. GH deficiency is rarely a cause of growth retardation in childhood. Hypoglycemia can be a manifestation of GH deficiency in both children and adults.

IV. **Diagnostic Tests**

A. The diagnosis of hypopituitarism rests on the demonstration of diminished tropic hormone reserve. In the simplest sense, the demonstration of a low (or inappropriately low) tropic hormone level in conjunction with a low target hormone level is diagnostic of pituitary hormone deficiency; however, in some cases, dynamic tests may be required to document decreased reserve (see Table 118-2).

B. After establishing the presence of hypopituitarism, the next step is to exclude a tumorous etiology. This is best accomplished by MRI of the pituitary and the suprasellar region.

V. **Treatment**

Treatment of hypopituitarism consists of replacement of the hormonal deficiencies, as well as addressing the underlying etiology.

Sheehan's Syndrome

I. **Definition**

This syndrome results from postpartum necrosis of the pituitary gland. The exact incidence of Sheehan's syndrome is not known, but clearly the condition is underrecognized.

II. **Pathophysiology**

The pituitary gland enlarges during pregnancy, predominantly due to hyperplasia of the lactotropes, with maximal enlargement occurring in the third trimester. The development of hypotension during pregnancy, delivery, or in the postpartum period leads to a cascade of events resulting in severe arteriolar spasm of the portal vessels that supply the anterior pituitary. This results in ischemia that can be severe enough to completely eliminate pituitary function.

III. **Clinical Features**

A. A classic picture of bleeding or obstetric shock is obtainable in 90% of patients.

B. The immediate effects of this phenomenon include the development of acute adrenal insufficiency in the postpartum period. Inability to lactate and failure to resume normal menses following delivery are classic historical clues to the diagnosis.

C. The hypopituitarism that results can be partial or complete, with varying degrees of tropic hormone deficiency.

D. Rarely, hypothalamic involvement may be seen in Sheehan's syndrome with diabetes insipidus and, paradoxically, galactorrhea.

E. The hypopituitarism that results from Sheehan's syndrome can manifest as late as 15 years after the original vascular insult. An autoimmune pathophysiology may be involved in such cases.

IV. **Diagnosis**

The same diagnostic approach used for hypopituitarism is employed. The size of the sella is often reduced in patients with Sheehan's syndrome.

V. **Treatment**

Appropriate replacement of the deficient hormones (i.e., levothyroxine, cortisone acetate, and sex steroids as indicated).

Bibliography

Abboud CF. Laboratory diagnosis of hypopituitarism. *Mayo Clin Proc* 61:35–48, 1986.

Fraioli B, Esposito V, Palma L, et al. Hemorrhagic pituitary adenomas: Clinicopathological features and surgical treatment. *Neurosurgery* 27:741–748, 1990.

Frohman L. Clinical review 22: Therapeutic options in acromegaly. *J Clin Endocrinol Metab* 72:1175–1181, 1991.

Klibanski A, Zervas NT. Diagnosis and management of hormone-secreting pituitary adenomas. *N Engl J Med* 324:822–831, 1991.

Molitch ME, Elton RL, Blackwell RD, et al. Bromocriptine as primary therapy for prolactin-secreting macroadenomas: Results of a prospective multicenter study. *J Clin Endocrinol Metab* 60:698–705, 1985.

Molitch ME, Russell EJ. The pituitary "incidentaloma." *Ann Intern Med* 112:925–931, 1990.

CHAPTER 119

Disorders of the Thyroid

Arcot Dwarakanathan, M.D.

Introduction

The thyroid gland is one of the largest endocrine organs. It is located in the neck and is closely affixed to the anterior and lateral aspects of the trachea. It consists of left and right lobes, each measuring about 2–2.5 cm in thickness and width and about 4 cm in length, connected in the middle by a thin band of tissue, the isthmus.

I. Embryology

A. The thyroid starts as a budding growth from the pharynx and elongates into the neck, becoming bilobar.

B. The structure connecting the thyroid to the pharynx, called the *thyroglossal duct*, is normally absent in most people. Remnants of this duct may persist and present as a thyroglossal cyst.

C. Neural crest cells that migrate into the fourth brachial pouches and ultimobranchial bodies become the parafollicular "C" cells of the thyroid that secrete calcitonin.

D. The thyroid gland becomes active by the 10th week of fetal development.

E. There are four parathyroid glands, two behind each thyroid lobe, normally located at the upper and lower poles of each lobe. The parathyroid glands and the parafollicular C cells are involved in calcium and bone homeostasis.

F. Blood supply: The superior thyroid artery arises from the external carotid artery. The inferior thyroid artery arises from the thyrocervical trunk of the subclavian artery.

II. Histology

Thyroid cells are arranged in a follicular pattern, and the follicles are lined by cuboidal cells. The lumen of the follicles contains the colloid. Here the nascent thyroid hormone is stored as an integral part of thyroglobulin.

III. Physiology

A. Thyroid hormones

1. Single amino acids and the only iodine-containing molecules in the human body.

2. Necessary both in utero and during the neonatal period for normal development of the central nervous system.

3. Essential for normal growth and development.

4. Through the effects on calorigenesis, play a pivotal role in temperature regulation.

5. Several specific enzyme systems are dependent on thyroid hormones for induction.
6. Thyroxine (T_4) is tetraiodothyronine. T_3 is triiodothyronine (Figure 119-1). Reverse T_3 is biologically inactive. Deiodination of T_4 at the 5' position produces T_3, and the same process at the 5 position results in reverse T_3.
B. Synthesis and secretion of thyroid hormones
   1. The first step is active uptake of iodide from the circulation by the thyroid gland. This is an active process, and the iodide concentration can reach 500 times that of plasma.
   2. Iodide is oxidized by thyroid peroxidase located at the apical membrane.
   3. This active form of iodide immediately binds to the tyrosyl groups within the thyroglobulin molecule. This process may produce monoiodotyrosine (MIT) or diiodotyrosine (DIT). This step is called *organification*.
   4. Two molecules of DIT may combine to form T_4, or MIT and DIT may combine to form T_3. This step is termed *coupling*.
   5. Mobilization and secretion of thyroid hormone from thyroglobulin begins with endocytosis of the colloid by the follicular cell. The resultant endocytotic vesicles fuse with the lysosomes to form phagolysomes. Proteolysis of the thyroglobulin releases T_3, T_4, MIT, and DIT as the phagolysomes migrate to the base of the follicular cell. Thyroid hormones diffuse into the circulation, while MIT and DIT are dehalogenated and iodide molecules are reclaimed. A small amount of iodide leaks out of the gland.
   6. Thyroid-stimulating hormone (TSH) stimulates all the above steps in thyroid hormone synthesis and release while also promoting growth of the thyroid cells.
   7. Iodide is also an important regulator of the above steps. Large doses of iodide can inhibit release of thyroid hormones (this effect is useful clinically), and it can also temporarily inhibit the organification process (Wolf-Chaikoff effect).
   8. Antithyroid drugs, which are thionamide derivatives, exert their effect by inhibiting thyroid peroxidase activity.
   9. Lithium can inhibit thyroid hormone release, an effect similar to that produced by iodide.
C. Thyroid hormone regulation and metabolism
   1. Both T_4 and T_3 exert their effect by binding to nuclear receptors.
   2. These receptors bind more avidly to T_3, explaining the increased bioactivity of T_3.
   3. T_4 may well be viewed as a prohormone. Fully 80% of the circulating T_3 is derived from the peripheral deiodination of T_4,

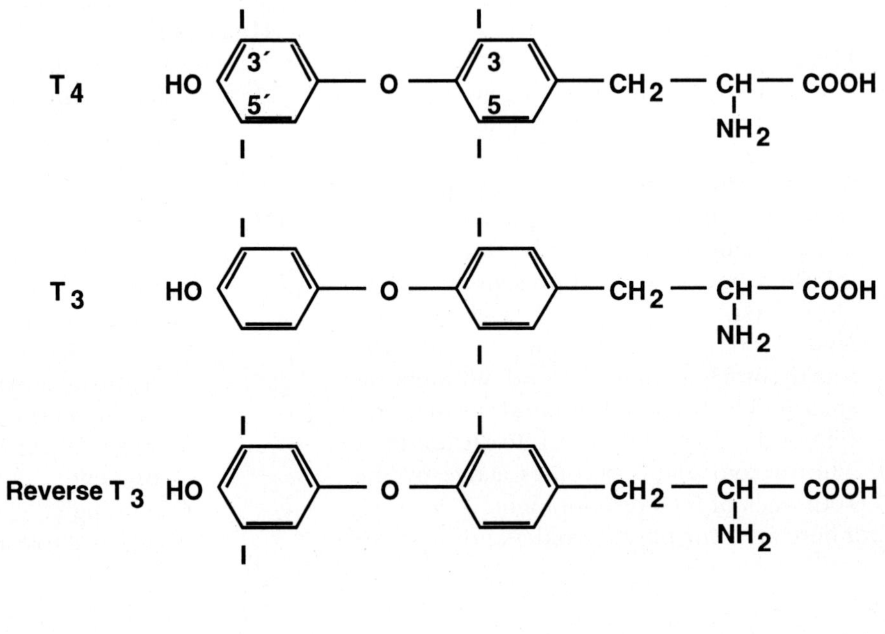

Figure 119-1.

and only 20% is directly secreted from the gland.

4. Both T_4 and T_3 are transported in the blood bound to protein; only 0.02% of T_4 and 0.3% of T_3 exist in the free form. This free form is the biologically active portion.

5. This extensive binding to serum proteins serves as a reservoir of thyroid hormones and prevents excretion of these small molecules by the kidney.

6. The major binding protein is thyroid-binding globulin (TBG), a 63,000-dalton glycoprotein. A small portion of the thyroid hormones bind to prealbumin and albumin.

7. The binding affinity of TBG for T_4 is 10 times that for T_3.

D. Regulation: There are two important steps regulating the level of biologically active thyroid hormone.

1. The hypothalamus secretes a tripeptide called *thyrotropin-releasing hormone (TRH)* that acts on the anterior pituitary thyrotrophs to release thyroid-stimulating hormone (TSH). This glycoprotein, in turn, influences the thyroid gland, regulating its growth, as well as thyroid hormone synthesis and release. The free fractions of T_4 and T_3 that are present in the circulation influence hypothalamic TRH and pituitary TSH secretion by a feedback mechanism. This feedback loop serves to maintain thyroid hormone levels in the physiologic range (Figure 119-2).

2. Peripheral conversion of T_4 to T_3 is also a regulatory step. Normally, 35% of circulating T_4 undergoes 5′ deiodination to form T_3, and 45% of T_4 is deiodinated at position 5 to form reverse T_3 (biologically inactive). In situations of calorie deprivation or illness, formation of reverse T_3 increases further.

IV. **Thyroid Function Tests**

A. Peripheral blood tests

1. T_4: Direct radioimmunoassay of T_4 in the blood. Simple, well standardized, least expensive, and a good screening test. Alterations in TBG will affect the test. An increase in TBG (as in pregnancy or estrogen treatment) will increase T_4; conversely, a decrease in TBG (congenital, nephrotic syndrome,

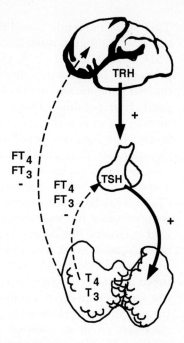

Figure 119-2. TRH and TSH in a stimulatory role. Free T_4 and T_3 in a feedback inhibitory role.

anticonvulsant drug use) will decrease T_4.

2. T_3: Direct radioimmunoassay of T_3 in the blood. Useful in diagnosing T_3 toxicosis. Levels fluctuate more rapidly than those of T_4. Changes in TBG level will alter T_3, just as in the case of T_4.

3. T_3 resin uptake (T_3 RU): Measurement of the percentage of labeled T_3 that is bound to the resin after being exposed to the test serum (TBG). If TBG (serum) is increased, a smaller percentage will bind to the resin, and vice versa.

4. Free thyroxine index (FTI) = $T_4 \times T_3$ RU (patient) divided by T_3^{RU} (mean control) will correct for changes in TBG. In some instances, this may not fully correct for the change in TBG.

5. Free T_4: Measurement of the free bioactive portion of T_4. The gold standard is the test performed by equilibrium dialysis. However, free T_4 is most often measured by a commercial kit utilizing two antibodies rather than by equilibrium dialysis; consequently, it is not as accurate.

6. Free T_3: Measurement of the free bioactive portion of T_3. Same problems occur as in free T_4.

7. TSH: The currently available, highly sensitive radioimmunoassay assay for TSH is very useful. It is elevated in primary hypothyroidism, normal in euthyroid patients, and suppressed in hyperthyroid patients. There are some normal patients with suppressed TSH levels. The significance of very slight elevations of TSH in otherwise euthyroid individuals is not known.

8. Thyroid-stimulating immunoglobulin (TSI): This IgG-class immunoglobulin is responsible for stimulating the thyroid in Graves' disease and is measured by increased cyclic adenosine monophosphate (AMP) generation in cultured thyroid cells when exposed to the test serum. Expensive and must be performed in a reputable laboratory. Not necessary in most cases of hyperthyroidism. Useful in pregnant hyperthyroid patients to predict neonatal hyperthyroidism.

9. Thyrotropin-binding inhibiting immunoglobulin (TBII): In vitro measurement of inhibition of thyrotropin binding to cultured thyroid cells by the test serum. Not necessary in most hyperthyroid patients.

10. TBG: A direct radioimmunoassay is done. Not necessary in most cases. TBGs of different binding characteristics are now being described.

11. Thyroglobulin: A direct radio immunoassay of thyroglobulin. A useful tumor marker which is used in follow-up of thyroid cancer patients in conjunction with ^{131}I scans. Slight elevations may be seen in other benign thyroid disorders like thyroiditis and Graves' disease.

12. Antithyroid antibodies (antithyroglobulin and antimicrosomal): Antimicrosomal antibodies are more sensitive, and high titers indicate lymphocytic thyroiditis (Hashimoto's thyroiditis). Slight elevations can be seen in Graves' disease.

13. Dynamic testing: TRH test: Measurement of TSH before and 30 min after administering 500 µg TRH by the intravenous route. A normal response indicates normal pituitary thyrotroph and thyroid function. An exaggerated response indicates underlying primary hypothyroidism with a resultant decrease in the negative feedback loop. Blunted or no response indicates hyperthyroidism (with resultant feedback suppression of TSH) or hypopituitarism. However, the clinical usefulness of this test is limited by frequent exceptions to the predicted responses, especially in hospitalized patients.

B. Imaging studies
   1. Technetium thyroid scan: Simple and easy to perform, with minimal radiation exposure.
   2. Iodide uptake: Measured in percentage terms; useful in the differential diagnosis of hyperthyroidism and in calculating the dose of ^{131}I for the therapy of hyperthyroidism.
   3. Ultrasonography: Simple, easy, noninvasive method used to evaluate thyroid nodules and differentiate cystic and solid lesions.

Hyperthyroidism

I. **Definition**
   This clinical condition is caused by any disorder of thyroid function that leads to increased levels of thyroid hormone in the bloodstream.

II. **Etiology**
   A. Graves' disease (most common).
   B. Hyperfunctioning thyroid nodule.
   C. Multinodular goiter.
   D. Jod-Basedow, or iodide induced.
   E. Iatrogenic.
   F. Subacute thyroiditis.
   G. Silent thyroiditis.
   H. Trophoblastic tumor.
   I. Ectopic thyroid tissue (struma, ovarii, functioning metastatic thyroid cancer).
   J. TSH-producing pituitary tumor.

III. **Pathophysiology**
   A. Graves' disease: Autoimmune disease with IgG antibodies against the TSH receptor on the thyroid cells. These immunoglobulins stimulate thyroid cell growth and the synthesis and release of thyroid hormone through their agonistic effect on the thyroid cells. Graves' disease is also associated with exophthalmos and infiltrative dermopathy, which are unique to this autoimmune disease.
   B. A single thyroid nodule may become auton-

omous and overwhelm the normal feedback control mechanism, leading to hyperthyroidism.

C. Multinodular goiter with multiple hyperfunctioning nodules may also lead to hyperthyroidism.

D. Jod-Basedow, or iodide-induced, hyperthyroidism is usually seen in patients with multinodular goiter when exogenous iodide is administered, usually during an iodide contrast x-ray study. It is usually self-limited and requires observation or temporary treatment only.

E. Patients may, intentionally or by prescription, take higher than usual replacement doses of iodide and manifest hyperthyroidism.

F. Subacute thyroiditis, also termed *viral thyroiditis*, usually follows an upper respiratory infection. It is characterized by mild to moderate hyperthyroidism and a painful, tender thyroid that is minimally enlarged. Hyperthyroidism is temporary, and patients recover completely. Mumps, coxsackie, influenza, ECHO, and adenoviruses have all been implicated.

G. Silent thyroiditis, another self-limited cause of hyperthyroidism with a histologic picture of lymphocytic infiltration. The thyroid is usually not enlarged or is just palpable, but there is no pain or tenderness.

H. Patients with molar pregnancy, may exhibit elevated levels of thyroid hormones secondary to extremely high levels of human chorionic gonadotropin that interacts with the TSH receptor on the thyroid cells. Symptoms of hyperthyroidism are usually mild or even absent. The condition resolves after removal of the trophoblastic tumor.

I. Ectopic thyroid tissue, as in metastatic follicular thyroid cancer, may not only take up iodide but also synthesize and release enough thyroid hormone to produce hyperthyroidism. Struma ovarii is an extremely rare disorder, with ectopic thyroid tissue in the ovary causing uncontrolled thyroid hormone production and hyperthyroidism.

J. TSH-producing pituitary tumors are rare and cause hyperthyroidism by continued stimulation of thyroid, wherein the usual feedback inhibitory action of thyroid hormones is not operative.

IV. **Diagnosis**
A. History: The symptoms commonly encoun-

tered in hyperthyroid patients are nervousness, increased sweating, heat intolerance, palpitations, insomnia, fatigue, weight loss (in spite of increased appetite and normal to increased food intake), muscle weakness, frequent bowel movements, and menstrual disturbance (usually decreased flow or oligomenorrhea). Patients with Graves' disease may also report bulging of the eyes and sometimes nodular skin changes, characteristically over the anterior surface of both lower extremities.

B. Clinical signs and physical findings: Increased pulse rate, warm moist hands, tremor, eye signs of lid lag, stare and eyeball lag, Plummer's nails, enlargement of the thyroid, bruit over the thyroid, and infiltrative dermopathy and ophthalmopathy in Graves' disease.

C. Diagnostic tests: Elevated levels of T_4 and T_3 RU; suppressed or undetectable TSH in all hyperthyroid patients except in rare cases of pituitary thyrotroph tumors. See Fig. 119-3.

V. **Differential Diagnosis**
A. Anxiety disorders may present with some of the well-known symptoms that are often associated with hyperthyroidism.

B. Other conditions with unexplained weight loss, including malabsorption syndromes, may pose a diagnostic problem.

C. Elderly patients with hyperthyroidism may not manifest the classic clinical signs and symptoms. They may present with muscle weakness, a worsening cardiac condition, or simply unexplained weight loss. The term *apathetic hyperthyroidism* is used to describe this clinical presentation in some elderly patients with hyperthyroidism.

D. Menopausal women with anxiety, hot flashes, and attendant heat intolerance may mimic a hyperthyroid condition.

E. Pregnancy sometimes presents a difficult problem because the hyperdynamic circulatory state of pregnancy is similar to the hyperthyroid condition. When to this is added the enlargement of the thyroid that occurs in normal pregnancy, it is understandable why it is sometimes difficult to establish the clinical diagnosis in this setting.

F. Pheochromocytoma with excessive catecholamine levels may be confused with hyperthyroidism.

G. Uncontrolled diabetes mellitus with weight loss, muscle weakness, and sometimes diar-

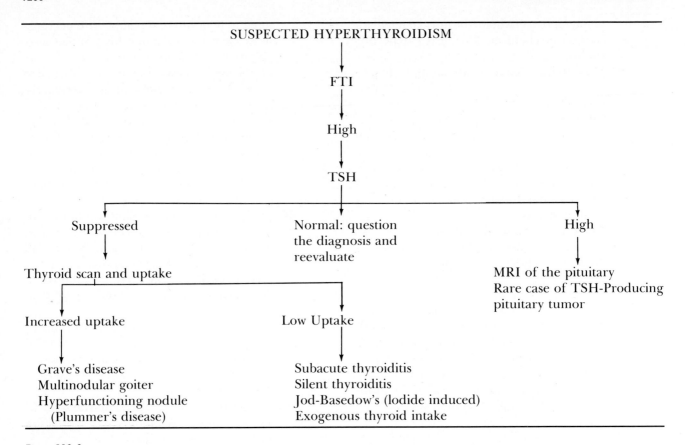

SUSPECTED HYPERTHYROIDISM

FTI

High

TSH

Suppressed   Normal: question   High
                              the diagnosis and
                              reevaluate

Thyroid scan and uptake   MRI of the pituitary
                                                                  Rare case of TSH-Producing
                                                                  pituitary tumor

Increased uptake   Low Uptake

Grave's disease   Subacute thyroiditis
Multinodular goiter   Silent thyroiditis
Hyperfunctioning nodule   Jod-Basedow's (Iodide induced)
   (Plummer's disease)   Exogenous thyroid intake

Figure 119-3.

rhea may pose a diagnostic problem. Thyroid function tests should solve the problem.

VI. Treatment

    A. Symptomatic: Propranalol or other β-blockers are used to control the symptoms of anxiety, palpitations, and increased sweating. Tranquilizers may be necessary in some cases.

    B. Definitive

        1. Antithyroid drugs

            a. Thiourea compounds, propylthiouracil or methimazole, work by inhibiting thyroid peroxidase, thereby decreasing the synthesis of thyroid hormones. Propylthiouracil also has the added effect of inhibiting peripheral conversion of T_4 to T_3.

            b. Even though treatment with antithyroid drugs is quite effective in controlling the hyperthyroidism of Graves' disease, the underlying autoimmune process continues, resulting in only temporary suppression. In 70% or more of the patients, the hyperthyroidism returns once the drugs are discontinued, even after 1 year of such treatment. The most frequent adverse reaction to the thiourea compounds is an allergic rash, which occurs in about 5% of such patients. The most serious reaction is agranulocytosis, which occurs in about 0.1–0.4% of patients and is reversible.

        2. Iodides in the form of Lugol's solution or a saturated solution of potassium iodide work very well by inhibiting thyroid hormone release and are useful in urgent situations. However, there is "escape" from this effect in a few weeks; therefore, iodides are not suitable for long-term treatment of hyperthyroidism.

        3. Lithium controls hyperthyroidism in a manner similar to that of iodide by inhibiting release of thyroid hormone. However, because of its inherent toxicity, it is not suitable for regular use in hyperthyroidism.

        4. Radioactive iodine: Administered in the form of ^{131}I, it is safe, effective, and economical in achieving control of hyper-

thyroidism. Ablation of the thyroid is achieved, as in surgery, without the need for anesthesia, avoiding the complications inherent in such surgery. An estimated dose of 50–100 μc per gram of thyroid tissue administered as a single oral dose. Attempts to use smaller dosages usually result in persistent hyperthyroidism, requiring repeat administration of ^{131}I. Subsequent hypothyroidism occurs in about 30% of patients within 5 years. A continued increase in the incidence of hypothyroidism at the rate of 3% per year is the main adverse effect of ^{131}I treatment. No increased incidence of thyroid carcinoma, leukemia, or transmissible genetic damage has been noted in approximately 40 years of observation of patients treated with ^{131}I. This treatment is definitely contraindicated in pregnant women because of damage to fetal thyroid tissue.

5. Surgery: Subtotal thyroidectomy, by removing a good portion of the thyroid, achieves rapid control of hyperthyroidism. The amount of thyroid tissue removed not only determines the cure rate but also accounts for the incidence of subsequent hypothyroidism. As with ^{131}I treatment, the more aggressive the surgery, the greater the incidence of subsequent hypothyroidism. Patients must be prepared preoperatively, over several weeks with antithyroid drugs, iodine, and propranalol, to avoid exacerbation of hyperthyroidism following surgery that may result in thyroid storm. Damage to the recurrent laryngeal nerve and parathyroid glands, as well as complications related to general anesthesia, are also to be considered before surgery is contemplated.

VII. Patient Monitoring

A. Patients treated with thionamide compounds should be monitored closely and have the medication dosage adjusted frequently, based on serum levels of thyroid hormone. After a year of such therapy, medication can be discontinued to assess for potential remission.

B. Patients treated with radioactive iodine or surgery require long-term periodic clinical evaluation and tests of serum thyroid hormone levels to detect subsequent hypothy-

roidism. It is important to note that the risk of hypothyroidism continues indefinitely.

VIII. Prognosis

Prognosis for life is excellent in the absence of serious complications like thyroid storm or cardiac disease, provided that the diagnosis is made promptly and hyperthyroidism controlled.

IX. Special Circumstances

A. Thyroid storm is a condition characterized by extreme hyperthyroidism often associated with fever, tachycardia (with or without signs of congestive heart failure), tremor, restlessness, and, in some cases, frank psychosis. Nausea, vomiting, and abdominal pain may be present. As the condition progresses, apathy, stupor, coma, and hypotension leading to shock may supervene. The usual precipitating factors are infection, trauma, surgery, and sometimes conditions like diabetic ketoacidosis, toxemia of pregnancy, and parturition. Proper preoperative preparation has virtually eliminated subtotal thyroidectomy as a leading cause of thyroid storm. Early recognition and prompt fluid resuscitation, treatment of the underlying precipitating factors, and immediate antithyroid therapy have decreased the overall mortality considerably. Antithyroid measures include iodides (oral or intravenous), antithyroid drugs (preferably propylthiouracil because of its inhibitory action on peripheral deiodination of T_4 to T_3), β-blockers (orally or intravenous), and the use of stress doses of glucocorticoids. Overall mortality, however, still remains at 20%.

B. Hyperthyroidism in pregnancy

1. This is almost always due to Graves' disease. Increased fetal wastage occurs in untreated patients. Radioactive iodine is contraindicated. Subtotal thyroidectomy in the second trimester is utilized by some, but the risks of anesthesia and surgery are unnecessary.

2. Antithyroid treatment with propylthiouracil is the preferred treatment. Since the drug crosses the placenta and can affect the fetal thyroid, caution is advised and the smallest effective dose is used, maintaining the FTI at or slightly above the upper normal range.

3. Measuring TSI close to delivery is useful to predict the possibility of neonatal hyperthyroidism. This condition occurs mainly because of the stimulation of the

infant thyroid by the passively transferred maternal TSI. This self-limited
condition can be managed with either
Lugol's solution or β-blockers administered over a few weeks.

Hypothyroidism

I. Definition

This condition is characterized by inadequate or
low levels of thyroid hormone. Since thyroid
hormones influence the function of nearly all
organ systems in the body, manifestations are
widespread.

II. Etiology

A. Currently, the most common cause of hypothyroidism is damage to the thyroid, either by radioactive iodine or surgery.

B. The most common cause of naturally occurring hypothyroidism is autoimmune destruction. The incidence of spontaneous
overt hypothyroidism is about 2 per 1,000
per year.

C. Congenital hypothyroidism is now being
recognized promptly due to routine neonatal screening. If untreated, this condition
leads to impaired growth, as well as impaired neurologic and intellectual development. The incidence is about 1 in 4,000 live
births.

D. Endemic iodide deficiency presents with goitrous hypothyroidism. Iodide supplementation of bread and salt has virtually eliminated this condition.

E. Defects in the enzyme systems involved in
thyroid hormonogenesis are inherited and
cause goitrous cretinism.

F. Rare instances of peripheral thyroid hormone resistance have been described.

G. Secondary hypothyroidism can occur due to
deficient production of TSH from the pituitary gland. Milder degrees of hypothyroidism, the presence of a pituitary tumor
(in some cases), and association with deficiencies of other pituitary tropic hormones
differentiate this entity from the more common primary hypothyroidism.

H. Tertiary hypothyroidism, caused by deficient TRH production by the hypothalamus, may occur and can sometimes be differentiated from the secondary form by a
delayed TSH response to intravenous TRH.
Since the subsequent treatment is the same
as that of the secondary form, this diagnosis

is not absolutely essential for patient management as long as the rest of the pituitary
function in adequately tested.

III. Pathophysiology

Autoimmune destruction of the thyroid by infiltration with cytotoxic lymphocytes is the most
common cause of spontaneous primary hypothyroidism in the general population. Damage by ^{131}I or surgery in the treatment for
hyperthyroidism usually accounts for the rest of
the primary hypothyroid patients.

IV. Diagnosis

A. History

1. Symptoms involve multiple organ systems and are due to the hypometabolic
state. The gradual onset of these manifestations explains the delay in diagnosis.

2. Weakness, lethargy (and in some cases
frank somnolence), cold intolerance, dry
skin, dry brittle hair, hoarseness, facial
puffiness, shortness of breath, increasing
pallor, paresthesias, muscle cramping,
weight gain, constipation, fatigue, menstrual irregularity (mainly menorrhagia),
slow mentation, depression, and in some
cases frank psychosis.

B. Physical findings

1. The chronic insidious onset and the nonspecific nature of the usual symptoms
account for the initial difficulty and some
delay in the diagnosis. However, the classic signs include puffy dry face, dry brittle hair, large tongue, hoarse voice with
slow speech, galactorrhea (in some cases),
pleural or pericardial effusions, and anemia (usually normocytic normochromic);
however, iron deficiency secondary to
menorrhagia or vitamin B_{12} deficiency
from malabsorption may be seen. Hyper-
carotenemia leadng to the characteristc
skin color may be present.

2. Bradycardia, narrow pulse pressure,
and, in some cases, hypertension underlying coronary artery disease may pose a
serious problem in the subsequent treatment.

3. Nerve entrapment syndromes like bilateral carpal tunnel syndrome or diminished hearing. Characteristic hung reflexes from prolongation of the relaxation
phase during a deep tendon reflex. Mild
hypothermia may be present. Extreme
cases of hypothyroidism may lead to
coma. In children with hypothyroidism,

retardation of growth may be the first sign. Impaired free water excretion by the kidneys may lead to hyponatremia. Patients with secondary or tertiary hypothyroidism may manifest symptoms and signs of deficiency of other trophic hormones.

C. Diagnostic tests

1. Demonstration of a low thyroid hormone level, as evidenced by a low FTI, is important, as many of the manifestations may be nonspecific.

2. Measurement of TSH is imperative to establish the nature of the underlying hypothyroidism. A clearly elevated TSH level indicates primary thyroid failure, and a low TSH level in the hypothyroid patient signifies pituitary or hypothalamic disease.

3. In patients with low TSH levels, testing for other pituitary hormones and imaging studies looking for pituitary or hypothalamic lesions are indicated. In elderly patients, evaluation of the heart for underlying coronary artery disease is essential prior to initiation of treatment.

V. Differential Diagnosis

Frank myxedema poses little difficulty in diagnosis. However, in milder cases, the symptoms are nonspecific and common, leading to delay in diagnosis. The important clinical clue is any change in the patient's usual condition—for example, if a patient who is always warm develops cold intolerance or if a patient who usually has regular bowel movements develops unexplained constipation. A history of previous goiter or treatment of hyperthyroidism would be extremely useful. The diagnostic dilemma is more evident in a seriously ill patient. Hypothermia, a thyroidectomy scar, presence of effusions, or hung-up reflexes may be helpful in supporting the diagnosis of hypothyroidism in such patients.

VI. Treatment

A. Administration of levothyroxine or T_4 is preferred. Circulating T_3 will be derived from peripheral deiodination of T_4, and this deiodinase activity is closely regulated according to the metabolic needs of the body. This, therefore, is the most physiologic way of replacing thyroid hormones. Preparations that contain a mixture of T_4 and T_3 or T_3 alone are not recommended for the routine treatment of hypothyroidism, as the onset of action may be abrupt and T_3 bypasses the regulatory deiodinase step described previously.

B. Measurement of currently available, highly sensitive TSH has greatly facilitated evaluation of the adequacy of thyroid replacement. Demonstration of elevated TSH prior to initiation of thyroid replacement is mandatory to avoid misdiagnosis of secondary or tertiary hypothyroidism. Addisonian crisis may result in secondary hypothyroidism and adrenocorticotropic hormone (ACTH) deficiency if thyroid replacement is initiated without hydrocortisone administration. In elderly patients, one must be extremely cautious and assume that underlying coronary artery disease is present, even in the absence of overt signs or symptoms. Replacement is started with very small doses of T_4 (25 μg) and gradually increased by 25 μg every 3–4 weeks until a replacement dose of 75–100 μg is achieved. In some cases, the underlying coronary artery disease has to be treated, either by angioplasty or bypass surgery, before replacement can be initiated.

VII. Patient Monitoring

Measurement of highly sensitive TSH has simplified such monitoring. Maintenance of this level within the normal range indicates physiologic replacement. Following ablative treatment of thyroid cancer patients, the T_4 dosage is adjusted to achieve undetectable levels of TSH. Despite the accuracy of the TSH measurement, the patient's symptoms may dictate a change in dosage in some instances.

VIII. Prognosis

In the usual case of primary hypothyroidism from autoimmune thyroiditis, and in cases caused by ablative treatment for hyperthyroidism, prompt diagnosis and treatment result in an excellent prognosis. In advanced cases of myxedema and in cases complicated by underlying coronary artery disease, the prognosis is less certain.

IX. Special Circumstances

Myxedema coma: Characterized by extreme hypothyroidism and a high mortality rate. Coma, hypothermia, hypotension, hypoglycemia, hyponatremia, and respiratory failure, either alone or in combination, may occur. Therapy should be prompt and should not wait for laboratory confirmation. Supportive measures include mechanical ventilation, passive warming with blankets, glucose infusion for hypoglycemia, free water restriction for hyponatremia, and cautious fluid and electrolyte replacement to combat hypotension. Prompt intravenous administration of 300–500 μg of T$_4$, followed by 50–100 μg daily, is recommended. Intravenous hydrocortisone in doses of 400 mg/day is also administered to combat potential adrenocortical deficiency.

Thyroid Nodule and Goiter

I. Definition

Enlargement of the thyroid, usually multinodular, is also called *goiter* and occurs at a rate of 4–7% in the general population. The nodules may be single or multiple and are usually not associated with hyperthyroidism, hence the term *nontoxic goiter*. Endemic iodide deficiency is no longer a common cause of goiter as a result of iodide supplementation of salt and water.

II. Etiology and Pathophysiology

The precise etiology of nodular thyroid disease is unknown. Some patients with Hashimoto's thyroiditis (autoimmune chronic lymphocytic thyroiditis) may present with a multinodular goiter. In most instances, the underlying mechanism leading to nodule formation is unknown. Local production of growth-promoting factors (immunoglobulin?) causing single or multiple nodules is an attractive hypothesis but is still unsubstantiated.

III. Diagnosis

A. History and physical findings: The diagnosis of an enlarged thyroid or thyroid nodule is usually made during a routine examination. Occasionally, the patient, a relative, or a close friend may bring attention to the enlarged thyroid. Thyroid function abnormalities are uncommon; hence no history to suggest hyperthyroidism or hypothyroidism is noted. Some patients with large or rapidly growing goiters may complain of local pressure symptoms. There may be a strong family history of goiters or other thyroid disorders. A past history of head and neck irradiation has been implicated in the increased incidence of thyroid nodules 5–35 years after exposure. The presence of single or multiple nodules should be noted. Thyroid nodules are more common in women than in men (10:1), so this presentation in a man requires closer scrutiny. Hoarseness, with vocal cord paresis or paralysis, indicates recurrent laryngeal nerve involvement by the enlarged thyroid, usually malignant in nature. Local lymph node enlargement is also a useful clinical sign indicating possible local malignant spread.

B. Diagnostic tests

1. Thyroid function tests, including FTI and TSH, may be indicated to ascertain the thyroid status of the patient. Antithyroid antibodies may be positive in the peripheral blood, suggesting goitrous Hashimoto's thyroiditis. Elevated calcitonin at baseline or after pentagastrin stimulation is necessary to diagnose early medullary thyroid cancer in a patient with family history of multiple endocrine neoplasia (MEN) II. However, in the vast majority of patients with nodular thyroid disease, all the above tests are usually normal.

2. Thyroid scan: Technetium thyroid scan is a safe, noninvasive test to evaluate thyroid enlargement. However, this test is not required to evaluate the great majority of patients with goiter. Approximately 90% of thyroid nodules are hypofunctioning.

3. Ultrasonography is another safe, noninvasive test that is most useful in distinguishing cystic from solid nodular lesions. However, this test is not routinely required. The majority of nodules are solid or mixed (solid with cystic components).

4. Fine needle aspiration biopsy: This technique, used to aspirate thyroid nodules, is a simple and safe office procedure. It is performed with a syringe and a 22- to 20-gauge needle and yields direct cytologic information. A wide variety of pathologic lesions including papillary thyroid cancer, medullary cancer, anaplastic cancer, Hashimoto's thyroiditis, and subacute thyroiditis can be readily diagnosed by examining the aspirated material. Simple cysts can be diagnosed instantly and resolved by aspiration. The major limitation of aspiration biopsy is the inability to distinguish benign from malignant follicular adenomas. Pathologists utilize clues such as vascular, lymphatic, or capsular invasion to diagnose malignancy in follicular lesions. Such information is obviously not available in a

specimen obtained by fine needle aspiration biopsy.

IV. **Treatment**

Since the majority of nodules are benign and since most patients are euthyroid, no further measures are necessary other than periodic follow-up examinations. Figure 119-4 summarizes the most cost-effective and efficient method of evaluation and follow-up of patients with thyroid nodules.

Thyroid Cancer

I. **Definition**

Malignant lesions of the thyroid are almost always epithelial in origin and are therefore carcinomas. Classification:

A. Epithelial cell tumors
   1. Follicular in origin
      a. Papillary thyroid cancer
      b. Follicular thyroid cancer
      c. Anaplastic thyroid cancer
   2. Parafollicular in origin
      a. Medullary cancer
   3. Metastatic extrathyroid cancers
B. Nonepithelial cell tumors
   1. Fibrosarcoma
   2. Angiosarcoma
   3. Lymphoma
   4. Plasmacytoma
   5. Teratoma
   6. Other sarcomas

II. **Clinical Features**

A. Papillary carcinoma: The most common thyroid cancer, accounting for 50–80% of all thyroid cancers. It presents as a solitary thyroid nodule. Histologic examination reveals a well-encapsulated nodule with columnar epithelium that is thrown into folds, forming papillary projections with connective tissue stalks. The nuclei may have an optically clear appearance or a "ground glass" chromatin pattern. Psammoma bodies (concentrically laminated microcalifications) are frequently seen in papillary carcinomas of the thyroid. Occasionally, papillary cancer may be multicentric. This is the least lethal thyroid cancer, and long survival is the rule. Older patients may exhibit more aggressive tumors with a slightly worse prognosis. A mortality rate of approximately 10% over several decades has been reported.

B. Follicular carcinoma: May or may not be encapsulated. It accounts for about 20–30% of thyroid carcinomas. It is composed of follicles made up of neoplastic epithelial cells. Capsular, vascular, or lymphatic invasion may be evident on examination of the

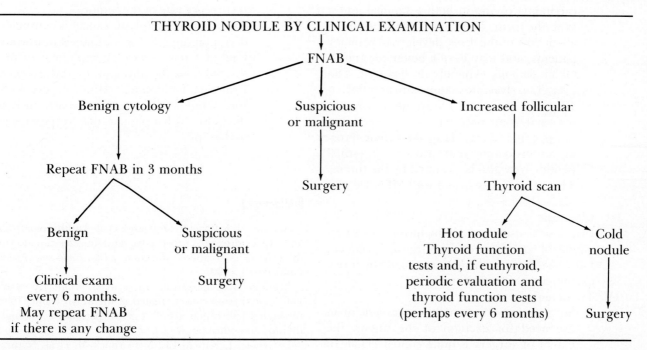

THYROID NODULE BY CLINICAL EXAMINATION

FNAB

Benign cytology → Repeat FNAB in 3 months → Benign → Clinical exam every 6 months. May repeat FNAB if there is any change / Suspicious or malignant → Surgery

Suspicious or malignant → Surgery

Increased follicular → Thyroid scan → Hot nodule Thyroid function tests and, if euthyroid, periodic evaluation and thyroid function tests (perhaps every 6 months) / Cold nodule → Surgery

Figure 119-4.

tumor. Papillary elements may also be present. The degree of invasiveness, which increases with advancing age, determines the prognosis. Ten-year survival with minimally invasive follicular cancers averages about 86%. In more invasive follicular cancers, the average survival rate is about 44%. The clinical presentation is predominantly that of a thyroid nodule. Metastatic lesions may accumulate iodine; rarely, the functioning metastatic lesions may produce sufficient thyroid hormone to cause hyperthyroidism.

C. Anaplastic carcinoma: Anaplastic thyroid cancers are rare, comprising only 5–10% of all thyroid carcinomas. This highly malignant tumor is composed of spindle cells and giant cells and usually occurs in older patients. It is a very aggressive tumor and is uniformly fatal in a few months.

D. Medullary carcinoma: Medullary thyroid carcinoma arises from the parafollicular C cells. It accounts for about 5–10% of all thyroid cancers. Histologically, it is composed of relatively uniform ovoid to spindle-shaped neuroendocrine cells that can occur as either nodules or trabeculae. Amyloid may be demonstrable in the tumor. Calcitonin, secreted by the tumor, serves as a marker and permits early detection and documentation of cure in some cases. Medullary carcinoma occurs in both a familial and a sporadic form. The familial form occurs in about 20% of the cases, develops in younger patients, and may have a better prognosis. Older patients generally do less well. The overall survival rate is approximately 66% at 10 years. Carcinoid syndrome and Cushing's syndrome may occur due to secretion of serotonin or ACTH by the tumor. Prostaglandins, kinins, and vasoactive intestinal peptide may also be secreted by the tumor. This tumor is associated with MEN IIa and MEN IIb.

III. **Diagnosis**

Diagnosis is usually made by histologic examination of an aspirated or surgical specimen. Final histologic confirmation is made by direct examination of excised tumor.

IV. **Treatment**

A. Surgery: Even though there is agreement on the need for excision of the tumor, the extent of surgery is quite controversial. In papillary thyroid carcinomas that are localized, well encapsulated, without signs of invasion, and 2 cm or less in size, surgical removal is considered curative. Larger tumors or tumors with signs of invasion, and all medullary carcinomas, require near-total thyroidectomy to achieve a maximal chance of cure. This also facilitates subsequent ^{131}I treatment of papillary and follicular cancers by removing thyroid tissue in the neck and enhancing iodide uptake by metastatic lesions. Surgery is the mainstay of treatment of medullary carcinoma. Locally recurrent lesions and some accessible distant metastatic lesions should be surgically removed.

B. Radioactive iodine: This is a useful adjunct to thyroid surgery in papillary and follicular thyroid cancers, as iodide is also accumulated by these tumors, thereby facilitating localized radiotherapy to metasteses. Approximately 100 mCi of ^{131}I is administered when the patient is hypothyroid postthyroidectomy in order to maximize iodide uptake by the tumor. Patients are scanned periodically, and residual tumor can be retreated with ^{131}I.

C. Thyroid hormone treatment: T_4 in doses sufficient to suppress TSH to an undetectable level is central to the successful treatment of thyroid cancer (papillary and follicular). This treatment markedly reduces the recurrence rate of the tumor.

D. Treatment of anaplastic cancer is extremely disappointing, and this tumor is uniformly fatal in a few months. Lymphomas of the thyroid may be difficult to differentiate from anaplastic cancer. However, every effort should be made to establish such a diagnosis, as lymphomas may respond well to therapy.

Bibliography

Allannic H, Fauchet R, Orgiazzi J, et al. Antithyroid drugs and Graves' disease. A prospective randomized evaluation of the efficacy of treatment duration. *J Clin Endocrinol Metab* 70:675–679, 1990.

Brennan MD, Bergstralh EJ, Van Heerden JA, et al. Follicular thyroid cancer treated at the Mayo Clinic, 1946 through 1970. Initial manifestations, pathologic findings, therapy and outcome. *Mayo Clin Proc* 66:11–22, 1991.

DeGroot LJ, Kaplan EL, McCormick M, et al. Natural

history, treatment and course of papillary thyroid carcinoma. *J Clin Endocrinol Metab* 71:414–424, 1990.

Singer PA. Thyroiditis acute, subacute and chronic. *Med Clin North Am* 75:16–75, 1991.

Staren ED, Dwarakanathan A, Miller AW, et al. *Percuta-* *nuous Needle Aspiration Biopsy of Thyroid Masses. Adjuncts to Cancer Surgery.* Philadelphia, Lea & Febiger, 1991, p 141.

Surks MI, Chopra IJ, Mariash CN, et al. American thyroid association guidelines for use of laboratory tests in thyroid disorders. *JAMA* 263:1529–1532, 1990.

CHAPTER 120

The Adrenal Gland

Ludwig Kornel, M.D., Ph.D.

Diseases of the Adrenal Cortex

Introduction

Three major groups of adrenal steroids are glucocorticoids, mineralocorticoids, and adrenal androgens. Glucocorticoids control the metabolism of carbohydrates, proteins, and lipids; mineralocorticoids
control the metabolism of minerals, chiefly sodium
(Na^+) and potassium (K^+). The functions of adrenal
androgen are not yet completely understood.

Chronic Adrenocortical Insufficiency

I. Definition
The clinical syndrome of adrenal insufficiency
results from deficient production of cortisol and,
less commonly, aldosterone.

II. Etiology
A. Primary chronic adrenocortical insufficiency
(Addison's disease) is characterized by insidious onset, caused by gradual destruction of
the adrenal gland by a disease process. There
are several potential etiologic factors (Table
120-1):

1. Autoimmune destruction, usually associated with autoimmune destruction of
other endocrine glands (so-called polyen-
docrine deficiency syndromes).
2. Granulomatous diseases of the adrenal
gland.
3. Human immunodeficiency virus–related
destruction of the adrenal gland.
B. Secondary chronic adrenocortical insufficiency is due to abnormalities of the hypothalamus or pituitary gland, leading to deficiency of adrenocorticotropic hormone
(ACTH) or is iatrogenic due to pituitary suppression by exogenously administered glucocorticoids.

III. Pathophysiology
The symptoms and signs of both primary and
secondary adrenocortical insufficiency are the
result of inadequate glucocorticoid activity and
sometimes inadequate mineralocorticoid activity
as well.
A. The rate of gluconeogenesis is decreased.
B. Insulin-promoted glucose transfer into cells
is not adequately counterbalanced by glucocorticoids: hypoglycemia ensues.
C. Since high intra-adrenal concentrations of glu-

Table 120-1. Causes of Primary Adrenocortical Insufficiency

Major causes
    Autoimmune (about 80%)
    Tuberculosis (about 20%)
Rare causes
    Adrenal hemorrhage and infarction
    Fungal infections
    Metastatic and lymphomatous replacement
    Amyloidosis
    Sarcoidosis
    Hemochromatosis
    Radiation therapy
    Surgical adrenalectomy
    Enzyme inhibitors (metyrapone,
      aminoglutethimide, trilostane)
    Cytotoxic agents (mitotane; o,p'-DDD)
    Congenital (enzyme defects, hypoplasia, familial
      glucocorticoid deficiency)

Source: From Tyrrell JB, Aron DC, Forsham PH. Glucocorticoids and adrenal androgens, in Greenspen FS (ed), *Basic and Clinical Endocrinology,* ed 3. Norwalk, Conn, Appleton and Lange, 1991, p 340. Reprinted with permission.

cocorticoid are necessary for production of medullary catecholamines, the response of the adrenal medulla to stress is attenuated. This deepens hypoglycemia (inadequate epinephrine) and hypotension (inadequate norepinephrine).

D. Since both mineralocorticoids and glucocorticoids are necessary for the maintenance of proper tissue and extracellular sodium concentrations, the total amount of extracellular sodium is reduced and intravascular volume decreases; hypovolemia and hypotension ensue. The latter is also caused by a decreased intracellular concentration of sodium in vascular smooth muscle, which decreases the tone of the muscle and its responsiveness to vasoconstrictive stimuli.

E. Hypovolemia and reduced cardiac output also lead to decreased renal perfusion pressure. This results in decreased renal excretion of metabolic waste products in the urine. Consequently, serum creatinine and blood urea are elevated (so-called prerenal azotemia). This leads to nausea and vomiting, with additional loss of fluid and more shrinkage of the circulating plasma volume.

F. In primary adrenocortical insufficiency, the decreased inhibition of pituitary corticotropes by low cortisol levels leads to excessive ACTH secretion. Secretion of ACTH is usu-

ally coupled with that of β-lipotropin and β-melanocyte stimulating hormone (βMSH) accounts for most of the hyperpigmentation of skin and mucous membranes encountered in patients with Addison's disease.

IV. **Diagnosis**

A. History

1. The prominent complaint is fatigue and weakness, steadily increasing over periods of months or even years, sometimes precipitated by a stressful event or intercurrent illness.

2. Additional complaints are anorexia, nausea, vomiting, abdominal pain, and diarrhea.

3. Weight loss occurs.

4. In primary adrenocortical insufficiency, skin pigmentation gradually increases.

5. In adrenocortical insufficiency, as part of the polyglandular syndrome, there may be a history of hypofunction of other involved endocrine glands (i.e., the thyroid, parathyroid, and pancreas).

B. Clinical signs and physical findings:

1. The gradual development of adrenal insufficiency may go unnoticed by the patient or physician until a large majority of adrenocortical function is lost. The most distinctive clinical signs in primary adrenocortical insufficiency are:

a. Weight loss.

b. Diarrhea and vomiting, causing dehydration.

c. Hypotension, orthostatic hypotension, and even orthostatic syncope.

d. Hyperpigmentation in skin areas exposed to sunlight, in the palmar creases and at the pressure points, breast areolae, cutaneous scars, and mucous membranes; it may begin so subtly that it may be mistaken for a normal suntan, except that it fails to fade. In secondary adrenocortical insufficiency, hyperpigmentation is absent and there is a grayish pallor of the skin characteristic of hypopituitarism.

e. Vitiligo, which is a manifestation of autoimmune destruction of skin melanocytes, occurs in about 15% of patients with autoimmune Addison's disease.

f. Anemia: Some patients have macrocytic megaloblastic anemia, which is the manifestation of coexisting autoimmune destruction of gastric parietal cells resulting in achlorhydria, which impairs folic acid and/or vitamin B_{12} absorption. Otherwise, patients with primary and secondary adrenal insufficiency develop a mild to moderate normocytic or microcytic anemia due to decreased iron utilization.

2. The diagnosis of primary adrenocortical insufficiency is easier than that of the secondary type. It is strongly suggested by the presence of muscular weakness and fatigability, anorexia and weight loss, and hyperpigmentation of the skin.

3. The clinical features of ACTH and, consequently, glucocorticoid deficiency are less specific than those of the primary adrenocortical insufficiency. They consist mainly of weakness, fatigability, anorexia, nausea, and, less frequently, vomiting and various degrees of lethargy. Arthralgia and myalgia are frequent.

C. Diagnostic tests

1. The classic triad is hyponatremia, hyperkalemia, and azotemia; it exists in 80–90% of patients with Addison's disease but is rarely encountered in patients with secondary adrenocortical insufficiency. Clinical features of mineralocorticoid deficiency are usually absent in secondary insufficiency.

2. The crucial laboratory test is demonstration of the lack of response in plasma cortisol level to exogenous ACTH. The basal levels of plasma cortisol or urinary 17-hydroxycorticosteroids (17-OHCS), may be normal since various degrees of adrenocortical deficiency occur. Synthetic ACTH is given as a 250-μg bolus intravenous injection, and blood is drawn 30 and 60 min after the injection for the measurement of plasma cortisol.

3. Plasma ACTH levels in patients with primary adrenal insufficiency are high (200–2,000 pg/ml); in secondary adrenal insufficiency due to pituitary ACTH deficiency, they are low (0–50 pg/ml).

4. In secondary adrenocortical insufficiency, the patient should also be evaluated for other pituitary deficiencies and for the presence of pituitary or hypothalamic tumors (see Chapter 118).

5. Serologic studies for antibodies to adrenal tissue confirm the autoimmune pathogen-esis of the disease; however, antiadrenal antibodies may occasionally occur and disappear from serum of patients with no evidence of adrenal insufficiency.

6. Mild to moderate hypercalcemia occurs in about 10% of patients with primary adrenocortical insufficiency. Hypocalcemia and hyperphosphatemia are present in patients with associated hypoparathyroidism.

7. The differential white blood cell count shows neutropenia, a relative lymphocytosis, and eosinophilia.

V. Differential Diagnosis

A. The most common symptoms—tiredness, increased fatigability on exertion, and weight loss—are present in a whole range of chronic disorders and may result from diseases of many different organ systems, as well as from psychological causes (e.g., neurasthenia, chronic depression). The hyperpigmentation of Addison's disease must be distinguished from that encountered in some patients with ectopic ACTH syndrome (compare below) or in idiopathic hemochromatosis.

B. The prerenal azotemia in patients with fatigue and weight loss but without hyperpigmentation encountered in secondary adrenocortical insufficiency must be differentiated from the azotemia of renal origin.

VI. Treatment

A. Treatment of primary chronic adrenocortical insufficiency: Maintenance therapy with 25–30 mg hydrocortisone per day (or its equivalent) plus 0.05–0.1 mg of fluorohydrocortisone if severe hypotension or electrolyte abnormalities persist. Half of the patients do not need the mineralocorticoid supplement. If a patient with Addison's disease on replacement combined therapy with a glucocorticoid and a mineralocorticoid develops heart disease and cardiac failure, the administration of mineralocorticoid may have to be discontinued or substantially reduced to avoid cardiac overload. In the case of an intercurrent infection or any prolonged psychological or physical stress, the glucocorticoid dose should be increased; as a rule, doubling of the dose suffices. In severe, major acute illness or if surgery is required, doses as high as 100–200 mg hydrocortisone should be administered orally or intramuscularly (cortisone acetate) and intravenously during surgery (hydrocortisone hemisuccinate). The oral administration is resumed when normal gastrointestinal function is reestablished. The dose is then gradually tapered to a normal maintenance dose.

B. Treatment of secondary chronic adrenocortical insufficiency depends on the diagnosed etiology. The most common cause, withdrawal after prolonged glucocorticoid therapy for chronic inflammatory or autoimmune disorders, requires a gradual, slow tapering of the dose, monitored by plasma steroid level, and, at the end, testing of the adrenal response with the ACTH stimulation test. Complete recovery of the adrenal after prolonged suppression may take as long as 6 months to 1 year. Replacement with mineralocorticoid is usually not needed. If secondary adrenocortical insufficiency is due to pituitary ACTH deficiency, the treatment is that of the pituitary and/or hypothalamic disorder; if this necessitates ablation of the pituitary, the treatment of adrenal insufficiency is the same as that of primary insufficiency (i.e., chronic replacement with a glucocorticoid). The replacement of mineralocorticoids is usually not needed.

Acute Adrenocortical Insufficiency

I. Definition
An acute, life-threatening condition due to inadequate secretion of cortisol, with or without aldosterone deficiency, at a time when the organism needs to respond to an acute stress.

II. Etiology
A. Acute adrenal insufficiency may develop in an individual with borderline chronic adrenocortical insufficiency subjected to acute stress when the condition was not previously known ("limited adrenocortical reserve") or when acute stress in an addisonian patient was not accompanied by an appropriate increase in the steroid maintenance dose.

B. Initiation of thyroid replacement therapy in a patient with long-standing hypothyroidism and hypoadrenocorticism.

C. Fulminating adrenal destruction by a disseminated infectious process or bilateral intraadrenal hemorrhage (seen with anticoagulation or in acute septicemia).

D. Sudden withdrawal of chronic exogenous steroid therapy. In such a case, acute adrenal insufficiency requires a coincidental acute stressful condition.

III. Pathophysiology
The pathophysiology of acute adrenal insufficiency is very similar to that described above for chronic adrenocortical insufficiency, except that the signs and symptoms develop very rapidly and are very severe.

IV. Diagnosis
A. History: This is described in Section II above.
B. Clinical signs and physical findings
1. Hypotension and hypoglycemia are the dominant signs. In an untreated patient, the former progresses rapidly to cardiovascular collapse.
2. Fever, frequently high, even with negative bacterial cultures. Its pathogenesis is not clear.
3. Nausea, vomiting, diarrhea, and severe dehydration with profound volume depletion.
4. Abdominal or flank pain together with abdominal distention, particularly in patients with bilateral adrenal hemorrhage. Unilateral adrenal hemorrhage may also present as an acute abdomen.
C. Diagnostic tests
1. The most specific diagnostic test is the level of plasma cortisol. Since in individuals with normal adrenal function plasma cortisol concentrations range between 20 and 120 μg/dl during severe stress or shock, levels of plasma cortisol below 20 μg/dl favor the diagnosis of adrenal insufficiency. It is also desirable to determine the cortisol level after ACTH administration (as described for chronic adrenocortical insufficiency). However, it is not safe to await the results of steroid determinations in the patient suspected of being in acute adrenal crisis. After specimens have been obtained for diagnosis, hormone substitution and fluid restoration must be instituted as quickly as possible.
2. Hyponatremia and hyperkalemia are present; the latter is frequently severe.
3. Adrenal hemorrhage can be detected by ultrasonography or computed tomography (CT). The appearance of the hemorrhage on CT scan is usually diagnostic.
4. Blood should be drawn for bacterial culture.

V. Differential Diagnosis
Disorders which must be differentiated from

acute adrenal insufficiency are septic shock without adrenal insufficiency and acute cardiovascular collapse from other causes. Levels of plasma cortisol and the response to exogenous ACTH are unequivocally diagnostic.

VI. Treatment

A. Regardless of the cause, acute adrenal insufficiency, once suspected, demands immediate treatment. If the rapid ACTH test is to be carried out, the initial treatment should be with 10 mg dexamethasone phosphate or 20 mg methyl prednisolone phosphate intravenously. After the test, treatment should be continued with 100 mg hydrocortisone hemisuccinate or hydrocortisone phosphate intravenously every 6–8 hr, for the first 24 hr. If the patient responds favorably, the dose is reduced to 50 mg every 6 hr and then tapered gradually to the maintenance oral dose by the fifth day. The recommended treatment regimen is outlined in Table 120-2. Mineralocorticoid therapy is usually required when the cortisol dose is decreased below 50 mg/day. Fluid replacement should commence at the same time as the initial steroid injection, using isotonic saline and glucose. Severe hyperkalemia and/or acidosis may occasionally require specific therapy.

B. Patients with septicemia should be vigorously treated with antibiotics.

Selective Hypoaldosteronism

I. Definition

A condition resulting from deficient secretion of aldosterone in the face of normal secretion of other adrenal steroids (glucocorticoids, androgens).

Table 120-2. Treatment of Acute Adrenocortical Insufficiency (Adrenal Crisis)

---

1. Cortisol, 100 mg IV, every 6 h for 24 h. Reduce to 50 mg every 6 h if progress is satisfactory and then taper to oral maintenance dose by day 4 or 5. Maintain or increase dosage to 200 to 400 mg/24 h if complications persist or occur.
2. IV saline and glucose.
3. Correction of precipitating factors.
4. General supportive measures.

Source: Baxter JD, Tyrrell JB. The adrenal cortex, in Felig, P, Baxter JD, Broadus AE, et al (eds), *Endocrinology and Metabolism*, ed 2. New York, McGraw-Hill, 1987, p 594. Reprinted with permission.

II. Etiology

A. Primary selective hypoaldosteronism: This can result from congenital enzyme abnormalities in the zona glomerulosa of the adrenal cortex. The family history should suggest an autosomal recessive genetic lesion.

B. Secondary hypoaldosteronism

1. This may be iatrogenic when it occurs during prolonged administration of large doses of angiotensin-II antagonists or angiotensin converting enzyme (ACE) inhibitors. Hyporeninemia is the important defect in most cases of hypoaldosteronism. The most common conditions associated with hyporeninemia are diabetes mellitus and renal disease (glomerulonephritis, interstitial nephritis, chronic pyelonephritis, diabetic or hypertensive nephropathy). Acute hyporeninemic hypoaldosteronism may be iatrogenic due to administration of cyclooxygenase inhibitors. This condition is fully reversible when the drug is discontinued.

2. Hyporeninemic hypoaldosteronism occurs in 70% of patients with chronic renal insufficiency and hyperkalemia. Transient hypoaldosteronism has also been described after surgical removal of an aldosternoma. The remaining zona glomerulosa is atrophic and responds poorly to exogenous angiotensin-II or ACTH. Patients with autonomic insufficiency manifested as postural hypotension may also exhibit hypoaldosteronism, which is due to inadequate neurogenic renin stimulation.

III. Pathophysiology

Inadequate secretion of aldosterone accounts for all signs and symptoms. However, since cortisol exhibits high affinity for mineralocorticoid receptors and is capable of activating them if sufficient intracellular levels exist, about 40% of patients with selective hypoaldosteronism may be normokalemic and asymptomatic.

IV. Diagnosis

A. History

1. In patients with hyporeninemia, this relates mostly to the underlying disorder. Most patients with hyporeninemic hypoaldosteronism are elderly, with mild nonoliguric renal disease and asymptomatic hyperkalemia. Therefore, hyperkalemia in the absence of overt renal failure should alert one to the possibility of hypoaldosteronism.

2. In iatrogenic hypoaldosteronism, a history of drug use inhibiting renin or aldosterone synthesis is prominent. Patients' complaints may be similar to those of patients with chronic adrenocortical insufficiency: weakness, volume depletion, and hypotension.

B. Clinical signs and physical findings

1. Volume depletion and low intracellular concentration of sodium ions in vascular smooth muscle result in a decreased tone of these muscles and, consequently, decreased responsiveness to vasoconstrictive stimuli. This may result in orthostatic hypotension and is improved with the administration of fluorocortisol. Cardiac conduction disturbances—arrhythmias, asystole, and syncope—may occur as a consequence of hyperkalemia. In general, however, the patient is much less severely ill than the one with glucocorticoid deficiency.

2. Up to 75% of patients with hyporeninemic hypoaldosteronism may have diabetes mellitus at the time of diagnosis. Hyperchloremic metabolic acidosis is seen in about 50% of patients.

C. Diagnostic tests

1. Demonstration of low aldosterone levels in the presence of normal cortisol levels and a normal cortisol response to exogenous ACTH.

2. Demonstration of the lack of response of aldosterone levels to stimuli which usually elevate aldosterone: upright position for 4 hr and/or sodium depletion with furosemide injection. The latter should be performed only in equivocal cases (borderline hypoaldosteronism) and with great caution.

3. Hyporeninemic hypoaldosteronism is diagnosed by low levels of plasma renin activity and aldosterone and by the patient's failure to respond to known stimulatory maneuvers.

V. Differential Diagnosis

The following disorders must be distinguished from primary or secondary selective hypoaldosteronism:

A. Primary chronic adrenocortical insufficiency with hypoaldosteronism.

B. Orthostatic hypotension due to autonomic nervous system insufficiency without hypoaldosteronism.

VI. Treatment

The treatment consists of mineralocorticoid replacement. Fluorohydrocortisone, 0.1–0.4 mg/day, is the drug of choice.

VII. Prognosis

The prognosis in primary hypoaldosteronism with proper mineralocorticoid replacement is very good. In secondary hypoaldosteronism, although exogenous mineralocorticoids will correct abnormalities stemming from hypoaldosteronism, the prognosis depends on the treatability of the underlying disorder (e.g., diabetes mellitus, renal disease, hypertensive nephropathy).

Chronic Hypercortisolism: Cushing's Syndrome

I. Definition

A disorder of adrenocortical function resulting in the elevated secretion of cortisol. Iatrogenic Cushing's syndrome results from chronic administration of pharmacologic doses of cortisol or synthetic glucocorticoid

II. Etiology

A. Endogenous Cushing's syndrome may be either ACTH dependent or ACTH independent.

B. The ACTH-dependent disease is caused by excessive secretion of ACTH by the pituitary or by ectopic nonendocrine ACTH-secreting tumors. Chronic overstimulation with ACTH results in adrenocortical hyperplasia.

C. The pituitary form can be due to oversecretion of ACTH by a pituitary tumor (in most cases a microadenoma) or by corticotrope hyperplasia. Either one is responsive to corticotropin-releasing hormone (CRH). The pituitary-dependent Cushing's syndrome is often referred to as *Cushing's disease*. One-third of pituitary ACTH-secreting tumors are chromophobe adenomas. They are usually much larger than the basophilic ones.

D. The second cause of adrenocortical hyperplasia is secretion of ACTH by a nonendocrine tumor. In this form of ACTH-dependent Cushing's syndrome, plasma levels of ACTH are usually much higher than those in the pituitary disease (200–2,000 vs. 50–200 pg/ml). Various ACTH-secreting tumors are listed, in their order of prevalence, in Table 120-3. Ectopic CRH production is much more rare and has been reported from metastatic carcinoma of prostate and from medullary thyroid carcinoma.

Table 120-3. Tumor Most Frequently Causing the Ectopic ACTH Syndrome

Oat cell carcinoma of the lung
Thymoma
Pancreatic islet cell carcinoma
Carcinoid tumors (lung, gut, pancreas, ovary)
Thyroid medullary carcinoma
Pheochromocytoma and related tumors

Source: Baxter JD, Tyrrell JB. The adrenal cortex, in Felig P, Baxter JD, Broadus AE, et al (eds), *Endocrinology and Metabolism,* ed 2. New York, McGraw-Hill, 1987, p. 604.

E. The source of ACTH-independent Cushing's syndrome is an autonomous tumor of the adrenal cortex hypersecreting cortisol, with or without hypersecretion of other adrenal steroids. As a rule, adenomas secrete only cortisol; carcinomas frequently secrete androgens and mineralocorticoids.

F. Pituitary-dependent Cushing's syndrome (Cushing's disease) constitutes 68% of all cases of endogenous disease; the disorder due to autonomous adrenal tumor, 17% (adenoma, 9%; carcinoma, 8%); and adrenal hyperplasia due to ectopic ACTH secretion from nonendocrine tumors, 15%.

G. A small percentage of patients (~15%) with ACTH-dependent disease exhibit a nodular hyperplasia of the adrenal cortex. The nodules may vary in size and are usually bilateral; they are associated with the simple hyperplasia of nonadenomatous cells (as a result of ACTH stimulation). Nodular hyperplasia is more common in children than in adults (roughly 50% of pituitary-dependent Cushing's syndrome of childhood).

III. **Pathophysiology**
A. All signs and symptoms of Cushing's syndrome are due to hypercortisolemia. In some patients with Cushing's disease, morning levels of plasma cortisol may be within the normal range, but there is a marked increase in the afternoon levels. The latter contributes significantly to the elevation of total 24-hr secretion of cortisol.

B. Patients with ectopic ACTH syndrome usually have much higher production rates of both ACTH and cortisol than do those with pituitary-dependent disease. Cortisol secretion is also higher in the disease due to autonomously secreting adrenocortical tumors than in the pituitary-dependent disease; the diurnal rhythm is also missing.

C. Chronic hypercortisolemia leads to:
1. Overall decrease in the rate of protein synthesis, resulting in overall protein depletion. This leads to muscle weakness, thinning of extremities, and inadequate formation of subcutaneous tissue and bone matrix. This last process results in a decrease in the rate of calcium deposition in bones, which, together with glucocorticoid-induced diminished calcium ion reabsorption in the gut, leads to osteoporosis.
2. An increased rate of gluconeogenesis, which, coupled with decreased glucose uptake by all tissue, with the exception of the liver, results in impaired glucose tolerance, hyperglycemia, and, very frequently, overt diabetes (steroid-induced).
3. Sodium and water retention due to glucocorticoid action in the kidneys (probably through mineralocorticoid receptors) and, more important, an enhanced rate of sodium and calcium entry into vascular smooth muscle cells, and, consequently, their increased tone and responsiveness to vasoconstrictive stimuli; this results in hypertension.
4. Characteristic deposition of fat in the abdominal region (centripetal or truncal obesity), in the posterior cervical region ("buffalo hump"), and in the buccal areas ("moon facies"). The reason for this topographically selective fat accumulation is not clear.
5. Increased susceptibility to infection as a result of the immunosuppressive action of glucocorticoids.
6. Increased bruising due to a decrease in the wall thickness of blood vessels and the loss of elasticity of subcutaneous connective tissue (both are the result of protein depletion); another factor contributing to the increased tendency to bruise is a prolonged bleeding time due to a down-regulated rate of thromboxane production.

D. When adrenal androgen secretion is also enhanced (which almost always occurs in Cushing's syndrome due to adrenocortical carcinoma but also in some patients with Cushing's disease), manifestations of hyperandrogenism occur in female patients: hirsutism, sometimes masculinization, acne, and amenorrhea. In male patients, a decrease in the testicular production rate of testosterone by glucocorticoids may lead to decreased libido and impotence.

E. Markedly elevated levels of ACTH in ectopic ACTH syndrome result in hyperpigmentation of the skin. Nonendocrine ACTH-secreting tumors usually secrete other cleavage products of the ACTH prehormone: pro-opiomelanocortin and β-MSH, among others.

IV. **Diagnosis**

A. History

1. The disease is about nine times more common in women than in men.

2. The onset of the disease is usually gradual over a period of 1–2 years. In women, the first noted abnormality is frequently a change in the menstrual cycle, which may progress to amenorrhea.

3. Early symptoms are lassitude and loss of muscle strength, sometimes profound.

4. Often the patient reports a change in general physical appearance (see Section IV, B).

5. The patient's family usually notices a change in mood and sometimes incapacitating emotional disturbances such as paranoid and psychotic reactions.

6. Some patients with ectopic ACTH syndrome may show weight loss instead of weight gain and may even be emaciated due to debilitating effects of the tumor.

B. Clinical signs and physical findings

1. Physical examination reveals rounding of the face and fullness of the cheeks (moon facies) and increased deposition of fat in the lower posterior cervical region and supraclavicular fossae (buffalo hump) and around the girdle (centripetal obesity). The arms and legs are usually thin, but in some patients the typical truncal pattern of obesity may be less accentuated.

2. The skin is atrophic and nonpliable and manifests purple striae. The latter are usually found in the lower abdominal and bilateral hip regions. Facial plethora is present in most patients.

3. Hypertension is found in over 80% of patients and may be severe. Left ventricular hypertrophy is present, and congestive heart failure is found in about 20% of patients.

4. Various degrees of hirsutism may be present in female patients, ranging from a mild increase in facial hair to a male pattern of abdominal and thoracic hair. This is rarely present in patients with pituitary-dependent Cushing's syndrome but is very common in the syndrome due to adrenocortical carcinoma.

5. Various degrees of hyperglycemia are present in most patients, ranging from slightly impaired glucose tolerance to overt diabetes. Patients with long-standing, severe hypercortisolemia have hypercalciuria and an increased incidence of renal stones.

C. Diagnostic tests: Crucial to the diagnosis of Cushing's syndrome is the demonstration of chronic hypercortisolemia and impaired suppressibility of pituitary ACTH secretion.

1. The most reliable test is the measurement of urinary 24-hr excretion of free (non-protein-bound) cortisol. Free cortisol excretion is significantly elevated in 98% of patients with Cushing's syndrome of any of the discussed etiologies. This is due to an increased level of cortisol which exceeds the binding capacity of transcortin. The unbound steroid filters easily through kidney glomeruli.

2. Another screening test consists of administration of 1 mg dexamethasone at midnight and estimation of the plasma cortisol level next morning (at 11:00 A.M.). Cortisol values above 5 mg/dl are considered abnormal. This test is less specific than measurement of urinary cortisol.

3. If the screening tests confirm the presence of Cushing's syndrome, the next step is to determine if the syndrome results from pituitary ACTH production, ectopic ACTH production, or an adrenal tumor. There is considerable diversity in the recommended approach for making this determination. One approach is to measure ACTH levels next. These will be very low in primary adrenal disease (less than 50 pg/ml), very high in ectopic ACTH (more than 200 pg/ml), and intermediate in pituitary Cushing's syndrome. A relatively recently described suppression test has also been found to be useful. This involves the administration of an 8-mg dose of dexamethasone at 2300 hr. A subsequent 8 A.M. cortisol level which falls by more than 50% compared to control levels supports a diagnosis of pituitary Cushing's syndrome.

4. It is important to recognize that no test or combination of tests are infallible for the differential diagnosis of Cushing's syndrome. Additional tests which may be employed in complex cases include CRH testing with inferior petrosal sinus sampling, metapyrone testing, more prolonged suppression tests, and selective venous sampling for ACTH.

5. CT scan and magnetic resonance imaging (MRI): If biochemical tests suggest pituitary Cushing's syndrome, abnormalities of the sella turcica can be demonstrated on CT or MRI scans of the sella. From 30% to 60% of patients with Cushing's disease have a detectable pituitary adenoma on CT scanning. However, 10–25% of normal subjects may harbor a small nonfunctioning pituitary tumor. "Empty sellas" diagnosed by the routine skull film or by CT scan have been found to harbor pituitary adenomas.

6. Adrenal hyperplasia can be identified by CT scanning, but false-positive identification is not uncommon. Adrenal tumors are detected by CT or MRI scanning with more than 90% sensitivity if they are >2 cm in diameter.

V. Differential Diagnosis

A. Obesity with hypertension is the most common diagnostic problem in Cushing's syndrome. Thirteen percent of obese patients have abnormal responses to the overnight 1-mg dexamethasone suppression test. However, urinary free cortisol excretion is almost always within the normal range.

B. Patients with chronic alcoholism may have both clinical and biochemical features of Cushing's syndrome (alcohol-induced pseudo-Cushing's syndrome). All abnormal steroid tests revert to normal 3–4 weeks following cessation of alcohol intake. In view of the frequency of excessive alcohol use, this possibility should be considered whenever hypercortisolism is suspected.

C. Patients with depression frequently have abnormal steroid levels—increased cortisol secretion with elevated plasma cortisol levels, absence of diurnal variation, increased urinary free cortisol, and impaired suppressibility to dexamethasone. These patients do not have physical cushingoid features, but they may be obese and hypertensive. Responses to metapyrone and CRH help to differentiate depressed patients from those with true Cushing's syndrome.

D. Patients with anorexia nervosa also have steroid dynamics similar to those of Cushing's disease. These patients are easily distinguished from the latter by their clinical presentation. The differentiation from emaciated patients with the ectopic ACTH syndrome may be more difficult, particularly from those with a rapid onset of the disease and a rapid course due to a fulminating malignancy and, consequently, total absence of the cushingoid appearance and of hyperpigmentation. However, almost all anorectics suppress with high-dose dexamethasone, whereas most patients with ectopic ACTH syndrome do not. Abnormal steroid dynamics revert to normal on psychological recovery.

E. Patients with so-called cyclic Cushing's disease may present serious diagnostic problems, particularly during the periods when their adrenal cortisol secretion is normal. These patients may have Cushing's disease, the ectopic ACTH syndrome, or adrenal tumors. They have cushingoid features which do not recede during the short periods of normalization of cortisol levels (exceptions have been described). Repeated evaluations and use of the localizing procedures described above are necessary to establish the correct diagnosis. The cause of the "cycling" of these patients is not clear.

VI. Treatment

A. Surgical treatment
   1. Transsphenoidal adenomectomy is the appropriate treatment of a patient with Cushing's disease with identified and lateralized pituitary microadenoma. The success of this operation by an experienced neurosurgeon is almost 90% when the tumor is identified preoperatively. Large tumors, such as ACTH-secreting chromophobe adenomas, usually require a transfrontal approach.
   2. Bilateral total adrenalectomy as a treatment of Cushing's disease, commonly performed in the past, has been now abandoned. It is, however, reserved for those patients in whom florid symptoms of hypercortisolism are present and who do not have a demonstrable adrenal tumor, but in whom neither an ectopic ACTH-producing tumor nor a pituitary adenoma can be localized.

3. In Cushing's syndrome due to adrenocortical adenoma, the surgical removal of the adenoma is the only rational treatment. Carcinomas should be also removed surgically. Unfortunately, most adrenocortical carcinomas are discovered in an invasive stage. As much malignant tissue as possible should be removed, followed by medical treatment (see below).

4. Treatment of ectopic ACTH syndrome consists of localization of the tumor and its surgical removal before it metastasizes. If the tumor cannot be removed in toto, the surgery should be followed not only by tumor chemotherapy but also by administration of one of adrenolytic agents (see below).

5. To prevent acute adrenal crisis during or immediately after any surgery for hypercortisolism, the patient should be premedicated with a preparation of soluble cortisol (phosphate or hemisuccinate), 200 mg in 500 ml 5% dextrose intravenously every 6 hr; this dose should be continued during the operation and tapered off to 50 mg every 6 hr beginning on the second postoperative day, followed by intramuscular injections of cortisol, until the patient can take a normal maintenance dose of cortisol or an equivalent preparation.

B. Medical treatment
1. Pharmacologic agents which inhibit adrenal steroidogenesis are useful only as adjunctive therapy.
   a. To decrease the catabolic effects of glucocorticoids prior to surgical treatment.
   b. In combination with radiation treatment (see below) when surgery is not possible or not successful.
   c. When a malignant steroid-producing adrenal tumor cannot be removed in toto or is inoperable.
2. Drugs available
   a. Mitotane, the strongest in the series of adrenolytic drugs, not only inhibits cortisol synthesis but also causes adrenal atrophy, predominantly of the zonae fasciculata and reticularis. It induces remissions in 80% of patients with Cushing's disease, but 60% relapse following cessation of therapy. In an effective dose (8–12 g/day), mitotane causes serious side effects: various

gastrointestinal symptoms, sometimes very severe (nausea, vomiting, diarrhea), somnolence, depression, and skin rash. These frequently necessitate discontinuation of treatment.
   b. Aminogluthetimide inhibits cortisol synthesis through inhibition of the conversion of cholesterol to pregnenolone. Aminogluthetimide causes somnolence, skin rash, and goiter (as a result of the inhibition of thyroid hormone synthesis).
   c. Metapyrone inhibits cortisol synthesis through inhibition of the 11β-hydroxylation step. Metapyrone causes mainly gastrointestinal side effects.
   d. Ketoconazole (an imidazole derivative) blocks adrenal steroidogenesis and acts as a peripheral cortisol antagonist.

C. Radiotherapy
1. The adrenal gland is insensitive to radiotherapy. However, the pituitary is radiosensitive. Pituitary radiotherapy is therefore recommended as second-line therapy for pituitary Cushing's syndrome when pituitary surgery fails to yield positive results.

VII. Prognosis
A. Untreated Cushing's syndrome is a fatal illness. The mortality may be due to the underlying tumor, as in adrenal carcinoma or ectopic ACTH syndrome, or to the end result of a prolonged hypercortisolism, such as cardiovascular disease, hypertension, stroke, renal failure, thromboembolism, or susceptibility to infection. If untreated, 50% of patients will die within 5 years of the onset of the disease.

B. If properly treated, the morbidity and the mortality are reduced significantly. The prognosis of patients with adrenal adenomas treated by resection is excellent. Patients with Cushing's disease due to pituitary microadenoma treated by transsphenoidal adenomectomy carried out by an experienced neurosurgeon have a good prognosis. Patients with Cushing's disease who have large pituitary tumors have a markedly less favorable prognosis. They may die as a consequence of tumor invasion of brain structures adjacent to the pituitary or due to persisting hypercortisolism.

C. In adrenal carcinoma, the prognosis is universally poor. In spite of the available treatment regimens, the survival period is usually less than 4 years.

D. The prognosis for patients with ectopic ACTH syndrome due to malignant tumors depends on the developmental stage of the tumor and the success of its resection. In patients with ectopic ACTH syndrome due to a benign tumor, the prognosis is good provided that the tumor is completely removed.

Primary Aldosteronism: Conn's Syndrome

I. Definition

A disorder in the function of the adrenal zona glomerulosa resulting in hypersecretion of aldosterone, characterized by hypokalemia, alkalosis, and hypertension.

II. Etiology

A. Seventy percent of patients with primary hyperaldosteronism have an aldosterone-producing adenoma (APA).

B. The second most frequent cause of primary aldosteronism is hyperplasia of the zona glomerulosa (HZG). The original stimulus which results in HZG is not known.

C. The third cause of primary aldosteronism is a persistence, beyond the fetal period, of an intermediate zone of the adrenal cortex, between the zona glomerulosa and zona fasciculata. The persistent transitional zone possesses enzymes responsible for the last step in aldosterone biosynthesis, which, unlike the mature zona glomerulosa, are under the control of ACTH. Thus, suppression of ACTH secretion with an exogenous glucocorticoid (e.g., dexamethasone) results in the cessation of excessive aldosterone secretion. This pathogenetic form of hyperaldosteronism has been named *dexamethasone-remediable aldosteronism (DRA)*. DRA is a familial disorder inherited as an autosomal dominant trait and occurs primarily in young men.

D. Finally, the source of hypersecretion of aldosterone may be a malignant adrenocortical tumor. Such tumors also usually produce glucocorticoids and androgens. Malignant adrenal tumors producing only aldosterone have been described but are extremely rare.

III. Pathophysiology

All signs and symptoms of hyperaldosteronism are due to excessive mineralocorticoid activity.

A. Hypokalemia and alkalosis are the prominent features of hyperaldosteronism. The former is due to excessive renal excretion of potassium; the latter is due to an increased rate of renal excretion of hydrogen ion promoted by the action of aldosterone on the renal distal tubule. Hypokalemia results in muscle weakness (and occasionally muscle paralysis).

B. About half of the patients with hyperaldosteronism also exhibit hypomagnesemia due to excessive excretion of magnesium ion by the distal tubule. Intracellular hypokalemia and hypomagnesemia are responsible for tetany clinically identical to that due to hypocalcemia, which is encountered in about 20% of patients with hyperaldosteronism.

C. Hyperaldosteronism causes increased Na^+ ion and water reabsorption in distal tubules. This leads to an increased circulating plasma volume, an increased extracellular fluid volume, and an increased exchangeable sodium pool. Together with an aldosterone-induced increase in the rate of sodium influx into the arterial smooth muscle cells, this leads to the increased peripheral resistance and hypertension present in 98% of patients with primary hyperaldosteronism. It should be stressed that unlike hypokalemia, which is present in 90% of patients with aldosteronism, hypernatremia is seen in less than 15% of patients. This probably relates to the fact that a sodium "escape" phenomenon occurs when extracellular fluid has been expanded by approximately 500 ml. Normokalemic patients have also been reported. In these patients, hypokalemia can be unmasked by normalization of sodium intake (120 mEq/day). When the concentration of Na^+ ion in the renal tubular lumen is low, as in patients on restricted sodium intake, renal tubular cells do not substantially increase K^+ ion excretion in response to aldosterone.

D. The direct action of aldosterone on the hypothalamic thirst center (via its receptors) leads to polydypsia, which leads to polyuria. The second cause of polyuria is the impairment of the urinary concentrating ability secondary to potassium depletion.

IV. Diagnosis

A. History: The most common complaints are muscle weakness, lassitude (both due to potassium depletion), and headaches. The last are caused by high blood pressure. The patient may have been treated for hypertension for some time but, characteristically, treatment with diuretics will aggravate hypokalemia and thus lassitude and muscle weakness. An occasional patient may complain of periodic muscle paralysis and muscle cramps, as in tetany. Complaints of polydipsia and polyuria are present in about 15% of patients. In some patients (who are diagnosed as having DRA), there is a family history of similar symptoms.

B. Clinical signs and physical findings
1. Frequently, hypertension is the only sign. The severity of hypertension is mild to moderate. Severe hypertension is present in fewer than 10% of patients. As a rule, edema is absent.
2. With long-standing, untreated hypertension, left ventricular hypertrophy and signs of congestive heart failure may be present, but these are rare and complicate the diagnosis because of secondary hyperaldosteronism (see below).
3. In patients with pronounced hypokalemia, neurologic examination reveals decreased muscle strength and signs of tetany—positive Chvostek and Trousseau signs, the latter particularly when hypomagnesemia is present.
4. Decreased carbohydrate tolerance (shown by an abnormal glucose tolerance test) and resistance to antidiuretic hormone (nephrogenic diabetes insipidus) occur even with moderate potassium depletion. Severe potassium depletion blunts baroreceptor function, which may lead to postural hypotension.

C. Diagnostic tests
1. The hallmarks of primary aldosteronism are hypertension, hypokalemia, suppression of the renin-angiotensin system, and increased aldosterone production in the presence of normal cortisol secretion. A diagnostic screening procedure consists of a number of consecutive steps, which are outlined in Figure 120-1. Care must be taken to control sodium intake before serum electrolyte levels are measured. On sodium intakes greater than 120 mEq/day, hypokalemia should be apparent in most patients with primary aldosteronism by the fourth day. Previous diuretic therapy is the most common cause of hypokalemia in patients with hypertension. Therefore, for the demonstration of hypokalemia as a sign of primary hyperaldosteronism, the

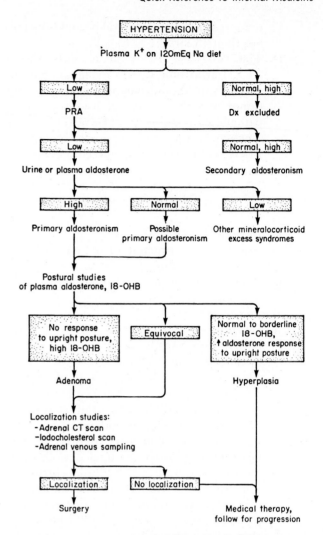

Figure 120-1. Flow diagram for diagnosis of primary aldosteronism and differentiation of adrenal adenoma from hyperplasia. (From Baxter, JD, Perloff D, Hsueh W, et al. The endocrinology of hypertension, in Felig P, Baxter JD, Perloff D, et al., eds., *Endocrinology and Metabolism.* New York, McGraw-Hill, 1987, p 754. Reprinted with permission.)

patient should be off diuretics for at least 3 weeks.
2. Demonstration of suppressed plasma renin activity (PRA) and an increased plasma level and/or 24-hr urinary excretion of aldosterone confirm the diagnosis. The PRA level should be determined in the morning, while the patient is in a recumbent position following a night of sleep, and then after 4 hr of ambulation. The lack of increase in PRA is suggestive of primary aldosteronism. Additional evidence is obtained by repeating the PRA measurement when the patient is depleted of sodium by the diet (1 week on a 10-mEq

intake) or after intravenous administration of 40–60 mg furosemide.

3. Plasma aldosterone can also be determined before and following sodium loading (intravenous infusion of 2 liters of normal saline over 4 hr) or after administration of 11-deoxycorticosterone acetate (DOCA) (10 mg intramuscularly every 12 hr) for 3 days. Lack of suppression identifies primary aldosteronism. Once the diagnosis of primary aldosteronism has been established, it is of the utmost importance to determine the etiology of the disease, since totally different therapeutic approaches are applied to adenomatous versus hyperplastic disease.

V. Differential Diagnosis

A. Differentiation of APA from HZG and from DRA and lateralization of APA.

1. APA usually secretes significantly larger amounts of aldosterone and of aldosterone percussor, 18-hydroxycorticosterone (18-OH-B) than does HZG. Plasma 18-OH-B is invariably above 100 ng/dl in patients with adenoma, and there is no overlap with only slightly elevated levels of this steroid in patients with hyperplasia, measured at 8 A.M. after overnight recumbency.

2. Postural testing: This is performed as described in Section IV, C. The plasma aldosterone level in patients with APA does not change, while that in patients with HZG increases (although not to the same extent as that in normal subjects). PRA does not respond to this maneuver and remains suppressed, while in HZG there is a slight to moderate increase in PRA.

3. CT and MRI scans: Most nodules more than 1.5 cm in diameter and 50% of nodules 1.0–1.4 cm in diameter are identified by CT OR MRI scan. Nodules less than 1.0 cm in diameter are usually not recognized. Thus, almost 80% of patients with APA will be identified. Hyperplasia of the zona glomerulosa is not identifiable by CT.

4. Iodocholesterol scan: Adrenal scintigraphy may sometimes be useful in the preoperative localization of aldosteronoma.

5. Bilateral adrenal vein catheterization: This procedure is used in patients with biochemical evidence of an adenoma which is not identifiable by CT scanning or when scintiscanning does not give clear-cut results.

6. Dexamethasone suppression test: This is used to identify the subgroup of patients with DRA among those with hyperplasia of the zona glomerulosa.

B. Differentiation of primary aldosteronism from low renin essential hypertension

1. Unmasking of hypokalemia with normalization of sodium intake (as described in Section IV, C), will identify aldosteronism.

2. A single dose of converting enzyme (ACE) inhibitor (50 mg captopril orally) can discriminate between hyperaldosteronism and low renin essential hypertension. Plasma aldosterone increases more dramatically in essential hypertension than in HZG, whereas it is unchanged in APA.

3. The saline infusion test or DOCA administration clearly distinguishes hyperaldosteronism from essential hypertension. Plasma or urinary aldosterone, compared with pretreatment values, is suppressed minimally or not at all by DOCA treatment or by saline infusion in patients with APA or HZG but is reduced markedly in essential hypertension.

C. Differentiation of primary from secondary aldosteronism: The main laboratory finding differentiating the two is plasma renin. It is high in secondary aldosteronism but low (suppressed) and nonresponsive to the usual stimuli in primary aldosteronism.

VI. Treatment

This depends on the cause of hyperaldosteronism.

A. The treatment of choice for patients with diagnosed and properly lateralized APA is surgical removal of the adenoma. APAs are usually small, and there is no certainty that they can be properly and completely dissected. Moreover, not infrequently, there are one or two even smaller "satellite" adenomas. For all of these reasons, total unilateral adrenalectomy is performed in most cases. The cure rate of hypokalemia is 100%; that of hypertension is only about 80%. Hypertension in the remaining 20% of unilaterally adrenalectomized patients often persists, but in most patients it is appreciably lower than it was prior to removal of the adenoma. The proper assessment of the effect of surgery on hypertension can be done only 1 year after the operation. Those patients in whom hypertension persists are treated with the usual antihypertensive medications but require lower doses of drugs than they did before adrenalectomy. The persistence of hypertension in 20% of unilaterally adrenalectomized APA patients is likely to be due to a concomitant essential hypertension since most of these patients have a family history of hypertension.

B. Medical treatment

1. The patients who cannot undergo surgery for various reasons are treated with spironolactone. This compound acts as a competitive inhibitor of aldosterone binding to the mineralocorticoid receptors, thereby antagonizing the action of mineralocorticoids in target tissues. The dosage of spironolactone ranges from 50 mg once daily to 100 mg twice daily. This aldosterone antagonist also has antiandrogenic and progestagenic activities (side effects: decreased libido and gynecomastia in about 50% of male patients; menometrorrhagia and mastodynia in an equal number of female patients).

2. Spironolactone is also used as a short-term treatment to assess the anticipated benefit of the surgical treatment of APA. Spironolactone is administered for 4–8 weeks in a dose of 200–400 mg/day. Reversal of hypokalemia and normalization of blood pressure are excellent predictors of the success of unilateral adrenalectomy. A similar dosage of spironolactone is also used as preoperative treatment. It is then reduced to 100–150 mg/day until the time of surgery. The important desirable effect of such preoperative preparation is the activation of the suppressed renin-angiotensin system. This stimulates the suppressed zona glomerulosa of the nonadenomatous adrenal gland, which markedly decreases the postoperative hypoaldosteronism with hyperkalemia.

3. Two potassium-sparing antidiuretics, amiloride (20–40 mg/day) and triamterene, may also be used for the medical treatment of APA. They oppose the effect of aldosterone on the renal tubule by inhibiting sodium reabsorption and potassium secretion through a direct effect on the transmembrane transport systems for these electrolytes in the tubular cell.

4. Nifedipine and other calcium channel blockers also yield beneficial effects in the medical treatment of hyperaldosteronism.

In addition to their antihypertensive action through a decrease in the rate of Ca^{2+} influx into vascular smooth muscle cells and central nervous system neurons, nifedipine decreases the rate of sodium reabsorption from the tubular lumen into the tubular cell and reduces the rate of aldosterone synthesis. A combined treatment with small doses of potassium-sparing diuretics and calcium channel blockers probably constitutes the optimal alternative to the surgical treatment of APA.

C. Treatment of hyperaldosteronism caused by HZG is primarily medical since adrenalectomy, even bilateral, does not correct hypertension in patients with HZG, except in rare cases. These patients should be treated with an ACE inhibitor or a calcium channel blocker. If hypokalemia persists, the addition of amiloride or triamterine is helpful.

D. The treatment of DRA consists of a permanent replacement dosage of 1–2 mg dexamethasone daily. This will abolish hypokalemia and reduce blood pressure within 3–4 weeks. Upon withdrawal of treatment, all signs and symptoms recur.

VII. Prognosis

The prognosis for patients with APA properly identified, lateralized, and surgically treated is excellent. The prognosis for patients with HZG treated medically (as described above) is also very good. Since medical treatment will correct both hypokalemia and hypertension in these patients, surgical treatment should not be performed. The prognosis for patients with DRA is excellent, provided that they are treated with a permanent replacement dose of dexamethasone or another glucocorticoid analog.

Congenital Adrenal Hyperplasia (CAH)

I. Definition

Cellular hyperplasia of the adrenal cortex resulting from congenital defects of any of the adrenal enzymes catalyzing various steps in the biosynthetic pathways of adrenal steroids.

II. Etiology

The enzymatic defects are genetic due to mutational alterations in the encoding genes. The hyperplasia is the result of an inadequate inhibition of secretion of ACTH due to deficient biosynthesis of cortisol, the steroid which provides inhibition.

III. Pathophysiology

The deficient functioning of the affected enzyme leads to a block in the synthesis of steroids produced in the part of the biosynthetic pathway distal to this enzyme. The steroid precursors proximal to the block accumulate and lead to clinical symptoms characteristic of a given enzymatic deficiency. The extent of the enzyme deficiency may be variable; consequently, the extent of deficiency of steroid biosynthesis varies; the severity of clinical expression of a given enzymatic defect differs accordingly. The end result of most of these defects is a deficient secretion of cortisol.

A. 21-Hydroxylase deficiency
1. The most common type of adrenal enzymatic defect, present in 90% of patients with CAH. It is inherited as autosomal recessive trait. The gene locus is linked closely to the human leukocyte antigen (HLA) region on chromosome 6.
2. The steroids secreted in excess (synthesized proximally to the block) are 17α-hydroxyprogesterone and progesterone. Their accumulation in the adrenal cortex leads to an increased rate of conversion to the androgenic steroids androstenedione and testosterone.

B. 11B-Hydroxylase deficiency
1. The second most frequent enzymatic defect in CAH. Inherited as an autosomal recessive trait, it is due to defective function of the cytochrome $P-450_{11B/18}$ gene.
2. The steroids secreted in excess are 11-desoxycortisol (compound S_R) and 11-desoxycorticosterone (DOC). The latter, being a mineralocorticoid, causes sodium retention and hypertension. Accumulating steroid precursors are converted to the androgenic steroids androstenedione and testosterone.

C. 17α-Hydroxylase deficiency.

D. 3β-Hydroxysteroid dehydrogenase (3β-HSD) deficiency.

E. Cholesterol side-chain cleavage enzyme deficiency.

F. Corticosterone methyl oxidase deficiency.

These enzymatic defects are rare and will not be discussed here.

IV. Diagnosis

A. History and clinical signs
1. With sodium retention and hypertension: 11β-hydroxylase deficiency.
2. With sodium wasting: 21-hydroxylase deficiency (if severe).

3. With hyperproduction of potent androgens: 11β-hydroxylase and 21-hydroxylase deficiency.

B. Severe enzyme deficiencies are manifested early in life, frequently at birth.

C. Specific clinical findings
1. 21-Hydroxylase deficiency
   a. In the severe form, signs of adrenal insufficiency include anorexia, failure to gain weight, vomiting, and dehydration. If not treated immediately, death occurs from shock and cardiovascular collapse.
   b. In female infants, ambiguous genitalia develop (as a result of hyperandrogenization in utero); in milder forms, only clitoral hypertrophy occurs.
   c. With milder defects, children are normal at birth and there is no evidence of adrenal insufficiency. Hyperandrogenism is manifested as accelerated growth. At puberty there are no menses, underdeveloped breasts, facial hirsutism, and sometimes virilization.
   d. With very mild defects (so-called late-onset or attenuated forms), development throughout childhood is normal; at puberty hirsution may develop, but infertility is usually present.
2. 11β-Hydroxylase deficiency
3. The severe form is manifested in early childhood.
4. Signs of virilization similar to those present in 21-hydroxylase deficiency occur, but are usually less severe.
5. Hypertension, sodium retention, and hypokalemia are classic manifestations but are not always present in early childhood.
6. In late-onset forms, hirsutism with menstrual irregularities develop at puberty in females and pseudoprecocious puberty occurs in males.

D. Diagnostic tests
1. Determination of the plasma ACTH level (grossly elevated in severe forms, less so in milder forms).
2. Determination of the levels of urinary 17-ketosteroids.
3. Determination of the plasma cortisol level.
4. Determination of the levels of pathognomonic steroids in plasma and/or urine.
   a. 21-Hydroxylase defect: Plasma: 17-hydroxyprogesterone, urine pregnanetriol. HLA typing is used for detection

of heterozygous carriers and for prenatal diagnosis. In the so-called cryptic variant of the late-onset form, intramuscular administration of 50 U ACTH will uncover the enzymatic defect by producing a dramatic increase in plasma 17-hydroxyprogesterone.

   b. 11β-Hydroxylase defect: Plasma; DOC, 11-desoxycortisol (compound S_R).

V. Differential Diagnosis

Forms of CAH with increased secretion of androgens and clinical signs of virilization should be differentiated from other causes of "adrenogenital syndrome," such as benign and malignant androgen-producing tumors and Cushing's syndrome with hyperproduction of androgens. The size of these tumors permits their detection by CT scanning of the adrenals; the steroid pattern is quite different from that described above for the virilizing form of CAH.

VI. Treatment

   A. In most forms of CAH, treatment with cortisol replacement corrects all abnormalities.

   B. Patients with severe forms of 21-hydroxylase deficiency should be treated also with mineralocorticoid replacement (Fluorinef, 0.05–0.2 mg/day).

VII. Prognosis

Excellent in most forms.

Disease of the Adrenal Medulla

Introduction

The common precursor of all catecholamines is tyrosine. This is either derived directly from the diet or is formed in the liver from the amino acid phenylalanine. Through a number of consecutive enzymatic steps, hydroxylations, decarboxylation, and methylation, tyrosine is transformed into dopamine, norepinephrine, and epinephrine. Norepinephrine is methylated to epinephrine in chromaffin tissues such as adrenal medulla. However, this conversion also takes place in some neurons of the central nervous system.

The initial step in the mechanism of action of catecholamines is their binding to specific receptors, named *adrenergic receptors*, on the membrane of the target cells. There are two types of adrenergic receptors, α and β. Each one is subdivided into two subtypes, α_1 and α_2 and β_1 and β_2. Epinephrine has higher affinity for all adrenergic receptors than norepinephrine.

In vascular smooth muscle, activation of α_1 receptors leads to general vasoconstriction, whereas activation of β_2 receptors leads to vasodilation. Activation of β_1 receptors in the heart promotes the inotropic and chronotropic effects of the agonists. Table 120-4 presents the adrenergic responses of various tissues to catecholamine stimulation.

Pheochromocytoma

I. Definition

Pheochromocytomas are tumors arising from chromaffin cells in the sympathetic nervous system, most frequently from the adrenal medulla, causing hypertension.

II. Etiology

   A. Neoplastic growth of chromaffin cells. Most frequently, the tumors are benign; fewer than 10% are malignant. Over 95% of pheochromocytomas are found in the abdomen, 85% of them in the adrenal.

   B. Hyperplasia of the adrenal medulla, which frequently develops into a tumor, occurs as a heritable disorder in association with other endocrine tumors (see Chapter 124).

III. Pathophysiology

   A. Pheochromocytomas synthesize and release epinephrine or norepinephrine or both. Occasionally, dopamine is also released in appreciable amounts. Excessive levels of catecholamines cause hypertension. About 0.1% of patients with diastolic hypertension have pheochromocytomas. In about half of them, hypertension is not sustained but occurs episodically. This *paroxysmal hypertension* is caused by sudden increase in the release of epinephrine and/or norepinephrine by the tumor.

   B. Symptoms other than hypertension (see Section IV, B) also stem from excessive levels of catecholamines and vary in their intensity, depending on the relative amounts of epinephrine and norepinephrine secreted.

IV. Diagnosis

   A. History: There is a history of hypertension, with the attending symptoms. In patients with paroxysmal symptoms, attacks occur several times a week, frequently two or three times in one day or more often. Paroxysms may consist of palpitations, headache, and diaphoresis. They usually last for 15 min or less.

   B. Clinical signs and physical findings: These

Table 120-4. Adrenergic Response of Selected Tissues

Organ or Tissue	Receptor	Effect
Heart (myocardium)	β_1	Increased force of contraction
		Increased rate of contraction
Blood vessels	α	Vasoconstriction
	β_2	Vasodilation
Kidney	β	Increased renin release
Gut	α, β	Decreased motility and increased sphincter tone
Pancreas	α	Decreased insulin release
		Decreased glucagon release
	β	Increased insulin release
		Increased glucagon release
Liver	α, β	Increased glycogenolysis
Adipose tissue	β	Increased lipolysis
Most tissues	β	Increased calorigenesis
Skin (apocrine glands on hands, axillae, etc.)	α	Increased sweating
Bronchioles	β_2	Dilation
Uterus	α	Contraction
	β_2	Relaxation

Source: Goldfien A, Adrenal Medulla, in Greenspan FS (ed.), *Basic and Clinical Endocrinology*, ed 3. Norwalk, San Mateo, Appleton & Lange, 1991, p. 387. Reprinted with permission.

pertain mostly to hypertension but also to signs of sympathetic hyperactivity: tachycardia (sometimes reflex bradycardia), sweating, tremor, fatigue, nausea, vomiting, and abdominal or chest pain. The physical findings depend on:

1. The duration and severity of hypertension.
2. Paroxysmal versus sustained character of the symptoms.
3. The ratio of norepinephrine to epinephrine secreted by the tumor.

C. Diagnostic tests

1. Clinical and biochemical suspicion of pheochromocytoma should be high before performing adrenal imaging procedures. Biochemical tests include determination of plasma epinephrine, norepinephrine and dopamine levels, as well as measurement of the urinary excretion of catecholamines or metanephrines. Each of these tests has a number of drawbacks which could lead to misleading results. It is therefore often necessary to perform multiple tests on several occasions. In most patients, the measurement of 24-hr urine for metanephrine excretion is the most reliable screening test.
2. The clonidine suppression test is sometimes helpful in confirming biochemically the presence of a pheochromocytoma. Patients with pheochromocytoma do *not* suppress plasma norepinephrine to the normal range. In normal subjects, clonidine suppresses plasma norepinephrine by stimulating central α-adrenergic receptors.
3. Localization of tumors: CT and MRI scanning give good results. Adrenal medullary scintigraphy with a labeled precursor for catecholamine synthesis may also be necessary in difficult cases.

V. Differential Diagnosis

The diagnosis of pheochromocytoma should be considered in all patients with paroxysmal symptoms; in hypertensive patients with diabetes and hypermetabolism; in patients in whom change of position precipitates hypertension; in severe hypertensives not responding to therapy; and in all hypertensive children in whom the cause of hypertension cannot be identified. Common disorders sometimes confused with pheochromocytoma include thyrotoxicosis, anxiety attacks, and menopause in women with essential hypertension.

VI. Treatment

A. Adrenergic antagonists are used for preparation for surgery (phentolaminine, prazosin, phenoxybenzamine). This preparation minimizes the hazards of anesthesia and surgery.

B. Surgical resection of the tumor usually results in a dramatic cure. This is the only effective treatment of pheochromocytoma.

C. Postoperative hypotension may require blood volume expansion. Pressor therapy should not be substituted for volume expansion.

D. Patients with nonresectable malignant tumors can be managed medically for prolonged periods. They are treated with phenoxybenzamine and/or metyrosine (which blocks conversion of tyrosine to catecholamines).

VII. Prognosis

A. Excellent in benign tumors with proper localization and extirpation of the tumor. If not treated, severe hypertension develops, with fatal complications.

B. In malignant pheochromocytomas, the prognosis is poor; however, with the use of a combination of chemotherapeutic agents (such as cyclophosphamide, vincristine, and dacarbazine), adrenergic antagonists, and metyrosine, survival may be prolonged for several years.

Bibliography

Baxter JD, Tyrell JB. *The Adrenal Cortex.* in *Endocrinology and Metabolism*, ed 2. New York, McGraw-Hill, 1987, pp. 511–630.

Biglieri E, Melby J. *Endocrine Hypertension* in *Comprehensive Endocrinology.* Revised Series, Burger H, DeKretser D (eds). New York, Raven Press, 1989.

Gomez-Sanchez CE, Gill JR, Ganguly A, et al. Glucocorticoid-suppressible aldosteronism: A disorder of the adrenal transitional zone. *J Clin Endocrinol Metab* 67:444–448, 1988.

Kaye TB, Crapo L. The Cushing's syndrome: An update on diagnostic tests. *Ann Intern Med* 112:434–444, 1990.

Kornel L. Steroids, in Dulbecco R (ed), *Encyclopedia of Human Biology*, vol 7. San Diego, Calif, Academic Press, 1991, pp 257–283.

Macdougall IC, Isles CG, Stewart H, et al. Overnight clonidine suppression test in the diagnosis and exclusion of pheochromocytoma. *Am J Med* 84:993–1025, 1988.

New MI, Levine LS. *Congenital Adrenal Hyperplasia.* New York, Springer-Verlag, 1984.

Sheps SG, Jiang NJ, Klee GG, et al. Recent developments in the diagnosis and treatment of pheochromocytoma. *Mayo Clin Proc* 65:88–95, 1990.

CHAPTER 121

Disorders of the Female and Male Reproductive Organs

Gretajo Northrop, M.D., Ph.D.

Hirsutism

I. Definition

Hirsutism results from exposure of the female body to excessive levels of male sex hormones. Increasing exposure, longer duration, or higher concentrations of male sex hormones eventually results in virilization and defeminization.

A. The term *hirsutism* is reserved for excessive androgen-dependent hair growth on one or more regions of the body and is usually the initial event.

B. *Virilization* encompasses not only hirsutism but also more severe androgen-induced events such as deepening voice, recession of the temporal scalp hairline, and clitoral hypertrophy.

C. *Defeminization* denotes menstrual disturbance, decrease in breast size, excessive muscular development, and loss of female hair pattern.

D. *Hypertrichosis* is the increased growth of hair in non-androgen-dependent areas such as the ears, nose, and interphalangeal joints.

II. Etiology

Androgen production is elevated in virtually all hirsute women in whom the condition has been studied.

A. Diseases of the ovary
  1. Polycystic ovary disease (PCOD): Chronic anovulation due to any cause in a women with adequate pituitary hormonal reserve may lead to PCOD.
  2. Hyperthecosis (similar to PCOD).
  3. Luteoma of pregnancy.
  4. Neoplasms of the ovary.

B. Diseases of the adrenal glands
  1. Congenital adrenal hyperplasia (CAH): A group of hereditary diseases in which one or several enzymes required for cortisol synthesis are deficient, resulting in excessive adrenocorticotropic hormone (ACTH) stimulation of adrenal androgen synthesis.
  2. Cushing's syndrome.
  3. Neoplasms of the adrenal glands.

C. Other diseases occasionally associated with increased body hair
  1. Anorexia nervosa and starvation: Fine

lanugo hair may cover most of the body, but not in the male hair pattern distribution.

2. Hypothyroidism.

3. Intersexuality

   a. Female pseudohermaphroditism: Intrauterine exposure of a 46 XX fetus to excessive androgens due to CAH, maternal tumor, or excessive drug ingestion.

   b. Male pseudohermaphroditism: Androgen resistance syndromes, CAH, and gonadal dysgenesis of the 46 XY fetus. Phenotypic females (genetic males) may appear hirsute at or before puberty.

4. Rare diseases and syndromes: There are many syndromes associated with hirsutism whose etiology remains unknown. Hirsutism in some of these may be related to insulin-like factors which are known to stimulate the ovary to produce excess androgens.

   a. Achard-Thiers syndrome
   b. Bird-headed dwarf of Seckel
   c. Cornelia de Lange's syndrome
   d. Gangliosidosis
   e. Hypertrichosis lanuginosa
   f. Leprechaunism
   g. Lipodystrophy

5. Drugs

   a. ACTH
   b. Methyldopa
   c. Minoxidil
   d. Anabolic steroids
   e. Diazoxide
   f. Phenytoin
   g. Glucocorticoids
   h. Oral contraceptives
   i. Phenothiazines
   j. Spironolactone
   k. Streptomycin
   l. Cyclosporine

III. **Pathophysiology**

   A. Androgens are produced by the gonads, adrenal glands, and placenta and transported in the blood, bound to sex-hormone-binding-globulin (SHBG). Only 1% of testosterone (T) is transported in the free (unbound), biologically active form, which can cross the cell membrane and bind to intracellular receptors, where it causes the biologic response characteristic of the cell type that is stimulated. Androgens cause collagen formation in the skin, oiliness, hyperhidrosis, increased sebum production, and hair growth, depending on the type of skin cell stimulated.

   B. When T production exceeds the metabolic capacity of the liver (approximately 400 g/day), increased androgen metabolism in peripheral (nonhepatic) cells occurs with the above-mentioned clinical findings, including hirsutism. When androgen production exceeds both hepatic and nonhepatic cellular metabolism, the plasma androgen concentrations increase. Elevation of T also causes a decrease in SHBG, which results in a relative increase of free T. Thus increased T production, resulting in nonhepatic cell metabolism as well as relatively increased free T, may together result in a normal total plasma level of T in a hirsute woman with increased T production and clinical hyperandrogenism (Figure 121-1).

IV. **Diagnosis**

   A. History

      1. Age of onset: The age of onset of symptoms may provide some clues to the likely diagnosis (Table 121-1).

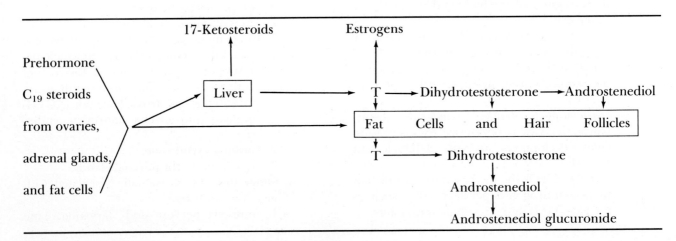

Figure 121-1. Summary of androgen formation and disposition in women.

Table 121-1. Etiology of Hirsutism by Age Group

Age Group	Cause of Hirsutism

Birth to puberty	Genetic syndromes
	    Congenital adrenal hyperplasia (classical form)
	    Leprechaunism
	    Gangliosidosis
	    Bird-headed dwarf of Seckel
	    Cornelia de Lange's syndrome
	    Hypertrichosis lanuginosa
	Starvation syndromes
	Precocious puberty
	    Idiopathic
	    Tumors (see below)
	Tumors
	    Pituitary
	    Ovaries
	    Adrenal glands
	    Ectopic hormone producing tumor sites
	        Lung
	        Liver
	        Pancreas
	        etc.
	Drugs
	    Hormones: oral contraceptives
	    Phenytoin
	    Diazoxide

Puberty to menopause	PCOD
	Hyperandrogenemia without evidence of PCOD (hyperthecosis)
	Genetic syndromes
	    Intersex problems
	    Male pseudohermaphroditism
	Gonadal dysgenesis
	Congenital adrenal hyperplasia (nonclassical form)
	Pregnancy: Luteoma
	Tumors
	    Pituitary
	        Adrenomas associated with Cushing's disease
	    Acromegaly
	    Adrenal glands
	    Adenomas and carcinomas
	Drugs
	    Hormones: Oral contraceptives, ACTH, anabolic steroids, androgens, progestogens
	    Phenytoin
	    Diazoxide (rarely in adults)
	    Streptomycin
	    Cyclosporin
	    Minoxidil, methyldopa
	    Phenothiazines
	Miscellaneous: Conditions of localized hypervascularity may be associated with localized hirsutism (e.g., chronic skin irritation, chronic osteomyelitis, severe varicose veins, stasis ulcers). Increased localized hair growth following inguinal lymphadenopathy for melanoma.
	Unilateral facial hair growth was reportedly associated with ipsilateral Dilantin-induced gingival hyperplasia, and in another woman it occurred without known cause.

Postmenopause	Ovary: With aging, the numbers of ova and presumably of granulosa cells decline. The presence of excessive theca cells in relation to granulosa cells results in an elevated androstenedione/estradiol ratio. The extragonadal metabolism of androstenedione (principally in adipose tissue) accounts for increases in estrone and 3-androstenediol glucuronide, as well as in the more biologically active androgens, T and dihydrotestosterone.

2. Symptoms: The severity and rapidity of progression of symptoms and signs may provide a clue to the cause of hyperandrogenemia.

3. Reproductive history: Frequently, menstrual cycles are long and occur irregularly in PCOD. Fertility is usually impaired with increasing androgen concentration.

4. Obesity or difficulty with weight control: The anabolic effect of androgens results in increased muscle mass. Hyperinsulinism associated with obesity and hyperandrogenemia promotes fat accumulation, particularly in the upper trunk regions.

5. Hypothyroidism: This results in impaired metabolic clearance of T due to decreased 5α reductase.

6. CAH: Enzyme deficiency may result in increased use of alternate steroid metabolic pathways and hyperandrogenemia.

7. PCOD: Hyperandrogenemia is frequently associated with this disease.

B. Physical findings related to hyperandrogenemia

1. Skin

a. Hair: The male pattern of hair distribution includes hair on the face, neck, shoulders, abdomen, and presacral area, as well as heavy growth on the arms and legs to the dorsum of the hands and feet. Thinning or balding of scalp hair may be noted, usually in the frontal or temporal region.

b. Acne: Acne may vary in severity from pimples to boils or abscesses on the face or in inguinal and axillary skin folds.

c. Hyperhidrosis: Excessive sweating may be the patient's only complaint.

d. Acanthosis nigricans: A black, velvety pigmentation may be noted on the neck, axilla, and in flexor skin folds. It is associated with obesity, hirsutism, PCOD, and insulin resistance.

2. Breasts: Breast size may decrease in women with hyperandrogenemia.

3. Clitoris: Clitoral enlargement is associated with long duration and high concentrations of plasma androgens.

4. Ovary: In some patients, enlarged ovaries with multiple cysts and thick capsules are noted.

5. Muscle: Muscle mass may be increased in women when androgen exposure has been prolonged at high concentrations.

C. Laboratory examination and diagnostic procedures

1. General principles

a. Most women who seek medical advice because of mild to moderate hirsutism do not require an exhaustive search for the etiology if they report the gradual onset of hirsutism or acne and absence of drug use. However, the primary reason for failure to diagnose and successfully treat the hirsute patient is inadequate laboratory evaluation. Abbreviated androgen blood profiles may be initially obtained, but if no elevation of androgen intermediates is detected or if the patient does not respond to treatment, a complete profile is essential.

Blood Test	Significance of Elevation in Peripheral Blood
Dehydroepiandrosterone (DHEA), Dehydroepiandrosterone sulfate (DHEAS)	Excessive adrenal cortical secretion
Androstenedione (A) Testosterone (T)	Excessive adrenocortical or ovarian secretion
Dehydrotestosterone (DHT)	Excessive conversion of DHEA, DHEAS, A, or T by tissue 5α reductase
3-Androstenediol glucuronide	Excessive conversion of androgens in peripheral tissues
Luteinizing hormone (LH)/Follicle-stimulating hormone (FSH)	Ratios above 2 or 3 are suggestive of PCOD
Sex hormone-binding globulin (SHBG)	Low concentrations permit a greater percentage of the total T or DHT to remain unbound and therefore biologically active

b. Dynamic testing protocols for localization of androgen secretion are time-consuming, expensive, and ineffective. Excessive androgen comes from the adrenal glands in about one-third of all patients; in another one-third, it comes from the ovaries and in the remaining third, it comes from both the adrenals and ovaries.

2. Specific tests for localization of the sources of circulating androgens when the peripheral blood concentration approaches twice normal are indicated.

a. Ultrasonography: Ultrasonography is particularly useful in evaluating pelvic structures. Ovarian size may be estimated, and cystic tumors may be differentiated from solid ones.

b. Computed tomography (CT): CT is appropriate to search for tumors in the head, neck, chest, and abdomen. Bilateral adrenal hyperplasia can be distinguished from solitary tumors that are at least 7 mm in diameter. Nonfunctional adrenal tumors of up to 4 cm are reported as incidental findings in healthy adults.

c. Magnetic resonance imaging (MRI): MRI provides another method for evaluation of possible head or body tumors. Controversy exists as to whether MRI or CT is best for detection of pituitary tumors, but adrenal cortical tumors are probably best detected by CT.

d. Selective catheterization to obtain blood from either adrenal or ovarian veins may be helpful when noninvasive methods have failed to locate the tumor.

e. Laparoscopy: Laparoscopy is particularly helpful in hirsute women when the ovaries differ widely in size. Small tumors and lipid cell tumors may be missed when ovarian biopsy is performed with the laparoscope.

V. **Management**

Most hirsute women do not have a tumor or classic congenital adrenal hyperplasia. The majority of hirsute women have mild hyperandrogenemia and/or PCOD, which usually responds to medical management. Depending on the results of blood testing, suppression of either the ovaries or adrenal glands, or both, along with simultaneous electrolysis to damage the hair follicles, will lead to successful treatment. Either suppression or electrolysis alone is *not* likely to be successful.

A. Corticosteroids are appropriate for hirsute women who likely have PCOD with elevated DHEA and/or DHEAS. Most women respond to prednisone, 2.5 mg at bedtime, with a lowering of DHEAS to low normal levels in 4–6 weeks. Rarely is a full suppressive dose of 7.5 mg required to normalize DHEA and DHEAS. The long biological half-life of dexamethasone produces more side effects and it should not be used.

B. Oral contraceptives are used for suppression of excessive androgen secretion of ovarian origin. In addition, these agents increase SHBG levels so that the biologically active free hormone is reduced.

C. Spironolactone may be used in combination with oral contraceptives and/or corticosteroids to potentiate these agents or as the only agent in women who are not candidates for other agents, such as postmenopausal women and women with a history of thromboembolic disease. In addition to blocking steroid synthesis, spironolactone blocks the steroid receptor in the hair follicle and thus decreases the effect of androgens on the target cell.

D. Surgery has a place in patients with PCOD who are not candidates for medical management. Hirsutism is a profound psychological burden to some women. If medical management cannot be employed, ovarian stromal tissue can be markedly decreased (androgen levels lowered) by cautery or laser via the laparoscope. Ovarian wedge resection to facilitate pregnancy has sometimes been used. It results in lower androgen levels, with subsequent pregnancy and decreased hirsutism. The laparoscope accomplishes the same effect without adhesions and abdominal surgery.

VI. **Prognosis**

Successful treatment of hirsutism requires discovery of the cause of the excessive androgen secretion, with reduction to low normal blood levels by medical suppression or surgical removal of the androgen-producing tissue. In the majority of cases, and when hair has been present for more than 12 months, electrolysis is necessary until follicles are destroyed. Constant suppression may be required for long periods of time to prevent new growth. Most cases can be managed quite successfully if both patient and physician are compulsive and diligent.

Amenorrhea

I. **Definition**
  A. The term *primary amenorrhea* is reserved for girls 14 years or older who have never had spontaneous menses. In 14-year-old girls with secondary sex characteristics, complete evaluation may be delayed until age 16.
  B. Secondary amenorrhea is used to denote nonpregnant women who have previously had spontaneous periods and have stopped having menstrual cycles for at least 6 months.

II. **Etiology**
  A. A normal physiologic process, pregnancy, or menopause.
  B. Anatomic absence of the uterus or its lining, endometrium, or vagina. Blockade of the genital tract, as in congenital malformation, cervical or vaginal stenosis, or imperforate hymen.
  C. Ovarian pathology including chromosomal abnormalities, agenesis, and tumors.
  D. Pituitary-hypothalamic disease, including tumors, arrested maturation, congenital defects, stress, and psychosis.
  E. Systemic disease may result in amenorrhea. Systemic conditions include malnutrition, obesity, infections, cancer (including chemotherapy), or dysfunction of other endocrine glands.

III. **Pathophysiology**
  Any changes which result in interruption of the hormonal cycling mechanism, destruction of the endometrium, or blockade of the outflow tract will lead to absence of menses.
  A. During pregnancy the fetal, placental, and maternal compartments combine to produce hormone levels sufficiently elevated to prevent maternal gonadotropin cycling and amenorrhea.
  B. Absence of adequate endometrium to respond to estrogen stimulation is the cause of amenorrhea in müllerian developmental defects such as agensis or atresia of the uterus.
  C. Removal of the endometrium during curettage (iatrogenic) or secondary to infection (schistosomiasis, tuberculosis, etc.) may lead to Asherman's syndrome. Imperforate hy-

men and vaginal agenesis prevent demonstrable menstrual outflow.
  D. Abnormal or absent DNA in ova prevents completion of the normal developmental cycle.
    1. Absence of DNA (Turner's syndrome, 45 XO) results in incomplete granulosa cell formation around the ova and streak ovaries. Rarely, mosaicism may permit menses and even pregnancy in women with Turner's syndrome.
    2. Phenotypic females with a male karyotype (Swyer's syndrome, 46 XY) have normal müllerian-derived organs but streak ovaries. A high malignancy rate makes gonadal removal necessary as soon as the diagnosis is made. The etiology of this syndrome and of gonadal agenesis are unknown.
    3. Premature ovarian failure may be due to deletion of one short or long arm on the X chromosome. Premature ovarian failure may also be due to an autoimmune or infectious process, thereby resulting in destruction of the ova containing follicles.
  E. Androgen excess syndromes occasionally result in either primary or secondary amenorrhea, depending on when the process is initiated. Excessive blood levels of androgen arising from the ovaries, from the adrenal glands, or from conversion of steroids in the fat cells may prevent ovulation, with modest elevation of androgens or amenorrhea if the levels are high (see the discussion of hirsutism).
  F. Miscellaneous
    1. Resistant ovary syndrome, defined at laparoscopy in women with ovarian follicles, elevated gonadotropins, and no evidence of lymphocytic infiltration, or autoimmune disease affecting the ovaries.
    2. Radiation and chemotherapeutic agents are destructive to ovaries. Children and younger women have a larger number of ova than older women. This may be the reason why the younger the patient, the more likely menses or even pregnancy may ensue, sometimes many years after treatment.
    3. Pituitary destruction by prolactin-secreting adenoma and craniopharyngioma, as well as postpartum hypotension (Sheehan's syndrome), are examples of amenorrhea secondary to low gonadotropin secretion.

IV. Diagnosis

A. The patient's history permits separation of primary from secondary amenorrhea, and the physical examination provides anatomically distinguishing characteristics of many abnormalities related to reproductive failure. Regardless of the history, pregnancy must always be ruled out.

B. In the absence of spontaneous initiation of menses, the history should include a family history of similar problems, participation in sports, eating disorders, treatment for tumors, and treatment for acne or hirsutism. Determine if the patient has had drug-induced menses or surgical repair of a hernia.

   1. Testes feminization and androgen resistance syndromes are sometimes familial. A history of bilateral herniorraphies in phenotypic females is almost pathognomonic of this syndrome.

   2. Medical treatment for severe acne or hirsutism is suggestive of PCOD beginning at an early age before puberty. CAH should also be considered. A patient who reports previous drug-induced periods due to oral contraceptives or medroxyprogesterone use has clearly demonstrated a functional outflow tract.

   3. Women who have been treated for eating disorders or who have avidly pursued sports such as ballet, gymnastics, or running may have too small a body mass to initiate cyclic menses.

   4. Children treated for tumor with chemotherapy or radiation therapy to the brain, including the upper face and orbits and lower abdomen, may begin menses later than normal or never.

C. In women who have had cyclic menses which subsequently stopped, the outflow tract has been proven to be intact at one time.

   1. A history of irregular menses accompanied by acne, hirsutism, or scalp hair loss is suggestive of PCOD.

   2. Oligomenorrhea accompanied by a history of galactorrhea is suggestive of a pituitary adenoma. Drug use (such as psychotropic medications or marijuana) must also be considered.

   3. Amenorrhea following a complicated pregnancy, particularly if documented hypotension or transfusions were given intra- or postpartum, is highly suggestive of Sheehan's syndrome, particularly if there was absence of postpartum breast milk.

   4. Premature menopause due to autoimmune disease is suggested by other autoimmune diseases resulting in loss of function of the β cells, parathyroids, or adrenal glands. Resistant ovary syndrome gives no histologic clues.

D. Physical findings suggest or confirm the historical information. All patients do not have all the characteristics listed.

   1. Turner's syndrome: Short stature, shield chest, low cervical hairline, aortic abnormalities, minimal to absent pubic hair, no breast development, and no evidence of estrogen stimulation on pelvic organs.

   2. Swyers syndrome: Eunuchoid stature, shortened fourth and/or fifth metacarpals, evidence of minimal estrogen stimulation on pelvic organs, and no breast stimulation.

   3. Testicular feminization: Prominent breast development, absent axillary and pubic hair, absent cervix.

   4. Prolactin-secreting adenoma: Galactorrhea.

   5. Androgen excess syndromes: Facial, neck, chest, nipple, abdominal, presacral, forearm (with extension above the elbow and dorsum of the hands), thigh, and buttock hair. Scalp hair decreased in temporal and frontal areas. Oily skin, hyperhydrosis, and acne may be present.

   6. Eating disorder syndromes: Extreme thinness or gross obesity. Women with anorexia nervosa have extremely coarse, dry, flaky skin.

E. Laboratory tests

   1. Human chorionic gonadotropin: The most frequent cause of amenorrhea is pregnancy. Regardless of the history, this must be ruled out.

   2. FSH and LH
      a. FSH and LH, both low, suggest that the patient is prepubertal or has hypogonadotropic hypogonadism.
      b. LH/FSH ratio between 1 and 2.5 is normal.
      c. LH/FSH ratio below 1: Hypothalamic disease likely.
      d. LH/FSH ratio above 2.5: PCOD likely.
      e. FSH and LH elevated: Ovarian failure likely (e.g., menopause).

   3. Estradiol (E_2) is elevated just prior to the

LH midcycle spike at ovulation. E_2 is elevated in some obese patients and in the presence of some ovarian tumors.

4. Estrone (E_1) is elevated with obesity and some ovarian tumors.

5. Prolactin is elevated minimally in some patients with PCOD but usually less than 60 mg/ml. When a prolactin-secreting pituitary microadenoma is present, levels usually exceed 60 mg/ml. The higher the level, the larger the tumor. Primary hypothyroidism with elevated thyroid-stimulating hormone (TSH) may induce hyperprolactinemia due to thyrotropin-releasing hormone (TRH) stimulation of TSH and prolactin. Prolactin levels in this situation are rarely higher than 100 mg/ml.

6. Elevated TSH may be diagnostic if amenorrhea is associated with galactorrhea and thyroid disease.

7. An androgen screen is essential in androgen excess syndromes if evaluation is to be optimal. Shortcuts such as ordering only T and DHEAS miss the diagnosis in a considerable number of patients.

   a. The following tests should be ordered: T (total and free), androstenedione, dihydrotestosterone, DHEA, DHEAS, 3-androstenediol glucuronide.

8. Free cortisol in a 24-hr urine collection is an excellent screening test for Cushing's syndrome.

9. 17-Hydroxyprogesterone is rarely helpful in evaluation of amenorrhea.

10. CT and MRI are used when tumor is suspected in the pituitary, ovaries, or adrenal glands.

11. Pelvic ultrasound permits better ovarian evaluation than CT and MRI.

V. Differential Diagnosis

Amenorrhea associated with normal menopause occurs between 45 and 55 years of age. As the amenorrheic woman approaches age 45, the likelihood of ovarian failure as the etiology increases. Middle-aged women with elevated FSH and LH, low estradiol levels (below 20 pg/ml), and hot flashes likely have normal menopause. In younger women, increasing concern should be directed toward amenorrhea, and a search for another nonphysiologic cause should be initiated.

VI. Treatment

Management of amenorrhea is directed at diagnosing and correcting the cause where possible. In women with menopause the goal should be to correct the expected or demonstrated physiologic changes associated with estradiol deficiency.

A. Amenorrhea due to chromosomal defects requires long-term estrogen replacement for urogenital and pelvic structure maintenance. Breast development will proceed with estrogen and progesterone replacement.

1. Oral contraceptives may be used.

2. Cyclic estrogen-progestin therapy

   a. Premarin, 1.25 mg/day or from day 6 to the end of the month.

   b. Provera, 10 mg/day, for the last 12 days of the month.

   c. In patients with a Y component in the karyotype, gonadoectomy is required because of the high malignancy rate in these organism in the abdominal area.

   d. The vagina will usually accommodate sexual activity in patients with testicular feminization, so surgical intervention is generally not necessary.

B. Hyperprolactinemia can usually be managed with bromocriptine, 2.5 mg one to three times a day (See Chapter 118.)

C. Androgen excess syndromes can be managed by suppression of the site producing the androgen, with simutaneous electrolysis to remove the hair-producing follicles (see the section on hirsutism).

D. Ovarian suppression is accomplished with oral contraceptives. For adrenal suppression with prednisone at bedtime, give 2.5 mg; rarely, 5 or 7.5 mg is required. Spironolactone, 50–200 mg/day, blocks receptor uptake of androgen and androgen synthesis.

E. Weight loss in the obese patient is encouraged through diet and exercise. Nutritional counseling and psychiatric consultation are essential in anorexics. Bone density should be evaluated and maintenance estrogen and progestin given if appropriate. Os Cal 500 and multivitamins are also appropriate in amenorrhea including sports related amenorrhea.

VII. Patient Monitoring

Successful treatment is demonstrated by initiation and/or continuation of menses. Whatever condition was discovered to be the cause of amenorrhea must be monitored in the future.

A. Patients with abnormal chromosomes will require hormone replacement therapy indefinitely. Pap smears, as well as blood pressure and blood glucose monitoring, will be required.

B. Depending on the level of prolactin and the presence of a macroadenoma, testing of blood levels of prolactin and visual fields, as well as pituitary MRI, are required to monitor these patients.

C. Patients with androgen excess need continued suppression of the ovaries, the adrenal glands, or both. Once abnormal values are lowered to normal and the electrolysist reports a hair decrease, with less time required for effective control, yearly monitoring of the patient for maintenance care is appropriate. See Chapter 120 on the adrenal glands, for monitoring of patients with Cushing's syndrome and congenital adrenal hyperplasia.

D. Patients who have eating disorders will always require monitoring to keep weight off or to put weight on, as these problems are chronic. Bone density measurement requires yearly monitoring for improvement.

VIII. **Prognosis**

Amenorrhea is either treated successfully, with continuation of spontaneous menses, or medication is required to induce menses on a cyclical basis. In either case, the amenorrhea is usually cured.

Testis

I. **Function**

The testes serve two major functions:
A. Production of androgens.
B. Production of spermatozoa.

II. **Anatomy**

A. Paired structures measuring 5 × 3 cm, with a volume of 25 ml, located in the scrotum.
B. Functional regions
1. Interstitial: Leydig cells are stimulated by LH to produce T.
2. Seminiferous tubule
a. Germinal epithelium under the influence of FSH and T produces spermatozoa.
b. Sertoli cells: Surround the germ cells and, under FSH stimulation, create the environment necessary for the maturation of sperm.

III. **Hormonal Control**

A. Hypothalamus: Releases gonadotropin-releasing (GnRH) in a pulsatile manner.

B. Pituitary GnRH acts on gonadotropin cells to produce pulsatile release of FSH and LH.
C. Testis: LH acts predominantly on Leydig cells to produce T. FSH acts on the Sertoli cells to create the environment for spermatozoa to develop. Both FSH and T are required for the formation of mature sperm.
D. Sertoli cells: Produce inhibin, which acts at the pituitary to inhibit FSH secretion.

Hypogonadotropic Hypogonadism

I. **Definition**

Low gonadotropin levels and impaired testicular function as a result of injury to the pituitary or hypothalamus.

II. **Etiology**

A. Congenital factors
1. Kallman's syndrome: Isolated gonadotropin deficiency; can be X-linked or autosomal dominant
2. Congenital hypopituitarism
3. Genetic syndromes
a. Prader-Labhart-Willi syndrome
b. Laurence-Moon-Biedl syndrome
B. Infections
1. Bacterial
2. Fungal
3. Protozoan
C. Inflammatory diseases
1. Sarcoidosis
2. Connective tissue diseases
3. Histiocytosis X
D. Neoplasms
1. Dysgerminoma
2. Craniopharyngioma
3. Prolactinoma
4. Other pituitary adenomas
E. Metabolic diseases
1. Hemochromatosis
2. Malnutrition
3. Liver disease
4. Renal disease

III. **Pathophysiology**

Any process that affects hypothalamic secretion of GnRH or pituitary secretion of LH and FSH will render the individual hypogonadotropic. Without LH and FSH stimulation, the testis will become atrophic, and spermatozoa and T will not be produced.

IV. **Diagnosis**

A. History
1. Prepubertal: Young men with congenital

hypopituitarism may come to the doctor's attention because of severe growth retardation, as evidenced by markedly abnormal growth charts. Young men with Kallman's syndrome present with delayed puberty.

2. Postpubertal men will present with complaints of impotence, headaches, visual field disturbances, or infertility. Most men are reluctant to discuss sexual dysfunction in the presence of their partners.

B. Clinical signs and physical findings
1. Prepubertal
   a. Evaluation of growth charts reveals a flattening of the growth curve in children with congenital hypopituitarism
   b. Kallman's syndrome (may also be detected postpubertally)
      (1) Eunuchoid proportions (arm span greater than height)
      (2) Anosmia or hyposmia
      (3) Cleft lip or palate
      (4) Cryptorchidism
      (5) Congenital deafness
   c. Signs of other congenital syndromes
2. Adult
   a. Evaluate for signs of puberty.
      (1) Testicular size: Enlargement of the testes is the earliest sign of puberty. The measurement can be made with an orchidometer or ruler. Normal testes are approximately 4 cm in diameter (seminiferous tubules account for 95% of the volume).
      (2) Penis size: Look for developmental abnormalities such as hypospadia or microphallus.
      (3) Virilization: If patients have not had adequate T, they will have poor development of skeletal muscle and sexual body hair.
      (4) Gynecomastia.
C. Diagnostic tests
1. Seminal fluid analysis: Fluid should be obtained after masturbation into a glass or plastic container. Collection should take place after 48 hr of continence but no longer than after 7 days of continence.
   a. Normal volume is 2–6 ml. Specimens should be examined within 1 hr of collection.
   b. Motility should be evaluated; normally, 60% of the sperm should be motile.

   c. Sperm density: More than 20 million/ml is normal.
   d. Sperm morphology: More than 60% normal morphology is normal.
   e. Acute illness or medications can affect seminal fluid analysis. It is therefore mandatory to evaluate three samples over a 2- to 3-month period before considering the fluid.
2. Visual field evaluation: Defects in visual fields can be seen in patients with prolactinomas and other pituitary tumors. Young men with prolactinomas may have expressible galactorrhea, where as older men with prolactinomas may not.
3. Basal levels of LH, FSH, and T: These may not be sufficient by themselves, as FSH and LH are pulsatile and T undergoes diurnal variation. An abnormally low value may be seen on the nadir of the curve of a normal person.
4. GnRH test: Evaluates the capacity of gonadotropin to release FSH and LH. If gonadotropins are functional, a 100-μg bolus of GnRH produces a 2- to 3-fold rise in LH at 30 min, and a 1.5- to 2-fold increase is seen in FSH at 60 min.
5. Clomiphene test: Clomiphene is given after an estrogen antagonist and exerts an antiestrogen effect at the level of the hypothalamus. Clomiphene, 100 mg/day for 7 days, produces a 100% rise in LH and a 50% rise in FSH.

V. Differential Diagnosis
A. Physiologic delayed puberty: A Diagnosis of Exclusion
   1. Usually familial.
   2. Does not display the abnormalities seen in the other processes.
   3. Puberty usually takes place between 14 and 18 years but may occur late.
B. Diseases associated with low total T with normal free T levels (caused by a low SHBP level)
   1. Hypothyroidism
   2. Obesity
   3. Acromegaly
C. Other systemic diseases, including sarcoidosis, connective tissue increases, and hemochromatosis.

VI. Treatment
A. Identify any systemic disease and treat it.
B. Prolactinoma: Give Bromocriptine at bedtime.
C. T injections can be administered to ensure

virilization; give T cypionate, 200 mg intramuscularly, for 2 weeks.

D. The use of T alone will not allow spermatogenesis to occur. Spermatogenesis can occur in an environment where FSH or FSH and B-HCG are administered with T.

E. GnRH agonist therapy may be useful in Kallman's syndrome.

VII. Prognosis

Since testes are intact, proper stimulation may allow spermatogenesis and fertility.

Hypergonadotropic Hypogonadism

I. Definition

Hypergonadotropic hypogonadism is a primary testicular process leading to small testicular size, low T levels, absent spermatogenesis, and high FSH and LH levels from lack of feedback inhibition.

II. Etiology

A. Congenital causes

1. Klinefelter's syndrome: The most common disorder causing male hypogonadism. It is characterized by extra X chromosomes; the most common karyotype is 47 XXY.

2. Down's syndrome.

3. XYY syndrome.

4. Male Turner's syndrome.

B. Infection

1. Mumps orchitis: Testes may show germ or Leydig cell destruction in 25% men, rarely prepubital boys. Atrophy may be noted in one or both testes.

C. Neoplasms

1. Acute lymphocytic leukemia

a. Direct infiltration of tumor cells.

b. Ionizing radiation

(1) A dose of 600 rads can destroy spermatogenesis.

(2) Leydig cell dysfunction is seen after a dose of more than 800 rads.

D. Metabolic conditions

1. Hormone resistance: Androgen insensitivity may lead to phenotypic femaleness in a 46 XY individual.

2. Enzymatic deficiencies

a. 17-Hydroxylase deficiency

b. 17-Ketoreductase deficiency

3. Marijuana and alcohol can interfere with steroidogenesis.

III. Pathophysiology

Any process that leads to primary gonadal failure will result in impaired to absent T and spermatogenesis. The lack of T and inhibin leads to nonsuppressed FSH and LH secretion. Hence FSH and LH will be markedly elevated.

IV. Diagnosis

A. History: The patient presents with complaints of delayed puberty, impotence, or infertility.

B. Clinical signs and physical findings: The most common finding is small, firm testicles on a routine physical exam (less than 2.0 cm in length); some patients may present with azoospermia.

1. Klinefelter's syndrome

a. Klinefelter's syndrome: Patients present with eunuchoid stature (arm span more than 2 cm longer than height).

b. Gynecomastia is usually present.

c. Mean intelligence is below average.

d. Such chronic diseases as diabetes mellitus are prevalent.

C. Diagnostic tests

1. FSH and LH are markedly elevated.

2. Inhibin levels are very low.

3. T levels are low.

4. In the presence of an enzymatic deficiency, precursors are elevated.

a. Increased progesterone in 17-hydroxylase deficiency.

b. Increased androstenedione in 17-ketoreductase deficiency.

V. Treatment

A. Patients with hypergonadotropic hypogonadism will not be able to produce spermatozoa because their germ cell pool is either absent or destroyed.

B. T cypionate can be given intramuscularly every 2 weeks to maintain normal androgen functions.

VI. Prognosis

Klinefelter's syndrome patients must be evaluated for possible breast cancer. Fertility cannot be restored.

Germinal Cell Failure

I. Definition

Involves abnormalities in spermatogenesis, with either normal or subclinical Leydig cell dysfunction. These patients present with infertility.

II. Etiology

A. Infections

1. Genitourinary infections
   a. Ureaplasma urealyticum
   b. *Escherichia coli*
2. Sinopulmonary: Infertility syndrome
   a. Immotile cilla syndrome: Presents with abnormal sperm and cilia structure.
   b. Cystic fibrosis: Congenital malformation of the vas deferens; sperm and cilia ultrastructure are normal.
   c. Young's syndrome: Inspissated secretion in the vas deferens associated with azoospermia.
B. Idiopathic causes
   1. Varicocele.
   2. Arrest of germinal cell maturation.
   3. Generalized hypospermatogenesis.
   4. Sertoli cell only syndrome: Loss of germinal cell function with preservation of Leydig cell function.
   5. Idiopathic seminiferous tubule dysfunction with hyalinization.

III. Pathophysiology

The underlying processes seen in these conditions are azoospermia and infertility, either secondary to abnormal germinal cell function or due to anatomic abnormalities, obstruction, or infection.

IV. Diagnosis

A. History: Inquire about a history of respiratory illnesses. A detailed reproductive history is necessary. Ask for a history of venereal disease or urethral discharge.
B. Clinical signs and physical findings
   1. Examine scrotal veins during the Valsalva maneuver to rule out a varicocele. Examine the testes for size.
   2. Perform genital and rectal exams to evaluate potential abnormalities of the vas deferens, epididymis, and prostate.
C. Diagnostic tests
   1. Measure FSH, LH, T, and prolactin.
   2. Culture seminal fluid to rule out infection.
   3. Semen analysis will document azoospermia.
   4. If FSH is normal, testicular biopsy may be helpful to evaluate the extent of germinal cell failure.

V. Treatment

A. Varicocele: A urologist can ligate the testicular veins.
B. Infections: Can be treated with appropriate antibiotics.

VI. Prognosis

Many long standing or non-infective cases will not have adequate spermatogenesis and will not be able to conceive.

Gynecomastia

I. Definition

An increase in glandular and stromal tissue in men. This increase may be unilateral or bilateral.

II. Etiology

A. Physiologic
   1. Neonatal
   2. Pubertal
B. Congenital
   1. Cryptorchism
   2. Klinefelter's syndrome
   3. Vanishing testes syndrome
   4. Defect in T biosynthesis or androgen resistance
C. Infection
   1. Mumps
   2. Leprosy
D. Neoplasm
   1. Producing B-HCG
      a. Testicular
      b. Lung
   2. Estrogen-producing
      a. Adrenal feminizing tumor
      b. Testicular
E. Metabolic
   1. Drugs
      a. Estrogens
      b. Digitalis
      c. Cimetidine
      d. D-Penicillamine
      e. Marijuana
      f. Spironolactone
      g. Phenytoin
      h. Sulindac
      i. Alkylating chemotherapeutic agents
      j. Tricyclic antidepressants
      k. Ketoconazole
   2. Renal failure
   3. Hepatitis
   4. Thyrotoxicosis
   5. Cirrhosis
   6. Refeeding after starvation
F. Trauma
   1. Testicular trauma
   2. Radiation therapy
   3. Surgery

III. Pathophysiology

A. Normal breast development
   1. Composed of lobules connected by a ductal system.
   2. Lobules consist of:
      a. Areolar cells.
      b. Myoepithelial cells.

3. Lobules are connected by ducts, which, in turn, connect to the nipple and areola.

4. Breast tissue is covered by a layer of adipose tissue.

5. Breast development in women is categorized according to the stages of Tanner:

   a. Stage I: No breast tissue or nipple, and areola less than 2 cm in diameter.

   b. Stage II: Breast tissue palpable, with an increase in areola diameter.

   c. Stage III: Growth and elevation of the breast.

   d. Stage IV: Secondary mound above breast contour.

   e. Stage V: Adult breast.

B. Breast development is dependent on estrogen stimulation

   1. Any process that increases the estrogen level can cause gynecomastia.

      a. Estrogen-producing tumor.

      b. Exogenous estrogen use (for prostate cancer).

   2. It is known that disorders of androgen deficiency in the presence of normal estrogen levels can produce gynecomastia. This implies that it is the relative estrogen/androgen ratio that is important in the development of gynecomastia rather than an absolute increase in estrogen level.

C. Congenital: Results in a low T level with a normal estrogen level, causing a increase in the estrogen/androgen ratio and resultant gynecomastia.

D. Drugs

   1. Gynecomastia caused by increased estrogen production/action

      a. Exogenous estrogens: Used for treatment of prostate cancer and found in foods from estrogen-treated animals.

      b. Marijuana: Interacts with estrogen receptor; there may be increased estrogen material in crude extracts.

   2. Gynecomastia caused by decreased androgen production/action

      a. Ketoconazole: Inhibits T production.

      b. Cimetidine: Blocks androgen receptors.

      c. Spironolactone: Decreases androgen production and blocks androgen receptors.

      d. Alkylating agents: Cause Leydig cell damage, leading to elevated LH to maintain the T level. The elevated LH leads to increased estrogen production and to an elevation in the estrogen/androgen ratio and gynecomastia.

E. Infection: Mumps results in testicular failure and decreased T.

F. Neoplasms

   1. Estrogen-producing: Adrenal, Testicular

   2. B-HCG-producing tumor: Acts like LH and stimulates estrogen production, resulting in an elevated estrogen/androgen ratio.

G. Metabolic

   1. Rental failure: Gynecomastia results from primary gonadal failure with uremia, decreasing T production.

   2. Cirrhosis: Increased estrogen production leads to increased peripheral conversion of androgen precursors to estrogen.

   3. Thyrotoxicosis: Enhances peripheral conversion of androgens to estrogens.

IV. **Diagnosis**

A. History

   1. Ask the patient about medications; ask about cosmetics because they may contain estrogenic material.

   2. Look for symptoms of hypogonadism.

   3. Ask about a history of fertility/infertility.

   4. Look for symptoms of systemic disease (e.g., liver disease, kidney disease).

B. Physical exam

   1. Evaluate for secondary sexual characteristics.

   2. Evaluate testicular size.

   3. Look for possible abdominal mass (possible adrenal tumor).

   4. Breast exam: Distinguish pseudogynecomastia from true gynecomastia. Pseudogynecomastia is breast enlargement secondary to fatty deposits. Look for palpable breast tissue that can be palpated near the nipple; the areoa will be enlarged and convex in true gynecomastia.

C. Diagnostic tests

   1. Measure LH, FSH, T, estradiol, prolactin, BHCG; perform liver function tests, kidney function tests, and, if indicated, thyroid function tests.

   2. If there is an elevated estradiol level with an elevated B-HCG or low LH level, a testicular or adrenal tumor must be considered.

V. **Differential Diagnosis**

A. Pseudogynecomastia

B. Breast carcinoma

VI. **Treatment**

A. Stop giving any drug that may be responsible for gynecomastia.

B. Treat any underlying disease (e.g., thyrotoxicosis).

C. In primary gonadal failure, T shots may help treat gynecomastia.

D. Mammoplasty may be necessary, especially if gynecomastia is long-standing.

Bibliography

Barth JH, Cherry CA, Wojnarowska F. Spironolactone is an effective and well tolerated systemic antiandrogen therapy for hirsute women. *J Clin Endocrinol Metab* 68:966–970, 1989.

Braunstein GD. Current concepts: Gynecomastia. *NEJM* 328(7):490–495, 1993.

Emans SJ, Mansfield MJ. Anorexia nervosa, athletics and amenorrhea. *Pediatr Clin North Am* 36:533–549, 1989.

Erkkola R, Ruutiainen K. Hirsutism: Definitions and etiology. *Ann Med* 22:99–103, 1990.

Kirschner MA. Hirsutism and virilism in women. Special topics in *Endocrinol Metab* 6:55–93, 1984.

Lloyd T, Myers C, Buchanan JR, et al. Collegiate women athletes with irregular menses during adolescence have decreased bone density. *Obstet Gynecol* 72:639–642, 1988.

Ludmerer KM, Kissane JM. Hirsutism with virilization. *Am J Med* 89:794–804, 1990.

McKenna TJ. Pathogenesis and treatment of polycystic ovary syndrome. *N Engl J Med* 318:558–562, 1968.

Northrop GJ. *Hirsutism, Defeminization, and Virilization.* New York, 1991, pp 376–400.

Santen RJ. The testis, in Felig P (ed), *Endocrinology and Metabolism*, ed 2. St Louis, McGraw-Hill, 1987, pp 821–905.

Veldhuis JD. Management of amenorrhea. *Hosp Pract* 23:40–56, 1988.

CHAPTER 122

Parathyroid Hormone, Calcitonin, Vitamin D, Minerals, and Metabolic Bone Disease

Will G. Ryan, M.D.

Introduction

The following fundamental facts are helpful in understanding the disorders discussed in this chapter.

Calcium

This measures 1 kg in adult humans: 99% in skeleton, 1% in extracellular fluid. One gram is ingested per day; 0.1–0.3 g is absorbed by the gut and excreted in urine when the individual is in calcium balance. Calcium has both structural (skeleton) and metabolic functions (cell and neuromuscular activity, blood coagulation, etc.). The serum level is 8.6–10.5 mg/dl, 50% of which is normally ionized (not bound to albumin, etc.) and therefore is metabolically important.

Phosphorus

This measures 600 g in adult humans: 80–90% in the skeleton, the rest in tissues and serum. It is one of the major intracellular anions; 1 g is ingested per day, two-thirds of which is excreted in urine. The adult serum level is 2.5–4.0 mg/dl; that of the growing child is 4.5–6.0 mg/dl.

Vitamin D

Sources are dietary (fortified dairy products) or sunlight irradiation of 7-dehydrocholesterol in skin (hydroxylated at the 25 position in the liver and further hydroxylated at the 1 position in the kidney). 1,25 $(OH)_2$ vitamin D is the most potent naturally occurring form. Its major activity is enhancement of intestinal calcium absorption, but it has less well defined activity in bone as well.

Calcitonin

This is a peptide hormone secreted by medullary cells of the thyroid; it is a potent suppressor of osteoclastic activity. Its role in human physiology is not well defined, but it may help prevent hypercalcemia after ingestion of calcium. Measurement of serum levels is most useful for detection of medullary carcinoma of the thyroid, particularly in patients at risk of developing multiple endocrine neoplasia type II syndrome.

Pharmacologic doses are useful in the treatment of Paget's disease of bone and osteoporosis.

Parathyroid hormone

This is a peptide hormone secreted by the parathyroid glands. Its major role is regulation of serum calcium within a very narrow range (approximately 8.5–10.5 mg/dl). Further description of its activity is presented in the section on primary hyperparathyroidism.

Bone

Matrix is 90% type I collagen; other components are osteocalcin, osteonectin, and others. Noncalcified matrix is known as *osteoid* and comprises 30% of dry body weight. Hydroxyproline is a major component of collagen, and measurement of urinary hydroxyproline excretion is helpful in estimating matrix degradation. The crystalline component is calcium phosphate; 70% of dry weight occurs as hydroxyapatite.

Osteoclast

This resorbs mineral and matrix of bone. It is derived from the macrophage cell line. It appears in bone as multinucleated giant cells and is rich in tartrate-resistant acid phosphatase.

Osteoblast

This builds collagen matrix and possibly facilitates the transport of calcium and phosphorus into bone. It is rich in alkaline phosphatase. The serum level is normally derived half from bone and half from liver. It is a useful measure of metabolic bone activity, as osteoclastic and osteoblastic activities tend to be tightly coupled.

The following sections discuss common disorders.

Hypercalcemia

I. **Definition**

Increase in serum calcium to levels above the normal range of approximately 8.5–10.5 mg/dl. Levels below 12 mg/dl are considered mildly hypercalcemic; 12–14 mg/dl, moderately hy-

percalcemic; 14–16 mg/dl, severely hypercalcemic; and above 16 mg/dl, extremely hypercalcemic.

II. **Etiology**

A. Primary hyperparathyroidism is the most common etiology, usually leading to mild hypercalcemia.

B. Malignancy-associated hypercalcemia is the second most common form and is usually more severe.

C. Miscellaneous types: Granulomatous disease, vitamin D intoxication, milk alkali syndrome, hyperthyroidism, tertiary hyperparathyroidism of renal disease, and prolonged immobilization (especially in children and others with accelerated bone turnover).

III. **Pathophysiology**

A. Primary hyperparathyroidism

B. Malignancy associated

1. Metastatic: Local dissolution of bone by tumor-elaborated substances, causing release of calcium into the circulation and overwhelming the normal homeostatic mechanism. The same is true of multiple myeloma, but the factors elaborated may differ.

2. Nonmetastatic or humoral hypercalcemia of malignancy (HHM): Elaboration of parathyroid hormone-related peptide (PTHRP) by various tumors, the most common being squamous cell carcinoma of the lung, head, or neck.

3. Miscellaneous

a. Granulomatous diseases and certain lymphomas produce excess 1,25 $(OH)_2$ vitamin D by transformed macrophages or lymphocytes.

b. Medications or vitamin D intoxication: Ingestion of excessive amounts of vitamin A or D or their active metabolites. Thiazide decreases renal excretion of calcium. Lithium may lead to stimulation of parathyroid hormone secretion by the parathyroid glands.

c. Milk alkali syndrome (now uncommon): Ingestion of excessive amounts of calcium in milk or antacids along with excess alkali, resulting in nephrocalcinosis—the combination resulting in hypercalcemia from both excessive intake and the inability to excrete calcium.

d. Nonparathyroid endocrine disorders: Hyperthyroidism—pathophysiology unclear, but may result both increased metabolic activity of bone and parathyroid glands. Pheochromocytoma, adrenal insufficiency, VIPoma—pathophysiology also unknown.

e. "Tertiary" hyperparathyroidism of renal disease may result from prolonged secondary hyperparathyroidism as a result of the kidney's inability to excrete adequate amounts of ingested phosphorus, which leads to sustained hyperphosphatemia and hypocalcemia. The parathyroid glands become autonomous after variable periods of time.

f. Immobilization: Results in inadequate stimulation of bone formation and excessive bone resorption, which overwhelm the normal homeostatic mechanisms.

g. Familial hypercalcemic hypocalciuria: Reduced renal excretion of calcium and stimulation of parathyroid glands for unknown reasons. Characterized by elevation of serum calcium and magnesium, as well as hypocalciuria.

h. Parenteral nutrition: Mechanisms obscure.

IV. Diagnosis

A. History: Anorexia, constipation, nausea, vomiting, lassitude, weakness, polyuria, mental aberration, or obtundation, depending on the severity of hypercalcemia.

B. Clinical signs and physical findings: Usually signs of dehydration in moderate hypercalcemia and mental obtundation in more severe cases.

C. Diagnostic tests: Serum PTH calcium, phosphorus, creatinine. See specific related disorders for other diagnostic tests.

V. Differential Diagnosis

None of particular note.

VI. Treatment

A. Acute: Rapid hydration with normal saline (4–6 liters/day) plus a loop diuretic (furosemide, 80 mg every 4–6 hr or its equivalent) to avoid volume overload and promote calciuresis. If the response is inadequate (and depending on the severity), add subcutaneous salmon calcitonin (Calcimar), 100 U every 4–6 hr; or plicamycin (Mithracin), 15–25 μg per kilogram of body weight by intravenous injection; or pamidronate (Aredia), 60 mg/24 hr intravenous infusion; or gallium nitrate (Ganite), 300 mg/day as a 24-hr intravenous infusion for 5 days.

1. Varying combinations of the above drugs may be used in refractory cases.

B. Subacute or chronic: Glucocorticoids (prednisone, 10–40 mg/day) for granulomatous disease. Also useful for vitamin D intoxication.

1. Treatment of various malignancies when implicated.
2. Stop ingesting excess milk and alkali.
3. Treatment of hyperthyroidism.
4. Mobilize if possible.
5. Remove hyperplastic or adenomatous parathyroid glands.

VII. Patient Monitoring

Frequent determination of serum electrolytes, calcium, and creatinine is necessary in those undergoing rehydration and diuresis. Electrocardiographic monitoring is advisable as well. Mental status exam is needed in more severe cases. Milder cases may require only serial determinations of serum calcium and creatinine, along with discontinuing offending medications or excessive calcium intake.

VIII. Prognosis

Generally good except for cases associated with malignancy (life expectancy, 3 months). Prognosis of other cases is generally good if hypercalcemia is corrected early enough to avoid significant renal damage.

Primary Hyperparathyroidism

I. Definition

A state of primary hyperactivity of one or more parathyroid glands (usually due to a benign adenoma or hyperplasia) resulting in chronic excessive secretion of parathyroid hormone with attendant abnormalities, depending on the extent and duration of the condition.

II. Etiology

Unknown; may occasionally be related to prior radiation exposure to the neck; rarely, due to carcinoma.

III. Pathophysiology

Consequences of increased parathyroid hormone secretion.

A. Increased conversion in the kidney of 25 OH vitamin D to $1,25(OH)_2$ vitamin D, which acts on an intestinal receptor to increase absorption of calcium and phosphorus.

B. Increased osteoclastic resorption of bone and increased osteoblastic bone formation.

C. Increased kidney tubular resorption of calcium; decreased tubular resorption of phosphorus and bicarbonate.

IV. Diagnosis

A. History: Often asymptomatic. Symptoms of hypercalcemia (unless severe) are relatively nonspecific (constipation, anorexia, nausea, polyuria, depression, etc.). Severe hypercalcemia unusual except with parathyroid carcinoma.

B. Clinical signs and physical findings: Usually none. Band keratopathy always mentioned but rarely seen. Occasionally, kidney stones; rarely, kidney failure. Occasionally, fracture secondary to bone disease.

C. Diagnostic tests

1. Elevated serum calcium in the presence of elevated serum parathyroid hormone is almost certainly diagnostic. Mild forms may have high normal serum parathyroid hormone, but this will be inappropriately high for the level of serum calcium. Low serum phosphorus and mild hypercholeremic acidosis may also be seen.

2. Radiographs may show subperiosteal resorption, particularly in phalanges.

3. Advanced cases may show classic osteitis fibrosa cystica. Nephrocalcinosis and stones also may be seen. Bone scan may show generalized increased uptake of radioisotope.

V. Differential Diagnosis

All other causes of hypercalcemia (malignancy is most common), but these are almost invariably associated with a low (or low normal) serum parathyroid hormone level.

VI. Treatment

A. Removal of one or more enlarged parathyroid glands.

B. Medical management: Careful observation with avoidance of dehydration, estrogen replacement in postmenopausal women, and oral phosphorus supplements in hypophosphatemic patients. Used mainly for very mild hypercalcemia or when surgery is contraindicated.

VII. Patient Monitoring

A. Essentially none in patients successfully operated on.

B. Serum calcium determinations about every 3 months in patients under medical management, with approximately yearly serum creatinine determinations.

VIII. Prognosis

A. Excellent in patients successfully operated on.

B. May be problematic in those who have had unsuccessful surgery and in those under medical management if serum calcium exceeds 12 mg/dl.

Hypocalcemia

I. Definition

A total serum calcium level of less than 8.5 mg/dl. Approximately 7.5–8.5 mg/dl is mild hypocalcemia; 6.5–7.5 mg/dl is moderate hypocalcemia; and below 6.5 mg/dl is severe hypocalcemia. In some cases, it may be necessary to measure ionized calcium in order to distinguish between true hypocalcemia and a change in binding to albumin.

II. Etiology

A. Hypoparathyroidism: Partial or total destruction of parathyroid glands. Accidental destruction during surgery is the most common cause; autoimmune disease, infiltrative disease, ionizing radiation, and chemotherapy are unusual or rare causes. Congenital absence of the parathyroid glands (Di George syndrome) is rare.

B. Miscellaneous: Acute pancreatitis, acute increase in serum phosphate (rhabdomyolysis chemotherapy, toxic shock—release of intracellular phosphate), severe hypo- or hypermagnesemia, osteoblastic metastases, multiple citrated blood transfusions, states of $1,25 (OH)_2$ vitamin D deficiency, some vitamin D–resistant states.

C. Pseudohypoparathyroidism, types I and II.

D. Artifactual: Hypoalbuminemia or severe alkalosis.

III. Pathophysiology

A. Hypoparathyroidism: Inadequate function (either absolute or relative) to maintain serum calcium in the normal range. (See the section on hypercalcemia for the functions of parathyroid hormone.)

B. Pseudohypoparathyroidism: Genetic disorder; type 1—results from generalized deficiency of G proteins responsible for transmission of receptor signal to cyclic AMP; type II—cause unknown.

IV. **Diagnosis**
   A. History: Circumoral or distal extremity paresthesia usually described as "tingling"; muscular excitability usually described as twitching or cramping; difficulty or inability to breathe due to airway obstruction in severe forms.
   B. Clinical signs and physical findings: Chvostek's sign (twitching of the lip or other facial muscles elicited by tapping the facial nerve just anterior to the ear); Trousseau's sign (cramping of the hand elicited by pumping a blood pressure cuff to halfway between systolic and diastolic blood pressures for several minutes; laryngeal stridor or complete airway obstruction with cyanosis (due to tetany of vocal chords) and convulsive seizures in severe forms.
   C. Diagnostic tests: Low serum calcium and often high serum phosphorus; sometimes basal ganglia calcification or cataracts in the chronic state.

V. **Differential Diagnosis**
   Conditions mentioned above.

VI. **Treatment**
   Acute intravenous injection (over 1–5 min) of calcium gluconate (1 g contains 100 mg ionized calcium) is sufficient to relieve symptoms; repeat as necessary. Laryngeal spasm may require emergency tracheostomy. Chronic: Vitamin D: generally 50,000–200,000 U/day (or an equivalent dose of bioactive metabolites; see Table 122-1) and oral calcium: generally 1–3 g/day is sufficient to maintain serum calcium in the low normal range.

VII. **Patient Monitoring**
   Serum calcium determinations generally every several hours in acute states; generally about monthly in chronic states. Caution: Brief periods of serum calcium in excess of 12 mg/dl can cause permanent renal damage.

VIII. **Prognosis**
   Generally good with appropriate therapy and monitoring.

Osteoporosis

I. **Definition**
   Loss of skeletal mass sufficient to result in increased susceptibility to fracture. Usually generalized but may be localized. Type I osteoporosis refers to bone loss predominantly in trabecular bone (vertebral and femoral). Type II refers to predominant cortical bone loss.

II. **Etiology**
   A. Advanced age is most common cause.
   B. Loss of estrogen after menopause is second cause.
   C. Drugs: Glucocorticoids, alcohol, methotrexate.
   D. Inadequate dietary calcium, particularly during childhood and adolescence, may be a major contributing factor.
   E. Other causes much less common.

III. **Pathophysiology**
   A. Progressive loss of skeletal mass (trabecular bone usually lost before cortical bone).
   B. When sufficient, results in fracture with minor trauma.
   C. Residual bone usually thought to be of normal quality.
   D. Areas of skeleton containing mostly trabecular bone (vertebrae) usually fracture first (type I); areas with more cortical bone usually fracture later (type II).

IV. **Diagnosis**
   A. History
      1. Asymptomatic until fracture occurs.
      2. Back pain common with vertebral fracture.
      3. Usual symptoms of other fractures, often with minor or sometimes no apparent trauma.

Table 122-1. Forms of Vitamin D

Preparation	Usual Dose	Serum Half-Life	Time to Correction of Hypercalcemia	How Supplied
Vitamin D_3	1.25–2.5 mg/day	Months	Weeks–months	1.25-mg tabs (50,000 U)
25OH D_3	20–50 μg/day	16 days	Usually 2–3 weeks	20- + 50-μg tabs (Calderol)
1,25 $(OH)_2$ D_3	0.25–1.0 μg/day	36 hr	Usually a few days	0.25- + 0.50-μg tabs (Rocaltrol)

B. Clinical signs and physical findings
 1. None until fracture occurs.
 2. Minor fractures of vertebrae may result in progressive vertebral deformity, usually resulting in kyphosis or sometimes scoliosis.
 3. Wrist and hip fractures also common.
C. Diagnostic tests
 1. Serum chemistries usually normal.
 2. Sometimes minor elevation of serum alkaline phosphatase.
 3. Radiographs detect vertebral deformity; density of bone may appear decreased, but this is often unreliable except in advanced stages.
 4. Bone scan helpful in determining whether or not vertebral fracture is recent.
 5. Bone density determinations most helpful for quantitation of severity; those measuring primarily trabecular bone are generally most sensitive.

V. Differential Diagnosis
A. Usually none.
B. Osteomalacia may sometimes be contributory.
C. Determination of the cause may be most problematic, but advanced age and postmenopausal state are by far the most common causes.

VI. Treatment
A. Prevention is much better than treatment.
B. Approved treatments
 1. Estrogen (conjugated—Premarin), 0.625 mg/day orally, plus medroxyprogesterone (Provera), 2.5 mg/day orally (the latter needed only in patients with a uterus).
 2. Adequate calcium intake (1,000–1,500 mg/day, either dietary or in combination with a supplement).
 3. Calcitonin: Salmon (Calcimar), 100 U/day, or human (Cibacalcin), 0.5 mg/day subcutaneously, decreasing to 3 times per week after 1–2 months.
 4. Moderate exercise (without spine flexion).
C. Investigational but widely used treatments
 1. Sodium etidronate (Didronel), 400 mg/day for 2 weeks of 15 weeks cyclically.
 2. Sodium fluoride, 25 mg twice daily with meals; stimulates osteoblastic activity (always give with at least 1,000 mg/day supplemental calcium; otherwise, may it cause osteomalacia).

VII. Patient Monitoring
A. Bone density determinations: Lumbar spine and proximal femur, approximately yearly.
B. Radiographs or bone scan for suspected fracture.

VIII. Prognosis
A. Mild to moderate osteoporosis: Good prognosis for prevention of future fracture.
B. Severe osteoporosis: Generally not good, but some patients may respond unusually well to therapy.

Renal Osteodystrophy

I. Definition
A complex metabolic bone disease which encompasses a variety of abnormalities, ranging from parathyroid-induced bone disease to osteomalacia.

II. Etiology
Failure of renal function preventing adequate excretion of ingested phosphorus, as well as poorly understood abnormalities comprising uremia.

III. Pathophysiology
A. Inability to excrete phosphorus adequately results in inadequate renal production of 1,25 dihydroxy vitamin D ($1,25 (OH)_2 D$) to sustain adequate intestinal calcium absorption.
B. Inadequate calcium absorption combined with hyperphosphatemia results in a decreased serum calcium level, which, in turn, results in increased secretion of parathyroid hormone (secondary hyperparathyroidism).
C. Increased secretion of parathyroid hormone stimulates the production of $1,25 (OH)_2 D$ and osteoclastic resorption of bone, which temporarily corrects the serum calcium level. In addition, the phosphaturic effect of parathyroid hormone helps to lower the serum phosphorus level.
D. As renal function declines further, the above homeostatic mechanisms arc overwhelmed. Serum phosphorus continues to rise and serum calcium decreases to a slightly low range. Continued hyperparathyroidism results in bone disease (osteitis fibrosa cystica). Absorption of aluminum-containing compounds to help lower serum phosphorus causes aluminum deposition in bone, resulting in osteomalacia. Subcutaneous calcification and gangrene of skin or

various portions of the body results from inadequate serum phosphorus control.

IV. Diagnosis

A. History: Asymptomatic in early stages. Bone pain and easy fracturing in more advanced stages.

B. Clinical signs and physical findings: Usually none unless fracturing or deformation of bone.

C. Diagnostic tests: Elevated serum creatinine, blood urea nitrogen, and parathyroid hormone; normal to elevated serum phosphorus; normal to low serum calcium. Radiographs generally show subperiosteal resorption. Bone scan may show a generalized increase in uptake of isotopically labeled bisphosphonate. Calcification of blood vessels seen in advanced cases when serum phosphorus is inadequately controlled.

V. Differential Diagnosis

Secondary hyperparathyroidism or osteomalacia due to other causes; generally, calcium malabsorption or renal phosphorus wasting.

VI. Treatment

Low-phosphorus diet, oral calcium supplements (carbonate or acetate) to improve calcium absorption and bind phosphorus in the gut. Use aluminum-containing antacids as sparingly as possible if necessary for more gut phosphorus binding. Give intravenous 1,25 $(OH)_2$ D to suppress parathyroid and improve calcium absorption (oral form generally results in excessive calcium absorption, leading to hypercalcemia). Kidney transplantation is the most satisfactory solution in advanced cases.

VII. Patient Monitoring

Serum calcium, phosphorus, parathyroid hormone: Try to maintain these in the normal range. Selected radiographs. Bone biopsy with tetracycline labeling and quantitative histomorphometry in selected cases.

VIII. Prognosis

Generally poor in advanced cases unless renal transplantation done.

Pagets' Disease of Bone

I. Definition

A chronic skeletal disorder, usually discovered in middle to old age, resulting in various deformities, susceptibility to fracture, and various disabilities, *depending on the extent and strategic location* in the skeleton.

II. Etiology

A. Unknown; possibly "slow virus" (nucleocapsid of measles or respiratory syncytial virus or a hybrid).

B. Also genetic, as this disease has some familial tendency and is seen primarily in subjects of British descent; common in Great Britain and in most countries colonized by the British (e.g., United States, Australia); rare in Asia.

III. Pathophysiology

A. Primary increase in the number and activity of osteoclasts in the areas of skeleton involved.

B. Compensatory increase in osteoblastic activity in the same areas.

C. Results in greatly accelerated bone turnover.

D. Rapid remodeling results in bone of poor structural quality, deformity, and increased vascularity.

IV. Diagnosis

A. History: Many patients asymptomatic; often bone pain, fracture, arthropathy, or symptoms due to neural compression.

B. Clinical signs and physical findings
   1. Usually deformity of bones involved.
   2. Neural compression signs (often deafness if disease affects the base of the skull).
   3. Warmth of skin if bone near the surface is involved (tibia).

C. Diagnostic tests
   1. Usually elevated serum alkaline phosphatase (reflects increased osteoblastic activity).
   2. Elevated urinary hydroxyproline (reflects increased osteoclastic activity degrading the collagen matrix of bone), the degree depending on the extent and activity of the disease.
   3. Bone scans have a characteristic appearance and are most sensitive for diagnosis.
   4. Radiographs of involved areas usually have a diagnostic appearance but may be mistaken for osteoblastic prostatic carcinoma.

V. Differential Diagnosis

A. Elevated serum alkaline phosphatase may be mistaken as indicating liver disease.

B. Osteoblastic metastases may mimic skeletal changes of Pagets' disease.

VI. Treatment

    A. Calcitonin: salmon [Calcimar], 100 U/day, or human [Cibacalcin], 0.5 mg/day—both subcutaneously). These agents are primarily indicated for patients with severe disease in weight-bearing bones or with impending fracture.

    B. Sodium etidronate (a bisphosphonate Didronel^r), 400 mg/day orally on an empty stomach; otherwise, poorly absorbed.

        a. Limit courses to 6 months, with 3–6 months off therapy; Otherwise, osteomalacia may result.

        b. Use cautiously in patients with disease in weight-bearing bones (femur or tibia).

    C. Plicamycin: Reserved for resistant cases because of toxicity (liver, kidneys, platelets).

VII. Patient Monitoring

    A. Serial serum alkaline phosphatase determinations most convenient and inexpensive.

        1. Progressive decrease indicates a successful response; nonresponse or a plateau indicates resistance to treatment; increase after decrease indicates relapse.

    B. Serial bone scans also helpful but expensive.

    C. Radiographs may sometimes show regression or progression and complications such as fracture, neural compression, or sarcoma.

VIII. Prognosis

    A. Generally good if there is a good response to therapy.

    B. If not, continued bone pain, progressive deformity, or neural compression. Osteosarcoma develops in less than 1% of cases.

Bibliography

Bilezikian JP. Hypercalcemia. *Disease a Month* 34:741–799, 1988.

Favus M (ed). *Primer on the Metabolic Bone Diseases and Disorders of Mineral Metabolism.* Kelseyville, Ca., American Society for Bone and Mineral Research, 1990.

Mundy GR. Hypercalcemia of malignancy revisited. *J Clin Invest* 82:1–6, 1988.

Raisz LG. Local and systemic factors in the pathogenesis of osteoporosis. *N Engl J Med* 318:818–828, 1988.

Reichel H, Koeffler HP, Normon AW. The role of the vitamin D endocrine system in health and disease. *N Engl J Med* 320:980–991, 1989.

Singer FR, Wallach S (eds). *Pagets Disease of Bone: Clinical Assessment, Present and Future Therapy.* New York, Elsevier, 1991.

CHAPTER 123

Diabetes Mellitus and Adult Hypoglycemia

David Baldwin, Jr., M.D.
John D. Blackman, M.D.

I. **Definition**

Diabetes mellitus is a collection of diseases in which abnormalities in insulin secretion and/or insulin action lead to chronic hyperglycemia and disordered lipid metabolism. Most diabetic patients can be classified as having either type I or type II diabetes; generally, these correspond to youth and adult ages of onset, respectively. Each type will be discussed separately.

Chronic hyperglycemia is associated with the chronic microvascular complications of diabetes: retinopathy, nephropathy, and neuropathy. These and macrovascular atherosclerosis constitute the morbidity and mortality of diabetes, and they will be discussed in the concluding section.

II. **Etiology and Pathophysiology**

Type I diabetes is a chronic autoimmune disease.

A. Peak incidence occurs at age 15.

B. Most patients have developed hyperglycemia by age 30, but a few patients may present at any older age.

C. Certain human leukocyte antigen (HLA)-DR and -DQ genotypes are strongly associated with susceptibility to type I diabetes.

D. The incidence in the general population of the Western world is 1:400; the disease is much less common in Africa and Asia.

E. The risk of developing the disease among first-degree relatives of a type I diabetic is 1:20. The risk in a monozygotic twin approaches 1:2.

F. An unidentified agent (environmental? infectious?) triggers a lymphocytic infiltration of the pancreatic islets.

G. These lymphocytes mediate a cytotoxic attack on the insulin, producing β-cells.

H. When more than 90% of the β-cell mass has been destroyed, severe insulin deficiency and hyperglycemia supervene.

I. Antibodies directed at islet cells and at human insulin are present in the plasma of patients many years prior to the development of overt hyperglycemia (Fig. 123-1).

J. Patients have a progressively defective insulin response to intravenous glucose.

K. Although islet cell antibodies and reduced insulin secretion are reliable premonitors of the clinical expression of type I diabetes, there is no successful therapy to arrest the immune destruction of islet cells.

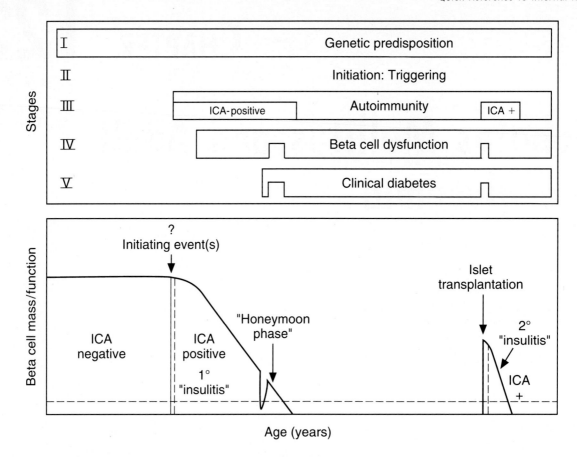

Figure 123-1.   Pathogenetic scheme. Autoimmune β-cell destruction and insulin-dependent diabetes mellitus. (Reprinted with permission from Vardi et al., *Diabetes Care*, Vol. 10, 1987. Copyright 1987 by American Diabetes Association, Inc.)

L. Pancreatic transplants in type I diabetics suffer the same fate as the native islets unless immunosuppressive therapy is employed.

M. In most children with type I diabetes, all capacity for insulin and glucagon secretion is destroyed within 5 years of the onset of hyperglycemia. Many type I diabetics with onset of hyperglycemia after age 25 will have permanently preserved residual secretion of insulin, enabling smoother control of hyperglycemia with injected insulin.

N. It is common for children with type I diabetes to have other coexisting chronic autoimmune endocrinopathies, such as hypothyroidism, hypoadrenalism, and hypogonadism.

III. **Diagnosis**

The diagnosis of type I diabetes should be suspected in any patient with a typical history, especially if a parent or sibling is a preexisting type I diabetic.

A. History
1. Polyuria
2. Polydipsia
3. Polyphagia
4. Weight loss
5. Frequent bacterial/fungal mucocutaneous infections
6. Blurred vision
7. Coma (ketoacidosis)

B. Physical findings
1. Dehydration (orthostatic hypotension)
2. Coexisting infection
3. Odor of acetone on breath

C. Diagnostic tests: Generally, the diagnosis of type I diabetes may be confirmed immediately in the outpatient setting by fingerstick blood glucose and dipstick urine ketone testing.
1. Blood or serum glucose is usually significantly elevated (greater than 250 mg/dl).
2. Ketosis is often present in the urine on qualitative dipstick testing.
3. Evidence of acidemia (low blood pH and bicarbonate level) must be sought immediately in all patients with newly diagnosed hyperglycemia and ketonuria.

4. Occasionlly, type I diabetics will present with ketoacidosis and normal or near-normal blood glucose levels. Thus outpatient evaluation must always include *both* blood glucose and urine ketone testing.

5. There is no place for oral glucose tolerance testing in the diagnosis of type I diabetes.

6. Although the glycohemoglobin (see Section VI) may be elevated, the short duration of hyperglycemia in many type I diabetics prior to diagnosis precludes this test from being reliably helpful.

IV. Differential Diagnosis

A. The only two common causes of chronic hyperglycemia are type I and type II diabetes mellitus. They are generally distinguished by the presence or absence of ketosis/ketoacidosis.

B. Age of onset is a less reliable indicator, as a subset of type II diabetics present as teenagers and type I diabetes may present at any age.

C. Black Americans may have an atypical form of diabetes in which diabetic ketoacidosis may be present on occasion and yet hyperglycemia and insulin dependence may wax and wane over many years. Islet cell antibodies are absent in this group.

D. Specific markers of type I diabetes, such as near-zero insulin secretion and islet cell antibodies, are rarely necessary to test for in the clinical care of diabetic patients but may occasionally be helpful.

E. The differential diagnosis of ketosis and ketoacidosis is interesting because all causes of ketoacidosis may be associated with mild hyperglycemia (100–300 mg/dl) and thus may be confused.

1. Starvation ketosis
2. Type I diabetic ketoacidosis
3. Alcoholic ketoacidosis
4. Toxic salicylism—associated ketoacidosis

V. Treatment

A. A primary difference between type I and type II diabetes is that all type I patients are dependent on injected exogenous insulin for their survival. Without daily hormone replacement therapy, ketoacidosis and death would rapidly ensue. While some type II diabetics may benefit from insulin therapy, they are not truly dependent on insulin for daily survival. Thus the terms *insulin-dependent diabetes mellitus (IDDM)* and *non-insulin-dependent diabetes mellitus (NIDDM)* have become synonymous with types I and II diabetes, respectively.

B. All type I diabetics should immediately be started on insulin injection as soon as this diagnosis is made. There is never a role for dietary modification or oral hypoglycemic agents in their treatment.

C. The general goal of insulin therapy is to control the blood glucose at a level as close to normal as is possible in the individual patient without incurring a significant risk of dangerous hypoglycemia. Except in patients with end-stage renal failure, where the half-life of insulin is prolonged, it is rarely possible to meet this goal without two or three injections per day. It is never possible without home blood glucose monitoring.

D. Intensive insulin therapy aimed at tight glucose control rarely normalizes blood glucose levels. There is not yet proof that tight control or even normalization of glucose levels will completely prevent the chronic microvascular complications of diabetes. However, the body of indirect evidence linking glucose control and these complications is compelling enough to allow us to recommend the above-mentioned goal to all patients except the following:

1. Unreliable patients.
2. Patients who are unwilling or unable to perform home blood glucose monitoring.
3. Patients with diabetic autonomic neuropathy and "hypoglycemic unawareness" due to loss of glucagon and epinephrine counterregulatory responses.

E. Ideally, home blood glucose measurements should be taken before each meal and at bedtime. In properly instructed patients, these readings can be highly accurate. Target readings are 80–120 mg/dl fasting in the morning and 100–150 mg/dl 4–6 hr after each meal. Patients with hypoglycemic unawareness should have 100 mg/dl higher than these ranges.

F. There are two common approaches to insulin therapy in type I diabetes:

1. NPH mixed with regular insulin is injected 0–30 min prior to breakfast. Lente insulin is not used, as it mixes poorly with regular insulin. The patient is instructed to split the total daily calorie intake into 20% at breakfast, 30% at lunch, 40% at supper, and 10% for a bedtime snack

consisting largely of protein. Lunch must be eaten on time, and occasionally midmorning and/or midafternoon snacks are necessary to avoid hypoglycemia. The dose of morning regular insulin is adjusted according to the prelunch blood glucose level. The dose of morning NPH is adjusted according to the presupper blood glucose level. Mixed NPH and regular insulin is injected again with supper, and the doses are adjusted from the bedtime and next morning glucose levels. In some patients whose breakfast and supper are closer together than 10 hr during the day, the evening NPH should be delayed 3–4 hr and injected at bedtime.

2. Ultralente may be injected each evening. It is long-lasting enough to provide a steady basal level of insulin adequate to meet fasting needs. Its dose is adjusted according to the fasting morning blood glucose level. The patient then takes regular insulin with each meal. The third injection of regular insulin may be mixed with the daily dose of ultralente at supper. The three-injection program of ultralente and regular insulin allows more flexibility in the timing and content of meals than the two-injection NPH and regular insulin program. The continuous subcutaneous insulin pump is analogous to the ultralente and regular program and has not been shown to be superior to it.

VI. **Patient Monitoring**

A. Urine glucose testing is no longer an acceptable technique for type I diabetics to monitor daily blood glucose control. Multiple studies have shown a poor correlation with actual blood glucose measurements, and hypoglycemia will never be detected.

B. Daily home blood glucose monitoring has become the standard of care for nearly all type I diabetics. Patients should be instructed to keep an ongoing diary of two to four tests per day. Simple, accurate devices for the measurement of blood glucose are widely available and are the most significant advance in diabetic care since the discovery of insulin. At the time of diagnosis, patients should be taught how to use their daily results to make changes in their doses of regular insulin according to predetermined algorithms.

C. Glycosylated hemoglobin

1. Hemoglobin A_1 is slowly glycosylated by an irreversible reaction throughout the 120-day life of erythrocytes.

2. The percentage of hemoglobin A_1 molecules which are glycosylated is dependent on the mean blood glucose level to which erythrocytes are exposed during their life span.

3. The percentage of glycosylated hemoglobin is a reliable marker of the mean blood glucose concentration during the previous 60–120 days.

4. It is recommended that all diabetic patients have a glycohemoglobin measurement two to four times per year.

VII. **Diabetic Ketoacidosis**

Diabetic ketoacidosis (DKA) is the acute decompensation of type I diabetes. Infection and omission of insulin are common etiologies of DKA.

A. Metabolic alterations

1. Usually severe hyperglycemia.

2. Fifteen percent of patients have normal or near-normal blood glucose levels—"euglycemic" DKA.

3. β-Hydroxybutyric acid (the dominant ketone body) accumulates, causing metabolic acidosis; other ketone bodies (acetoacetate and acetone) are often but not invariably present in blood and are detected by the nitroprusside reaction.

4. Patients are usually dehydrated secondary to the osmotic diuresis induced by hyperglycemia and/or the emesis induced by ketoacidosis itself.

5. Initially, hyperkalemia may be present due to the intra- to extracellular shift to potassium in acidosis. However, most patients have a total body depletion of potassium stores secondary to prehospital osmotic diuresis.

6. A normal blood glucose level or a negative serum acetone level in an acidotic diabetic should not dissuade the treating physician from the correct diagnosis of DKA.

B. Treatment

1. Perform a thorough and rapid history and physical exam; focus on possibilities of infection.

2. Establish reliable intravenous access; measure serum glucose, acetone, electrolytes, blood urea nitrogen, and creatinine; perform a complete blood count, arterial blood gas determination, and urinalysis.

3. Begin volume repletion with 0.9% normal saline (NS) at a rate of 200–500 ml/hr.

4. Begin a continuous intravenous insulin infusion. Add 100 U regular insulin to 100 ml 9% NS and begin at 5–10 U/hr (0.1 U/kg/hr).

5. Begin empiric antibiotics if infection is suspected after cultures are obtained.

6. Sodium bicarbonate therapy has been shown not be be helpful in the management of DKA unless acidosis is severe enough to be immediately life-threatening.

7. While hypophosphatemia may occur in DKA, its correction has not been shown to be helpful.

8. Blood glucose should be measured every 1–2 hr; when it reaches 200–250 mg/dl, intravenous fluid must be changed to 5% dextrose and 0.45% NS at a rate of 100–200 ml/hr.

9. Patients with euglycemic DKA should be initially hydrated with 5% dextrose and 0.9% NS.

10. After the blood glucose level drops below 250 mg/dl, the insulin infusion may be reduced to 2–4 U/hr but then must be continued for another 24 hr to allow full resolution of the ketoacidotic state.

11. Serum bicarbonate and acetrone should be monitored every 6–12 hr. In patients whose glucose or bicarbonate concentrations are not beginning to correct after 6 hr, the rate of insulin infusion should be doubled.

12. Serum potassium should be measured every 3 hr, and potassium replacement should begin after the level falls below 4–4.5 mEq/liter. Patients with potassium levels less than 3.0 mEq/liter may require replacement rates of 10–20 mEq/hr and very close monitoring of the electrocardiogram (ECG) and serum potassium.

13. NPH and regular insulin therapy may be resumed after ketoacidosis is resolved. Since the half-life of intravenous regular insulin is 5 min, the insulin infusion must continue for 2 hr after the first subcutaneous injection of NPH and regular insulin.

C. Complications
1. Cerebral edema may uncommonly occur in children with DKA. Its exact etiology and optimal therapy are unknown.

2. Undiagnosed infection: Rhinocerebral mucormycosis is an opportunistic infection which may complicate DKA. Patients have tissue necrosis and inflammation within the nose or mouth. All comatose patients with DKA who do not awaken with the normalizaton of blood glucose should have a careful ear, nose, and throat evaluation, as well as computed tomography/magnetic resonance imaging (CT/MRI) brain scan and, if cerebral edema is absent, a lumbar puncture to seek evidence of meningitis.

3. Unrecognized hypokalemia or hyperkalemia may cause cardiac or respiratory arrest.

4. Failure to maintain continuous intravenous insulin infusion, balanced by 5% dextrose infusion, for 24 hr after blood glucose has normalized is a common error in the management of DKA.

Type II Diabetes Mellitus

I. Etiology and Pathophysiology

A. Most patients are over age 50, are overweight, and have a strong family history of type II diabetes.

B. The incidence of type II diabetes in the Western world is 1:20 but rises to 1:2 in certain populations, such as the Pima Indians of Arizona.

C. Type II diabetes represents 90% of all diabetes in the Western world. It is estimated that 50% of all type II diabetics are currently undiagnosed.

D. Insulin resistance is likely to be the first defect chronologically in type II diabetes. It is present in most obese patients and in most normoglycemic patients who are destined to develop type II diabetes (Fig. 123-2).

E. Defects in insulin receptor number and affinity, as well as postreceptor and glucose transporter function, have been described in obesity and type II diabetes.

F. Nondiabetic patients with insulin resistance are hyperinsulinemic in order to maintain euglycemia.

G. In the genetically susceptible patient, insulin secretion eventually falls and hyperglycemia develops. Whether this is due to "β-cell exhaustion" or chronic glucose toxicity to the β-cell is unknown.

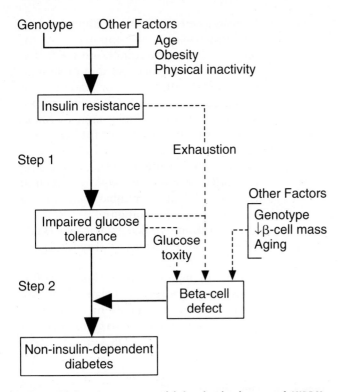

Genotype   Other Factors
                        Age
                        Obesity
                        Physical inactivity

Insulin resistance ┄┄┄┄┄┄┄┄

Step 1   Exhaustion

                                    Other Factors
                                    Genotype
Impaired glucose ┄┄┄┄┄   ↓β-cell mass
tolerance   Glucose ┄   Aging
                    toxity

Step 2   Beta-cell
                           defect

Non-insulin-dependent
diabetes

Figure 123-2.   A two-step model for the development of NIDDM. Dotted lines imply hypothetic possibilities. (From SAAD MF, Knowler WC, Pettitt DJ, et al. A two-step model for development of non-insulin-dependent diabetes. *Am J Med* 90:230, 1991. Reprinted by permission of *Yorke Medical Journal* and the authors)

H. Inadequate activation of skeletal muscle glucose uptake by insulin causes postprandial hyperglycemia. The failure of insulin to inhibit hepatic glucose output causes fasting hyperglycemia.

I. Eventually the islets of type II diabetics have a decreased number of β-cells, fibrosis, and amyloid deposition.

II. **Diagnosis**

A. The history is much less sensitive in suggesting the diagnosis of type II diabetes compared with type I. Although polyuria, weight loss, and blurred vision are common, complete lack of symptoms is common as well. Many patients are hyperglycemic several years prior to diagnosis. A chronic complication of diabetes such as neuropathy may be the first clue to the underlying hyperglycemia.

B. A few fasting serum glucose values in excess of 140 mg/dl or random serum glucose values in excess of 200 mg/dl will establish the diagnosis of diabetes.

C. A glycosylated hemoglobin more than 3 SD above the mean of normal will establish the diagnosis of diabetes. A glycosylated hemoglobin less than the mean of normal rules out the diagnosis of diabetes.

D. The diagnosis of type II diabetes can be established without oral glucose tolerance testing (OGTT) in most patients by (B) or (C) above. Rarely, the OGTT is performed by administering 75 g of glucose, and diabetes is diagnosed when the 60-min *and* 120-min serum glucose values both exceed 200 mg/dl.

E. Screening of asymptomatic individuals for diabetes has not been recommended except possibly for obese patients with a family history of type II diabetes.

F. Conversely, all nondiabetic pregnant women should be screened for gestational diabetes (type II diabetes presenting during pregnancy) between the 24th and 28th weeks of gestation by a 50-OGTT. This form of transient type II diabetes is present in 3% of all pregnant women and is a harbinger of chronic type II diabetes later in life in up to one-half of such patients.

III. **Differential Diagnosis**

A. Type I diabetes is distinguished from type II by the young age of onset and by the production of ketones.

B. Type II diabetes may occur in young patients as well. Maturity-onset diabetes of the young (MODY) is inherited by autosomal dominance and usually presents in the second decade of life. In some families, obesity and insulin resistance play a dominant role, whereas in other families, impaired insulin secretion is more evident. Islet cell antibodies and ketosis are absent. All patients may be treated successfully with oral hypoglycemic agents.

C. MODY patients are as susceptible to the chronic complications of diabetes as other type I or type II patients.

IV. **Treatment**

A. Diet: Dietary modification is generally the first step in controlling hyperglycemia and reducing the risk of accelerated atherosclerosis in type II diabetes.

   1. Total daily calories:
      a. Carbohydrate, 50%
      b. Fats, 30%
      c. Protein, 20%
   2. Complex carbohydrates are preferred to simple concentrated sugars.

3. Saturated fats (animal, dairy) are to be avoided. Cholesterol intake should be reduced to less than 300 mg/day.
4. Caloric intake should be uniformly spread throughout the day, usually among breakfast, lunch, supper, and a bedtime snack.
5. For most type II diabetics a hypocaloric weight reduction diet is of key importance. Caloric restriction and subsequent weight loss will ameliorate insulin resistance. Patients should be referred to a program utilizing dietary and behavior modification and providing adequate encouragement and support.

B. Exercise: Moderate regular physical exercise is beneficial in preventing or reducing glucose intolerance.
1. Weight loss is facilitated.
2. Insulin sensitivity is improved even prior to weight loss.
3. Blood pressure may be lowered.
4. Low density lipoprotein cholesterol may be lowered and high density lipoprotein cholesterol may increase.

C. Oral hyperglycemic agents: When modifications of diet and exercise fail to control hyperglycemia, oral hypoglycemic agents or insulin are indicated. Approximately three-quarters of all type II diabetics will respond well to oral agents, at least initially. Thus a trial of these agents is indicated in all type II patients prior to insulin therapy.
1. Mechanisms of action
   a. Acute and chronic stimulation of insulin release.
   b. Insulin sensitivity may be increased by augmentation of insulin receptors and postreceptor insulin action.
2. Specific drugs
   a. Tolbutamide and acetohexamide are relatively weak drugs with short half-lives requiring dosing two or three times per day.
   b. Tolazamide is also a weak agent which may be given one or two times per day.
   c. Chlorpropamide is a more potent agent with a long half-life. It should always be given once per day. It may cause inappropriate antidiuretic hormone secretion and hyponatremia.
   d. Glyburide and glipizide are newer potent drugs which may be given one or two times per day. They have significant renal clearance and may accumu-

late in renal failure, causing prolonged hypoglycemia.
   e. Glyburide, glipizide, or chlorpropamide may often be more effective than tolbutamide, acetohexamide, or tolazamide.
   f. All oral hypoglycemic agents have the potential to cause serious hypoglycemia, especially in the elderly and those with concurrent illness.
   g. Generally, patients are begun on glyburide (2.5 mg), glipizide (5 mg), or chlorpropamide (100 mg) given as a single daily dose. The dose may be slowly increased over weeks to 10 mg twice per day, 20 mg twice per day, or 500 mg/day, respectively, according to the blood glucose response.
   h. Failure to respond to the more potent drugs reflects severe β-cell exhaustion or continued consumption of excess calories and indicates the need to initiate insulin therapy.

D. Insulin therapy
1. Many overweight type II diabetics will respond adequately to NPH or regular insulin and NPH each morning.
2. The majority of thin type II patients who have failed with oral hypoglycemic therapy have severe insulin secretion defects. Thus they will require NPH and regular insulin both in the morning and at night, similar to type I diabetics.
3. Insulin doses should be adjusted according to home blood glucose monitoring data and glycohemoglobin testing.

E. Combination insulin and oral hypoglycemic agent therapy: A variety of studies have shown minimal improvement in diabetic control when oral hypoglycemic agents are added to insulin therapy. This approach is occasionally helpful in the obese diabetic resistant to more than 150 U of human insulin per day. In most other patients, the small potential benefit could more easily be accrued by a modest increase in their insulin dose. Thus combination therapy is not generally recommended.

F. Diabetogenic drugs
1. Glucocorticoids have the potential to worsen glucose tolerance dramatically in type II diabetics or patients with risk factors for type II diabetes (obesity, family history).

2. Oral hypoglycemic agents are typically ineffective in treating steroid-induced diabetes; insulin is usually required.

3. Thiazide diuretics can be significantly diabetogenic in the susceptible elderly patient. They should be used with caution and avoided if possible in this population.

V. Patient Monitoring

A. Most stable type II diabetics treated with oral hypoglycemic agents may be adequately monitored with daily urine glucose testing and quarterly glycohemoglobin testing. Some patients may benefit from home blood glucose monitoring.

B. Most insulin-treated type II diabetics should perform daily home blood glucose testing. Stable patients may be adequately monitored by one test per day performed at rotating times. The more labile the patient's blood glucose level is, the more often per day testing is advised.

C. All type II diabetics should be followed quarterly with glycohemoglobin testing. Significant improvement in diabetic control may be guided by these data; often these changes would otherwise be inapparent.

Acute Complication

I. The Hyperosmolar Nonketotic Syndrome

A. This severe decompensation of type II diabetes usually occurs in the elderly and has a mortality of 10–30%.

B. Patients may have no prior history of diabetes. Hyperglycemic osmotic diuresis causes dehydration, but residual insulin secretion prevents ketoacidosis.

C. Lethargy, focal or generalized seizures, and coma are common clinical presentations.

D. Mental status is closely related to serum osmolarity. Patients who do not develop compensatory hyponatremia in response to hyperglycemia are most likely to be in a coma.

E. The precipitating cause of hyperosmolar coma is infection in 50% of cases; 25% of patients have an iatrogenic etiology such as unmonitored initiation of glucocorticoid or thiazide therapy or withdrawal of an oral hypoglycemic agent or of insulin.

F. Treatment of hyperosmolar coma is similar to that previously outlined for diabetic ketoacidosis.

1. The intravascular volume deficit must be replaced carefully, according to direct measurements of right- or left-sided cardiac filling pressures.

2. NS, 0.9%, should be given initially but should be changed to 0.45% NS or 5% dextrose in water in patients with significant hypernatremia. Additional volume deficits may be corrected with salt-poor 25% albumin or packed red blood cells. In this manner, the adverse neurologic consequences of worsening hypernatemia may be avoided while correcting tissue hypoperfusion.

3. Most comatose patients should be electively intubated to control oxygenation and ventilation and to protect against aspiration of gastric contents.

4. Most patients should be given empiric broad-spectrum antibiotics after obtaining cultures, whether or not infection is immediately obvious.

5. Continuous intravenous insulin infusion at 0.05 U/kg/hr is appropriate for most patients. Many patients may not require chronic insulin therapy.

6. The complications of hyperosmolar coma include seizures, adult respiratory distress syndrome, lactic acidosis, rhabdomyolysis, vascular thrombosis, and aspiration pneumonia. These and occult infections must be watched for in the diagnosis and therapy of these patients.

Chronic Complications of Diabetes Mellitus

I. Biochemical Basis of Microvascular Complications of Diabetes

A. Sorbitol may accumulate in diabetic nerves and in retinal and glomerular capillaries. It is derived from glucose via aldose reductase. Excess sorbitol may be chronically toxic, and inhibition of aldose reductase may prevent some injury to these tissues in diabetics.

B. Nonenzymatic glycosylation of cellular proteins in diabetic tissues may be more important than sorbitol accumulation. This reaction was first shown in the glycosylation of hemoglobin A. Accumulation of long-lived protein glycosylation products in thickened basement membranes of diabetic cells may play a pivotal role in the etiology of diabetic complications.

II. Risk of Diabetic Microvascular Complications

Is the risk related to long-term control?

A. Long-term (25- to 40-year) prospective non-randomized studies of diabetic control and complications have shown a 10-fold increase in the prevalence of retinopathy, neuropathy, and nephropathy in poorly versus well-controlled patients. Assessment of control in these studies was rather crude, however.

B. Several prospective randomized short-term (1- to 3-year) trials have assessed the effects of near normalization of blood glucose on the progression of established diabetic complications. Benefits have not consistently been shown.

C. The Diabetics Control and Complications Trial (DCCT) is a 7-year prospective randomized trial currently being carried out. Patients with and without objective evidence of established complications have been randomized to a intensive insulin near-normoglycemic group or to an average control group. Glycosylated hemoglobin, as well as retinal, glomerular, and nerve functions, are being serially assessed. Intensively treated patients have a threefold increase in severe hypoglycemia. Hopefully, this large trial will clarify the risks and benefits of intensive insulin therapy.

D. The risk of developing diabetic complications seems to have a strong genetic component as well. Twenty percent of all diabetics will never develop complications despite poor control.

III. Diabetic Retinopathy

A. Background retinopathy can be found in most diabetics after 15 years of hyperglycemia.

1. Microaneurysms
2. Dot hemorrhages
3. Hard exudates (extravasated protein)
4. Macular edema

Macular edema is the only form of nonproliferative diabetic retinopathy which may lead to loss of vision.

B. Proliferative retinopathy begins after 10–15 years of diabetes. Fifty percent of patients may develop proliferative changes after 30 years of disease. Diabetic control in the 5 years prior to the development of proliferative retinopathy is closely associated with its risk of development. It is not halted by a successful pancreas transplant.

1. Neovascularization

2. Vitreous hemorrhage

Proliferative retinopathy is the leading cause of blindness in diabetes; up to 10% of type I diabetics may eventually become blind.

C. Diagnosis and treatment: Studies have shown that nonophthalmologists correctly diagnose only one-half of patients with proliferative retinopathy. Thus it is recommended that all diabetics be examined annually by an experienced ophthalmologist.

1. Laser photocoagulation
2. Vitrectomy

IV. Diabetic Nephropathy

The risk of developing diabetic nephropathy begins after 5 years of disease and peaks at 15–20 years. Thereafter the risk diminishes; only 25–30% of diabetics will eventually develop nephropathy. There is a genetic susceptibility of diabetic nephropathy which is linked to a familial predisposition to hypertension. From 80% to 90% of diabetics who develop nephropathy will also have proliferative retinopathy.

A. Diabetic nephropathy develops in stages.

1. Stage 1: Renal hypertrophy and hyperfiltration. These changes are closely and reversibly related to glycemic control.

2. Stage 2: Mild elevation of urine albumin excretion (microalbuminuria). Preliminary studies suggest that intensive diabetic control with insulin or a pancreas transplant may halt the progression of microalbuminuria. In the absence of near normoglycemia, most patients with microalbuminuria will progress to gross proteinuria and hypertension.

3. Stage 3: Clinical nephropathy with heavy proteinuria. Once this stage is reached, improved diabetic control fails to retard the inevitable progression by all patients to end-stage renal failure. Hypertension develops in most patients.

4. Stage 4: End-stage renal failure. Most diabetics will progress from dipstick-positive albuminuria to end-stage renal failure in 10 years or less. At this stage, coronary atherosclerosis is accelerated and the annual mortality of a diabetic on dailysis increases dramatically.

B. Treatment

1. Various therapies have been shown to retard the progression of the stages of diabetic nephropathy. In stages 1 and 2, improved diabetic control and treatment of hypertension may be helpful. In stage

3, treatment of hypertension is critical. Angiotensin-converting enzyme inhibitors may be more effective than other agents at slowing the progressive increase in albuminuria and serum creatinine. Dietary protein restriction (0.6 g/kg/day) has also been shown to retard the progression of diabetic nephropathy.
2. Chronic hemodialysis.
3. Chronic ambulatory peritoneal dialysis.
4. Kidney transplantation (cadaver or living related).
5. Combined kidney-pancreas transplantation (cadaver).

V. Diabetic Neuropathy
Up to 50% of diabetics will develop one or more types of neuropathy after 30 years of hyperglycemia.
   A. Symmetric distal sensory polyneuropathy
      1. Painful paresthesias.
      2. Loss of pain and temperature.
   B. Symmetric proximal motor neuropathy
      1. Proximal weakness of legs.
      2. Involved muscles may be painful.
   C. Focal motor neuropathy
      1. Foot drop.
      2. Wasting of hand muscles.
      3. Wasting of thigh muscles.
      4. Cranial nerve (III, VI) ophthalmoplegia.
   D. Acute painful neuropathy
      1. Lower extremity.
      2. Thoracoabdominal radiculopathy.
      3. Weight loss and depression often accompany the pain.
      4. Radiculopathy may be misdiagnosed as angina or abdominal malignancy.
      5. CT/MRI is required to rule out spinal cord compression.
      6. A self-limited course and spontaneous recovery are common.
   E. Autonomic neuropathy
      1. Fixed heart rate (R-R interval).
      2. Orthostatic hypotension.
      3. "Silent," painless myocardial ischemia.
      4. Hypoglycemic unawareness.
      5. Gastroparesis.
      6. Diarrhea.
      7. Constipation.
      8. Impotence.
      9. Cystoparesis.
   F. Treatment of diabetic neuropathy
      1. Antidepressants, carbamazapine, and capsaicin cream may be useful in alleviating painful neuropathy.

2. Improvement in diabetic control with intensive insulin or pancreas transplantation may stabilize or improve motor and sensory neuropathy. Autonomic neuropathy is not likely to be helped.
3. Orthostatic hypotension usually responds to fluorohydrocortisone (Florinef, 0.1–0.3 mg/day).
4. Gastroparesis usually responds to metoclopramide and may be helped by erythromycin, cisapride, bethanecol, or dromperidon. Nuclide gastric emptying scanning is useful for diagnosis. Upper endoscopy should be performed, as esophagitis, gastritis, and bezoars are common contributors to nausea and vomiting. They usually respond to H_2 blockers or omeprazole.
5. After other etiologies have been ruled out, chronic diarrhea in the diabetic may be treated with empiric courses of tetracycline (? bacterial overgrowth), opiates, oral or transdermal clonidine, or octreotide.
6. Cystoparesis with urine retention, stasis, and infection may be helped by bethanecol, intermittent catheterization, and antibiotics.

VI. Infections in the Diabetic
   A. Malignant otitis externa
      1. Elderly type II diabetics are at greatest risk.
      2. Otalgia, drainage, facial nerve paralysis, cranial osteomyelitis.
      3. *Pseudomonas aeruginosa* is the dominant pathogen and is treated with appropriate intravenous antibiotics.
   B. Rhinocerebral mucormycosis
      1. Type I diabetics in ketoacidosis are at greatest risk.
      2. Nasal pain, discharge, and necrosis are present.
      3. Surgical drainage and amphotericin B are necessary for successful treatment.
   C. Diabetic foot infections
      1. Risk factors
         a. Sensory neuropathy
         b. Macrovascular disease
         c. Microvascular disease
         d. Uncontrolled hyperglycemia
      2. Clinical stages
         a. Superficial ulcer without infection
         b. Deeper ulcer with soft tissue infection
         c. Ulcer with underlying osteomyelitis
         d. Gangrene

3. Clinical evaluation
   a. Plain x-ray (most will be negative in early osteomyelitis).
   b. Bone scan (positive scan is not very specific for osteomyelitis).
   c. Indium-labeled white blood cell scan is the most accurate test for osteomyelitis.
   d. Bone biopsy and culture provide important microbiologic and histologic information to guide antibiotic choice and duration of therapy.
   e. Noninvasive arterial evaluation will help select those patients who may require arteriography.

4. Treatment
   a. Necrotic soft tissue or bone should be debrided if possible.
   b. All patients with significant cellulitis or osteomyelitis should be hospitalized and treated with intravenous antibiotics active against *Staphylococcus aureus* and gram-negative rods.
   c. Macrovascular ischemia should be corrected with angioplasty or bypass surgery if possible.
   d. Classic therapy for diabetic osteomyelitis is 4–6 weeks of intravenous antibiotics. Recent studies indicate that 10 weeks of oral antibiotics may be effective if preceded by surgical resection of infected bone and 7–10 days of intravenous antibiotics.
   e. Amputation is necessary when extensive necrosis and gangrene are present.

Hypoglycemia

I. Definition

A. Most laboratories place the normal glucose level at 60–100 mg/dl after an overnight fast and at 60–140 mg/dl in the nonfasting state.

B. Using the above criteria, a value below 60 mg/dl would be considered low. However, some individuals, especially females, may have fasting glucose levels as low as 45 mg/dl in the absence of organic pathology.

II. Etiology

A. Fasting hypoglycemia
   1. Islet cell tumor or hyperplasia
      a. Insulinoma—benign or malignant
      b. Nesidioblastosis
   2. Abnormalities of counterregulation
      a. Growth hormone deficiency
      b. Adrenal axis abnormalities
         (1) Isolated adrenocorticotropic hormone deficiency
         (2) Hypopituitarism
         (3) Addison's disease
   3. Nonpancreatic tumors
      a. Retroperitoneal sarcomas
      b. Heptomas
      c. Leukemia or lymphoma
      d. Carcinoid tumors
   4. Renal disease
   5. Hepatic disease
      a. Cirrhosis
      b. Metastatic tumor
      c. Ethanol consumption
      d. Sepsis
   6. Autoimmune disease
      a. Antibodies to insulin
      b. Antibodies to the insulin receptor
   7. Drug induced
      a. Salicylate
      b. Propranolol
      c. Sulfonamides
      d. Lidocaine
      e. Can be seen with sulfonylureas plus nonsteroidal anti-inflammatory drugs
   8. Exercise induced

B. Stimulated hypoglycemia
   1. Alimentary hypoglycemia
   2. Early type II diabetes
   3. Idiopathic

C. Factitious hypoglycemia
   1. Factitious use of insulin
   2. Factitious use of sulfonylureas

III. Pathophysiology

A. Fasting hypoglycemia: Normal glucose homeostasis requires a balance between ingested glucose, glycogen formation, glycogenolysis, and gluconeogenesis.
   1. Normal glucose level is maintained at between 60 and 140 mg/dl. If there is not enough ingested glucose to maintain this level, the liver can break down its store of glycogen via glycogenolysis. The counterregulatory hormones glucagon, epinephrine, growth hormone, and cortisol facilitate this process.
   2. The normal glycogen stores in the liver are able to supply fuel for only a short period of time. Once glycogen stores are utilized, blood glucose is kept stable by gluconeogenesis—the formation of glucose-6-phosphate via precursors. This

control occurs under the same hormonal process that governs glycogenolysis.

3. Increased insulin levels from an insulinoma will decrease glycogenolysis and gluconeogenesis despite a fall in blood glucose.

4. Abnormalities in counterregulation will also prevent appropriate glycogenolysis and gluconeogenesis when glucose is reduced.

5. Nonpancreatic tumors may produce an insulin-like substance that has the same effects on glucose homeostasis as excess insulin. These factors do not cross-react with insulin in assays, and insulin levels will be low.

6. Renal disease
   a. Commonly associated with malnutrition and therefore with decreased precursors for gluconeogenesis.
   b. Glycogenolysis is also decreased.

7. Hepatic disease
   a. Any process that prevents normal liver function will prevent appropriate glycogenolysis and gluconeogenesis.
   b. Ethanol
      (1) Chronic alcoholics will have a poor nutritional status as one contributing factor to hypoglycemia.
      (2) Ethanol intake and subsequent metabolism increase the hepatic reduced nicotinamide-adenine dinucleoide/nicotinamideadenine dinucleotide (NADH/NAD) ratio, which will decrease gluconeogenesis.
      (3) This process usually occurs with ketosis.

8. Autoimmune disease
   a. Antibodies to insulin—autoimmune insulin syndrome (AIS)
      (1) By binding to the insulin receptor, these antibodies can mimic the hypoglycemic action of insulin.
      (2) Patients who have never been exposed to exogenous insulin will have antibodies to insulin.
      (3) Antibodies alternately bind and release. If the unbound portion is increased and not enough glucose is present, blood sugar will drop in the face of the increased insulin level.

9. Drug induced
   a. Seen in patients with poor nutritional status.
   b. The mechanism varies: increasing insulin secretion or increasing glucose uptake.

10. Exercise induced
    a. During exercise, glucose is taken up by the muscle in a insulin-independent manner.
    b. Under normal conditions, the liver will be able to supply enough glucose to prevent hypoglycemia. If the demand cannot be met, hypoglycemia will occur.

B. Stimulated hypoglycemia
   1. Alimentary hypoglycemia: Seen after gastric surgery; there is rapid gastric emptying leading to excessive glucose absorption. The absorption leads to increased insulin release and hypoglycemia.
   2. Early type 1: The postprandial insulin secretion is delayed, and blood glucose will increase transiently. The insulin secretory burst increase is seen later, and hypoglycemia develops.

IV. Diagnosis
A. History
   1. The first step is to determine whether the hypoglycemia occurs in a fasting or postprandial state. This can be done with careful questioning regarding the timing of symptoms in relation to meals.
   2. Symptoms can be divided into two categories
      a. Adrenergic
         (1) Tremor
         (2) Palpitations
         (3) Diaphoresis
         (4) Anxiety
         (5) Hunger
      b. Neuroglycopenic
         (1) Headache
         (2) Confusion
         (3) Blurred vision
         (4) Dizziness
         (5) Seizures
         (6) Unconsciousness
   3. A history of known renal disease, liver disease, autoimmune disease, alcohol abuse, or prior gastric surgery and medications can guide the workup. The presence of cachexia and weight loss may point

to malnutrition or a non–islet cell tumor as a cause.

4. Hypoglycemia in a health care worker or patient with a family member using insulin or sulfonylurea may suggest factitious disease.

B. Clinical signs and physical findings
1. Look for signs of possible liver disease.
   a. Hepatomegaly or splenomegaly
   b. Palmar erythema
   c. Caput medusa
   d. Spider angiomas
   e. Gynecomastia
2. Look for signs of related autoimmune diseases.
   a. Systemic lupus erythematosus
   b. Hashimoto's thyroiditis
   c. Pernicious anemia
   d. Primary biliary cirrhosis
3. Look for signs of adrenal insufficiency.
   a. Increased gingival pigmentation
   b. Increased axillary pigmentation
   c. Weight loss
   d. Nausea and vomiting
   e. Hypotension
4. If the patient experiences severe neuroglycopenia, he or she may have focal neurologic deficits that may make the physician think of cerebrovascular accident. These deficits may be reversed if the hypoglycemia is corrected.

C. Diagnostic tests
1. Document the glucose level. Once it has been documented that the glucose level is low, document that symptoms occur with a low glucose level. Once these findings are confirmed, demonstrate that symptoms resolve after returning the glucose to normal.
2. Consider checking the cortisol level or a cortrosyn stimulation test to rule out adrenal insufficiency.
3. Obtain simultaneous glucose, insulin, and C-peptide levels. Proinsulin may also be helpful. When blood glucose is low:
   a. If insulin is increased and C-peptide is normal or decreased, suspect surreptitious insulin use (Table 123-1).
   b. If insulin is normal or decreased and C-peptide is normal or decreased, suspect a non–islet cell tumor or antireceptor antibody.
      (1) A CT scan of the abdomen may reveal a retroperitoneal sarcoma.

(2) In the proper clinical setting, assaying for antireceptor antibodies will help make the diagnosis.
   c. If both insulin and C-peptide are increased, suspect either an islet cell tumor or surreptitious use of sulfonylurea.
      (1) Urinary sulfonylurea assays are available to help with the diagnosis.
      (2) If insulinoma is suspected, a CT scan of the abdomen may well be negative, as these tumors are very small when hypoglycemia develops. Some investigators suggest doing selective celiac angiography; others believe that the most sensitive test is intraoperative ultrasound.
   d. If a simultaneous glucose, insulin, and C-peptide levels cannot be obtained when the patient is hypoglycemic or nondiagnostic, a 72-hr fast can be instituted in order to make the diagnosis of islet cell tumor.
      (1) At the start, glucose, insulin, and C-peptide samples are obtained every 6 hr. The patient is observed, and any symptoms are recorded.
      (2) If the patient reports any symptoms, glucose, insulin, and C-peptide measurements are performed at that time.
      (3) Most patients with islet cell tumors develop symptomatic hypoglycemia within the first 24 hr, and nearly all do by 72 hr.

V. **Differential Diagnosis of a "Hypoglycemic" Episode**
   A. Angina pectoris
   B. Hyperthyroidism
   C. Pheochromocytoma
   D. Anxiety attack
   E. Temporal lobe seizures
   F. Hyperventilation syndrome
   G. Menopausal hot flashes
   H. Stroke

VI. **Treatment**
   A. Acute therapy
   1. Mild to moderate hypoglycemia: Usually seen with blood sugar levels of 45–60 mg/dl; the patient will usually be able to take carbohydrates; any candy or simple sugar will rapidly raise the blood sugar.

Table 123-1. Autoimmune Diabetes: Immunotherapy

	BB Wistar Rat	Nonobese Diabetic Mouse	Human
Glucocorticoids	X*[89]	X	X[82, 99, 101]
Azathioprine			X[85]
Cyclosporin A	X*[89, 92]	X	X[80, 81, 98]
Ciamexone			X[114]
Anti-lymphocyte serum/globulin	X*[89, 93]	X*	X[99]
MoAb T12			X
MoAb anti-Ia	X*		
MoAb anti-interleukin 2 receptor		X	
Antibody-Anti-ICSA		X	
Neonatal thymectomy	X*[94]	X*	
Irradiation (WB, TLI)	X*[96]	X*	
Ultraviolet light		X*	
Plasmapheresis			X[86]
Silica	X*[97]		
Bone marrow transplantation	X*[91]	X*	
Blood transfusions	X*[90]		X[115]
Lymphocyte infusions	X*[95]		
Dialyzable lymphokine	X[119]		
Interferon			X[111]
Levamisole			X[112]
Methisoprinol			X
OK-432		X*[118]	
Monosodium L-glutamate		X*	
Nicotinamide		X*[117]	X
Hypoglycemia (insulin)	X*[113, 116]		
Modified diet	X*[87]		

MoAb, monoclonal antibody; WB, whole body; TLI, total lymphoid irradiation.

*Prophylactic/therapeutic effect, in terms of amelioration of diabetes.

Source: Reprinted with permission from Vardi et al., *Diabetes Care*, Vol. 10, 1987. Copyright 1987 by American Diabetes Association, Inc.

2. More profound hypoglycemia will usually present emergently. The patient can be given ampules of 50% dextrose intravenously until blood sugar returns to normal. If necessary, maintenance infusions of 10–20% dextrose can be given until euglycemia established.

B. If counterregulatory deficiency occurs: Replace absent hormone (e.g., cortisone acetate, 25 mg in the morning and 12.5 mg in the evening).

C. Stop any medication that may be contributing to hypoglycemia.

D. Small, frequent meals may decrease the occurrence of alimentary hypoglycemia.

E. Provide psychiatric therapy for factitious use of insulin or sulfonylurea.

F. Non–islet cell tumors: Identify and treat with either chemotherapy or radiation therapy.

G. Autoimmune diseases: Corticosteroids may be helpful; dilantin or diazoxide may also be useful.

H. Islet cell tumor: Surgery should be performed for insulinoma; if the patient is not a surgical candidate, diazoxide may be helpful.

Bibliography

Eisenbarth GS. Type I diabetes mellitus. A chronic autoimmune disease. *N Engl J Med* 314:1360–1368, 1986.

Field J. Hypoglycemia. Endocrinology and metabolism. *Med Clin North Am* 18:1–257, 1989.

Gerich JE. Oral hypoglycemic agents. *N Engl J Med* 321:1231–1245, 1989.

Nelson RL. Hypoglycemia: Fact or fiction? *Mayo Clin Proc* 60:844–850, 1985.

Singer DE, Coley CM, Samet JH, et al. Tests of glycemia in diabetes mellitus: Their use in establishing a diagnosis and in treatment. *Ann Intern Med* 110:125–137, 1989.

Zinman B. The physiologic replacement of insulin: An elusive goal. *N Engl J Med* 321:363–370, 1989.

CHAPTER 124

Ectopic Hormone and Multiple Endocrine Neoplasia Syndromes

Will G. Ryan, M.D.

Ectopic Hormone Syndromes

I. **Definition**

Peptide or glycopeptide hormone production by nonendocrine gland tumors (often malignant) resulting in clinical manifestations resembling classic hypersecreting endocrine gland syndromes.

II. **Etiology**

Generally malignant transformation of the cells of certain tumors, possibly resulting in gene derepression such that they produce various hormones.

III. **Pathophysiology**

Overproduction of various hormones (see Table 124-1 for the best-described syndromes).

A. Adrenocorticotropic hormone (ACTH): Small cell cancer of lung, carcinoid tumors.

B. Antidiuretic hormone: Small cell cancer of lung.

C. Parathyroid hormone-related protein: Squamous cell cancers of the lung, head, and neck; hypernephroma; and others.

D. Gonadotropins (principally human chorionic gonadotropin): Various types of lung carcinoma, hepatic carcinoma, and others.

E. Other less common factors: trophoblastic thyrotropin, hypoglycemia with non–islet cell tumors, calcitonin, erythropoietin, placental lactogen, prolactin, growth hormone and growth hormone-releasing hormone, vasoactive intestinal polypeptide, renin, hypophosphatemic osteomalacia factor.

IV. **Diagnosis**

A. History: Similar to that of classic endocrine syndromes but tend to follow a more fulminant course.

B. Clinical signs and physical findings: As above.

C. Diagnostic tests: As above. Various imaging procedures necessary to localize the offending tumor.

V. **Differential Diagnosis**

That of the classic endocrine syndrome it may be mimicking.

VI. **Treatment**

Surgical removal of the offending tumor if

Table 124-1. Ectopic Hormone Syndromes

Type	Tumor	Humoral Substance	Remarks
Humoral hyper-calcemia of malignancy	Most often squamous cell cancer of the lung, head or neck; also renal or ovarian cancer, etc.	Parathyroid hormone-related protein (18,000 daltons)	Usually more severe hypercalcemia than that seen with hyperparathyroidism. Specific assay becoming available. Parathyroid hormone levels suppressed.
Hypercortisolism	Most often small cell carcinoma of the lung; also carcinoid tumors, etc.	ACTH	Usually more fulminant hypercortisolism with electrolyte disturbance and hyperpigmentation due to very high level of ACTH. Carcinoid tumors tend to produce the more classic Cushing syndrome.
Hypoglycemia	Usually hepatomas or large mesenchymal tumors such as fibrosarcomas, leiomyosarcomas, etc.	Possibly IGF I or II	Insulin levels usualy suppressed.

Table 124-2 MEN Syndromes

MEN Type I	MEN Type IIa	MEN Type IIb
Pituitary (65%)*	Medullary thyroid (100%)	Medullary thyroid (100%)
Pancreas (75%)	Pheochromocytomas (50%)	Pheochromocytomas (50%)
Parathyroid (90%)	Parathyroid (20%)	Mucosal neuromas with marfanoid habitus (100%)

Pituitary tumors (MEN type I): Usually benign, most often growth hormone, prolactin, or ACTH producing.

Pancreatic tumors (MEN type I): Usually gastrinomas (30% malignant) or insulinomas (sometimes malignant). Other tumors occasionally (somatostinomas, glucagonomas, pancreatic peptidomas).

Parathyroid adenomas or hyperplasia (MEN I and IIa): When hypercalcemia occurs, removal of at least three and one-half glands with autotransplantation of the remaining one-half indicated to prevent recurrent hypercalcemia. Rare malignancies reported.

Medullary thyroid carcinoma (often preceded by hyperplasia (MEN IIa and IIb): Multicentric and total thyroidectomy is indicated as son as the diagnosis is made. Annual screening of first-degree relatives, including small children with serum calcitonin concentration (preferably with pentagastrin or calcium stimulation), indicated for early diagnosis. Medullary carcinoma may be quite indolent or very aggressive. Those in MEN IIb are generally quite aggressive. This tumor has been associated with the production of over 20 bioactive substances ranging from calcitonin to chromogranin A.

Pheochromocytomas (MEN IIa and IIb): Tendency to be epinephrine rather than norepinephrine producing; most are bilateral; hyperplasia precedes tumor.

Other tumors (lipomas, carcinoid, adrenocortical adenomas, vipomas, etc.) may be seen occasionally, particularly in MEN I.

*Percentage numbers in parentheses refer to approximate incidence of the various syndromes.

possible; chemotherapy or radiation therapy of nonresectable tumors.

VII. Patient Monitoring

Generally as for classic endocrine syndromes.

VIII. Prognosis

Good if the tumor can be completely eradicated, poor if this cannot be done.

Multiple Endocrine Neoplasia (MEN) Syndromes

A group of hereditary autosomal dominant disorders with a high degree of penetrance and variable expression resulting in hyperplasia and/or tumors of various glands. Highlights of the syndromes are delineated in Table 124-2.

Bibliography

Blackman MR, Rosen SW, Weintraub BD. Ectopic hormones. *Adv Intern Med* 23:85–113, 1978.

Brandi ML. Familial multiple endocrine neoplasia Type I: A new look at the pathophysiology. *Endocinol Rev* 8:391–405, 1987.

Felig P, Baxter JD, Broadens AE, et al. (eds). *Endocrinology and Metabolism,* ed 2. New York, McGraw-Hill, 1987.

Gagel RF, Levy ML, Donovan DT, et al. Multiple endocrine neoplasia type 2a associated with cutaneous lichen amyloidosis. *Ann Intern Med* 111:802–806, 1989.

Grauer A, Raue F, Gogel RF. Changing concepts in the management of hereditary and sporadic medullary thyroid carcinoma. *Endocinol Metab Clin Am* 19:613–635, 1990.

Sipple JH. The association of pheochromocytoma with carcinoma of the thyroid. *Am J Med* 31:163, 1961.

Wermer P. Genetic aspects of adenomatosis of endocrine glands. *Am J Med* 16:363–371, 1954.

CHAPTER 125

Blood Lipid Disorders

John D. Bagdade, M.D.

I. Definition

Dyslipidemia is defined as an increase in plasma triglyceride, cholesterol, or both or an isolated reduction in high density lipoprotein C (HDL-C). Patients with these disorders demonstrate increased concentrations of one or more of the following major lipoprotein classes (A, B below) or a reduction in HDL-C (C, below) in plasma obtained after a 12-hr fast:

A. Triglyceride-rich lipoproteins: Occasionally, chylomicrons formed in the gut in response to the ingestion of dietary fat, but more often very low density lipoproteins (VLDL) which are being continuously synthesized and secreted by the liver.

B. Cholesterol-rich lipoproteins: Low density lipoproteins (LDL), which are normally a product of the catabolism of VLDL but which in certain abnormal conditions may also be produced de novo by the liver.

C. HDL: Produced in nascent form by the liver and intestine but acquire surface constituents from the catabolism of triglyceride (TG)-rich lipoproteins during their delipidation by lipoprotein lipase.

II. Etiology

Dyslipidemia results when there is an imbalance between the production and removal of these lipoprotein classes.

A. Hypertriglyceridemia may be due to:
  1. Increased VLDL production.
  2. Decreased removal of VLDL and chylomicrons, which is mediated by the tissue lipoprotein lipase (LpL) enzyme system.
  3. A combination of the above.

B. Hypercholesterolemia may be due to:
  1. Increased LDL production.
  2. Decreased LDL uptake.

C. Low-HDL syndromes may result from:
  1. Rare inherited disorders in which the synthesis of apoprotein-A-I, the principal apoprotein of HDL, is reduced or its catabolism is accelerated.
  2. Impairment in the function of LpL in the delipidation cascade of the triglyceride-rich lipoproteins (chylomicrons, VLDL, intermediate density lipoprotein [IDL]) which leads to a decrease in the availability of lipoprotein surface lipids (phospholipid, free cholesterol) and apoproteins (A-II, E,

C) that are essential for the maturation of HDL in plasma.

III. Pathophysiology

A. VLDL overproduction
1. Primary (inherited) forms: Familial hypertriglyceridemia, familial combined hyperlipidemia.
2. Secondary: Alcohol, hyperinsulinemic states/obesity, estrogen, non-insulin-dependent diabetes mellitus (NIDDM), acromegaly.
3. Findings: Elevated plasma TG, reduced HDL-C.

B. Reduced LpL activity.
1. Primary (inherited) forms: Deficiency of the enzyme or its activator, apoprotein C-II.
2. Secondary: Poorly controlled diabetes mellitus (untreated), uremia, hypothyroidism, autoimmune disease.
3. Findings: Elevated plasma TG, reduced HDL-C.

C. Impaired removal of remnant lipoproteins.
1. Primary (inherited) form: Broad beta disease (type III) resulting from a mutation in the primary structure of apoprotein E.
2. Secondary: Liver disease, hypothyroidism.
3. Findings: Increased triglyceride and cholesterol levels, reflecting the accumulation of remnant particles.

D. LDL overproduction.
1. Primary: (Inherited) familial combined hyperlipidemia, familial hypercholesterolemia.
2. Secondary: Nephrotic syndrome, glucocorticoid treatment.
3. Findings: Elevated total plasma and LDL cholesterol.

E. Impaired catabolism of LDL.
1. Primary (inherited): Deficient or dysfunctional LDL receptors can cause familial hypercholesterolemia.
2. Secondary: Hypothyroidism (since thyroxine is required to regulate LDL receptor function), insulin-deficient diabetes mellitus.

IV. Diagnosis

Dyslipidemia should be suspected in individuals who have evidence of coronary heart disease before the age of 55 or who have first-degree relatives with premature cardiovascular disease.

A. Historical data
1. Premature atherosclerotic heart disease has been associated with all of the above disturbances except the inherited form of LpL deficiency.
2. Presence of other cardiac risk factors (smoking, obesity, hypertension, diabetes mellitus, male gender) increases the cardiovascular risk geometrically.
3. Previous unexplained recurrent pancreatitis raises the possibility of LpL deficiency.
4. Medications can exacerbate dyslipidemia: thiazide diuretics, β-blockers, estrogens, anabolic steroids, isoretinoin.

B. Physical findings attributable to a specific alteration in lipoprotein transport are generally not present unless the disturbance in lipid transport is marked.
1. Chylomicronemia syndromes cause abdominal pain, lipemia retinalis, and eruptive xanthoma on the buttocks, elbows, and knees.
2. Broad beta disease is associated with palmar, planar, and tuberous xanthomas.
3. Hypercholesterolemia, when severe, can cause xanthomata in extensor and Achilles tendons.

C. Tests: Laboratory data should confirm the impression derived from the history and physical exam. Reliable measurements of plasma lipids (TG, cholesterol, HDL-C) are essential in establishing the correct diagnosis.
1. Plasma lipid measurements after a 12- to 14-hr overnight fast are most important, and abnormalities should be confirmed by repeat testing.
   a. When TG is increased with normal cholesterol, VLDL is increased.
   b. When chylomicronemia is present, TG usually exceeds 2,000 mg/dl; cholesterol may be moderately elevated when TG is very high because of the minor cholesterol content of chylomicrons and VLDL.
   c. When plasma cholesterol is elevated with a normal plasma TG, the LDL concentration is usually increased, although occasionally it may reflect marked increases in HDL.
   d. When plasma TG and cholesterol are both increased significantly, a combined elevation of VLDL and LDL is usually present. Occasionally, this profile reflects the accumulation of remnant particles in patients with dysbetalipoproteinemia.
2. Apoprotein studies: May be useful in spe-

cial situations, such as in establishing the diagnosis of broad beta disease (by confirming the presence of an abnormal isoform of apoprotein E) or quantitating lipoprotein a in patients with unexplained premature coronary artery disease. In most cases at present, the measurement of apoproteins B and A-I provides information that is no more useful than reliable plasma lipid measurements (TG, cholesterol, HDL-C).

V. Differential Diagnosis

Dyslipidemia can be a manifestation of another systemic disease or can result from various medical therapies.

A. Medical causes (hypothyroidism, nephrotic syndrome, chronic uremia, diabetes mellitus, particularly NIDDM, obesity).

B. Iatrogenic (oral contraceptives, glucocorticoid and anabolic steroids, isoretinoin, thiazide diuretics, β-blockers).

VI. Treatment

A. Rationale: It is now well established that elevated TG or cholesterol and decreased HDL-C all increase the cardiovascular risk, and that reversing these abnormalities through aggressive intervention reduces this risk. Moreover, lipid-modifying treatments have now been shown not only to arrest the progression but also to reverse preexisting coronary lesions. Since not all patients are likely to benefit to the same degree, individual strategies need to be developed for their control in each patient to achieve these goals. In patients with severe triglyceride elevation, the goal is to prevent pancreatitis.

B. Goals: Goals of therapy for each lipid abnormality should be established, taking into account the presence of other risk factors.

1. In the presence of coronary heart disease (CHD) or two or more risk factors, LDL-C should be less than 130 mg/dl, triglycerides less than 150 mg/dl, and HDL-C greater than 45 mg/dl.

2. In the absence of CHD or other risk factors, LDL-C should be less than 160 mg/dl triglycerides under 200 mg/dl, and HDL-C greater than 40 mg/dl.

C. Approach

1. Diet: The American Heart Association (AHA) "Step" diets are useful not only for patients with high cholesterol, but also for those with high triglyceride levels. In the elderly and in pregnant women with in-

creased nutrient requirements, adjustments may need to be made.

a. Step one diet: Total dietary fat below 30% of total calories, saturated fat below 10% of calories, cholesterol intake below 300 mg/day (restricting egg yolks and organ meats such as liver, kidney, brains, and sweetbreads), polyunsaturated fat less than 10%, and monounsaturated fat 10–15% of total calories.

b. If the goal is not met after 6–12 weeks, continued regular visits with the dietitian may be helpful for ensuring compliance. Alternatively, further restricting dietary fat in a Step two diet (saturated fat below 7% of calories and daily cholesterol intake less than 200 mg/day) may be necessary.

c. Duration of diet therapy alone may be up to 6 months, with monitoring of responses at 6- to 8-week intervals; for patients with other risk factors or evidence of CHD, this period may be shortened considerably.

d. Special considerations

(1) Chylomicronemia syndrome patients may require severe restriction of dietary fat (10–20% of total calories as fat). LPL deficiency in its inherited form can only be treated with diet, as drugs have no effect.

(2) Hypertriglyceridemic patients will respond to caloric restriction but may need to reduce ingestion of simple sugars and alcohol.

(3) Exercise is useful adjunctive therapy because it may facilitate weight loss, reduce triglycerides, and increase HDL-C.

2. Drug therapy: Indicated if the desired directional change in plasma lipids has not been achieved after an appropriate trial of diet and (where indicated) exercise and weight reduction. Treatment goals with regard to specific plasma lipid levels are the same as for diet therapy (see Section VI, A above). Diet therapy must be continued. Drug choices: only three drugs (niacin, cholestyramine, and gemfibrozil) have been shown to lower the cardiovascular risk in large clinical trials. Though they are widely used, no comparable information is available in patients treated with the

(HMGCoA) reductase inhibitor lovastatin or with probucol.

a. Specific low-density lipoprotein (LDL)-lowering agents

(1) Bile acid binding resins: Cholestyramine (initial dose, 4 g twice per day) and cholestipol (initial 5 g twice per day) bind bile acids in the intestine. By preventing their resorption, hepatic cholesterol is diverted to bile acid synthesis and LDL receptors are up-regulated. Total plasma cholesterol declines about 5% with each packet or scoop of resin. Compliance is enhanced by starting with low doses.

(a) Side effects: mainly gastrointestinal (constipation, bloating, heartburn, flatulence). Resins after the absorption of thiazides, warfarin, thyroxine, and digoxin, which should be taken 1 hr before or 4 hr after resins. VLDL levels may increase.

(2) Niacin: This water-soluble vitamin is a broad-spectrum, lipid-modifying drug. The key to successful treatment is to start with low doses and increase slowly. Since untoward effects with niacin and other lipid-lowering drugs are dose related, raising doses above 2–2.5 g/day may not be prudent. Initial dosage should be 250 mg/day of niacin before meals for 1 week, increasing by 250 mg/week until the dose is 1.5 g/day. At that time the plasma lipid response should be evaluated. Liver function tests should also be monitored on a regular basis. Aspirin (325 mg) taken once daily about 30 min before niacin will attenuate the prostaglandin-mediated flush reaction, which subsides without aspirin in 1–2 months.

(a) Side effects limit the use of niacin in one-third of patients. These include nausea, dyspepsia, activation of peptic ulcer, anorexia, dizziness, hypotension, and gout. Laboratory abnormalities include hyperuricemia, liver dysfunction (with actual hepatitis), and glucose intolerance.

(b) Contraindications: Gout, peptic ulcer disease, inflammatory bowel disease, cardiac arrhythmias. NIDDM is a relative contraindication.

(3) Probucol (Lorelco) is the only lipid-modifying drug that is an antioxidant and, as such, may be anti-atherogenic. Its mechanism for lowering LDL (approximately 20%) is unknown but appears not to require the LDL receptor, since it lowers LDL in receptor-deficient patients and animals. Its low incidence of side effects makes it useful in combination therapy. Probucol has not been prescribed widely in the United States because of concern about its lowering of HDL-C (approximately 15–20% reduction), but it has been used effectively throughout the world and there is no clinical evidence that this decrease is deleterious.

b. Lovastatin: This HMGCoA reductase inhibitor is widely used in the United States (20 mg/day with the evening meal) because of its effective LDL-lowering properties (−25%) and favorable profile of short-term side effects. In certain hypercholesterolemic patients, it also appears to lower triglycerides and raise HDL-C. Because there is no evidence from clinical trials that lovastatin reduces the cardiovascular risk, and because no information is available about its possible long-term side effects, the use of lovastatin should be confined to high-risk patients or those unable to tolerate the other available drugs.

(1) Side effects: Are dose dependent, and it is questionable whether increasing the dose beyond 20 mg twice per day results in any further lowering of LDL. Lovastatin is generally well tolerated, but it may cause a variety of transient gastrointestinal symptoms and insomnia. Mild abnormalities in liver function are common and, as with niacin, usually decrease with continued therapy. Myalgias, myositis, and elevated creatine phosphokinase levels occur in 2% of patients.

Liver function tests should be monitored during initiation of therapy.

c. Specific VLDL-lowering drugs

(1) Gemfibrozil (Lopid) lowers plasma triglyceride levels by decreasing VLDL production and enhancing LPL-related triglyceride removal. Gemfibrozil (600 mg twice per day with meals) raises HDL-C both by improving the delipidation of VLDL and by directly stimulating the synthesis apoprotein A-I, the principal apoprotein of HDL. Like cholestyramine and niacin, gemfibrozil has been shown in a large clinical trial to decrease the cardiovascular risk.

(a) Side effects: Nausea, bloating, abdominal pain, diarrhea, and headache are infrequent, and the drug is generally well tolerated. After initiating therapy, liver function should be monitored. Gemfibrozil may be used effectively but with caution in hyperlipidemic transplant patients in combination with lovastatin (no more than 20 mg/day) and alone at a markedly reduced dosage in patients with end-stage renal disease. The effects of warfarin are potentiated by gemfibrozil.

d. Specific HDL-raising drugs

(1) Niacin at relatively low doses (1–2 g/day) may raise HDL-C.

(2) Gemfibrozil (600 mg twice per day; see above) appears to have salutary effects on HDL by two different mechanisms.

Bibliography

Brown MS, Goldstein JL. A receptor-mediated pathway for cholesterol homeostasis. *Science* 232:34–47, 1986.

Frick MH, ELO O, Haapa K, et al. Helsinki Heart Study: Primary prevention trial with gemfibrozil in middle-aged men with dyslipidemia: Safety of treatment changes in risk factors, and incidence of coronary heart disease. *J Engl J Med* 317:1237–1245, 1987.

Havel RJ. Lowering cholesterol, 1988. Rationale, mechanisms, and means. *J Clin Invest* 81:1653–1660, 1988.

Lipid Research Clinics Program. The Lipid Research Clinics Coronary Primary Prevention Trial results II. The relationship of reduction in incidence of coronary heart disease to cholesterol lowering. *JAMA* 251:365–374, 1984.

Stampfer MJ, Sacks FM, Salvini S, et al. A prospective study of cholesterol, apolipoproteins, and the risk of myocardial infarction. *N Engl J Med* 325:373–381, 1991.

The Expert Panel: Report of the National Cholesterol Education Program Expect Panel on Detection, Evaluation and Treatment of High Blood Cholesterol in Adults. *Arch Intern Med* 148:36–39, 1988.

SECTION 13

Neurology

CHAPTER 126

The Approach to the Patient with a Neurologic Problem

Barry J. Riskin, M.D.
Michael C. Smith, M.D.

Many physicians are uncomfortable when caring for patients with neurologic problems. Most do not know how to organize and perform the neurologic examination. In this section, we will attempt to simplify and organize the approach to patients with neurologic problems. deficiency

I. Step I

To begin with, one must recognize that despite the complexity of the nervous system and the many etiologies and mechanisms of nervous system disease, there are a limited number of ways in which disease processes manifest themselves in terms of their pattern of nervous system dysfunction. The first step, therefore, in the approach to the patient with a neurologic problem is to *recognize* the type or pattern of nervous system dysfunction.

A. Changes in the level of consciousness
   1. Delirium.
   2. Stupor and coma.
B. Abnormalities of cognitive function
   1. Impairment of memory (e.g., dementing illnesses).
   2. Impairment of language (e.g., aphasia).
   3. Impairment of attention (e.g., neglect).

C. Abnormalities of motor function
   1. Loss of strength (i.e., weakness).
   2. Changes in muscle tone (e.g., spasticity, flaccidity).
   3. Abnormal involuntary movements
      a. Tremor.
      b. Chorea.
      c. Myoclonus.
      d. Motor manifestations of seizures (e.g., automatism).
   4. Abnormal posture
      a. Decorticate, decerebrate.
      b. Opisthotonic.
D. Sensory impairment
   1. Loss of sensation, numbness, tingling.
E. Loss of coordinated movement
   1. Observed as dyssynergia, dysmetria, and dysdiadochokinesia of the arms and legs.
   2. Nystagmus of the eyes.
F. Gait abnormalities
   1. Impairment of gait can include difficulty initiating walking, loss of postural or "righting" reflexes, or difficulty maintaining balance.
G. Abnormal reflexes
   1. Extensor toe sign (Babinski), clonus, or loss of reflexes.

II. Step 2

The next important step in the care of patients with a suspected neurologic problem is to match the *type* of dysfunction with the *level* within the nervous system in which the dysfunction has occurred. This process is called *localization*.

A. Lesions localized to the cerebral hemispheres
1. Focal versus global lesions
a. Focal lesions lead to discrete dysfunction (e.g., visual field deficits, aphasia, hemiparesis).
b. Global disturbances lead to widespread dysfunction (e.g., delirium, stupor, coma).

B. Lesions localized to the brain stem
1. Cranial nerve dysfunction is the most important localizing sign.
2. Often produce "crossed" syndromes (e.g., ipsilateral cranial nerve III dysfunction with contralateral hemiparesis).

C. Lesions localized to the spinal cord
1. Often localized by the level of sensory dysfunction.
2. Loss of vibration, position sense, and strength with increased reflexes are observed ipsilateral to the side of the lesion.
3. Pin and temperature sense are affected contralateral to the side of the lesion.

D. Lesions localized to the peripheral nerve
1. Lead to loss of strength, sensation, and reflexes.
2. Can lead to abnormal sensation (e.g., burning, tingling).

E. Lesions localized to the neuromuscular junction
1. Weakness is the chief complaint, especially with the repetitive use of muscles.
2. Can produce other symptoms by virtue of muscle weakness, but weakness is often not the chief complaint (e.g., double vision, difficulty swallowing, shortness of breath).

F. Lesions localized to muscle
1. Lead to loss of strength, most often in the proximal muscles.
2. Can produce symptoms of pain, swelling, or cramping.

III. History

Emphasis must be placed on the history.

A. Besides obtaining the history of the patient, corroborative histories should be obtained (e.g., from family members, emergency personnel, other treating physicians and health care workers).

1. Attention should be paid to the timing of all symptoms.
a. Episodic or persistent (e.g., transient cerebral ischemia vs. cerebral infarction).
b. Onset: Sudden or slowly developing (e.g., acute headache from aneurysmal subarachnoid hemorrhage vs. migraine headache).
c. Frequency: Increasing, decreasing, staying the same (e.g., weakness of myasthenia gravis after repetitive muscle use).
d. Duration of symptoms: Confusion lasting for several minutes in a postictal state vs. lengthy confusion in encephalopathic states.
e. Specific time of day: Headache worse in morning often secondary to increased intracranial pressure.
f. Associated with specific activity (e.g., radicular back pain made worse by coughing, sneezing, straining to stool—Valsalva maneuver).

2. Determine the quality of the symptoms.
a. Are there single or multiple symptoms (e.g., pure hemiplegia of lacunar infarction vs. hemiparesis with vertigo and double vision indicative of brain stem dysfunction)?
b. Are there associated nonneurologic symptoms that occur before, during, or after the neurologic symptoms (e.g., diaphoresis, palpitations, and/or nausea associated with cardiac arrhythmia)?
c. What improves or worsens symptoms (e.g., positional sensitivity in various types of benign vertigo)?

3. Has there been any previous medical investigation of current symptoms?
a. What did past workup consist of, including diagnostic tests (e.g., magnetic resonance imaging, computed tomography, electromyography/nerve conduction velocity)?
b. Were previous diagnoses made surrounding current symptoms (e.g., atrial fibrillation, carotid stenosis)?

4. Determine pertinent points from the general history.
a. All past medical conditions and current medical illnesses; identify significant risk factors.
b. Recent or past surgeries: Carotid en-

darterectomy, coronary artery bypass graft, cardiac valve replacement, any surgery where the position of the arms and legs may have caused peripheral nerve or plexus injury.

c. Past and current medications (e.g., antiplatelet agents, anticoagulants, past anticonvulsants tried, sedatives, other neurotropic medications).

d. Allergies to medication.

e. Recent and past trauma, with attention to head, neck, and back injuries.

f. Childhood or birth-related disorders (e.g., perinatal hypoxia, childhood seizures, developmental delay, meningitis-encephalitis).

g. Family history of similar complaints (e.g., neoplasms of the nervous system in neurofibromatosis).

h. Alcohol, tobacco, and illicit drug use; risk factors for malignancies, trauma, withdrawal states.

i. Occupational and toxic exposure (e.g., risk factors in neuropathies).

j. Travel history (e.g., endemic areas for Lyme disease, neuroborreliois, neurocystericosis).

IV. Physical Examination

The purpose of the physical examination is to confirm the suspected level of dysfunction. If the findings of the physical exam are unexpected, the history should be reviewed.

A. Initial assessment includes the patient's general appearance and vital signs.

B. The neurologic examination should be complete but should focus on the suspected level of dysfunction.

1. Cerebral hemispheric testing
   a. Level of spontaneous and sustained arousal.
   b. Ability to maintain attention.
   c. Language
      (1) Fluency: Number of words per minute spoken.
      (2) Comprehension: Ability to follow commands.
      (3) Repetition: Repeat "No ifs, ands, or buts."
      (4) Naming, pointing to object and asking: "What would you call this?"
   d. Memory
      (1) Immediate
         (a) Verbal: Remember three words at 5 min.
         (b) Spatial: Remember the location of three hidden objects in 5 min.
      (2) Remote: Events of the past.
   e. Judgment, insight, and overall fund of knowledge.

2. Cranial nerve testing
   a. Visual acuity with and without corrective lenses.
   b. Visual fields to confrontation.
   c. Extraocular movement.
   d. Pupillary size and reactivity.
   e. Facial symmetry, spontaneous and on command.
   f. Facial and corneal sensation.
   g. Gross hearing.
   h. Tongue and oropharyngeal movement.

3. Motor testing
   a. Strength, major muscle groups.
   b. Muscle bulk, presence of tenderness, swelling.
   c. Tone of extremities to passive movement.
   d. Presence of abnormal movements, postures.

4. Sensory testing
   a. Primary sensory modalities
      (1) Vibratory and position sense.
         (a) Romberg test.
      (2) Pin and temperature.
      (3) Light touch.
   b. Cortical sensation
      (1) Graphaesthesia.
      (2) Stereognosis.
      (3) Double simultaneous stimulation.
      (4) Neglect.

5. Cerebellar testing
   a. Finger to nose.
   b. Heel to shin.
   c. Rapid alternating movements.
   d. Testing eye movements for nystagmus.

6. Gait testing
   a. General appearance of gait: Speed, direction, degree of difficulty.
   b. Stance: Narrow versus wide base.
   c. Associated movements (e.g., arm swing).
   d. Tests of strength
      (1) Toe walking.
      (2) Heel walking.
   e. Tandem gait: Walk heel to toe.
   f. Postural reflex: Ability to remain upright despite perturbation backward.

7. Reflexes
   a. Deep tendon reflexes.

b. Abnormal reflexes.
  (1) Extensor toe on plantar stimulation (i.e., Babinski's sign).
  (2) Snout, grasp, and sustained blinking on glabellar tapping.
  (3) Crossed adduction on stimulation of the deep tendon reflex of the knee.

V. Diagnostic Testing

Diagnostic testing focuses on the suspected level of dysfunction.

  A. Neuroimaging tests
    1. Magnetic resonance imaging: Advantages include excellent visualization of the posterior fossa (cerebellum and brain stem), temporal lobes, and spinal cord. Disadvantages include high cost and inability to visualize bony structures.
    2. Computed tomography: Advantages include short duration of the test and excellent visualization of bone and acute blood. Disadvantages include poor visualization of temporal lobes and the structures of the posterior fossa.
    3. Cerebral angiography: Used to visualize the vascular tree that supplies the cranium. The test usually includes both the intracerebral and extracerebral vasculature.
  B. Electrodiagnostic tests
    1. Electroencephalography: This test is used to characterize and localize any abnormal brain wave activity. It can be used for both focal and global disorders. It is most often used to document the presence of epileptiform activity.
    2. Electromyography and nerve conduction study: These tests are often performed in tandem to evaluate the integrity of the peripheral nervous system: nerve, muscle, and neuromuscular junction.
    3. Evoked potentials
      a. Three types of evoked potential testing
        (1) Visual
        (2) Somatosensory
        (3) Brain stem auditory
        (4) Long latency (P300)
          (a) Used today for investigational purposes.
          (b) May one day be utilized in diagnosing certain dementing illnesses (e.g., Alzheimer's disease).
      b. These tests can evaluate the integrity of the peripheral and central pathways used in somatic sensation, vision, and hearing. Evoked potentials may help to differentiate central from peripheral nervous system dysfunction.
  C. Lumbar puncture: Cerebrospinal fluid obtained after lumbar puncture can be used to test for evidence of hemorrhage, inflammation, infection, or malignancy in the central nervous system.

VI. Summary of the Diagnostic Approach

  A. In order to diagnose correctly and treat disorders of the nervous system (either primary or secondary), one must first elicit a careful and thorough history. Then one must perform the physical examination, with emphasis on the suspected level of dysfunction.
  B. One must be able to recognize the pattern of nervous system dysfunction, localize the anatomic level of the dysfunction, and focus the diagnostic tests at the suspected level.
  C. The remainder of this section will describe the types of neurologic disorders, their manifestations of dysfunction, and ways to approach their respective diagnoses and treatments.

Bibliography

Adams RD, Victor M. Principles of Neurology, ed 5. McGraw Hill, New York, 1993.

Merritt HH. Merritt's Textbook of Neurology, ed 8. Lea and Febiger, Philadelphia, 1989.

CHAPTER 127

Diagnostic Procedures

Joseph J. Jares III, M.D.
Robert B. Wright, M.D.

I. General
  A. Diagnostic procedures are not a substitute for basic clinical skills of history taking and neurologic examination.
  B. They are best utilized when a specific hypothesis needs testing.

II. Specific Diagnostic Procedures
  A. Lumbar puncture (LP) and cerebrospinal fluid (CSF) examination
    1. Technique
      a. Best performed with patient in lateral decubitus position, with hips and knees flexed; may also be performed in sitting position.
      b. Lumbar interspaces are identified; L3–L4 interspace is perpendicular to the spinal column at the superior iliac.
      c. The skin is cleansed with antiseptic solution; using sterile technique, the lumbar region is draped.
      d. Local anesthetic is infused into skin, subcutaneous, and deeper regions at L3–L4 interspace.
      e. Spinal needle is inserted in L3–L4 interspace, with stylet in place, and slowly advanced until lumbar subarachnoid space is entered.
      f. The stylet is removed and a three-way stopcock connected to a spinal fluid manometer is connected to the hub of the spinal needle.
      g. Patient's legs and neck are extended; CSF is allowed to flow into manometer, and opening CSF pressure measurement to be made. If patient is in a sitting position, after spinal needle is inserted into lumbar subarachnoid space, the patient is first placed in the lateral decubitus position.
      h. After the opening pressure is measured, collect the CSF samples in sterile tubes.
      i. After CSF specimen is obtained, the stopcock is repositioned to direct flow back into manometer and the closing pressure is measured.
      j. The stopcock and manometer are removed, the stylet is reinserted into the cannula, and the spinal needle is removed. A sterile bandage is placed over the puncture site.

2. Indications
   a. Nervous systems infections: Meningitis, encephalitis, and rarely, abscesses after computed tomography (CT) scanning.
   b. Inflammatory disorders: Chemical meningitis, encephalitis secondary to systemic inflammatory or neoplastic disorders, demyelinating diseases, inflammatory neuropathies, vasculitides.
   c. Neoplastic processes: Neoplastic meningitis, cranial neuropathies, paraneoplastic encephalitis, radiculopathies, peripheral neuropathies, and after chemotherapy for malignancies.
   d. Subarachnoid hemorrhage (SAH)
      (1) Diagnosis of SAH in CT-negative cases.
      (2) Repeated LP to treat obstructive hydrocephalus after SAH.
   e. Disturbances of CSF pressure dynamics
      (1) Diagnosis and therapy of pseudotumor cerebri (benign intercranial hypertension).
         (a) Elevated CSF pressure (greater than 180 mm H_2O) with normal CSF constituents in the absence of intracranial mass lesion.
      (2) Therapy for normal pressure hydrocephalus
         (a) Reduction of CSF volume may improve clinical signs.
         (b) May be used to prognosticate likelihood of improving with shunting.
3. Potential findings (Table 127-1)
   a. Elevated CSF pressure
      (1) Defined as opening pressure above 180 mm H_2O (when patient is in lateral decubitus position).
      (2) Seen in some meningitides and encephalitides, SAH, pseudotumor cerebri, and spinal subarachnoid block (e.g., epidural spinal cord compression).
   b. Abnormal cellular constituents
      (1) Leukocytosis: Not specific for etiology but extremely elevated white blood cell (WBC) count (suggestive of infectious process, particularly bacterial).
         (a) Significantly elevated polymorphonuclear cells: Bacterial infections.
         (b) Mildly elevated polymorphonu-clear cells: Bacterial, fungal, or parasitic infections; viral meningitides; encephalitides; early brain abscesses.
         (c) Slightly elevated polymorphonuclear cells: Early bacterial infections; fungal, viral, or parasitic infections; inflammatory diseases; neoplastic processes.
         (d) Elevated lymphocytes: Mycobacterial infections, viral infections, brain abscesses, other inflammatory processes.
      (2) Erythrocytosis
         (a) Red blood cell (RBC) count that decreases significantly from the first tube to the last tube is highly suggestive of a traumatic tap.
         (b) Persistently elevated RBCs in CSF sample, without clot, highly suggestive of hemorrhage.
         (c) Mild to moderately elevated RBCs with increased protein and increased WBCs suggestive of hemorrhagic encephalitis (e.g., herpes encephalitis).
      (3) Abnormal WBC morphology. Abnormal forms highly suggestive of a neoplastic process such as neoplastic meningitis.
   c. Protein content
      (1) Normal protein value increases steadily with age.
      (2) Mild to moderate elevation in protein nonspecific; may be seen in infectious, inflammatory, or neoplastic processes.
      (3) Massive elevation in protein (several hundred to several thousand milligrams per deciliter) highly suggestive of obstruction to CSF flow, either due to obstructive hydrocephalus or spinal epidural block (Froin syndrome).
      (4) Reduced protein content has no pathologic significance but may be seen in pseudotumor cerebri.
   d. Protein composition
      (1) Increased IgG level, IgG synthesis rate, and IgG/albumin ratio nonspecific finding: may occur in syphilis, meningitis, and sarcoidosis but is typical of demyelinating processes (e.g., multiple sclerosis).

Table 127-1. CSF Composition

	Appearance	Opening Pressure	Red Blood Cells	White Blood Cells	Glucose	Protein	Smears Cultures
Normal	Clear, colorless	<180 mm H$_2$O	0/µl	Mononuclear ≤5/µl	≥45 mg/dl	≤45 mg/dl	—
Bacterial meningitis	Cloudy	↑	Normal	↑↑ (Polymorphonuclear)*	↓↓	↑↑	Gram stain (+) Cultures (+)
Tuberculous meningitis	Normal or cloudy	↑	Normal	↑ (Mononuclear)†,‡	↓	↑	ABF stain (±) Cultures (±)
Fungal meningitis	Normal or cloudy	Normal or ↑	Normal	↑ (Mononuclear)	↓	↑	Indian ink (+) *Cryptococus* cultures (±)
Viral meningitis/ encephalitis	Normal	Normal or ↑	Normal§	↑ (Mononuclear)‡	Normal	Normal or ↑	—
Carcinomatous meningitis	Normal or cloudy	Normal or ↑	Normal	Normal or ↑ (mononuclear)	Normal or ↓	Normal or ↑	Cytology (+)
Subarachnoid hemorrhage	Diur-red (supernatant yellow)	↑	↑	Normal or ↑ (polymorphonuclear)	Normal	↑	—
Cerebral lupus erythematosus	Normal	Normal or ↑	Normal	Normal or ↑ (Mononuclear)	Normal	Normal or ↑	—

Source: Simon RP, Aminoff MJ, Greenberg DA. *Clinical Neurology.* Norwalk, Conn., Appleton and Lange, 1989.
*Polymorphonuclear predominance.
†Mononuclear predominance.
‡Polymorphonuclear predominance may be seen early in course.
§Elevated RBCs seen in herpes encephalitis.

(2) Presence of oligoclonal IgG subtypes (*oligoclonal bands*) nonspecific; may occur in infections and inflammatory disorders but is also frequently seen in multiple sclerosis.

(3) Abnormal antigens: Used in rapid diagnosis of bacterial, treponemal, fungal, and viral processes.

e. Glucose content

(1) Normal ratio of CSF glucose to serum glucose is 0.6. Elevated glucose content is seen in diabetics. Elevated glucose concentration alone is not suggestive of a pathologic process other than reflecting the presence of hyperglycemia. Thus when the CSF glucose is of great diagnostic importance, CSF and blood glucose levels should be obtained simultaneously, with the patient in a fasting state for at least 4 hr.

(2) Reduction of CFS glucose to less than 30% of the serum value is seen in many processes, particularly bacterial and fungal, as well as in neoplastic meningitis.

(3) Severe reduction of glucose is seen in fulminant bacterial meningitis and active tuberculous meningitis.

f. Microbiologic techniques

(1) Gram stain: Extremely useful for rapid identification of causative organisms of bacterial meningitis.

(2) Fungal and mycobacterial smears.

(3) Bacterial antigen assays: Counterimmunoelectrophoresis or latex agglutination tests are useful for the diagnosis of *Haemophilus influenzae* and *Neisseria meningitides*, *Streptococcus pneumoniae*, β-hemolytic streptococci, and *Escherichia coli*. The tests may be useful for the detection of gram-negative infections such as *H. influenzae*; they may on occasion be positive with *Candida* or *Aspergillus* infection.

(4) Treponemal antigen assays: Useful for the diagnosis of neurosyphilis and Lyme disease.

(5) Viral antigen assays: Early reports suggest the polymerase chain reaction to be sensitive and specific in the early diagnosis of herpes encephalitis.

(6) Culture studies: Necessary for precise identification of suspected pathogens (bacterial, fungal, viral, microbacterial, parasitic).

4. Limitations of LP and CSF analysis

a. In the diagnosis of nervous system infections, no other techniques are as important and useful.

b. In inflammatory conditions, findings are often nonspecific (e.g., mild protein elevation, mild CSF leukocytosis) and do not provide definitive diagnosis.

5. Contraindications to LP

a. Intracranial or intraspinal mass lesion

(1) LP contraindicated due to risk of decompression and brain or spinal cord herniation.

(2) Exclude by neurologic exam, fundoscopic exam, CT or magnetic resonance imaging (MRI) scan.

b. Coagulopathy

(1) Check routine coagulation studies prior to performing LP.

(2) If a coagulopathy is detected, correct in advance of LP (e.g., if prothrombin time/partial thromboplastin time is abnormal, infuse fresh frozen plasma. If there are fewer than 60,000 platelets, give platelet transfusion).

(3) If the patient is on anticoagulants, stop the drugs well in advance of LP if possible and check coagulation studies to see if normalized.

(4) If coagulopathy develops after LP, treat aggressively due to risk of delayed hemorrhage.

c. Local infection

(1) Contraindicated if there is skin, subcutaneous, or deeper infection at puncture site due to risk of introducing bacteria into the subarachnoid space.

(2) Consider a cervical puncture by an experienced practitioner if CSF studies are deemed essential.

6. Complications

a. Precipitation or exacerbation of brain or spinal cord herniation.

(1) Most important complication.

(2) Maintain high index of suspicion; treat aggressively to lower intracranial pressure or reduce spinal cord swelling if this occurs.

b. Headache

      (1) Most common complication.

      (2) Pathophysiology uncertain; probably due to a persistent dural leak of CSF.

      (3) Worse with upright position.

      (4) Can last for weeks after LP.

      (5) Treat with strict bed rest, mild analgesics, fluids. Reserve blood patch for intractable cases.

      (6) Avoid, if possible, by using 20-gauge needles, fewest possible puncture attempts, smallest possible CSF sample, and prone position after LP.

  c. Hemorrhage

      (1) May be epidural at LP site, resulting in spinal root compression manifested by back or lower extremity pain or sensory disturbance, with or without lower extremity weakness. This may become a surgical emergency.

      (2) May be subarachnoid, which may result in altered mental status, with or without focal neurologic deficits.

  d. Diplopia

      (1) Due to cranial nerve VI palsy presumably secondary to changes in intracranial pressure.

      (2) Usually transient.

  e. Infection

      (1) Theoretical risk of inducing central nervous system (CNS) infection via inoculation of skin organisms or introduction of blood-borne organisms into subarachnoid space.

      (2) Especially important in immunocompromised patients.

B. Electroencephalography (EEG)

  1. Description

    a. An EEG is performed by recording the naturally occurring electrical potentials of the brain, using electrodes placed on the head in standardized fashion.

    b. Electrical activity is recorded during quiet wakefulness, drowsiness, and sleep. Occasionally, oral sedation is necessary to obtain sleep. A complete EEG includes a recording during sleep.

    c. Activation procedures such as hyperventilation and photic stimulation are used to enhance detection of abnormalities.

    d. Portable 24-hr recording equipment is available for recording over long periods of time.

    e. The EEG is interpreted based on the age of the patient, prior medical history, and medication used. Attempts are made to characterize the global activity and to discover any focal abnormalities.

  2. Indications

    a. Assessment of CNS physiology

      (1) Globally: Seizure disorders, encephalopathies, degenerative conditions, brain death.

      (2) Focally: Seizure disorders or focal pathologic lesions.

    b. Evaluation of paroxysmal disorders such as seizures, syncope, dizziness, or migraine.

  3. Potential findings

    a. Seizure disorders

      (1) Certain seizure disorders have characteristic EEG patterns which allow classification of the seizure type.

      (2) If the patient experiences a clinical seizure during EEG, valuable information may be gained regarding seizure type, location of onset, and degree of spread. This information may influence therapy.

      (3) EEG may be nonspecifically abnormal or normal even in patients who have clinical seizures.

    b. Encephalopathies

      (1) Abnormal toxic or metabolic states may affect the EEG background activity diffusely.

      (2) EEG may provide a semiquantitative means of estimating the degree of CNS disturbance (e.g., metabolic coma, encephalitis).

    c. Dementia

      (1) Useful in assessing the degree of CNS dysfunction.

      (2) Helpful in excluding Jakob-Creutzfeldt disease as a cause of dementia, as this disease usually has a characteristic EEG pattern.

    d. Behavioral disturbances: May be useful in excluding an ictal cause of behavioral abnormalities.

    e. Brain death

      (1) Not a substitute for neurologic examination in the determination of brain death.

      (2) Does not directly reflect brain stem activity, the absence of which correlates with clinical brain death.

(3) EEG subject to artifact, which may lead to false-positive interpretation.

(4) If performed, should be done in the absence of hyposedative drugs (e.g., barbiturates) and hypothermia, which may give false-negative results.

f. Paroxysmal disorders

(1) Seizures: See Section B,3,a.

(2) Syncope

(a) Limited usefulness; must be interpreted with caution (see Section B,4).

(b) Very rarely, may be supportive of an ictal etiology of syncope.

(3) Dizziness: Rarely helpful; rarely, may exclude an ictal etiology.

(4) Migraine

(a) Controversial association of migraine and seizure disorders.

i) Increased incidence of EEG abnormalities in patients with migraine.

ii) Increased incidence of clinical seizures in patients with migraine.

(b) Abnormalities may point to a shared pathophysiology (if it exists) of migraine and epilepsy.

(c) Not useful in the diagnosis of headaches.

4. Limitations

a. Seizure disorders

(1) Significant percentage of normal persons have mild, nonspecific abnormalities on EEG and never suffer a clinical seizure.

(2) Interictal EEG in many patients with seizures may be normal or may show only slight, nonspecific abnormalities.

(3) Thus, a normal EEG does not exclude a diagnosis of seizure and an abnormal EEG does not confirm the diagnosis. Seizures remain a clinical diagnosis.

b. Brain death.

(1) As above.

(2) High potential for technical inadequacy for interpretation.

5. Contraindications

a. Absolute: None exist for EEG.

b. Relative

(1) Maximal information obtained from cooperative patients; less useful information obtained from combative or confused patients.

(2) Skin conditions affecting scalp

(a) May be aggravated by electrode conductivity gel.

(b) May prevent adequate contact between electrode and scalp.

6. Complications

a. No significant complications exist.

b. Minor transient scalp discomfort when surface electrodes attached.

c. Patients with hyperventilation-induced or photoconvulsive seizures have risk of having a seizure during activation procedures.

7. Risks/benefits

a. Provides useful information about physiologic function of CNS at little to no risk to patients.

b. Findings must be interpreted in the setting of clinical data.

C. Electromyography (EMG) and nerve conduction studies (NCS)

1. Description

a. EMG is performed by inserting needle electrodes into selected muscles and recording the electrical signals generated at rest and during voluntary muscle activation.

b. NCS are performed by transcutaneous stimulation of cranial or peripheral nerves and recording and interpreting the potentials generated.

2. Indications

a. Evaluation of motor weakness.

(1) Generalized: Anterior horn cell and other motor neuron diseases; peripheral neuropathies, neuromuscular junction diseases, and myopathies.

(2) Focal disorders of names, roots, and plexus.

b. Sensory disturbances: Radiculopathies, peripheral neuropathies, mononeuropathies (e.g., entrapment neuropathies).

c. Neck, back, or extremity pain.

3. Limitations

a. Radiculopathies

(1) Abnormalities may be detected only when there has been significant radicular injury; that is, radicular dysfunction may exist but may not be detected by EMG/NCS if it is either mild or of recent onset (less than 2–3 weeks).

(2) May be falsely negative in chronic radicular process if abnormalities have had sufficient time to be corrected.

b. Peripheral neuropathies

(1) NCS techniques assess only the larger, more heavily myelinated fibers. Small-fiber neuropathies are not well assessed by current NCS methods. A patient may have a significant small-fiber neuropathy with little abnormality on NCS.

(2) Early or mild entrapment neuropathies may not produce detectable abnormalities on EMG/NCS until a significant percentage of the nerve fibers are dysfunctional.

c. Neuromuscular junction disorders

(1) Assessment of neuromuscular transmission depends on many variables, including therapy with anticholinesterase drugs. Repetitive stimulation may be falsely negative if performed while the patient is on anticholinesterase medications.

(2) Neuromuscular transmission studies show a higher rate of abnormalities on stimulation of more proximal sites. If distal stimulation alone is performed, the result may be falsely negative.

d. Myopathies

(1) Due to the patchy nature of some myopathic processes and the possibility of sampling errors, EMG studies may be falsely negative in myopathies.

(2) The inability of the patient to tolerate muscular activation during EMG will greatly influence the diagnostic yield.

4. Contraindications

a. EMG studies

(1) In patients who are receiving anticoagulant medications or who have underlying coagulopathies, needle EMG studies are contraindicated due to the risk of deep and hard-to-detect hemorrhages.

(2) Patients with valvular heart disease or with prosthetic heart valves or other structural cardiac defects (atrial or ventricular septal defect) should receive antibiotic prophylaxis

prior to needle EMG studies because of the small risk of bacterial endocarditis.

b. NCS: No significant medical contraindications.

5. Complications.

a. EMG studies

(1) Hemorrhage, bruising

(a) Deep, paraspinal

(b) Superficial

(2) Infection (local or hematogenous)

(3) Pain

(a) Immediate, usually transient.

(b) Persistent; suspect hematoma or infection.

(4) Elevated creatine phosphokinase due to muscle cell trauma.

b. NCS: No significant complications.

6. Risk/benefits

a. Mild to moderately invasive means of assessing weakness, sensory disturbance, and pain.

b. Helpful in localizing level of disturbance in peripheral nervous system and classifying type of dysfunction.

c. Not helpful in assessing upper motor neuron processes.

d. Although patients vary substantially in their tolerance, the usefulness of information gained must be weighed against degree of discomfort experience by the patient during the test.

D. Radiologic evaluation.

1. Technical description

a. MRI

(1) Examination of hydrogen nuclear protons within tissues by assessing energy state of protons following radiofrequency pulse.

(2) Comparison of "proton density" between normal and abnormal tissues.

(3) Computer-assisted generation of multiplanar images.

(4) Gadolinium-DTPA, an intravenous contrast agent, useful in increasing diagnostic sensitivity and specificity.

b. CT

(1) Mathematical reconstruction of tissue densities of brain, skull, and spinal column using x-rays.

(2) Typically performed in axial plane.

(3) Intravenous contrast agents used to improve sensitivity and specificity.

c. Myelography

(1) Similar to LP, except that after small amount of CSF is removed, a small quantity of radiopaque contrast agent is instilled into the spinal subarachnoid space and allowed to flow around the spinal cord.

(2) Radiologic images are obtained, outlining the spinal cord and permitting characterization of lesions as intramedullary, intradural, or extradural.

(3) May be performed by the cervical approach as well if the suspected lesion lies in the cervical or thoracic region.

(4) Often followed by CT of the spine to increase diagnostic yield and specificity.

d. Angiography

(1) Consists of direct radiography visualization of cranial vessels following percutaneous infusion of arterial contrast agents.

(2) Rapid-sequence x-rays are obtained to assess circulation.

2. Indications

a. MRI

(1) Cranial: Excellent visualization of brain parenchyma, especially middle and posterior fossa structures.

(a) Vascular: Ischemic strokes; hemorrhages: intraparenchymal, subdural, epidural; vessel abnormalities; aneurysms, arteriovenous malformations (AVMs), vessel thrombosis, stenosis.

(b) Neoplastic: Intra-axial: primary CNS tumors, metastases; Extra-axial: meningiomas; neoplastic meningitis.

(c) Inflammatory: Multiple sclerosis plaques, encephalitis, vasculitis.

(d) Degenerative: Dementia, other degenerative disorders (e.g., Parkinson's disease, Huntington's disease).

(e) Trauma: CT more useful in assessment of acute head trauma because bony abnormalities and acute hemorrhages better visualized on CT.

(f) Infections: Abscess, encephalitis, meningitis.

(2) Spinal

(a) Spinal cord: Visualization of spinal cord parenchyma plus surrounding structures; neoplasms: intramedullary, intradural, extramedullary; inflammatory lesions, multiple sclerosis; vascular: ischemic, hemorrhagic, AVM; traumatic: syringomyelia, hematomyelia; degenerative.

(b) Vertebral column, discs; Degenerative: spondylosis, spinal stenosis, disc herniation; Neoplastic: bony-based lesions, metastases; infections: epidural abscess, diskitis, osteomyelitis of vertebral bodies.

b. CT

(1) Cranial

(a) Similar to MRI but less sensitive for small lesions, particularly those affecting deeper structures or posterior fossa.

(b) More sensitive than MRI in detecting subarachnoid hemorrhage or other acute hemorrhages.

(c) Useful for imaging cranial bony abnormalities, especially at base of skull.

(d) Necessary in patients with pacemakers or ferromagnetic aneurysm clips who cannot undergo MRI.

(2) Spinal

(a) Better assessment of bony degenerative change than that of MRI, especially when performed after myelography.

(b) Poorer visualization of spinal cord than that of MRI.

c. Myelography: Best assessment of spinal subarachnoid block, seen as limitation of flow of contrast column.

(1) Intramedullary

(a) Neoplastic: Astrocytomas, ependymomas.

(b) Inflammatory: Transverse myelitis, postradiation myelitis.

(c) Infection: Abscess, myelitis.

(d) Traumatic: Hematomyelia, syringomyelia.

(e) Degenerative: Syringomyelia.

(2) Intradural

(a) Neoplastic: Meningioma, neurofibroma.

(3) Extradural

(a) Neoplastic: Metastases.

(b) Infection: Epidural abscess.

(c) Degenerative, traumatic: Spondylosis, herniated disc.

d. Angiography

(1) Vascular: Gold standard, more sensitive than noninvasive techniques (carotid Doppler, transcranial Doppler, MRI, angiography).

(a) Carotid stenosis.

(b) Carotid or vertebral dissection.

(c) Intracranial atheromatous disease.

(d) Cerebral embolism, thrombosis.

(e) Vasculitis.

(f) Aneurysms.

(g) AVM

(2) Neoplastic: MRI/CT more sensitive and specific in detecting abnormalities of brain parenchyma.

(a) Meningioma.

(b) Primary brain tumors.

(c) Particularly useful in preoperative assessment of blood supply to tumors.

(3) Inflammatory: Vessel beading in vasculitis.

(4) Traumatic: Large vessel dissection.

3. Potential findings

a. MRI: See Section D,2,a.

(1) Cranial: Detection of ischemic, hemorrhagic, neoplastic, inflammatory, and infectious lesions and degenerative changes.

(2) Spinal: Degenerative, neoplastic, inflammatory, and traumatic lesions.

b. CT: See Section D,2,b. Similar to MRI but provides better definition of bony abnormalities of skull and spine.

c. Myelopathy: See Section D,2,c. Primarily, helps to distinguish between intramedullary, intradural, and extradural lesions.

d. Angiography: See Section D,2,d.

4. Limitations

a. While these techniques are often very sensitive, particularly MRI, they are often nonspecific. For example, multiple areas of high signal on MRI may represent ischemic infarction or multiple foci of inflammation; an intraparenchymal

mass on MRI/CT may represent a tumor, an abscess, or a vascular lesion.

b. Increasing technological sophistication allows better prediction of pathologic nature of lesions, but assumptions regarding etiology are perilous.

c. Often histologic examination is required to produce the correct diagnosis.

5. Contraindications

a. MRI

(1) Ferromagnetic foreign objects (e.g., metal filings in orbits, aneurysm clips, certain prostheses) may become displaced during MRI.

(2) Pacemakers, defibrillators, or other electronic implanted devices may become deprogrammed due to the magnetic field.

(3) Infusion pumps cannot operate within the MRI suite.

(4) Severe renal insufficiency precludes use of gadolinium-DTPA as a contrast agent.

(5) An uncooperative, confused, or combative patient may not be able to lie still for the length of time required for MRI.

(6) Claustrophobia.

b. CT: Allergy to intravenous contrast agents precludes use in CT studies.

c. Myelography: Similar to LP.

(1) Increased intracranial pressure due to risks of herniated brain or spinal cord.

(2) LP below level of cord compression may cause worsening of clinical signs or herniation of spinal cord; therefore, myelogram should be performed above the suspected level (e.g., using a cervical approach).

(3) Coagulopathies.

(4) Local infection.

(5) History of allergic reaction to myelographic contrast agents.

d. Angiography

(1) History of allergic reaction to contrast agents.

(2) Renal insufficiency.

(3) Coagulopathy.

(4) Peripheral vascular lesions (e.g., severe atherosclerotic lesions of the femoral artery) may necessitate use of an alternative percutaneous site.

6. Complications

a. MRI
  (1) No known biological risk to humans.
  (2) Gadolinium-DPTA may exacerbate renal insufficiency.
  (3) Risk of displacement of ferromagnetic objects such as orbital metal filings, surgical clips, prostheses; risk of electrical dysfunction of pacemakers.
b. CT
  (1) Biological risk of radiation exposure.
  (2) Risk of allergic reaction to contrast agents.
  (3) Worsening of renal insufficiency due to contrast agents.
c. Myelography
  (1) Headache.
  (2) Back pain.
  (3) Traumatic herniated intervertebral disc.
  (4) Vasovagal reactions: Hypotension, nausea, vomiting, dizziness, lightheadedness, diaphoresis, fainting.
  (5) Transection of nerve filaments.
  (6) Arachnoiditis.
d. Angiography
  (1) Death.
  (2) Stroke.
  (3) Seizure.
  (4) Transient ischemic attack, transient visual loss, change in mental status.
  (5) Headache.
  (6) Nausea, vomiting, diaphoresis, chest pain, dizziness, hypotension, fainting.
  (7) Hematoma, vessel dissection, transection.
  (8) Infection.
  (9) Allergic dye reaction.

7. Risks/benefits
  a. MRI/CT offer excellent, noninvasive means of visualizing CNS anatomy at relatively little risk to patients. MRI is preferred imaging method for most situations requiring assessment of brain and spinal cord. CT also provides similar information but with less sensitivity and specificity.
  b. MRI, while more expensive than CT, provides greater yield.
  c. Myelography and angiography are more invasive than MRI/CT and carry greater potential risk. Often sufficient diagnostic information can be obtained by noninvasive techniques, but occasionally myelography and angiography are necessary. With equivocal findings on spinal MRI, myelography may be necessary.

Bibliography

Aminoff MJ. *Electrodiagnosis in Clinical Neurology*, ed 2. New York, Churchill Livingstone, 1986.

Bleck TP. Clinical use of neurologic diagnostic tests, in Weiner WJ, Goetz CG (eds), *Neurology for the Non-Neurologist*, ed 2. Philadelphia, Lippincott, 1989.

Fishman RA. *Cerebrospinal Fluid in Diseases of the Nervous System*. Philadelphia, Saunders, 1980.

Mayo Clinic and Mayo Foundation. *Clinical Examinations in Neurology*, ed 6. St Louis, Mosby, 1991.

Ramsey RG. *Neuroradiology*, ed 2. Philadelphia, Saunders, 1987.

CHAPTER 128

Coma

Barry J. Riskin, M.D.
Michael C. Smith, M.D.

Alteration in the level of consciousness is a common problem that occurs in hospitalized patients. The prognosis is determined by early recognition of the disease state, rapid identification of the underlying pathophysiologic mechanism, and institution of correct therapies. Change in mental status implies a wide range of clinical states. Coma is the most severe change in the level of consciousness.

This chapter will list some of the etiologies and pathophysiologic mechanisms of coma, highlight important considerations when performing the history and physical exam, and propose some guidelines for diagnostic testing and treatment. Of note, these principles can be generalized for all patients with a change in mental status, not just for those in coma.

I. **Definition**
Consciousness is the state of awareness of the self and the environment; coma is the total absence of awareness of self and the environment even when the subject is externally stimulated. Loss of consciousness has many potential causes, but the pathophysiologic mechanisms that underlie coma are more limited.

II. **Etiology**
There are two major groups of potential etiologies of coma. One group is disorders that cause structural disruption (injury) of nervous tissue. The other is disorders that cause diffuse metabolic derangements and secondary neuronal dysfunction.

A. Structural lesions can be further subdivided.
  1. Destructive lesions
    a. Cerebral infarction.
    b. Penetrating brain injury.
  2. Space-occupying lesions
    a. Primary brain tumors (e.g., glioma).
    b. Metastatic brain tumors (e.g., carcinoma of the lung or breast).
    c. Intracranial hemorrhage: intraparenchymal (primary), subdural, subarachnoid with intraparenchymal extension.
    d. Abscess.
    e. Hydrocephalus.
B. Metabolic derangements
  1. Hypernatremia, hyponatremia.
  2. Hypercalcemia, hypocalcemia.
  3. Uremia—renal failure.
  4. Hepatic failure.
  5. Intoxication (drugs, ethanol).
  6. Central nervous system infection, sepsis.

III. Pathophysiology

Coma can result from either bilateral cerebral hemispheric dysfunction, dysfunction of the brain stem's reticular activating system (RAS), or both.

A. The experience of consciousness can be divided into two components: arousal and content.

1. Arousal is the ability of the organism to awaken, either spontaneously or with stimulation.

2. Arousal is a function primarily of the RAS. The RAS is chiefly located within the midline deep gray matter (periaqueductal gray) of the mesencephalon (midbrain).

3. Content of consciousness is provided and maintained by the cerebral hemispheres.

4. Cortical functions of language, insight, judgment, memory, emotion, and attention are therefore absent when coma is due to bilateral hemispheric dysfunction.

5. Some patients, despite having bilateral hemispheric dysfunction, can have preserved sleep-wake cycles, eye opening and closing, yawning, smiling, and other facial expressions without any demonstrable interaction with the examiner or the environment.

IV. Diagnosis

A. Emphasis in the diagnosis of coma should be placed on the patient's history. The history should be obtained carefully and completely.

1. Attention should be paid to significant past medical history.

   a. Heart disease.

   b. Previous neurologic disorders.

   c. Liver or kidney disease.

   d. Bleeding diathesis.

   e. Use of prescription medications, illicit drugs, and alcohol.

   f. Recent or past trauma.

B. The clinical exam should focus on the level of arousal, breathing patterns, eye positions and movement, pupil size, spontaneous movement of the extremities, and specific reflexes. The neurologic exam should be performed in a serial fashion, and all findings should be carefully documented to permit rapid recognition of any deterioration. Documentation using the Glasgow Coma Scale can be helpful.

1. On noting the level of arousal, it is more important to describe the patient's clinical state than to ascribe a name to the patient's clinical condition. For example, state that "The patient required repeated verbal and tactile stimulation to remain awake. Once awake, the patient responded appropriately and followed all commands correctly," rather than "The patient appeared lethargic."

2. Spontaneous breathing patterns should be recorded. If the patient is intubated and being mechanically ventilated, this may not be possible.

3. Pupil size and reactivity must be carefully noted.

   a. Small, reactive pupils suggest either a diffuse metabolic encephalopathy, a narcotic overdose, or a diencephalic lesion as the cause of coma.

   b. Midposition, nonreactive pupils approximately 4–6 mm in diameter suggest midbrain dysfunction.

   c. Pinpoint pupils are seen with pontine lesions.

   d. Large, unreactive pupils more than 6 mm in diameter are often seen in agonal or pre-agonal states.

   e. A unilateral, large, unreactive pupil suggests compression of the third cranial nerve and is seen in herniation syndromes.

4. The position of the eyes at rest and during movement must be noted.

   a. Conjugate eye deviation is described as a preference of the eyes to remain toward one side, not readily crossing the midline. This is seen commonly in patients in coma.

      (1) Hemiparesis ipsilateral to the side of conjugate eye deviation suggests a pontine lesion on the side opposite the eye deviation.

      (2) Hemiparesis contralateral to the side of conjugate eye deviation suggests a lesion in the cerebral hemisphere on the same side as the eye deviation.

      (3) Eyes can also deviate as a result of an irritative process (seizure) of the cerebral cortex. In this case, the eyes conjugately deviate away from the side of seizure discharge. Often twitching or other repetitive movements will be seen on the

side of the body ipsilateral to the side of eye deviation.

  b. Dysconjugate gaze is defined as a condition in which eye movements are no longer "yoked" together and each eye assumes its own relative position.

    (1) Dysconjugate gaze, either with movement or at rest, suggests a brain stem lesion.

    (2) Skew deviation of the eyes suggests a lesion in the posterior fossa, either the brain stem or cerebellum.

5. Movement of the extremities, either spontaneously or in response to stimuli, can be used to judge the integrity of the motor system.

  a. Abnormal movements or postures often occur in patients with coma.

    (1) Decorticate posture (obligate flexion of the upper extremities and extension of the lower extremities) and decerebrate posture (obligate extension and supination of the upper extremities and extension of the lower extremities) occur in association with diencephalic and midbrain lesions, respectively.

    (2) Myoclonus (brief, repetitive, lightning-like, arrhythmic, asynchronous movements of the limbs) and seizure activity may occur in metabolic and hypoxic-ischemic encephalopathies.

6. Besides the pupillary light reflex, cervico-ocular and vestibulo-ocular reflex testing should be performed in all patients in coma.

  a. The cervico-ocular reflex (oculocephalic), or "doll's-eye" maneuver, is performed by passively moving the patient's head back and forth, and up and down, with the patient's eyes gently held opened. If the brain stem centers that control eye movement are intact, the eyes will move freely and completely in the direction opposite to the passive head movement. This test should *not* be performed in patients in whom there is uncertainty about the stability of the cervical spine until the possibility of cervical fracture or dislocation has been ruled out radiographically (e.g., a trauma victim in coma).

  b. The vestibulo-ocular (vestibulocephalic) reflex similarly tests the integrity of the brain stem centers that control gaze. This maneuver is a stronger stimulus for eye movement than the cervico-ocular test. After the inner ear canal and tympanic membrane have been inspected for obstruction or perforation, and with the head of the patient at 30 degrees above horizontal, up to 100 ml of ice water should be injected slowly into each ear, one at a time, separated by 5 min between each side. If the brain stem centers for gaze and peripheral vestibular function are intact, the eyes should deviate conjugately *toward* the ear receiving the cold water.

  c. In patients in hysterical unresponsive states, and in patients in more mildly impaired states, the presence of (correcting) nystagmus is evidence of intact cerebral cortical bulbar activity.

C. Laboratory tests

1. The laboratory findings will depend on the underlying etiology of the loss of consciousness. The following should be a guide to the tests ordered in the comatose patient when the etiology is unknown.

  a. Electrolyte and serum chemistries, with attention to glucose, serum sodium, osmolality, blood urea nitrogen, creatinine, and serum calcium.

  b. Evidence of a coagulopathy may not be clinically evident; therefore, attention should focus on prothrombin time (PT), activated partial thromboplastin time (PTT), platelet count, and, as necessary, fibrinogen and fibrin split products.

  c. Complete blood cell count (CBC), leukocyte differential.

  d. Blood and urine cultures if infection is suspected.

  e. Serum or urine toxicologic screening, as well as serum alcohol levels in all patients in coma of unknown etiology.

D. Diagnostic tests

1. A cranial computed tomography (CT) or magnetic resonance imaging (MRI) scan should be obtained to identify and characterize any intracranial mass or mass effect or detect the presence of intracranial bleeding.

2. An electroencephalogram can provide evidence of ongoing seizure activity, demonstrate focal slowing indicating focal anatomic pathology, and at times give insight into the cause of the coma. Examples include fast activity in barbiturate coma and triphasic waves in metabolic encephalopathy.

3. If the loss of consciousness is suspected to have been preceded by some type of cardiac dysfunction, the workup should include continuous electrocardiographic monitoring and echocardiogram, as well as cardiac enzymes to rule out evidence of myocardial ischemia.

4. Lumbar puncture should be performed to rule out central nervous system infection or subarachnoid hemorrhage. Lumbar puncture should be performed after intracerebral mass effect or the presence of a posterior fossa mass has been ruled out. This usually requires cranial CT or MRI scans to be performed prior to the lumbar puncture.

   a. Cerebrospinal fluid (CSF) should be sent for a cell count and differential in the first as well as the last tube, for glucose and protein, and for Gram stain and culture.

5. Cerebral angiogram should be considered in patients in whom intracranial bleeding, specifically aneurysmal subarachnoid hemorrhage, or arterial dissection is suspected if the neuroimaging and CSF studies are unrevealing.

V. Treatment

Treatment of any state of altered consciousness encompasses treatment of the underlying condition(s) or disorder(s) that led to the concurrent neurologic dysfunction.

A. As with all medical emergencies, the first objective of treatment is to secure the airway, maintaining breathing and circulation. This includes all measures to ensure hemodynamic stability: oxygen therapy, intravenous fluids, antiarrhythmic drugs, and pressor agents if needed.

B. Obtain serum blood and urine samples for laboratory investigation.

C. Administer 50% glucose (D50), naloxone, and intravenous thiamine. Naloxone is used to reverse the effects of opiates. Thiamine should be used in patients if recent or past ethanol abuse is suspected, in patients with suspected nutritional deficiencies (e.g., malignancies), and in coma of unknown etiology. Where available, flumazenil should similarly be employed to reverse the effects of benzodiazepines.

D. Correct all serum electrolyte and osmolarity values where possible. Caution should be used to prevent overly rapid correction of serum hypo-osmolality to avoid the possibility of central pontine myelinolysis.

E. If a space-occupying lesion or hydrocephalus is discovered, or if there is a history of craniocervical trauma, neurosurgical consultation should be obtained. Removal of the cause of the increased intracranial pressure and potential herniation may prove to be lifesaving.

F. All infections should be treated accordingly. Special attention should be paid to suspected cases of herpes simplex encephalitis, with expedient treatment with acyclovir.

G. All seizures need appropriate treatment with anticonvulsants and, when possible, correction of any identifiable etiology of seizure (e.g., hypoglycemia). Myoclonus is often mistaken for seizure activity. Multifocal myoclonus is seen frequently in hypoxic-ischemic encephalopathy.

H. Regional poison control centers should be consulted when there is suspicion of hazardous exposure, drug overdose, or accidental ingestion of toxic material. Treatment in these settings should focus on decontamination, enhanced elimination, and specific antidotes where indicated. In the case of iron overdose, for example, this would include gastric lavage, cathartic use, and deferoxamine, respectively.

VI. Patient Monitoring

All patients who acutely lapse into coma or in whom the etiology of the coma is unknown should be placed in an intensive care unit. If no such unit exists, cardiac monitoring (telemetry), blood pressure monitoring, and frequent neurologic and general physical examinations should be provided.

VII. Prognosis

The prognosis of coma depends on the underlying cause and depth of coma, as well as the duration of the state of unconsciousness.

A. As a general rule, lesions that cause structural brain injury (cerebral infarction, subarachnoid hemorrhage) have a worse prognosis than those that cause diffuse (hypoxic-ischemic encephalopathy) or metabolic dysfunction (hepatic encephalopathy).

B. The probability of regaining independent functioning is inversely proportional to the duration of coma.

C. The prognosis should be estimated as soon as possible.

1. Accurate prognosis can be made by performing repeated (serial) examinations of the patient, first as a baseline and then at 24, 48, and 72 hr.

2. All confounding variables must be accounted for and eliminated (e.g., benzo-

diazepines can suppress the oculovestibular response).

3. Determination of prognosis is important to formulate appropriate comprehensive therapeutic treatment plan.

Bibliography

Levy DE, Prognosis in nontraumatic coma. *Ann Intern Med* 94(3):293–301, 1981.

Plum F, Posner JB. *The Diagnosis of Stupor and Coma*, ed 3. Philadelphia, Davis, 1986.

CHAPTER 129

Vascular Disorders of the Brain and Spinal Cord

Steven Brint, M.D.

Cerebrovascular diseases encompass a broad spectrum of pathologies. Symptoms usually result from brain ischemia, whether due to thrombosis, embolism, or vasospasm (Table 129-1).

The precise clinical localization of disease within the cerebrovascular tree often cannot be determined on the basis of physical examination alone. Neither can the differentiation of infarction, hemorrhage, and hemorrhagic infarction. Newer imaging methodologies such as magnetic resonance imaging (MRI), MRI-angiography (MRA), single photon emission computed tomography (SPECT), positron emission tomography (PET), and transcranial Doppler imaging, in addition to conventional angiography, are becoming increasingly important.

Within the past decade, therapeutic nihilism regarding cerebrovascular diseases, particularly stroke, has been replaced with cautious optimism as several promising lines of attack have been developed, including newer antithrombotics (low molecular weight heparinoid), thrombolytics (tissue plasminogen activator, streptokinase, urokinase), and receptor-activated ionic channel blockers (calcium channel blockers, N-methyl-D-aspartate (NMDA) blockers, etc).

In addition, more rational attempts to ameliorate ischemia physiologically are being developed, particu-larly with regard to optimizing blood pressure, blood glucose, and oxygen delivery.

Stroke

I. Definitions

A. Stroke is a fixed focal neurologic deficit which results from ischemia in a recognizable vascular distribution.

B. Transient ischemic attack (TIA) is a short-lived focal brain or ocular dysfunction secondary to ischemia, with rapid onset and resolution and without a clinically detectable deficit after 24 hr. Recent evidence suggests that most TIAs actually last for less than 30 min and although they may leave no clinical residual, they may cause persistent changes on MRI.

C. Reversible ischemic neurologic deficit (RIND) is a TIA-like dysfunction persisting for more than 24 hr but completely resolving within days.

D. Stroke in evolution is a stroke-like deficit which has a fluctuating intensity or steady progression over minutes to several hours. In the past, it was felt to be amenable to conventional anticoagulation; however, this is not currently clear.

1385

Table 129-1.   Classification of Cerebrovascular Diseases

I. Developmental
   A. Aneurysms
      1. Berry
      2. Fusiform
      3. Giant
   B. AVMs
      1. Isolated
      2. In association with diseases such as Von Hippel-Lindau disease
   C. Fibromuscular dysplasia
   D. Atresias
      1. Moya-moya
      2. Individual vessels
II. Inflammatory
   A. Systemic vasculitis with CNS involvment (e.g., lupus, Behçet's disease, polyarteritis nodosa, temporal arteritis, Takayasu's disease)
   B. Isolated CNS vasculitis (e.g., granulomatous angiitis)
   C. Infectious (e.g., syphilis, fungal, ?viral)
III. Occlusive
   A. Atherosclerotic disease causing:
      1. Artery-to-artery emboli
      2. In situ thrombosis
   B. Dissection
   C. Systemic embolic occlusion: clot originating in
      1. Heart
      2. Deep veins or lung with paradoxical communication
   D. Venous occlusion causing secondary ischemia
      1. Sagittal sinus thrombosis
      2. Large cortical vein thrombosis
IV. Hemorrhagic
   A. Ruptured aneurysm
   B. Bleeding AVM
   C. Lobar hemorrhage
      1. Spontaneous
      2. Hypertensive
      3. Amyloid angiopathy
   D. Hypertensive hemorrhage
   E. Coagulopathy

E. Crescendo TIAs are increasingly frequent TIAs over a short period (e.g., several days) despite antiplatelet therapy.

F. Delayed ischemic deficit (DID) is neurologic deterioration occurring usually within 14 days after subarachnoid hemorrhage.

Note: The temporal cutoffs for defining TIA, RIND, and stroke have been arbitrary and not based on actual pathophysiology. As such they appear to have less and less practical importance. Permanent injury is dependent on the duration, magnitude and frequency of focal ischemia.

II. Risk Factors for Ischemic Stroke
   A. Strong risk factors in the adult
      1. Age
      2. Hypertension
      3. Cardiac disease
      4. Prior stroke*
      5. Prior TIA (the risk of stroke after a TIA is about 4–7% per year)
   B. Minor adult risk factors
      1. Diabetes mellitus
      2. Smoking
      3. Binge drinking
      4. Hyperlipidemia

C. Risk factors in the young adult
1. Drug abuse
2. Hypertension
3. Blood dyscrasias
4. Cardiac disease
5. Smoking and birth control pill usage
6. Complicated migraine
7. Cervical trauma (dissection)
8. Sickle cell disease

*Note: The major causes of death in stroke patients are, first, myocardial infarction and, second, recurrent stroke.

III. Pathophysiology of Cerebrovascular Disease
A. Focal brain ischemia
1. Description
   a. Normal mean cerebral blood flow (CBF) is about 50 ml/min per 100 g of tissue. Gray matter has four times the CBF of white matter. During ischemia, normal vascular autoregulation is dysfunctional; therefore, flow becomes dependent on systemic blood pressure.
   b. CBF in the range of 8–23 ml/min per 100 g of tissue causes synaptic failure, flattening of the electroencephalogram, and functional impairment.
   c. CBF less than 8 ml/min per 100 g of tissue usually causes membrane failure and irreversible cell injury. In addition to membrane failure, uncontrolled local release of excitatory neurotransmitters (glutamate, aspartate) may contribute to acute and/or delayed neuronal death.
   d. Maximal injury of cerebral cortex occurs within 3–8 hr of focal ischemia. Therapeutic interventions are most likely to succeed when begun early.
   e. Regions of tenuous but viable circulation occurring around an ischemic core may persist for hours to days. They may be amenable to therapy even after the acute ictus in a number of patients. (This is the so-called ischemic penumbra).
2. Etiology
   a. Embolic occlusion
      (1) Embolic occlusion often results from artery-artery embolization of platelet fibrin debris or fresh clot from a mature atherosclerotic plaque. The most common plaque locations are the proximal internal carotid and vertebrobasilar system. Less common is carotid siphon and middle cerebral artery stem.
      (2) The heart is the source of up to one-third of all cerebral emboli. Atrial fibrillation (intermittent or chronic) is the main risk factor (5–7 times), especially in a setting of rheumatic heart disease (17 times). Lone atrial fibrillation (atrial fibrillation without proven cardiac disease) may not pose a threat for stroke. Recent transmural infarction (mostly within 3 months) and infective or noninfective bacterial endocarditis are other common sources of emboli (Table 129-2).
      (3) Cerebral emboli present with an abrupt deficit (seconds to minutes). Symptoms often persist, but most emboli lyse within 2 weeks, many within several days.
      (4) Amaurosis fugax (transient monocular blindness) often presents as a veil or shade descending over one eye and is strongly correlated with cervical atherosclerotic disease in the adult.
      (5) Eighty percent of embolic occlusions involve the middle cerebral artery. The most common sites in the posterior circulation are the posterior cerebral arteries.
      (6) Ulceration of the internal carotid artery alone, without significant luminal narrowing, is rarely responsible for embolization.
   b. Thrombosis
      (1) In situ arterial thrombosis usually occurs in the setting of underlying atherosclerotic narrowing of the cervical internal carotid, carotid siphon, proximal middle cerebral, or basilar arteries.
      (2) Hypercoaguable states may cause arterial thrombosis in the absence of atherosclerosis, especially in the young stroke patient (see Table 129-2).
      (3) Small arteries or end arterioles may thrombose secondary to:
         (a) Hypertension-induced endarteritis obliterans. This may result in characteristic lacunar syndromes (Table 129-3B).
         (b) Vasculitis.
            Note: Stroke in systemic lupus

Table 129-2. Cardiac and Hematologic Etiologies of Stroke

I. Cardiac abnormalities
  A. Heart wall abnormalities
    1. Acute myocardial infarction
    2. Ventricular aneurysm or akinesis
    3. Cardiomyopathy
    4. Atrial myxoma
    5. Septal defects—paradoxical embolism
  B. Valvular disease
    1. Rheumatic mitral stenosis/regurgitation
    2. Aortic sclerosis
    3. Infective endocarditis
    4. Nonbacterial thrombotic endocarditis
    5. Prosthetic heart valves
    6. Mitral valve prolapse (small percentage of cases)
  C. Arrhythmias
    1. Atrial fibrillation (acute, chronic, intermittent)
    2. Sick sinus syndrome
  D. Other cardiac sources
    1. Postcardiac catheterization
    2. Postaortic cross-clamping release (heart surgery)
    3. Cardiac surgery
    4. Aortic disease (dissection, atherosclerosis)
II. Hematologic disorders
  A. Red blood cell
    1. Sickle cell disease
    2. Malaria
    3. Polycythemia (hyperviscosity)
  B. White blood cell
    1. Leukemias
  C. 1. Thrombocytosis (thrombosis)
    2. Thrombocytopenia (hemorrhage)
  D. Procoagulant factors
    1. Protein S deficiency
    2. Protein C deficiency
    3. Antithrombin III deficiency
    4. Circulating "anticoagulant" (e.g., lupus anticoagulant)
  E. Other hematologic factors
    1. Drug effects (anticoagulants—warfarin, heparin, aspirin; procoagulants—aminocaproic acid, estrogens)
    2. Secondary effects of alcoholic binge drinking
    3. Hyperviscosity states (lymphoma, myeloma)

erythematosus may actually be related to circulating factors which are procoagulants and produce in situ thrombosis.

(4) Cerebral venous thrombotic occlusions may occur secondary to extensive dural sinus occlusion and may result in hemorrhagic infarction. Often the patient presents with protracted headache, seizures, or focal neurologic symptoms. Elevated intracranial pressures may contribute to the hemorrhagic infection. Cerebral venous infarction may occur in hypercoaguable states:
  (a) Postpartum
  (b) Severe dehydration
  (c) Infection
  (d) Cancer
c. Vasospasm may occur after:

Table 129-3A. Common Symptoms of Stroke

Vessel	Possible Symptoms	Brain Region Involved
1. L middle cerebral	R hemiparesis, R hemisensory defect, Quadrant or hemianopia, aphasia	Frontal/parietal cortex, basal ganglia, internal capsule.
upper division	Anterior—expressive	
lower division	Posterior—receptive	
2. R middle cerebral	L hemiparesis, L hemisensory defect, sensory neglect syndrome, asomatognosia, spatial disorientation, quadrant or hemianopsia	Frontal/parietal cortex, basal ganglia, internal capsule
3. Unilater anterior cerebral	Contralateral leg weakness	Frontal cortex
4. Bilateral anterior paraplegia, incontinence	Gait apraxia, abulia,	Frontal cortex
5. L internal carotid	(1) and (3)	
6. R internal carotid	(2) and (3)	
7. Vertebral	Vertigo, ataxia, dysarthria, contralateral hemisensory defect	Lateral medulla, cerebellum
8. Basilar	Diplopia, quadriparesis, alteration of consciousness, visual field defect, memory impairment	Pons, midbrain, occipital cortex, mesial temporal lobes
9. L posterior cerebral	R homonymous hemianopsia, unformed visual hallucinations	Occipital cortex
10. R posterior cerebral	L homonymous hemianopsia, unformed visual hallucinations	Occipital cortex

Table 129-3B Lancunar Syndromes

Type	Brain Region Involved
Pure motor: hemiparesis	Internal capsule, pons
Pure sensory: hemisensory defect	Thalamus
Sensorimotor stroke: hemisensory and pyramidal signs	Thalamus and posterior (ipsilateral) internal capsule
Ataxic hemiparesis	Pons, midbrain or capsule
Clumsy hand-dysarthria syndrome	Pontine tegmentum

(1) Subarachnoid hemorrhage: This often occurs within 5–12 days post-bleed and may cause a delayed ischemic deficit which often improves with hypertensive therapy.

(2) Cerebral embolization of vasoactive debris.

(3) Prolonged, complicated migraine resulting in stroke, usually involving the occipital lobes.

  d. Low flow state

(1) This may occur in a setting of multiple large-vessel extracranial disease, poor intracranial collateralization, and/or systemic hypotension. Ischemic injury occurs in the border zone region between two major arterial supplies (e.g., middle cerebral artery, posterior cerebral artery).

(2) Symptoms may begin with multiple stereotypic, transient deficits or vague complaints involving graying of vision, numbness of the face, hand, and/or tongue, loss of control of the hand or arm, buckling of the leg, jerking of an extremity, or inability to speak.

B. Intracerebral hemorrhage

  1. Clinical presentation

    a. Intracerebral hemorrhages may be difficult to distinguish clinically from ischemic stroke.

b. The deficit may have a more prolonged evolution, often up to several hours to a maximum deficit.

c. Most (70%) hemorrhages occur in a setting of hypertension.

d. Hemorrhages may cause:
   (1) Secondary mass effects such as brain herniation.
   (2) Seizures from local cortical irritation.
   (3) Secondary hydrocephalus from ventricular compression or intra-ventricular hemorrhage.
   (4) Secondary brain edema.

2. Etiology
   a. Rupture of microaneurysms secondary to hypertension.
   b. Rupture of an arteriovenous malformation (AVM).
   c. Rupture of a diseased, brittle cerebral vessel, as seen in congophilic angiopathy (amyloid angiopathy).
   d. cocaine/amphetamine abuse

3. Treatment
   a. Elevation of the head (30°) to prevent aspiration and to help control intracranial pressure (ICP).
   b. Correction of coagulopathies.
   c. Monitoring and treatment of elevated ICP.
   d. Shunting for acute hydrocephalus.
   e. Anticonvulsants in selected cases.
   f. Surgical decompression for cerebellar hemorrhages and certain select cases of lobar hemorrhage with mass effect.

4. Delayed complications
   a. Seizures.
   b. Hydrocephalus.
   c. Syndrome of inappropriate antidiuretic hormone.

C. Subarachnoid hemorrhage
   1. Subarachnoid hemorrhage may result from trauma or rupture of aneurysms or angiomas.
   2. Ruptured aneurysms
      a. These usually present as sudden severe headaches. Occasionally, there is transient loss of consciousness and, rarely, seizures. Focal deficits (e.g. third nerve palsy) may help to localize the site of bleeding. Associated cardiac arrhythmias are common due to high circulating catecholamine levels.
      b. Sentinel (warning) bleeds may occur in up to 50% of patients with aneurysm.

c. Aneurysmal size and the presence of hypertension or immediate prior activity may influence the risk of bleeding. Twenty-five percent of aneurysm patients have multiple aneurysms.

d. The Hunt-Hess system is commonly used to grade patients clinically.

   Grade I: Asymptomatic; minimal headache, slight neck stiffness

   Grade II: Moderate to severe headache; no neurologic deficit other than cranial nerve palsy

   Grade III: Alteration of mental status (drowsiness, confusion) or mild focal deficit

   Grade IV: Stupor or severe hemiparesis or early decerebration

   Grade V: Coma; decerebration; moribund

3. AVMs typically present with intracerebral bleeding or seizures. Prognosis after AVM bleeding is much better than after aneurysmal bleeding.

4. The risk of recurrent bleeding after:
   a. An aneurysmal bleed is about 2–3% per year if there has been no rebleeding by 6 months; it is about 30% within 14 days after a bleed; it may be greatest within 24 hr.
   b. An AVM bleed is about 4% per year.

5. Most centers operate early on ruptured aneurysms which are grade I or II. Early surgery offers the advantage of preventing early rebleeding, washing clean bloody cisterns, and utilizing more aggressive hypertensive therapy should vasospasm develop. The disadvantage is that the surgery is technically more difficult in swollen brain.

6. Calcium channel blockers such as nimodipine seem to offer mild protection against DID. Aminocaproic acid's side effects appear to outway its theoretical benefit.

7. Delayed hydrocephalus and syndrome of inappropriate diuretic hormone (SIADH) are frequent delayed complications.

IV. **Diagnosis**
   A. CT is the most sensitive means of detecting acute hemorrhage (less than 24 hr). Most ischemic infarctions are not detected on CT until 20–24 hr after onset.

B. MRI is the most sensitive means of detecting acute focal ischemia since it can detect subtle water changes in damaged tissue as early as 4 hr. Brain stem and cerebellum can be well visualized with MRI but not with CT. MRI is particularly sensitive in detecting:

1. Small focal subcortical strokes (lacunes).
2. Dural sinus and venous thrombosis.
3. AVMs.
4. Evidence of old hemorrhage.

C. Noninvasive Doppler studies are a sensitive means of detecting vessel stenosis. In the cervical region, carotid duplex Doppler studies may be as sensitive as angiography. Intracranially, transcranial Doppler may be useful for identifying focal stenosis, spasm, or occlusion.

D. Conventional cerebral angiography after stroke is generally warranted if carotid artery surgery is being considered, when there is a diagnostic dilemma (e.g., possibility of angiitis), or when stroke has occurred in a young person. Increasingly used selective catherterization studies reduce radiologic dye loads.

E. Conventional transthoracic cardiac ultrasonography (i.e., cardiac echocardiography) does not appear to be as sensitive in detecting cardiac thrombus as transesophageal echocardiography or ultrafast cardiac CT scanning.

F. Laboratory tests including complete blood count, coagulation profile, sed rate, Venereal Disease Research Laboratory (VDRL), autoimmune profile, lupus anticoagulant, antithrombin III, protein C and protein S activities, lipid profile, and blood and toxicologic screens may be helpful in the appropriate setting.

V. **Treatment**

A. Ischemic stroke
1. Prevention
a. Treat risk factors and hypertension.
b. Antiplatelet agents appear to reduce the risk of stroke about 20% in patients with prior minor stroke or TIAs. The most efficacious dosage has yet to be determined; however, 325 mg/day is associated with fewer side effects than those revealed in studies originally utilizing 325 mg four times per day. Ticlopidine appears to offer greater protection than aspirin; however, it may produce diarrhea and neutropenia and needs to be given, BID.
c. Carotid endarterectomy for symptom-

atic internal carotid disease (greater than 70% stenosis) with symptoms within the prior 3 months.
d. Most physicians treat symptomatic atrial fibrillation chronically with warfarin. Strokes are prevented in asymptomatic, nonvalvular atrial fibrillation by treatment with warfarin or aspirin (with risk reduction up to 80%).
e. Many physicians prophylactically anticoagulate patients with large transmural anterior myocardial infarctions for 3 months.
f. Full anticoagulation with heparin followed by warfarin is usually indicated after a stroke secondary to cardiac thrombus embolization. Hemorrhage must first be ruled out by head CT. Anticoagulation should probably be delayed 48–72 hr after a large ischemic stroke. The duration of treatment is uncertain.

2. Acute stroke management
a. Avoid hypotension (this worsens perfusion to areas with borderline perfusion).
b. Minimize hyperglycemia during the first 24 hr.
c. Avoid hyperthermia.
d. Correct hematocrit elevations greater than 55% (oxygen delivery decreases due to hyperviscosity).
e. Consider delaying full anticoagulation for the first 48–72 hr in the setting of a large cortical stroke of suspected embolic origin.
f. Provide anticoagulation with heparin followed by warfarin in selected cases of cerebral embolism.
g. Consider hypertensive therapy in selected patients (ex. vasospasm).

3. Promising new therapies
a. Acute thrombolysis (e.g., r-tpa).
b. Calcium blockers with good central nervous system (CNS) penetration (nimodipine currently approved for prevention of DID after subarachnoid hemorrhage.
c. Excitatory amino acid antagonists.

B. Hemorrhagic stroke
1. Elevate head to decrease ICP; consider ICP monitoring.
2. Correct coagulation abnormalities.
3. Control hypertension.
4. Treat elevated ICP (hyperventilation, mannitol).

5. Treat secondary obstructive hydrocephalus with ventriculostomy.
   C. Subarachnoid hemorrhage
   1. Calcium channel blocker with CNS penetration (e.g., nimodipine to ameliorate DID.
   2. Hypertensive therapy to treat DID.
   3. Surgical clipping of aneurysms.
   4. Ventriculostomy for secondary hydrocephalus (recent data suggest that risk of rebleeding is less in nonshunted patients).
   5. Treatment of SIADH.
   6. Treatment of pain and nausea.
   D. Treatment of CNS vasculitis
   1. Glucocorticoids are the initial therapy.
   2. Long-term immunosuppressive therapy (usually cyclophosphamide).

Vascular Disease of Spinal Cord

I. **Introduction: Spinal Cord Circulation**
   A. Circulation to the anterior two-thirds of the spinal cord is from the anterior spinal artery, which varies in caliber along the cord. Its cervical and upper thoracic feeders are branches of the vertebral arteries and cervical branches of the subclavian artery and provide good collateral circulation.
   B. The anterior spinal artery in the lower thoracic and lumbosacral cords is supplied predominantly by more or less well-developed branches off the aorta. The lumbosacral cord's major feeder is the segmental artery of Adamkiewicz.
   C. The posterior spinal artery is formed off the vertebrals or posterior inferior cerebellar artery, runs posteriorly along the cord, and joins the anterior spinal artery in the sacral region. The posterior circulation to the cord is much less frequently affected by intrinsic disease.
   D. The mid-lower thoracic aorta has the most marginal collateral blood supply and thus is most susceptible to aortic disease and hypotension.

II. **Definition of Spinal Cord Infarction**
   Cerebrovascular diseases affecting the spinal cord usually result in occlusion of the anterior spinal artery, thereby producing injury to the anterior two-thirds of the cord and sparing the posterior columns. Initially, the diagnosis is often difficult to confirm.

III. **Etiology**
   A. Infarction may result from ischemia secondary to:
   1. Interruption of feeders (e.g., aortic dissection, spinal trauma).

2. Occlusion of the anterior median spinal artery secondary to arteritis, infection, or embolus.
   3. Small-vessel occlusion (air embolism, radiation myelopathy).
   4. Vascular malformations may rarely produce chronic cord ischemia, which presents as a progressive spastic paraparesis.
   B. In general, the most common cause of acute cord ischemia is compression secondary to spinal metastasis.
   C. Cord ischemia usually presents as paraplegia. Sensory exam may show a level to pinprick. A less common presentation is a Brown-Séquard syndrome.

IV. **Treatment of Acute Spinal Cord Ischemia**
   A. Initially, the acutely paraplegic patient should probably be presumptively treated for spinal cord trauma with high-dose corticosteroids (methylprednisolone, 30 mg/kg).
   B. Hypotension should be avoided.
   C. Blood tests, spinal MRI, CSF analysis, and a search for possible embolic sources may all aid in the diagnosis of acute paraplegia.
   D. Compressive lesions should be sought utilizing spinal MRI, myelography, and/or plain films. Surgical decompression or emergency radiation therapy may be indicated when spinal cancer is diagnosed.
   E. Infection should be sought (syphilis, human immunodeficiency virus, herpes, tuberculosis, paravertebral abscess, etc.) and treated when possible.
   F. No efficacious therapy is currently recommended to augment or reconstitute cord blood flow.

Spontaneous Spinal Cord Hemorrhage

I. **Clinical Presentation**
   Most spinal hemorrhages are extradural or, less often, intradural. The onset of back pain followed several hours later by paraplegia and loss of sphincter control suggests spinal hemorrhage. These conditions are seen in a setting of coagulopathy, thrombocytopenia, and/or trauma. Lumbar puncture in the setting of coagulopathy may produce a spinal subdural hematoma.

II. **Treatment**
   Treatment requires medical correction of the blood abnormality and neurosurgical consultation.

AVMs

I. Clinical Presentation

A. Spinal AVMs are usually intradural.

B. They may present as subarachnoid hemorrhage, cord compression, or chronic ischemia.

C. Hemorrhages may cause meningeal irritation, myelopathy, or radiculopathy.

D. Unruptured AVMs may cause chronic and progressive myelopathy on an ischemic basis. They may also compress the spinal cord or roots and cause intermittent radicular pain symptoms.

II. Treatment

Unruptured symptomatic spinal AVMs may be treated with selective embolization and/or surgery.

Bibliography

Anderson CA. Progress report of the stroke prevention in atrial fibrillation study. *Stroke* 21(Suppl III):III-12–III-17, 1990.

Antiplatelet Trialists' Collaboration. Secondary prevention of vascular disease by prolonged antiplatelet treatment. *Br Med J* 296:320–331, 1988.

Caplan LR, Stein RW. *Stroke: A Clinical Approach.* Butterworth-Heinemann, Boston, 1986.

Hass WH. A randomized trial comparing ticlopidine hydrochloride with aspirin for the prevention of stroke in high risk patients. *N Engl J Med* 321:501–507, 1989.

Kistler JP. Therapy of ischemic cerebral vascular disease due to atherothrombosis. Parts 1 and 2. *N Engl J Med* 311:27–34, 99–105, 1984.

NASCET Collaborators. Beneficial effect of carotid endarterectomy in symptomatic patients with high-grade carotid stenosis. *N Engl J Med* 325:445–453, 1991.

Olsen TS. Regional cerebral blood flow after occlusion of the middle cerebral artery. *Acta Neurol Scand* 73:321–337, 1986.

Chapter 130

Seizure Disorders

Steven L. Meyers, M.D.
Serge J.C. Pierre-Louis, M.D.

I. Definition

The epilepsies are a group of disorders of diverse etiologies all characterized by recurrent seizures. Seizures are the behavioral manifestations of abnormal synchronized electrical discharges of groups of neurons. The first step in understanding seizure disorders is to classify the type of seizure. Seizures are divided into two main categories.

A. Partial (focal, localization related) seizures arise in one portion of one cerebral hemisphere. They are further subdivided on the basis of alteration in consciousness.
   1. Simple partial: No alteration in consciousness.
   2. Complex partial: Impairment or loss of consciousness.
   3. Secondarily generalized: Partial seizures that become generalized.
B. Generalized seizures arise simultaneously in both cerebral hemispheres. They are further subdivided based on the clinical manifestations.
   1. Tonic-clonic
   2. Absence
   3. Myoclonic

4. Tonic
5. Clonic
6. Atonic

II. Etiology

The etiologies of the various seizure disorders are as varied as their clinical manifestations. Although an exhaustive evaluation may fail to reveal a specific etiology in up to one-half of patients, finding an etiology may significantly alter therapeutic decisions. The possible etiologies vary with the age of the patient.

A. Infants and children
   1. Birth and perinatal injuries
   2. Cerebrovascular injuries
   3. Congenital malformations
   4. Metabolic derangements/inborn errors of metabolism
   5. Head injuries
   6. Central nervous system (CNS) infections
   7. Neoplasms
   8. Idiopathic (genetic predisposition)
B. Adults
   1. Cerebrovascular diseases
   2. Head trauma
   3. Drugs and alcohol
   4. Neoplasms

5. CNS infections

6. Idiopathic (genetic predisposition)

III. Pathophysiology

Seizures represent an abnormal, hypersynchronous activation of large populations of cortical neurons. It is likely that different mechanisms subserve the various etiologies. However, it is generally believed that an interplay between altered excitability, altered inhibition, and hypersynchrony, superimposed on a genetic predisposition, is responsible for the abnormal behavior of neurons. Fundamental features that have been partially explained include the following:

A. The interictal electroencephalographic (EEG) spike is a marker of areas of hyperexcitable cortex. The paroxysmal depolarizing shift (PDS) is the intracellular event that underlies the EEG spike.

  1. The PDS is a sustained membrane depolarization with a superimposed burst of action potentials.

  2. The development of the PDS appears to depend on a combination of excitatory synaptic inputs and various voltage-dependent membrane currents that serve to amplify and sustain these inputs.

    a. Membrane currents implicated include slowly inactivating sodium and calcium currents and a sustained calcium current that appears to be necessary for the action potential burst.

    b. *N*-methyl-D-aspartate (NMDA)-mediated excitatory channels are important in the maintenance of the PDS and in calcium-mediated cytotoxicity.

B. Failure of normal inhibitory inputs plays a role in the conversion from interictal spike to seizure discharge.

  1. Normal inhibition is ensured by several mechanisms which depend mainly on gamma-aminobutyric acid (GABA)-mediated synaptic inputs.

  2. GABA-mediated inhibition declines rapidly with repeated neuronal activation; this decline has been implicated in the spread of seizure activity.

  3. Excessive inhibition, by facilitating synchronous activation of cortical neurons, may be the underlying mechanism associated with the 3-Hz spike wave discharges of childhood absence.

C. Synchronization of large neuronal populations is essential for the development of a seizure focus.

  1. Recurrent synaptic excitation via recurrent collateral fibers is thought to play an important role in the development of synchrony.

  2. Electrical fields created by the flow of current within neurons can influence adjacent neurons.

  3. The changes in extracellular ionic concentrations that occur during seizures make surrounding neurons more excitable and may lead to synchrony.

IV. Diagnosis

The diagnosis of epilepsy is made on historical grounds; the neurologic exam and laboratory tests help define the seizure type and its etiology.

A. History

The diagnosis of epilepsy should be considered in patients who complain of recurrent paroxysmal attacks of a stereotyped nature. Historical data of importance include the age of onset, the presence of an aura, a detailed description of the attack and the immediate postictal period, the frequency of attacks, and any precipitating or predisposing factors.

  1. Generalized seizures are seen predominantly in children and young adults, whereas partial seizures are more evenly distributed. A positive family history is more frequent with generalized epilepsy.

  2. An aura is a sensation or psychic phenomenon experienced by the patient at the onset of the seizure.

    a. The aura has great localizing value. It represents the focus of onset and defines a seizure as partial.

    b. Common auras include epigastric sensations, visual or auditory phenomena, gustatory or olfactory sensations, somatic sensations, and psychic phenomena such as déja vu or fear.

  3. A description of the attack should be obtained from eyewitnesses, as the patient is frequently amnestic for the event.

  4. Postictal neurologic deficits (Todd's paralysis) are clues to both the focus of onset and the underlying CNS pathology.

  5. Precipitating factors include sleep deprivation, stress, alcohol or drug use, head trauma, and febrile illnesses.

  6. The previous medical history (e.g., febrile convulsions, meningitis or encephalitis, head injury, stroke, intracranial sur-

gery) occasionally points to the etiology and the type of seizure.

B. Neurologic examination is frequently normal. Focal findings suggest an underlying cerebral structural pathology. Specific areas of the exam should be emphasized.

1. General cognitive function should be assessed, since there is an association between certain types of epilepsy and mental dysfunction.

2. A discrepancy between verbal (dominant hemisphere) and spatial (nondominant hemisphere) memory may be of lateralizing value.

3. Fundoscopic exam may reveal findings suggesting an inborn error of metabolism or a phakomatosis.

4. A search for distinctive skin lesions may lead to the diagnosis of a phakomatosis.

5. Cardiac abnormalities may suggest an etiology and help in the differential diagnosis.

6. An ocular bruit may be associated with an intracranial vascular malformation causing seizures.

C. Diagnostic testing may give clues to the etiology, but it can neither prove nor exclude the diagnosis of epilepsy.

1. Laboratory testing is used mainly to screen for metabolic derangements and inborn metabolic errors.

a. All patients should be screened for electrolyte imbalance, hypoglycemia, hepatic and renal function, and toxic or drug exposures.

b. Children, in addition, may need special metabolic and chromosomal analyses.

2. Two forms of neurologic imaging are currently used in routine evaluation: computed tomography (CT) and magnetic resonance imaging (MRI).

a. MRI is the study of choice. Compared to CT, it gives better anatomic and pathologic details, especially in imaging the temporal lobes.

b. MRI is clearly superior in detecting low-grade gliomas and mesial temporal sclerosis, two frequent etiologies.

c. Drawbacks include the long scan times required, poor visualization of calcifications, inability to scan patients with implanted metal devices (pacemakers, prosthetic valves), and high cost.

d. CT is relatively inexpensive and fast. It is extremely sensitive to acute hemorrhage and is the procedure of choice in an emergency setting.

e. All adult patients and children with partial seizures should undergo scanning.

3. The EEG remains of paramount importance in the evaluation.

a. Certain EEG patterns are highly suggestive of specific seizure types or syndromes that have typical etiologies or responses to therapy.

b. The EEG is a sensitive detector of focal slowing, which suggests focal pathology.

c. A normal EEG during a clinical spell is highly suggestive of, though not definite proof of, a nonepileptic event.

d. A normal routine EEG never excludes the diagnosis of epilepsy.

(1) Approximately one-half of epileptics will have a normal first EEG.

(2) Repeated EEGs raise the yield of abnormalities to about 80%.

(3) The yield can be increased by the use of activation procedures such as hyperventilation, photic stimulation, sleep deprivation, and special recording techniques.

(4) Single photon emission tomography (SPECT) scan, positron emission tomography (PET) scan, and neuropsychological testing are used experimentally or when patients with refractory partial seizures are being evaluated for epilepsy surgery.

V. Differential Diagnosis

A. There are many nonepileptic paroxysmal disorders that may mimic seizures. These vary with age (see Table 130-1).

B. Details of events during the preictal, ictal, and postictal periods will frequently clarify the diagnosis. The mode of onset and cessation of the attack, as well as its duration, should be ascertained.

C. Clonic limb movements are frequently seen in syncopal attacks (syncopal seizures), especially if the patient is held upright.

D. In patients who do not respond to standard anticonvulsant therapy, consider a nonepileptic condition.

Table 130-1. Differential Diagnosis of Paroxysmal Disorders

Children	Adults
Apneic spells	Migraine
Sleep myoclonus	Transient ischemic attacks
Breath-holding spells	Vertebrobasilar insufficiency
Gastroesophageal reflux	Movement disorders
	Narcolepsy
Shivering attacks	Syncope
Movement disorders	Hyperventilation attacks
Migraine	Psychogenic seizures
Syncope	
Hyperventilation attacks	
Psychogenic seizures	

E. Epilepsy is an infrequent cause of syncope.

VI. **Treatment** (see also Chapter 138 for specifics on medications)

   A. Basic principles

     1. Monotherapy (use of a single drug) is usually as effective as polypharmacy, and results in fewer side effects and better compliance.

     2. Choice of the initial drug is guided by the seizure type.

       a. Carbamazepine, phenytoin, primidone, and phenobarbital may each be effective in treating partial seizures, although one may be more effective in a given patient. Carbamazepine or phenytoin is usually tried first.

       b. Valproate is used mainly in the treatment of generalized seizures; more recently, it has been tried in partial seizures, with some success.

       c. Ethosuximide is the treatment of choice for pure absence epilepsy.

       d. Benzodiazepines are used in myoclonic seizures and as an adjunct in other seizure types.

     3. Since the drugs used for partial seizures are equally effective, the initial drug is chosen based upon pharmacologic and side effect profiles.

     4. There are three ways of initiating drug therapy. The method chosen depends primarily on the drug and, to some extent, on the patient's circumstances.

       a. Start an assumed effective dose initially.

       b. Start a subtherapeutic dose and slowly increase over time to an effective dose.

       c. Give a large loading dose to achieve an effective serum level quickly.

         (1) The second method is usually safest and best tolerated, although it leaves the patient unprotected longer. The method chosen should take into account the pharmacokinetics of the drug.

     5. Standard therapeutic levels are only guidelines.

       a. Some patients are controlled at low drug levels, while others may show signs of toxicity at these levels.

       b. Many patients require toxic drug levels for adequate control and will not show side effects.

       c. In general, any given drug should be pushed to the point of seizure control or clinical toxicity prior to discarding it, regardless of the serum level.

   B. The decision to start therapy following a single seizure remains controversial. The decision is based on several factors.

     1. Risk of recurrence versus risk associated with chronic drug use.

       a. The risk of recurrence following a single seizure at 5 years is approximately 35%. This risk can be altered based on the presence or absence of various factors.

         (1) Previous CNS injury

         (2) Sibling with epilepsy

         (3) Abnormal EEG

         (4) History of febrile convulsions or status epilepticus

         (5) Postictal Todd's paralysis

         (6) Abnormal neurologic examination

         (7) An obvious precipitating factor

       b. About 35% of patients experience medication side effects that require a change in therapy.

     2. Effects of further seizures on the patient's life (e.g., driving, employment).

     3. Probability that drug therapy will reduce the risk of future seizures. Several studies have failed to demonstrate substantial remission rates, although some controversy remains.

   C. Seizures that do *not* require therapy

     1. Alcohol withdrawal seizures are generalized convulsions that occur 6–36 hr after cessation of drinking. Anticonvulsants are not useful in this situation, and the

combination of certain anticonvulsants (barbiturates and benzodiazepines) and alcohol is dangerous.

2. Simple febrile convulsions are brief (≤ 15 min), generalized, nonrepetitive seizures that occur in children between the ages of 3 months and 5 years during a febrile illness not associated with CNS infection. About 3% will later develop epilepsy. Prophylactic medication is not indicated.

3. Other seizures that are *reactive* to specific metabolic derangements (sodium, calcium, glucose), to drugs that lower seizure threshold (see Table 130-2), and to special situations (reflex epilepsies) may require only correction or removal of the precipitating factor.

4. Temporary use of anticonvulsant drugs may occasionally be appropriate even with *reactive* seizures (e.g., when the underlying condition cannot be quickly controlled or when repeated seizures are deemed deleterious).

D. Status epilepticus (SE) is defined as a seizure lasting ≥ 20 min or recurrent seizures without full return of consciousness between seizures. SE is a medical emergency, as permanent neuronal damage and death may occur.

1. Basic life support is the first step, with paramount attention to airway protection. Hypotension is rarely secondary to SE and should suggest cardiac dysfunction or hypovolemia. Give dextrose and thiamine.

2. Termination of SE may require several drugs but is usually easy to accomplish.
   a. Benzodiazepines, especially lorazepam (2–8 mg in adults), are the drugs of first choice. Diazepam's antiseizure effect lasts for only 10–20 min.
   b. Phenytoin should be given at a dose of 18–20 mg/kg by slow intravenous injection (50 mg/min). An additional 10 mg/kg may be given if necessary. Blood pressure and the electrocardiogram should be monitored during infusion.
   c. Barbiturates (phenobarbital or pentobarbital) are the next drugs used in refractory seizures. The patient must be intubated at this point.
   d. EEG monitoring is usually necessary during the initial therapy of complex partial and absence SE.

3. Recurrence is prevented by initiating maintenance anticonvulsant therapy at the time of cessation of SE.

Table 130-2. Management of Status Epilepticus

1. Basic life support
   A. Protect airway.
   B. Assess vital signs. Hypotension is rarely secondary to SE and suggests cardiac dysfunction or hypothermia.
   C. Place two IV lines and draw blood for electrolytes, calcium, magnesium, blood urea nitrogen, glucose creatinine, anticonvulsant levels, and alcohol and toxic screen when indicated.
   D. Give thiamine, 100 mg, and glucose.
2. Termination of SE
   A. Lorazepam (0.05–0.2 mg/kg at 2 mg/min); maximal dose, 8 mg.
   B. Phenytoin (18 mg/kg at 50 mg/min); may produce hypotension or arrhythmias. ECG monitoring recommended.
   C. If above fails to terminate SE, several options remain:
      1. Phenobarbital (5–10 mg/kg IV).
      2. Paraldehyde (0.1–0.2 ml/kg per rectum (PR) in oil).
      3. Midazolam (0.05–0.20 mg/kg intravenous push (IVP) followed by 0.05–0.1 mg/hr).
   D. If SE continues, begin pentobarbital (10–12 mg/kg at 50 mg/min, then 0.25–1.0 mg/kg/hr).
      1. Terminates all seizures.
      2. Requires EEG monitoring to ensure burst suppression pattern.
      3. Frequently produces hypotension, requiring blood pressure support, and hypothermia.
      4. Maintain pentobarbital for 12 hr; then taper over another 12–24 hr or longer.
3. Prevention of recurrent seizures: Continue phenobarbital and/or phenytoin; maintain therapeutic blood levels.

E. Discontinuation of therapy may be considered in patients who have been seizure free for 2–4 years. This is especially true of the primary generalized epilepsies.

VII. Patient Monitoring
  A. When to check serum levels
    1. During initiation of therapy.
    2. When seizures recur after adequate control has been achieved.
    3. When toxic symptoms appear in patients on more than one drug.
    4. In patients on polypharmacy; more frequent determinations may help prevent side effects due to drug interactions.
    5. In patients with liver or kidney disease who may have unusual pharmacokinetics.
    6. During pregnancy, when drug levels may fluctuate.
  B. Anticonvulsants can have significant liver or hematologic toxicities; routine evaluation of liver function by prothrombin time/partial thromboplastin time and blood counts are often suggested. It is not clear that such monitoring actually prevents serious toxicity, most of which is idiosyncratic.
  C. Reevaluation of the diagnosis should always be considered in patients refractory to standard therapy.
  D. The development of a new seizure pattern may indicate the presence of a progressive disease and warrants reevaluation.

VIII. Prognosis
The prognosis for seizure control in the majority of patients is excellent. However, certain seizure disorders have a better prognosis than others.
  A. In general, childhood-onset generalized seizures are better controlled than adult-onset seizures.
  B. Factors that worsen the prognosis include partial seizures, multiple seizure types, underlying CNS pathology, and the number of seizures prior to initiating therapy.
  C. Although spontaneous remission is uncommon, approximately 80% of patients sustain a prolonged remission once therapy is initiated. This may be permanent in a significant number.

Bibliography

Commission on Classification and Terminology of the International League Against Epilepsy. Proposal for revised classification of epilepsies and epileptic syndromes. *Epilepsia* 30(4):389–399, 1989.

Hauser WA, Rich S, Annegers J, et al. Seizure recurrence after 1st unprovoked seizure: An extended follow-up. *Neurology* 40:1163–1170, 1990.

Johanessen S, Loyning Y, Munthe-Kaas A. General aspects of medical therapy, in Dam M, Gram L (eds), *Comprehensive Epileptology*. New York, Raven Press, 1991, pp 505–524.

Mattson R, Cramer J, Collins J, et a. Comparison of carbamazepine, phenobarbital, phenytoin and primidone in partial and secondarily generalized tonic clonic seizures. *N Engl J Med* 313:145–150, 1985.

Niedermeyer E. *The Epilepsies: Diagnosis and Management.* Baltimore, Urban and Schwarzenberg, 1990, pp 219–237.

Scheuer M, Pedley T. The evaluation and treatment of seizures. *N Engl J Med* 323:1468–1474, 1990.

CHAPTER 131

Medical Consequences of Nervous System Trauma

Steven B. Wilkinson, M.D.

Cranial Trauma

I. Definition

A classification system for different types of cranial trauma follows. Most medical consequences of central nervous system (CNS) trauma can occur with any of the following types of trauma.
A. Skull fractures
1. Simple skull fractures are nondisplaced, linear fractures of the cranial vault.
2. Basilar skull fractures occur through the cranial base, which is a more sturdy portion of the skull. Consequently, the force required to produce such a fracture is greater and leads to more neurologic sequelae.
3. Compound fractures have several fracture lines, creating free fragments of bone. These may be either open (in which the integrity of the skin is lost) or closed and either depressed (pushed below the inner table of the surrounding skull) or nondepressed.
B. Traumatic intracranial hematomas
1. Subdural hematoma (SDH) has blood

that lies on the surface of the brain between the arachnoid and the dura.
   a. Acute SDH occurs within 3 days of the injury and is composed of thick, clotted blood.
   b. Chronic SDH is sometime seen after 3 days. Usually it becomes symptomatic 2–4 weeks after the injury. It is composed of a mixture of solid clot and liquified blood, and the older ones have a membrane that encases them.
2. Epidural hematoma (EDH) has blood that lies between the dura and the cranial vault. EDH is frequently associated with skull fractures.
3. Intraparenchymal hematomas form within the substance of the brain. Cerebral contusion is a form of intraparenchymal hematoma that occurs when the brain strikes the cranial vault.
4. Subarachnoid hemorrhage has blood that lies between the surface of the brain and the arachnoid. In most cases, it is clinically silent. It is the most frequent form of traumatic intracranial hemorrhage.
C. Diffuse axonal injury is thought to occur

due to rotational injuries with shearing of the nerve fibers. This state leads to severe neurologic injury, usually without dramatic findings on computed tomography (CT) scan.

D. Open cranial injuries other than fractures occur with gunshot or missile injuries and rare cranial stab wounds. These are usually associated with quite severe brain injury.

E. Concussion, which is a brief loss of consciousness following trauma, is the most common and mild form of head injury. By definition there are no residua after a concussion.

II. **Pathophysiology**

A. The brain is housed in a nonexpansile chamber (the skull).

B. The contents of the skull include the brain, cerebrospinal fluid (CSF), and intravascular fluid. In traumatic lesions with an essentially intact skull, any additional volume (i.e., hematoma) will be added at the expense of CSF and intravascular fluid. When these two fluids can no longer compensate, a rise in intracranial pressure occurs.

C. The brain is protected and bathed in CSF. Sudden acceleration of the skull will cause the brain (which lags slightly behind because of inertia) to be forced into the inner surface of the skull. (The same holds true for sudden deceleration.) The vector and force of the impact will determine the type and degree of injury.

III. **Medical Complications**

The balance of the chapter covers a group of common medical complications of cranial trauma. Most of these complications can also be seen in spinal cord injuries. A unique group of medical complications particular to spinal cord injury will be discussed at the end.

Coagulopathy

I. **Definition**

Coagulopathy is an abnormality in the ability to clot blood that may present clinically as bleeding or be reflected in particular coagulation tests. There is a strong association between significant head injury and coagulopathy.

II. **Etiology**

This condition is felt to be secondary to a release of fibrinolytic substances from injured brain.

III. **Pathophysiology**

Fibrinolytic substances such as tissue thrombo-

plastin are released into the systemic circulation in traumatic brain injury. This leads to a prolongation of the prothrombin time (PT) and the partial thromboplastin time (PTT) and, if severe enough, to disseminated intravascular coagulation (DIC).

IV. **Diagnosis**

A. History: Coagulopathy may occur with any type of CNS trauma but is most often seen in more severe types of trauma (e.g., SDH) and in open brain injuries.

B. Clinical signs: It may take many forms, ranging from frank DIC with diffuse bleeding to recurrent or delayed hematoma.

C. Diagnostic tests: The PT and PTT will be prolonged beyond normal, and the platelet count will usually be low. In more severe cases, fibrin split products will be elevated and fibrinogen will be low.

V. **Differential Diagnosis**

DIC may be seen in many medical and surgical disorders. In the setting of CNS trauma the etiology will be clear, but in cases of mild trauma other causes of coagulopathy need to be ruled out. These include sepsis, drug reaction, and congenital clotting disorder.

VI. **Treatment**

Fresh frozen plasma transfusion is the quickest and safest way to correct the problem. Platelet transfusions may be needed if the platelet count falls below 60,000. The PT/PTT should be corrected as soon as possible. Surgery on all but life-threatening lesions should be delayed until this step is completed.

VII. **Patient Monitoring**

All patients with severe head trauma, especially any open brain injuries, should have a complete set of coagulation function tests and a platelet count done on admission and repeated if abnormal or daily until the patient is stable. These tests should also be repeated on discovery of a delayed or recurrent hemorrhage.

VIII. **Prognosis**

Coagulation dysfunction is usually a bad prognostic sign. In general, the more severe the coagulopathy, the more severe the injury.

Pulmonary Complications

I. **Definition**

Pulmonary complications are quite frequent in CNS trauma and range from atelectasis to the adult respiratory distress syndrome (ARDS).

II. Etiology

After CNS trauma there may be a decreased level of consciousness, which may reduce respiratory movements and diminish airway protection, leading to pulmonary complications.

III. Pathophysiology

Decreased respiratory effort leads to atelectasis. In major trauma, blood and volume replacement and concomitant long bone injury are often predecessors of ARDS. Finally, neurogenic pulmonary edema (NPE) may occur in the setting of severe trauma. This is thought to be due to a massive sympathetic discharge initiated from the hypothalamus, which leads to increased filling pressures and then overload of the pulmonary vascular bed. Other studies suggest that pulmonary venoconstriction may produce fluid translation with pulmonary edema without raising filling pressures. In experimental animals, this can be blocked by cervical cord transection.

IV. Diagnosis

A. History: All patients with head trauma who have a decreased level of consciousness or inability to protect the airway are at risk for pulmonary complications.

B. Clinical signs: Tachypnea, abnormal breathing pattern (i.e. Cheyne-Stokes), inspiratory stridor, prolonged exhalation, and decreased breath sounds may be found.

C. Diagnostic tests: All patients seen with significant head trauma should have at least a baseline chest x-ray and an arterial blood gas determination.

V. Differential Diagnosis

The differential diagnosis of respiratory insufficiency is essentially the same in any patient.

A. Atelectasis may be seen secondary to poor ventilatory effort, mucous plugging, or both.

B. Pneumonia, as in other critically ill patients, is seen frequently and is most often due to aspiration of oral or stomach contents. Patients with unexplained fever should have a chest x-ray and sputum analysis to rule out pneumonia.

C. Pulmonary embolism (see section below)

D. NPE occurs in the setting of severe CNS injury and usually has a delayed onset after the injury. The differentiation from ARDS is difficult, but the same treatment measures apply. Airway pressures are higher in ARDS patients than in those within NPE.

E. ARDS needs to be differentiated from cardiogenic pulmonary edema; this is most often done with pulmonary wedge pressure determination to rule out increased filling pressures.

VI. Treatment

A. Therapy is directed at correcting hypoxemia and hypercarbia, both of which have an adverse effect on neurologic function and outcome.

B. Intubation and mechanical ventilation are needed for those patients who cannot protect the airway due to a decreased level of consciousness or who cannot maintain normocarbia. Intubation may also be required for hyperventilation as a treatment for increased intracranial pressure (ICP).

C. Early intubation and institution of positive end-expiratory pressure (PEEP) may be required for the treatment of ARDS and NPE. The amount of PEEP used must be carefully monitored since it may increase ICP. ICP monitoring is very useful in this situation.

D. Cardiogenic pulmonary edema may require fluid restriction, diuretics, and possibly inotropic agents.

E. Hospital-acquired pneumonia should be empirically treated with broad-spectrum antibiotics to cover gram-negative organisms and anaerobes. Bronchodilators may help to improve oxygenation.

F. Aggressive, good pulmonary toilet is necessary. Therapeutic bronchoscopy may be needed to clear plugged airways. Rotating beds may be a useful adjunct in some patients to aid in cleaning bronchial secretions.

VII. Patient Monitoring

A. Frequent arterial blood gas (ABG) determinations to assess oxygenation, carbon dioxide partial pressure, and pH are needed in patients with serious respiratory dysfunction. Pulse oximetry may be used as an on-line monitor of oxygenation. Daily chest x-rays to monitor for atelectasis and pneumonia should be obtained in critically ill patients.

B. Any time there is a fall in the oxygenation or an increase in the airway pressure, a chest x-ray is needed to rule out pneumothorax volume loss from a mucous plug or consolidating process.

C. Mixed venous oxygenation, as measured continuously via an oximetric pulmonary artery catheter, provides an indirect measure of adequacy of respiratory function.

D. An end-tidal CO_2 monitor may be useful in assessing the adequacy of ventilation.

VIII. **Prognosis**

Hypoxemia and hypercarbia may lead to an increase in neurologic dysfunction or neuronal injury. All attempts should be made to prevent this and to treat quickly when it occurs. Mortality from ARDS and NPE is quite high, approaching 70% in some studies.

Deep Venous Thrombosis and Pulmonary Embolism

I. **Definition**

Deep venous thrombosis (DVT) and pulmonary embolism (PE) are common in the trauma victim, especially in patients with neurologic injury. DVT may occur in up to 90% of patients with severe trauma and PE in up to 25%.

II. **Etiology**

Immobilization is one of the major risk factors in DVT. Patients with neurologic injury have decreased muscular function, leading to inadequate venous return and venous stasis.

III. **Pathophysiology**

Thrombi form in the major venous tributaries of the lower extremity and pelvis. These may break off, and pieces of the thrombus may travel to the lung. Depending on the size and number of these emboli, pulmonary injury may result. The embolus blocks pulmonary arterial flow to a segment of the lung. Secondary bronchoconstriction occurs, leading to ventilation-perfusion mismatch and worsening pulmonary function.

IV. **Diagnosis**

A. History: Dyspnea, chest pain, and hemoptysis may occur, but these features may not be evident in the brain-injured patient. Lower extremity pain, redness, and tenderness are the classic findings of DVT, but they may not be present.

B. Clinical signs and physical findings

1. Homan's sign is an unreliable indication of a DVT. Its absence, especially in a neurologically impaired patient, does not rule out DVT. Increase in calf width, warmth, tenderness, and palpable thrombosed veins are also suggestive, but their absence does not rule out DVT.

2. Tachypnea, hypotension, fever, hemoptysis, decreased breath sounds on auscultation, and pleural friction rub may all be seen with PE but are not diagnostic.

C. Diagnostic tests

1. Chest x-ray is also nonspecific but may show pleural effusion or a pulmonary infiltrate. ABG determination may show hypoxemia and hypocarbia or, in more severe insults, hypercarbia. Unfortunately, physical exam and chest x-ray changes are nonspecific and do not usually rule out DVT or PE, making other tests necessary.

2. The gold standard for diagnosis is contrast venography for DVT and pulmonary arteriography for PE. These tests are invasive, have complications, and are difficult to perform in the neurologically impaired patient. Impedance plethysmography, Doppler ultrasonography, and ^{125}I fibrinogen uptake are other screening tests for DVT. Unfortunately, there is quite a bit of technical variability among different institutions, making accuracy difficult to evaluate. Deciding on which test or combination of tests to use will therefore depend on their performance accuracy in any given institution. Ventilation-perfusion scans are up to 80% accurate in suggesting a low or high probability of PE. This test is difficult to perform and interpret in an intubated patient. The most important point in the diagnosis of DVT or PE in a neurologically compromised patient is a high clinical suspicion, since the signs and symptoms of PE are nonspecific.

V. **Differential Diagnosis**

DVT should be anticipated in all patients with neurologic injury or immobilization, and steps should be taken for its prevention (see Section VI,B). The diagnosis of PE should be entertained in all cases of unexplained tachycardia, tachypnea, hypoxia, respiratory distress or failure, or hemodynamic collapse. Other entities, such as atelectasis, pneumonia, and ARDS, need to be excluded.

VI. **Treatment**

A. Anticoagulation, initially with heparin and then chronically with coumadin, is the standard treatment.

1. In patients with head injury, full anticoagulation is contraindicated in most circumstances.

2. Delay the use of anticoagulants in head injury for 3 days to 2 weeks, depending on the injury suggested.

3. During initial anticoagulation, frequent clinical exams and possibly CT scans need to be repeated to detect intracranial hemorrhage.

4. The duration of anticoagulation should be 4–6 months.

5. Vena cava interruption should be considered in head injury patients with significant DVT or PE. This may provide protection from recurrent PE until anticoagulation can safely be started.

6. Fibrinolytic agents are contraindicated in serious head trauma but can be used once the risk of recurrent hemorrhage has abated.

B. The best treatment for DVT and PE is prevention.

1. Patients with significant head injury should have pneumatic compression devices placed. In some studies, this has been shown to decrease significantly the incidence of DVT.

2. Low-dose heparin (5,000 U subcutaneously twice a day) has been shown to decrease the incidence of DVT, but its use in head-injured patients remains controversial, with some authors reporting its safety and others reporting adverse bleeding. It is probably safest to avoid the use of low-dose heparin during the first 3 days after head trauma.

VII. **Patient Monitoring**

A. Patients on heparin need to have the PTT checked routinely. Platelet counts should be checked periodically to rule out heparin-induced thrombocytopenia.

B. The PT should be kept 1.2–1.8 times the control value in patients on coumadin. It should be remembered that warfarin affects the metabolism of many medications, including most common anticonvulsants. The level of this medication should be checked routinely.

VIII. **Prognosis**

There may be up to 30% excess mortality from PE. Recurrent PE may lead to cor pulmonale. Following one episode of DVT, the involved extremity is at a higher risk for recurrent DVT.

Fluid and Electrolyte Disturbances

I. **Definition**

A. In head injury, the two most common fluid and electrolyte abnormalities are due to the syndrome of inappropriate release of antidiuretic hormone (SIADH) and to diabetes insipidus (DI).

B. SIADH leads to hyponatremia from continuous release of ADH, with absorption of free water in excess of sodium.

C. DI is a deficiency of ADH leading to renal loss of free water and resultant hypernatremia. Other causes of hypo- or hypernatremia will be discussed below.

II. **Etiology**

SIADH may be seen after any type of serious head trauma, but it may also occur as a side effect of some medications such as carbamazepine. Direct or secondary injury to the pituitary or the hypothalamus may lead to DI. This is seen occasionally in brain-dead patients.

III. **Pathophysiology**

A. ADH is released from the posterior pituitary and acts on the distal renal tubule of the collecting system in the kidney to increase free water absorption. The release of ADH is triggered by an increase in serum osmolality, as sensed by chemoreceptors in the hypothalamus. It may also be triggered by volume receptors in the left atrium of the heart to protect the circulating blood volume. This stimulus is actually a stronger influence on ADH release than is osmolality. Therefore, volume will be protected at the expense of low osmolality.

B. In SIADH there is an abnormal release of ADH despite a low serum osmolality; in DI there is inadequate release of ADH to keep serum osmolality from rising. Traumatic DI tends to have a triphasic pattern. Initial DI, which will resolve over several days as the pituitary releases stored ADH, is followed by a more long-lasting DI due to the lack of ADH production.

IV. **Diagnosis**

A. History

1. SIADH and hyponatremia may present with alteration in the level of consciousness, anorexia, weakness, dizziness, and even focal neurologic findings or seizures.

2. DI presents with polyuria and polydipsia, which may be missed in the neurologically injured patient. Inadequate intake in a neurologically impaired patient with DI may lead to hypovolemia and then hypotension.

B. Clinical signs and physical findings: There

are no specific findings to indicate hypo- or hypernatremia.

C. Diagnostic tests

   1. For the diagnosis of SIADH the following are found:

     a. Serum Na^+: <135 mEq/liter

     b. Urine Na^+: >25 mEq/liter

     c. Serum osmolality: <280 mOsm/kg

     d. Urine osmolality inappropriately concentrated for the degree of serum osmolality.

   2. For the diagnosis of DI the following are found:

     a. Urine specific gravity: <1.003

     b. Urine output: >300 ml/hr

   3. Frequently found in DI but not necessary for the diagnosis are:

     a. Serum Na^+: >145 mEq/liter

     b. Serum osmolality: >290 mOsm/kg

V. Differential Diagnosis

A. Replacement of fluid losses with hypotonic fluid is probably the most common iatrogenic cause of hyponatremia. These patients will not have inappropriately high urine osmolalities. An adverse effect of carbamazepine is SIADH, but this is seldom seen in the first few months of treatment. Cerebral salt wasting may be seen after head injury or other major CNS insults. This condition has all the laboratory findings of SIADH, but since the blood volume is contracted, the urine osmolality is appropriately elevated. It is secondary to central release of atrial natriuretic factor.

B. The differential diagnosis of hypernatremia should include excess free water loss from osmotic therapy (mannitol) and inappropriate fluid replacement with hypertonic solutions. In patients receiving enteral feedings, hypernatremia may result from the hyperosmolar feedings.

VI. Treatment

A. The first step in the treatment of SIADH is fluid restriction, usually to about 1 liter/day. For patients with seizures or other severe symptoms, cautious replacement of serum Na^+ with saline solutions (500 ml over 6–12 hr) along with furosemide (which increases free water loss) may be needed. Hypertonic saline is rarely needed. Vigorous replacement of sodium has been associated with central pontine myelinolysis. In chronic cases of SIADH, demeclocycline in a dose of 600–1,200 mg/day may be employed.

B. In patients who are awake and alert and who can tolerate oral intake, allowing drinking to thirst is the best initial management of DI. In comatose patients, aqueous vasopressin, 5–10 U subcutaneously every 4–6 hr, may be needed to control urine output. Appropriate replacement of urine losses with hypotonic fluid will be needed. Use of longer-acting compounds such as vasopressin in oil should be avoided initially because of the changing course of traumatic DI (see above). For chronic DI, intranasal 1-deamino-(8-D-arginine)-vasopressin (DDAVP), 10–20 μg once or twice a day, can be used to control urine output.

VII. Patient Monitoring

Abnormalities of electrolytes, serum osmolality, and excessive urinary output with frequent measurement of serum electrolytes are detected and monitoring of fluid balance. The early recognition of these problems will help prevent severe complications. Any significant change in the neurologic exam should prompt a determination of the serum electrolyte levels. Posttraumatic patients with DI should have a complete workup of pituitary function to detect other pituitary deficiencies.

VIII. Prognosis

Except for the grave indicator of DI in the brain-dead patient, these abnormalities in themselves are not predicative of the neurologic outcome. While some studies suggest that posttraumatic DI predicts poorer ultimate neurologic progress, this conclusion has not been universally accepted.

Miscellaneous Complications

There are several other significant medical complications of head injury.

I. Head Injury

A. Gastritis occurs in up to 75% of patients with significant head injuries. This may be due to hypersecretion of gastric acid or decreased mucosal blood flow. Treatment with antacids and H-2 blockers decreases the risk of hemorrhage but unfortunately increases the risk of pneumonia from aspiration (this mechanism is debatable).

B. After head injury, the caloric requirement may rise to 200% of normal. This should be kept in mind when determining nutritional replacement.

C. Infections may be seen in any critically ill patient. Basilar skull fractures, open cranial wounds, and patients after neurosurgery are all at increased risk of meningitis. In this setting, meningitis is usually due to *Staphylococcus aureus* or streptococcus pneumonia.

D. Patients who are neurologically impaired are at risk for skin breakdown. These patients should have frequent turning and special vigilance by the nursing staff for early signs of breakdown.

II. Spinal Cord Injury

Patients with spinal cord injury (SCI) are at risk for the development of all of the complications seen in head injury except for coagulopathy. Several consequences unique to SCI will be mentioned here.

A. Cardiovascular

1. Spinal shock, which may occur acutely, is defined as a loss of deep tendon reflexes, muscle tone, and autonomic function below the level of the injury. Since the vagus nerve carries most of the parasympathetic fibers and is not involved in spinal cord injury, a "vagal" state ensues.

2. These patients are at risk for hypotension and bradycardia. These problems seldom manifest as long as the patient is supine.

3. Autonomic dysreflexia is the chronic consequence of spinal shock. It is usually triggered by bladder or bowel distention. Hypertension, headache, and sweating and flushing above the level of the injury are seen.

4. Autonomic dysreflexia is initially treated by elevating the head of the bed, ensuring that bladder outflow is not obstructed and that there is no fecal impaction.

5. Nifedipine, 10 mg by mouth, may be used if the hypertension persists.

B. Gastrointestinal: Because SCI patients do not have normal sensation and cutaneous reflexes, the detection of abdominal pathology is difficult and a high index of suspicion is needed. Gallstones are three times as common in SCI patients as in the general population, and the rate of colorectal carcinoma may also be higher. Chronic rectal problems such as anal fissures and hemorrhoids are common in these patients.

C. Genitourinary

1. In acute spinal injury the bladder is atonic and flaccid, which leads to urinary retention and an increased risk of infection. Intermittent catheterization should be initiated early to improve bladder tone and prevent bladder distention. As reflexive emptying of the bladder returns, it may be accompanied by vesicoureteral reflux. These patients shoulds have a urologic consultation to study the urinary dynamics, follow the bladder training program, and help treat infection.

2. Squamous bladder carcinoma may occur in patients with SCI. Urologic consultation and monitoring of indwelling catheters and urine cytology, along with cystoscopy as needed, will prevent some of these complications.

D. Metabolic: Initially after SCI, hypercalcemia and hyperphosphatemia may be seen; these conditions usually resolve spontaneously. Chronic hyponatremia may also be found.

Bibliography

Foo D. Management of acute complications of spinal cord injury. *Spine: State Art Rev* 3(2):211–219, 1989.

Foo D. Management of chronic complications of spinal cord injury. *Spine: State Art Rev* 3(2):221–230, 1989.

Marion DW. Complications of head injury and their therapy. *Neurosurg Clin North Am* 2(2):411–424, 1991.

Ratcheson RA, Wirth FP (eds). *Neurosurgical Critical Care.* Baltimore, Williams and Wilkins, 1989.

Wilkins RH, Rengachary SS (eds). *Neurosurgery.* New York, McGraw-Hill, 1985.

CHAPTER 132

Movement Disorders

Melanie Brandabur, M.D.
Cynthia Comella, M.D.

The term *movement disorders* encompasses a variety of neurologic conditions in which there is a disturbance of normal volitional movement and/or the presence of abnormal, involuntary movements (see Table 132-1). There may also be associated changes in muscle tone, but there is no substantial change in muscle strength. These disorders are all thought to arise from dysfunction of the basal ganglia and other deep gray matter structures such as the subthalamic nucleus and substantia nigra, but they are not necessarily limited to these regions. Included in this category are various disorders of involuntary motor control such as parkinsonism, dystonia, tics, and chorea. Maladies of the upper and lower motor neurons, spinal cord, peripheral nerves, and musculature, as well as "pure" cerebellar diseases, are generally excluded.

Parkinsonism

I. Definition

Parkinsonism is a clinical syndrome with four cardinal manifestations and several associated findings. Not all need be present for the clinical diagnosis.

A. Tremor: Usually occurs predominantly at rest, lessening with action or on assuming a posture.

B. Cogwheel rigidity: Increased tone with a ratchety component detected on passive range of motion.

C. Bradykinesia: Difficulty initiating movement and slowness of movement.

D. Postural reflex impairment: Inability to compensate for a postural threat. Tested by standing behind the patient and administering a firm push on the back or pull on the shoulders.

E. Associated findings: Micrographia, masked face, drooling, stooped posture, difficulty with fine motor movements (e.g., buttoning buttons), difficulty getting out of low chairs, rolling over in bed, freezing.

F. *Significant objective motor weakness is not associated with parkinsonism.*

II. Etiology

The etiology of Idiopathic Parkinson's disease remains unknown.

III. Pathophysiology and Differential Diagnosis

Parkinsonism results from underactivity of a specific neuronal system, which involves a pathway from the substantia nigra to the striatum. This

Table 132-1. Definition of Movement Disorders

Disorder	Definition
Tremor	A rhythmic, sinusoidal, oscillating movement
Chorea	Irregularly timed, randomly distributed, abrupt, spontaneous movements
Dystonia	Sustained muscle contractions, frequently resulting in twisting and repetitive movements with abnormal postures
Myoclonus	Brief, shock-like muscle jerks originating in the CNS and often repetitive in the same muscles
Tics	Stereotypic, repetitive movements that can be slow or fast, simple or complex, and are partially suppressible
Akathisia	Restlessness that is relieved by purposeful movement
Ballismus	Proximal, violent throwing movements, usually unilateral

system uses the neurotransmitter dopamine, so that a reduction in the activity of dopamine or dopamine receptors leads to parkinsonism.

A. The loss of dopamine-producing neurons in the substantia nigra, with loss of pigmented nuclei and Lewy body formation. This constellation describes idiopathic Parkinson's disease (IPD). IPD usually begins in the fifties, although earlier onset IPD also occurs. It affects approximately 500,000 individuals in the United States. The etiology of IPD remains unknown, but much research is in progress.

B. The blockade of dopamine receptors: This is usually the result of antipsychotic drugs (haloperidol, thioridazine, thorazine), but it also occurs with agents typically used to treat gastrointestinal complaints such as metoclopramide (Reglan).

C. The loss of dopamine receptors at the level of the striatum instead of the substantia nigra. This results in the parkinson-plus syndromes (progressive supranuclear palsy, olivopontocerebellar atrophy, cortical-basal ganglionic degeneration, and multiple systems atrophy [Shy-Drager]), as well as ischemic damage to the striatum (arteriosclerotic parkinsonism).

D. Other drugs causing parkinsonism and/or resting tremor: methyldopa, tetrabenazine, reserpine.

IV. Treatment of IPD

A. Prevention of progression: Selegiline (Eldepryl) is an irreversible monoamine oxidase (MAO)-B inhibitor that slows the progression of diability due to IPD in patients with early, mild disease. The dose is 5 mg in the morning and at noon.

B. Symptomatic treatment
1. Anticholinergic drugs (trihexyphenidyl, benztropine) are useful for tremor and rigidity. Begin with low doses and gradually increase. Side effects: dry mouth, urinary retention, memory loss, confusion, hallucinations. Use with caution in elderly patients.
2. Amantadine: Indirect dopamine agonist useful for all cardinal manifestations of IPD. The dose is 100–300 mg/day. It is excreted unchanged through the kidney, so it is safest to use in patients without renal impairment. Side effects: confusion, hallucinations, myoclonus, toxic delirium.
3. Levodopa: Combined with carbidopa as Sinemet. It is converted centrally into dopamine and effectively treats most IPD symptoms. Start at a low dose and gradual increase. Side effects: nausea, hypotension, sleepiness, motor fluctuations, confusion, hallucinations, other psychiatric abnormalities.
4. Direct dopamine agonists (pergolide, bromocriptine) may be used alone or as adjuncts to Sinemet. Side effects: orthostatic hypotension and other dopaminergic effects.
5. Selegiline is often used with levodopa preparations to prolong the effect of dopamine and prevent fluctuations.

Chorea

I. Definition
Chorea is a term used to describe abnormal, involuntary, irregular, quick, jerky movements, typically involving the face (lip smacking, chewing, and grimacing), hands (irregular, continuous, fidgety movements of the fingers, hands, and/or wrists), legs, and feet (irregular, continuous movements of the toes, feet, or ankles and sometimes a dance-like gait).

II. Etiology
Chorea is a generalized term—numerous etiologies have been associated with its symptoms.

III. Pathophysiology

Chorea is usually associated with conditions in which there is relative overactivity of the dopaminergic system. This may be due to excessive dopamine, hypersensitivity of dopamine receptors, or a disruption of the acetylcholine–dopamine balance in which there is a relative reduction in the activity of acetylcholine.

IV. Differential Diagnosis

A. Huntington's disease (HD)
 1. A progressive degenerative disorder characterized typically by chorea, dementia, and psychiatric disturbances. HD is inherited in an autosomal dominant pattern with complete penetrance. Symptoms usually emerge in the fifth decade and consist of chorea, motor impersistence, dysarthria, abnormal gait, cognitive impairment, and psychiatric disturbances (depression, increased risk of suicide). Death is usually due to aspiration and occurs, on average, 15 years after the onset of symptoms.
 2. Treatment is symptomatic. Dopamine receptor blockers (haloperidol, pimozide) are used to control chorea. A variety of psychotropic agents have been used to treat the associated behavioral conditions, including neuroleptics, antidepressants, and anxiolytics. Genetic counseling of the patient and family is also important.

B. Tardive dyskinesia (TD)
 1. A syndrome of abnormal involuntary movements associated with chronic (at least 3 months) treatment with neuroleptics, metoclopramide (Reglan), or certain calcium channel blockers such as cinnarizine and flunarizine. About 10–20% of patients treated with neuroleptics will develop TD.
 2. Treatment involves withdrawal of the causative agent if possible. If the patient's psychiatric condition precludes discontinuation of the neuroleptic, then maintaining the patient on the lowest possible dose is generally advised. As neuroleptic agents are reduced or discontinued, mild TD may increase in severity or new dyskinetic symptoms may appear. This is an unmasking of the underlying TD. Indications for therapy should be frequently reevaluated. If treatment is required, low doses of benzodiazepines or phenobarbital may reduce mild dyskinesias. Dopamine depletion with reserpine may be required in severe cases.

C. Other drug-induced choreas
 1. Dopaminergic drugs
 2. Anticholinergics
 3. Antihistaminics
 4. Triazolam
 5. Oral contraceptives, estrogens
 6. Lithium
 7. Isoniazid
 8. Anticonvulsants
 9. Amphetamines, methadone
 10. Alcohol withdrawal
 11. Cimetidine

D. Chorea gravidarum (occurring with pregnancy)

E. Postinfectious: Group B streptococcus (Sydenham's chorea)

F. Metabolic: Hyperthyroidism

G. Neuroacanthocytosis

Dystonia

I. Definition

Dystonia is a slow, involuntary movement that leads to the assumption of an abnormal sustained posture, often with overlying spasms or tremor. Dystonia is categorized in several ways. One way is by the body areas affected.

A. Generalized dystonia: Involvement of several body areas. Idiopathic torsion dystonia is an inherited disorder that usually begins in childhood. The gene responsible for this disorder has been localized to chromosome 9. Initial involvement is typically in the foot, usually with generalized spread thereafter. Although the patient may become physically handicapped, cognition remains intact unless side effects of medicine intervene.

B. Focal and segmental dystonia: Involvement of a single body area (focal) or two contiguous body areas (segmental). This disorder typically begins in adulthood and rarely progresses to a generalized form. The etiology of adult-onset focal and segmental dystonia is unknown, although some cases may be an incomplete expression of the same abnormality as ITD or a related abnormality. A variety of clinical syndromes occur: blepharospasm (eye closing dystonia), oromandibular (jaw opening or closing dystonia), spasmodic torticollis (neck muscles with head turning), limb dystonia (involvement of the hand or foot), and occupational dystonia (occurring with a particular action, such as writing dystonia).

II. Pathophysiology and Etiology
  A. The pathophysiology of dystonia is unknown. Some have suggested that abnormalities of the basal ganglia or thalamus may be involved.
  B. Etiology
    1. Hereditary
    2. Idiopathic
    3. Wilson's disease
    4. Drug induced
       a. Neuroleptics: Acute dystonic reactions and tardive dystonia
       b. Dopaminergics in IPD
       c. Metoclopramide
       d. Antimalarial drugs
  C. Caution: Because dystonia may have superimposed muscle spasms or tremor (e.g., spasmodic torticollis), these patients sometimes receive a diagnosis of essential tremor, which is managed differently than dystonia.

III. Treatment
  A. Anticholinergics
  B. Baclofen
  C. Clonazepam
  D. Levodopa (Segawa syndrome)
  E. Other drugs: Lithium, tegretol, dilantin, etc.
  F. Botulinum toxin injections for focal dystonia
  G. Surgery

Tics

I. Definition
Tics are repetitive, brief, stereotypic movements or vocalizations that can be partially suppressed by the patient.
  A. Motor tics
    1. Simple: Consist of actions such as eye blinks, shoulder shrugs, facial grimaces, or jerking of the arms or legs.
    2. Complex: Involve a combination of more than one tic into a complex motor movement: jumping, smelling the hands, shaking the head, or hitting.
  B. Vocal tics
    1. Simple: Include grunts, barks, coughs, and throat clearing.
    2. Complex: Coprolalia, panting, belching, hiccoughs, echolalia, and stuttering.

II. Etiology
The etiology of tic disorders is not known at present.

III. Pathophysiology
The pathophysiology of tic disorders is poorly understood but an increased sensitivity of dopamine receptors has been suggested. Abnormalities involving acetylcholine, serotonin, norepinephrine, and gamma-aminobutyric acid (GABA) have also been proposed.

IV. Differential Diagnosis
  A. Transient tic disorder: A syndrome of multiple motor tics which begins during childhood and lasts for less than 1 year.
  B. Chronic motor tic disorder: A tic disorder lasting longer than 1 year in which no more than three muscle groups are involved at any one time.
  C. Gilles de la Tourette syndrome (GTS): Consists of multiple motor and vocal tics beginning in childhood or adolescence. GTS is usually a lifelong disorder and is thought to be inherited in an autosomal dominant manner with variable penetration. The syndrome is frequently accompanied by a variety of behavioral abnormalities, including:
    1. Obsessive/compulsive disorder
    2. Attention deficit disorder
    3. Learning disorders
    4. Hyperactivity
    5. Impulse control problems
  D. Tic disorders may also be seen in relation to the following drugs:
    1. Stimulants (possibly)
    2. Anticonvulsants
    3. Neuroleptics (late effects)
    4. Levodopa and dopaminergic agents
  E. Tics may develop in relation to cerebral insults such as head trauma, stroke, encephalitis, and carbon monoxide poisoning.

V. Treatment of GTS
  A. Treatment is indicated when tics interfere with normal intellectual and/or social functioning.
  B. Dopamine blockers
    1. Haloperidol: Initial daily dose of 0.25–0.5 mg, increasing as needed by 0.25–0.5 mg/week to a dose range of 4–6 mg/day. Possible side effects include parkinsonism, sedation, acute dystonic reaction, and tardive dyskinesia.
    2. Pimozide: Initial daily dose of 0.5–1.0 mg, increasing as needed by 0.5–1.0 mg/week to a dose range of 4–8 mg/day (average). There is generally less sedation, but otherwise the side effects are the same as those seen with haldoperidol.
    3. Other agents reported to be useful in some patients with GTS or the behavioral abnormalities associated with it include clonidine, clonazepam, and fluoxetine.

Table 132-2. Tremor Classification

Tremor Type	Description	Associated Disorders
Rest tremor	Large-amplitude; 4- to 6-Hz frequency; occurs at rest; decreased with action or posture	Parkinsonism, Rubral tremor, Wilson's disease
Postural tremor	Amplitude varies; 6- to 8-Hz frequency; occurs with assumption of posture	Essential tremor
Movement tremor	Large amplitude; 3- to 4-Hz frequency; occurs with movement of involved limb	Cerebellar tremor

Essential Tremor

I. Definition

A. Essential tremor (ET), the most common movement disorder, consists of a 4- to 12-Hz tremor with postural and kinetic components.

B. Categories

1. Familial: Inherited in an autosomal dominant pattern.

2. Benign: Sporadic occurrence with no family history.

3. Senile: Sporadic occurrence after age 65.

II. Clinical Characteristics

A. Usually involves the upper extremities and head (may also involve the voice, trunk, or legs).

B. May be unilateral at onset.

C. Onset varies from adolescence to adulthood.

D. Ameliorated with ingestion of ethanol in 50% of patients.

E. May be extremely disabling, especially if tremor interferes with tasks such as writing, eating, and drinking.

III. Differential Diagnosis (see also Table 132-2)

A. Physiologic tremor exaggerated by fatigue, emotion, and toxic-metabolic factors.

B. Parkinsonism.

C. Dystonic tremor.

D. Tremor occurring with a peripheral neuropathy (Roussy-Levy syndrome).

E. Cerebellar tremor.

F. Drugs including thyroxine, neuroleptics, reserpine, tetrabenazine, sympathomimetics, caffeine, amphetamines, tricyclics, steroids, lithium, nicotine, arecoline (betel nut), bethanechol, calcitonin, MSG, bismuth, amiodarone, and anticonvulsants.

G. Withdrawl of alcohol, β-blockers, benzodiazepines, or opiates.

IV. Treatment

A. Propranolol: Start at 20 mg three times per day, and increase gradually to 240 mg/day if there are no contraindications (asthma, congestive heart failure, atrioventricular heart block, diabetes mellitus). The long-acting preparation may also be used.

B. Primidone, in doses of up to 750 mg/day, may also be effective and is sometimes used in combination with propranolol.

C. Clonazepam and other benzodiazepines have also been used with moderate success.

Wilson's Disease

I. Definition

Also known as *hepatolenticular degeneration*, this autosomal recessive disorder is a rare but treatable cause of abnormal involuntary movements presenting before the age of 40.

II. Etiology

Wilson's disease is an inherited condition that is passed on to descendants through an autosomal-recessive pattern.

III. Pathophysiology

The pathophysiology involves excessive deposition of copper in the nervous system, liver, and other organs. There is also bilateral degeneration of the lenticular nuclei. Although most patients have ceruloplasmin deficiency, the significance of this condition is not completely understood.

IV. Clinical Manifestations

A. Wilson's disease can have a variety of neurologic manifestations, including chorea, tremor, rigidity, bradykinesia, dystonia, gait disorders, dysarthria, dysphagia, and cognitive changes.

B. An important associated ophthalmologic finding is the ring of gold or greenish brown around the lumbus of the cornea (Kayser-Fleischer ring), which often requires a slit lamp examination by an experienced ophthalmologist to detect.

C. In addition, there may be associated psychiatric and hepatic manifestations, as well as hypersplenism.

V. Diagnosis

Because the disease is fatal without treatment, it should be considered in all cases of movement disorders in young people by obtaining serum copper and ceruloplasmin levels and performing slit lamp evaluations.

VI. Treatment

Treatment consists of 1–1.5 of *d*-penicillamine daily. Copper-rich foods (nuts, shellfish, liver, chocolate, mushrooms) should be avoided.

Bibliography

Fahn S, Marsden CD, Calne DB (eds). *Advances in Neurology*, Vol 50, *Dystonia*. New York, Raven Press, 1988.

Fahn S, Marsden CD, Jenner P, et al (eds). *Recent Developments in Parkinson's Disease*. New York, Raven Press, 1986.

Goetz CG, Gilles de la Tourette syndrome, in Vinken PJ, Bruyn GW, Klawans HL (eds), *Handbook of Clinical Neurology*. New York, Elsevier, 1986, pp 627–640.

Goetz CG. *Iatrogenic Movement Disorders Course*. Miami, Fla, American Academy of Neurology, 1990.

Jancovic J, Tolosa E. *Parkinson's Disease and Movement Disorders*. Baltimore, Urban and Schwarzenberg, 1988.

Lees A. *Tics and Related Disorders*. New York, Churchill Livingstone, 1985.

Tanner CM. Drug-induced movement disorders, in Vinken PJ, Bruyn GW, Klawans HL (eds), *Handbook of Clinical Neurology*. New York, Elsevier, 1986, pp 185–204.

Weiner WJ, Lang AE. *Movement Disorders: A Comprehensive Survey*. New York, Futura, 1989.

CHAPTER 133

Disorders of Balance and Coordination

Judd Jensen, M.D.

Diseases affecting bipedal locomotion, spatial orientation, and extremity coordination result in a broad spectrum of clinical problems. This chapter divides these problems into three groups:

1. The vertigo syndromes.
2. The ataxia syndromes.
3. Gait disorders of the elderly.

While there may be considerable overlap among these syndromes, this separation reflects the common clinical presentations of these disorders.

Vertigo Syndromes

I. Definition

Vertigo is a false sensation of movement which is usually rotational but can be described as "tilting," "feeling pushed," or a "back-and-forth" sensation.

II. Etiology

Vertigo is produced when there is an *abrupt* change in the function of one of the paired vestibular apparatuses. Gradual disruption of one or both vestibular systems tends to produce a dysequilibrium or ataxia syndrome. Vertigo can be caused by a disturbance of either the periph-

eral or central components of the vestibular system (see below), although peripheral etiologies are much more common.

III. Vestibular Anatomy and Physiology

The vestibular system is divided into peripheral and central components. The peripheral component includes the labyrinth, which is located in the petrous portion of the temporal bone, and the vestibular portion of the eighth cranial nerve, which is located in the internal auditory canal and cerebellopontine angle adjacent to the brain stem. The central component includes the vestibular nuclei located in the lower pons and upper medulla of the brain stem and the connections of these nuclei with the cerebellum and other brain stem nuclei controlling eye movements. The paired labyrinths supply information to the vestibular nuclei regarding the position and movement of the head. The vestibular nuclei, in turn, send impulses to the cerebellum and eye movement centers so that appropriate responses can be mounted to whatever environmental challenge is present.

IV. Clinical Findings

A. History: As noted above, vertigo is produced by an abrupt change in vestibular function.

Thus, vertigo syndromes are typically paroxysmal in onset and present clinically as either a single, acute, episode or recurrent episodes of vertigo. Nausea and vomiting are frequent accompaniments to these episodes.

B. Physical examination: While appendicular and/or gait ataxia are common findings during an attack of vertigo, nystagmus is the hallmark of vertigo. Nystagmus is almost always present while the patient is experiencing vertigo. The character of the nystagmus seen in peripheral vestibular disorders is different from that seen in central vestibular disorders. The differences are often useful in determining the etiology of a patient's syndrome.

1. Nystagmus of peripheral vestibular origin
   a. Unidirectional: The fast component of the nystagmus always beats in the same direction, regardless of the direction in which the patient is looking.
   b. Mixed: Typically has both a horizontal and a rotatory component.
   c. Suppressed by fixation: As when the patient watches the examiner's finger as he or she moves it back and forth.

2. Nystagmus of central vestibular origin
   a. Multidirectional: The fast component of the nystagmus changes with the direction of gaze.
   b. Often purely horizontal, vertical, or rotatory (i.e., not mixed).
   c. Not suppressed by fixation.

3. Unfortunately, nystagmus of central origin can mimic a peripheral lesion by being unidirectional or mixed. In general, nystagmus from peripheral vestibular dysfunction is less prominent than central nystagmus. This contrasts with the patient's experience of vertigo, which is often more intense in peripheral disorders.

V. Clinical Syndromes
   A. Causes of recurrent episodes of vertigo
      1. Benign paroxysmal positional vertigo (BPPV): The single most common cause of vertigo.
         a. Definition: Recurrent, brief (seconds) attacks of vertigo associated with the attainment of a certain head position. Most commonly occurs when the patient is supine and turns the head to one side but can occur when sitting or standing. Characteristically, there is a brief *latency* to the onset of vertigo after the head position has been attained. In ad-

dition, the vertigo typically *fatigues* if the head is placed in the offending position repeatedly over a short period of time.
         b. Etiology: Most vertigo is idiopathic but can also be seen after head trauma, acute vestibulopathy (see Section V,B,1), labyrinthine infarction or in the setting of Ménière's disease (see Section V,A,2). This disorder is thought to be related to labyrinthine dysfunction.
         c. Clinical findings: Hearing loss and tinnitus are not present except in the rare cases associated with Ménière's disease. The standard neurologic examination is normal. However, when the patient is shifted from the sitting to the supine position with the head extended over the edge of the examining table or bed (Halpike or Neylan-Barany maneuver), vertigo and nystagmus with peripheral vestibular characteristics (see Section IV,B,1) are usually elicited.
         d. Test results: Computed tomography (CT) and magnetic resonance imaging (MRI) of the posterior fossa are normal and are not needed in the evaluation of patients with typical BPPV. Audiogram and brain stem auditory evoked responses (BAERs) are normal except in the unusual cases with hearing loss after an acute vestibulopathy or in patients with Ménière's disease. Electronystagmography (ENG) is typically abnormal during the sitting to supine positioning test.
         e. Therapy: Specific positioning exercises are the most effective treatment for this disorder. The patient is asked to sit on the edge of the bed and then quickly lie down on the side in the position that produces the vertigo. The patient holds the position until the vertigo subsides and then returns to the upright position. The maneuver is repeated until the vertigo fatigues. The exercise should be repeated two or three times daily. Meclizine and phenothiazines may be helpful during the exercises but are not otherwise useful in this syndrome.
         f. Prognosis: Most patients exhibit a waxing and waning course that can last for weeks, months, or years. Eventual remission occurs in the great majority.

2. Ménière's disease
   a. Definition: Recurrent attacks of vertigo and tinnitus, lasting for hours to days, superimposed on progressive hearing loss.
   b. Etiology: Endolymphatic hydrops—increased volume of endolymph and progressive dilation of the membranous labyrinth.
   c. Clinical findings
      (1) History: In addition to vertigo, tinnitus, and hearing loss, patients often describe pressure in one or both ears. Nausea and vomiting frequently accompany the episodes of vertigo.
      (2) Physical examination: Nystagmus with peripheral vestibular characteristics (see Section IV,B,1) is typically present during the attacks of vertigo. Hearing loss can usually be demonstrated, and ataxia (limb or gait) may be present during the vertigo.
   d. Test results: CT and MRI of the posterior fossa are normal. Audiogram demonstrates hearing loss, which may fluctuate early in the disease. BAERs are usually normal, and ENG typically shows unilateral or bilateral weakness in the response to calorics.
   e. Therapy: Meclizine, phenothiazines, and benzodiazepines are useful during the acute episodes of vertigo. Dietary salt restriction, acetazolamide, and thiazide diuretics may be helpful in reducing the frequency and severity of the attacks of vertigo. Shunt procedures and ablative procedures have been used with some success.
   f. Prognosis: A significant percentage of patients will experience spontaneous remission within 5 years. Patients may exhibit a persistent disequilibrium or an ataxic syndrome after an episode of vertigo has resolved.
3. Vertebrobasilar transient ischemic attacks (TIA): Vertebrobasilar vascular disease is discussed in more detail in Section V,B,2. Vertigo is a common symptom in this syndrome. It usually occurs with other signs of posterior circulation ischemia (i.e., bilateral visual blurring, homonymous hemianopsia, diplopia, slurred speech, ataxia, facial and/or extremity numbness, hemiparesis, quadriparesis, or paraparesis). However, vertigo can be seen in isolation. When repeated attacks of vertigo occur, there is usually a high-grade stenosis or "unstable" atherosclerotic plaque in the vertebrobasilar system. Episodes typically last for minutes but can persist for hours. Nausea, headache, or neck pain may also occur. If the patient is examined during an attack, limb and gait ataxia as well as nystagmus of central origin will be found. CT scan is usually normal. MRI scan may demonstrate areas of ischemia in the brain stem or cerebellum. Transcranial Doppler ultrasonography may be helpful in demonstrating stenosis in the large vessels of the vertebrobasilar system. Angiography remains the gold standard for demonstrating vertebrobasilar occlusive disease but is not necessary in most patients. Treatment is with antiplatelet agents or warafin. The prognosis in severe vertebrobasilar stenosis is guarded.
4. Migraine: Vertigo can result from migrainous vasospasm of the basilar artery and subsequent ischemia to the brain stem vestibular nuclei. In most patients, the accompanying vascular headache is the dominant clinical manifestation. However, some patients with a history of vertigo from basilar artery migraine will develop episodes of vertigo unassociated with headache. Other symptoms of basilar artery spasm (positive or negative visual scotoma, diplopia, slurred speech, ataxia, unilateral or bilateral facial and extremity numbness or weakness) may also be present. These episodes are called *acephalic migraine* or *migraine "equivalents."* The diagnosis rests on a history of similar symptoms associated with headache. Migraine equivalents do not usually require treatment. However, in the unusual patient with frequent episodes, propranolol can be tried.
5. Temporal lobe epilepsy: Vertigo can be produced by discharges from a temporal lobe seizure focus and thus can be experienced as an "aura" in patients with complex-partial seizures. However, such patients have other features of complex-partial seizures, such as altered consciousness, automatism, and postictal confusion or lethargy. Isolated vertigo is rarely, if

ever, a manifestation of epilepsy; thus, an electroencephalogram (EEG) is not indicated in the routine workup of patients with vertigo.

B. Causes of a single acute episode of vertigo

1. Acute peripheral vestibulopathy: This most common cause of a prolonged episode of vertigo occurs in all age groups. Because the pathophysiology of this disorder is poorly understood, a confusing nomenclature has persisted. *Labyrinthitis* and *vestibular neuronitis* are the terms commonly used to describe this syndrome.

   a. Definition: Acute or subacute onset of vertigo due to a peripheral vestibular disturbance. The symptoms last for hours to days, and some patients experience associated tinnitus and/or hearing loss.

   b. Etiology: Uncertain but thought to be viral or postviral.

   c. Clinical findings
      (1) History: Vertigo, nausea, and vomiting. Some patients have tinnitus or hearing loss.
      (2) Physical exam: Nystagmus with peripheral vestibular characteristics (see Section IV,B,1) and mild limb or gait ataxia.

   d. Differential diagnosis: This syndrome can be difficult to distinguish from the more serious vascular disorders of the posterior circulation (see Section V,B,2). In particular, labyrinthine infarction may be impossible to distinguish on clinical grounds and, thus, should be considered in older patients or in those with risk factors for atherosclerosis. Brain stem and cerebellar infarctions and hemorrhages can usually be distinguished by the presence of other neurologic findings (see Section V,B,2,c) and nystagmus of central origin. In addition, the ataxia associated with central vestibular disorders is typically much more prominent than that seen in peripheral vestibular disorders.

   e. Test results: Imaging studies of the posterior fossa are normal. Audiogram and BAERs are usually normal. ENG typically demonstrates a unilateral weakness to caloric stimulation.

   f. Therapy: Meclizine, phenothiazines, antiemetics, and benzodiazepines are given for symptomatic relief. Intravenous fluids should be given if vomiting is protracted.

   g. Prognosis: Many patients experience a disequilibrium or a mild ataxic syndrome that can persist for weeks to months after the acute vertigo has resolved. This can be treated with vestibular exercises. Otherwise, patients recover completely. A small number may experience subsequent episodes of vertigo.

2. Vertebrobasilar vascular disease (VBVD): This is the most serious but, fortunately, not the most common cause of vertigo.

   a. Definition: Acute onset of vertigo (usually with other neurologic findings) due to infarction or hemorrhage in the brain stem, cerebellum or labyrinth.

   b. Etiology: Atherosclerosis of the vertebrobasilar system is the most common cause of ischemic infarction in these areas. However, other causes include cariogenic embolus, arterial dissection, arteritis, and hypercoagulable states. Chronic hypertension is the most common cause of brain stem or cerebellar hemorrhage, but coagulation disorders, vascular malformations, central nervous system tumors, and sympathomimetic drugs are also causes of posterior fossa hemorrhage.

   c. Clinical findings
      (1) Wallenberg syndrome (lateral medullary infarction): The most common brain stem stroke. Symptoms and signs include vertigo, nausea, central nystagmus, gait and ipsilateral limb ataxia, loss of pain and temperature sensations on the ipsilateral face and contralateral body, dysphagia, hoarseness, hiccoughs, ipsilateral Horner's sign, and ipsilateral weakness of the soft palate. Partial syndromes are the rule.
      (2) Pontine infarction: Some combination of vertigo, nystagmus, ipsilateral facial weakness, facial sensory loss, and appendicular ataxia is present.
      (3) Cerebellar infarction: Early symptoms include vertigo, nausea and vomiting, central nystagmus, and prominent appendicular and gait

ataxia. If the area of infarction is large enough and significant edema ensues, signs of brain stem compression (deteriorating level of consciousness, cranial nerve palsies, and quadriplegia) can occur 24–72 hr after the initial symptoms.

(4) Labyrinthine infarction: Sudden onset of vertigo, nausea, nystagmus of peripheral origin, and mild ataxia. Hearing loss may be present and is often profound.

(5) Pontine hemorrhage: While vertigo and nausea may be early symptoms, the clinical picture is usually dominated by progressive alteration in consciousness, quadriplegia, and gaze palsies.

(6) Cerebellar hemorrhage: The clinical presentation varies with the size of the hemorrhage. Large lesions produce sudden headache, vomiting, and ataxia followed by rapidly progressive obtundation. Smaller lesions produce vertigo, nausea, central nystagmus, and ataxia. Occipital headache and neck stiffness are usually present and are important distinguishing factors (see Section V,B,2,d). Even patients with small hemorrhages can deteriorate in 24–72 hr because of resultant edema and brain stem compression.

d. Differential diagnosis: Acute peripheral vestibulopathy (APV) is the primary differential diagnostic entity to consider in evaluating patients with suspected VBVD. While VBVD is primarily a disease of the elderly and those with risk factors for vascular disease, APV is common in patients of all ages. The distinction must be made by other clinical clues. Patients with brain stem ischemic infarction usually have nystagmus of central origin and other neurologic signs, although those signs may be subtle at times, especially in the Wallenberg syndrome. Patients with cerebellar infarction can be distinguished by the prominence of limb and ataxia as well as central nystagmus. Brain stem and cerebellar hemorrhages usually provoke prominent headache, and alteration of consciousness is com-

mon. Labyrinthine infarction can be very difficult to distinguish from APV.

e. Test results: CT scan is usually normal in brain stem infarction, although it may demonstrate a cerebellar infarct. Pontine and cerebellar hemorrhages are usually seen with CT. MRI typically demonstrates both ischemic and hemorrhagic vascular lesions in the posterior fossa. Neither CT nor MRI demonstrates labyrinthine infarction. Transcranial Doppler (TCD) ultrasonography may demonstrate stenosis or occlusion in the large vessels of the vertebrobasilar system in patients with ischemic events. Carotid duplex scanning is usually not indicated in such patients. Transthoracic and transesophageal echocardiography may be helpful in patients suspected of having cariogenic embolus or patients without risk factors for atherosclerosis. A vertebrobasilar ischemic event in a young person should raise the questions of vertebral artery dissection or hypercoagulable state. TCD or cerebral angiography is helpful in the former; antiphospholipid antibodies should be sought in the latter. Temporal arteritis can occasionally affect the vertebral arteries. The Westergren sedimentation rate is usually elevated in such patients. Temporal artery biopsy and cerebral angiography may be helpful in confirming the diagnosis.

f. Therapy

(1) Antiplatelet agents are the rule in ischemic brain stem infarction. Anticoagulation with heparin or warfarin is generally not indicated in the Wallenberg syndrome or in pontine infarction causing vertigo. However, vertigo can be seen, along with other neurologic findings, in basilar artery thrombosis. If a fluctuating or progressive course occurs in such patients, anticoagulation may be indicated. Finally, warfarin therapy should be considered in all patients with ischemic stroke and a suspected cariogenic source of embolus.

(2) Patients with cerebellar infarction must be monitored closely for signs

of brain stem compression (i.e., obtundation and cranial nerve palsies). Surgical decompression may be necessary in such patients. Pontine hemorrhage is treated with the supportive measures afforded all stroke patients. Cerebellar hemorrhage was formerly considered an indication for immediate surgical decompression of the affected cerebellar hemisphere. However, small hemorrhages are now usually treated nonsurgically, although close clinical observation is required. While corticosteroids are often used in cerebellar hemorrhage, there is no proof of their efficacy. Steroids are not indicated in pontine hemorrhage or ischemic posterior circulation disease. Hyperventilation and osmotic agents are useful in the setting of brain stem compression from ischemic or hemorrhagic cerebellar lesions. However, their effect is temporary and cannot substitute for definitive surgical decompression. Patients with labyrinthine infarction are treated symptomatically as patients with acute peripheral vestibulopathy (see Section V,B,1,f).

g. Prognosis: Patients with Wallenberg syndrome and ischemic pontine infarction typically recover fairly well. Labyrinthine infarction often produces a disequilibrium syndrome that persists after the vertigo resolves and may last for weeks or months. Cerebellar infarction also often has a good prognosis (even after cerebellar hemispherec-

tomy), although the period of rehabilitation is usually longer. Rontine hemorrhage typically carries a poor prognosis for functional recovery. Cerebellar hemorrhage has a high mortality in the acute phase of the illness. However, if the syndrome is recognized early and treated appropriately, the long-term prognosis can be good.

3. Multiple sclerosis: Vertigo is a relatively common symptom in this disease and is usually present in the setting of other neurologic symptoms, past or present. However, vertigo can be seen in isolation and can be the initial symptom in multiple sclerosis (See Chapter 134). The vertigo is usually subacute in onset and is commonly associated with nausea and ataxia. Hearing loss and tinnitus are rare but do occur. The symptoms are due to areas of demyelination in the brain stem. Patients typically exhibit central nystagmus and mild to moderate limb and gait ataxia. The primary differential diagnostic entity is APV. The character of the nystagmus and the degree of ataxia (greater in multiple sclerosis) usually distinguish the two conditions. MRI may show characteristic white matter abnormalities in the cerebral hemispheres and brain stem, although if the episode of vertigo represents the first neurologic symptom of multiple sclerosis, the MRI may be normal. BAERs may be abnormal. Spinal fluid examination may demonstrate elevated IgG and the presence of oligoclonal bands. Treatment is primarily symptomatic, as for APV. Adrenocorticotropic hormone or corticosteroids may also be helpful in shortening the duration of symptoms.

Chapter 134

Demyelinating Diseases

Joan C. Murray, M.D.

Multiple Sclerosis

I. Definition

Multiple Sclerosis (MS) is an inflammatory disease of young adults affecting the central nervous system (CNS) characterized by primary destruction of myelin. The disease is characterized clinically by episodes of focal dysfunction of the optic nerves, brain, and spinal cord which remit to a varying extent and recur over many years.

II. Etiology

The cause of MS remains unknown. Many hypotheses have been investigated. The most widely accepted theories are that MS occurs secondary to a viral infection or is the result of altered immunity, probably genetically determined. All attempts to confirm the isolation of a virus or to detect viral antigens in tissue from MS patients have failed.

III. Epidemiology

A. Geographic distribution: MS is rare in equatorial regions and increases in frequency with latitude in the Northern and Southern hemispheres. The prevalence in the Northern United States and Europe is 30–80 per 100,000. The prevalence in Rochester, Minnesota, was 177 per 100,000 in 1985. Those who migrate to another area after the mid-teens do not alter their susceptibility pattern, whereas those migrating earlier seem to acquire the susceptibility pattern of the new region.

B. Genetic influence

1. The risk of MS in first-degree relatives of those with the disease is 15- to 20-fold greater than that of the general population. One study found a 2.3% concordance rate in dizygotic twins and a 26% concordance rate in monozygotic twins. Whether this represents hereditary factors or a common environmental exposure, or both, is unclear.

2. Certain human leukocyte antigen (HLA) types (HLA-A3, -B7, -DW2, -DR2) are overrepresented in northern whites, whereas the frequency of other HLA types is decreased.

C. Racial differences: Whites are affected more frequently than blacks; however, blacks in the United States show similar geographical differences in prevalence. Persons of Asian descent are infrequently affected.

D. Age: The usual onset is between 20 and

40 years of age. Onset after the age of 60 is rare.

E. Sex: Females are affected more frequently than males, with an approximate female:male ratio of 1.5:1.

IV. Pathology

The term *multiple sclerosis* was initially used to describe the wide distribution of discrete lesions scattered throughout the white matter of the CNS. These plaques range from 1 to 4 mm in diameter and are characterized by breakdown of the myelin sheath with relative sparing of axons. They have a perivenous distribution. Early plaques contain macrophages, lymphocytes, and plasma cells, which are eventually replaced by extensive gliosis resulting in the characteristic sclerotic appearance.

V. Pathophysiology

A. Denuded axons conduct slowly, and if the demyelinated area is too long, conduction fails. Conduction block in demyelinated axons is due to a critical decrease in current resulting from short-circuiting through bare axonal internodes. Marginal conduction through demyelinated areas may fail in the presence of increased body temperature, increased calcium concentration, and fatigue.

B. Mechanical stimulation of denuded axons can generate axonal action potentials de novo, causing symptoms such as Lhermitte's sign, an electrical sensation felt down the spine on cervical flexion. Spontaneous generator potentials have been demonstrated in demyelinated axons and may explain paroxysmal positive symptoms such as trigeminal neuralgia, myokymia, and visual phosphenes. Nerve transmission might also be affected by edema or toxic factors liberated by immunocompetent cells in the plaque and periplaque regions. The rapid improvement in symptoms seen with steroid therapy may be due to decreased edema, pH changes, and reduction in cellular infiltrates, whereas delayed recovery may reflect utilization of alternative axonal pathways, a shift in sodium channels to internodal regions enhancing conduction, or possibly remyelination.

VI. Clinical Presentation

A. Signs and symptoms: Although MS is classically described as a relapsing-remitting disease of the CNS white matter in young adults, it displays marked heterogeneity, reflecting the multifocal areas of CNS myelin destruction. For unknown reasons, some areas of the CNS are involved more frequently than others. The optic nerves, brain stem, cerebellum, and spinal cord, particularly the corticospinal tracts and posterior columns, are among the most frequently affected sites.

1. Presenting symptoms and signs: The most common presenting symptoms and signs are weakness or sensory changes in one or more limbs which occur in approximately one-half of patients. Optic neuritis occurs as the initial symptom in 20–25% of patients. The remainder present with various symptoms including ataxia, incontinence, Lhermitte's sign, diplopia, and vertigo.

2. Established disease: Approximately one-half of patients have a mixed or generalized disease with variable involvement of the optic nerves, brain stem, cerebellum, and spinal cord. From 30% to 40% of patients have predominantly spinal cord disease; 5% have predominantly cerebellar disease; and 5% have primarily visual disturbances.

B. Clinical course

1. Relapsing-remitting: Relapses, one of the most characteristic clinical features, may have an acute or subacute onset and peak over several weeks. During remission, the symptoms abate to a variable degree and may resolve completely. Thirty-five percent of MS patients have a relapsing-remitting course. Relapse frequency averages 0.4–0.6 attacks per year, and relapses are generally more frequent earlier in the disease and tend to decrease in later years. Symptoms lasting for hours to days and occurring after febrile illness, physical exertion, and metabolic abnormalities, probably result from conduction block in previously demyelinated axons and are referred to as *pseudoexacerbations*.

2. Progressive: Twenty percent of MS patients experience a progressive course from the disease onset. These patients tend to develop the disease later, in their thirties or forties, and more commonly have a chronic, progressive, spastic paraparesis.

3. Relapsing and progressive: Forty-five percent of patients fall into this category and experience relapses in addition to progressive disability.

VII. Diagnosis

A. History and physical exam

1. MS is a clinical diagnosis based on histori-

cal and physical evidence of CNS white matter lesions disseminated in time and space. An attack, or exacerbation, is defined as neurologic symptoms, with or without objective confirmation, lasting for at least 24 hr. Two attacks have occurred when different, noncontiguous parts of the CNS have been affected, and these episodes were separated by at least one month.

2. In 1982, before there was much experience with magnetic resonance imaging (MRI), a new set of diagnostic criteria was developed. This was done primarily to aid in the diagnosis of patients included in research protocols, but these criteria can also be helpful for the clinician (Table 134-1).

B. Laboratory studies
1. Cerebrospinal fluid (CSF)
   a. Cell count
      (1) The CSF abnormalities found in MS are nonspecific and may be seen in other inflammatory neurologic diseases such as Guillain-Barré syndrome, subacute sclerosing panencephalitis, Lyme disease, neurosyphilis, herpes encephalitis and others.
      (2) Approximately one-third of all patients with MS, especially during exacerbations, have a slight to moderate pleocytosis, usually less than 50 cells/mm^3. These cells are predominantly T lymphocytes.

b. Protein: CSF protein is mildly increased in 25–40% of patients. CSF protein is generally less than 80 mg/dl, and a protein level of 100 mg/dl or greater should raise doubts about the diagnosis.
c. IgG/Alb index: Gamma globulin is increased in roughly two-thirds of patients. The CSF IgG index is more sensitive and reflects synthesis within the CNS. Approximately 70% of patients have increased IgG/Alb.

$$\text{CSF IgG index} = \frac{\text{CSF IgG/CSF Alb}}{\text{Serum IgG/serum Alb}}$$

d. Oligoclonal bands: The CSF gamma globulins migrate in agarose electrophoresis as abnormal discrete populations representing "nonsense antibody" produced by a few clones of plasma cells and are referred to as *oligoclonal bands*. Approximately 90% of patients with MS have oligoclonal bands. The oligoclonal banding tends to remain constant in an individual throughout the course of the disease and is not related to exacerbations, although additional bands may appear with time.
e. Myelin basic protein: Myelin basic protein is a breakdown product of myelin and may be transiently increased in up to 90% of patients after acute episodes. These levels return to normal over the

Table 134-1. Classification of MS

1. Clinically definite MS
   a. Two attacks and clinical evidence of two separate lesions
   b. Two attacks with clinical evidence of one lesion and paraclinical evidence of another (separate) lesion
2. Laboratory-supported definite MS
   a. Two attacks with either clinical or paraclinical evidence of one lesion and demonstration in CSF of IgG oligoclonal bands (OB) or increased CNS synthesis of IgG
   b. One attack, clinical evidence of two separate lesions, and demonstration of CSF OB/IgG
   c. One attack, clinical evidence of one lesion, paraclinical evidence of another (separate) lesion, and demonstration of CSF OB/IgG
3. Clinically probable MS
   a. Two attacks and clinical evidence of one lesion
   b. One attack and clinical evidence of two separate lesions
   c. One attack, clinical evidence of one lesion, and paraclinical evidence of another (separate) lesion
4. Laboratory-supported probable MS
   a. Two attacks and the presence of CSF OB/IgG

Source: Posner et al (1983).

next 2 weeks. The level in chronic disease is usually normal.

C. Neurophysiologic tests: The visual, auditory, and somatosensory pathways can be investigated with evoked potentials. Stimulation of a sensory pathway that is recorded through surface electrodes, amplified, and averaged, results in an evoked potential (EP). These techniques may detect lesions but do not delineate the cause of the lesion. EPs may confirm lesions in patients with unusual symptoms or equivocal deficits or demonstrate clinically silent abnormalities.

D. Neuroimaging

1. MRI: MRI, first reported for use in MS during 1981, is currently the most sensitive scanning technique for demonstrating areas of CNS demyelination. Typically, MRI demonstrates multiple discrete or coalescent lesions in the periventricular white matter of the cerebral hemispheres as high-signal lesions on the T_2-weighted scan. There may also be associated decreased signal areas on the T_1-weighted scans. The MRI lesions have been shown to correlate with plaques observed at autopsy. Lesions may also be seen in the brain stem and cervical spinal cord. Demonstrable lesions in the cerebellum, optic nerves, and thoracolumbar spinal cord are less common. In clinically definite MS, the MRI is abnormal in approximately 90% of patients. The duration of MS and patient disability has been associated with the number of lesions and the presence of confluent periventricular lesions, although many MRI lesions are clinically silent. In patients with clinically active disease, some MRI lesions on T_1-weighted images are enhanced by gadolinium contrast and are, thus, thought to correlate with acute breakdown of the blood-brain barrier.

2. Computed tomography (CT): CT is not nearly as sensitive as MRI in detecting demyelinating lesions, but it may demonstrate hypodense lesions in the periventricular and deep white matter. Hypodense lesions on noncontrast CT may be seen in approximately one-third of patients with clinically definite MS.

VIII. Differential Diagnosis

Numerous diseases may be misdiagnosed as MS. The following features should suggest the need for a more extensive diagnostic workup:

(1) absence of optic nerve involvement or ocular motility disorders; (2) absence of clinical remissions (especially in a younger patient); (3) localized disease (posterior fossa, craniocervical junction, spinal cord); (4) atypical clinical features (absence of sensory findings and bladder involvement); (5) absence of CSF abnormalities; and (6) onset of symptoms after age 60.

A. See Table 134-2 for a list of conditions that can mimic multiple sclerosis.

IX. Treatment

There is no current treatment that will significantly alter the course of MS. Current management of MS encompasses treating exacerbations, halting progression, and symptomatic treatment.

A. Exacerbating-remitting disease

1. Corticosteroids or adrenocorticotropic hormone (ACTH): These remain the mainstay of therapy for acute MS exacerbations that involve significant impairment. A double-blind, cooperative study demonstrated that ACTH administration shortened the duration of acute exacerbations; however, it had no significant effect on the long-term course. Similar improvement in symptoms during MS attacks has been reported in studies comparing high-dose intravenous (IV) methylprednisolone to placebo. Whether high-dose methylprednisolone is more effective than ACTH is controversial, and contradictory results have been reported by several groups.

a. The rapid improvement with adrenocorticosteroids or ACTH is probably secondary to their anti-inflammatory and antiedema effects, whereas the persistent improvement after discontinuation of the drug is probably due to immunosuppressive effects.

b. The current regimen for adrenocorticosteroids is 1 g methylprednisolone IV daily for 5–7 days followed by an oral prednisone taper for 2–14 weeks. Some patients have recurrence of symptoms with the more rapid steroid tapers and may require an individualized withdrawal schedule.

c. Common protocols for ACTH are 80 U/day IV for 10 days and intramuscular (IM) ACTH gel tapered over 14 days. Despite hastening recovery from acute MS exacerbations, ACS and ACTH do not appear to prevent future

Table 134-2. Categories of Conditions That May Be Mistaken for MS

Diseases capable of causing multiple lesions of the CNS, often with a relapsing-remitting course
    Vasculitides (systemic lupus erythematosus and polyarteritis nodosa)
    Behçet's disease
    Sarcoidosis
    Acute disseminated encephalomyelitis
    Subacute myelo-optic neuritis
    Cerebrovascular occlusive disease
    Meningovascular syphilis
    Paraneoplastic effects of malignant disease
    Migrant sensory neuritis of Wartenburg
Systematized CNS diseases often causing multiple lesions in the CNS but in a more orderly, symmetric
pattern and with a progressive course
    Hereditary spinocerebellar ataxia
    Subacute combined degeneration of the spinal cord (vitamin B_{12} deficiency)
    Myelopathies due to infections, primarily viral (e.g. retroviruses)
Single lesions of the CNS with a relapsing-remitting course
    Brain tumors, especially extramedullary tumors in the region of the foramen magnum
    Primary CNS lymphoma
    Arteriovenous malformations of the brain stem and spinal cord
    Spinal cord tumors
Single lesions with a progressive course
    Arnold-Chiari malformation
    CNS neoplasms, especially in the posterior fossa and spinal cord
    Arachnoid cyst
Nonorganic (psychiatric) disorders

Source: Swanson (1989).

attacks or the development of further disability.

2. Copolymer I: Copolymer, a synthetic peptide which simulates myeln basic protein and suppresses experimental allergic encephalomyelitis in several species, has recently been reported to decrease the number of exacerbations in patients treated for a 2-year period. The initial reports are encouraging but need confirmation by larger multicenter clinical trials.

3. 4-Aminopyridine: This potassium channel blocker reportedly improves symptoms in MS, presumably by restoring conduction in blocked, demyelinated nerve. Further studies are necessary to assess the efficacy and safety of long-term administration.

B. Chronic progressive disease: The treatment of chronic progressive MS is controversial. Various immunosuppressive therapies are under investigation, including cyclophosphamide, azathioprine, plasmapheresis, β-interferon, total lymphoid irradiation, cyclosporin A, and monoclonal antibodies.

1. Cyclophosphamide: Cyclophosphamide, an alkylating agent acting mainly on proliferating cells and a potent inhibitor of B-cell activity, has been used widely in the treatment of MS in Europe for many years. Whether cyclophosphamide stabilizes the disease is controversial, according to recently published reports, and its use is limited by clinical toxicity.

2. Azathioprine: Similarly, azathioprine, a purine analog with a cytolytic effect on replicating lymphocytes, has not been convincingly shown to alter the course of the disease and is associated with significant toxicity.

3. Plasmapheresis: Plasmapheresis, still an investigative procedure, has been associated with transient improvement in symptoms, but its use is limited by risks, expense, and time.

4. Cyclosporine: Reports regarding delay of progression are contradictory, and many study patients dropped out because of side effects.

5. Interferon

a. α-Interferon: Systemic α-interferon has no clear therapeutic effect.

b. β-interferon: Subcutaneous β-interferon has recently been shown to reduce exacerbation rates, severity of exacerbations, and accumulation of MRI abnormalities in patients with relapsing-remitting MS.

c. γ-Interferon: γ-Interferon is a lymphokine that acts as an immune enhancer. Intrathecal administration results in MS exacerbations.

6. Total lymphoid irradiation: This is still experimental but has been reported by one group to result in less disease progression.

7. Monoclonal antibodies: These have been effective in treatment of experimental allergic encephalomyelitis (EAE) but have thus far been used only in pilot trials in MS.

C. Symptomatic treatment

1. Fatigue: Some patients have a modest improvement in their fatigue, a poorly understood symptom, with amantadine.

2. Spasticity: Spasticity, if troublesome, may be lessened with baclofen or a benzodiazepine.

3. Cerebellar tremor: Cerebellar tremor, often disabling, is infrequently improved with propranolol, primidone, or isoniazid.

4. Bladder function: Urinary urgency and incontinence may be controlled with anticholinergics such as propantheline, oxybutynin, or imipramine. Urinary retention may be improved with cholinergics such as bethanecol and intermittent catheterization if postvoid residual urine volumes exceed 100 ml.

5. Bowel function: MS patients frequently complain of constipation. Conservative measures such as high-fiber diet, increased fluid intake, regular exercise, and stool softeners or bulk laxatives are effective in most patients.

6. Paroxysmal manifestations: Painful tonic spasms, trigeminal neuralgia, and transient motor and sensory phenomena often respond to carbamazepine in doses of 200–800 mg/day.

7. Sexual dysfunction: Female patients usually retain sexual function. A penile implant may be used in men with impaired erections.

X. **Patient Monitoring**

A. Debilitated patients need frequent changes of position and skin monitoring to prevent de-

cubiti formation. Patients with urinary retention and those newly taking anticholinergics for urinary frequency and urgency need postvoid residual urine volumes measured. If volumes are 100 ml or more, intermittent catheterization may be employed to avoid urinary tract infections.

B. Serial MRI scanning, which has been reported to reveal new asymptomatic lesions, may be used in the future as an indicator of disease activity and of the efficacy of treatment in controlled studies.

XI. **Prognosis**

The long-term outcome of MS patients is highly variable, with some remaining asymptomatic and a small number having a fulminant progression to death. Approximately 20% of patients have a benign course for 15 or more years. Onset at an early age has a more favorable prognosis than later onset. Initial sensory or cranial nerve symptoms have a better prognosis than motor or cerebellar abnormalities. MS seems to progress more slowly in women than in men. It does not seem to affect the life span appreciably. In one study, the 25-year survival was 77%, with expected survival based on an age- and sex-matched control group of 82%. Two-thirds of surviving patients remained ambulatory for 25 years after onset of the disease.

Optic Neuritis (ON)

ON is acute or subacute visual loss resulting from optic nerve demyelination. There is often associated eye pain accentuated by ocular movements. The degree of visual loss is variable and affects mainly central vision. When the head of the optic nerve is involved, papillitis (disc edema) is seen. Usually the lesion is retrobulbar, and the funduscopic exam is normal. Later in the course, optic disc pallor may be seen. Simultaneous bilateral involvement of the optic nerves is infrequent. Subsequent development of MS after an initial episode of ON is reported to occur in 20–80% of patients. ON has also been reported after measles, mumps, rubella, and varicella. The majority of patients recover their vision, with one-third recovering completely. ACTH and ACS appear to shorten the course of ON but do not influence the degree of ultimate visual recovery.

Neuromyelitis Optica (Devic's disease)

Devic's disease is the clinical syndrome of acute bilateral optic neuritis and transverse myelitis. Most cases occur as part of MS but may be seen as a manifestation of postinfectious encephalomyelitis. The prognosis is poor because of the frequency of necrotizing pathology involving the affected structures.

Acute Disseminated Encephalomyelitis (ADEM)

ADEM is an uncommon uniphasic demyelinating disease of the brain and spinal cord occurring in association with immunization, vaccination, or systemic viral infection. The disease is characterized by encephalopathy, seizures, and focal signs reflecting cerebral, brain stem, and spinal cord involvement. Recovery usually occurs over weeks to months, with complete recovery occurring in approximately 50%. Mortality varies from 10% to 30%. No specific laboratory or imaging abnormalities are pathognomonic of ADEM. Corticosteroids are felt to reduce the severity of the disease, although no clinical controlled studies have been reported.

Transverse Myelitis

Transverse myelitis is the development of isolated spinal cord dysfunction over hours to days in the absence of a compressive lesion. Approximately one-third of patients report a preceding febrile illness. The prognosis is good in roughly one-third, fair in one-third, and poor in one-third. Some patients later develop MS.

Concentric Sclerosis of Balo

Balo's disease is considered by most to be a variant of MS. This is a histopathologic diagnosis characterized by concentric areas of demyelination alternating with bands of preserved myelin.

Diffuse Sclerosis of Schilder

Diffuse sclerosis is a rare progressive disease most frequently seen in children or young adults with clinical manifestations of dementia, homonymous hemianopsia, cortical blindness and deafness, varying degrees of hemiplegia and quadraplegia, and pseudobulbar palsy. Most patients die within a few months or years. The characteristic pathologic lesion is a large, asymmetric focus of demyelination often involving an entire lobe or cerebral hemisphere, typically with extension across the corpus callosum affecting the opposite hemisphere. Diffuse sclerosis must be differentiated from adrenoleukodystrophy by eliminating those cases with other lesions demonstrated by clinical or imaging studies, involvement of peripheral nerve or adrenal glands, absence of very long chain fatty acids of cholesterol esters, or histologic findings identical to those of MS.

Multiple Sclerosis with Demyelinative Peripheral Neuropathy

Reports have suggested that peripheral nervous system involvement in MS may be more frequent than was previously thought. Prospective studies may be able to define the incidence and prevalence of peripheral nerve disease more accurately in MS patients.

Bibliography

Adams RD, Victor M. *Principles of Neurology*, ed 4. New York, McGraw-Hill, 1989, pp 756–774.

Bradley WG, Daroff RB, Fenichel GM, et al (eds). *Neurology in Clinical Practice*. Boston, Butterworth-Heinenmann, 1991, pp 1131–1166.

Davis FA, Stefoski D, Rush J. Orally administered 4-aminopyridine improves clinical signs in multiple sclerosis. *Ann Neurol* 27:186–192, 1990.

Eblen F, Poremba M, Grodd W, et al. Myelinoclastic diffuse sclerosis (Schilder's disease): Cliniconeuroradiologic correlations. *Neurology* 41:589–591, 1991.

Matthews WB, Acheson ED, Batchelor JR, et al. *McAlpine's Multiple Sclerosis*. New York, Churchill Livingstone, 1985.

McFarlin DE, McFarland HF. Multiple sclerosis. *N Engl J Med* 307:1183–1188, 1982.

McFarlin DE, McFarland HF. Multiple sclerosis. *N Engl J Med* 307:1246–1251, 1982.

Meyers LW. Management of multiple sclerosis. *Autoimmunity Forum—neurology* 2:3–11, 1990.

Poser CM, Paty DW, Scheinberg L, et al. New diagnostic criteria for multiple sclerosis: Guidelines for research protocols. *Ann Neurol* 13:227–231, 1983.

Rodriguez M. Multiple sclerosis: Basic concepts and hypothesis. *Mayo Clin Proc* 64:570–576, 1989.

Rowland LP (ed). *Merritt's Textbook of Neurology*. Philadelphia, Lea and Febinger, 1989, pp 741–765.

Stefoski D, Davis FA, Faut M, et al. 4-Aminopyridine improves clinical signs in multiple sclerosis. *Ann Neurol* 21:71–77, 1987.

Swanson JW. Multiple sclerosis: Update in diagnosis and review of prognostic factors. *Mayo Clin Proc* 64:577–586, 1989.

The IFNβ Multiple Sclerosis Study Group. Interferon beta-1β is effective in relapsing-remitting multiple sclerosis. *Neurology* 43:655–661, 1993.

Tourtelotte WW, Pick PW. Current concepts about multiple sclerosis. *Mayo Clin Proc* 64:592–596, 1989.

Willoughby EW, Grochowcki E, Li DKS, et al. Serial magnetic resonance scanning in multiple sclerosis: a second prospective study in relapsing patients. *Ann Neurol* 25:43–49, 1989.

Wynn DR, Rodriguez M, O'Fallon WM, et al. Update on the epidemiology of multiple sclerosis. *Mayo Clin Proc* 64:808–817, 1989.

CHAPTER 135

Peripheral Nerve and Muscle Diseases

Robert B. Wright, M.D.
Joseph J. Jares III, M.D.

The peripheral nervous system (PNS) reaches from the anterior horn cell in the spinal cord, via spinal nerve roots, through the course of peripheral nerves, across the neuromuscular junction to muscle. It carries motor instructions to muscles and sensory information from various receptors back to the spinal cord. Diseases of the PNS are diagnosed by localizing signs and symptoms and then establishing their etiology, which may, in turn, suggest means of treatment.

Anterior Horn Cell Diseases

I. **Definition**
   A. The anterior horn cell is the cell body of the motor neuron. The anterior horn cell is influenced by information from the corticospinal tracts. Its output is also regulated by reflex sensory feedback mechanisms. Diseases of the anterior horn cell lead to degeneration of the axon and the motor nerve and to secondary atrophy of the muscles serves by the motor neuron.
   B. The motor unit consists of the anterior horn cell, its axonal projection, and the muscle fibers it innervates.

II. **Symptoms**
   A. Anterior horn cells control motor activity. Loss of this control leads to weakness. Initially, the patient may note difficulty with fine motor movements involving the use of many motor units.
   B. Later the patient notes that these small, precisely controlled distal muscles lose mass (atrophy) due to loss of the trophic influences of the motor nerve on muscle. This distal motor atrophy may be accompanied by the bulbar symptoms of dysarthria and dysphagia from loss of anterior horn cells in the lower brain stem.
   C. Higher brain stem functions such as eye movements are almost always spared.
   D. Loss of anterior horn cells controlling respiratory muscles leads to dyspnea.

III. **Signs**
   A. The cardinal signs on physical examination are distal weakness and atrophy of muscles; later in the course of the disease, fasciculations may be seen.
      1. Fasciculations are small, involuntary twitches of muscle fibers caused by the simultaneous spontaneous contractions of

multiple fibers reinnervated by a single anterior horn cell after loss of their original individual sources of innervation.

B. Loss of the motor component of the reflex pathways of the PNS can produce decreased deep tendon reflexes (hyporeflexia).

C. If the process destroying anterior horn cells in the spinal cord also damages the long corticospinal tracts, a mixed picture of hypo- and hyperreflexia may be seen.

IV. Pathology

Anterior horn cell diseases produce degeneration and loss of motor neuron cells in the spinal cord.

V. Examples

A. Amyotrophic lateral sclerosis (ALS)
  1. Etiology
     a. The etiology of ALS has not been proven. Links to toxins such as lead have been postulated.
     b. Antibodies against motor neurons have been suggested.
     c. The occasional development of ALS in prior victims of poliomyelitis, a viral disease of anterior horn cells, suggests an infectious etiology.
  2. Clinical features: ALS is a motor neuron disease involving both anterior horn cells and corticospinal tracts.
     a. ALS produces weakness, atrophy, fasciculations, and a mixture of hypo- and hyperreflexia but spares the ocular muscles.
     b. Bladder and bowel control are usually maintained.
     c. Progressive weakening of respiratory and swallowing muscles usually leads to death in about 3 years, although survival for up to 30 years has been reported.
  3. Diagnosis
     a. The diagnosis of ALS is made by the cardinal signs of weakness, atrophy, fasciculations with mixed hypo- and hyperreflexia, and electromyographic studies showing evidence of denervation in three out of four limbs studied.
     b. Rarely, cervical spine disease may show a similar combination of denervation and mixed hypo- and hyperreflexia. This must be excluded in most cases by cervical spine magnetic resonance imaging (MRI) or myelography.
  4. Treatment
     a. Experimental treatments of ALS have

included thyroid-releasing hormone and branched chain amino acids.
     b. Steroids and plasmapheresis have not shown any benefit.
     c. Major modalities of treatment include assistive and orthotic devices, wheelchairs, respiratory management, and nutritional assistance.
        (1) Thickened liquids may improve swallowing.
        (2) Gastrostomy may improve the nutritional status, and cricopharyngeal myotomy may improve passage of food through a hypertonic pharynx.
        (3) Amitriptyline in small doses may help by decreasing oral secretions and modulating the emotional incontinence (laughing and crying without appropriate emotional content) sometimes seen in ALS patients with bulbar symptoms.

B. Other Anterior Horn Cell Diseases
  1. Other diseases of the anterior horn cell include the pediatric spinal muscular atrophies characterized by hyporeflexia without hyperreflexia.
  2. Hexosaminidase deficiency may also produce a motor neuron disease.

Radiculopathy

I. Definition

Radiculopathy is damage to the nerve root of either the motor neuron or a sensory nerve.

A. Damage can occur at the level of the neural foramina as the nerve passes through the bony spine to or from the spinal cord.

B. Damage to the dorsal nerve root produces sensory symptoms, while damage to the ventral nerve root produces motor deficits.

C. Although radiculopathy can occur anywhere along the spine, the cervical and lumbosacral segments seem most likely to be affected.

II. Symptoms

A. Pain is a cardinal symptom of irritation of the dorsal nerve root.
  1. The pain usually radiates along the territory of the sensory root involved, allowing localization by dermatonal distribution.
  2. Anesthesia (loss of sensation) may also occur in the same distribution.

B. Weakness is a primary symptom of damage to the ventral root.

1. The weakness is confined to the muscles innervated by the nerve root involved, again allowing localization of the root pathology.

III. Signs

1. Since damage to either the sensory or the motor nerve root will disrupt the spinal reflex arc, hyporeflexia is a cardinal sign of radiculopathy on neurologic examination. The hyporeflexia is limited to the distribution of the involved nerve root.
2. Sensory loss and motor weakness can also be elicited in the territory of the involved root.

IV. Examples

A. Etiology

1. Etiologies of radiculopathy may include disc herniation.
2. Hypertrophic bony changes of the neural foramen may also cause radiculopathy by narrowing the opening through which the root passes, causing compression when the nerve root exits.
3. Other etiologies of radicular symptoms include metabolic processes which cause microinfarctions of the nerve root (e.g., diabetes mellitus).
4. Radiculopathy may affect only one level of the spine or may present as a polyradiculopathy with pathology at multiple spinal nerve roots. Polyradiculopathy may be caused by metabolic processes such as diabetes or by structural disease at multiple levels.

B. Clinical features

1. Herniation of the nucleus pulposus through the annulus fibrosus of an intervertebral disc may compress a nerve root in the neural foramina of the spine. This mechanical irritation of the root may lead to pain, loss of sensation, weakness, and hyporeflexia.
   a. For example, if the C6 root is damaged, sensory loss may be noted in the thumb and second finger. Motor weakness may be seen in the biceps brachii. An absent or weak biceps reflex may also be noted.

C. Diagnosis

1. Diagnosis of radiculopathy is made by localization of the symptoms of pain and weakness of hyporeflexia, sensory loss, and motor weakness to one or several nerve roots. Straight leg raising produces radicular symptoms by stretching the nerve root.

Sparling's maneuver (rotation and hyperextension of the neck) causes the nerve roots to be compressed by bony spurs or disc material and reproduces the radicular pain.

2. This can be confirmed by needle electromyography (EMG), which demonstrates denervation in the distribution of particular nerve roots. These electrical changes of abnormal spontaneous activity, such as positive sharp waves of fibrillation potentials, probably reflect the hypersensitivity of muscle fibers deprived of their usual motor nerve innervation. These changes may take up to 2 weeks to be seen.
3. Radiologic studies of the anatomy of the region of the suspected nerve root pathology complement the electrophysiologic findings of EMG.
   a. Computed tomography (CT) may be helpful in visualizing the bony structures surrounding the nerve root.
   b. Myelography introduces contrast into the subarachnoid space surrounding the spinal cord and the nerve roots. Structural disease compressing nerve roots may therefore be demonstrated by the contrast medium. The combination of myelography followed by CT may be particularly helpful in demonstrating bony spurs such as osteophytes or herniated disc material impinging on nerve roots.
   c. Magnetic resonance imaging (MRI) may also allow resolution of the nerve roots and their pathology without requiring the invasive procedure of introducing myelographic contrast agents into the subarachnoid space.

D. Treatment

The treatment of radiculopathy depends on establishing its etiology

1. Structural damage to the root may be treated by surgical removal of compressive osteophytes, widening of the neural foramen, or eliminating herniated disc material. In some cases, attempts may be made to dissolve extruded disc with enzymes such as chymopapain injected in proximity to the disc. In other cases, excision of the disc is performed directly.
2. In many cases, conservative therapy aimed at reducing the inflammation at the site of the nerve root damage is all that is necessary.

a. This may be attempted by oral nonsteroidal anti-inflammatory drugs or by injections of steroids at the involved root.

b. Analgesics may reduce pain while inflammation is decreasing.

c. Physical therapy may provide relief from pain and spasm, as well as maintaining mobility and reconditioning muscles damaged by radiculopathy.

3. Metabolic diseases of the nerve roots, such as diabetes, may present with signs and symptoms of either a polyradiculopathy or a monoradiculopathy.

a. EMG will show evidence of radicular damage, but radiologic examinations will be normal.

b. Diabetic radiculopathy may be treated with management of the diabetes.

c. Also frequently required are measures for chronic pain, such as low doses of amitriptyline. Fortunately, the pain of diabetic radiculopathy is often self-limited and resolves over several months to a year.

Peripheral Neuropathies

I. Definition

Peripheral neuropathy is dysfunction of the nerves outside of the spine and spinal roots.

A. Motor neuropathies affect motor nerves.

B. Sensory neuropathies impair sensation.

C. Large-fiber sensory neuropathies damage the large, heavily myelinated nerves that carry rapidly conducted information such as vibration and proprioception.

D. Small-fiber sensory neuropathies affect the smaller, less myelinated fibers responsible for sensations of pain.

E. Autonomic neuropathies affect the portions of the PNS dealing with autonomic functions such as control of vasodilation, blood pressure, and sweating.

F. A polyneuropathy affects many nerves in a diffuse, frequently symmetrical fashion.

G. A mononeuropathy affects an individual motor sensory nerve.

H. Neuropathy may affect the myelin covering of peripheral nerves, producing demyelinative pathology. Damage to the axon itself causes an axonopathic neuropathy.

II. Signs and Symptoms

A. A diffuse *polyneuropathy* usually produces symmetrical, distal symptoms. The motor symptom consists of weakness. Sensory symptoms include a distal stocking-and-glove loss of sensation and may also produce abnormal spontaneous sensations such as burning or tingling. Normal sensory inputs such as touch may be misinterpreted as noxious stimuli.

B. If the autonomic nervous system is involved, symptoms such as lightheadedness on standing may develop.

C. A *mononeuropathy*, such as a median neuropathy, will produce sensory and motor symptoms solely in the distribution of that nerve.

D. Signs of peripheral neuropathy

1. A diffuse peripheral neuropathy will produce distal loss of motor strength and loss or reduction of sensations such as vibration, proprioception, and sharpness.

2. Because the sensory and motor components of the reflex arc may both be affected, peripheral neuropathy usually produces hyporeflexia.

3. Autonomic neuropathy may produce signs such as an orthostatic drop in blood pressure.

III. Examples

A. Carpal tunnel syndrome (CTS)

1. Etiology

A common mononeuropathy consisting of median nerve dysfunction at the level of the wrist.

a. CTS results from compression of the median nerve, usually by the thickened flexor retinaculum covering the carpal tunnel, through with the median nerve travels with numerous tendons and blood vessels. The retinaculum can be thickened by repeated trauma from repetitive motion at the wrist, by rheumatoid inflammatory processes, or by edema associated with pregnancy.

b. Metabolic processes such as diabetes can produce microinfarctions of the nerve, preferentially at sites of frequent irritation such as the carpal tunnel.

2. Clinical features

a. CTS produces numbness and tingling in the first three and one-half fingers which may be exacerbated by flexion of the wrist during sleep. This produces the characteristic "wake and shake" phenomenon in which the patient

wakes from sleeps to shake the numbness from the hand.
    b. Weakness may be noted by the patient in fine motor activities such as writing or buttoning. On examination, weakness is usually most prominent on abduction of the thumb.
3. Diagnosis
    a. Diagnosis of CTS is made by the characteristics signs and symptoms of motor and sensory loss in the distal distribution of the median nerve.
    b. Nerve conduction studies may initially show slowing of sensory impulses and then of motor impulses across the median nerve at the wrist. Early compression of the median nerve preferentially damages the myelin insulating sheath of the nerve, producing slowing of conduction velocities. If damage worsens to involve the axon within the nerve, as well as the myelin surrounding it, the amplitude of the recorded nerve responses becomes small. *Demyelinative neuropathies* produce slowed conductions. *Axonopathic neuropathies* cause small amplitudes on conduction studies.
    c. Needle EMG of the abductor pollicis brevis (APB) will show little or no change if only the myelin sheath of the median nerve is affected; however, abnormal spontaneous activity will be seen in muscles when the axon supplying them is damaged. As the pathology of CTS worsens, denervation potentials may be seen in the (APB), which moves the thumb and receives its innervation by the portion of the median nerve which pass through the carpal tunnel.
    d. Irritability of the damaged median nerve may also be demonstrated by percussing the nerve at the wrist and reproducing the patient's abnormal sensations with Tinel's sign.
4. Treatment
    a. Treatment of a mononeuropathy such as CTS is initially aimed at reducing inflammation and eliminating trauma to the nerve. A splint for the wrist worn especially at night or during repetitive wrist activity may protect the median nerve from further trauma. Nonsteroidal anti-inflammatory drugs may reduce inflammation.
    b. If the EMG demonstrates denervation in the APB, significant damage may already have occurred, suggesting that surgical decompression of the nerve may be necessary.
B. Diabetic polyneuropathy
    1. Etiology
       Diabetic polyneuropathy is probably caused by metabolic insults to the blood vessels serving nerves.
    2. Clinical features
       a. Diffuse peripheral polyneuropathies may be of gradual or rapid onset. Diabetes may cause diffuse damage to multiple nerves, producing a slow, progressive impairment of distal motor and sensory function in the arms and legs.
       b. It may also damage autonomic fibers, leading to abnormal digestive motility and problems such as sexual dysfunction and orthostatic hypotension.
    3. Treatment
       a. While control of the diabetes is the main focus of therapy, symptomatic measures also may be needed.
       b. Amitriptyline in low doses may alter perceptions of pain and abnormal sensation. It may also produce mild analgesia by its effects on serotonin.
       c. Capsaicin topical analgesic cream may cause depletion of substance P with continued and repeated use, producing a reduction in pain and noxious sensations mediated by substance P in diabetic neuropathy.
C. Guillain-Barré syndrome
    1. Etiology
       Guillain-Barre syndrome is caused by a misdirected immune attack on peripheral nerves.
    2. Clinical features
       a. A rapidly progressive diffuse polyneuropathy also known as *acute inflammatory demyelinating polyneuropathy (AIDP)*.
       b. AIDP initially may present with symptoms of minor sensory disturbances such as tingling, with little objective evidence on neurologic examination of sensory loss.
       c. It frequently progresses to demyelinate multiple motor nerves, producing rapidly spreading weakness of the limbs, facial musculature, and respiratory muscles.

d. On examination, this loss of motor strength is accompanied by the disappearance of deep tendon reflexes.

e. Autonomic nerve demyelination can produce blood pressure and heart rate fluctuations.

3. Diagnosis

a. Electrophysiologic studies early in AIDP may be normal or show only prolongation of conduction times with special late-response techniques such as F-waves.

b. As demyelination progresses, slowing of conduction velocities over multiple motor nerve segments becomes obvious electrically, although sensory conduction may remain largely normal.

c. If this autoimmune-mediated attack on peripheral motor and autonomic nerves continues, the axon as well its myelin coating may be damaged. This leads to small amplitudes on motor nerve conductions and denervation potentials in muscles sampled by needle EMG.

4. Treatment

a. Treatment of AIDP consists of protecting respiratory function by monitoring vital capacities and mechanical ventilation if necessary.

b. Monitoring of autonomic function and gentle control of blood pressure and fluids will help the autonomic problems associated with AIDP.

c. Other causes of rapid diffuse motor neuropathy such as acute intermittent porphyria, tic paralysis, and botulism should be excluded.

d. If the patient has developed severe weakness with potential respiratory compromise, plasmapheresis may speed recovery from AIDP.

e. The addition of steroids probably is not helpful in these circumstances.

f. Physical and occupational therapy are necessary to maintain and restore muscle function in the AIDP patient.

g. Frequent turning to maintain skin integrity in these immobile patients and measures to prevent the development of peripheral venous clots are also necessary.

h. AIDP is usually a monophasic illness associated with a recent infection, surgery, or stress. Recovery frequently is excellent if the patient can be adequately maintained throughout the period of acute weakness and autonomic instability.

D. Other peripheral neuropathies

1. As with the CTS and the polyneuropathies of diabetes and AIDP, diagnosis is dependent on physical signs and symptoms localizing the pathology to specific sites on individual nerves or to a diffuse process affecting multiple nerves.

2. Nerve conduction studies and needle EMG may be particularly useful extensions of the physical examination, not only to determine the location of the pathology but also to show whether it is preferentially sensory, motor, demyelinative, axonopathic, or mixed.

3. As a general principle, inflammatory neuropathies are more likely to appear demyelinative on nerve conduction studies, while most toxic neuropathies are more likely to appear axonopathic.

4. Metabolic neuropathies such as diabetes may show mixed demyelinative and axonopathic features.

5. Local trauma to nerves, when limited to the myelin sheath initially, appears demyelinative. As the axon also becomes damaged, it will take on axonopathic electrical features.

Neuromuscular Junction (NMJ) Diseases

I. Definition

Nerve impulses travel to the muscles from peripheral nerves across the synapse from the motor nerve as quanta of acetylcholine to postsynaptic acetylcholine receptors on muscle.

A. Impaired release of acetylcholine from the motor neuron may cause weakness that at least transiently improves with repeated releases triggered by further exercise. This is the *myasthenic syndrome of Eaton-Lambert (ELS)*.

B. Damage to the acetylcholine receptors leaves fewer receptors available for quanta of acetylcholine released by normal motor nerves. As more acetylcholine is released by further exercise, some receptors are bound and blocked by acetylcholine, further reducing available normal receptors. This worsening fatigue of motor strength with repetitive activity is *myasthenia gravis (MG)*, a usually autoimmune disease of acetylcholine receptors.

II. Symptoms

The chief symptom of neuromuscular junction disease is weakness.

III. Signs

The primary sign of NMJ disease is weakness.

IV. Examples

A. Myasthenia gravis

    1. Etiology

        a. MG is usually caused by a defect in neuromuscular transmission associated with acetylcholine (AChR) receptor antibodies.

        b. These antibodies block and increase the degradation rate of nicotinic AChR. Autonomic innervated muscles are usually not involved.

        c. The blockade of AChR in patients with already reduced numbers of receptors may be precipitated by various medications that can bind to the receptors. While these agents usually do not produce weakness in normal people with adequate neuromuscular transmission safety factors, that may trigger myasthenic weakness in patients with subclinical MG.

        d. Drugs that have been reported to trigger MG include antibiotics (especially aminoglycosides), local anesthetics, β-blockers, neuromuscular blocking agents (e.g., pancuronium), iodinated contrast agents, and corticosteroids.

    2. Clinical features

        a. Symptoms of Myasthenia Gravis
The cardinal feature of MG is fatigue with exercise and improvement in strength with rest.

            (1) Characteristically, muscles which are used most frequently are most affected, so patients note extraocular muscle symptoms such as double vision, weak voice, shortness of breath, weakness of hand muscles, and increasing fatigue with walking. Chewing and swallowing may also be affected.

            (2) Symptoms improve with rest and generally are better after sleep. They worsen with continued activity through the day.

            (3) Sensory symptoms are quite unusual.

        b. Signs of Myasthenia Gravis

            (1) On physical examination, patients with MG frequently show weakness of extraocular muscles, with intermittent dysconjugate gaze and ptosis of eyelids. These signs worsen with continued activity of the muscles.

            (2) Neck flexors, used continuously to maintain head posture, may show weakness.

            (3) Ability to count for long periods of time on a single breath may be impaired, as well as more conventional measures of vital capacity such as spirometry.

            (4) The voice may be nasal, breathy, or increasingly low in volume.

            (5) Facial muscles may be weak, producing a "myasthenic sneer."

            (6) Arm and leg muscles may show fatigue with repeated use.

            (7) Reflexes and sensory examination are usually normal in MG.

    3. Diagnosis

        a. Approximately 80–90% of patients will show AChR antibodies in their blood on conventional testing. AChR antibody levels are therefore the usual confirmatory test when a patient's signs and symptoms suggest the intermittent weakness of MG.

        b. Unfortunately, a significant minority of MG patients lack detectable antibodies. A few of these patients have familial protein defects in the structure of AChR.

        c. Further testing for MG includes repetitive electrical stimulation recording the amplitude of evoked motor responses. Since MG is a disease characterized by fatigue with exercise, in up to 50–60% of these patients a decrement in motor amplitudes will be seen on repetitive stimulation.

        d. An edrophonium chloride (Tensilon) test may be helpful to demonstrate a response to drugs which increase the amount of acetylcholine at the synapse by inhibiting the breakdown of acetylcholine. Since this is a relatively short-acting agent, its beneficial or deleterious effects on the nicotinic receptor will be rapidly cleared. Its effects on autonomic muscarinic receptors can be reversed by atropine. While it may temporarily increase the strength of patients with MG, it is not specific for myasthenia. Autonomic side effects such as bradycardia and gastrointestinal distress are common. For maximum utility, it should be performed with a placebo injection, a small test dose, and then a full dose. An objective measure of strength, such as millimeters of eyelid ptosis or dynamometer grip strength recordings, should be used. Emergency management of respiratory collapse from cholinergic excess or cardiac rhythm disturbances must be immediately available when the edrophonium chloride test is performed.

   e. The ice pack test may be helpful if ptosis is present. Symptoms of MG frequently improve as neuromuscular transmission improves with cooling. An ice pack placed over the ptotic lid of an MG patient will frequently produce rapid but transitory reversal of ptosis.

4. Treatment

   a. The mainstays of treatment of MG are acetylcholinesterase inhibitor drugs and immune modulation.

   b. The most commonly used inhibitor drug is pyridostigmine bromide (Mestinon). This drug may be given orally or intramuscularly, but cholinergic muscarinic side effects (such as bradycardia, diarrhea, and cramps) are more common with the intramuscular route. The dosage of pyridostigmine bromide is determined for each patient by trial and error, titrating improvement in strength against muscarinic cholinergic side effects.

   c. Excessive doses of pyridostigmine bromide can produce blockade at the nicotinic skeletal muscle receptors, producing weakness and fasciculations.

      (1) Usually the muscarinic cholinergic symptoms occur before nicotinic *cholinergic crisis* occurs from overdose of acetylcholinesterase inhibitors.

      (2) If cholinergic crisis is suspected, usually the most prudent course of management is gradual lowering of medication dose, with facilities for immediate ventilatory support available.

   d. Immunotherapy of MG can be accomplished by corticosteroids, azathioprine, or plasmapheresis.

      (1) The most rapid response is to plasmapheresis, frequently within 24–48 hr but usually requiring multiple doses and having only temporary benefits, as the production of AChR antibodies is not blocked. Plasmapheresis is most useful for achieving a rapid response in myasthenic crisis, especially when respiratory strength is compromised.

      (2) Corticosteroids, when used continuously, may produce prolonged reduction in AChR antibody activity, thereby improving the signs and symptoms of MG. Initially, however, they may cause worsening of MG through neuromuscular blockade and are best introduced in an inpatient setting to observe for this usually self-limited adverse reaction. Long-term side effects of corticosteroids, include weight gain, elevated blood sugars, increased incidence of peptic ulcers, cataracts, and infections, are well described.

      (3) Azathioprine may require 4–6 months to become effective in MG, but it can then be used to reduce or eliminate the need for corticosteroids in some MG patients. The patient must be monitored regularly for leukopenia, macrocytosis, and liver dysfunction while on azathioprine. Malignancies have occasionally been reported.

   e. Up to 70–80% of MG patients will improve over 5 years after thymectomy. The procedure is probably best reserved for generalized MG patients whose age suggests that they will have a prolonged need for pharmacotherapy. About 5% of MG patients may harbor a thymoma. If this is demonstrated by CT or MRI, then thymectomy is mandatory.

B. Eaton-Lambert Syndrome

   1. Etiology
      Eaton-Lambert Syndrome is caused by a presynaptic autoimmune attack.

   2. Clinical features
      a. Symptoms of Eaton-Lambert syndrome

Patients with ELS notice weakness that initially improves with activity.
  b. Signs of Eaton-Lambert syndrome
    (1) Examination of ELS patients shows an initial improvement in baseline weakness with exercise.
    (2) Ocular muscles are frequently spared, and deep tendon reflexes may be decreased.
  3. Diagnosis of Eaton-Lambert syndrome
    In ELS an increment in amplitude is seen on rapid, repetitive stimulation.
  4. Treatment
    Treatment of Eaton-Lambert syndrome is done with pyrido stigmine bromide, steroids,3,4 diaminopyridine, and treatment of an underlying tumor if found.

Diseases of Muscle

I. Definition
Diseases of muscle may be primary myopathies due to inborn errors of muscle metabolism or other genetic factors or acquired due to inflammatory processes, infection, or systemic illnesses.
  A. Muscular dystrophies are diseases of muscle characterized by failure of muscle to maintain normal development and mass.
  B. A myositis is an inflammatory disorder of muscle.

II. Symptoms
  A. Muscle diseases characteristically produce weakness.
  B. They may sometimes be accompanied by cramps and pain, especially with exercise.
  C. Myopathies affecting the lower extremities produce complaints of difficulty rising from a chair or of walking problems.
  D. Myopathies affecting the upper extremities may produce symptoms of difficulty using the arms over the head or poor hand function.
  E. Respiratory, ocular, facial, pharyngeal, and even cardiac muscle may be affected.

III. Signs
  A. Muscle disease usually presents on physical examination as proximal weakness.
  B. In many advanced cases wasting may be seen, but in some dystrophies, such as Duchenne's, there may be pseudohypertrophy as muscle is replaced by fibrotic tissue.
  C. In myotonic dystrophy, the ability of muscle to relax from a contracted state is impaired.
  D. Deep tendon reflexes remain intact until muscles are severely wasted, at which time reflexes decrease.

IV. Examples
  A. Myotonic dystrophy
    1. Etiology
      The etiology of myotonic dystrophy is repetition of the CTG trinucleotide on chromosome 19.
    2. Clinical features
      a. Myotonic dystrophy is an autosomal dominant muscular dystrophy linked to a gene located on chromosome 19.
      b. Unlike the usual presentation of myopathy, it predominantly affects distal musculature.
      c. It is probably the most common muscular dystrophy of adults and usually presents in early adulthood.
      d. Facial weakness causes an elongated face, with wasting of temporal and masseter muscles and frontal balding.
      e. Cataracts and dysarthric, nasal speech are common.
      f. Cardiac conduction defects, hypersomnia, hearing loss, and endocrine dysfunction may all occur.
      g. A delay in relaxation of percussed muscle gradually gives way to weakness and wasting as the disease progresses.
    3. Diagnosis
      a. EMG demonstrates spontaneous waxing and waning of the motor unit amplitude and frequency. The amplified sound of this myotonic muscle's electrical activity is reminiscent of the sound of starting a motorcycle.
      b. The clinical picture is usually so characteristic that EMG is usually the only confirmatory test necessary.
    4. Pathophysiology
      a. While goat hereditary myotonia is associated with abnormalities in cell membrane chloride conductance, chloride conductance is normal in patients with myotonic dystrophy.
      b. Myotonia may occur in several illnesses, including Thomson's disease, which is associated with true muscular hypertrophy producing a Herculean physique.
      c. The drug 20, 25 diazacholesteral may also produce myotonia.
    5. Treatment
      a. Orthotic devices to correct distal hand and foot weakness may be helpful.

   b. Quinine, phenytoin, and carbamazepine have all been helpful in alleviating myotonia but do not reverse the weakness associated with myotonic dystrophy.

B. Dermatomyositis

   1. Etiology

   The etiology of dermatomyositis is an autoimmune attack on skin and muscle.

   2. Clinical features

      a. Dermatomyositis is an acquired inflammatory disease associated with a blotchy, purplish rash over the maxilla and eyelids. Erythematous changes may be seen over the chest, and calcified nodules may occur under the skin.

      b. Many patients complain of aching muscles, but dermatomyositis may occur without muscle pain.

      c. Proximal weakness may develop suddenly, limiting the ability to hold up the head, rise from a chair, or lift the arms.

      d. Some patients have a recurrent form of the disease, with relapses and remissions.

      e. Approximately one-half of patients recover completely after a single attack.

      f. A few may develop a chronic form which may progress to difficulty swallowing and maintaining respiratory function.

      g. Approximately 10–20% of dermatomyositis patients harbor a malignancy; the breast, gastric, lung, and ovary are the most common sites.

   3. Diagnosis

      a. Dermatomyositis may be confirmed in patients with characteristic rash and weakness by measurement of serum creatine kinase (CK), EMG, and muscle biopsy.

      b. Serum CK is usually elevated during acute phases of the illness.

      c. EMG shows brief small-amplitude polyphasic motor unit potentials typical of myopathy on activation of the muscle. At rest, EMG detects muscle membrane irritability with positive sharp waves, fibrillation potentials, and bizarre, high-frequency discharges.

      d. Muscle biopsy shows inflammatory changes in most patients, abnormalities on ATPase staining, and atrophy of fibers at the outside margin of muscles fascicles.

      e. Curiously, patients with symptoms similar to those of dermatomyositis but lacking the rash (i.e., polymyositis) often lack this perifascicular atrophy as well.

   4. Pathophysiology

   Some experimental evidence suggest that most of the inflammatory damage is due to humoral factors attacking muscle fibers on an autoimmune basis.

   5. Treatment

      a. Dermatomyositis patients are managed with high-dose steroids, azathioprine, plasmapheresis, and no immunosuppression at all.

      b. Generally, patients do better with higher doses of steroids, started early in the course of the disease, and maintained for up to 1 year until improvement in muscle strength is no longer seen.

      c. The usual gastric, ophthalmologic, infectious, bony, and endocrinologic complications of chronic corticosteroid use can be expected.

      d. Most aspects of the classification and treatment of dermatomyositis/polymyositis remain controversial.

Bibliography

Brooke MH. *A Clinician's View of Neuromuscular Diseases,* ed 2. Baltimore, Williams and Wilkins, 1986.

Schaumburg HH, Berger AR, Thomas PK. *Disorders of Peripheral Nerves,* ed 2. Philadelphia, Davis, 1992.

Wright RB. Myasthenia, in Klawans HK, Goetz CG, Tanner CM (eds), *Textbook of Clinical Neuropharmacology and Therapeutics,* ed 2. New York, Raven Press, 1992, pp 505–516.

CHAPTER 136

Somatoform Disorders

Donald A. Misch, M.D.

I. Definition

A. The somatoform disorders (Table 136-1) encompass a group of psychiatric syndromes characterized by preoccupation with physical symptoms and disease. In each of these disorders, true organic pathology is absent and there is no known pathophysiologic mechanism to explain the symptom; or, if an underlying physical disorder is present, the patient's perception of its severity is grossly out of proportion to demonstrable physical findings. Patients with somatoform disorders are believed to express psychological distress through physical symptoms (somatization), but these symptoms are not under conscious, voluntary control. In contrast, patients with factitious disorders or malingering consciously fabricate their difficulties.

B. It is important that the clinician be aware of, and properly diagnose, somatoform disorders. Failure to do so may result in serious difficulties or complications.

1. Wasteful use of medical resources and adverse consequences to the patient through unnecessary, needlessly expensive, prolonged, and potentially dangerous medical testing, hospitalization, and invasive procedures.

2. Addiction to various psychoactive drugs such as pain medications (including narcotic analgesics) and anxiolytics (such as benzodiazepines), as well as exposure to disturbing and potentially dangerous side effects of unwarranted medications.

3. Frustration and anger on the part of both patients and their physicians, which may result in unpleasant relations between doctor and patient as well as potential danger for the patient. The intensity of such feelings is likely to be reduced if the clinician is aware that he or she is dealing with a somatoform disorder.

II. Etiology

Many theories have been advanced to explain the behavior of patients suffering from somatoform disorders. It is important to remember that multiple etiologic factors may be involved in the genesis of a somatoform disorder for any given patient. Therefore, it is essential to explore carefully with each patient those factors that are relevant to him or her.

Table 136-1. Somatoform Disorders

Disorder	Epidemiology	Presentation	Associated Features	Course
Somatization disorder (Briquet's syndrome): Prolonged history of recurrent, multiple somatic complaints for which no organic pathology or known pathophysiologic mechanism can be found. If there is related organic pathology, symptoms and resulting impairment are grossly in excess of what would be expected from the physical findings.	Most common in women, usually beginning before age 30. Lifetime prevalence in women: 0.2–2%	Complaints presented in a dramatic, vague, or exaggerated way. Complicated medical history with many treating physicians and multiple diagnoses.	Frequent anxiety, depression, suicide threats and attempts. Occupational, interpersonal, and marital difficulties. Increased risk of unnecessary medical procedures and drug/medication (e.g., anxiolytic) dependence.	Chronic with fluctuating severity; rarely remits spontaneously.
Hypochondriasis: Preoccupation with fear of having, or belief that one has, a serious disease even though medical evaluation does not support a diagnosis of any physical disorder. Fear of having, or belief that one has, a disease persists despite medical reassurance.	Equal sex ratio; common in general medical practice. Onset most frequent in the twenties.	Focus on bodily functions (e.g., heartbeat, peristalsis), minor physical abnormalities (e.g., occasional cough), or organ systems (e.g., cardiac neurosis). Medical history presented in great detail. "Doctor shopping" is common, as is frustration and anger between patient and physician.	Anxiety, depression, obsessive-compulsive traits. Impairment in social and occupational functioning.	Chronic with waxing and waning of symptoms; recovery occurs in many cases.

Disorder	Definition	Epidemiology	Associated features	Complications	Course
Somatoform pain disorder:	Preoccupation with pain for which appropriate evaluation uncovers no organic pathology or pathophysiologic mechanism. If there is related organic pathology, the complaint of pain and resulting social or occupational impairment is grossly in excess of what would be expected from the physical findings.	Twice as frequent in females as in males; common in general medical practice. Onset most frequent in the thirties and forties.	Symptom is inconsistent with anatomic distribution of nervous system; or if it mimics a known disease entity, no organic pathology can be found. Frequent visits to physicians, "doctor shopping," excessive analgesic use, and requests for surgery.	Depression, incapacitation, and invalid role are common. Frequent iatrogenic complications (analgesic and anxiolytic dependence, repeated unsuccessful surgeries).	Onset often sudden, with increase in severity over weeks or months; often persists for years.
Conversion disorder:	An alteration or loss of physical functioning which suggests a physical disorder but which is caused by unconscious psychological factors and not intentionally produced. No organic pathology or pathophysiologic mechanism can be found to explain the symptom. There is a temporal relationship between a psychosocial stressor and initiation or exacerbation of the symptom.	Sex ratio is unknown but disorder may be more common in women; onset is often in adolescence or early adulthood. Much less prevalent now than decades ago.	Symptoms often suggest neurologic disease such as paralysis, seizures, blindness and other sensory disturbances. Other organ systems may be involved, including pseudocyesis (false pregnancy). Antecedent physical disorders, exposure to other persons with physical disorders as role models, severe psychosocial stress, somatization disorder, and associated psychopathology are predisposing factors.	Impairment in life functioning is often marked. Prolonged loss of physical function may produce serious complications such as contractures or disuse atrophy.	Often of short duration, with abrupt onset and resolution. Recurrence predicts a chronic course.

Source: Adapted from *American Psychiatric Association–Diagnostic and Statistical Manual of Mental Disorders*, Third Edition, Revised, Washington, DC, American Psychiatric Association, 1987. Used with permission.

A. Neurophysiologic and cognitive-perceptual theories have focused on the perception and interpretation of normal bodily functions and pain. Neurophysiologic hypersensitivity to sensory stimulation and abnormal cognitive processing may lead to misperception and amplification of normal bodily sensations and pain.

B. Many patients with somatoform disorders are both linguistically and psychologically unsophisticated, such that they are unable to recognize, label, and verbally express emotional states and needs. Instead, they communicate their feelings and wishes through relatively primitive means such as the use of physical symptoms.

C. Behavioral and family dynamic theories have emphasized the importance of environmental reinforcement for the production and maintenance of somatic symptoms. Such symptoms may be used to gain attention, support, physical well-being, and release from usual responsibilities at school, work, or home. Positive environmental reinforcement of this type leads to "secondary gain" from the somatic symptoms. Conversely, environmental intolerance of emotions may leave a person with little choice but to express feelings by other, primitive and indirect means such as somatization.

D. Somatic symptoms may be strongly influenced by cultural factors. Some cultures do not allow direct verbal expression of feelings or conflicts, while others condone or even foster such behavior. Somatoform disorders may be more common among persons from lower socioeconomic classes, rural areas, and certain ethnic groups, as well as those who are less educated.

E. Persons with certain personality disorders, such as borderline, histrionic (hysterical), antisocial, dependent, and passive-aggressive, may be more prone to somaticize. This is presumably related to (B) above, as well as to the indirect expression of pressing unconscious, unmet dependency needs, anger, sexual urges, and guilt. Not all persons with somatoform disorders suffer from personality disorders, however.

III. **Evaluation and Diagnosis**
A. The diagnosis of somatoform disorders can be made only if (1) the patient fits the clinical picture of one of the disorders and (2) relevant organic pathology has been investigated and ruled out.

B. Diagnosis may be difficult and prolonged. Complicated medical histories with multiple or uncertain diagnoses, frequent office visits with normal examinations and laboratory testing, and an increasing sense of frustration and/or anger on the part of the physician should raise one's index of suspicion for these disorders.

C. The clinician will need to take a careful and extensive history and perform an appropriate physical exam. Often it is crucial to obtain previous medical records and test results.

D. Laboratory tests should be carefully and appropriately chosen to avoid subjecting the patient to unnecessary, needlessly expensive, or dangerous tests or procedures.

E. Patients with somatoform disorders need to be taken seriously and appropriately evaluated medically so as to not miss underlying physical or psychiatric pathology. The development of new symptoms or significant changes in previous symptoms may warrant further medical investigation.

1. A significant number of patients thought to have somatoform disorders will go on, over time, to develop diagnosable organic illnesses (e.g., multiple sclerosis, connective tissue disorders like systemic lupus erythematosus) that, in retrospect, can be shown to account for the earlier somatic symptoms. Thus, the clinician must remain alert to the possibility that such patients may, in fact, have an underlying or occult organic illness that will become manifest over time.

2. Patients with somatoform disorders may suffer from (a) concurrent related organic disease (e.g., patients with "hysterical" pseudoseizures often have an associated true seizure disorder), (b) concurrent unrelated organic disease (e.g., pneumonia, myocardial infarction, rheumatoid arthritis), or (c) concurrent psychiatric illness (e.g., depression, anxiety, panic attacks, personality disorders). A valid diagnosis of a somatoform disorder does not exclude the possibility that the patient may really be suffering from another illness as well.

IV. **Differential Diagnosis**
Somatoform disorders can be confused with almost any physical or psychiatric illness.
A. True illness of any organ system, including diseases that may present initially with ill-defined and confusing symptoms (e.g., multi-

ple sclerosis, seizure disorders, autoimmune diseases).

B. Side effects, intoxication, and withdrawal from nonprescription and prescription medications.

C. Chemical dependency (alcohol and other recreational substances).

D. Primary psychiatric illnesses

1. Depression: Somatic complaints are frequent presenting symptoms in depression, and some patients, especially the elderly, may present only with physical complaints and deny having a depressed mood altogether.

2. Anxiety disorders, including generalized anxiety and panic disorder.

3. Psychotic disorders, including schizophrenia (in which the somatic complaints may be of delusional intensity and quite bizarre: "I feel as though worms are eating my brain.").

4. Obsessive-compulsive disorder.

5. Personality disorders, especially borderline, histrionic (hysterical), antisocial, dependent, and passive-aggressive.

6. Factitious disorder (Table 136-2).

7. Malingering (Table 136-2).

V. Treatment

Treatment of patients with somatoform disorders requires understanding, patience, and sound medical judgment. A multidisciplinary, biopsychosocial approach is often necessary. Management is most effective in the medical setting, and many such patients refuse psychiatric referral.

A. The patient needs a primary care physician willing to work long term and to coordinate actively all aspects of care, including diagnosis, treatment, and rehabilitation. This physician should be the one to initiate appropriate subspecialty referrals and should be in frequent communication with chosen subspecialists. It is often helpful if test and procedure results, even those obtained by subspecialists, are explained to the patient by the primary care physician.

B. Be open, supportive, and empathic. Even though the patient may not have true organic pathology, he or she is truly suffering and is deserving of consideration and appropriate medical evaluation. It may be helpful to speak frankly with the patient about the diagnosis and its implications, although direct confrontation (e.g., in patients with conversion disorder) is often counterproductive.

C. Office vists should be scheduled on a regular, relatively frequent basis, and they should not be contingent on the development of new or worsened symptoms. They may be brief, but with appropriate attention and concern for the patient's physical complaints. Often a short exploration of current symptoms with a brief, relevant physical exam will be sufficient. Thereafter, it can be helpful to direct the conversation tactfully to exploration of other important areas of the patient's life (e.g., family, marriage, other interpersonal relationships, work). Exploration of the latter subjects may help to identify psychosocial precipitants or exacerbating factors in the patient's somatic symptoms, as well as to change the focus gradually from the patient's physical to his or her emotional distress.

D. Avoid unnecessary, needlessly expensive, and dangerous medical tests without clear indications. Similarly, hospitalization and operative procedures should be carefully considered and sparingly used.

E. Treatment of specific symptoms should be judiciously chosen, with emphasis on measures that are relatively safe and inexpensive (e.g., physical therapy, vitamins). Minimize the use of any medications, and avoid dangerous or addictive medications (including narcotic analgesics, anxiolytics, and sedatives). If such medications must be used, be careful to clarify their specific purpose and the likely duration of treatment. By clarifying initial plans and expectations, and by promptly discontinuing treatment if it is not effective, the physician is less likely to be pushed into an addictive or dangerous treatment program.

F. Be alert to concurrent primary or secondary psychopathology (e.g., depression, anxiety, chemical dependency, or medication abuse) and treat appropriately with psychotropic medications or refer the patient for psychiatric evaluation. Individual, marital, family, or group psychotherapy may also be indicated in addition to relaxation and other stress-reduction techniques. Behavioral interventions with family members and others are useful in decreasing secondary gain.

G. Clinicians must monitor their own feelings in dealing with patients with somatoform disorders. Frustration, anger, resentment, a sense of depletion, and a wish to avoid or be rid of the patient are common. An understanding of the nature of these disorders and frank dis-

Table 136-2. Factitious Disorder and Malingering

Factitious Disorder	
Intentional production or feigning of physical symptoms in the absence of external incentives (such as economic gain or avoidance of unwanted responsibilities). The unconscious goal is to satisfy the psychological need to assume the sick role.	History is dramatic, vague, and inconsistent. Pain complaints and analgesic requests are common. Often eager to undergo invasive procedures but may be noncompliant with hospital routine. Few visitors while in hospital. When confronted, patients often deny their actions and leave hospital against medical advice.
Often present in relatively young women with history of employment in medically related fields who have extensive knowledge of medical terms and procedures. As compared to Munchausen patients, occupational and social functioning is relatively intact.	Munchausen syndrome is a chronic form of factitious disorder associated with pathological lying and recurrent hospitalizations across the city or country. Patients are more likely to be men who have antisocial personality traits and suffer extreme incapacitation in work and interpersonal relationships. Onset of Munchausen syndrome is often in early adulthood.
Presentation patterns include (1) simulated illness (e.g., feigning acute abdominal pain when none exists, thermometer manipulation to suggest fever, falsifying medical records), (2) self-inflicted illness (e.g., injection of saliva to cause skin abscess, self-medication with thyroid hormone to cause hyperthyroidism or with anticoagulants to cause bleeding), or (3) exaggeration or exacerbation of a preexisting physical condition (e.g., surreptitious manipulation of surgical incision to prevent healing or accepting penicillin injection with history of penicillin allergy and anaphylaxis).	Multiple hospitalizations lead to iatrogenic complications (e.g., from invasive procedures or medications). Analgesic and anxiolytic abuse common.

Malingering	
Intentional production of false or grossly exaggerated physical symptoms, motivated by external incentives (secondary gain) such as avoiding military duty or work, obtaining financial compensation, evading criminal prosecution, obtaining drugs, or securing better living conditions.	May present with any type of physical symptom or sign. Note medicolegal context of presentation (e.g., patient referred for evaluation by his attorney, impending or ongoing lawsuit), marked discrepancy between claimed disability and objective findings, lack of cooperation with diagnostic evaluation or treatment, presence of antisocial personality traits.

Source: Adapted from American Psychiatric Association-Diagnostic and Statistical Manual of Mental Disorders, Third Edition, Revised, Washington, DC, American Psychiatric Association, 1987. Used with permission.

cussion with the patient contribute to an increase in physician equanimity and a reduction in avoidance behavior and unnecessary referrals.

VI. Prognosis

Contrary to the opinion of many, patients with somatoform disorders can often be helped to lead happier and more productive lives, and their overutilization of medical resources can be controlled.

Bibliography

American Psychiatric Association. *Diagnostic and Statistical Manual of Mental Disorders*, Third Edition, Revised, Washington, DC, American Psychiatric Association, 1987, pp 255–267, 315–318, 360.

Barsky AJ. Somatoform disorders. in Kaplan HI, Sadock BJ (eds): *Comprehensive Textbook of Psychiatry*, ed. 5. Baltimore, Williams and Wilkins, 1989, pp 1009–1027.

Morrison J. Managing somatization disorder. *Disease-a-Month* October, 1990, pp 539–591.

CHAPTER 137

Headache, Facial Pain, and Chronic Pain

Michael G. Chez, M.D.

Headache and Facial Pain

Since recorded history, headache and facial pain have been reported. Ancient and more recent physicians have compiled elegant descriptions of migraine and other types of facial pain. Famous persons have also left us descriptions of their personal suffering, including Sigmund Freud and Thomas Jefferson.

I. **Definition**
   A. Headaches can be difficult to classify. A reclassification of headache types was published in 1988 by the International Headache Society. For the practicing primary physician, however, a more simplified classification may be more useful.
      1. Migraine or vascular headache.
      2. Cluster headache.
      3. Chronic daily tension or stress headache, including psychosomatic headaches and those secondary to depression.
      4. Sinus headache.
      5. Somatic head and facial pain, including tic douloureux, occipital neuralgia, cervical pain, temporal-mandibular joint (TMJ) pain, and giant cell arteritis.
      6. Headache from increased intracranial pressure.
   B. Classification of headaches can often be determined by a careful clinical history and physical examination. Pain remains poorly understood, but several working hypotheses have allowed both symptomatic and prophylactic treatments to be developed.
II. **Frequency and Factors**
   A. Frequency: Headache affects a large percentage of the population. Only a minority report never having headaches. As many as 75–85% of population groups studied in the United States have some type of headache, with severe or disabling headaches affecting 20–45% of the population.
   B. Sex, race, and age
      1. Headache occurs in men slightly less often than in women, according to various surveys; subtypes such as cluster headaches seem much more prevalent in men.
      2. Race seems not to play a major role in headache except, again, in cluster headache, which black women seem to suffer more frequently than white women.
      3. Cultural differences in pain tolerance may

account for some racial or sexual differences in the reporting of headache frequency or severity.

4. Hormones do not play a significant role except in a small percentage of women migraine suffers who report increased frequency during menstruation.

5. Age does not affect the onset of vascular headaches, since children suffer migraine, as do adults. Those over 65 years of age show a decreased incidence of vascular headache, perhaps due to vasomotor changes or the use of cardiac and antihypertension medications.

III. Pathophysiology and Clinical Presentation

The underlying mechanisms of headache and facial pain depend on the type of headache. Therefore, each type will be discussed separately.

Pain can be experienced through a variety of mechanisms. These include:

1. Pressure due to edema or displacement of cranial or intracranial structures.
2. Perivascular sterile inflammation.
3. Inflammation secondary to infection or arthritic conditions.
4. Pain due to direct compression of peripheral or cranial nerves.
5. The role of central neurochemicals, such as serotonin, norepinephrine, prostaglandin, and histamine, are postulated to play a role in headache pain.

A. Migraine is classified as either common or classic.

1. Classification
   a. Classic migraine has a triad of unilateral throbbing pain, visual scotoma, and nausea and/or vomiting.
   b. Common migraine may have some of these components.
   c. Complex or atypical migraine may have transient neurologic deficits, unusual paroxysmal symptoms without headache pain, or intermittent loss of neurologic function or consciousness without any other etiology.

2. Pathophysiology
   a. Vascular component: Direct effects of vasoconstriction or vasodilation are felt to play a role in migraine. Cerebral blood flow changes have been noted by transcranial Doppler, single photon emission computed tomography (SPECT) scanning, and magnetic resonance imaging (MRI). Electroencephalography (EEG) may show transient focal slowing if performed within 24 hr of the development of migraine symptoms. Vasomotor changes may be influenced by β- and α-norepinephrine receptors, as well as by serotonergic receptors. This may affect local neuronal function, causing clinical symptoms such as visual scotoma or other sensory or motor impairment.
   b. Nausea and vomiting may be due to an effect on serotonergic receptors within the area postrema.
   c. Painful sensation may be regulated by prostaglandin synthesis and direct serotonergic mechanisms within the perivascular region, as well as by more distant central nervous system pain pathways. Scalp localization of headache pain may switch sides and does not always correlate with underlying pathophysiology. Perivascular sterile inflammation is seen in severe migraine. This may be related to activation of serotonin receptors in the vascular smooth muscle, which then increases prostaglandin release.

3. Clinical presentation and course
   a. Migraine typically is characterized as an intermittent headache occurring every 1–4 weeks with severe pain and at times incapacitation of the patient. Migraines may occur any time of the day or night, but awakenings from sleep are atypical. Symptoms usually last for a few hours and resolve within 12–24 hr. Sleep, quiet, and a dark room all provide symptomatic relief. Medical intervention is discussed in Section V.
   b. Unusual migraine patterns do occur, such as clustering of migraines lasting for more than 24 hr. Migraine rarely occurs daily, usually for only brief periods (less than 5–7 days). Illness, stress, menstruation, and eating of foods rich in tryptophan or sulfites may induce migraines. Neurologic complications such as sensory loss, hemiplegia, or pupillary defects are usually transient, but if significant focal ischemia occurs, a more delayed recovery or mild permanent deficit may persist. Seizures and stroke have been reported as sequelae to migraine.

B. Cluster headache: Cluster headache is a unilateral, periocular, painful headache with several postulated pathophysiologic mechanisms. These headaches differ from migraine and chronic tension headaches in presentation and clinical course.
  1. Pathophysiology
    a. Vascular changes: Abnormal extracranial and regional cerebral blood flow changes have been noted, with increased dilation of the ipsilateral ophthalmic artery. Occasional compression of the carotid sympathetic plexus may occur, with ipsilateral Horner's syndrome noted if there is relative edema of the carotid in the petrous canal. Impaired vascular autoregulation seems to be present.
    b. Cyclic hormone changes/chronobiologic factors
      (1) Cluster headaches tend to occur with the onset of rapid eye movement (REM) sleep.
      (2) Serum testosterone levels are lower than normal during cluster attacks, with other abnormalities noted in levels of prolactin, cortisol, and endogenous endorphins.
      (3) Altered circadian rhythms for blood pressure and temperature have been noted.
      (4) These alterations suggest hypothalamic or pituitary involvement in cluster headache.
    c. Serotonin, histamine, and autonomic factors
      (1) Serotonin: Increased cerebrospinal fluid (CSF) and platelet tryptophan and serotonin levels were found during attacks.
      (2) Histamine: H1 and H2 blockers have no clear effect, but increased mast cells in temporal skin biopsies of cluster headache patients have been reported.
      (3) Autonomic factors: Both parasympathetic and sympathetic systems have been implicated.
        (a) Surgical ablation of cranial nerve VII, with disruption of parasympathetic input to the petrosal and sphenopalatine ganglia, has relieved cluster headaches.
        (b) Decreased pupillary responses to sympathometic agents have been demonstrated in cluster headache patients.
  2. Clinical description
    a. Episodic cluster: Represents 80% of cluster headache sufferers.
      (1) Patients are susceptible to attacks every 6–12 months, with approximately 1–3 months of headaches during these cycles.
      (2) Headaches typically consist of a boring, sharp pain in the periocular region unilaterally. Pain may radiate to occipital-temporal, frontotemporal, and maxillary regions.
      (3) Headaches last for 45–60 min (range, 10 min–3 hr). Attacks occur daily and occur two times a day in approximately 80% of sufferers. Twenty percent may suffer more frequent daily attacks. These headaches differ from migraine and tension headaches because they commonly awaken patients from sleep and are of short duration. Onset typically occurs during the first REM sleep cycle.
      (4) Associated signs include lacrimation, nasal congestion and rhinorrhea, conjunctival irritation, and, rarely, an ipsilateral Horner's syndrome.
    b. Chronic cluster: This headache is clinically similar to episodic cluster, but there are no typical headache-free remission periods. These headaches may be primary or evolve as a secondary type from initial episodic headaches.
    c. Remission: This occurs when headaches are no longer present and cannot be provoked. Usually these periods are intermittent, lasting for less than 2 years in 70% of patients.
C. Tension (muscle contraction, stress, or somatiform) headache
  1. Pathophysiology: The exact etiology remains uncertain. Underlying depression or other psychiatric conditions may be present.
    a. Muscle spasm: Occasionally secondary to neck or head injury.
    b. Electromyographic (EMG) data demonstrating muscle contraction are often

contradictory, with no clear association with pain.

c. Serotonin may play a role in central pain mechanisms in tension headache.

2. Differential diagnosis

a. Mood or anxiety disorders are often associated with or result in headache symptoms.

b. Cervical spine disease must be excluded as an etiology of tension headache.

c. Occipital neuralgia will often present with a trigger point that elicits the pain.

d. Dental or infectious processes: Included in these categories are TMJ disease, dental infection, and chronic sinusitis.

3. Clinical course and symptoms

a. Daily or frequent headaches occur, with no clear underlying neurologic disease.

b. Dull ache or pressure sensation, often bifrontal, bioccipital, or band-like, encircling the head, may be present.

c. Absence of vascular headache symptoms, such as intermittent frequency, throbbing, or neurologic symptoms.

d. Chronic fatigue, vague dizziness, altered affect, or weakness may be present in chronic headache sufferers. Other etiologies may need to be ruled out.

D. Headache due to elevated intracranial pressure (ICP)

1. Tumor, trauma, infection, hydrocephalus, and pseudotumor cerebri are the most common etiologies.

2. Course of the headache is usually progressive in acute, subacute, or indolent fashion until ICP reaches a critical level where focal neurologic signs may be present.

3. Papilledema, pupillary, or cranial nerve deficits may be early findings on examination.

4. Headache pain typically progresses over a period of weeks or months. Early morning awakening with headache, nausea, or vomiting is a sensitive sign to possible elevated ICP. Headaches typically lessen after the patients rises due to a relative decrease in ICP in the erect position.

5. Treatment varies and is aimed at the underlying pathology. Treatable conditions include infection, pseudotumor cerebri, resectable tumors, and superficial or drainable fluid collections. Hydrocephalus can be treated by CSF shunt procedures.

E. Facial pain

1. Disorder of cranial, sinus, dental, or neck structures include the following:

a. Cranial bones: Fracture or inflammatory process (neoplasms rarely present with pain in cranial bones).

b. Cervical spine disorders that cause pain most commonly projecting to the forehead, temples, vertex, occiput, or orbits. Pain is increased with change of position or movement. Retropharyngeal inflammation may also result in headaches.

c. Acute ophthalmologic disorders, especially inflammatory conditions such as glaucoma or uveitis, may cause facial pain. Occasionally, headache due to refractive errors in vision and secondary squinting is seen.

d. Sinuses: Acute and, rarely, chronic sinus infection produces bifrontal facial pain.

e. Dental: TMJ, abscess, and toothache are the most common causes of dental-induced facial pain.

2. Cranial nerve and peripheral nerve pain, both chronic and intermittent (tic-like):

a. Compression syndromes: Seen with compression of trigeminal, facial, glossopharyngeal, or vagal nerves. This may be seen with neoplasm, aneurysm, or basilar meningitis.

b. Demyelination: Optic neuritis. Visual symptoms can be present, often associated with eye pain.

c. Infarction of cranial nerves: Most common in diabetic cranial neuropathy or vasculitic conditions which may cause facial pain. Cranial nerve III is the nerve most commonly affected, with changes in ocular motility and pupillary sparing.

d. Inflammatory conditions

(1) Commonly seen with herpes zoster: Trigeminal distribution (80% ophthalmic division). Ramsey Hunt syndrome may involve the external auditory canal with unilateral facial weakness.

(2) Gradenigo syndrome: Pain with palsy of cranial nerves VII and VI that usually follows chronic mastoiditis.

(3) Tolosa-Hunt syndrome: Granulomatous lesion in the cavernous sinus

causes ocular pain and damage to cranial III, VI, and IV.

   (4) Raeder's paratrigeminal neuralgia: May mimic cluster headache symptoms.

e. Cranial neuralgias

   (1) Trigeminal neuralgia (*tic douloureux*): This presents with lancinating, paroxysmal, electric shock-like pain lasting for seconds. Affects the maxillary and mandibular branches of cranial nerve V in 95% of cases and in 97% is unilateral. Symptomatic forms are associated with intracranial organic lesions such as meningitis, aneurysms, tumors, and demyelination. Idiopathic forms have no clear etiology but may be seen with tortuous arteries compressing cranial nerve V in the posterior fossa.

   (2) Glossopharyngeal neuralgia: Pain similar to trigeminal pain but occurs at base of tongue.

   (3) Geniculate neuralgia: Pain may be more prolonged and occurs deep in the middle ear.

   (4) Occipital neuralgia: Usually less severe than above neuralgias, with a more prolonged dull type of headache pain in distribution among the greater and lesser occipital nerves. Entrapment of the nerve is a common etiology.

f. Central facial pain

   (1) Thalamic pain: Facial dysesthesia secondary to infarction or similar injury to the thalamus or trigeminothalamic pathway.

   (2) Atypical facial pain: Usually associated with depression or psychosomatic disorders.

IV. Treatment

A. Migraine: Treatment is divided into abortive therapy, and prophylaxis.

   1. Abortive therapy

   a. Intermittent migraines are usually treated with a variety of agents, usually involving either nonsteroidal anti-inflammatory drugs (NSAIDs) or ergotamines. These agents are now being augmented by specific serotonin receptor agents such as sumatriptan.

   b. Ergotamines: These agents act to vaso-
constrict peripheral vessels and also seem to decrease firing of midbrain raphe nuclei, releasing serotonin. Oral and sublingual forms are available under various names. An intravenous ergotamine, DHE-45, is very potent at both midbrain raphe nuclei serotonin receptors and also in peripheral vascular serotonin binding sites. Side effects include severe nausea, abdominal pain, vomiting, diarrhea, and vasoconstriction.

   c. NSAIDs: These drugs are useful due to their inhibiting action at sites of peripheral prostaglandin synthesis, which can produce vasodilation and perivascular sterile inflammation, as well as the pain response. In addition, central serotonergic receptors appear to be a site of action of NSAIDs. These sites are probably responsible for the main analgesic properties of these drugs.

   (1) Naprosyn: This NSAID is very effective in migraine abortive therapy. Dosages are 500–750 mg orally initially, with subsequent doses of 500–550 orally every 6–8 hr.

   (2) Ketorolac (Toradol): The only currently available parenteral NSAID. This agent has been useful in acute migraines with intramuscular injection at a dose of 30–90 mg. An oral preparation is expected.

   (3) Other oral NSAIDs used for migraine include ibuprofen, fenuprofen, and aspirin.

   d. Meclopramide (Reglan): Several reports have documented the usefulness of this agent in relieving symptoms of nausea or vomiting. Prochlorperazine has also been used for this purpose. Central action or serotonin receptors in the region of the area postrema in the medulla is responsible for the antiemetic action.

   e. Narcotics: Oral, intramuscular, and intravascular administration has been useful for severe pain during the acute attack. These drugs act by breaking the pain cycle and promoting sleep. Side effects include anticholinergic action, sedation, and potential for addiction and abuse.

   f. Serotonin (5HT) agonists: Sumatriptan

given intravenously, subcutaneously, or by inhalation act on 5HT-1D receptors of central nervous system (CNS) arteries to cause vasoconstriction. In addition, it decreases the firing rate of midline raphe nuclei by binding to 5HT-1A receptors, which alters serotonin action carefully.

2. Migraine prophylaxis:
   a. β-Blockers: Agents such as Inderal and atenolol act by binding CNS 5HT receptors. The most widely studied is Inderal, which is used in dosages of 60–240 mg/day as tolerated. Sedation, mood swings, cardiovascular and sympathetic instability, and other side effects may limit its usage.
   b. Calcium channel blockers: These prevent excessive vasoconstriction-vasodilation by acting on arterial calcium receptor channels. In addition, central serotonergic action is postulated. The best-studied drugs are verapamil and diltiazem.
   c. Anticonvulsants: Phenytoin, carbamazapine, and valproic acid have all been studied, and for some patients with atypical or complicated migraine they may be beneficial.
   d. Cyproheptadine (Periactin): This serotonergic agonist acts centrally and peripherally. The major side effect is weight gain, which is secondary to appetite stimulation.
   e. Methysergide: This is another prophylactic agent that acts on central serotonergic receptors. Retroperitoneal fibrosis has been reported after chronic, uninterrupted use.
   f. Antidepressants: Amitriptyline and other tricyclics act by suppressing the activity of midline raphe nuclei, binding 5HT-1A receptors, and preventing serotonergic stimulation of the prostaglandin/arachidonic acid pathways to prevent sterile inflammation.
   g. Corticosteroids: For patients with intractable migraine or frequent clustering of migraine attacks, a brief course of prednisone, 60–80 mg/day with tapering over 1–3 weeks, may be helpful in decreasing the severity and frequency of the attacks.

B. Cluster headaches: Both prophylactic and symptomatic treatments have been described.
   1. Prophylactic treatment:
      a. Ergotamine: 2 mg prior to sleep can prevent REM-associated cluster attacks.
      b. Calcium channel blockers: Verapamil, 80 mg four times per day, has been useful and may be combined with qHS ergotamines. Verapamil is helpful in up to 70% of cluster headache patients. The precise site of action is unknown, but it may be the effect on arterial vasoactive properties, as well as some low affinity binding to various 5HT receptors centrally.
      c. Lithium: 300 mg twice a day may be useful in 70–80% of patients who fail calcium channel blockers or ergotamine treatment. The mechanism of action is unclear.
      d. Methysergide is useful in younger patients suffering from only one or two headaches per cluster attack. It is less useful in patients with frequent attacks.
      e. Prednisone: 40–60 mg/day for 1–3 weeks has been used for refractory cluster headaches resistant to the therapies mentioned above.
   2. Symptomatic treatment
      a. Oxygen: Early use of oxygen in the cluster attack is effective in aborting the attack. Oxygen flow at 7 liters/min via facial mask to an upright or seated patient is suggested. Action is presumed to be via vasoconstriction of arteries.
      b. Sublingual or inhaled ergotamines: Vasoconstriction appears to be the mechanism of these agents.
      c. Sumatriptan: When studied for acute attacks, this serotonergic agent has proven useful, presumably by binding a 5HT-1D and 5HT-1A receptors.

C. Tension headache/chronic headache
   1. Symptomatic treatment of acute headache
      a. NSAIDs are useful for acute or semiacute flareup of these headaches. Ibuprofen and Naprosyn are most commonly used.
      b. Acetaminophen and aspirin: These agents are generally useful for mild-moderate relief of acute headaches.
      c. Pressure applied to the scalp, often with warmth, has been useful in some clinical trials.
      d. Biofeedback or relaxation techniques are often useful in more chronic headaches.
   2. Treatment of chronic headache

a. Tricyclics are often useful for their central serotonergic action of pain relief, as well as treatment of possible underlying depression. Anticholinergic properties may limit their use. Amitriptilene is the most commonly used agent.

b. Psychotherapy/biofeedback: These techniques and supportive therapy are often useful in relief of underlying anxiety or depression. They are often used in combination with NSAIDs or tricyclics.

c. Avoid opiates, benzodiazepines, and sedatives because of their addictive properties. Patients should be instructed to avoid alcohol, excessive caffeine, and tobacco use.

D. Facial pain

1. Tic douloureux/trigeminal or other cranial neuralgias

   a. Carbamazapine or phenytoin provide effective relief from neuropathic pain. These compounds decrease repetitive neuronal firing, a possible cause of neuropathic pain.

   b. Tricyclic treatment may be useful for central pain relief.

   c. Surgical decompression of the nerve from a tortuous vessel is often successful in the treatment of intractable tic-like pain.

2. Arthritic conditions are usually treated symptomatically with NSAIDs.

3. Sinusitis should be treated with appropriate antibiotics and decongestants.

4. TMJ: Treatment of the underlying jaw misalignment is often successful in eliminating the pain of TMJ. NSAIDs are helpful for pain. Other dental problems are treated symptomatically.

E. Elevated ICP: This condition is treated symptomatically. Decadron, diuretics, hyperventilation, and surgical decompression are useful in acutely elevated ICP. Pseudotumor cerebri (benign intracranial hypertension) may benefit from serially repeated lumbar puncture, with some patients requiring carbonic anhydrase inhibitors or oral steroid therapy as well.

Chronic Pain

I. Definition

An unpleasant sensory or emotional experience which persists beyond an arbitrary period, usually 3–6 months. This may have an identifiable cause or may be idiopathic. Further subdivisions of chronic pain are made by the presence or absence of disability. Our discussion will focus mainly on nonmalignant, idiopathic pain.

A. Chronic pain with a known etiology is usually due to a systemic or local response to inflammatory, myopathic, neuropathic, arthritic, traumatic, malignant, or other such conditions that are diagnosable.

B. Idiopathic chronic pain may occur in 10–20% of chronic pain sufferers and in as much as 1–2% of the general population.

C. Chronic pain due to similar pathology may vary among individuals.

D. Idiopathic chronic pain may be from secondary or primary pathology, psychological causes, or other etiologies.

II. Patient Evaluation

A. The physician must rule out a diagnosable primary cause of pain whenever possible.

B. Psychosocial factors, as well as individual personality traits and coping skills, must be evaluated.

C. Concurrent psychiatric illness, most commonly subclinical, and clinical depression must be ruled out.

III. Modification of Chronic Pain

A. Circumstances surrounding the onset of chronic pain may alter perception (i.e. a battle wound vs. a job-related injury).

B. Individual variation in pain perception exists, so treatment must be modified for each patient.

C. Social support systems may modify pain in a positive or negative manner.

IV. Treatment Strategies

A. Always focus on the treatment of primary or secondary causes of pain that may be the result of insufficient healing or complications of the primary injury.

B. If no tissue or somatic source of pain is identified, then the approach should be multifaceted, including medication, psychological counseling, and rehabilitative efforts to help the patient function.

C. Medications should be used only to help patients cope in reasonable comfort. Medications alone will probably fail to help those with chronic pain and disability.

V. Medication

A. NSAIDs

1. The agents found to be useful include ibuprofen, aspirin, ketoprofen, and Naprosyn.

2. These agents are useful for inflammatory

pain or pain from old injuries. Their side effects include gastric irritation, bleeding anomalies, renal fibrosis, and rare allergic reactions. Side effects are worse with chronic use.

3. An important advantage is that they are nonaddictive.

4. They act on prostaglandin synthesis and the subsequent inflammatory cycle of pain.

B. Tricyclic agents

1. The most widely used agents are amitriptyline, nontriptyline, fluoxetine, and others.

2. They may help with sleep problems and with underlying or secondary depression.

3. The side effects that limit their use are mainly anticholinergic, including rare cardiac arrhythmia.

4. They are nonaddictive.

5. They act by modifying serotonergic receptors centrally and therefore dampening pain perception. In addition, underlying depression is relieved simultaneously, which may modify coping skills in a positive manner.

C. Anticonvulsants

1. Carbamazapine and phenytoin are the most widely used agents. Phenobarbital is rarely used for its sedative effect.

2. These agents are used mainly for neuropathic pain related to nerve injury. However, carbamazapine is related structurally to tricyclics and may be useful for central pain as well.

3. Both phenytoin and carbamazapine bind to serotonin receptors and may act centrally or at the spinal level to modify pain as well.

4. Major side effects include toxic reactions, allergic reactions, bone marrow or leukocyte suppression, and liver dysfunction.

D. Antianxiety medications (benzodiazepines)

1. These act to reduce anxiety, coping problems, and agitation related to chronic pain.

2. For acute or semiacute flareup, they may help calm the patient and decrease the severity of pain.

3. The risks of abuse, overdose, and addiction must be monitored.

4. The main agents used are diazepam, clonazepam, and aprazolam.

E. Narcotics

1. Both oral and parenteral agents are available. These are never recommended except for acute use or during a flareup of acute pain associated with chronic illness (e.g., sickle cell crisis).

2. The risks of abuse and addiction are high, but selective monitored use may still allow these agents to play a role in breaking pain cycles.

3. There is no major role between acute severe pain cycles.

F. Other agents or techniques useful in pain control

1. Lithium and valproic acid: May be useful in chronic cluster headache, patients with bipolar disorder and pain, or other refractive pain conditions.

2. Stimulants such as dexedrine and methylphenidate: May play a role in pain inhibition via modification of the norepinephrine concentrations in the CNS.

3. Acupuncture may modify pain, but the exact mechanism of action remains unclear.

4. Biofeedback helps patients relax and modify pain stressors.

5. Psychotherapy: May help with coping skills and underlying issues related to depression.

Bibliography

Diamond S (ed). Headache. *Med Clin North Am* 75(3): , 1991.

Headaches Classification Committee of the International Headache Society. Classification and diagnostic criteria for headache disorder, cranial neuralgias, and facial pain. *Cephalgia* 8(Suppl 7):9–96, 1988.

Matthew NT (ed). Headache. *Neurol Clin North Am* 8(4): 1990.

McGrath PJ, Unruh AM, Branson SM. Chronic nonmalignant pain with disability. *Adv Pain Res Ther* 15:255–271, 1990.

Raskin NH. Serotonin receptors and headaches. *N Engl J Med* 325(5):353–354, 1991.

Silberstein SD (ed). Intractable headaches: Inpatient and outpatient treatment strategies. *Neurology* 42(Suppl 2):1–51, 1992.

The Subcutaneous Sumatriptan International Study Group. Treatment of migraine attacks with sumatriptan.

The Sumatriptan Cluster Headache Study Groups. Treatment of acute cluster headache with sumatriptan. 325(5): 322–326, 1991.

CHAPTER 138

Drugs Used by Neurologists

Paul Evans Later, M.D.

This chapter presents an overview of the drugs commonly used by neurologists. The drugs are organized according to disease processes. Problems commonly encountered clinically are emphasized, including side effects, drug interactions, and dosage guidelines.

I. Anticonvulsants
   A. Phenytoin (Dilantin)
   1. Classification: An anticonvulsant with a chemical structure similar to that of the barbiturates.
   2. Mechanism of action
      a. Inhibits sustained high-frequency neuronal firing.
      b. Posttetanic potentiation is strongly inhibited, limiting the stimulation of neighboring cortical areas by seizure focus.
   3. Indications: Simple partial seizures, complex partial seizures, and primarily generalized tonic/clonic seizures.
   4. Dosage: Parenteral or oral route.
      a. Loading dose: 13–18 mg/kg
      b. Maintenance dose: 5 mg/kg/day; if given intravenously (IV), must be given every 8 hr.

   c. Depending on the imminent risk of further seizures, phenytoin can be rapidly loaded by the IV route, orally loaded over 4–6 hr, or gently loaded orally over days.
   d. Close observation, including frequent blood pressure checks and electrocardiographic (ECG) monitoring for a prolonged QTC interval, are necessary with IV infusion. The parenteral form must be given in a glucose-free solution in order to prevent precipitation.
   e. The rate of infusion must be *limited to less than 25–50 mg/min* to avoid cardiovascular side effects, especially in older or cardiovascularly compromised patients. The dosage requirements may be drastically affected by a low albumin, elevated serum blood urea nitrogen, or other protein bound substances.
   5. Interactions (see Table 138-1).
   6. Complications: Physical findings indicate dose-dependent toxicity. Nystagmus, which may be present without toxicity, can appear at a serum level of about 20 μg/ml,

Table 138-1.   Changes in Anticonvulsant Concentration with the Addition of a Second Agent

First Drug	Second Drug Added	Effect on First Drug
Carbamazepine	Phenobarbital	Decrease
	Phenytoin	Decrease
	Primidone	Decrease
Phenobarbital	Carbamazepine	No change
	Phenytoin	Increase
	Valproic acid	Increase
Phenytoin	Carbamazepine	Increase
	Phenobarbital	Decrease, increase, or no change
	Primidone	No change
	Valproic acid	Decrease
Primidone	Carbamazepine	Increased phenobarbital
	Phenytoin	Increased phenobarbital
	Valproic acid	Increase
Valproic acid	Carbamazepine	Decrease
	Phenobarbital	Decrease
	Phenytoin	Decrease
	Primidone	Decrease

Source: Brown TR, Feldman RG. *Epilepsy: Diagnosis and Management.* Boston: Little, Brown, 1983, p 155. Used with permission

ataxia at about 30 μg/ml, and decreased level of consciousness at about 40 μg/ml.

a. Other reversible side effects
   (1) Encephalopathy.
   (2) Gastric upset.
   (3) Total ophthalmoplegia following large loading doses.
b. Idiosyncratic reaction or effect of chronic toxicity (some of which may require stopping diphenylhydantoin)
   (1) Lupus-like syndrome with positive antinuclear antibody titer.
   (2) Predominantly axonal sensory poly-neuropathy.
   (3) Hepatic transaminase elevations up to two to three times normal but generally not requiring discontinu-ation. Rarely, more significant liver dysfunction occurs in association with signs of systemic allergic reac-tion (serum sickness).
   (4) Hypocalcemia and osteomalacia due to vitamin D deficiency.
   (5) Dermatologic: Hirsutism, gingival hypertrophy, acneiform lesions, coarsening facies.
   (6) Blood dycrasias: Leukopenia, agranulocytosis, thrombocytopenia, aplastic anemia, pseudolymphoma, and megaloblastic anemia.
B. Carbemazepine (Tegretol)

1. An anticonvulsant structurally related to the tricyclics.
2. Mechanism of action: Reduces posttetanic potentiation and polysynaptic responses.
3. Indications: Partial seizures, complex par-tial seizures with or without generalization, and generalized tonic/clonic seizures.
4. Dosage: Poor patient tolerance is most fre-quently a result of increasing starting doses too rapidly.
   a. Give 100 mg twice a day (or 200 mg q HS) for 2–3 days, adding 100 mg/day every 3–4 days
   b. Total of 7–15 mg/kg/day on a twice daily or three times daily schedule.
   c. Carbemazepine induces its own enzy-matic clearance, so the dosage may need to be increased over the first 6 weeks to maintain a therapeutic level.
5. Interactions: When carbemazepine is initi-ated in the presence of phenytoin, there may be increased sensitivity to the toxic effects of both drugs (see Table 138-1).
6. Complications
   a. Often associated with transient mild leukopenia, which is usually not a prob-lem. Very rare cases of aplastic anemia occur, which led to the warning in the PDR recommending very close moni-toring of the complete blood count (CBC).

b. Acute dose-related toxicity: Diplopia, drowsiness, nausea, vomiting, and ataxia.

c. Serious side effects: Rash in 3%, often with other signs of allergic reaction (Stevens-Johnson syndrome and photosensitivity have been reported), hepatotoxicity, pseudolymphoma, and lupus-like syndrome.

d. Chronic use may result in hyponatremia after several months.

C. Valproic acid (Depakene and Depakote)

1. Classification: A dicarboxylic acid chemically unrelated to other anticonvulsants.

2. Mechanism of action: Appears to be related to sodium and potassium channel inhibition.

3. Indications: Drug of choice in patients with multiple primary generalized seizures; also used in those with atypical absence, myoclonic seizures, and complex partial seizures and in those with many different types of seizures.

4. Dosage: 15–60 mg/kg/day in three to four divided doses.

5. Complications

a. Common side effects: Gastrointestinal upset, which is generally less with Depakote than with Depakene, skin rash, weight gain, alopecia, peripheral edema, fine (essential-like) tremor, drowsiness, hyperactivity, and ataxia.

b. Uncommon serious side effects: Encephalopathy, bone marrow suppression resulting in thrombocytopenia, pancreatitis, and rare cases of fatal liver failure have been reported in children less than 3 years old on multiple anticonvulsant medications.

c. Follow serum glutamic-oxaloacetic transaminase (SGOT), serum glutamic-pyruvic transaminase (SGPT), CBC, and platelet counts prior to initiation of therapy and at intervals. The first indications of liver dysfunction are prolonged prothrombin time and elevated ammonia. These generally normalize with a decrease in the daily dosage.

6. Contraindications: Valproate should be used with caution in women of childbearing age because of the risk of neural tube defects. This has been seen in up to 1% of infants born to mothers taking the drug during their first trimester.

D. Phenobarbital

1. Classification: A barbiturate whose anticonvulsant properties are more potent than its sedating properties compared to other barbiturates.

2. Mechanism of action: Phenobarbital prolongs the open time of the chloride channel coupled to the gamma aminobutyric acid (GABA) A receptor.

3. Indications: Primary generalized tonic/clonic seizures and all forms of partial seizures, either added as a second agent or used as a single agent in certain patients who have difficulty with first-line agents. Phenobarbital monotherapy at high doses (40 mg/ml) is useful in difficult-to-control simple partial seizures of neocortical origin.

4. Dosage: Range: children, 3–5 mg/kg; adults, 60–120 mg/day

5. Complications

a. Its dose-limiting side effect is sedation. This is primarily a problem early in treatment. A significant percentage of children have behavioral problems such as hyperactivity.

b. Rare side effects: Teratogenicity, maculopapular rash, toxic epidermal necrolysis, Dupuytren's contracture, folate- and vitamin B_{12}-responsive megaloblastic anemia, and osteomalacia due to vitamin D deficiency.

c. Risk of withdrawal seizures from stopping the medication too quickly. Phenobarbital can be decreased by one-third and then by 15 mg every 2 weeks; it may have to be decreased more slowly with certain sensitive patients.

E. Primidone (Mysoline)

1. Classification: Metabolized to phenobarbital and phenylethylmalonamide (PEMA), both with independent anticonvulsant effects.

2. Mechanism of action: Resembles phenobarbital in many ways but is somewhat more selective in modifying the maximal electroshock seizure pattern in animals.

3. Indications: It may be more effective as a second drug in preventing generalized tonic/clonic convulsions if phenobarbital fails.

4. Dosage: Initially, a test dose of 50 mg should be given, looking for an idiosyncratic hypersomnolent reaction; then give

125 or 250 mg/day, increasing by 250 mg every 5–7 days until an effective dose is reached or toxicity occurs.

5. Interactions: Phenytoin increases the conversion of primidone to phenobarbital; otherwise, interactions are similar to those of phenobarbital.

6. Complications: Similar to phenobarbital except for acute cerebellar ataxia and vertigo, which sometimes occur in the first few days of treatment and which generally resolve.

II. Movement Disorders

A. Parkinson's disease (see Table 138-2)

1. Levodopa, carbidopa, and levodopa/carbidopa (Sinemet)

a. Mechanism of action: Levodopa (L-3,4-dihydroxyphenylalanine), given orally, crosses into the central nervous system and is converted into dopamine, which is deficient in Parkinson's disease. Dopamine cannot be given directly because it does not cross the blood-brain barrier. If given alone, levodopa is mainly converted to dopamine in the periphery and causes peripheral side effects. Carbidopa is given to minimize peripheral conversion of levodopa to dopamine. It decreases the dose of levodopa needed for therapeutic effect and reduces the peripheral side effects of dopamine. To block peripheral conversion, 75–100 mg of carbidopa is needed per day.

b. Indications: Levodopa is used effectively in extrapyramidal disorders including Parkinson's disease, dystonia, and neuroleptic malignant syndrome.

c. Dosage: In the treatment of Parkinson's disease, an initial dose of 25/100 of carbidopa/levodopa (Sinemet R) should be given two to three times per day, either 30 min before or 1 hr after meals for more consistent absorption. The dosage must be increased *slowly* to avoid toxicity. Give the last evening dose early (approximately 7 P.M.) to avoid sleep disturbance.

d. Complications: Side effects are generally dose dependent and reversible.

(1) Early side effects: Nausea and vomiting, which are reduced by taking medication with food, by a more gradual increase in the Sinemet R dose, or by a higher dose of carbidopa.

(2) Later effects: Dyskinesias or dystonic involuntary movements affecting the limbs, neck, and face.

(3) Psychiatric disturbances can also be quite frequent and dose limiting. Frank psychosis is usually preceded by a progression from altered sleep patterns to vivid dreams to nonthreatening visual daytime hallucinations to a schizophreniform psychosis.

2. Selegiline (Deprenyl, Eldepryl)

a. Classification: A highly selective monoamine oxidase (MAO)-B inhibitor.

b. Mechanism of action

(1) Selegiline inhibits the metabolism of dopamine and presumably enhances and prolongs the effect of endogenous and exogenous dopamine in the basal ganglia.

Table 138-2. Drugs Used for the Treatment of Parkinson's Disease

Drug	Generic Name	Dosage	Mechanism
Carbidopa/levodopa	Sinemet	25/100 TID up to 8 tabs per day	Neurotransmitter precursor
Bromocriptine	Parlodel	2.5 mg/day slowly up to 50 mg/day	Direct-acting dopamine agonist
Pergolide	Permax	0.1 mg/day up to 1–4 mg/day	Direct-acting dopamine agonist
Amantadine	Symmetrel	100 mg BID	Increases synaptic dopamine
Selegiline	Eldepryl	5 mg in the morning and at noon	MAO-B inhibitor
Trihexyphenidyl	Artane	1.0–5.0 mg TID	Anticholinergic
Benztropine	Cogentin	0.5–4.0 mg BID	Anticholinergic
Ethopropazine	Parsidol	10–20 mg TID	Anticholinergic

(2) In an experimental form of parkinsonism caused by a toxic metabolite of the chemical methyl phenyl tetra hydropyridine (MPTP), selegiline inhibits the conversion by MAO-B of MPTP to its toxic metabolite (MPP+), which is capable of inducing parkinsonism in animals and humans. Thus, by inhibiting MAO-B in parkinsonian patients, disease progression may be slowed if an unknown toxic substance is involved. Selegiline also appears to benefit parkinsonian patients symptomatically.

  c. Indications: Parkinson's disease.

  d. Dosage: 5 mg in the morning and at noon (to avoid insomnia), with a gradual reduction in the dosage of levodopa by 10–30% beginning 2–3 days after starting selegiline. Further reductions may be made if evidence of levodopa toxicity develops, such as hallucinations or dyskinesias.

  e. Complications: Generally a safe drug; the main side effect is exacerbation of the effects of toxic levodopa, which is generally apparent in the first 24–48 hr and responds quickly to a decrease in the levodopa dose. A relative contraindication is peptic ulcer disease, which may be worsened by selegiline.

3. Direct-acting dopamine agonists: Bromocriptine (Parlodel) and pergolide (Permax)

  a. Classification: Ergot alkaloids. Pergolide is a semisynthetic ergot which was developed after bromocriptine and is about 10 times more potent.

  b. Mechanism of action: These agents directly stimulate postsynaptic dopamine receptors. In this way, they avoid levodopa's failure to produce dopamine when neurons (which contain dopa-decarboxylase) have degenerated.

  c. Indications: See Section II,A,1.

  d. Dosage: Agonists have long half-lives, which avoids some of the variation in effectiveness of levodopa, smoothing out its action.

    (1) Bromocriptine: Initially, give 2.5 mg/day, *slowly* increasing by one 2.5-mg tablet per week. Optimal benefit may lag behind dosage increases by weeks or months. Maximal dosage is 50–60 mg/day.

    (2) Pergolide: Mean effective dose is 1–4 mg/day. The starting dose is 0.1 mg and is increased slowly, as with bromocriptine. Attention to the frequent occurrence of orthostatic hypotension is especially necessary with pergolide.

  e. Interaction: When used in combination with levodopa, the incidence of psychiatric/cognitive disturbance is greater and the incidence of dyskinesia is less than with the use of levodopa alone.

  f. Complications: Postural hypotension is the most important side effect, occurring in 33% in one series. This usually improves after the first few doses. In patients with more severe Parkinson's disease, mental status changes are the most frequent reason for discontinuing the drug.

4. Amantadine (Symmetrel)

  a. Classification: Introduced as an antiviral agent, amantadine produced serendipitous improvement in parkinsonism.

  b. Mechanism of action: The mechanism of action is not known, but amantadine is thought to release dopamine from central neurons and delay reuptake of dopamine; it may have some anticholinergic effects as well.

  c. Indication: Used as a single agent in mildly parkinsonian patients or as a mild agonist with Sinemet. It must be used cautiously in demented patients or those with renal insufficiency, as it is excreted unchanged in urine and may cause confusion and hallucinations.

  d. Dosage: 100 mg twice a day; may be increased to three times a day if renal function is adequate. Serum concentrations should be obtained at a high dose in elderly patients.

  e. Complications: Side effects occur much more commonly at dosages above 200 mg/day. Hallucinations, confusion, and memory impairment are seen with toxic doses or if the drug is given concomitantly with anticholinergics. Long-term use may lead to livedo reticularis in the lower extremities, but discontinuation is not necessary.

5. Anticholinergics

  a. Classification: Centrally acting muscarinic antagonists.

b. Mechanism of action: Due to the deficiency of dopamine in the striatum in Parkinson's disease, the cholinergic system is relatively overactive. These drugs act at the central muscarinic receptors to maintain dopamine–acetylcholine balance.

c. Indications: Parkinson's disease and acute or chronic dystonia. These drugs are most useful for the relief of parkinsonian tremor but rarely affect other manifestations of the disease.

d. Dosage
(1) Trihexyphenidyl (Artane): 1.0–5.0 mg three times a day.
(2) Benztropine mesylate (Cogentin): 0.5–4.0 mg twice a day.
(3) Ethopropazine (Parsidol): 10–20 mg three times a day.
The dosage is increased *slowly* to avoid side effects. The above dosages are usual for Parkinson's disease, but much higher doses are often tolerated in dystonic patients.

e. Complications: Frequently these medications are poorly tolerated by elderly patients. Check for evidence of urinary retention, prostatic hypertrophy, or narrow angle glaucoma.
(1) Common side effects: Dry mouth, blurred vision, and dizziness.
(2) More serious side effects: Acute confusion, constipation, urinary retention, and precipitation of narrow-angle glaucoma.

B. Essential (postural) tremor: A common disorder involving tremor of the hands, voice, and sometimes the legs. A fine, rapid tremor is present when maintaining a position (postural) or precision movements (kinetic).

1. Primidone (Mysoline): The drug of choice for patients who can tolerate it. The main reaction is an ill feeling with nausea, ataxia, and malaise. Most patients tolerate this if warned of the side effects. Give an initial dose of 50 mg at night and then 125–250 mg qHS after a few weeks. If this dose is ineffective it may be discontinued and propranolol may be tried. If there is some effect but some tremor remains, propranolol may be added to primidone. (See the full description of primidone in Section I,E)

2. Beta blockers: Propranolol: 40–320 mg/

day. One may start with 80 mg of the long-acting form and work up. Rarely does propranolol alone abolish the tremor. If the patient has contraindications to propranolol, other β-blockers such as metoprolol (Lopressor) in asthmatics or nadolol, (Corgard), with a longer half-life, can be used. The patient who does not respond to propranolol will not respond to other β-blockers. The β-2 selectivity of these agents is not absolute; patients should be carefully observed for signs of reactive airway disease.

3. Other agents used include phenobarbital, with less efficacy and more sedation. Alprazolam (Xanax) may be effective in some cases where primidone or propranolol is not.

C. Acute dystonic reactions
1. Benztropine (Cogentin): 1.0 mg IM or IV initially, followed by 1–2 mg three times a day orally for the next 48 hr. If possible, the offending agent should be discontinued and the benztropine tapered.
2. Diphenhydramine (Benadryl): 50 mg IV initially, followed by 25 mg orally three times a day for 48 hr, and then tapered.

III. **Myasthenia Gravis** (see Table 138-3)
A. Cholinesterase inhibitors
1. Classification: Pyridostigmine bromide (Mestinon), neostigmine bromide (Prostigmine), and ambenonium chloride (Mytelase) are the clinically used cholinesterase inhibitors. Pyridostigmine is most frequently used, with fewer gastrointestinal side effects than the other drugs.
2. Mechanism of action: Reversibly inhibit acetylcholinesterase enzyme (AChE), preventing the hydrolysis of acetylcholine (ACh), allowing the accumulation of ACh in the synapse, and prolonging its action. This action is aimed at the motor end plate

Table 138-3. Anticholinesterase Drugs Used for Myasthenia

Drug	Route	Adult Dose	Frequency
Pyridostigmine	PO	60 mg	Up to every
(Mestinon)	IM, IV	2 mg	3–4 hr
Mestinon Timespan	PO	180 mg	Every 8–10 hr
Neostigmine	PO	15 mg	Up to every
(Prostigmine)	IM, IV	0.5 mg	2–3 hr

but autonomic cholinergic synapses are affected, leading to side effects.

3. Indications: The first-line therapy for myasthenia, causing dramatic improvement in some patients. Combination therapy with corticosteroids is sometimes necessary.

4. Dosage: The dosage and schedule of administration are dictated by the severity of disease symptoms and the side effects experienced by a given patient. This schedule may vary from day to day and in response to many factors. The usual starting dose of pyridostigmine is 30–60 mg orally every 4–6 hr. Adjustments are then based on the patient's symptomatic response to the drug versus the reported side effects. The parenteral form may be needed in an acute exacerbation if dysphagia is significant.
   Note: The dose of the parenteral form is 1/30th the oral dose for pyridostigmine and neostigmine.

5. Interactions: Atropine may mask the symptoms of cholinergic excess.

6. Complications: Excessive cholinergic side effects include nausea, vomiting, diarrhea, abdominal cramps, increased salivation, diaphoresis, increased bronchial secretions, miosis, fasciculation, muscle cramps, and weakness.

B. Tensilon (edrophonium) test
1. Developed to determine whether a clearly observable sign of weakness such as ptosis, extraocular muscle function, diplopia, or hypoventilation is due to myasthenia gravis.

2. Other disease processes have shown a positive response to edrophonium, Lambert-Eaton syndrome, motor neuron disease, diabetic third nerve palsy, or a third nerve palsy secondary to cerebral aneurysms.

3. Patients with asthma or cardiac arrhythmia should not be tested. Hypotension and/or bradycardia are rare reactions if these patients are not given the test. Cardiac monitoring is recommended. If bradycardia is observed, atropine (0.6 mg) can be given to reverse this effect. An increase in oral secretions is another potential danger and can also be prevented or treated with atropine.

4. A placebo should be used, with the observers blinded to maintain objectivity. Edrophonium may also be given during EMG testing or spirometry to measure improvement.

C. Drugs which may precipitate myasthenic weakness
1. Antibiotics: Aminoglycosides: streptomycin, kanamycin, neomycin, gentamicin, tobramycin, tetracyclines.

2. Quinine and related agents: Antimalarial drugs (e.g., chloroquine), antiarrhythmics (e.g., procainamide and quinidine), antihelminths (e.g., piperazine), and local anesthetics (e.g., lidocaine).

3. Psychotropic drugs: Benzodiazepines, chlorpromazine, phenelzine, and lithium carbonate.

4. β-Blockers.

5. Anticonvulsants: Phenytoin, diazepam, trimethadone.

6. Corticosteroids and adrenocorticotropic hormone: May cause deterioration at the onset of treatment.

7. D-Penicillamine.

8. Diuretics: Acetazolamide.

Bibliography

Brodie MJ. Epilepsy octet: Established anticonvulsants and treatment of refractory epilepsy. *Lancet* 336:350–354, 1990.

Delgago-Escueta AV, Treiman DM, Walsh GO. The treatable epilepsies. *N Engl J Med* 308(25):1508–1515, 308(26):1576–1584, 1983.

Gilman AG, Rall TW, Nies AS, et al. *Goodman and Gilman's The Pharmacological Basis of Therapeutics,* ed 8. New York, Pergamon Press, 1990.

Klawans HL. Emerging strategies in Parkinson's disease. *Neurology* 40(Suppl 3), 1990.

Klawans HL, Goetz CG, Tanner CM. *Textbook of Clinical Pharmacology and Therapeutics,* ed 2. New York, Raven Press, 1992.

SECTION 14

Geriatric Medicine

CHAPTER 139

Assessment of the Older Patient

Steven Rothschild, M.D.

Any review of the care of the elderly must begin with a caveat: The older patient is *not* fundamentally different from other adults. However, physiologic changes which occur with age, the increased prevalence of multiple chronic conditions, declines in function, and a unique set of psychological and social issues require that physicians modify the traditional model of history taking and physical examination.

In forming diagnoses of the older patient, keep in mind that multiple simultaneous conditions are the rule. Seeking a single pathologic process to explain a patient's signs and symptoms is often inappropriate in the geriatric population. A multidisciplinary approach must be used in the diagnosis and treatment of older patients.

I. **The Successful Interview of the Older Patient**
   A. Optimize environmental factors and allow for sensory deficits. For the hard-of-hearing, make eye contact, speak clearly, lower the pitch of the voice, and eliminate background noise.
   B. Be respectful.
      1. Do not condescend to the patient.
      2. Never use the patient's first name unless told to do so.
      3. If the patient is cognitively intact and able to speak, obtain the history directly from the patient.
      4. Allow adequate time for the exam.
      5. The patient may downplay important symptoms. Ask specific questions. Listen for hesitancy.

II. **Focus of the History**
   A. Atypical or nonspecific presentations of acute illness are common, especially over age 80.
   B. Illness often presents as a change in the level of function. Systematically inquire about baselines for:
      1. Activities of daily living (ADLs)
         a. Bathing
         b. Dressing
         c. Toileting/continence
         d. Transfer into and out of bed and chair
         e. Ambulation
         f. Feeding
      2. Instrumental activities of daily living: higher-level activities required for independent living.
         a. Use of the telephone
         b. Traveling via own car, bus, or taxi
         c. Shopping
         d. Handling money, paying bills

e. Preparing meals
f. Doing housework
g. Management of medications

C. Past medical history
1. Obtain complete old records.
2. Assess medications via the "brown bag test"; have the patient/family bring in any medications found in the home.
3. Determine immunization status, including polyvalent pneumonia vaccine, annual influenza vaccine, and tetanus status. Almost all elderly women, and men who have not been in military service, will need a primary tetanus immunization series.
4. Obtain a history of tobacco, alcohol, and drug use. Alcoholism is prevalent in older adults, just as in the general population.

D. Social history is critical.
1. Persons with whom the patient lives, family/friends.
2. Formal/informal support systems.
3. Housing: Stairs, distance to bathrooms, floor surfaces, other factors affecting mobility.
4. Economic supports: Most older persons live on fixed incomes. Medicare (Part A) pays most hospital costs; outpatient costs are paid largely out of pocket, especially if the person does not have Medicare (Part B). Outpatient medications are never paid for by Medicare.

E. Attitudes regarding cardiopulmonary resuscitation should be sought. This query is almost always well received by the older patient. Laws of individual states should be consulted regarding documentation of advance directives.
1. Living wills allow patients to specify treatments they wish performed or withheld in a terminal illness. This document goes into effect only when a terminal condition has been diagnosed and the patient can no longer communicate preferences. It may not cover such situations as withholding food and fluids, dependent on individual state laws.
2. A durable power of attorney for health care decision making allows patients to designate spokesperson(s) as their proxy in making health care decisions. This document goes into effect when the patient can no longer communicate wishes personally, even if a terminal condition is not diagnosed. It can include the patient's personal guidelines to aid the proxy in decision

making. The designated spokesperson can make decisions about any medical questions, including resuscitation and tube feeding.

III. Changes in the Physical Exam
A. Vital signs
1. Temperature
a. Ability to generate a fever diminishes with age.
b. Hypothermia more frequent.
2. Blood pressure
a. Systolic blood pressure increases throughout life. Diastolic blood pressure increases into the seventh decade; after this time, diastolic pressure gradually declines, with loss of elastic compliance in the great vessels.
b. Orthostatic hypotension due to loss of autonomic tone is more common with age. Orthostasis is more pronounced with diabetes, Parkinson's disease, and with the use of a wide range of medications.
3. Pulse
a. No change in rate with age.
b. Pulse rates above 100 may indicate acute illness or infection.
4. Respirations
a. No change with age
b. Respiratory rates >28/min indicate acute illness or pulmonary infection, even if no fever/typical symptoms are present.

B. Skin
1. Loss of subcutaneous fat is the norm. Skin turgor is an unreliable marker of hydration.
2. Systematically inspect all areas, focusing on:
a. Pressure points
b. Feet
c. Sun-exposed areas: Actinic keratoses or squamous cell carcinomas.
d. Other: Basal cell carcinomas or petechiae or ecchymoses suggesting coagulopathy or physical abuse

C. Head and neck
1. Skull: Nodularity of metastatic bone disease or Paget's disease
2. Eye (see Chapter 140D)
3. Ear
a. Inspect for internal auditory canal obstruction with cerumen.
b. Assess function by using whispered speech, not lower-pitched tuning forks.

    c. Refer any patients with impairment.
4. Nose and throat
    a. Inspect condition and fit of dentures; loose fit occurs with as little as a 15-kg. weight loss.
    b. Always remove dentures to inspect the oral mucosa.
D. Lungs
  1. Inspect chest configuration: note if kyphosis is present.
  2. Bibasilar crepitance or rales are the norm with advanced age due to atelectasis and decreased chest wall elasticity.
E. Heart
  1. S4 may be chronic; if new, then evaluate.
  2. S3 always pathologic.
F. Breast exam annually.
G. Abdomen
  1. Palpate for abdominal aortic aneurysm.
  2. Acute abdomen can exist without classic signs.
H. Genital and rectal exam
  1. Rectal exam must be performed at least annually. It should include palpation of the prostate, evaluation for masses, stool exam for occult blood, and assessment of sphincter tone.
  2. An estimated 40% of women over the age of 65 have never had a pelvic exam and Pap test, yet they remain at risk for cervical cancer. Any women with a history of postmenopausal bleeding may need referral for endometrial sampling.
I. Neurologic exam
  1. Mental status exam: Standardized mental status evaluations (see Chapters 140A, 140B).
  2. Peripheral neuropathies: Test proprioception and vibratory sensation. Isolated bilateral loss of Achilles tendon reflex frequent among normal elderly persons.
  3. Gait analysis includes observing the patient:
    a. Getting up from a hard chair without the use of the upper extremities.
    b. Walking forward approximately 10 ft.
    c. Turning around and returning to the chair.
    d. Sitting down again.

Bibliography

Lachs MS, et al. A Simple Procedure for General Screening for Functional Disability in Elderly Patients *Annals of Internal Medicine,* 112:699–706, 1990.

Levkoff SE, et al. Illness Behavior in the Aged: Implications for Clinicians, *Journal of the American Geriatrics Society,* 36:622–629, 1988.

Robbins AS, Rubenstein LZ. Communicating with the Elderly Patient *Medical Times,* 115(10):81–98, 1987.

Dementia

David A. Bennett, M.D.
Judith Heyworth, M.D.

I. **Definition**
    A. Dementia is a syndrome of acquired, persistent deterioration in intellectual function. To distinguish dementia from more focal lesions, there must be compromise of at least two of the six major spheres of mental activity in an adult:
        1. Memory
        2. Language
        3. Visuospatial skills
        4. Emotion
        5. Personality
        6. Other higher cortical functions such as aphasia, apraxia, and agnosia
    B. The *Diagnostic and Statistical Manual of Mental Disorders* (DSM-III) currently requires that the loss of these cognitive abilities be of sufficient severity to interfere with daily function. The National Institute of Neurological and Communicative Disorders and Stroke (NINCDS) does not make this stipulation, requiring only that function be decreased relative to a previous level of performance.
    C. Dementia is a collection of symptoms, not a disease. To say that someone has a dementia is not a diagnosis. A complete workup should be done in order to reach a diagnosis and to determine whether or not there is a treatable or reversible component to the dementia.
    D. Many of the diseases underlying a dementia are terminal. The patient and family deserve to have the most correct clinical diagnosis possible so that they know what to expect and can be advised to do some advance planning.

II. **Epidemiology**
    A. Dementia is not considered a normal part of aging.
    B. Dementia is prevalent with aging, affecting approximately 10% of persons over age 65 and nearly 50% of those over age 85.
    C. In 1950 only 8% of the U.S. population (i.e., 12 million persons) were over age 65; this proportion will grow to 20% (or 50 million people) by the year 2025.

III. **Diagnosis**
    A careful history, a complete physical exam, a mental status exam, and some laboratory tests are all needed. Together they can lead to an accurate diagnosis in over 90% of those suffering from a dementia.

A. History
   1. First, review any active medical problems or complaints. Second, seek specific information relating to cognitive function. Remember that dementias are common, but do not confuse common with normal. Allow time for the patient to respond, and attempt to be nonthreatening in your approach.
   2. An acute event may be superimposed on a background of dementia, and this may be what has caused the family/patient to seek help. Both the acute problem and the underlying dementia need to be investigated.
   3. A history must be obtained from someone familiar with the patient. It is never adequate to rely solely on the patient's account. There is always someone else with whom you can talk.
      a. History of the present illness should include:
         (1) The time course of onset (gradual/insidious, sudden/abrupt).
         (2) The duration (days, years).
         (3) The rate of any deterioration (slow, rapid).
         (4) The usual course (continuous decline, stepwise decline with "plateau" periods of stability, or variable periods in which there may even be some improvement over weeks, months, or years).
         (5) Associated signs and/or symptoms, specifically depression, altered mood, agitation, self-neglect (hygiene, food intake), confusion, memory loss, getting lost in familiar surroundings, difficulty driving, problems with language (e.g., naming) or speech, personality changes, behavior or thought disturbance including delusional thinking, paranoid ideation, social disinhibition, obsessions and compulsions, or hallucinations.
      b. Medication review, with attention to all drugs taken or discontinued in the last year. Include over-the-counter medications, ophthalmics, and topical drugs.
      c. Past medical history, focusing on pertinent negative events including stroke, transient ischemic attacks, headache/migraine, seizures, falls, head trauma with or without loss of consciousness, syncope, palpitations, hypertension, diabetes, hypercholesterolemia, thyroid disease, syphilis, cancer, and any other known disease processes including cardiovascular, neurologic, infectious, rheumatologic, or autoimmune disease and any prior psychiatric illness.
      d. Family history, focusing on blood relatives with known cardiovascular, neurologic, psychiatric, or genetic disease. Specifically, ask about others in the family who may have had a dementia. Ask about Down syndrome.
      e. Social history, focusing on:
         (1) Level of education and occupational skills attained, since these will partly influence the performance on neuropsychiatric testing.
         (2) History of alcohol use.
         (3) Basic and instrumental activities of daily living, since the presence and time course of changes in these activities are significant diagnostic clues.
         (4) Potential and actual support systems, including paid help, should be documented.
      f. Review of systems should be completed as usual, but information about weight change, sleep patterns, incontinence, falls, and gait disturbance should be particularly stressed.
B. Examination should include a complete physical exam, as well as a mental status exam.
   1. Physical exam: Pay special attention to the cardiovascular and neurologic systems.
   2. Mental status examination should include:
      a. Your own (and possibly a neuropsychologist's) documented observations of the patient's appearance, mood, speech, and responses to specific questions about delusions and hallucinations.
      b. The result of a standardized cognitive screening test, noting that no one test or result is specifically diagnostic; one such useful test is the Folstein Mini-Mental Status Examination.

IV. Differential Diagnosis

There are over 100 causes of dementia. These can be broken down in many different ways for classification.

A. Degenerative Dementias: Involve alteration in the structure, function, and number of neurons in certain parts of the brain. These include:

1. Primary degenerative dementia (Alzheimer's disease): A diagnosis of exclusion, yet still the most frequent cause of dementia.
2. Lobar dementias; Due to intrinsic pathology (Pick's disease) or acquired (e.g., dementia pugilistica—boxer's dementia).
3. Parkinson's disease.
4. Subcortical gliosis, including thalamic dementia.
5. Progressive supranuclear palsy.
6. Amyotrophic lateral sclerosis.

B. Vascular dementias: This category is second in frequency only to Alzheimer's disease.

1. Multi-infarct dementia, associated with cardiovascular disease.
2. Binswanger's disease, including lacunar dementias, often associated with hypertension.
3. Anoxic encephalopathy due to either acute or chronic brain insult.
4. Vasculitis, including association with lupus, polyarteritis nodosa, and granulomatous angiitis.

C. Potentially treatable and reversible dementias

1. General paresis (syphilis).
2. Normal pressure hydrocephalus.
3. Space-occupying lesions, including frontal meningiomas, subdural hematomas (acute and chronic), and central nervous system lymphoma.
4. Depression (known as *pseudodementia*).
5. Drug toxicity, including but not limited to:
   a. Hypnotics (benzodiazepines, barbiturates).
   b. Antihistamines.
   c. Anticholinergics (artane, cogentin).
   d. Analgesics (both narcotic and nonnarcotic).
   e. Cardiac medications (digoxin).
   f. Diuretics and antihypertensives.
   g. Antibiotics (gentamicin, isoniazid).
   h. Psychotropics.
   i. H-2 blockers.
   j. Steroids.
6. Nutritional/vitamin deficiencies (e.g., vitamin B_{12} deficiency, as in pernicious anemia, or folate deficiency, as in pellagra).
7. Metabolic and endocrine disorders, including thyroid disease, parathyroid disease, liver or kidney failure, hypoglycemia, and hyponatremia.

D. Infectious etiology (dementias from a transmissible cause)

1. Creutzfeldt-Jakob disease.
2. Human immunodeficiency virus encephalitis (acquired immunodeficiency syndrome dementia).
3. Progressive multifocal leukoencephalopathy.
4. Syphilis.

E. Inherited dementias, including:

1. Some forms of Alzheimer's disease, both early and late onset.
2. Huntington's disease.
3. Wilson's Disease.
4. Leukodystrophies.

V. Dementia Workup

A. The basic laboratory evaluation should include:

1. Blood work: Complete blood count, chemistry and electrolyte profile, thyroid function tests, vitamin B_{12} and folate levels, syphilis serology, Westergren erythrocyte sedimentation rate.
2. Urinalysis.
3. Electrocardiogram.
4. Chest x-ray.
5. Brain scan: Computed tomography (CT) or magnetic resonance imaging (MRI).
   a. MRI is more sensitive but less specific for vascular disease.
   b. Mass lesions to be ruled out inlcude primary brain tumors such as subfrontal meningiomas and butterfly gliomas; metastatic brain tumors such as those from the lung or breast; subdural hematomas, which may be acute or chronic; and cerebral abscesses.
      (1) CT is good for imaging acute subdural hematomas.
      (2) CT may miss chronic or bilateral subdural hematomas.
   c. Normal pressure hydrocephalus.
   d. Demyelinating diseases such as multiple sclerosis, for which MRI is far superior.

B. Additional testing, as indicated, might include:
   1. Lumbar puncture for suspected meningitis, positive syphilis serology, suspected demyelinating disease or vasculitis.
   2. Electroencephalography for suspected Creutzfeld-Jakob disease or to assess temporal lobe status or adult-onset petit mal status.
   3. Heavy metal screens (e.g., lead, arsenic, mercury).
   4. Long chain fatty acids (as in adrenoleukodystrophy).
   5. Urinary arylsulfatase A (as in metachromatic leukodystrophy).
   6. Formal neuropsychiatric examination.
   7. Psychiatric evaluation for depression and/or behavior management.
   8. Angiography in some cases of vasculitis.
   9. Cerebral biopsy in rare cases.

VI. **Alzheimer's Disease (AD)**
   A. Diagnosis
      1. NINCDS/Alzheimer's Disease and Related Disorders Association (ADRDA) criteria; note that the diagnosis is clinical in almost all cases, since the only positive diagnostic test currently is to examine brain tissue pathology.
      2. History: AD is typically insidious in onset, with steadily progressive memory loss, either verbal or spatial. General health is usually excellent. Peak incidence is in the seventh decade.
      3. Neurologic examination is typically normal.
      4. Routine laboratory workup should be normal.
      5. Several investigational diagnostic tests are being researched, including p300 measuring event–related cortical potentials; extracerebral amyloid deposits in skin and/or spinal fluid; specific abnormal proteins [A68, Alzheimer's Disease Related Protein (ADAP)] in spinal fluid; RFLP markers in familiar cases.
   B. Genetic studies
      1. Early-onset familial AD is linked to chromosome 21. Late-onset familial AD has not been so linked.
      2. Most cases of AD are sporadic, with age being the only known risk factor.
      3. Nearly all persons with Down syndrome will develop the pathology of AD by ages

35–40 and will be clinically demented by ages 50–60.
   C. Etiology is unknown.
   D. No treatment for the underlying process exists.
      1. Deficits in cholinergic function correlate roughly with the severity of dementia and the degree of pathology. Several cholinergic strategies have been employed experimentally:
         a. Cholinergic precursors (lecithin, acetyl carnitine).
         b. Direct agonists (intraventricular bethanacol).
         c. Antiacetylcholinesterases (Tetrahydroaminoacridine THA/Cognex, physostigmine).
      2. Metabolic enhancers: Piracitam, hydergine.
      3. Other: Adrenergic agents, serotonergic agents, neuropeptides (somatostatin, gamma-aminobutyric acid agents); in the future, trials will likely include nerve growth factor, l-deprenyl, and glutaminergics.
      4. Treatment of behavioral symptoms (aggression, paranoia, delusions, hallucinations)
         a. Low-dose thioridizine (10 mg/day, increasing weekly); low-dose haloperidol (0.5 mg/day, increasing weekly).
      5. Reversed sleep-wake cycles may respond to:
         a. Low-dose thioridizine or mesoridizine.
         b. Maprotiline (antidepressant with low anticholinergic properties).
         c. Low-dose, short- or medium-acting benzodiazepines.
      6. Education, supportive counseling, assistance in maintaining good general health, referral to a support group, highlighting community support systems including the Alzheimer's Association, and advising that advance directives be executed (wills, living wills, durable power of attorney), if desired, are among the most useful management strategies.
   E. Prognosis
      1. Alzheimer's disease is a terminal illness.
      2. Duration is typically 1–20 years, with an average of 5–10 years; rate of progression is highly inidividual.
   F. Pathology

1. Neuritic plaques (NP) and neurofibrillary tangles (NFT) are the hallmark of AD and are most easily seen on silver staining. They are most often found in the hippocampus, amygdala, temporal neocortex, and neocortical association cortices.

2. The exact number/density of NP and/or NFT necessary to make a pathologic diagnosis of AD was determined by a National Institute on Aging (NIA)-sponsored workshop group.

VII. Vascular Dementias

These are the second most common cause of dementia. Their incidence peaks in the seventh and eighth decades, and they are more common in males. Both multiple cortical strokes and multiple subcortical strokes can cause dementia. Simply demonstrating that a person has had a stroke does not prove that the stroke caused the dementia. Most patients diagnosed with vascular dementia actually have both AD and a vascular component.

A. Diagnosis: To date there are no good clinical or pathologic criteria.
1. History
   a. Virtually all patients have some vascular risk factors such as hypertension, diabetes, and hyperlipidemia.
   b. Dementia often has abrupt onset with stepwise deterioration.
   c. There is often a history of stroke.
   d. Memory may or may not be affected first.
   e. Depression tends to be more common than in AD.
   f. Paranoia is not usually an early feature.
   g. Gait disorders, extrapyramidal rigidity, and incontinence are common earlier in the course.
2. Routine laboratory workup
   a. Blood work may show abnormal blood glucose and cholesterol levels and abnormal kidney function.
   b. Chest x-ray and electrocardiogram may be consistent with cardiovascular disease.
   c. Brain scan will demonstrate multiple strokes with varying amounts of hydrocephalus. MRI is more sensitive than CT, but not every lesion on MRI is an infarct. The brain scan is not meant to be used as a diagnos-

tic tool except in a negative sense (i.e., if the clinical diagnosis is of a vascular dementia, then some evidence of this must appear on the MRI scan).

B. Treatment: There is no proven therapy. Aggressive management of cardiovascular risk factors seems prudent but should be individualized. Four aspirin daily is recommended if the patient is able to tolerate it.

VIII. Pick's Disease

A. Clinical features: Personality changes often precede intellectual decline. Language is affected more than memory. Visuospatial skills are preserved early. Extrapyramidal signs occur earlier than in AD. The typical course is 10–12 years.

B. Laboratory findings: Predominantly frontal and temporal atrophy on brain scan.

IX. Hydrocephalic Dementias

These account for fewer than 5% of dementias in adults.
A. Clinical characteristics
1. Patient is often quiet, withdrawn, slow, and depressed, in addition to having dementia.
2. Gait disorder and incontinence occur early.
B. Laboratory findings
1. Hydrocephalus on brain scan.
2. Cisternography and diagnostic lumbar punctures are not reliable predictors of the response to treatment.
C. Treatment: Cerebrospinal fluid shunting.

X. Thiamine Deficiency

Up to 50% of chronic alcoholics have impaired cognition, accounting for about 5% of dementia patients. It is not known whether alcohol causes a dementia distinct from Korsakoff's syndrome. Korsakoff's syndrome is a dietary deficiency and may be seen with any malabsorption syndrome.
A. Clinical characteristics
1. A classic Wernicke's encephalopathy with nystagmus, ophthalmoplegia, ataxia, and confusion.
2. If the patient is treated with thiamine early, the ocular signs resolve within hours and the ataxia within days.
3. Memory difficulties become apparent as the confusion clears; confabulation is common early.
4. A peripheral neuropathy may be present.

5. Twenty percent of patients have no documented clinical signs.
6. Many of these patients have had prior head injury, seizures, and small strokes.

B. Laboratory findings
1. Blood work may show associated hepatic and hematologic abnormalities.
2. Brain scans show atrophy; strokes may have occurred.

C. Treatment: In the acute phase, give thiamine IV for at least three days along with multivitamins in every IV bag. Also give B complex vitamins.

Bibliography

Folstein MF, Folstein SE, McHugh PR. "Mini Mental State." A practical method for grading the cognitive state of patients for the clinician. *J Psychiatric Research* 12:189–198, 1975.

Delirium in the Elderly Hospitalized Patient

Mark Overton, M.D.

I. Definition

The term *delirium* and *acute confusional state* are quite similar. The term *delirium* suggests a well-defined clinical syndrome, as in DSM-III-R:

A. Attentional deficit.

B. Thought disorder/disorganized thinking.

C. At least two of the following:
1. Reduced level of consciousness.
2. Perceptual disturbances/hallucinations/delusions.
3. Disturbance of the sleep-wake cycle.
4. Increased or decreased psychomotor activity.
5. Disorientation.
6. Memory impairment.

D. These features develop over a short time period.

E. Either evidence of a specific organic cause or assumed organic etiology if the disturbance is not related to a nonorganic mental disorder.

II. Common Clinical Presentations

A. Agitation
1. Often associated with combativeness and hyperarousal; fear and rage common.

2. Frequently associated with medication or alcohol withdrawal.
3. Drowsiness/sleeping more than usual.
4. Often missed; quietly delirious.
5. Associated with a poorer outcome.
6. Commonly seen with systemic illness affecting the central nervous system.

B. Drowsiness/sleeping more than usual.
1. Often missed; quietly delirious.
2. Associated with a poorer outcome.
3. Commonly seen with systemic illness affecting the central nervous system.

C. Clearly fluctuating states of arousal
1. Sleep/wake cycle problems.
2. Common in intensive care unit (ICU), as well as with drug withdrawal and medication toxicity.
3. Often seen postoperatively.
4. May be the first manifestation of delirium in dementia.

III. Epidemiology

A. Prevalence data
1. Geriatric unit: 35–80% of patients are either hospitalized with confusion or develop it while hospitalized

2. Acute medical and surgical wards: 20% of those over age 65 are delirious at any time.

B. Incidence data: questionable, poorly documented.

1. Postoperative: commonly within 1–7 days.

a. Incidence of 10–35% on general surgery ward.

b. Fifty percent or more after heart surgery.

c. Forty percent or more of hip fracture patients on an orthopedic service.

2. During acute medical hospitalization

a. ICU: up to 100% of patients become transiently delirious.

b. Ward settings: 5–15% have a new delirium not noted on admission.

C. Risk factors: SUNDOWNERS mnemonic

1. *Sick*: Multiple comorbid medical problems.

2. *Urinary* retention or fecal impaction.

3. *New* environment or sensory deprivation/isolation.

4. *Dementia*: or depression and cognitive impairment.

5. *Older* people more at risk.

6. *Writhing* in pain.

7. *Not* adequately evaluated.

8. *Eyes* and ears: Sensory impairment (especially visual impairment combined with hearing loss).

9. *Rx*: Medication effects, polypharmacy.

10. *Sleep* deprivation.

These risk factors are not clearly causative. See Section IV,B.

IV. Etiology

A. Detection

1. Clinical picture may resemble dementia, may not be considered as an acute illness. (refs)

2. Delay in diagnosis associated with poorer outcome.

3. See Table 140B-1.

4. Brief clinical instruments used to assess mental status

a. Mini-Mental State Exam.

b. Short Portable Mental Status Questionnaire.

c. Reaction times.

d. Mental control.

e. Trail Making Test.

5. Adequate history is crucial for diagnosis; seek historical information from any possible source.

B. Differential diagnosis

1. Primary intracranial diseases

a. Dementia, as above

b. Catatonia (relatively uncommon in the elderly)

c. Depression with pseudodelirium

d. Schizophrenia

e. Cerebrovascular events

f. Brain trauma

Table 140B-1.   Delirium versus Dementia

	Delirium	Dementia
Onset:	Rapid	Insidious
Duration:	Hours–weeks	Months–years
Course:	Fluctuating	Steady
Attention:	Impaired	Usually normal
Orientation:	Impaired	Often intact or mild impairment, may be some confabulation
Memory:	Recent and immediate impaired, long-term fund of knowledge intact	Recent and remote impaired, usually some loss in fund of knowledge
Thinking:	Slow or accelerated, "dream-like"	Poor abstraction, impoverished
Misperception:	Often visual, some auditory	Often absent
Sleep–wake:	Always disrupted cycle	Often fragmented
Acute illness:	Usually identifiable	Often absent
Drug toxicity:	Often present	Usually absent

After Lipowski, 1989.

g. Neurodegenerative diseases (Parkinson's disease, etc.)

2. Systemic illnesses affecting the brain secondarily
   a. Infectons
   b. Congestive heart failure/acute myocardial infarction
   c. Cancers and cancer treatments
   d. Diabetes mellitus (especially hypoglycemia)
   e. Thyroid disease (hyper- or hypothyroidism)
   f. Malnutrition
   g. Volume depletion/dehydration
   h. Hyponatremia

3. Medications (for a more complete list, see Dicks et al., 1989).
   a. Anticholinergics/antihistaminics
   b. Antipsychotics and antidepressants
   c. Sedative/hypnotics
   d. Antihypertensives
   e. Diuretics
   f. Digoxin/digitalis preparations
   g. Antiarrhythmics
   h. Nonsteroidal anti-inflammatory drugs
   i. Some H_2 blockers
   j. Steroids
   k. Anticonvulsants
   l. Medications for parkinsonism
   m. Stimulants/psychostimulants/decongestants

4. Toxic-metabolic encephalopathies
   a. Acute intoxication: Alcohol, sedative-hypnotics, narcotics, street drugs/cocaine.
   b. Withdrawal states: alcohol, barbiturates, benzodiazepines/sedating medications, narcotics/opiates.
   c. Environmental toxins: Lead, mercury, arsenicals, solvents/hydrocarbons.

V. Pathophysiology

A. The anticholinergic hypothesis, supported by clinical observations that:
   1. Impairment of cerebral metabolism from hypoxemia or hypoglycemia impairs the synthesis of acetylcholine.
   2. Anticholinergic intoxication produces a delirium that is reversible with cholinesterase inhibitors.

B. Other theories
   1. Cortisol/stress psychosis: Circadian pattern different postoperatively and in ICU; catecholamine excess may play a role.

2. Endogenous opiates
   a. β-endorphins elevated in postoperative delirium but not in delirium tremens.
   b. Sensitivity to these substances increased in elderly patients.

3. Mediators of the inflammatory response: Interleukins, tumor necrosis factor.

VI. Diagnostic Testing

A. History
   1. Time course of the cognitive impairment.
   2. Exacerbating or alleviating events or medications.
   3. Functional limitations caused by the impairment.
   4. Use of restraints.
   5. Medication profile.
   6. Drowsiness or poor participation in therapies.
   7. Family's or friend's interpretation of events.

B. Physical examination
   1. Postural blood pressure and pulse.
   2. Complete, careful neurologic examination.
   3. Skin examination to rule out infectious processes.
   4. Cooperation of the patient; the patient who is difficult to examine may have a delirium.
   5. Look for other potential infectious illnesses such as pneumonitis, cystitis, pyelonephritis, etc.
   6. Cardiac and vascular examinations to look for possible poor cardiac output states or arterial insufficiency.

C. Mental status testing
   1. Clinical interpretation of the above tests.
   2. Serial brief tests.
   3. Neuropsychiatric tests.
   4. Full mental status/psychiatric evaluation.

D. Electroencephalogram
   1. Not diagnostic!
   2. May be helpful if atypical seizure disorder is suspected.

E. Blood tests of relevance
   1. Levels of appropriate therapeutic medications.
   2. Metabolic screening: Glucose, calcium, magnesium.
   3. Fluid balance, renal function, electrolytes.

F. Brain imaging

1. Seldom diagnostic.
2. CT is of value if acute hematoma is suspected.
3. MRI may support clinically suspected vascular problems or reveal clinically silent ones.
4. Positron emission tomography (PET) and single photon emission computed tomography (SPECT) scanning if metabolic causes suspected, but these remain mostly research tools.

VII. **Treatment and Management**
  A. Find and treat the underlying problems; at least 2 weeks may be needed for recovery.
  B. "Generic" treatments
    1. Nonpharmacologic techniques.
       a. Night light, controlled environment.
       b. Fewer stimuli.
       c. Hearing aids in place and working.
       d. Glasses if needed.
       e. Physical activity important: *Get patients up and about!*
          (1) Bed rest often inappropriate.
          (2) Restraints may worsen behavior.
          (3) Sitters often helpful, especially at night or after procedures.
          (4) Objects from home, tapes of people in the family talking or reading.
       f. Foley catheters: Only if there is a good reason; toileting involves more work but is usually better.
       g. Signs, frequent reorientation.
    2. Pharmacologic therapies
       a. Review medications list daily.
          (1) Almost always better to delete than add medications.
          (2) Pay special attention to drug interactions.
          (3) Avoid anticholinergics if possible.
          (4) Pharmacology consultation necessary.
       b. Behavior-modifying medications: *Generally a two-edged sword*, since they adversely affect cognition.
          (1) Major tranquilizers (neuroleptics, phenothiazines)
              (a) Affect dopamine (dopa blockers).
              (b) Work well for hyperalert and hyperacute patients and for those with SUNDOWNERS risk factors.
              (c) In very low doses, may be useful to decrease agitation and restlessness (0.25–0.5 mg haloperidol or 5–10 mg mesoridazine PO or IM).
              (d) May require very frequent dosing intervals.
          (2) Benzodiazepines
              (a) Frequently are excitatory (15–30%).
              (b) Use least metabolized drugs (oxazepam, 10–15 mg PO, or lorazepam, 0.25–1 mg PO, IM, or IV up to every 4 hr).
              (c) Most useful in toxic/withdrawal states.
          (3) Anticonvulsants
              (a) Diphenylhydantoin: Seldom helpful; useful in complex partial seizures.
              (b) Carbamazepine: 100–200 mg up to twice a day; usefulness limited by sedation.
              (c) Clonazepam: Seldom helpful; may be a useful sedative if others are ineffective.
          (4) β-Blockers
              (a) Propranolol is the only agent studied.
              (b) Titration necessary; side effects commonly limit usefulness.
              (c) Effective only when β-blockade is complete.
          (5) Sedatives
              (a) Barbiturates: Very seldom useful; may worsen confusion and contribute to problems with sleep cycle.
              (b) Chloral hydrate: Short-acting, good sedative, little interaction; may not reverse sleep cycle problems.
          (6) Physostigmine
              (a) Still experimental; has been used in anticholinergic overdoses.
              (b) Used with success in other toxic states (benzodiazepines, delirium tremens).
              (c) β-Endorphin: no clear data available.

VIII. **Prognosis**
  A. Epidemiology
    1. In-hospital and postdischarge mortality

rates are higher in patients identified as delirious; mortality rates vary from 10% to 65%.
2. Survivors
   a. Likely to be discharged to nursing homes.
   b. Residual cognitive deficits common (up to 50%).
B. Clinical concerns include ongoing cognitive impairment: unmasked dementia, perioperative insults, ongoing illnesses/infections.

Bibliography

Dicks R, Besdine RW, Levkoff SE. Delirium. *Geriatric Med Annual* 1989, 117–136.

Francis J, Kapoor WN. Delirium in hospitalized elderly. *J Gen Intern Med* 5(1):65–79, 1990.

Lipowski ZJ. Delirium in the elderly patient. *N Engl J Med* 320(9):578–581, 1989.

CHAPTER 140-C

Incontinence

Steven Rothschild, M.D.

I. Definition

Urinary incontinence is the involuntary loss of urine in sufficient amount or frequency to constitute a social and/or health problem. It affects at least 10–20% of all community-dwelling persons over the age of 65.

A. Incontinence can result in shame, depression, social withdrawal, and even nursing home placement.

B. Medical complications
1. Pressure ulcers
2. Urinary tract infection, sepsis
3. Catheterization

C. Costs related to incontinence care in nursing homes in the United States total over $8 billion per year.

D. Key concepts
1. Incontinence of urine with aging is neither normal nor inevitable.
2. Incontinence of urine is not a diagnosis; it is a symptom.
3. Indwelling urinary catheters, condom catheters, and adult diapers have a role but are not treatments. Utilize them only after careful evaluation and trials of intervention.
4. In up to 70% of cases, systematic evaluation can lead to diagnosis and effective treatment.

II. Pathophysiology

The micturition cycle can be considered in three stages:

A. Phase of passive filling (0–200 ml)
1. Bladder detrusor contraction is inhibited due to:
   a. Direct β-adrenergic stimulation from the hypoglastic plexus (T11, T12, L1, L2).
   b. Inhibition of parasympathetic innervation from the sacral micturition center (S2, S3, S4).
2. The internal urethral sphincter is contracted by α-sympathetic stimulation and the pudendal nerve.

B. Phase of voluntary postponement (200–500 ml): As the bladder begins to fill, stretch receptors in the bladder detrusors stimulate reflex bladder contractions. This causes awareness of the need to void. Volitional activities include increased urethral sphincter tone and initiation of washroom-seeking behaviors. Continued inhibition of parasympathetics and maintenance of β-adrenergic tone follow.

C. Phase of bladder emptying
1. Increased parasympathetic tone via the sacral micturition center causes bladder detrusors to contract and the urethral sphincter to relax simultaneously.
2. Relaxation of the pelvic floor via the pudendal nerve.
3. Decreased α-sympathetic tone to the urethral sphincter.

III. Evaluation

A. A careful history and physical examination should seek to identify acute medical illnesses that could precipitate incontinence. Among the most common medical etiologies are:
1. Urinary tract infections.
2. Fecal impaction.
3. Medications (e.g., diuretics, anticholinergic drugs).
4. Acute confusional states or delirium.
5. Decreased mobility due to arthritis, stroke, or mechanical abnormalities (e.g., hyperglycemia, hypercalcemia).

B. In the absence of such acute illnesses, the physician must look for abnormalities in the micturition cycle to help explain the incontinence.

1. Key questions to ask in this evaluation include:
   a. What are the frequency and pattern of the incontinence?
   b. Is the voided volume large (>200 ml) or relatively small and frequent?
   c. Does the patient leak urine with coughing, sneezing, or laughing?
   d. Is the patient aware of the need to void? Does the patient feel the urge to void prior to the incontinence episode?
2. A voiding chart, with the patient, family, or nurse recording information about incontinence episodes, can be illuminating.
3. Physical examination must include:
   a. Pelvic examination.
   b. Rectal examination.
   c. Neurologic assessment, focusing especially on sacral reflexes and perineal sensation.
   d. Measurement of postvoid residual volume.
4. Laboratory studies
   a. Urinalysis, dipstick, and microscopic.
   b. Urine culture and sensitivity.
   c. Blood urea nitrogen, creatinine, glucose, calcium.
5. Invasive studies will be required for only a few selected patients:
   a. Cystometrics.
   b. Urine flowmetry.
   c. Cystoscopy.
   All patients, including long-term nursing home residents, deserve an evaluation of incontinence and a trial of intervention. See Algorithm.

IV. Differential Diagnosis and Treatment

A. Stress incontinence: Dysfunction of the bladder outlet resulting in inadequate sphincter pressure to maintain continence in the presence of increased intra-abdominal pressure.
   1. The most common form of incontinence.
   2. Patient reports leakage with cough, sneeze, laugh, etc. The volume of urine leaked is generally small. The problem can be demonstrated in the examination room by asking the patient with a full bladder to cough or bear down while in a standing position.
   3. Causes:
      a. Altered anatomy: Loss of posterior urethrovesicular angle due to laxity of the pelvic floor or cystocele.
      b. Neurologic conditions that diminish α-sympathetic tone to the urethral sphincter.
      c. Local urethral inflammation, most commonly from atrophic vaginitis/urethritis.

   d. Treatment
      Step 1
      (1) Treatment of atrophic vaginitis can be extremely effective in the correction of stress incontinence.
          (a) Topical estrogen cream, 0.5–1.0 g intravaginally daily.
          (b) Conjugated estrogens, 0.625 mg orally each day.
      (2) Restriction of fluids and a frequent voiding schedule.
      (3) Kegel exercises: Controversy exists regarding the efficacy of these exercises. The patient must be thoroughly educated in the technique. This can be done during routine pelvic examination; the patient is instructed to tighten the pelvic floor musculature on the examiner's fingers. Patients must be encouraged to perform Kegel exercises as frequently as possible (up to 100 or 200 times a day).
      (4) Biofeedback-aided bladder retraining.
      Step 2
      (1) Increase α-adrenergic tone: Sudafed, 15–30 mg three times a day. Phenylpropanolamine, 25–50 mg twice a day.
      (2) Imipramine, 10–25 mg three times a day.
      Step 3
      (1) Surgical options
          (a) Bladder suspension procedures (e.g., Marshall-Marchetti-Krantz) to restore the posterior vesicouretheral angle.
          (b) A vaginal sling can be created to lift the bladder neck in patients with a defective urethral wall.
      (2) Implantable prosthetic sphincter.
      (3) A pessary can be readily fitted for the patient who is not a surgical candidate and can be extremely effective.
      (4) Electrical stimulation of sphincter tone.

B. Urge incontinence: Failure to inhibit bladder contractions.
   1. Although most patients report feeling an urgent need to void, some patients will lack the sensation of urgency.
   2. Incontinence is of moderate to large volume (greater than 200 ml) and occurs every few hours.

3. Catheterization of the patient after urination (postvoid residual) will reveal small volumes of urine.
4. Causes:
   a. Failure of frontal lobe inhibition of the detrusor nucleus in the brain stem due to tumor, stroke, Parkinson's disease or other central nervous system (CNS) disease.
   b. Interruption of the spinal cord above S2, resulting in loss of ability of the CNS to inhibit the sacral micturition center.
   c. Hyperexcitable afferent pathways due to stimulation from:
      (1) Urinary tract infection.
      (2) Bladder tumor.
      (3) Stones.
   d. Deconditioned voiding reflexes, often as a result of hospitalization or institutionalization.
   e. Idiopathic detrusor instability
5. Treatment
   a. Correct any underlying pathology, such as urinary tract infections, inflammation or neoplasm, or spinal cord compression.
   b. As with stress incontinence, behavioral modification should be attempted first. These techniques are always safe and are frequently effective in the patient with urge incontinence. The patient should be encouraged to restrict fluids modestly, to schedule voiding at 1- to 2-hour intervals, and to void at the first sensation of a full bladder.
   c. Anticholinergics can be effectively utilized to diminish detrusor contractions.
      (1) Propantheline, 7.5–30.0 mg three times a day.
      (2) Imipramine, 25 mg at bedtime to 50 μg three times a day.
   d. Other medications
      (1) Direct smooth muscle relaxants
         (a) Oxybutinin, 5 mg three times a day.
         (b) Flavoxate, 100 mg three times a day.
      (2) Calcium channel blockers
         (a) Nifedipine, 10–20 mg three times a day.
C. Overflow incontinence: Failure of the bladder to empty normally, with resulting overdistention and urine leakage.
   1. The patient presents with frequent, nearly constant urine loss.
   2. Abdominal or suprapubic pain may or may not be present.

3. Causes
   a. Impairment of detrusor contractile capacity
      (1) Spinal cord lesion (sacral).
      (2) Prolonged bladder distention.
      (3) Peripheral neuropathy due to diabetes mellitus, alcoholism, or vitamin B_{12} deficiency.
   b. Outlet obstruction.
      (1) Fecal impaction is very common and is often overlooked.
      (2) Benign prostatic hypertrophy.
      (3) Bladder tumor.
      (4) Urethral stricture.
   c. Medications, especially any agents with anticholinergic properties.
      (1) Over-the-counter cold medications.
      (2) Antihistamines.
      (3) Tricyclic antidepressants.
      (4) Medications for Parkinson's disease.
      (5) Neuroleptic agents (thioridazine, chlorpromazine).
4. Treatment
   a. Treat the underlying illness; discontinue any medications which may aggravate the problem.
   b. Perform fecal disimpaction.
   c. Surgically correct any obstructing mass; perform resection of enlarged prostate.
   d. Intermittant self-catheterization (ISC) can be performed by many older persons without complications and has a high success rate.
   e. Cholinergic agonists augment detrusor function: Bethanechol, 10–30 mg three or four times a day
   f. α-Blockade can be used to relax the urethral sphincter: Phenoxybenzyline, 20–400 mg four times a day.
D. Functional and/or iatrogenic incontinence
   1. Structure/function of lower urinary tract is normal. Other factors interfere with the patient's ability to get to a bathroom prior to voiding.
      a. Mobility problems from stroke, arthritis, amputations, etc.
      b. Delirium or dementia.
      c. Use of restraints by health care workers.
      d. Obstacles in the patient's home or the long distance to the nearest bathroom.
   2. Treatment
      a. Move the patient closer to the bathroom or use a bedside commode.
      b. Recondition the voiding response in the patient. Do not place the patient who has just been incontinent of urine on the

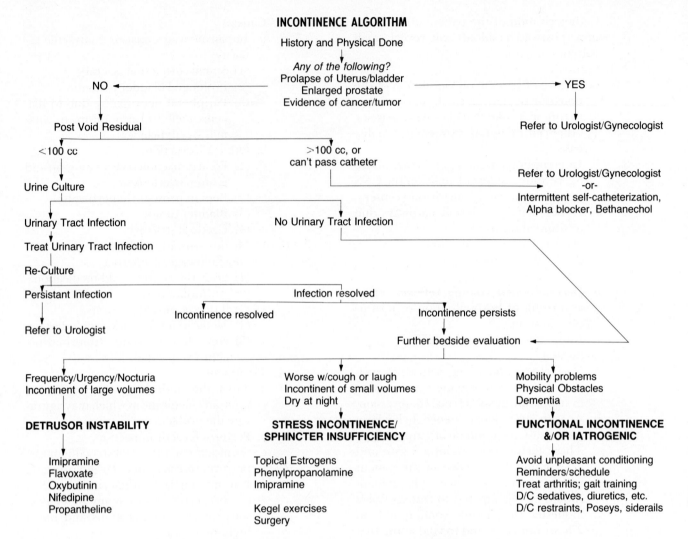

INCONTINENCE ALGORITHM

History and Physical Done

Any of the following?
Prolapse of Uterus/bladder
Enlarged prostate
Evidence of cancer/tumor

NO ← | → YES

Post Void Residual

Refer to Urologist/Gynecologist

<100 cc | >100 cc, or can't pass catheter

Urine Culture

Refer to Urologist/Gynecologist
-or-
Intermittent self-catheterization,
Alpha blocker, Bethanechol

Urinary Tract Infection | No Urinary Tract Infection

Treat Urinary Tract Infection

Re-Culture

Persistant Infection | Infection resolved

Incontinence resolved | Incontinence persists

Refer to Urologist

Further bedside evaluation

Frequency/Urgency/Nocturia
Incontinent of large volumes

Worse w/cough or laugh
Incontinent of small volumes
Dry at night

Mobility problems
Physical Obstacles
Dementia

DETRUSOR INSTABILITY

**STRESS INCONTINENCE/
SPHINCTER INSUFFICIENCY**

**FUNCTIONAL INCONTINENCE
&/OR IATROGENIC**

Imipramine
Flavoxate
Oxybutinin
Nifedipine
Propantheline

Topical Estrogens
Phenylpropanolamine
Imipramine

Kegel exercises
Surgery

Avoid unpleasant conditioning
Reminders/schedule
Treat arthritis; gait training
D/C sedatives, diuretics, etc.
D/C restraints, Poseys, siderails

toilet, as this creates unpleasant or even painful associations with voiding.

  c. Provide bladder training, as discussed earlier.

  d. Discontinue any sedatives or other medications which may cloud sensorium.

  e. Reduce the use of diuretics.

  f. Avoid the use of restraints, vests, and side rails whenever possible.

E. Mixed incontinence: In many older patients, the pattern of incontinence is not suggestive of any one category (e.g., cognitive impairment can coexist with peripheral neuropathy). These patients may be more difficult to assess and will benefit from studies such as cystometrics or urine flow studies.

V. Patients Refractory to Treatment

A. Chronic indwelling catheterization carries a high rate of morbidity and should be avoided if possible.

B. Highly absorbent pads and so-called adult diapers can help the incontinent patient maintain normal social activities.

C. Support groups exist for chronically incontinent persons and can provide useful information, as well as reducing the shame and isolation due to incontinence:

  1. HIP: Help for Incontinent People
P.O. Box 544
Union, SC 29379
(803) 579-7900 (Quarterly newsletter; publications or incontinence)

  2. The Simon Foundation
Box 835Z
Wilmette, IL 60091
(800) 237-4666 (free information packet and quarterly newsletter)

Bibliography

Ouslander JG, Leach GE., Staskrin DR. Simplified Tests of Lower Urinary Function in the evaluation of Geriatric Urinary Incontinence. *J Am Geriatr Soc* 37:706–714, 1989.

US Department of Health and Human Services. Clinical Practice Guideline: Urinary Incontinence in Adults. Agency for Health Care Policy and Research, Publication No. 92-0038, Rockville MD, March 1992.

CHAPTER 140-D

Special Sense Impairment

Jack Bulmash, M.D.

The Aging Eye

Major changes to the aging eye are due to age-related alterations in the eye's structural support, to changes in light transmission and accommodation, and to changes in the retina and nervous system.

I. **Changes in the support structures mainly alter the appearance of the eyes but can also result in vision changes and in increased susceptibility to injury and infection. These include:**
   A. Reduction in pupillary size, requiring more light to see.
   B. Lipid deposits in the sclera.
   C. Loss of extrabulbar and intraorbital fat.
   D. Loss of pigment in the iris.
   E. Lid laxity.
   F. Decreased production of tears and pooling of tears below the punctum.

II. **Changes in the transmission of light and in accommodation begin at ages 35 to 45.**
   A. Accommodation is the ability to focus on objects at different distances.
      1. The loss of accommodation is called *presbyopia*.
         a. Normal aging process.
         b. Manifested by the inability to see close objects sharply.
         c. Due to age-related change in the crystalline lens and its inability to change its refractory power with the proximity of objects.
         d. Can be corrected in people not originally nearsighted with weakly magnifying glasses.
      2. Persons unable to see distant objects initially improve their vision with normal aging.
   B. The crystalline lens yellows and darkens with age.
      1. Reduces intensity of the retinal image.
      2. Filters violet and blue light.
         a. Vision often improved with fluorescent light rich in blue light.
         b. Lens remits violet light in the form of green fluorescence, causing a haze in the retinal image.
         c. As the eye ages, the vitreous humor partially liquefies and droplets passing close to the retina are seen as "floaters."

III. **The gradual decline in retinal function and in other central nervous system functions affecting**

eyesight becomes important starting between 55 and 65 years of age.

A. Decrease in visual acuity and visual fields.
B. Reduction in intrinsic visual thresholds.
C. Poor adaptation to darkness.
D. Reduction in recovery from glare.
E. Increased sensitivity to flicker.

Cataracts

I. Definition

Cataracts are the loss of transparency of the crystalline lens. To some degree, cataracts are found in 50% of Americans between 65 and 74 and in 70% of those over the age of 75. They are an infrequent cause of blindness, and cataract removal is the most frequent surgical procedure performed in Americans over the age of 65.

II. Etiology

The lens, which accounts for 25% of the eye's refractive power, is made up of a nucleus and a cortex encased in a clear, elastic capsule. It is located between the posterior surface of the iris and the anterior surface of the vitreous humor, supported by zonular fibers attached to the ciliary body.

A. Cataract formation is poorly understood and is multifactorial.
1. The cortex is formed by bundles of lens fibers arranged in flat layers called *lamellae*. The oldest fibers are located most deeply within the lens.
2. Age reduces the water content of the lens and increases the amount of insoluble proteins and the calcium content. The nucleus becomes discolored and denser. Eventually, the transparent lens opacifies and forms a cataract.
3. Many other factors may contribute to cataract formation.
   a. Diabetes mellitus.
   b. Trauma.
   c. Glaucoma with therapy.
   d. Previous intraocular surgery.

B. Cataracts are classified according to location or by stage of development.
1. Nuclear sclerosis involves the nucleus, with clouding and discoloration. It is considered a cataract when it reduces visual acuity.
   a. Most common form of cataract.
   b. May be correctable with lenses.
2. Posterior subcapsular cataract usually begins in the visual axis of the posterior cortex just beneath the capsule. Less common is an anterior subcapsular variant.
   a. Often associated with chronic inflammation and chronic use of topical steroids.
   b. Usually clinically significant.
   c. Initially, may be treated with dilating drops.
3. Cortical cataract develops in the body of the lens.
   a. Often associated with acquired hyperopia.
   b. May progress rapidly.
4. Cataracts can be classified as:
   a. Immature when opacities are separated by areas of clear lens.
   b. Mature when the entire lens is opacified.
   c. Intumescent when the lens is swollen and blocks the flow of aqueous humor, resulting in acute angle closure glaucoma.
   d. Hypermature, with shrinkage of the anterior lens from liquefaction of lens cortex and leakage of fluid through the lens capsule.
   e. Morgagnian, with total liquefaction of the lens cortex.

III. Clinical Presentation and Diagnosis

Cataracts can cause a wide range of visual losses.

A. Symptoms are largely dependent on the size, location, and density of the opacity.
1. Visual acuity declines for distance but, paradoxically, near vision may improve.
2. Patients complain of seeing halos, glare, spots, and fog.
3. Monocular diplopia (double vision in one eye) may develop.

B. Full evaluation of cataracts requires a routine procedure to measure visual acuity and ocular power, as well as examination of the lens and of the anterior and posterior chambers.
1. Requires the services of an ophthalmologist.
2. Internist can usually detect the presence of a cataract with the use of a direct ophthalmoscope.

IV. Treatment

There is no medical regimen which will reverse or retard the progression of age-related cataracts.

A. Corrective lenses or a contact lens may occasionally improve visual acuity in early cataracts.
B. Surgery involves removal of the opacified lens

and its replacement. It is indicated when, after correction, the vision in the affected eye is 20/50 or worse and this is below the level acceptable for the patient.

1. With few exceptions, ophthalmologists prefer intraocular lens implants.
2. Surgery may be contraindicated in the presence of other eye diseases which preclude even limited improvement.
   a. Retinal detachment.
   b. Advanced glaucoma.
   c. Amblyopia.
   d. Optic atrophy.
3. Extracapsular extraction involves incision of the lens capsule and removal of the lens cortex and nucleus, leaving the posterior capsule and lens zonule in place.
4. Phacoemulsification is the fragmentation of the lens nucleus with ultrasonic energy and the subsequent aspiration of the lens material from the intact lens capsule.
5. Intracapsular extraction is the removal of the entire lens and capsule.
   a. The most common form of extraction in the 1950s to 1970s.
   b. Now reserved for cases of phacoanaphylaxis and subluxation of the lens.

Macular Degeneration

I. Definition
Macular degeneration is the loss of central vision due to damage of the macular photoreceptors (pigmented epithelium). It is the leading cause of permanent central vision loss in people over 65 years of age. Its prevalence increases with age and may affect 30% of people over 75 to some degree.

II. Etiology
The etiology is poorly understood.
A. Primary process of degeneration of retinal pigmented epithelium.
B. Disturbance in the metabolic interaction between the retinal pigmented epithelium and the photoreceptor cells.

III. Pathology
Pathologically, the condition has several hallmark features. These include the appearance of deposits of mucopolysaccharide and lipids called *drusen* between the plasma membrane of pigmented epithelium and its basement membrane, as well as between the basement membrane of the pigmented epithelium and the rest of Bruch's membranes (the next five layers of the retina).

A. Hard or nodular drusen appear as pinhead-sized, yellowish-white lesions.
   1. Membranous debris from retinal pigmented epithelium.
   2. Rarely accompanied by neovascularization.
B. Soft or granular drusen appear indistinct, are larger than hard drusen, and tend to become confluent.
   1. Collections of amorphous material, if confluent, are often associated with progressive degeneration of the pigmented epithelium.
   2. Predisposes to separation of the pigmented epithelium and its basement membrane from the rest of Bruch's membrane.
      a. Predisposes the eye to subretinal neovascularization.
      b. Serous or hemorrhagic detachment of the pigmented epithelium.
      c. Formation of fibrovascular scars.
      d. Atrophy of choroid.

IV. Clinical Presentation
Macular degeneration generally consists of two major clinical types.
A. Nonexudative or "dry" form, which accounts for 90% of all cases and causes a gradual loss of central vision.
   1. Usually involves both eyes.
   2. Drusen appear in the macula and can be hard, soft, confluent, or calcified.
B. Exudative or "wet" form, present in 80–90% of patients who lose central vision from macular degeneration.
   1. Serous or hemorrhagic separation of pigmented epithelium.
   2. Association with soft drusen carries a poor prognosis.
   3. Frequent formation of neovascular membrane under pigmented epithelium.
   4. Formation of disciform scars.

V. Diagnosis
Macular degeneration results in loss of central vision acuity.
A. Characteristically, this can be metamorphopsia (bending of straight lines), micropsia (reduced size of objects), or scotomata (localized central field defects).
B. Amsler grid test is used to detect these defects and to monitor patients.
C. Direct ophthalmoscopic exam
   1. Drusen in macula.
   2. Irregularity in color and transparency and increase in pigment or retina.

3. Subretinal hemorrhage.

4. Disciform scars.

D. Ophthalmologist will utilize other techniques, including slit lamp biomicroscopic examination and fluorescein angiography.

VI. Treatment

A. Early detection is necessary; all patients complaining of blurred or distorted near vision should be referred promptly to an ophthalmologist.

B. Patients will be instructed in the use of amsler grids.

C. No effective therapy or prevention is available for the dry form of macular degeneration.

1. Only 10% of patients progress to legal blindness.

2. Peripheral vision is preserved.

D. Wet macular degeneration has a poorer prognosis.

1. Daily self-testing with an amsler grid and immediate referral to an ophthalmologist for any visual disturbance.

2. Laser photocoagulation of choroidal neovascular membranes.

a. Must be more than 200 μm from the center of the foveal avascular zone.

b. Recurrences affect 25% of patients within 2 years after successful therapy.

3. Referral to low-vision specialist for visual aids.

Glaucoma

I. Definition

Glaucoma is progressive optic neuropathy resulting from increased intraocular pressure. It affects approximately 3% of the population over 60 and accounts for 12–15% of blindness in the United States; the prevalence rises with age.

A. Increased intraocular pressure above, on the average (90% of the population), 21 mmHg.

B. Optic disc cupping and pallor.

C. Loss of visual fields.

II. Etiology

Obstruction of the outflow of aqueous humor is the primary reason for the increased intraocular pressure.

A. Aqueous humor is produced by the ciliary body.

B. It moves from the posterior chamber via the iris to the anterior chamber.

C. It leaves the eye through the trabecular meshwork to the canal of Schlemm.

D. Sustained increase in intraocular pressure results in retinal nerve atrophy and chronic ischemia of the retina and optic nerve.

III. Forms

Primary adult glaucoma is of two varieties.

A. Open-angle glaucoma

1. Most common form, affecting 70% of patients with glaucoma; dominant hereditary pattern.

2. Cause is poorly understood, but aqueous flow is obstructed at the microscopic level in the trabecular network.

3. Can be asymptomatic until a great deal of vision is lost; central vision spared.

4. Diagnosis requires:

a. Elevated intraocular pressure.

b. Optic disc cupping.

c. Visual field losses.

5. Treatment

a. Drugs placed in the ocular cul de sac are systemically absorbed.

(1) Long-acting β-blockers Timolol maleate, which reduce aqueous formation, can cause bradycardia, bronchospasm, and confusion.

(2) Cholinomimetics (pilocarpine) causes miosis, with resultant reduction of aqueous inflow. Seriously reduces vision in patients with cataracts and at night.

(3) Sympathomimetics (epinephrine).

(4) Carbonic anhydrase inhibitors (acetazolamide) reduces aqueous production. Common side effects include fatigue, electrolyte imbalances, weight loss, and calcium phosphate nephrolithiasis.

b. Surgery: Usually used as second-line therapy but as first-line therapy in selected patients.

(1) Argon laser: Burns placed on or near trabecular network improve aqueous drainage.

(2) Filtration surgery creates a fistula between the anterior chamber and the subconjunctival space.

(3) Neodymium: Yttrium-aluminum-garnet (Nd:Yag) laser destruction of the ciliary body; rarely done.

B. Acute angle closure

1. Aqueous flow blocked by the iris, by scars secondary to inflammatory disease, or by trauma at the trabecular meshwork.

2. Often presents as an acute, red, painful

eye; pupil mildly dilated and fixed, with blurred vision; vomiting; and halos seen around lights.

3. Gonioscopy required to examine the angle of the anterior chamber.

4. An acute ophthalmologic emergency which requires immediate referral.

   a. Drugs are the initial therapy of choice.

   b. Surgery is used after the initial attack subsides. Nd:Yag laser, alone or in combination with the argon laser for iridectomies.

IV. Other Conditions

Other significant conditions which are more common in the elderly include vascular occlusion of the retina, retinal detachment, senile entropion and ectropion, senile ptosis, and dry eyes.

Olfaction and Taste

The senses of smell and taste are important because they determine the flavor of foods, which is a crucial factor in the maintenance of nutrition. In addition, olfaction provides warning of environmental dangers such as fires and gas leaks.

I. Assessment

Assessment of olfaction and taste requires a history, a physical examination with emphasis on the oral pharynx, and specific tests.

A. Early studies are based on simple detection or recognition thresholds.

B. Dynamic or suprathreshold studies are more revelant clinically and involve the ability to make distinctions among odorants and tastes with different qualities.

   1. Losses in suprathreshold ability can exist with or without changes in threshold levels.

   2. Deficiencies in suprathresholds among the elderly often result in the complaint that "everything tastes and smells the same."

C. Identification testing in the office can be used as a gross measurement of the patient's olfaction.

   1. Peanut butter, coffee, and chocolate are placed in small jars and covered with gauze.

      a. Patients are presented with an empty jar and one with an odorant and asked to choose the one with a smell.

      b. If the patient chooses the jar containing an odorant, then he or she is asked to identify the smell from a list of possibilities.

c. Each nostril should be checked separately.

2. Usually odor testing is combined with taste testing (see Section I,E).

D. Formal testing requires the skills of trained technical staff and includes:

   1. University of Pennsylvania smell inventory test.

   2. Gastrometer test.

   3. Henken's accusens T taste test.

   4. Unilateral carbinol test.

   5. University of Connecticut Home Olfactory test.

   6. Smell suprathreshold test.

   7. Full otolaryngology assessment.

E. Taste testing is more difficult and less standardized.

   1. Chemicals for the traditional primary tastes (sweet, sour, salt) plus amino acids are placed on 1- to 3-cm wafers or filter paper.

      a. Papers are placed on the tongue.

      b. Separate areas and sides of the tongue are tested to localize disorders.

      c. Different concentrations of chemical are used for thresholds.

   2. Commercial taste kits are available using the three-drop technique for testing.

II. Patterns of Impairment

Although studies have produced conflicting data, they do point to a marked decline in olfaction after the age of 65 years. Studies of taste are less clear-cut.

A. Ability to detect odors peaks between 40 and 60 years.

B. At equivalent ages, women are more accurate than men in identifying odors.

C. More than 80% of people over the age of 80 have major impairment in olfaction, with 50% being anosmic.

D. Sixty percent of people between 65 and 80 have major impairment in olfaction, with 25% being anosmic.

E. Thresholds for common flavors such as cherry, grape, and lemon are 11 times higher, on average, in the elderly.

F. Cooking gas cannot be detected at levels considered explosive by as many as 15% of people 70 years old or older.

G. Threshold taste tests comparing young and old people for salt, sugar, quinine, and hydrochloric acid have been equivocal.

H. Suprathreshold tests using salt, sucrose, citric acid, and quinine have failed to demonstrate differences with aging, though there seems to be a mild dysgeusia (background taste) in the elderly.

III. Etiology of Impairment

The anatomic and physiologic bases for age-related decline in olfaction and possibly taste are multiple and poorly understood. The number of taste buds declines significantly with age, with perhaps a reduction of 80% in functional units by age 85 years.

IV. Treatment

Treatment strategies for dysfunctional olfaction and taste are often unsatisfactory.

A. Many acute disorders (e.g., viral infections of the upper respiratory tract) are self-limited.

B. Oral zinc supplementation, though widely used, has failed to improve olfaction on double-blinded studies.

C. The flavor of food can be improved by the addition of commercially available, chemically simulated odors.

D. Mild background dysgeusia can be treated with chewing gum, ice, or rinses of sodium bicarbonate or potent long-acting sweeting agents.

E. Eating techniques such as thorough mastication and frequent food switching can be helpful.

F. Monosodium glutamate can enhance the taste of food but is high in sodium and has well-known side effects.

Hearing

Hearing impairment is the third most common condition affecting the elderly. Sixty percent of persons over 65 years of age and 90% of persons over 79 have some degree of hearing impairment. Among the elderly, 10–15% have severe or profound hearing loss, with a greater proportion of the seriously affected elderly population found in nursing homes.

I. Definition of the Human Auditory System

The human auditory system consists of the ear and associated neural pathways.

A. Afferent neural subsystem: Primary function is to transform acoustic stimulation into neural patterns and transmit them to the auditory cortex in the temporal lobe.

B. Efferent neural subsystem: Provides feedback control, either excitatory or inhibitory, or acoustic input (e.g., dampening the ossicles during sudden loud input).

C. With age, deterioration can occur in both systems at any level, as well as in the peripheral components of the ear dealing with sound transmission.

II. Age-Related Changes in the Structure of the Ear and in Hearing

A. Sound is described by frequency (Hertz [Hz]) and intensity (decibels [db]).

1. Audible frequencies for young adults range from 30 to 20,000 Hz. Aging produces progressive loss at the higher frequencies, so that over the age of 60 most people lose serviceable use of frequencies above 4,000 Hz. Speech usually occurs at 500–2,000 Hz at 50 db.

2. There are differences between the frequency and duration of vowels and consonants.

    a. Consonants are shorter sounds and occur at higher frequencies than vowels.

    b. Consonants, an essential part of words, are more difficult at all intensities for the elderly to hear.

3. Pitch discrimination declines as early as the fourth decade, and the rate of decline accelerates after the age of 55.

B. External auditory canal

1. Reduction in the number and activity of cerumen glands, atrophy of auditory canal epithelium and sebaceous glands, and increase in the length and tortuosity of the ear canal.

2. Increase in pruritus and in episodes of ceruminal impaction; the latter condition is a major contributor to reversible hearing loss.

C. Middle ear: Moderate to severe arthritic changes in the ossicles, which are usually symmetrical and which do not usually cause significant loss of conductive hearing.

D. Inner ear

1. Loss of vestibular nerve fibers and sensory cells in the cochlea, resulting in increased unsteadiness, disequilibrium, and vertigo.

2. Reduction in spiral ganglion cells in the cochlea and loss of functional neural units along the auditory pathway.

3. Atrophy and loss of hair cells in the organ of Corti; vascular sclerosis with calcification and atrophic changes in the stria vascularis.

Bibliography

Bartoshuk LM, Rifkin B, Marks LE, Bars P. Taste and Aging. *J Gerontol* 41:51–57, 1986.

Bienfang DC, Nicholson DH, Nussenblatt RB. Opthalmology. *N Engl J Med* 323(14):956–967, 1990.

Katsarkas A, Ayukawa H. Hearing loss due to aging (presbycusis). *The Journal of Otolaryngology* 15(4):239–244, 1986.

CHAPTER 140-E

Geriatric Nutrition

Susan Arendt, M.D., R.D.
Debra Syeluga, Ph.D., R.D.

I. Goals

   A. Determine whether or not the individual is at nutritional risk.

   B. Provide appropriate nutrition to maintain or improve status.

   C. Educate individual about diet.

   D. Monitor tolerance of prescribed diet.

II. Assessment (Nutritional Risk Factors)

   A. Anthropometry is not reliable in the elderly; check:

   1. Current weight.

   2. Usual weight; this may not be known.

   3. Clinically significant weight loss: 5% in 1 month, 7.5% in 3 months, 10% in 6 months.

   4. Ideal body weight (IBW) in this population is controversial. Traditional methods of arriving at IBW include:

      a. Formula

         (1) Females: 100 lb for first 5 ft in height and 5 lb for each additional inch.

         (2) Males: 106 lb for first 5 ft in height and 6 lb for each additional inch.

      b. Reference tables (e.g., from Metropolitian Life Insurance Company).

   B. Biochemical

   1. Albumin: $T_{1/2}$ = 14–21 days

      a. The best predictor of mortality.

      b. Provides early identification of those at nutritional risk (albumin <3.0/g/dl).

      c. Indicates visceral protein stores.

      d. Affected by hydration status.

   2. Hemoglobin/hematocrit: May be an indicator of malnutrition.

   3. Blood urea nitrogen/creatinine: Helps indicate hydration status and renal function.

   4. Cholesterol: Low serum cholesterol (<160 mg/dl) may be an indicator of morbidity.

   C. Other factors affecting intake

   1. Some medications and medical conditions alter the ability to taste, smell, swallow, or digest food.

   2. Psychological conditions may change appetite.

   3. Physical factors such as poor dentition, ill-fitting dentures, and decreased mobility may impair the ability to eat. Poor eyesight makes it difficult to shop for, prepare, see, and enjoy food.

   4. Social and economic factors of importance

a. Limited financial resources interferes with compliance/ability to purchase special foods.

b. Social isolation contributes to depression, decreased desire to shop, and reduced appetite.

5. Self-imposed restrictions are often unnecessary and may lead to inadequate intake. Strict diabetic, low-cholesterol, or other diets may result in insufficient intake.

D. Clinical

1. History should include documentation of:
   a. Weight loss.
   b. Nausea, vomiting, bowel habits, laxative use, and food intolerances.
   c. Chronic conditions which impact nutrition and are impacted by nutrition, such as heart failure, hypertension, arthritis, and osteoporosis.
   d. Medication use: Polypharmacy, whether prescribed or self-administered, and use of nutritional supplements (see Section VI).

2. Physical exam should focus on signs of nutrient deficiency, dehydration, malnutrition, and/or dysphagia.

III. **Nutritional Requirements**

A. Calories: 30 cal/kg needed for weight maintenance in a stressed patient.

B. Protein: 1 g protein per kilogram of body weight in a healthy elderly individual will achieve positive nitrogen balance. Protein needs must be individualized.

C. Fluid: 30–35 ml per kilogram of body weight should be adequate unless there are abnormal losses (e.g., fistula drainage) which must also be replaced.

D. Vitamins and minerals

1. Calcium: 1,500 mg/day in a postmenopausal woman.

2. Magnesium/phosphorus: Of particular concern when refeeding.

3. Iron: Decreased need compared to younger population.

4. Vitamin K must be considered if nutritional supplements are added, discontinued, or consumed sporadically by patients.

5. Vitamin B_{12}: Deficiency can be misdiagnosed as dementia. Intake in healthy elderly persons is often only marginally adequate.

IV. **Nutritional Therapy**

A. Oral intake: May be taken independently, taken with assistance such as cueing, or taken with spoon feeding.

1. Modified diets
   a. Diabetic diets
      (1) "No concentrated sweets" diet: Three balanced meals a day with limited simple sugars. Appropriate for most elderly diabetics.
      (2) American Diabetes Association (ADA) diet: Caloric level associated with diet. More strict than the "no concentrated sweets" diet. Appropriate for brittle diabetics on insulin. Base calorie intake on 30 calories per kilogram of body weight if the individual is not obese.
   b. Low-cholesterol diets: Of questionable benefit in this population. Not recommended for patients with fair to poor intake due to the limited calories this diet provides.
   c. Low-sodium diets: May not be appealing, particularly due to the taste changes associated with aging, and may decrease food intake.
   d. Others (including consistency modifications)
      (1) Pureed foods: May be used for patients with dysphagia but are not indicated solely on the basis of poor dentition.
      (2) Mechanical soft foods: May be useful for patients with dysphagia or poor dentition.

2. Supplements: Augment a patient's diet. Use special commercial products (Sustacal, Ensure, Osmolite, Citrotein) or high-calorie/high-protein snacks such as milk shakes.

B. Tube feeding

1. Indicated when there is a physical impairment preventing normal deglutition; in some hypermetabolic states or cases of maldigestion/malabsorption; in some postoperative cases; and in cases where inadequate calories are being ingested orally.

2. Commercially available formulas
   a. General purpose: Osmolite, Ensure, Enrich. Enrich contains fiber for constipation/diarrhea.
   b. Concentrated: Two Cal HN, Ensure Plus. Used when volume restriction is needed.
   c. High protein: Sustacal, Citrotein
   d. Elemental: Vital HN, Vivonex TEN, Portagen. Use if maldigestion/malabsorption is a problem.

e. Disease specific: Aminaid (renal failure), Hepatic aid (hepatic failure).
3. Additives (modules)
a. Protein (Promod): 0.75 g protein per gram of Promod. Used for patients with increased protein needs.
b. Fat (MCT oil/Microlipid): MCT oil: 7.7 kcal/ml; Microlipid: 4.5 kcal/ml. Used as a calorie source. medium chain triglycerides (MCT) do not contain essential fatty acids.
c. Carbohydrate (Polycose): 3.8 kcal/g or 2.0 kcal/ml. Used as a calorie source. Diabetics may need calorie supplementation with fat or a fat-carbohydrate combination if hyperglycemia is a problem
4. Complications of tube feeding
a. Mechanical: Tube occlusion/dislodgement.
b. Metabolic: fluid/electrolyte abnormalities, hyperglycemia.
c. Gastrointestinal: Diarrhea, constipation, malabsorption.
d. Aspiration/pneumonia.
5. Monitor tube feedings by checking:
a. Laboratory tests: albumin, electrolytes, magnesium, phosphorus, calcium.
b. Weight (daily)
c. Bowel function (daily).
d. Intake/output (daily).
e. Others: Residuals, blood sugar.
C. Parenteral nutrition can be supplied via:
1. Peripheral venous nutrition
a. When caloric depletion is not a problem.
b. If central venous nutrition is not possible.
c. To supplement either oral intake or tube feeding until goal is reached.
d. May be complicated by thrombosis.
e. Requires large volumes to meet complete nutritional requirements.
2. Central venous nutrition
a. To be used only when the gut is nonfunctional.
b. Used for cases of severe nutritional depletion, such as in sepsis, stress, or trauma.
c. May be complicated by:
(1) Catheter-related problems: Pneumothorax after insertion, air embolus, subclavian vein thrombosis, hemothorax, chylothorax, catheter malposition.
(2) Metabolic problems: Hypo- or hy-

perphosphatemia, hyperglycemia, volume overload or dehydration, mineral and electrolyte abnormalities.
(3) Infection: Particularly at entry and exit sites.
V. **Disease–Nutrition Interactions**
A. Cancer: Increases calorie/protein needs.
B. Pressure ulcers: Increase protein needs.
C. Sepsis: Increases calorie needs.
D. Postoperatively: Increases calorie/protein needs.
E. Dementias/depression: May require cueing the individual and/or spoon feeding. Tube feeding may become indicated.
F. Cerebrovascular accidents (CVA): Oral feedings may not be possible due to dysphagia or other problems. Consult speech therapist, occupational therapist, and dietitian for full evaluation.
G. Malabsorption/maldigestion.
VI. **Drug–Nutrient Interactions**
A. Over-the-counter medications
1. Antacids: Phosphorus depletion can be caused by antacids containing aluminum or magnesium hydroxide. Some antacids contain sodium bicarbonate.
2. Laxatives (see Section B,3).
3. Analgesics: Long-term use can cause erosion of the gastrointestinal mucosa, leading to blood loss and iron deficiency anemia. Folacin deficiency is more common among aspirin users.
4. Nutrient supplements: Usage is common among the elderly. If a well-balanced diet is consumed and no other confounding factors are present, a multivitamin is not needed. Megadoses are not recommended.
B. Prescribed medications
1. Cardiovascular agents
a. Antiarrhythmics.
b. Antihypertensives/diuretics: Potassium, magnesium, zinc, and sometimes calcium may be lost with diuretic use.
c. Cardiac glycosides: May cause decreased appetite.
d. Potassium supplements.
2. Anti-inflammatory agents
a. Corticosteroids: May increase blood sugar, sodium, and cholesterol while decreasing potassium and calcium. A low-sodium, high-potassium diet may be indicated.
b. Nonsteroidal anti-inflammatory drugs:

Increase potassium and decrease the absorption of amino acids.

3. Laxatives: Use increases with age. Side effects include decreased appetite, fluid/electrolyte imbalance, decreased fat-soluble vitamin absorption.

4. Diabetic agents

   a. Insulin: Follow appropriate diet as prescribed (ADA or "no concentrated sweets" diet).

   b. Oral hypoglycemic: Take before meals. Dietary compliance important. "No concentrated sweets" diet usually appropriate.

5. Nutrient supplements

   a. Calcium: Absorption dependent on source.

   b. Iron: Use may be indicated for iron deficiency anemia.

6. Antibiotics: Multiple effects. Most notable effects on the gastrointestinal tract and renal system. (May cause antibiotic-associated pseudomembranous colitis and increased blood urea nitrogen/creatine.)

7. Others

   a. Warfarin sodium: Foods high in vitamin K will decrease effectiveness.

   b. Phenytoin sodium: Tube feedings decrease bioavailability of the drug. To increase absorption, tube feeding may be done prior to and shortly after administration of the drug. In patients not receiving tube feeding, dilantin decreases folate absorption, and folic acid deficiency may be present

Bibliography

Fiatarone M. Nutrition in the geriatric patient. *Hosp Pract* 9A:38–54, 1990.

Morley J, Glick Z, Rubenstein L. *Geriatric Nutrition: A Comprehensive Review*, New York, Raven Press, 1990.

Roe DA. Geriatric nutrition. *Clin Ger Nutr* 6:319–334, 1990.

Rombeau J, Caldwell M. *Clinical Nutrition: Enteral and Tube Feeding*, ed 2. Philadelphia, Saunders, 1990.

CHAPTER 140-F

Falls

Jan Clarke, M.D., M.P.H.

I. **Definition and Epidemiology**
   A. A fall is an unintentional change in position, excluding overwhelming intrinsic or extrinsic events (e.g., stroke or motor vehicle accident). Thirty percent of community dwellers over 65 years of age and 40% of those over 80 fall yearly; the majority of these falls occur in the home. After the age of 75, the increased frequency of falls in women compared to men is no longer seen.
   B. Falls account for the majority of injury-related deaths—the sixth leading cause of death for the elderly. Vulnerability to injury is influenced by the presence of age-related changes (e.g., osteoporosis). Nonfatal injuries include fracture (5%; 1% are hip fractures) and serious soft tissue injury requiring medical care or prolonged immobilization. Recurrent falls is cited as contributing to 40% of nursing home admissions.

II. **Etiology**
   A single cause for a fall may be apparent, but frequently multiple elements that contribute to falling are identified.
   A. Intrinsic factors

1. Neurologic dysfunction (visual, auditory, vestibular, disturbed proprioception, muscle weakness. Increased muscle tone, cognitive dysfunction).
2. Musculoskeletal abnormalities (arthritis of peripheral or axial joints, foot disorders, joint contractures).
3. Acute or chronic systemic illness (including urinary tract infection, pneumonia, congestive heart failure, renal failure).
4. Medications (notably sedative/hypnotics, antidepressants, antihypertensives, antiarrhythmics, anticonvulsants, diuretics) and alcohol.
   B. The nature of the activity at the time of the fall may be mildly, moderately, or markedly displacing (e.g., standing still, maneuvering stairs, or climbing a ladder, respectively). Markedly displacing activities account for only a minority of falls in the elderly.
   C. Environmental factors that contribute to the risk of falling are common and include poor lighting, throw rugs, and slippery surfaces; loose or ill-fitting garments; and bed height. The degree to which environmental factors

pose a threat to safety is governed by individual frailty/disability and familiarity with the environment.

III. Evaluation and Prevention

Falls are often indicative of underlying conditions responsive to intervention. Careful evaluation includes assessment for the presence of risk factors, performance-oriented tests of gait and balance, and review of prior falls. Falls are underreported, so it is essential to make a specific inquiry.

A. The patient's history may be very useful and is best obtained soon after the event. Unfortunately, the patient's description may be vague or the symptoms may be nonspecific.

   1. Determine the time of the fall and premonitory symptoms.
   2. Review the activity associated with the fall, particularly association with change in position, difficulty walking, activities of daily living, or a new or strenuous activity.
   3. Review circumstances of previous falls.
   4. Determine the presence of any underlying chronic illness and degree of compensation.
   5. Identify symptoms of any new acute illness.
   6. Determine the names and doses of all prescribed and over-the-counter medications. Eliminate all nonessential medications and use the lowest effective doses of essential drugs.
   7. Determine the location of the fall and inquire about environmental hazards.

B. Physical findings

   1. Evidence of injury sustained during the fall (i.e., fracture, skin tear, hematoma).
   2. Signs of underlying conditions contributing to the event (e.g., reduced visual acuity, decreased hearing, orthostatic hypotension, cognitive dysfunction, muscle weakness, joint contractures).
   3. Balance abnormalities. Observe for trouble with or unsteadiness during:
      a. Rising from a chair or sitting down.
      b. Cervical rotation and extension.
      c. Sternal nudge.
   4. Gait disturbance: The gait of older persons is frequently slower, with shorter steps and a slightly broader base compared to younger adults, but gait disturbance may be detected by the presence of:
      a. Decreased lifting of the foot to step up.
      b. Unsteadiness on uneven surfaces.
      c. Unsteadiness with turning.
      d. Difficulty walking a straight line.

C. Diagnostic tests will be determined by the findings of the history and physical examination. *Routine* Holter monitoring is probably not indicated.

IV. Treatment

A. Treatment is dictated by the results of the assessment; it may involve medical treatment, rehabilitative interventions, and/or removal of environmental hazards. Treatment goals include prevention of future episodes and maintenance of patient autonomy.

B. Patient monitoring should include regular inquiry about recurrent falls and continued compliance with appropriate medical, rehabilitative, and environmental interventions, as well as evaluation for the emergence of new conditions that may increase the risk of falls.

V. Prognosis

Falls causing hip fracture and associated with "long lie" before discovery are associated with increased mortality. Fifty percent of patients surviving a fall resulting in hip fracture have a significant reduction in function. Even falls that do not cause direct injury may lead to fear of falling. Subsequent restriction of activity (by the patient or caregiver) is associated with immobility, functional decline, and the attendant complications. Recurrent falls frequently prompt institutionalization.

Bibliography

Kellogg International Work Group on the Prevention of Falls by the Elderly. The prevention of falls in later life. *Dan Med Bull* 34(Suppl 4):1–24, 1987.

Rubenstein LZ, Robbins AS, Josephson KR, et al. The value of assessing falls in an elderly population: A randomized clinical trial. *Ann Intern Med* 113:308–316, 1990.

Immobility

Jan Clarke, M.D., M.P.H.

I. Definition

a140g Immobility is a functional state in which an individual is confined to a wheelchair or bed and unable to take purposeful steps or to support significant body weight. Loss of mobility threatens independence and is a major reason for nursing home placement. Rapid functional decline with immobility may lead to a poor prognosis. Factors contributing to mobility are mental status; emotional state; sensory inputs; muscle strength, tone, and coordination; and axial and peripheral joint status.

II. Etiology

A. The most common causes of immobility are arthritis, cerebrovascular accident, hip fracture or other trauma, contractures, lower extremity amputation, and the pain of malignancy.

B. Unwillingness to ambulate is often seen and may be due to fear of falling, depression, dementia, a change in medical status (e.g., urinary tract infection), or a combination of factors.

C. Medications can impair balance and gait and contribute to immobility.

III. Complications

Particularly severe in the elderly, due to diminished physiologic reserve include the following complications:

A. Cardiovascular

1. Decreased cardiac output (contributes to decreased endurance).
2. Orthostatic hypotension
3. Increased risk of venous thrombosis.

B. Respiratory

1. Atelectasis.
2. Relative hypoxemia.
3. Impaired cough and pneumonia.

C. Musculoskeletal

1. Muscle atrophy, weakness, loss of oxidative capacity.
2. Osteoporosis (due to decreased bone formation and increased resorption).
3. Joint contractures (may begin within a week of immobility).

D. Gastrointestinal

1. Constipation.
2. Anorexia.

E. Genitourinary

1. Incontinence.
2. Hypercalciuria and renal calculi.

F. Skin: Pressure sores.

G. Neuropsychologic
   1. Changes in affect: Depression, anxiety, fear.
   2. Cognitive change: Poor concentration, disorientation.
   3. Reduced level of alertness: Apathy, stupor.

IV. **Evaluation and Treatment**
   A. Careful assessment for a new or newly active medical problem. Institute specific treatment.
   B. Review of all prescribed and nonprescribed medications; elimination all nonessential medications and reduction of essential medications to the lowest effective dose.
   C. Sensory stimulation and reorientation to the environment.
   D. Appropriate positioning and range-of-motion exercises—essential to prevent contractures and pressure sores.
   E. A graded program of active muscle exercise can be recommended by a physiatrist or physical therapist and can be initiated while still bed or chair bound.
   F. Breathing or coughing exercises.
   G. Adequate nutrition and fluid balance.

V. **Prognosis**
   Prognosis is dependent on prevention of the complications of immobility; the greater the functional reserve of the individual at the onset of the period of immobilization, the better the prognosis.

Bibliography

Harper CM, Lyles YM. Physiology and complications of bed rest. *JAGS* 36:1047–1054, 1988.

Chapter 140-H

Pressure Ulcers

Mark Overton, M.D.

I. **Definitions**
   A. Ulcer or sore: A break in the skin.
   B. Decubitus: Literally, "lying down," inadequate as a description or as a diagnosis.
   C. Pressure: What gravity does to something— force, or mechanical loading applied to a surface.
   D. Bed sore: Term no longer used.

II. **Etiology**
   A. Direct or primary (skin) factors
      1. Pressure
      2. Shearing forces
      3. Friction
      4. Moisture
   B. Systemic risk factors
      1. Fixed or unmodifiable
         a. Age; old skin
         b. Immobility, related to paralysis or fracture
         c. Severe illness
      2. Modifiable
         a. Nutrition
         b. Fecal incontinence
         c. Dementia/parkinsonism/delirium
         d. Immobility not related to paralysis or fracture

III. **Pathophysiology**
   A. Primary factors
      1. Pressure: Usually associated with weight bearing over a bony prominence. The exact pressure and time needed to cause damage are not known.
      2. Shearing forces: Occur when surfaces slide across one another.
      3. Friction: More superficial than shear; force created when two surfaces in contact move across each other.
         a. Alters the pressure–time relationship necessary for skin ischemia and necrosis.
         b. May cause skin tears, abrasions, blisters.
      4. Moisture
         a. Skin maceration; softens/disrupts skin's barrier.
         b. May cause local edema with surrounding dryness.
         c. Feces may lead to local irritation/abrasion; urine not a factor with intact skin.
   B. Other factors associated with pressure ulcer formation

1. Immobility
   a. Prolonged bed rest or sitting.
   b. Spinal stenosis, cerebrovascular accidents, especially in the presence of neglect, sensory impairment, or other neurologic problems.
   c. Arthritis, fractures, or trauma, especially of the back, spine, or lower extremities.
   d. Fatigue due to serious illness.
   e. Sedation/analgesia, especially if prolonged.
2. Malnutrition: Most frequently used predictor of risk is actual intake of protein.
3. Cognitive impairment.
   a. Dementia, especially when severe.
   b. Delirium.
   c. Cortical sensory impairment.
4. Infections.
5. Poor perfusion states, including poor cardiac output, prolonged hypotension, aortic balloons/pressors, spending more than 2 hr on a heart-lung machine, and edema.
6. Hospitalization
7. Postoperative states.
8. Contractures make positioning difficult.
9. Systemic medical illnesses
   a. Diabetes mellitus.
   b. Postphlebitic syndrome and other causes of venous stasis.
   c. Severe arteriosclerosis.
   d. Carcinoma.
   e. Autoimmune illnesses.
   f. Human immunodeficiency virus and other immune deficiency states.

IV. **Diagnosis (Risk Factor Assessment)**
   A. History
      1. Activity level of patient.
      2. Functional status/degree of dependency.
      3. Nutritional problems.
      4. Preexistent mobility problems.
      5. Altered skin integrity present/prior pressure ulcers.
   B. Clinical signs and physical findings (the Braden Scale; Table 140H-1)
      1. Assess mobility, especially in bed.
      2. Activities of daily living measures.

Table 140H-1. The Braden Scale*

Domain	Score			
	1	2	3	4
Sensory Perception (ability to respond meaningfully to pressure-related discomfort)	Completely limited	Very limited	Slightly limited	Not limited
Moisture (degree to which skin is exposed to moisture)	Constantly moist	Very moist	Occasionally moist	Not moist
Activity (degree of physical activity)	Bedfast	Chairfast	Occasionally walks	Walks frequently
Mobility (ability to change and control body position)	Completely immobile	Very limited	Slightly limited	Not limited
Nutrition (usual food intake pattern)	Very poor	Probably inadequate	Adequate	Excellent
Friction and Shear	Problems	Potential problems	No apparent problems	No apparent problems

Best total score possible = 23; at particular risk if score is < 16.

*The Braden Scale is used by permission from the authors, Bergstrom N, Braden BJ. *Nursing Research* 36:205–210, 1987.

3. Physical abnormalities
   a. Joint contractures, movement limitations.
   b. Loss of sacral lordosis.
   c. Amputations.
   d. Loss of subcutaneous fat pads over bony prominences or areas under braces/other supports.
C. Preventive techniques
   1. Mobilize patients as much as possible.
      a. *Bed rest only when clearly indicated.*
      b. Evaluation and treatment by physical therapist.
      c. Positioning techniques/devices to reduce pressure, especially on heels (bunny boots, etc.).
      d. Restraints and intravenous/other lines only when necessary for safety/treatment.
      e. Write turning orders if bed mobility is a problem.
      f. Avoid prolonged sitting; shift positions every 15–20 min.
      g. Use diapers and lifts to decrease friction.
      h. Keep head of bed below 30 degrees if possible.
   2. Ensure adequate nutrition.
      a. Obtain calorie counts, set nutritional goals, provide supplements.
      b. Monitor effectiveness of tube feedings.
      c. Hyperalimentation as necessary.
   3. Keep skin dry.
      a. Diapers and pads are not panaceas. Toileting reduces moisture and relieves pressure.
      b. Avoid chronic indwelling catheters for urinary or fecal incontinence if possible.
         (1) Urinary catheters increase the risk of urosepsis.
         (2) Indwelling rectal catheters carry a high risk of rectocolon necrosis and often leak.
         (3) Catheters decrease mobility.
         (4) Risk factor reduction (Table 140H-2 and the following guidelines).
      c. External condom catheters for male patients with urinary incontinence and potential for skin breakdown.
      d. Female patients with urinary incontinence may need timed voids (frequent toileting—e.g., every 2 hr) and/or straight catheterization, as well as diapering.
      e. Rectal pouches for recurrent diarrhea.
      f. Various cleansers, moisturizers, and barriers are available; none has established efficacy.
D. Staging of skin ulcers; staging system is not hierarchical; some pressure ulcers do not go through the unblanchable erythema/superficial defect stage.
   1. Stage I: Unblanchable erythema and/or superficial epithelial defect.
   2. Stage II: Full thickness of the skin to the subcutaneous fat.
   3. Stage III: Full thickness of the skin extending into subcutaneous fat, limited by deep fascia.
   4. Stage IV: Penetration of the deep fascia with extensive soft tissue spread; includes bone and joint involvement.

V. Differential Diagnosis

This is almost never a problem.
A. Neoplasia: Squamous cell carcinoma, skin involved by malignancy.
B. Infection: Abscesses, boils, furuncles; erythrasma; herpes simplex; syphilis.
C. Fissures/osteomyelitis may require sinograms for differentiation.
D. Other conditions: Psoriasis, dependent rubor, bullous skin disorders.

VI. Treatment (Table 140H-3)

A. Prevention: Only successful treatment method is to relieve pressure. Repositioning is the key (see Section IV,C).
B. Interventions by stage (Tables 140H-2 and 140H-3).
C. See Section VII.

VII. Patient Monitoring

A. Daily skin survey.
   1. Special attention to common problem areas.
      a. Bony prominences such as scapulae, greater trochanters, back of head, sacrum, iliac, and ischial tuberosities.
      b. Feet, especially heels, tips of toes, and lateral sides of the midfoot.
      c. Any neglected, denervated, or restrained limb.
   2. Skin tears are early warning signs; check forearms.
   3. Perineal, perianal, moisture-prone areas.
B. Parameters to follow in evaluating established pressure ulcers

Table 140H-2. Interventions by Braden Scale (For Predicting Pressure Sore Risk)

Domain	Interventions by Braden Scale Category
Sensory Perception or Mortality Score < 2	1) Schedule major position change every 2 hours (includes time spent in chair or in bed) 2) Place on pressure relieving device while lying in bed and sitting in chair 3) Avoid positioning on trochanter. 　　a) flex top knee 35 degrees 　　b) rest lower part of top leg on pillow behind midpoint of body 4) Use positioning devices (Bunny boots with frames, pillows, etc.) to keep feet and ankles off mattress
Activity Score < 2	1) If bedfast, encourage position change every 2 hours 2) If chairfast, encourage position change every 20–30 minutes
Moisture Score < 3	1) Determine source of moisture 2) If patient incontinent of urine and/or semi-formed stool: 　　a) cleanse area, rinse well, dry thoroughly 　　b) apply skin moisturizer, rub in thoroughly 　　c) apply moisture repellant, rub in thoroughly 　　d) repeat steps a–c after each incontinent episode 3) If the patient is incontinent of liquid stool, apply fecal incontinence pouch 4) If patient has drainage for tubes and/or open wounds, contact ET Nurse Consultation Services for pouching techniques 5) Place incontinence pad directly under patient and change as necessary
Nutrition Score < 2	1) Encourage patient to eat or help the patient to eat 2) Consult a dietician 3) Record amount eaten on menu and save for dietician
Friction/Shear Score < 2	1) Avoid elevating head of bed >30 degrees unless contraindicated by medical condition 2) Use trapeze or lifting sheets to facilitate movement 3) Decrease use of high friction materials (bath blankets, mattress pads) directly under patient 4) Apply transparent adhesive dressings to high-risk areas 5) If heels or elbows are at risk, cover with socks or heel/elbow protectors
<td colspan="1" style="text-align:center">**Other Interventions**</td>	
Stripping/tearing Score < 2	1) Keep skin moisturized 2) If skin is thin or tape is removed from one site frequently 　　a) cover area that will receive tape with a skin sealant and allow to dry before taping OR 　　b) tape onto skin barrier rather than directly onto skin

1. Document circumference of the defect and of any surrounding erythema or undermining.
2. Depth measurement not important; document tissue layers lost.
3. Stage ulcer per Section IV,D.
C. Provide local care; monitor effectiveness at least every other day
　1. Saline: "physiologic"; preferred for many stage II ulcers and for most stage III and IV ulcers. Maintains good pH and healing environment.

a. Wet to moist dressings (not wet to dry) preferred.
b. Change each shift or every 8 hr.
c. Low-pressure syringe irrigation may clean debris.
d. Can be used as filler; amount of moisture can be varied to absorb exudate.
e. Inexpensive
f. Lactated Ringer's solution may be used; more expensive.
　2. Special dressings: Protective, relatively inexpensive.

Table 140H-3. General Approaches to Therapy of Pressure Sores

Stage	Treat Wound-healing Retardant Factors	Eliminate Local Pressure	Clean and Remove Necrotic Tissue	Create a Tissue Growth Environment
1	Assess and support nutrition	Teach the patients to reposition themselves, or nursing staff should reposition the patient every 2 hours.	The surface should be washed every 8 hours with saline or a mild antibacterial skin cleanser	Expose to air or cover with hydrocolloid dressing or polyurethane film dressing.
	Treat complicating systemic diseases	Devices should be used to supplement repositioning maneuvers, e.g., overlays such as foam (eggcrate), gel, or air	Avoid excessive moisture or dryness of skin.	
	Improve mobility	Nursing staff should record turning the patient, and when possible use a turning or repositioning schedule		
2	Same as in Stage 1	Same as in Stage 1 Consider low air-loss bed (Flexicare) or water bed	Same as in Stage 1.	Apply adhesive hydrocolloid occlusive dressing every 3–5 days or film occlusive dressing every 2–3 days
3	Same as in Stage 1	Same as in Stage 1 Consider use of air flotation bed (Clinitron) or a low air-loss bed	*Debridement:* Surgical most effective, but often reserved for necrotic or heavily eschared wounds. *Enzymatic:* supplemental to surgical and Hubbard tank debridement (e.g. granulex, elase or santyl) will not clean the ulcer bed. *Hubbard tank:* hydrotherapy is often effective, especially for debris-	Once debridement and cleaning phases are completed, apply saline or Ringer's solution to clean necrosis-free ulcer every 6–8 hours or apply hydrocolloid dressing if wound is shallow enough.

(continued)

Stage	Treat Wound-healing Retardant Factors	Eliminate Local Pressure	Clean and Remove Necrotic Tissue	Create a Tissue Growth Environment
			filled wounds, but is costly, and often dehydrates skin. Any of these debridement techniques may remove granulation tissue or injure surrounding normal skin. *Cleaning:* after debridement, clean the ulcer every day or so with saline or very gentle washing with a mild skin cleanser (nontoxic). Hydrotherapy (Hubbard tank) for short intervals a few times each week effective for cleansing, but expensive and labor-intensive	
4	Same as in Stage 1	Same as in Stage 1	Follow steps in Stage 3 except *Debridement:* eschar (especially if black or tightly applied to the ulcer) must be surgically removed *Cleaning:* Follow the steps in Grade 3	Same as in Stage 3, but if deep, fillers may be needed, and gauze should be kept moist with saline or Ringer's solution. The surrounding normal skin must be protected; various devices are available. When the ulcer is clean, consider myocutaneous flap (general or plastic surgery).

a. Transparent films (operative site, tegaderm).
   (1) Gas and moisture permeable; keep out bacteria and dirt.
   (2) Used in stage I and stage II ulcers.
   (3) Change infrequently, not more than once a day; every 3 days is best.
   (4) Allows clinicians to see the ulcer.
   (5) Traps exudate against wound, creates a moist environment, promotes autolysis.
b. Hydrocolloid patches (restore, duoderm): Moderate in price; change every 3–5 days.
   (1) Adhesive, occlusive gel forms under areas exposed to exudate.
   (2) Same advantages as transparent films.
   (3) Used in stage II and some stage III ulcers.
   (4) Conform to contours; not helpful in deeper wounds, as contact with the wound exudate is critical for "occlusion."
c. Fillers and foams (duoderm granules, vigilon, lyofoam, seaweed): Not very useful, expensive.
   (1) Foams may help absorb exudate; used with wound fillers and in deep wounds with cellulitis.
   (2) Usefulness of seaweed and newer foams is unproven.

3. Topical agents
   a. Antibiotics
      (1) Seldom useful.
      (2) Sensitizing.
      (3) Necrotic, foul-smelling wounds may do well with metronidazole gel.
      (4) Adverse effects reported with most, including betadine, peroxide, and neosporin.
   b. Enzymes: Used in debridement of wounds where surgical debridement is difficult or unavailable.
      (1) Collagenase (Santyl).
      (2) Fibrinolysin-desoxyribonuclease (Elase).
      (3) Trypsin-papain (Granulex).
      (4) Will not treat black eschar.
      (5) Needs to be used for 5–7 days, followed by surgical debridement.
      (6) Surrounding normal skin *needs*

protection with a lotion and/or moisture barrier.
   c. Other substances (poor scientific substantiation)
      (1) Dermagran system.
      (2) *d*-Glucoside (Silvetti).
      (3) Local hyperalimentation.
      (4) Hirudoid (a leech-derived protein).

4. Special beds
   a. Flexicare or low-airless bed
      (1) Useful in stages II, III, and IV ulcers.
      (2) Good for pressure relief over trochanters.
      (3) Heels and sides of feet still at risk.
      (4) Does not replace good nursing care.
      (5) Moisture may become a problem.
   b. Clinitron or air flotation bed
      (1) Excellent for exudative, large ulcers.
      (2) Very drying, even of normal skin.
      (3) Most expensive bed to rent.
      (4) Nearly impossible to move around in it.

5. Surgical treatments
   a. Debridement
      (1) Serial debridement often required.
      (2) Atraumatic dissection preferred.
      (3) Surgical consultation recommended.
   b. Skin grafts: Seldom effective; may be useful in lower extremity stage II and III ulcers.
   c. Skin flaps: "Neurovascular"; contain arteries and nerves; effective but expensive.

6. Systemic antibiotics (usually intravenous): Indicated only for complications
   a. Fever/sepsis with no other source and worsening wound or exudative or necrotic ulcer.
   b. Underlying osteomyelitis; check plain film, erythrocyte sedimentation rate, white blood cell count; bone scan and/or gallium scan may be helpful.
   c. Cellulitis.

7. Antibiotic choices
   a. Clindamycin, aminoglycosides, and vancomycin known to penetrate pressure ulcers.
   b. Quinolones, third-generation ceph-

alosporins not well studied in pressure ulcers.

    c. Treat aggressively for an appropriate interval; usually more than two organisms; may have mixture of anaerobes and a gram-negative rod.

    d. Bone or deep tissue biopsy may be needed.

VIII. Prognosis

Depends on prevention of new ulcer formation.

A. Acquired during acute hospitalization

    1. As few as 12% of pressure ulcers heal during the incident hospitalization.

    2. Most patients discharged to nursing homes/intense home care.

B. Present at admission, complicated

    1. Associated with poor outcome, increased length of stay, and death.

    2. Often reflect failure of current treatment.

    3. Frequently require surgical intervention.

C. After surgical closure

    1. No data to predict prognosis; an interested, excellent surgeon and appropriate postoperative care needed.

    2. Myocutaneous flaps preferred to split or full-thickness skin grafts; appear to heal better.

Bibliography

Allman RM. Pressure ulcers among the elderly. *N Engl J Med* 320(13):850–853, 1989.

Longe RL. Current concepts in clinical therapeutics: Pressure sores. *Clin Pharmacy* 5:669–681, 1986.

Smith DM, Winsemius DK, Besdine RW. Pressure sores in the elderly: Can this outcome be prevented? *J Gen Intern Med* 6(1):81–93, 1991.

CHAPTER 140-I

Depression in the Elderly

Steven Rothschild, M.D.

I. Definition

A. Depression can be both a *symptom* and a *diagnosis*. It is critical that the physician make this distinction.

1. Depressed mood or feelings are referred to as *dysphoria*.

   a. Feelings in this category include hopelessness, helplessness, despair, gloom, frustration, or a decreased sense of self-worth.

2. Several depressive disorders are characterized in DSM-III-R. These include major depression, dysthymia, adjustment disorder with depressed mood, organic affective disorder, seasonal affective disorder, and uncomplicated bereavement.

3. Major depression is defined in DSM-III-R as requiring:

   a. A change from the previous level of functioning, with the presence of at least five of the following symptoms during the same 2-week period. At least one of the symptoms must be either (1) or (2).

     (1) Depressed mood.

     (2) Markedly diminished interest in or pleasure from most activities.

     (3) Significant weight loss or gain without dieting.

     (4) Insomnia or hypersomnia almost daily.

     (5) Psychomotor agitation or retardation.

     (6) Fatigue or loss of energy almost daily.

     (7) Feelings of worthlessness and/or inappropriate guilt.

     (8) Diminished ability to think, concentrate, or make decisions.

     (9) Recurrent thoughts of death.

   b. An organic cause cannot be established.

   c. The disturbance is not a normal reaction to death.

   d. At no time have there been delusions or hallucinations for as long as 2 weeks in the absence of prominent mood symptoms.

   e. The condition is not superimposed on schizophrenia, schizophreniform disorder, delusional disorder, or psychotic disorder NOS.

B. Depression is *not* a part of normal aging. The majority of older adults are in good mental health and are satisfied with their lives.

C. Studies indicate that depression is underdiagnosed (by as much as 50%) and undertreated. Every patient with depressive symptoms warrants careful evaluation. These symptoms should not be ignored.

II. **Epidemiology**
  A. Prevalence
    1. Community
      a. Symptoms of depression affect 10–15% of older persons.
      b. Prevalence of symptoms is greater among those persons >85 years old.
      c. Major depression: 1–2% of community-living elders; this prevalence is lower than that among younger adults.
      d. Dysthymia, neurotic depression: 2%
    2. Hospital
      a. Prevalence of symptoms of depression in older persons averages 38%.
      b. Major depression: Over 12%; some studies cite prevalences as high as 45%.
      c. High correlation between past psychiatric history and severity of medical illness with the prevalence of depressive symptoms.
    3. Nursing homes
      a. Prevalence is at least as high as that of patients hospitalized with medical illnesses, if not higher.
  B. Morbidity and mortality
    1. Death from all causes appears to be somewhat higher among depressed older persons, both in the community and in institutions. Considerable controversy regarding the causes for this situation. Likely to reflect factors such as poor self-care, increased carelessness, poor social support, and malnutrition, rather than direct effect of depression.
    2. Cycles of recovery and relapse are common.
    3. Suicide
      a. Persons >65 years old commit suicide at a higher rate than any other group! Increasing rate noted in 85+ age group. Suicide is among the top 10 causes of death in elderly persons of both sexes.
      b. Risk factors
        (1) Male sex.
        (2) Social isolation or living alone.
        (3) Concomitant physical illness.
        (4) Alcoholism.
      c. Unlike teenagers and young adults, the elderly make fewer attempts but are more likely to be successful (ratio of attempts to completed suicides = 4:1).

III. **Diagnosis**
Note that older patients are more likely to consult medical providers than psychiatrists/psychologists/mental health agencies for depression. As with other medical diagnoses (e.g., pulmonary embolism), you find depression only if you actively think about it.
  A. Presentation
    1. Physical symptoms and vegetative signs are common. Depression is the "great masquerader."
      a. Anorexia and weight loss are more common in older depressed patients than in younger ones.
      b. Sleep disturbance, especially insomnia.
      c. Pain: generalized or focused.
      d. Memory impairment.
    2. Psychological symptoms
      a. Withdrawal, social isolation, and loss of interest in regular activities are common.
      b. Agitation, anxiety.
      c. Hypochondriasis with numerous somatic complaints.
      d. Decreased sense of self-worth and guilt are less commonly seen in older persons with major depression.
  B. Screening: The Geriatric Depression Scale is a brief, self-administered instrument that has been validated in both medical inpatients and outpatients (Table 140I-1).

IV. **Differential Diagnosis**
  A. Medications (prescribed and over-the-counter)
    1. Antihypertensives: β-blockers, methyldopa, clonidine, prazocin, guanethidine.
    2. Sedative-hypnotics, major tranquilizers.
    3. Levodopa, amantadine.
    4. Corticosteroids.
    5. Digitalis.
    6. Narcotic analgesics.
    7. Cancer chemotherapeutic agents.
  B. Alcoholism or drug abuse
  C. Metabolic disturbances
    1. Hyponatremia or hypernatremia.
    2. Hypocalcemia or hypercalcemia.
    3. Hypoglycemia or hyperglycemia.
    4. Hypomagnesemia.
    5. Uremia, azotemia.
    6. Acid-base disturbances.
  D. Endocrinopathies
    1. Hypothyroidism and hyperthyroidism.

Table 1401-1. Geriatric Depression Scale (Short Form)

Choose the Best Answer for How You Felt Over the Past Week

1. Are you basically satisfied with your life? . . . . yes/no
2. Have you dropped many of your activities and interests? . . . . yes/no
3. Do you feel that your life is empty? . . . . yes/no
4. Do you often get bored? . . . . yes/no
5. Are you in good spirits most of the time? . . . . yes/no
6. Are you afraid that something bad is going to happen to you? . . . . yes/no
7. Do you feel happy most of the time? . . . . yes/no
8. Do you often feel helpless? . . . . yes/no
9. Do you prefer to stay at home, rather than going out and doing new things? . . . . yes/no
10. Do you feel you have more problems with memory than most? . . . . yes/no
11. Do you think it is wonderful to be alive now? . . . . yes/no
12. Do you feel pretty worthless the way you are now? . . . . yes/no
13. Do you feel full of energy? . . . . yes/no
14. Do you feel that your situation is hopeless? . . . . yes/no
15. Do you think that most people are better off than you are? . . . . yes/no

The following answers count one point; scores >5 indicate probable depression:

1. NO	6. YES	11. NO
2. YES	7. NO	12. YES
3. YES	8. YES	13. NO
4. YES	9. YES	14. YES
5. NO	10. YES	15. YES

Source: Reprinted with permission of Barbara J. Braden and Nancy Bergstrom.

2. Hyperparathyroidism.
3. Cushing's and Addison's diseases.
4. Hypopituitarism.
E. End-stage renal disease and hemodialysis
F. Cardiovascular disease: Congestive heart failure, cardiomyopathy, post-myocardial infarction
G. Chronic obstructive pulmonary disease
H. Malignancies (especially those involving the central nervous system)
I. Disorders associated with chronic pain
1. Polymyalgia rheumatica.
2. Arthritis.
3. Paget's disease.
4. Metastatic disease.
5. Osteoporosis.
J. Neurologic disorders
1. Alzheimer's disease—frequently complicated by depression in early stages.
2. Parkinson's disease.
3. Stroke.
4. Demyelinating disease.
5. Subdural hematomas.
K. Infections
1. Subacute bacterial endocarditis.
2. Encephalitis (especially viral).

3. Fungal meningitis.
4. Tuberculosis.
L. Other diseases
1. Anemia.
2. Vitamin deficiencies (B_{12}, folate).

V. Diagnostic Workup

Given the broad range of organic disorders which can cause signs and symptoms of depression, the physician is advised to perform a thorough history and physical exam prior to making a diagnosis of depression. Specific areas of attention are listed below.

A. History
1. Specific symptoms and their duration
   a. Note that excessive sleep often indicates a problem with medications rather than depression.
   b. Suicidal ideation must be assessed. Asking patients does not "put the idea into their head." Presence of suicidal ideation is an indication for immediate psychiatric referral.
2. Previous psychiatric history.
3. Review of medications.
4. Alcohol use history.

B. Physical examination

1. A complete physical exam is critical.
2. Neurologic exam, including mental status testing.

C. Laboratory tests
1. Complete blood count with indices.
2. Serum chemistries (electrolytes, blood urea nitrogen, creatinine, liver enzymes, glucose, calcium).
3. Serum vitamin B_{12} levels (especially in the presence of macrocytosis).
4. Thyroid function studies, including thyroid-stimulating hormone.

D. Biologic markers for depression
1. At this time, no valid biologic markers are found consistently among patients with depressive illness. The dexamethasone suppression test is widely used as a diagnostic tool, however.
2. Dexamethasone suppression test
   a. Dexamethasone, 1 mg orally at 11 P.M.
   b. Measure serum cortisol levels at 8 A.M., 4 P.M., and 11 P.M. the next day.
   c. Any cortisol level >5 µg/dl is considered positive for depression.
3. The dexamethasone suppression test has been noted by some authors to be helpful in evaluating depressive symptoms in medical inpatients and in persons with early Alzheimer's disease. Conflicting reports exist, however, with others reporting a high rate of false positives in patients with severe illness or weight loss and in patients with dementia without depressive symptomatology.
4. Electroencephalographic changes have been noted to distinguish depressed from nondepressed elderly persons in sleep studies, but such studies are not widely utilized.

VI. Treatment
A. Psychotherapy
1. The primary care physician can provide important support and counseling to the depressed patient.
   a. Active listening to the patient's concerns is critical; do not ignore, deny, or devalue the patient's problems.
   b. Provide information about the patient's diagnosis and treatment options. Whenever possible, involve the patient in the decision-making process.
   c. Prescribe daily physical activity such as short walks.
   d. Reduce social isolation; referral to se-

nior citizen's centers or day groups can be very helpful.
   e. Encourage activities of life review such as recording memories in a book or on an audiocassette. Calling old friends or taking trips to places of importance in the patient's life can be helpful.
2. Cognitive-behavioral therapies designed to encourage reduction of the patient's negative ideation and encourage new behaviors have been shown to be effective. Such therapy is more directive and educational than traditional psychotherapy with young adults and is usually limited in the number of sessions.

B. Pharmacotherapy: The medications listed below are not intended as an exhaustive list but comprise those which are widely utilized in the treatment of depression in older persons. Always begin with the lowest dose possible, and monitor side effects and outcomes. Consider possible adverse drug interactions.
1. Heterocyclic antidepressants: Keep in mind that these medications may require 4–6 weeks before therapeutic benefit is seen. After starting heterocyclics at a low dose, gradually increase at 5- to 7-day intervals.
   a. Doxepin
      (1) Starting dose: 10–20 mg at bedtime.
      (2) Very sedating
      (3) Anticholinergic side effects and orthostatic hypotension are common.
   b. Trazodone
      (1) Starting dose: 25–50 mg at bedtime.
      (2) Very sedating.
      (3) Almost no anticholinergic side effects make this drug particularly attractive; only mild orthostasis seen.
   c. Nortriptyline
      (1) Starting dose: 10–20 mg at bedtime.
      (2) Less sedating than doxepin or trazodone.
      (3) Moderate anticholinergic and orthostatic side effects.
      (4) Drug levels available associated with therapeutic response (50–150 ng/ml).
      (5) Long half-life in older patients (>50 hr).
   d. Desipramine
      (1) Starting dose: 25 mg every morning.
      (2) Minimally sedating; an excellent

choice for the patient with psycho-motor retardation, fatigue, or excessive sleep.

    (3) Minimal anticholinergic and orthostatic side effects.

    (4) Therapeutic drug level >125 ng/dl.

  e. Fluoxetine

    (1) Starting dose: 20 mg/day.

    (2) Lack of sedation is major advantage.

    (3) Relatively little experience in older patients to date.

2. Psychostimulants

  a. Methylphenidate, 2.5 mg at 8 A.M. and at noon, can be very effective, especially with apathetic or withdrawn inpatients.

  b. Has the advantage of inducing a response within a few doses; can be used concomitantly while starting a heterocyclic antidepressant.

  c. Monitor blood pressure carefully with first doses.

3. Monamine oxidase inhibitors

  a. Should probably not be used by the nonpsychiatrist unless one is very familiar with these medications.

  b. Advantages over heterocyclic antidepressants are less sedation and a more rapid response.

  c. Major disadvantage is the need for a strict tyramine-free diet. Eating cheeses, wines, chocolate, or other foods while taking these drugs can produce a hypertensive crisis.

C. Electroconvulsive therapy (ECT)

  1. ECT has a place in the treatment of older persons with severe psychotic depression refractive to psychotherapy and pharmacotherapy.

  2. Unilateral, nondominant hemisphere ECT, coupled with careful monitoring, produces relatively few injuries or adverse effects.

  3. Response is faster than with medications; may be a critical factor in treating actively suicidal patients.

  4. Memory impairment can be seen after ECT.

D. **Prognosis:** Over 80–90% of elderly exhibit positive response to medical treatments for depression.

Bibliography

Bienenfeld D. Verwoerdt's Clinical Geropsychiatry, ed 3. Williams and Wilkins, Baltimore, 1990.

Sadavoy J, Lazarus LW, Jarvik LF. Comprehensive Review of Geriatric Psychiatry. American Psychiatric Press, Washington, DC, 1991.

Spar JE, LaRue A. Concise Guide to Geriatric Psychiatry, American Psychiatric Press, Washington, DC, 1990.

Chapter 140-J

Sleep Disorders in the Elderly

Andrew Ripeckyj, M.D.

I. Definition

A. Sleep disorders are grouped on clinical grounds into:
   1. Insomnias: Disorders in initiating and maintaining sleep.
   2. Disorders of excessive somnolence.
   3. Disorders of the sleep-wake schedule.
   4. Parasomnias: Dysfunctions associated with sleep, such as sleepwalking, sleep terror, or sleep-related enuresis.

B. Prevalence data suggest that about 50% of the elderly (65 years or older) complain of a sleep problem. Sleep problems are more common in women. An association is suspected between complaints of insomnia and excess mortality in elderly populations.

II. Etiology

A. Primary sleep disorders
   1. Obstructive sleep apnea
      a. The occurrence of five or more 10-sec or greater cessations or two-thirds reduction of respiration per hour of sleep time.
      b. Occurs predominantly in men; incidence rises significantly with age.
      c. Usually presents with excessive daytime sleepiness.
   2. Nocturnal myoclonus
      a. "Restless leg syndrome": A presleep urge to move one's legs that interferes with initiation of sleep and periodic movements of one's legs during sleep that interfere with sleep maintenance.
      b. Common in the elderly; usually presents with daytime sleepiness.
   3. Central sleep apnea
      a. Identical to obstructive sleep apnea but with a different etiology.
      b. Presents with excessive daytime sleepiness.
   4. Persistent psychophysiologic insomnia (primary insomnia): Patients with persistent complaints of difficulty initiating or maintaining sleep in the absence of a specific sleep, medical, or psychiatric disorder are classified in this category.
   5. Narcolepsy
      a. Characterized by four major symptoms:
         (1) Excessive daytime sleepiness with sleep attacks.
         (2) Cataplexy.
         (3) Sleep paralysis.
         (4) Hypnagogic hallucinations.

  b. Usually begins in young adulthood, with rare onset after age 50. Tends to have a chronic course.
  6. Kleine-Levin syndrome: This has not been reported in elderly patients.
  7. Parasomnias: These are very rare in elderly patients.
  B. Sleep disorders occurring as secondary phenomena in patients with medical problems or medication side effects. Examples include:
  1. Patients with pain of any cause.
  2. Depression.
  3. Chronic obstructive pulmonary disease.
  4. Sedative/alcohol use.
  5. Use of stimulants such as caffeine and diuretics.
  C. Sleep disorders occurring in response to a problem with the sleep-wake schedule. A mismatch occurs between the person's sleep-wake schedule and environmental demands.

III. Pathophysiology
  A. Primary sleep disorders
  1. Obstructive sleep apnea
    a. Primarily mechanical; upper airway obstruction, commonly at the level of the pharynx; associated with obesity, hypertension, middle age, and male gender.
    b. Leads to increased respiratory effort, oxygen desaturation, cardiac arrhythmias, and multiple (hundreds) arousals from sleep nightly.
    c. Fragmentation of sleep leads to characteristic daytime somnolence.
  2. Nocturnal myoclonus
    a. Characterized by periodic leg twitches, especially during nonrapid eye movement sleep. Twitches associated with microarousals, leading to sleep fragmentation and subjectively nonrestorative sleep.
    b. Hereditary disease transmitted as an autosomal dominant trait.
    c. Pathophysiology poorly defined; probably secondary to central nervous system (CNS) dysfunction at the level of the brain stem.
  3. Central sleep apnea
    a. Characterized by the absence of both airflow and respiratory effort for at least 10 sec at a rate of five or more times per hour.
    b. Multiple etiologies; most common (in elderly patients) are:

      (1) Neurologic lesions due to cerebrovascular disease that affect the automatic respiratory control system.
      (2) Congestive heart failure via its effect of increasing circulation time, thus introducing a lag time in the readings made by peripheral oxygen partial pressure and carbon dioxide partial pressure chemoreceptors.
  4. Persistent psychophysiologic insomnia (primary insomnia)
    a. Most likely due to a conditioning or learning phenomenon.
    b. Patients tend to be more aroused (higher body temperature, heart and respiratory rates) before sleep than normal controls.
    c. Patients tend to misperceive the length of time they are asleep, usually underestimating their sleep time.
  5. Narcolepsy: No underlying mechanism known. Associated with reduced dopamine availability in the CNS, although cholinergic mechanisms are also probably involved.
  6. Parasomnias: Pathophysiology varies with the disorder.
  B. Secondary sleep disorders: Pathophysiology varies.
  C. Disorders of the sleep-wake schedule
  1. Transient sleep-wake schedule disorders, such as with jet lag or work shift changes.
  2. Persistent sleep-wake schedule disorders.
    a. Delayed sleep-phase syndrome.
    b. Irregular sleep-wake pattern.

IV. Diagnosis
  A. History: Elderly patients are less likely to volunteer information. Actively inquire as to:
  1. Quality and quantity of sleep at night.
  2. Daytime sleepiness/napping behavior.
  3. Satisfaction with sleep.
  4. Observation of the patient's bed partner regarding the above factors, as well as about snoring, movement, and kicking.
  5. Use of *all* medications, including alcohol, coffee, and over-the-counter medications.
  B. Clinical signs and physical findings
  1. Observed sleepiness while with the examiner.
  2. Risk factors such as obesity and hypertension.
  C. Diagnostic tests

1. Sleep-wake log over 2 weeks.
2. Sleep laboratory evaluation: Overnight recording of the electroencephalogram, electro-oculogram, chin electromyogram, and airflow at the mouth and nostrils.

V. Differential Diagnosis

A. Normal sleep changes associated with aging
1. Increased number of arousals (fragmentation of sleep).
2. Less total time in deep (stages II and IV) sleep and in rapid eye movement (REM) sleep.
3. Decreased REM sleep latency.
4. More total time spent awake (15–20% of total time in bed).
5. Increased sensitivity to environmental disruptions of sleep.

B. Secondary sleep disturbances
1. Medical and psychiatric illness (see Section II).
2. Early Alzheimer's dementia
   a. Significant reductions in depth and duration of sleep (relative to age-matched controls).
   b. Breakdown of sleep-wake cycle.

C. Primary sleep disturbances (Section II).

VI. Treatment

A. Obstructive sleep apnea
1. Weight reduction.
2. Smoking cessation.
3. Avoid CNS depressants.
4. Avoid the supine sleeping position.
   a. Position monitors alarm when patient is supine.
   b. A tennis ball sewn into the back of the pajama top helps the patient avoid the supine position.
5. Medications
   a. Protriptyline, a tricyclic antidepressant, appears to suppress REM sleep. Apneic episodes are reduced since most occur during REM sleep. Anticholinergic side effects are a drawback in the elderly.
   b. Medroxyprogesterone increases respiratory center chemosensitivity.
   c. Acetazolamide and L-tryptophan help only minimally.
6. Continuous positive airway pressure (CPAP)
   a. A nasal CPAP device can deliver a constant air pressure between 2 and 20 cm of water pressure. Optimal pressure must be determined in the sleep laboratory.

b. Poor long-term acceptance and compliance.
7. Surgery
   a. Appropriate for patients with localized upper airway lesions such as enlarged adenoids/tonsils.
   b. Concurrent tracheostomy in severe cases.
8. Airway patency devices
   a. Designed to prevent the tongue from occluding the posterior pharyngeal airway or to prevent the soft palate from occluding the upper airway.
   b. Usefulness severely limited; poorly tolerated.

B. Nocturnal myoclonus
1. Clonazepam, 0.5–2.0 mg at bedtime; Baclofen, 10–40 mg at bedtime; and bromocriptine mesylate, 2.5–5.0 mg at bedtime have been reported to be effective.
2. Low-dose opioid treatment may also be effective; concern about addiction limits use.

C. Central sleep apnea
1. Medical
   a. Treat underlying conditions such as heart failure.
   b. Weight loss, low-flow oxygen via nasal prong during sleep, and protriptyline have all been described as effective in some patients.
2. Surgical: Tracheostomy with nocturnal mechanical ventilation.
3. Mechanical: CPAP and intermittent positive-pressure ventilation effective.

D. Persistent psychophysiologic insomnia (primary insomnia)
1. Counseling critical. To improve sleep hygiene:
   a. Regular sleep and wakeup times important and should be adhered to 7 days a week.
   b. Restrict time in bed for sleep and sexual activity only. Do not stay in bed if unable to fall asleep.
   c. Regular exercise helps promote sleep.
   d. Avoid environmental intrusions (noise, light).
   e. Moderate temperatures are best.
   f. Eat and drink lightly before sleep.
   g. Avoid tobacco, alcohol, and stimulants.
   h. Associated psychosocial stressors require specific attention.
2. Use hypnotics sparingly.

a. Short-acting benzodiazepines best in elderly patients.

b. Tolerance may develop within 2 weeks.

c. Use lowest effective dose.

E. Narcolepsy

1. Medications have provided symptomatic relief for some of the disabling features.

a. Excessive daytime sleepiness responds to methylphenidate in divided doses of 10–40 mg/day. Dosage titrated to the clinical response. Other stimulants in use include pemoline and dextroamphetamine. Tolerance is occasionally a problem.

b. Cataplexy responds to protriptyline, 5–40 mg/day, and to other tricyclic antidepressants such as despiramine.

c. Hypnagogic hallucinations respond to imipramine, 25–100 mg at bedtime, or to protriptyline, 5–40 mg at bedtime.

2. Good sleep hygiene, a balanced diet, physical activity, and supportive counseling are also helpful.

Bibliography

Kuna, TS, Sant'Ambrogio G. Pathophysiology of upper airway closure during sleep. *JAMA* 266(10):1384–1389, 1991.

National Institutes of Health Consensus Development Conference Statement. The Treatment of Sleep Disorder of Older People, March 26–28, 1990. *Sleep* 14(2):169–177, 1991.

Reynolds, CF, Kupfer DJ. Sleep disorders, in Talbott JA, Hales RE, Yudofsky SC (eds), *Textbook of Psychiatry*. Washington, D.C., American Psychiatric Press, 1988, pp 737–752.

Vitiello MV, Prinz PN. Sleep and sleep disorders in normal aging, in Thorpy MJ (ed), *Handbook of Sleep Disorder*. New York, Marcel Dekker, 1990, pp 139–151.

CHAPTER 141

Clinical Pharmacology in the Elderly

Mark Overton, M.D.

I. **Classification**
The ideal drug factors to consider follow.
A. Efficacy
B. Patient profile
  1. Concomitant medical problems.
  2. Current medications.
  3. Allergies, idiosyncratic responses.
C. Possible adverse effects
  1. Side effect profile of the drug.
  2. Drug–drug interactions (medication list review).
  3. Drug–disease interactions (problem list).
  4. Drug–laboratory interactions.
  5. Drug–food/nutrient interactions.
  6. Up to 40% of hospitalizations in the elderly are related to adverse drug effects.
D. Costs
  1. Direct costs of the medication.
  2. Costs of monitoring treatment.
  3. Potential costs of alterations in life style.
  4. Costs of iatrogenic consequences.
E. Ease of administration
  1. Vehicle of administration
    a. Size: Pill, capsule.
    b. Taste and consistency, particularly if liquid.
    c. Color: Hard for elderly patients to see subtle shades of yellow, off-white, and green.
  2. Packaging.
  3. Frequency/timing of doses: Best rule is no more than five medications no more than three times a day.
F. Quality of life including general well-being, functional status, cognitive function, physical symptoms, sexual function, and life satisfaction.

II. **Mechanism of Action**
Alterations in pharmacokinetics and pharmacodynamics are considered (Table 141-1).
A. Pharmacokinetics: The study of drug absorption and distribution throughout the body, metabolism, and elimination.
  1. Absorption: Usually passive; changes with aging.
    a. May be increase in gastric pH, delayed gastric emptying, decrease in splanchnic blood flow and in first-pass effect.
    b. Active transport of iron, calcium, thiamine, and galactose decreases.
  2. Distribution changes with aging
    a. Decreased total body water and skeletal muscle.

Table 141-1. Parameters Affecting Drug Dosage in the Elderly

Parameters	Outcome
Decrease in renal function	Decrease in renal excretion and concomitant increase in plasma level
Decrease in hepatic function	Decrease in mixed function oxidase microsomal enzymes and concomitant increase in plasma level
Decrease in total serum protein and albumin	Decrease in binding of highly protein-bound drugs and plasma levels
Decrease in compliance	Decrease in plasma levels Decrease in therapeutic outcome
Decrease or increase in target organ sensitivity	Enhanced or decreased drug effect
Chronic administration	Accumulation and increase in plasma level
Multiple drug interactions	Increase or decrease in renal elimination and/or hepatic degradation of active metabolites

  b. Increased total body fat.
   (1) Increased volume of distribution for lipophilic drugs (diazepam, propranolol).
   (2) Higher blood levels of ethanol, etc.
   (3) Decreased skeletal muscle binding (digoxin).
  c. Protein binding: Changes in protein affinity and concentration may occur.
   (1) *Blood levels may thus underestimate the activity of a given drug.*
   (2) Albumin often decreased.
 3. Metabolism
  a. Liver factors
   (1) Liver microsomal metabolism, especially oxidation, decreased in activity.
   (2) Decreased inducibility of some enzymes.
  b. Renal excretion
   (1) Decrease in renal blood flow, in renal mass, and in the functional number of nephrons.
   (2) With decreased renal clearance:

$$\frac{(140 - \text{age}) \times \text{body wt (kg)}}{72 \times \text{serum creatinine (mg/dL)}}$$

   Multiply above by 0.8 for women.

  c. Sequestration/depots may be altered in adipose tissue and muscles.
 B. Pharmacodynamics: How a drug affects the body/organism.
  1. Receptor issues
   a. Reduced sensitivity to β-blockers secondary to decreased number and responses of β-receptors.

   b. Blunted baroreceptors.
   c. Slower receptor induction.
  2. Sensitivity
   a. Benzodiazepines have greater effects at the same blood levels.
   b. Warfarin more potent and prolongs prothrombin time more at the same doses; may be vitamin K metabolism dependent.
   c. Antagonism: Blocking drugs.
   d. Synergism: Uncommon in the medications used by the elderly.
III. **Indications** (the MASTER mnemonic)
 Minimize the number of drugs.
 Alternatives must be considered, both other forms of therapy or treatment and alternative medications.
 Safety comes first; do no harm.
 Titrate therapy to desired benefit or adverse effect; goal is to use the smallest effective dose.
 Educate the patient/family.
 Review entire medication list regularly.
IV. **Dosages**
 Start low and go slow. Some suggestions follow.
 A. Antihypertensives
  1. Calcium channel antagonists
   a. Currently the drugs of choice for the elderly; no single agent preferred.
   b. No effect on lipids, electrolytes, or glucose tolerance; reverse left ventricular hypertrophy (LVH).
   c. Less slowing of PR interval by diltiazem and verapamil, but still negatively inotropic.
   d. Expensive.
   e. Starting doses of a few selected agents:
    (1) *Nifedipine:* 10 mg three times a day or 30 mg/day SR

(2) *Verapamil:* 40 mg three times a day or 180 mg/day SR

(3) *Diltiazem:* 30 mg three times a day or 120 mg/day SR

(4) *Israpidine:* 2.5 mg twice a day.

(5) *Nicardipine:* 20 mg twice a day.

2. Thiazide diuretics

   a. Inexpensive; reduce cardiac output and renal blood flow (creatinine clearance).

   b. Often worsen underlying problems of hyperuricemia, hyperlipidemia, hypokalemia, impaired glucose tolerance, arrhythmias, and sexual dysfunction.

   c. Negative effect on LVH.

   d. Not synergistic with calcium channel antagonists when used in the elderly.

3. Other diuretic agents

   a. Loop diuretics

     (1) Renal clearance may be reduced by up to 40%.

     (2) Suggested starting doses

       (a) Furosemide: 10–20 mg/day; no more than twice daily for outpatients.

       (b) Bumetanide: 0.25–0.5 mg/day; may need to give twice a day for effect.

   b. Indapamide (related to thiazides)

     (1) Less effect on glucose tolerance, lipids, plasma volume.

     (2) Starting dose: 2.5 mg/day or every other day.

4. Angiotensin-converting enzyme (ACE) inhibitors

   a. No effects on lipids or glucose tolerance; may improve LVH.

   b. Diuretics enhance effect, but best to start ACE inhibitor 2 weeks before starting the diuretic.

   c. Drugs of choice in combined congestive heart failure and hypertension.

   d. May cause hyperkalemia even in mild renal insufficiency.

5. β-Blockers

   a. Less attractive in the elderly.

   b. β-Adrenergic responsivity decreases with aging.

   c. Many side effects; of note are depression, heart failure, fatigue, central nervous system disturbance, sexual dysfunction, bronchospasm, sleep disorders, impaired glucose tolerance, and decreased peripheral arteriolar perfusion.

   d. Suggested agents

     (1) Pindolol: 5–10 mg twice a day.

     (2) Labetalol: 100–200 mg twice a day.

     (3) Acebutolol: 200–400 mg/day.

B. Other cardiovascular agents

1. Digoxin

   a. Up to 60% of elderly patients taking digoxin are not being treated for an indicated problem.

   b. Same loading dose as in younger patients; usual starting dose is 0.125 mg/day.

2. Quinidine

   a. Adverse reactions lead to discontinuation in up to 30–50% of patients.

   b. Clearance is decreased, half-life prolonged, and distribution increased.

C. Central nervous system agents

1. Benzodiazepines (Table 141-2)

   a. Increased sensitivity; metabolism may be markedly altered.

   b. Dependency common even at appropriate doses.

   c. Suggested agents and starting doses

     (1) Oxazepam: 10–15 mg up to every 8 hr.

     (2) Lorazepam: 0.25–0.5 mg up to every 6 hr.

2. Narcotics

   a. Oversedation, confusion, respiratory drive problems common.

   b. Pain relief may be seen at low doses.

   c. Delirium and hallucinations may occur at low doses.

   d. Suggestions

     (1) Morphine: 2–4 mg SC, IM, or PO up to every 4 hr.

     (2) Meperidine: 25–50 mg IM.

     (3) Pentazocine: 30 mg IM, 50 mg PO up to every 4 hr.

3. Antiparkinson's drugs

   a. Brains in elderly are dopamine poor yet do not tolerate dopaminergic compounds well.

   b. Common adverse reactions include nausea, vomiting, anorexia, dyskinesias, headaches, agitation, delirium, irritability, vivid dreams, hallucinations, and various psychiatric manifestations.

   c. Suggested drugs

     (1) Selegiline (Eldepryl): 5 mg/day.

     (2) Levodopa/carbidopa: 12.5 mg/50 mg twice a day with gradual titration to 25/100 three times a day.

Table 141-2.   Benzodiazepine Anxiolytic/Hypnotic Agents

Generic Name	Trade Name	Geriatric Maximum Daily Dose (mg)	Rate of Onset	Elimination Half-Life (hr) Parent	Elimination Half-Life (hr) Metabolite
Hypnotics					
Flurazepam	Dalmane	15	Intermediate	1–4	100–200
Triazolam	Halcion	0.25	Fast	2–5	—
Temazepam	Restoril	15	Intermediate	9–16	—
Anxiolytics					
Lorazepam	Ativan	3	Intermediate	10–20	—
Prazepam	Centrax	30	Slow	—	30–200
Chlordiazepoxide	Librium	40	Intermediate	5–30	30–200
Diazepam	Valium	20	Fastest	20–70	30–200
Oxazepam	Serax	60	Intermediate	5–15	—
Chlorazepate	Tranxene	30	Fast	—	30–200
Alprazolam	Xanax	2	Intermediate	7–15	12–15

(3) Bromocriptine: 2.5 mg/day with increase to twice a day if well tolerated.
4. Antidepressants (Table 141-3)
  a. Increased risk of antidepressant toxicity including orthostatic hypotension, cognitive impairment, blurred vision, dry mouth, constipation, and urinary retention.

b. Drugs may be causative, particularly the antihypertensives, steroids, and sedatives.
c. Cyclic antidepressants: These drugs need 3–4 weeks at therapeutic doses to show their full effect. Drugs of choice include:
(1) Nortriptyline: 10–25 mg at bedtime; increase by 10 mg every 3–7

Table 141-3   Polycyclic Antidepressants

Generic Name	Trade Name	Geriatric Maximum Dose (mg)	Sedative Effects	Anticholinergic Effects	Hypotensive Effects	Cardiac Effects
First-Generation Antidepressants						
Tertiary amines						
Amitriptyline	Elavil	150	High	High	High	Moderate
Doxepin	Adapin, Sinequan	150	High	High	Moderate	Moderate
Imipramine	Tofranil	150	High	High	High	Moderate
Secondary amines						
Desipramine HCl	Norpramin	150	Low	Low	Moderate	Moderate
Nortriptyline HCl	Pamelor	75	Moderate	Moderate	Moderate	Moderate
Protriptyline HCl	Vivactil	30	Low	Low	Moderate	Moderate
Second-Generation Antidepressants						
Amoxapine	Ascendin	200	Moderate	Low	Moderate	Low
Maprotiline HCl	Ludiomil	150	Moderate	Low	Low	Low
Trimipramine	Surmontil	150	Moderate	Moderate	Moderate	Moderate
Trazodone HCl	Desyrel	300	High	None	Low	Low
Buproprion	Wellbutrin	150–450	Activating	None	Low	Low
Fluoxetine	Prozac	20–40	Low	Low	Low	Low

Note: Cardiovascular effects include sinus tachycardia, ventricular arrhythmias, conduction blocks, and myocardial infarction.

days up to 50 mg at bedtime; check blood level in 2 weeks.

(2) Desipramine: (more activating): 10–25 mg/day to start; increase by 10–25 mg every 3–7 days up to 75 mg/day; check blood level after 2 weeks.

(3) Trazodone (sedating): 10 mg at bedtime; increase by 10 mg every 5–7 days up to 50 or 100 mg; may need up to 200 mg.

(4) Fluoxitine (activating): 10 mg every morning with increase to 20 mg every morning after 7–10 days; maintenance dose may be 20 mg every other day.

d. Psychostimulants

(1) Activating; helpful in sick, poorly motivated patients who are not clinically depressed.

(2) Methylphenidate and D-amphetamine are most commonly used.

(3) Atrial tachyarrhythmias may occur.

(4) Methylphenidate as an example: Start with 2.5 mg after breakfast and increase the dose by 2.5 mg until an appreciable effect is seen, or toxicity is noted, or a dose of 10 mg twice a day is reached. Maintain the dose for 3–5 days. If there is no effect, increase up to 15 mg twice a day. If there is still no effect, discon-

tinue. If benefit occurs, continue for at least 3 months; attempt tapering or conversion to other maintenance therapy thereafter.

e. Monoamine oxidase inhibitors

(1) Work best for anergic, apathetic, withdrawn patients.

(2) May be helpful in mild-moderate dementia associated with depression.

(3) Drug–food interactions limit their usefulness.

(4) A tyramine-free diet is prerequisite.

(5) Suggestions

(a) Tranycypromine (activating): 2.5–5 mg/day; increase by 2.5 mg every 3 days to a maximum of 15 mg/day or until a beneficial effect is achieved.

(b) Phenelzine: 7.5 mg/day with increases of 7.5 mg every 3 days, ranging from 15 to 60 mg for effect. Watch for sedation, postural hypotension, and edema.

5. Antipsychotics (Table 141-4): The elderly tend to be more sensitive to these drugs, so lower doses should be used.

a. Clinical uses

(1) To increase logical thinking and to reduce thought disorder.

(2) To decrease loose associations.

(3) To diminish delusions and hallucinations.

Table 141-4. Antipsychotics

Generic Name	Trade Name	Geriatric Maximum Daily Dose (mg)	Sedative Effects	Anticholinergic Effects	Hypotensive Effects	EPS
High Potency (Low Dose)						
Haloperidol	Haldol	50	Low	Low	Low	High
Thiothixene	Navane	30	Low	Low	Low	High
Fluphenazine HCl	Prolixin	20	Low	Low	Low	High
Trifluoperazine HCl	Stelazine	40	Moderate	Low	Low	High
Moderate Potency (Medium Dose)						
Perphenazine	Trilafon	32	Moderate	Moderate	Low	High
Loxapine succinate	Loxitane	125	Moderate	Moderate	Low	High
Molindone HCl	Moban	112	Moderate	Moderate	Low	High
Low Potency (High Dose)						
Chlorpromazine	Thorazine	800	High	High	High	High
Thioridazine	Mellaril	400	High	High	Moderate	Low

(4) To control behaviors in delirium and dementia (wandering, agitation, etc.)

b. Side-effect profiles (see Table 141-4).

c. The higher the potency, the more extrapyramidal symptoms (EPS): the lower the potency, the more sedating and anticholinergic the drug.

(1) High-potency antipsychotics

(a) Haloperidol: 0.25–0.5 mg PO or IM. Not sedating, little effect on blood pressure. Increase by 0.25–0.5 mg per dose per day.

(b) Fluphenazine: 1 mg up to every 4 hr; available in depot (IM) form.

(2) Low potency.

(a) Thioridazine (sedating, more autonomic nervous system effects, little EPS): 10 mg initially; up to 10–25 mg/day may be added to achieve the desired effect.

D. Anticoagulants

1. Warfarin has a lower dosage requirement.

2. Heparin: 5000 U every 12 hr or adjust doses to keep the activated partial thromboplastin time (APPT) near twice normal.

E. Nonsteroidal anti-inflammatory drugs (NSAIDs)

1. Salicylates show no significant changes in metabolism with aging, but low albumin levels will leave a higher free fraction of drug.

2. Ibuprofen shows no age-related changes in metabolism.

3. General statements about NSAIDs

a. There is no ideal NSAID for use in the elderly.

b. Start at or below the lowest recommended dose and increase cautiously.

c. Gastric mucosal protectants not suggested for all elderly patients; give only to high-risk patients (e.g., those with a prior history of ulcer disease, NSAID-induced gastropathy, or present symptoms/signs of gastritis).

d. Discourage concomitant use of NSAIDs with acetylsalicylic acid, alcohol, and tobacco.

F. Selected over-the-counter drugs

1. Cold and sinus remedies: Should be avoided by elderly persons because of toxicities and likely interactions with their other medications and diseases.

a. Antihistamines: Anticholinergic effects, drowsiness, irritability, and confusion.

b. Decongestants: Anxiety, nervousness, and confusion.

2. Sleeping remedies commonly cause anticholinergic side effects and may further disturb the sleep cycle.

V. Complications (Polypharmacy and Compliance)

A. Epidemiology of drug taking in the elderly

1. The elderly comprise 12% of the U.S. population, yet they consume 31% of all prescription drugs.

2. They use an estimated 30–50% of all nonprescribed drugs.

3. Forty percent of persons over age 60 use a nonprescribed drug daily.

4. Over 60% of outpatient physician visits by elderly patients include prescription of a drug.

5. An average of three or four prescribed drugs are used regularly; one nonprescribed drug is used regularly.

6. On average, elderly persons fill 12–14 new prescriptions yearly.

7. Significant drug side effects occur in 4 of every 100 new prescriptions.

B. Definitions

1. Polypharmacy: The prescription of multiple drugs for a single illness or the prescription of multiple drugs for coexisting polymorbidities.

2. Adverse drug reaction (ADR) (from the World Health Organization): Any response to a drug which is noxious and unintended and which occurs at doses normally used in humans for prophylaxis, diagnosis, or therapy.

3. Compliance (adherence to a drug regimen): The degree or extent to which a patient follows instructions.

C. Potential risks and problems of polypharmacy

1. ADRs: Even one unnecessary drug may risk an avoidable ADR.

a. ADRs occur in:
4% of patients taking 5 drugs.
10% of patients taking 6–10 drugs.
28% of patients taking 11–15 drugs.
54% of patients taking >16 drugs.

b. Alcohol may interact adversely with up to 50% of the drugs commonly prescribed for the elderly.

2. Poor compliance/adherence.
D. Strategies to reduce noncompliance and polypharmacy
  1. Simplify the regimen as much as possible.
  2. Educate the patient.
  3. Compliance aids do exist, including pill boxes with alarms, counters on bottles, and prefilled medication weekly or daily boxes.
  4. Updated medication and problem lists that are reviewed regularly.

Bibliography

Beers MH, Ouslander JG. Risk factors in geriatric drug prescribing: A practical guide to avoiding problems. *Drugs* 37:105–112, 1989.

Gomolin IH, Chapron DJ. Rational drug therapy for the aged. *Compr Ther* 9(7):17–30, 1983.

Lamy PP (ed). Clinical pharmacology. *Clin Geriatr Med* 6(2):229–452, 1990.

Salzman C. *Clinical Geriatric Psychopharmacology.* New York, McGraw-Hill, 1984.

Index